D1761278

Video Contents

Hand and Wrist Surgery

OPERATIVE TECHNIQUES

Hand and Wrist Surgery

2nd edition

Kevin C. Chung, MD, MS
Charles B. G. de Nancrede, MD Professor
Section of Plastic Surgery
Department of Surgery
Assistant Dean for Faculty Affairs
Associate Director of Global REACH
University of Michigan Medical School
Ann Arbor, Michigan

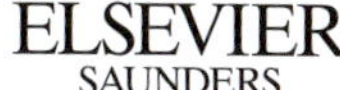

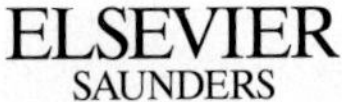

SAUNDERS

1600 John F. Kennedy Blvd.
Ste 1800
Philadelphia, PA 19103-2899

OPERATIVE TECHNIQUES: HAND AND WRIST SURGERY ISBN: 978-1-4557-4024-6

Copyright © 2012, 2008 by Saunders, an imprint of Elsevier Inc.

No part of this publication may be reproduced or transmitted in any form or by any means, electronic or mechanical, including photocopying, recording, or any information storage and retrieval system, without permission in writing from the publisher. Details on how to seek permission, further information about the Publisher's permissions policies, and our arrangements with organizations such as the Copyright Clearance Center and the Copyright Licensing Agency, can be found at our website: *www.elsevier.com/permissions.*

This book and the individual contributions contained in it are protected under copyright by the Publisher (other than as may be noted herein).

Notices

Knowledge and best practice in this field are constantly changing. As new research and experience broaden our understanding, changes in research methods, professional practices, or medical treatment may become necessary.

Practitioners and researchers must always rely on their own experience and knowledge in evaluating and using any information, methods, compounds, or experiments described herein. In using such information or methods they should be mindful of their own safety and the safety of others, including parties for whom they have a professional responsibility.

With respect to any drug or pharmaceutical products identified, readers are advised to check the most current information provided (i) on procedures featured or (ii) by the manufacturer of each product to be administered, to verify the recommended dose or formula, the method and duration of administration, and contraindications. It is the responsibility of practitioners, relying on their own experience and knowledge of their patients, to make diagnoses, to determine dosages and the best treatment for each individual patient, and to take all appropriate safety precautions.

To the fullest extent of the law, neither the Publisher nor the authors, contributors, or editors assume any liability for any injury and/or damage to persons or property as a matter of products liability, negligence or otherwise, or from any use or operation of any methods, products, instructions, or ideas contained in the material herein.

Library of Congress Cataloging-in-Publication Data

Hand & wrist surgery / [edited by] Kevin C. Chung — 2nd ed.
p. ; cm. — (Operative techniques)
Hand and wrist surgery
Rev. ed. of: Hand and wrist surgery / edited by Kevin C. Chung. c2008.
Includes bibliographical references and index.
ISBN 978-1-4557-4024-6 (hardcover : alk. paper)
I. Chung, Kevin C. II. Hand and wrist surgery. III. Title: Hand and wrist surgery. IV. Series: Operative techniques.
[DNLM: 1. Hand—surgery—Atlases. 2. Orthopedic Procedures—methods—Atlases. WE 17]
617.5′75059—dc23 2011042443

Acquisitions Editor: Dolores Meloni
Developmental Editor: Taylor Ball
Publishing Services Manager: Patricia Tannian
Senior Project Manager: Linda Van Pelt
Design Manager: Steve Stave
Illustrations Manager: Ceil Nuyianes
Marketing Manager: Tracie Pasker

Printed in United States of America
Last digit is the print number: 9 8 7 6 5 4 3 2 1

Working together to grow
libraries in developing countries

www.elsevier.com | www.bookaid.org | www.sabre.org

ELSEVIER BOOK AID International Sabre Foundation

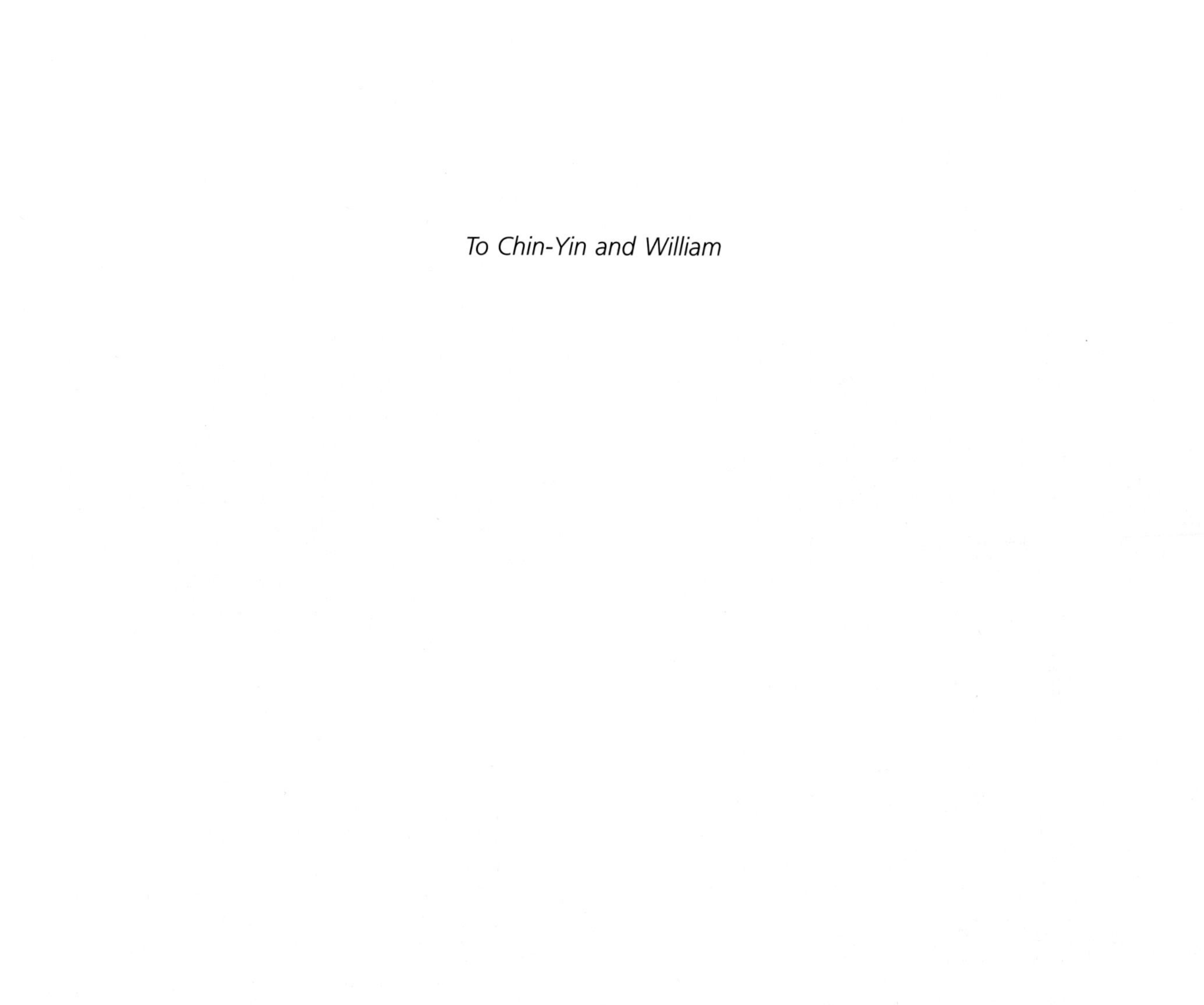

To Chin-Yin and William

Contributors

Naveen K. Ahuja, MD
Fellow, Plastic and Reconstructive Surgery, Division of Plastic Surgery, University of Medicine and Dentistry of New Jersey, Newark, New Jersey
Percutaneous Pinning of Distal Radius Fractures

Randy R. Bindra, MD, FRCS
Professor, Orthopaedic Surgery, Loyola University Medical Center, Maywood, Illinois
Metacarpophalangeal and Proximal Interphalangeal Joint Collateral Ligament Avulsion Fractures; Metacarpal Neck Fractures; Metacarpal Shaft Fractures

John T. Capo, MD
Professor, Department of Orthopaedics; Chief, Division of Hand and Microvascular Surgery, University of Medicine and Dentistry of New Jersey Medical School, Newark, New Jersey
Percutaneous Pinning of Distal Radius Fractures; Volar Plating of Distal Radius Fractures; External Fixation of Comminuted Intra-articular Distal Radius Fractures

Louis W. Catalano III, MD
Attending Hand Surgeon, CV Starr Hand Surgery Center, Roosevelt Hospital, New York, New York
Percutaneous Screw Fixation of Scaphoid Fractures; Vascularized Bone Grafting for Scaphoid Nonunion; Open Reduction and Acute Repair of Perilunate Fracture-Dislocations

Winston Y. C. Chew, FRCS
Senior Consultant and Head, Hand and Micro Surgery Section, Department of Orthopaedic Surgery, Tan Tock Seng Hospital; Adjunct Assistant Professor, Orthopaedic Surgery, Yong Loo Lin School of Medicine, National University of Singapore, Singapore
Open Reduction and Internal Fixation of Phalangeal Unicondylar Fractures; Open Reduction and Internal Fixation of Phalangeal Shaft Spiral or Long Oblique Fractures; Open Reduction and Internal Fixation of Phalangeal Shaft Comminuted Fractures; Arthrodesis of Finger and Thumb Interphalangeal and Metacarpophalangeal Joints

Kevin C. Chung, MD, MS
Charles B. G. de Nancrede, MD Professor, Section of Plastic Surgery, Department of Surgery, Assistant Dean for Faculty Affairs, Associate Director of Global REACH, University of Michigan Medical School, Ann Arbor, Michigan
Examination of the Hand and Wrist; Fasciotomy of the Upper Limb; Drainage of Purulent Flexor Tenosynovitis; Surgical Treatment of Trigger Digits; Surgical Treatment of de Quervain Tendovaginitis; Acute Repair of Zone 1 Flexor Digitorum Profundus Avulsion; Acute Repair of Zone 2 Flexor Tendon Injury; Staged Flexor Tendon Reconstruction; Extensor Tendon Repair in Zones 1 to 5; Endoscopic Carpal Tunnel Release; In Situ Cubital Tunnel Decompression; Distal Anterior Interosseous Nerve Transfer to Motor Branch of Ulnar Nerve; Treatment of a Nerve Gap in the Hand; Surgical Treatment of Neuromas in the Hand; Tendon Transfers for Carpal Tunnel Syndrome; Tendon Transfers for Ulnar Nerve Palsy; Tendon Transfers for Radial Nerve Palsy; Steindler Flexorplasty; Reconstruction of Key Pinch in Tetraplegia Patients; Flexor Carpi Ulnaris–to–Extensor Carpi Radialis Brevis Transfer; Pronator Teres Rerouting; Release of a Spastic Elbow Flexion Contracture; Synovectomy; Tendon Transfers for Extensor and Flexor Tendon Ruptures; Crossed Intrinsic Tendon Transfer; Silicone Metacarpophalangeal Joint Arthroplasty; Syndactyly Release; Duplicated Thumb Reconstruction; Reconstruction for Congenital Thumb Hypoplasia; Pollicization for Congenital Thumb Hypoplasia; Correction of Constriction Ring; Centralization for Radial Longitudinal Deficiency; Cleft Hand Reconstruction; Carpal Wedge Osteotomy for Congenital Wrist Flexion Contracture (Arthrogryposis); Dorsal Metacarpal Artery Perforator Flap; Dorsal Ulnar Artery Perforator Flap; Pedicled Groin Flap; Pyrocarbon Implant Arthroplasty of the Proximal Interphalangeal and Metacarpophalangeal Joints; Trapeziometacarpal Ligament Reconstruction; Trapeziectomy and Abductor Pollicis Longus Suspensionplasty; Trapeziometacarpal Fusion; Medial Femoral Condyle Vascularized Bone Flap for Scaphoid Nonunion; Dorsal Capsulodesis for Scapholunate Instability Using Suture Anchors; Scapholunate Ligament Reconstruction Using a Flexor Carpi Radialis Tendon Graft; Lunotriquetral Ligament Reconstruction Using a Slip of the Extensor Carpi Ulnaris Tendon; Ulnar Shortening Osteotomy; Radioulnar Ligament Reconstruction for Chronic Distal Radioulnar Joint

Instability; Darrach Procedure; Sauve-Kapandji Arthrodesis for Distal Radioulnar Joint Arthritis; Four-Corner Fusion Using a Circular Plate; Total Wrist Arthroplasty; Treatment of Mucous Cysts of the Distal Interphalangeal Joint; Excision of a Dorsal Wrist Ganglion; Digital Ray Amputation

Brent M. Egeland, MD
Resident Surgeon, Plastic Surgery, Department of Surgery, University of Michigan Health System, Ann Arbor, Michigan
Drainage of Purulent Flexor Tenosynovitis; Surgical Treatment of Trigger Digits; Surgical Treatment of de Quervain Tendovaginitis; Acute Repair of Zone 1 Flexor Digitorum Profundus Avulsion; Acute Repair of Zone 2 Flexor Tendon Injury; Staged Flexor Tendon Reconstruction

Safi R. Faruqui, DO
Mary S. Stern Hand Surgery Fellow, Hand Surgery Specialists, Cincinnati, Ohio
Dorsal Plate Fixation and Dorsal Distraction (Bridge) Plating for Distal Radius Fractures

Ramces Francisco, MD
Orthopaedic Hand and Microvascular Fellow, Department of Orthopaedics, University of Medicine and Dentistry of New Jersey Medical School, Newark, New Jersey
External Fixation of Comminuted Intra-articular Distal Radius Fractures

William B. Geissler, MD
Professor and Chief, Division of Hand and Upper Extremity Surgery, Chief, Arthroscopic Surgery and Sports Medicine, Director, Hand and Upper Extremity Fellowship, University of Mississippi Medical Center, Jackson, Mississippi
Diagnostic Wrist Arthroscopy; Arthroscopic Treatment for Septic Arthritis; Arthroscopic Ganglionectomy; Arthroscopic Triangular Fibrocartilage Complex Repair

Jeffrey A. Greenberg, MD, MS
Partner and Fellowship Director, Indiana Hand to Shoulder Center, Clinical Assistant Professor, Orthopaedic Surgery, Indiana University, Indianapolis, Indiana
Proximal Row Carpectomy; Four-Corner Fusion; Total Wrist Fusion

Harry A. Hoyen, MD
Associate Professor, Department of Orthopaedic Surgery, Case Western Reserve University, MetroHealth Medical Center, Cleveland, Ohio
Intrinsic Muscle Release for Thumb-in-Palm Deformity; Fractional Lengthening of the Flexor Tendons; Superficialis-to-Profundus Tendon Transfer; Flexor Pronator Slide

Christopher M. Jones, MD
Hand Surgery Fellow, CV Starr Hand Surgery Center, Roosevelt Hospital, New York, New York
Percutaneous Screw Fixation of Scaphoid Fractures; Vascularized Bone Grafting for Scaphoid Nonunion; Open Reduction and Acute Repair of Perilunate Fracture-Dislocations

Jesse B. Jupiter, MD
Hansjorg Wyss AO Professor of Orthopaedic Surgery, Harvard Medical School, Orthopaedic Hand Specialist, Department of Orthopaedic Surgery, Massachusetts General Hospital, Boston, Massachusetts
Corrective Osteotomy of Malunited Distal Radius Fractures

Jeffrey N. Lawton, MD
Associate Professor, Chief of the Division of Elbow, Hand and Microsurgery, Department of Orthopaedic Surgery, University of Michigan Medical Center, Ann Arbor, Michigan
Volar Plate Arthroplasty for Dorsal Fracture-Dislocations of the Proximal Interphalangeal Joint; Skier's Thumb: Repair of Acute Thumb Metacarpophalangeal Joint Ulnar Collateral Ligament Injury

Pao-Yuan Lin, MD
Assistant Professor of Surgery, Division of Plastic and Reconstructive Surgery, Department of Surgery, Kaohsiung Chang Gung Memorial Hospital and Chang Gung University College of Medicine, Taiwan
Fasciotomy of the Upper Limb; Nail Bed Repair; Extensor Tendon Repair in Zones 1 to 5; In Situ Cubital Tunnel Decompression; Distal Anterior Interosseous Nerve Transfer to Motor Branch of Ulnar Nerve; Steindler Flexorplasty; Reconstruction of Key Pinch in Tetraplegia Patients; Correction of Constriction Ring; Centralization for Radial Longitudinal Deficiency; Medial Femoral Condyle Vascularized Bone Flap for Scaphoid Nonunion; Digital Ray Amputation

Patrick J. Messerschmitt, MD
Fellow, Hand, Upper Extremity, and Microvascular Surgery, Department of Orthopaedics, Warren Alpert Medical School, Brown University, Providence, Rhode Island
Intrinsic Muscle Release for Thumb-in-Palm Deformity; Fractional Lengthening of the Flexor Tendons; Superficialis-to-Profundus Tendon Transfer; Flexor Pronator Slide

Akio Minami, MD, PhD
Professor and Chairman, Department of Orthopaedic Surgery, Hokkaido University Graduate School of Medicine, Sapporo, Japan
Correction of Swan-Neck Deformity in the Rheumatoid Hand; Reconstruction of the Central Slip with the Transverse Retinacular Ligament for Boutonnière Deformity; Scaphotrapeziotrapezoid Arthrodesis and Lunate Excision with Replacement by Palmaris Longus Tendon

Yoshitaka Minamikawa, MD
Chief of Hand Surgery, Tokyo Hand Surgery and Sports Medicine Institute, Tkatsuki Orthopaedic Shinbashi Clinic, Tokyo, Japan
Correction of Swan-Neck Deformity in the Rheumatoid Hand

Makoto Motomiya, MD, PhD
Hokkaido University Graduate School of Medicine, Orthopaedic Surgery, Sapporo, Japan
Reconstruction of the Central Slip with the Transverse Retinacular Ligament for Boutonnière Deformity

Shimpei Ono, MD, PhD
International Fellow, Section of Plastic Surgery, Department of Surgery, The University of Michigan Health System, Ann Arbor, Michigan, Department of Plastic, Reconstructive and Aesthetic Surgery, Nippon Medical School, Tokyo, Japan
Endoscopic Carpal Tunnel Release; Synovectomy; Tendon Transfers for Extensor and Flexor Tendon Ruptures; Crossed Intrinsic Tendon Transfer; Dorsal Capsulodesis for Scapholunate Instability Using Suture Anchors; Scapholunate Ligament Reconstruction Using a Flexor Carpi Radialis Tendon Graft; Lunotriquetral Ligament Reconstruction Using a Slip of the Extensor Carpi Ulnaris Tendon; Four-Corner Fusion Using a Circular Plate; Treatment of Mucous Cysts of the Distal Interphalangeal Joint

Jessica H. Peelman, MD
Mary S. Stern Hand Fellow, Department of Orthopaedic Surgery, University of Cincinnati College of Medicine, Cincinnati, Ohio
Wrist Denervation

Douglas Sammer, MD
Assistant Professor of Plastic Surgery, Co-director of Hand Surgery Fellowship, University of Texas Southwestern Medical Center, Dallas, Texas
Open Carpal Tunnel Release; Percutaneous Pinning of Bennett Fracture and Open Reduction and Internal Fixation of Rolando Fracture; Open Reduction of Metacarpophalangeal Joint Dislocation

Sandeep J. Sebastin, MCh (Plastic)
Consultant, Department of Hand and Reconstructive Microsurgery, National University Health System, Singapore
Examination of the Hand and Wrist; Fasciotomy of the Upper Limb; Nail Bed Repair; Drainage of Purulent Flexor Tenosynovitis; Surgical Treatment of Trigger Digits; Surgical Treatment of de Quervain Tendovaginitis; Acute Repair of Zone 1 Flexor Digitorum Profundus Avulsion; Acute Repair of Zone 2 Flexor Tendon Injury; Staged Flexor Tendon Reconstruction; Extensor Tendon Repair in Zones 1 to 5; Endoscopic Carpal Tunnel Release; In Situ Cubital Tunnel Decompression; Distal Anterior Interosseous Nerve Transfer to Motor Branch of Ulnar Nerve; Treatment of a Nerve Gap in the Hand; Surgical Treatment of Neuromas in the Hand; Tendon Transfers for Carpal Tunnel Syndrome; Tendon Transfers for Ulnar Nerve Palsy; Tendon Transfers for Radial Nerve Palsy; Steindler Flexorplasty; Reconstruction of Key Pinch in Tetraplegia Patients; Flexor Carpi Ulnaris–to–Extensor Carpi Radialis Brevis Transfer; Pronator Teres Rerouting; Release of a Spastic Elbow Flexion Contracture; Synovectomy; Tendon Transfers for Extensor and Flexor Tendon Ruptures; Crossed Intrinsic Tendon Transfer; Syndactyly Release; Duplicated Thumb Reconstruction; Reconstruction for Congenital Thumb Hypoplasia; Pollicization for Congenital Thumb Hypoplasia; Correction of Constriction Ring; Centralization for Radial Longitudinal Deficiency; Cleft Hand Reconstruction; Carpal Wedge Osteotomy for Congenital Wrist Flexion Contracture (Arthrogryposis); Dorsal Metacarpal Artery Perforator Flap; Dorsal Ulnar Artery Perforator Flap; Pedicled Groin Flap; Medial Femoral Condyle Vascularized Bone Flap for Scaphoid Nonunion; Dorsal Capsulodesis for Scapholunate Instability Using Suture Anchors; Scapholunate Ligament Reconstruction Using a Flexor Carpi Radialis Tendon Graft; Lunotriquetral Ligament Reconstruction Using a Slip of the Extensor Carpi Ulnaris Tendon; Ulnar Shortening Osteotomy; Radioulnar Ligament Reconstruction for Chronic Distal Radioulnar Joint Instability; Four-Corner Fusion Using a Circular Plate; Treatment of Mucous Cysts of the Distal Interphalangeal Joint; Excision of a Dorsal Wrist Ganglion; Digital Ray Amputation

Micah K. Sinclair, MD
Department of Orthopaedic Surgery, Loyola University Medical Center, Maywood, Illinois
Metacarpophalangeal and Proximal Interphalangeal Joint Collateral Ligament Avulsion Fractures; Metacarpal Neck Fractures; Metacarpal Shaft Fractures

Peter J. Stern, MD
Professor and Chairman, Department of Orthopaedic Surgery, University of Cincinnati College of Medicine, Cincinnati, Ohio
Hemi-Hamate Arthroplasty; Dorsal Plate Fixation and Dorsal Distraction (Bridge) Plating for Distal Radius Fractures; Wrist Denervation

Nathan S. Taylor, MD
Orthopaedic Surgery Associates of Marquette, Marquette, Michigan
Silicone Metacarpophalangeal Joint Arthroplasty; Pyrocarbon Implant Arthroplasty of the Proximal Interphalangeal and Metacarpophalangeal Joints; Trapeziometacarpal Ligament Reconstruction; Trapeziectomy and Abductor Pollicis Longus Suspensionplasty; Trapeziometacarpal Fusion; Darrach Procedure; Sauve-Kapandji Arthrodesis for Distal Radioulnar Joint Arthritis; Total Wrist Arthroplasty

Lam-Chuan Teoh, FRCS
Senior Consultant, Hand and Micro Surgery Section, Orthopaedic Surgery, Tan Tock Seng Hospital; Clinical Associate Professor, Yong Loo Lin School of Medicine, National University of Singapore, Singapore
Lateral Arm Flap for Upper Limb Coverage; Open Reduction and Internal Fixation of Phalangeal Unicondylar Fractures; Open Reduction and Internal Fixation of Phalangeal Shaft Comminuted Fractures; Arthrodesis of Finger and Thumb Interphalangeal and Metacarpophalangeal Joints

Christopher J. Utz, MD
Department of Orthopaedic Surgery, Cleveland Clinic Foundation, Cleveland, Ohio
Volar Plate Arthroplasty for Dorsal Fracture-Dislocations of the Proximal Interphalangeal Joint; Skier's Thumb: Repair of Acute Thumb Metacarpophalangeal Joint Ulnar Collateral Ligament Injury

Jennifer Waljee, MD
Hand Fellow, Section of Plastic Surgery, Department of Surgery, The University of Michigan Health System, Ann Arbor, Michigan
Syndactyly Release; Duplicated Thumb Reconstruction; Reconstruction for Congenital Thumb Hypoplasia; Pollicization for Congenital Thumb Hypoplasia; Ulnar Shortening Osteotomy; Radioulnar Ligament Reconstruction for Chronic Distal Radioulnar Joint Instability

Daniel C. M. Williams, MD
Department of Orthopaedic Surgery and Rehabilitation, University of Mississippi Health Care, Jackson, Mississippi
Diagnostic Wrist Arthroscopy; Arthroscopic Treatment for Septic Arthritis; Arthroscopic Ganglionectomy; Arthroscopic Triangular Fibrocartilage Complex Repair

Joyce M. Wilson, MD
Mary S. Stern Hand Fellow, Department of Orthopaedic Surgery, University of Cincinnati College of Medicine, Cincinnati, Ohio
Hemi-Hamate Arthroplasty

Lynda J. Yang, MD, PhD
Department of Neurosurgery, University of Michigan, Ann Arbor, Michigan
Nerve Transfer Techniques for Elbow Flexion in Brachial Plexus Palsy

Preface

The popularity of the first edition of *Operative Techniques: Hand and Wrist Surgery* has encouraged me to do even better with the second edition. The first edition has received international acclaim and was translated into the major languages of the world, including Spanish, Chinese, and Japanese. As I travel in the United States and abroad, I often see this book on the shelves of my hosts. I appreciate the feedback from many of the readers of the first edition regarding what they would like to see in the second edition.

My main wish for the second edition is to present added value by including more operative procedures as well as a richly organized video collection that surpasses the standards of the medical publishing world. I believe our team has accomplished just that. There are more than 90 entirely new chapters, including procedures that were not presented previously. Many of the procedures presented in the first edition were rewritten to improve upon certain features of the chapters. We meticulously planned the procedures to illustrate the technical sequences so as to help surgeons perform safe and predictable operations to the ultimate benefit of our patients. The combination of the first and second editions should encompass the majority of the operations that the hand surgeon must know to provide comprehensive care in hand surgery. With the addition of over 70 videos on the accompanying DVD, this volume justifies its title as a fully illustrated operative techniques book that promotes the art and science of hand surgery around the world.

Introducing a book of this caliber requires meticulous planning over a course of two years. My production team, which includes my international fellow from Singapore, Sandeep J. Sebastin, and my video coordinator, Pouya Entezami, have toiled tirelessly to make sure that this book is of the highest quality to impart my philosophy in hand surgery to you. I very much appreciate my many contributing authors, who were selected for their ability to share with you their experiences through techniques that they have found to be reliable in their practices. The reputation of Elsevier is fully displayed in this book. My developmental editor, Taylor Ball, is a great pleasure to work with and is fully committed to presenting you with the best product possible from Elsevier.

I am proud to offer this book to you. I am sure you will cherish it as much as I do. I also anticipate that there will be future editions as innovations in hand surgery continue to grow. I look forward to seeing this book on many shelves around the world to disseminate the principles of hand surgery and to serve as your companion in the care of your patients.

Kevin C. Chung, MD, MS

Foreword

I am pleased to write the Foreword for the second edition of my friend Dr. Chung's book, *Operative Techniques: Hand and Wrist Surgery.* I have accepted this task to honor the memory of our mutual friend, Dr. Paul Manske, who wrote the Foreword for the previous edition and has since passed away. Since its initial publication, this book has enjoyed international acclaim, having been translated into many major world languages.

This book provides a stunningly organized approach to common and complex surgical procedures for the hand. The illustrations are superbly done in a step-by-step fashion to guide surgeons of all abilities in the intricate execution of surgical procedures for the hand. The accompanying video series contains over 70 meticulously produced videos that are the pride and joy of Dr. Chung's effort over the course of 2 years. Each video is narrated by Dr. Chung and points out the essential components of the surgical procedure as well as the potential perils that need to be avoided. The pictures are elegantly presented to illustrate the methodical philosophy of hand surgery, which strives for perfection, artistry, and grace in the execution of a surgical procedure.

The second edition of *Operative Techniques: Hand and Wrist Surgery* will no doubt set the standard in the medical publishing world, and I am confident that this book will continue to enjoy national and international success. Although I just turned 90, I am still keen to learn and teach hand surgery. I look forward to reading this book in its entirety, for it will be the means of disseminating the principles of the unique specialty of hand surgery to all reaches of the world.

Adrian E. Flatt, MD (Cantab), FRCS, FACS
Chief Emeritus
George Truett James Orthopaedic Institute
Baylor University Medical Center
Dallas, Texas

Contents

Video Contents

OPERATIVE TECHNIQUES

Hand and Wrist Surgery

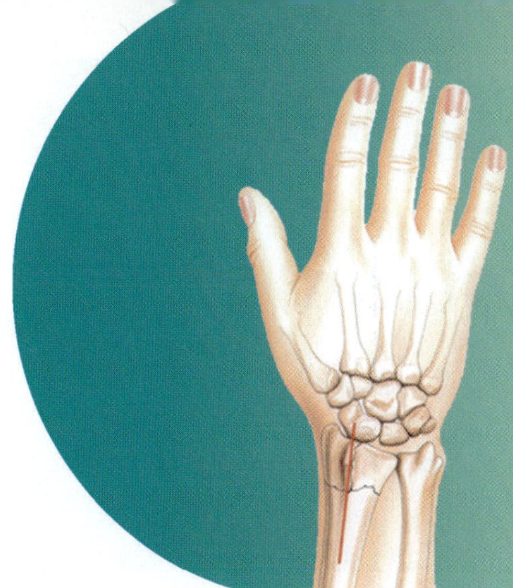

Section I

EXAMINATION AND EMERGENCY PROCEDURES

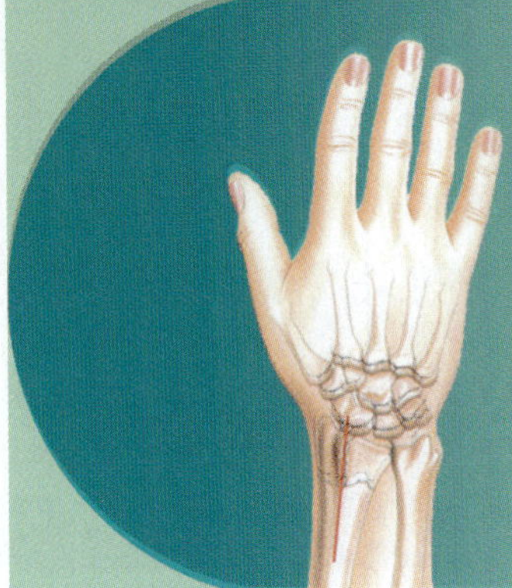

Examination of the Hand and Wrist

Sandeep J. Sebastin and Kevin C. Chung

> *"No organ, anatomical structure, or laboratory procedure can reveal as much practical information about a patient as can the hand."*
>
> Bruce W. Conolly, 1980

See Video 1: Clinical Examination of the Hand and Wrist

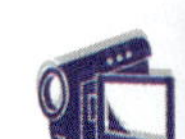

Man depends on his hands for work, recreation, and expression. The hand not only reflects emotional and physical character but also is a mirror of underlying systemic disease. An understanding of the basic functional anatomy of the hand is essential for examination, accurate diagnosis, and successful treatment of disorders of the hand. Standard terminology should be used when describing the anatomy and motion of the hand and wrist. This avoids confusion and compromised patient care when the pathology is described to colleagues.

The human hand consists of a broad palm with five digits, attached to the forearm at the wrist joint. The five digits include the thumb and the four fingers, namely the index (IF), long (LF), ring (RF), and small finger (SF) (Fig. 1-1). The long and small fingers are often called the middle and little fingers, respectively. We believe that the term *long finger* is more appropriate to avoid the ambiguity as to what constitutes the middle finger. The use of little finger and long finger confuses their acronyms (LF); hence, small finger is preferred.

The hand has two surfaces—dorsal and palmar. The use of the term *palmar* should be restricted to the area limited by the glabrous skin, and the term *volar* should be used for areas proximal to it (see Fig. 1-1). *Radial* is used to describe direction toward the thumb and *ulnar* to describe direction toward the small finger, rather than *lateral* and *medial* (see Fig. 1-1). The palm has two eminences: the thenar eminence, which contains the intrinsic muscles of the thumb; and the hypothenar eminence, which contains the intrinsic muscles of the small finger (see Fig. 1-1). The connotation of the word *intrinsic* is to describe muscles that originate and insert in the hand, whereas *extrinsic* indicates muscles that originate outside the hand, such as the extrinsic finger flexors. The three well-defined creases of the hand are the thenar crease (forms the boundary of the thenar eminence), the proximal and distal palmar creases, and the distal wrist crease (forms the boundary of the glabrous skin) (see Fig. 1-1).

Each finger has three phalanges, namely proximal, middle, and distal, and three joints, namely metacarpophalangeal (MCP), proximal interphalangeal (PIP), and

Figures 1-42 and 1-43 are from Chung KC, Yang L, McGillicuddy JE (eds). Practical Management of Pediatric and Adult Brachial Plexus Palsies. *Philadelphia: Elsevier; 2011.*

distal interphalangeal (DIP). The thumb has two phalanges, proximal and distal, and two joints, the MCP and the interphalangeal (IP). There are five metacarpals and five corresponding carpometacarpal (CMC) joints, which are numbered I to V from radial to ulnar. The first CMC joint is also known as the thumb basal joint (Fig. 1-2).

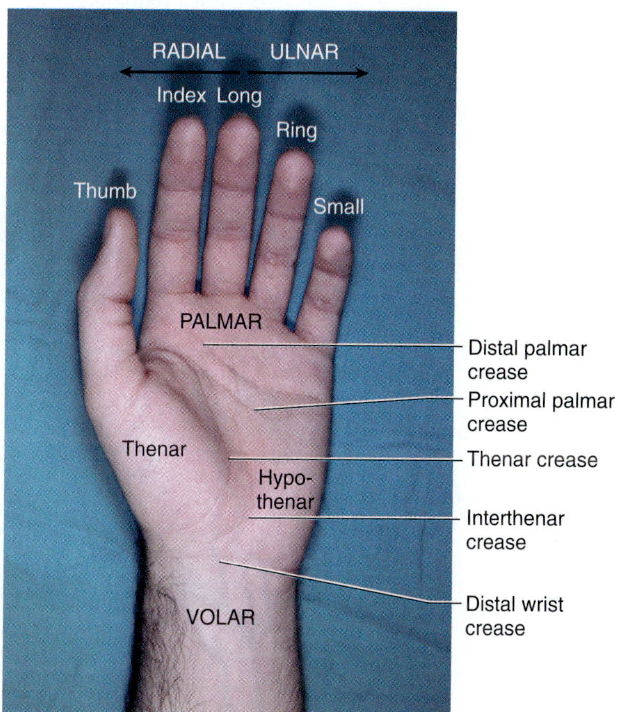

FIGURE 1-1

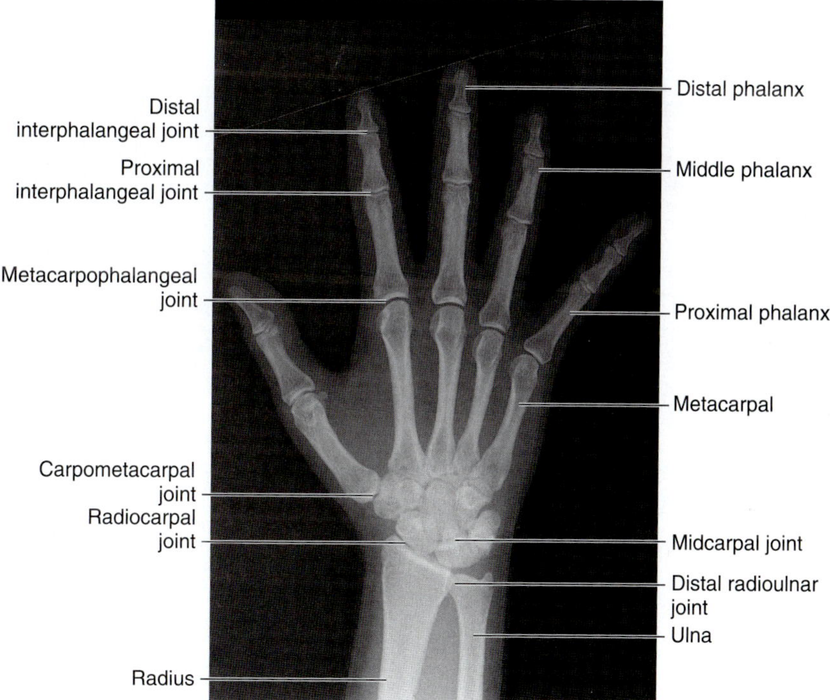

FIGURE 1-2

There are eight carpal bones arranged in roughly two rows. From radial to ulnar, the proximal row has the scaphoid, lunate, triquetrum, and pisiform, and the distal row has the trapezium, trapezoid, capitate, and hamate (Fig. 1-3). The bones of the distal row form the CMC joint with the base of the metacarpals and the midcarpal joint with the carpal bones of the proximal row. The proximal row articulates with the radius and the ulna. The palpable bony landmarks of the hand and wrist and their relation to the surrounding structures are depicted in Figure 1-4. The correct terminology to use when describing motion at the different joints of the hand is illustrated in Figure 1-5.

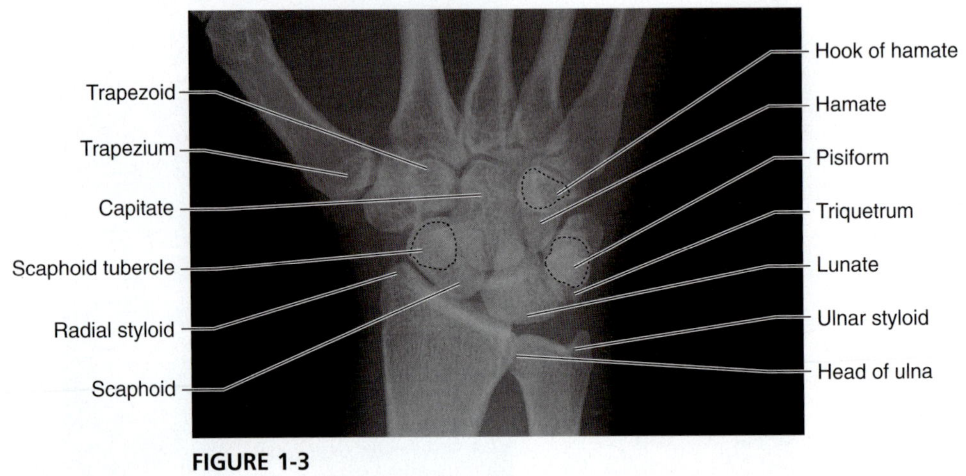

FIGURE 1-3

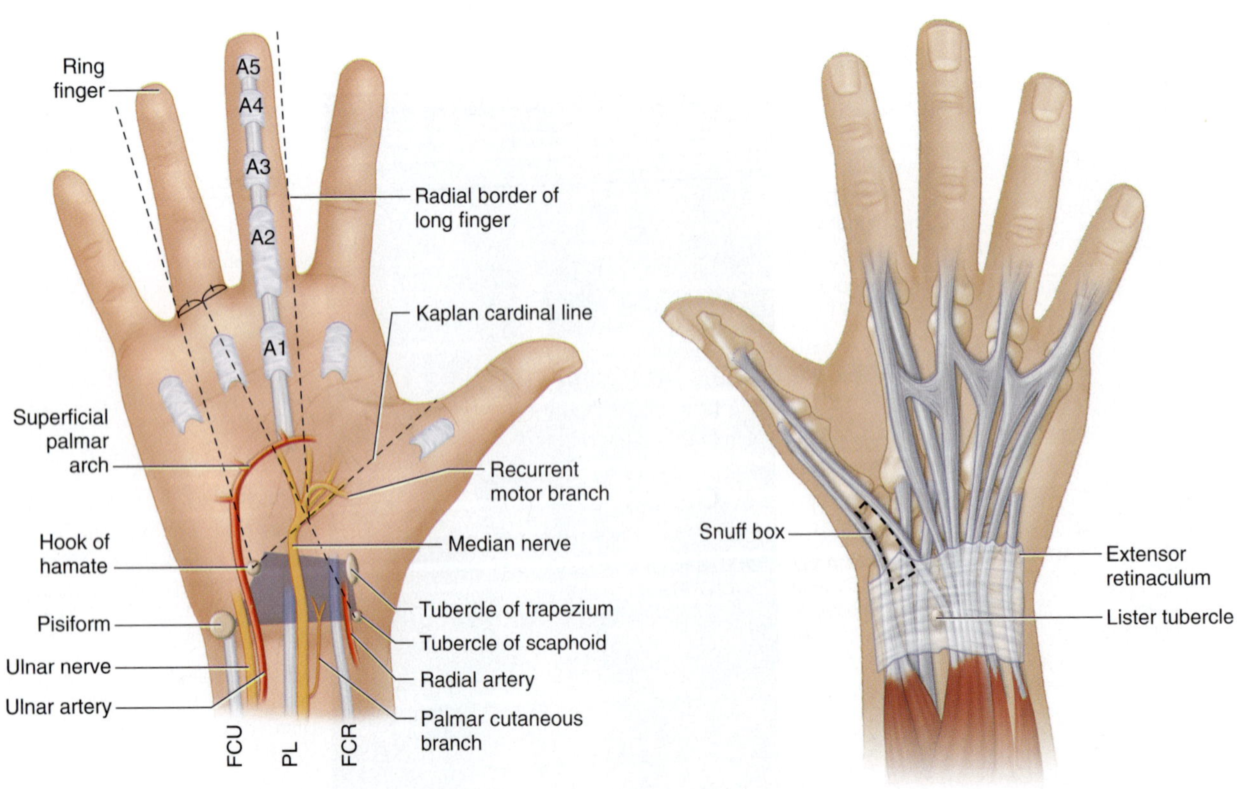

FIGURE 1-4

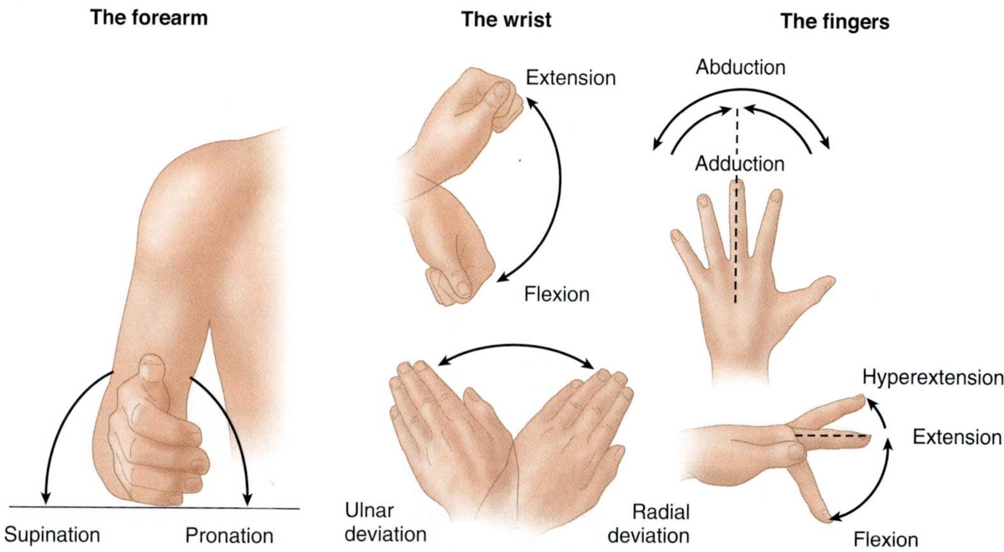

FIGURE 1-5

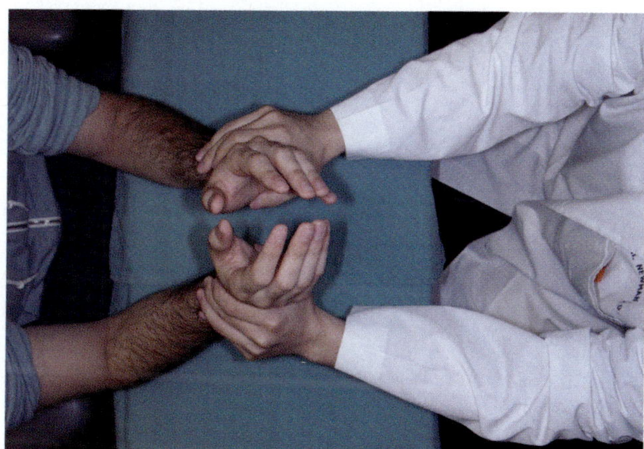

FIGURE 1-6

Examination/Imaging

Position

- The patient is examined in the sitting position with elbows exposed and resting on a table in front. The examiner sits opposite the patient across the table (Fig. 1-6).

Procedure

- We conduct our examination in stages (Table 1-1). In the first stage, we do a primary survey and focus on the hand as a whole, examining both hands. This stage begins by listening to the patient's complaints and obtaining relevant history. This is followed by the basic examination strategy of look (inspection), feel (palpation), and move (range of motion).

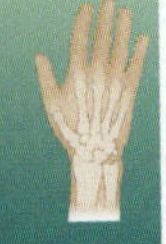

Table 1-1 Systematic Examination of the Hand and Wrist

I. Primary Survey (hand screen)—examine both hands
   1. Listen (patient complaints and history)
   2. Look
   3. Feel
   4. Move
II. Secondary Survey (system-specific examination)—examine involved hand
   1. Assessment of muscle and tendon function
   2. Assessment of nerve function
   3. Assessment of vascular function
   4. Assessment of bone and joint function
III. Preliminary Diagnosis and Differential Diagnosis
IV. Investigations
V. Tertiary Survey
VI. Final Diagnosis

- The second stage is a more focused examination of one or more specific systems limited to the involved hand. The system to be examined is derived based on the primary survey. At the completion of the secondary survey, we should have a preliminary diagnosis or a differential diagnosis. If a diagnosis is not apparent, one should not make up a nebulous diagnosis such as tendinitis or arthritis. These made-up diagnoses may satisfy the patient's need to have a reason for the discomfort but may label a patient erroneously when in fact there is no definite physiologic reason for the patient's complaint. It is suitable to note that the patient has hand pain or wrist pain and occasionally to tell the patient that you do not know what is wrong when it is indeed truthful. We can share with the patient that we do not understand or know everything and are not able to cure every ailment.
- Appropriate investigations are then ordered. The history and findings of the primary and secondary surveys are correlated with the investigations. If they do not match, a focused tertiary survey should be carried out to validate the investigation. A final diagnosis is then made and necessary treatment instituted.

Primary Survey

- The aim of the primary survey is to perform a rapid assessment of both hands to determine whether all is well.

Look

The following three regions are inspected in turn:

- Palmar aspect of hand and volar forearm (Fig. 1-7)
  - Fingers extended
    - Swelling, erythema, bruising, color changes, or scars
    - Deformity, abnormal finger posture, or amputation
    - Wasting (thenar, hypothenar, or forearm)
  - Fingers flexed
    - Active range of joint motion
    - Triggering
    - Abnormal finger posture
    - Scar adhesions during movement
- Dorsal aspect of hand and forearm (Fig. 1-8)
  - Hand
    - Swelling, erythema, bruising, color changes, or scars
    - Nail changes
    - Wasting (first web space and intermetacarpal space)

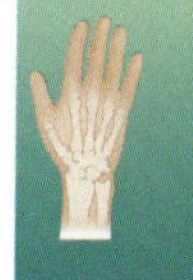

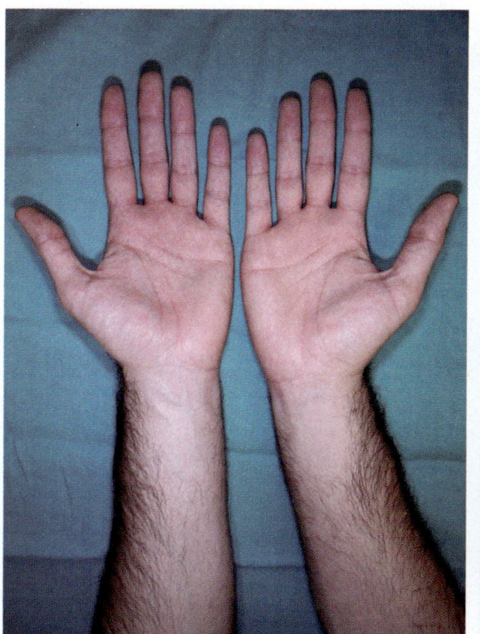

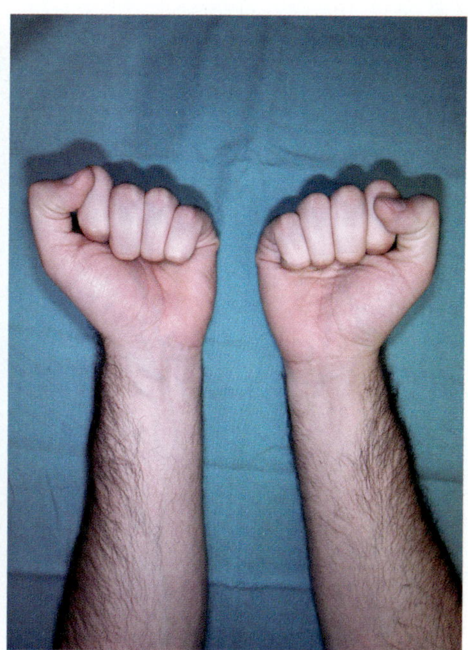

FIGURE 1-7

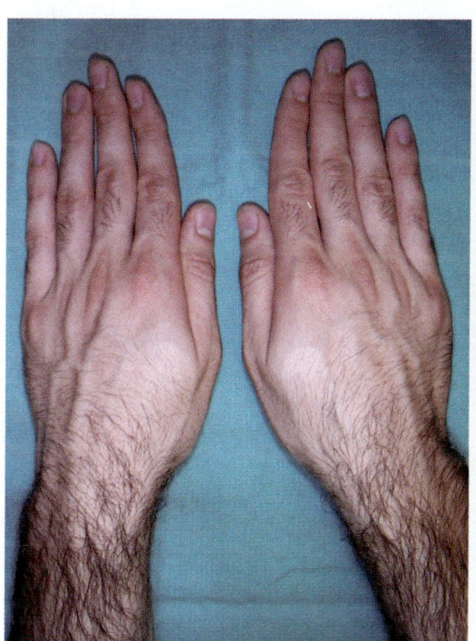

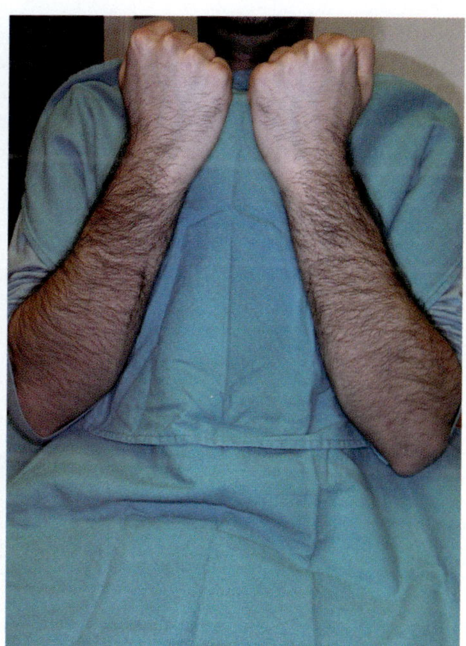

FIGURE 1-8

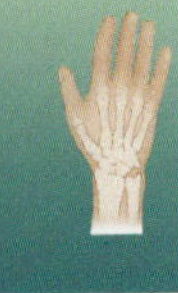

- Dorsal aspect of forearm and elbow
  - Swelling, erythema, bruising, color changes, or scars
  - Wasting
- Active range of wrist motion (flexion, extension, radial and ulnar deviation, and pronosupination)

Feel

- Vascularity
  - Do all digits feel warm?
  - Can you feel a radial pulse (Fig. 1-9)?
  - Check capillary refill
- Sensation (Fig. 1-10)
  - Lateral aspect of midarm (C5 dermatome)
  - Dorsum proximal phalanx of thumb (radial nerve, C6 dermatome)
  - Tip of long finger (median nerve, C7 dermatome)
  - Tip of small finger (ulnar nerve, C8 dermatome)
  - Medial aspect of elbow (T1 dermatome)
- Motor function (Fig. 1-11)
  - Palmar abduction of thumb—abductor pollicis brevis (APB) (median nerve)
  - Crossing long finger over index finger—interossei (ulnar nerve)
  - Raising thumb off table—extensor pollicis longus (EPL) (radial nerve)
- Autonomic function
  - Skin dry?
- Tenderness
  - Localization of specific points of tenderness

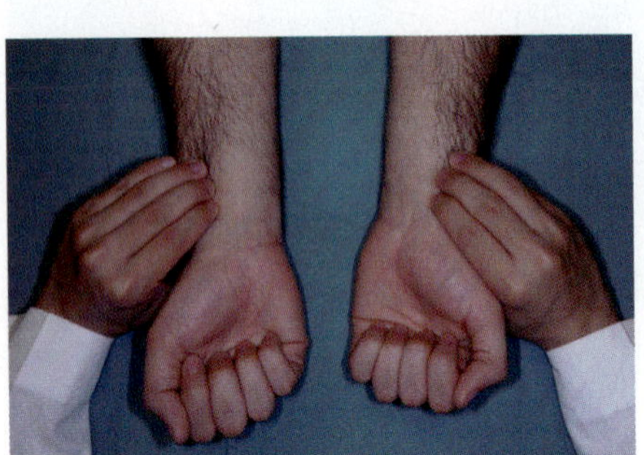

FIGURE 1-9

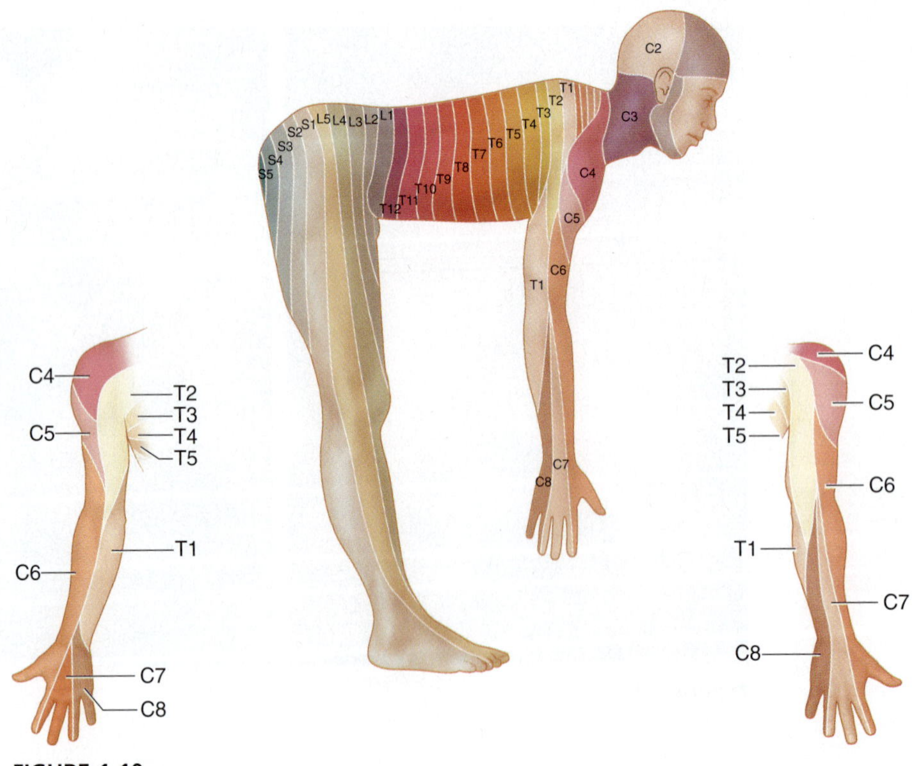

FIGURE 1-10

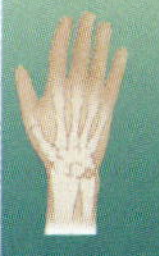

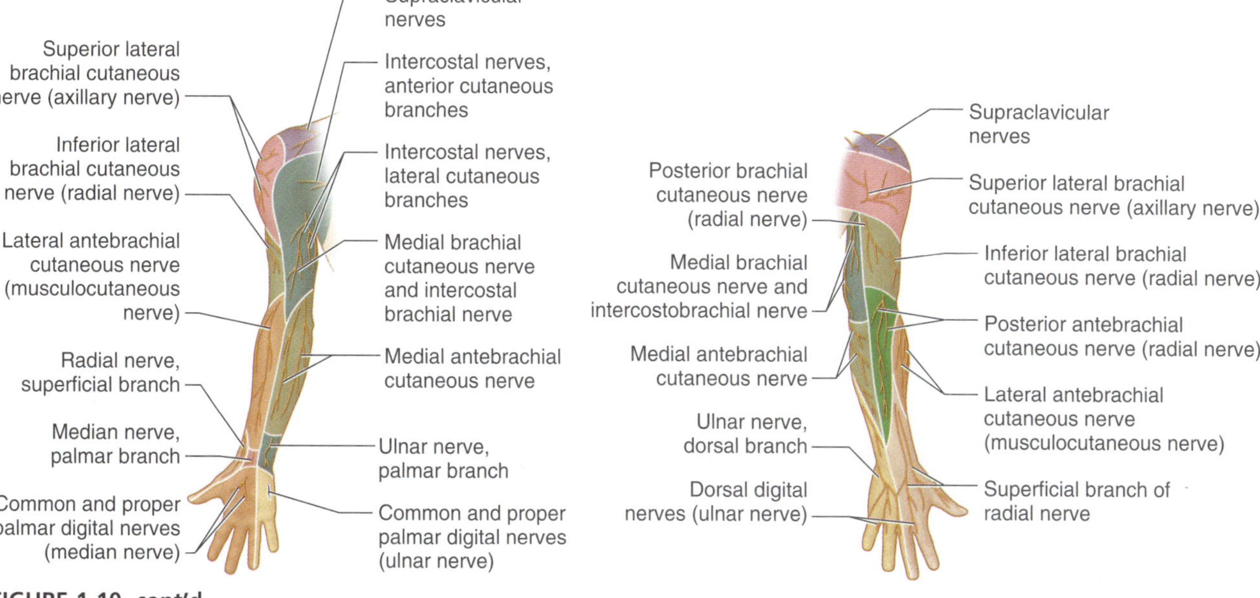

FIGURE 1-10, cont'd

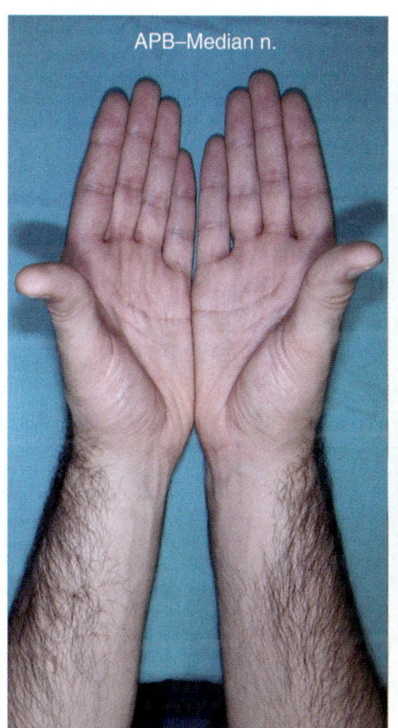

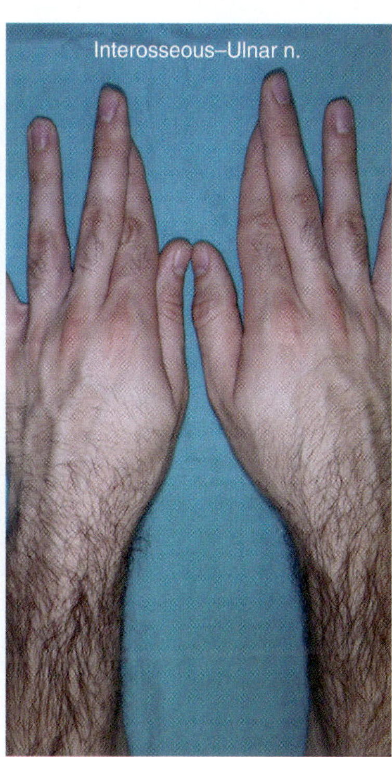

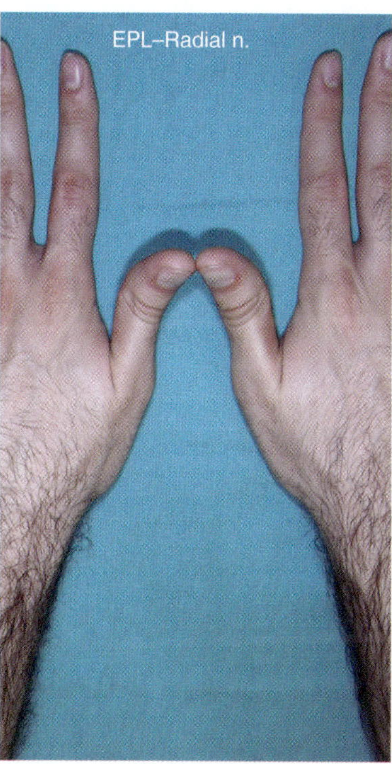

FIGURE 1-11

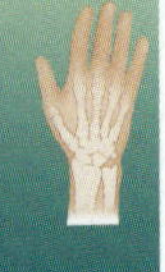

Table 1-2 Normal Range of Digital Motion

Digit	Distal Interphalangeal Joint	Proximal Interphalangeal Joint	Metacarpophalangeal Joint		Carpometacarpal Joint	
	Ext.-Flex.	*Ext.-Flex.*	*Ext.-Flex.*	*Add.-Abd.*	*Ext.-Flex.*	*Add.-Abd.*
Thumb	—	0-90 degrees	−10-70 degrees	−10-10 degrees	−10-30 degrees	0-50 degrees
Index finger	0-80 degrees	0-100 degrees	−20-90 degrees	−20-20 degrees	0 degrees	0 degrees
Long finger	0-80 degrees	0-100 degrees	−20-90 degrees	−20-20 degrees	0-10 degrees	0 degrees
Ring finger	0-80 degrees	0-100 degrees	−20-90 degrees	−20-20 degrees	0-20 degrees	0 degrees
Small finger	0-80 degrees	0-100 degrees	−20-90 degrees	−20-20 degrees	−10-30 degrees	0 degrees

Table 1-3 Normal Range of Wrist Motion

	Extension	Flexion	Radial Deviation	Ulnar Deviation	Pronation	Supination
Wrist	0-70 degrees	0-80 degrees	0-20 degrees	0-30 degrees	—	—
Motion at midcarpal joint	60%	67%	60%	60%		
Motion at radiocarpal joint	40%	33%	40%	40%		
Distal radioulnar joint	—	—	—	—	0-80 degrees	0-70 degrees

Move

- Assess passive range of motion
  - Thumb IP and MCP joints
  - Finger IP and MCP joints
  - Wrist (flexion, extension, radial and ulnar deviation, and pronosupination)
    - The normal range of motion at the different joints of the hand and wrist has been summarized in Tables 1-2 and 1-3, respectively. Extension should be measured with the goniometer placed palmar, whereas flexion is measured with the goniometer placed dorsally (Fig. 1-12). Radial and ulnar deviation of the wrist is measured with the goniometer placed along the long finger and dorsal aspect of the distal radius (Fig. 1-13). Pronation and supination should be measured with the elbow in 90 degrees flexion and the arms firmly pressed against the outer ribs (Fig. 1-14).
  - At the completion of the primary survey, if something appears abnormal, one should proceed to a secondary survey. The primary survey should be able to guide us toward the anatomic system that is problematic. For example, a patient presents with history of numbness of the left thumb and index finger, and the primary survey finds diminished sensation of the left long finger tip and weakness in palmar abduction of the left thumb. The secondary survey should therefore focus on examination of the left median nerve.

For an expanded version of this chapter, please see www.expertconsult.com.

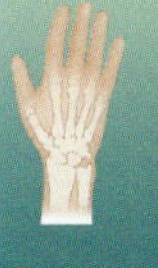

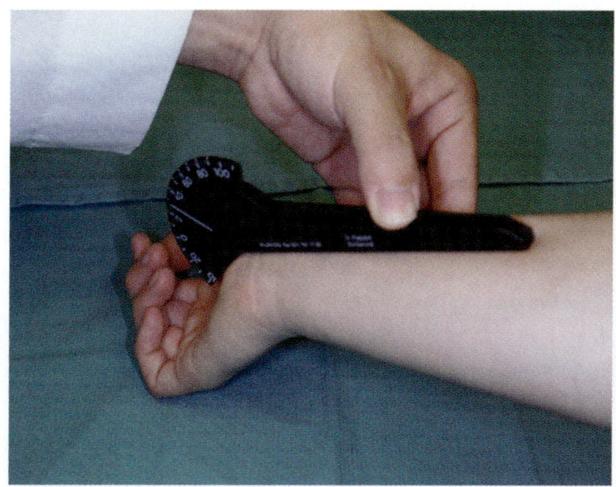

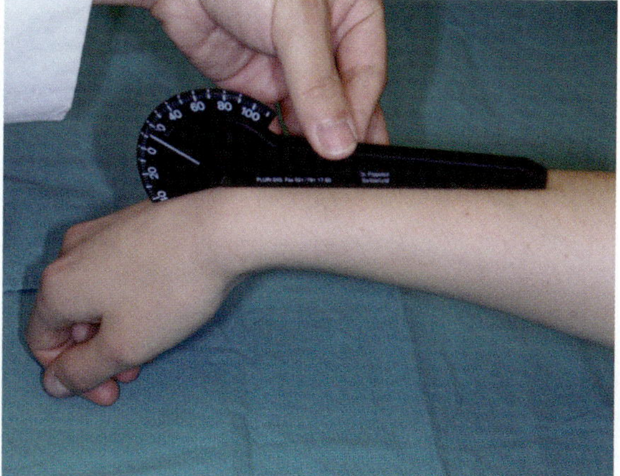

FIGURE 1-12

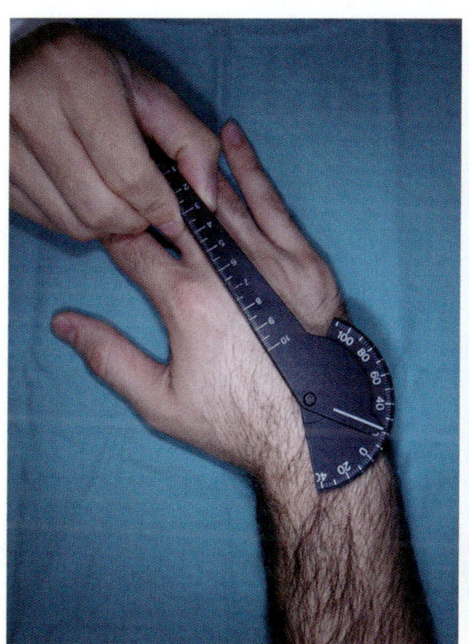

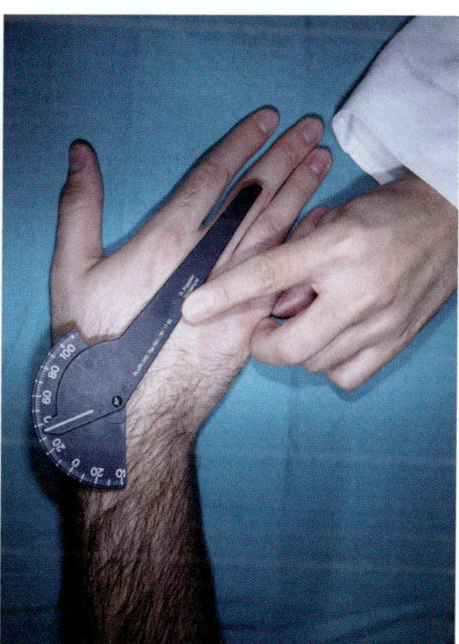

FIGURE 1-13

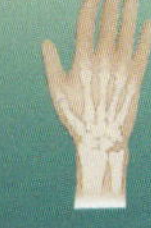

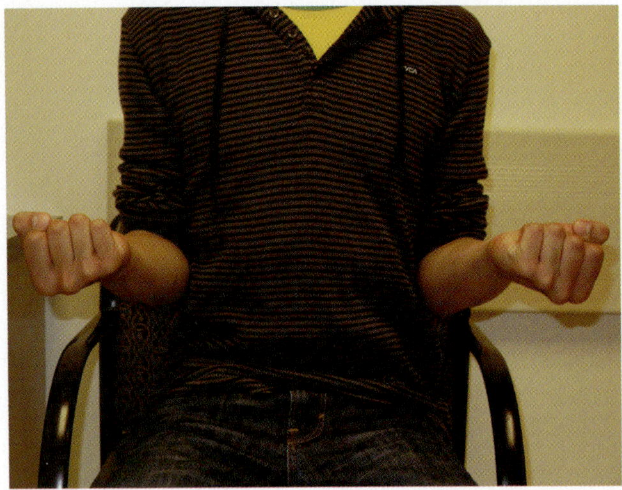

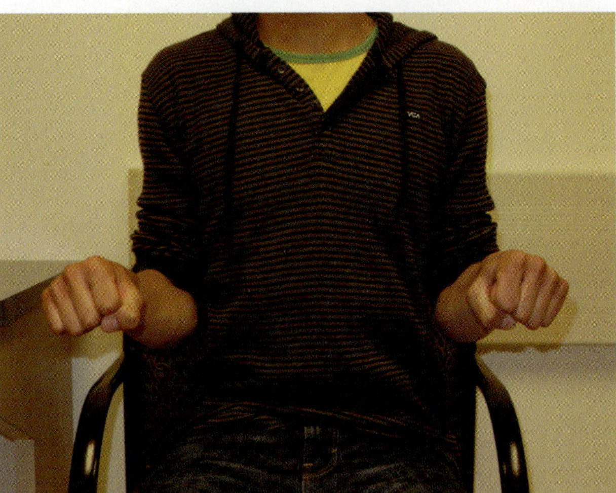

FIGURE 1-14

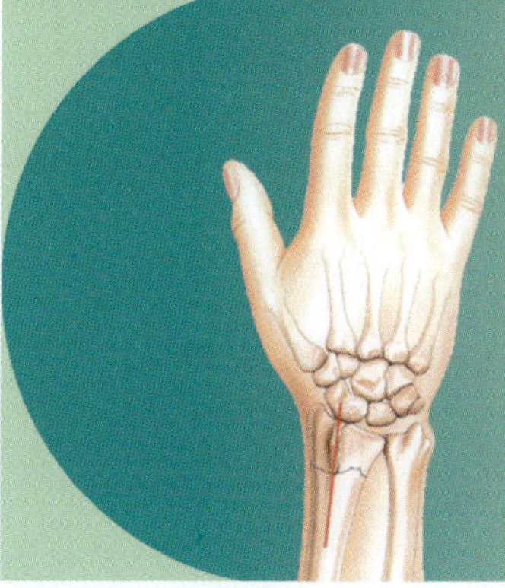

Fasciotomy of the Upper Limb

Pao-Yuan Lin, Sandeep J. Sebastin, and Kevin C. Chung

Indications

- Compartment syndrome
  - Circumferential thermal burns (Fig. 2-1A and B)
  - High-voltage electric burns (Fig. 2-2)
- Major limb (proximal to wrist) replantation/revascularization

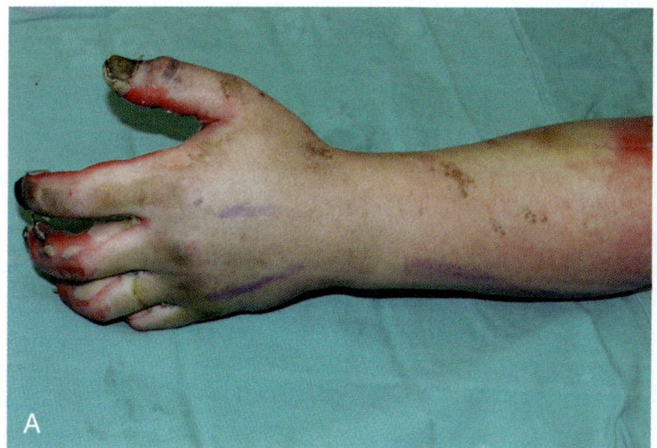

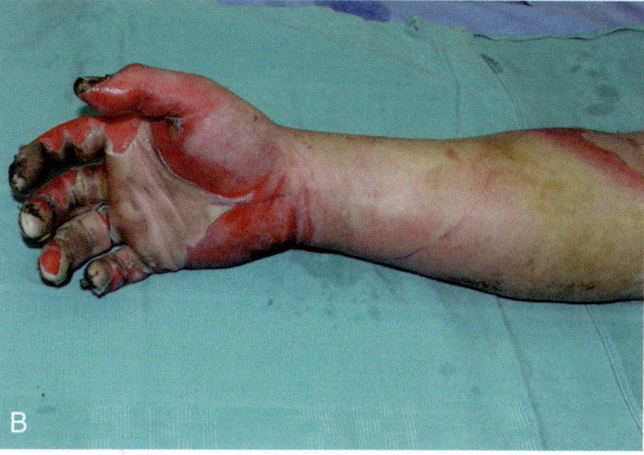

FIGURE 2-1

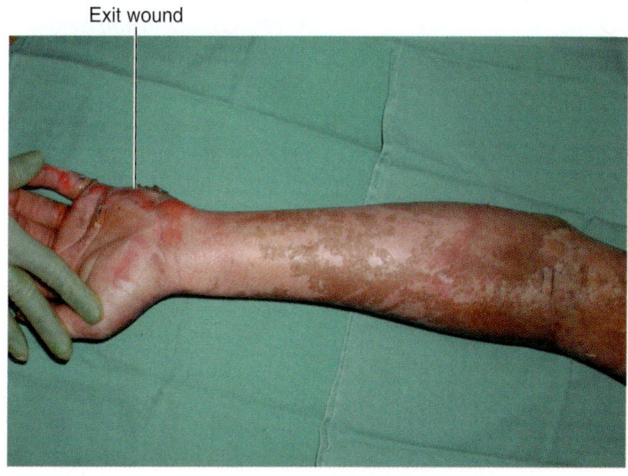

FIGURE 2-2

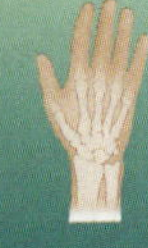

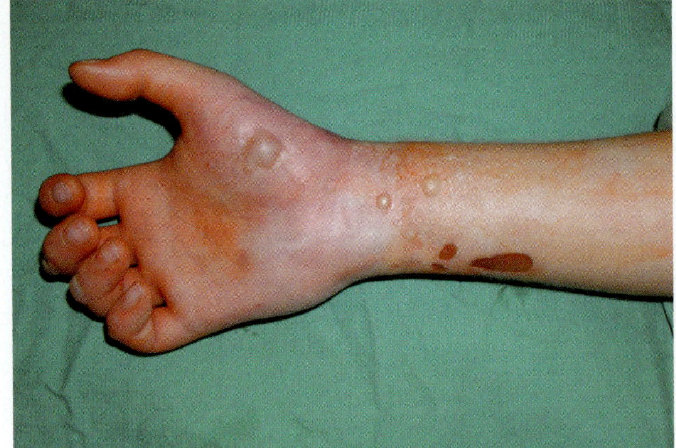

FIGURE 2-3

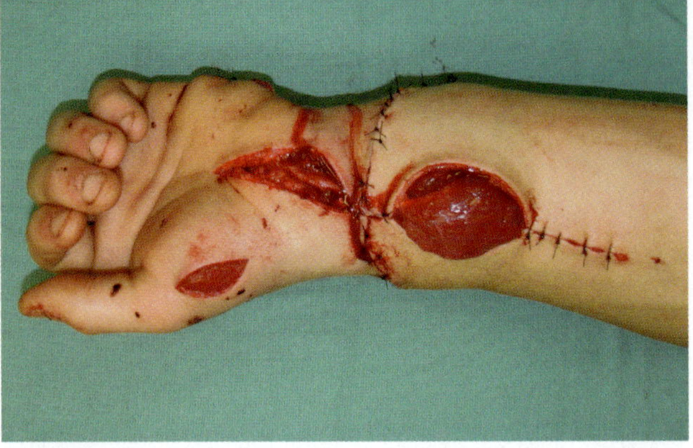

FIGURE 2-4

Examination/Imaging

Clinical Examination

- Compartment syndrome is caused by increased pressure within the myofascial compartments leading to a decrease in blood flow. Nerves followed by muscle are most sensitive to ischemia and undergo irreversible changes within 6 to 8 hours. It is therefore important to decompress the fascial compartment by performing a fasciotomy and to restore tissue perfusion as soon as possible.
- Compartment syndrome is a clinical diagnosis based on the features of ischemia of nerve (paresthesia, pain, and paralysis), muscle (pain on passive stretch), and vessel (pallor and pulselessness). All features may not be present in every patient, and a diagnosis is made based on the overall clinical scenario.
  - Paresthesia is the earliest symptom of nerve ischemia. Muscle paralysis develops after sensory loss.
  - Persistent pain disproportionate to the injury and not relieved by immobilization is the most important clinical feature. This pain characteristically increases on limb elevation and with passive stretch of the fingers. One must be careful in interpreting pain in patients who have a concomitant nerve injury or head injury, are intoxicated, or have not yet recovered from a regional nerve block.
  - Pallor and pulselessness are relatively late features and may not appear despite significant increase in compartment pressure.
  - The affected muscle compartment may be hard when palpated, and the overlying skin is shiny and has blisters (Fig. 2-3). Children may have profound anxiety and an increased need for analgesics.
  - Any casts and dressing should be removed and the patient examined frequently. One should be suspicious of this condition, and compartment pressure is obtained in equivocal cases.
- A prophylactic fasciotomy should be performed in all major limb replantations/revascularizations irrespective of the clinical appearance of the limb at the end of the procedure (Fig. 2-4). The limb is insensate and becomes progressively swollen as a result of diminished venous return and ischemia reperfusion injury. When a fasciotomy is not performed, the arterial inflow can be compromised, leading to failure of the replantation.

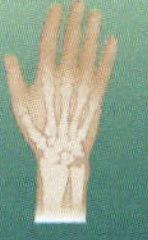

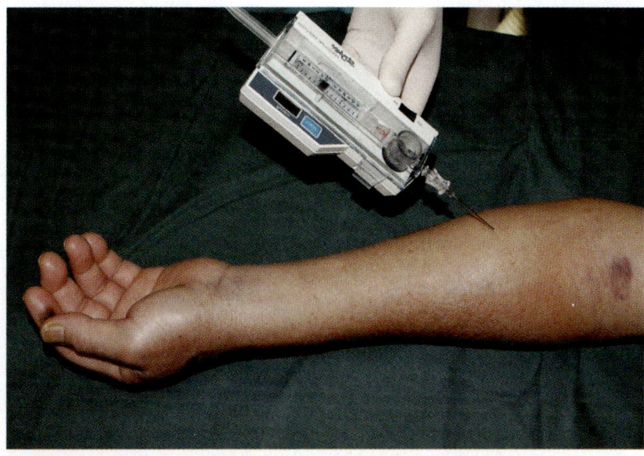

FIGURE 2-5

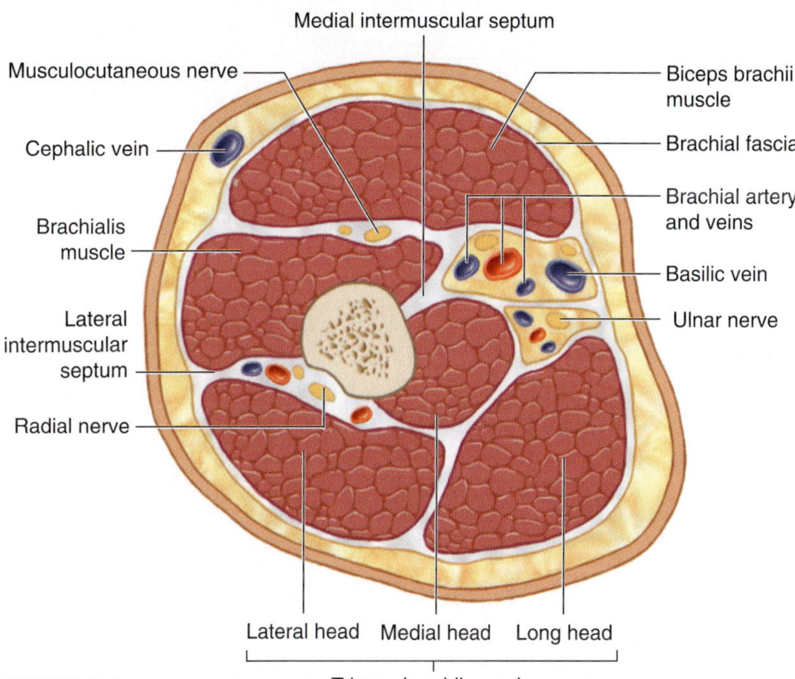

FIGURE 2-6

Investigations

- No investigations are required if a diagnosis of compartment syndrome is clinically apparent. Some laboratory studies (complete blood count, prothrombin time, partial thromboplastin time, serum and urine myoglobin, and creatinine phosphokinase) and imaging studies (radiographs, Doppler, and arteriography) can be used to complement the clinical findings.
- If a clinical diagnosis is equivocal, compartment pressure measurements should be obtained. We use a commercially available device (Stryker Intra-Compartmental Pressure Monitor) (Fig. 2-5). The normal tissue pressure is 0 to 8 mm Hg. A fasciotomy is recommended if the tissue pressure is higher than 30 mm Hg. Close monitoring, repeated clinical examination, and serial measurement of compartment pressures may be required for pressure measurements between 20 and 30 mm Hg.

Surgical Anatomy

- The myofascial compartments of the upper extremity may be divided into compartments of the arm, forearm, and hand (Figs. 2-6, 2-7, and 2-8). The compartments and their contents are listed in Table 2-1.

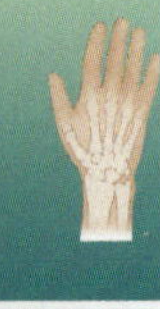

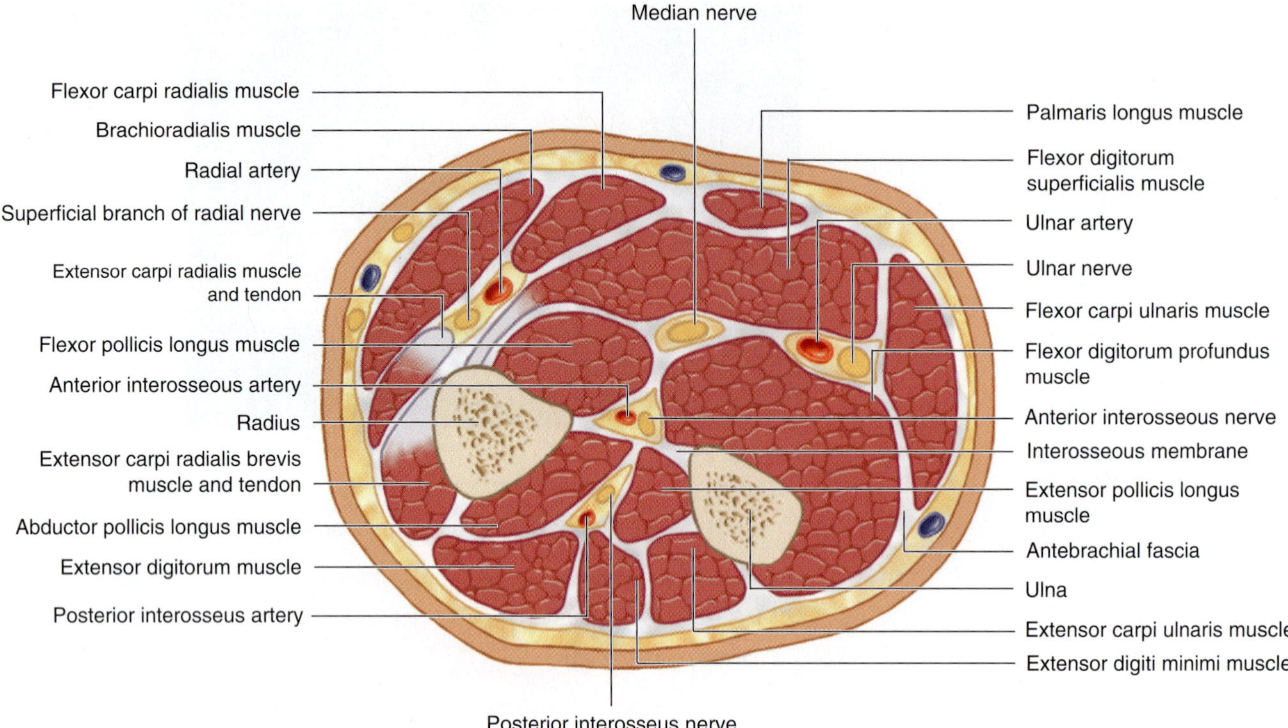

FIGURE 2-7

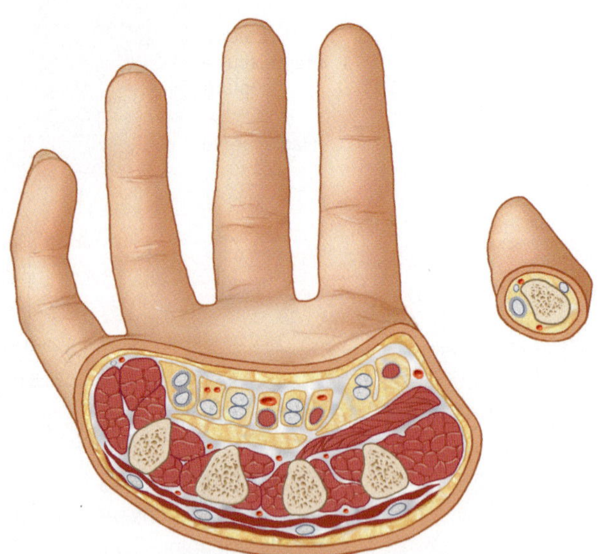

FIGURE 2-8

- The brachial fascia of the arm is thin and poorly defined compared with the fascia of the forearm; therefore, development of increased pressure in the arm is less likely. Although a distinct fascial layer has not been defined in the hand, the glabrous skin overlying the thenar and hypothenar muscle compartments is relatively unyielding and serves as a constricting layer.

Positioning

- The procedure is performed under tourniquet control and regional or general anesthesia. The patient is positioned supine with the affected extremity on a hand table. A fasciotomy is usually done at the end of major limb replantation, and a tourniquet is not used in this situation. An emergency escharotomy may be done at the bedside for a circumferential third-degree burn because such a burn is not painful.

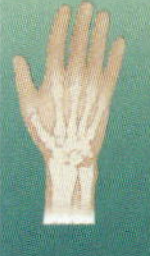

Table 2-1 Myofascial Compartments of the Upper Extremity and Their Contents

	Compartment	Muscle	Artery	Nerve
Arm	Anterior	Biceps, brachialis, coracobrachialis	Brachial	Musculocutaneous
	Posterior	Triceps	Profunda brachii	Radial
	Deltoid	Deltoid	—	Axillary
Forearm	**Volar**		Radial & ulnar	Median, ulnar, & anterior interosseous
	Superficial	Pronator teres, flexor carpi radialis, palmaris longus, flexor digitorum superficialis, flexor carpi ulnaris		
	Deep	Flexor pollicis longus, flexor digitorum profundus, pronator quadratus		
	Dorsal		Pos. interosseous	Pos. interosseous
	Superficial	Extensor digitorum communis, extensor digiti minimi, extensor carpi ulnaris		
	Deep	Abductor pollicis longus, extensor pollicis brevis, extensor pollicis longus, extensor indicis proprius, supinator		
	Mobile wad	Brachioradialis, extensor carpi radialis longus, extensor carpi radialis brevis	—	Radial
Hand	Thenar	Abductor pollicis brevis, opponens pollicis, flexor pollicis brevis	Digital	Recurrent motor
	Hypothenar	Abductor digiti minimi, opponens digiti minimi, flexor digiti minimi	—	Ulnar
	Adductor	Adductor pollicis	—	Ulnar
	Interosseous	4 dorsal and 3 palmar interosseous muscles	—	Ulnar
	Carpal tunnel	Flexor digitorum profundus, flexor digitorum superficialis, flexor pollicis longus	—	Median
	Digit		Digital	Digital

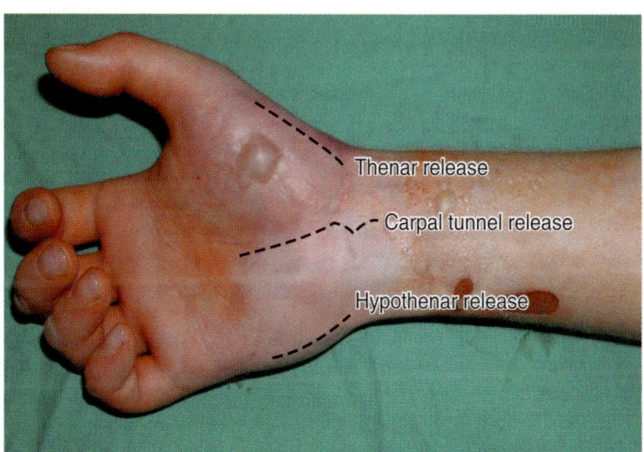

FIGURE 2-9

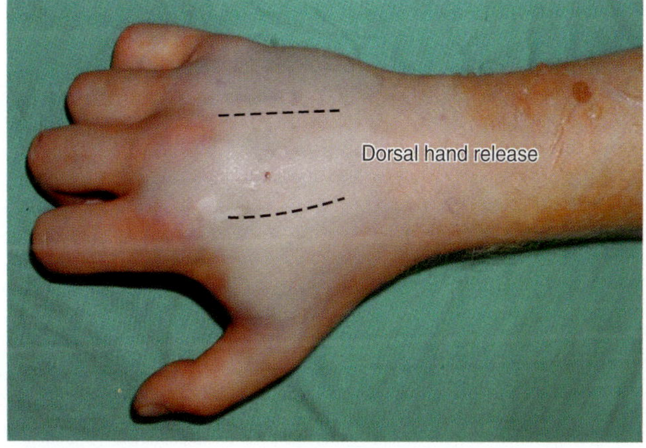

FIGURE 2-10

Exposures

Hand

- The carpal tunnel is decompressed by a single incision between the thenar and hypothenar muscles in line with the third web space (Fig. 2-9).
- The thenar compartment is decompressed by an oblique longitudinal incision along the radial margin of the thenar eminence (see Fig. 2-9).
- The hypothenar compartment is released via a longitudinal incision along the ulnar aspect of the palm (see Fig. 2-9).
- The dorsal compartments are released by two longitudinal incisions parallel to the radial border of the index and ring metacarpals (Fig. 2-10).
- Finger decompression is done by a midaxial incision on the noncontact side of the fingers (ulnar side of index and long finger and radial side of thumb, ring, and small fingers) (Fig. 2-11).

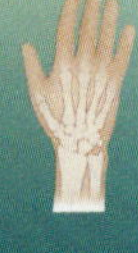

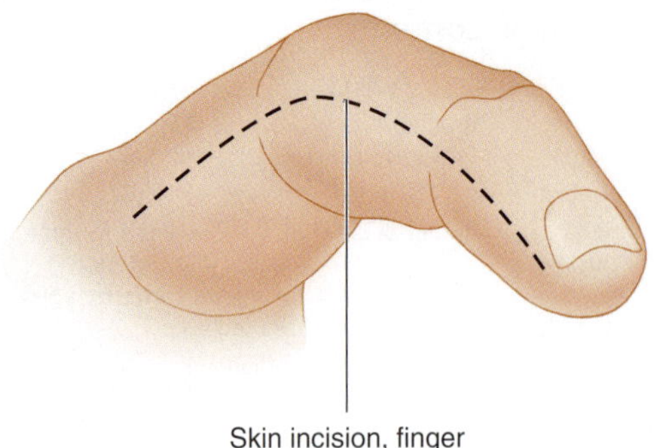

FIGURE 2-11

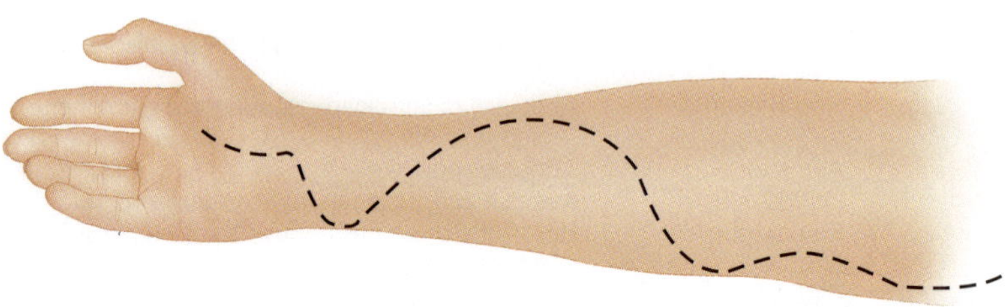

FIGURE 2-12

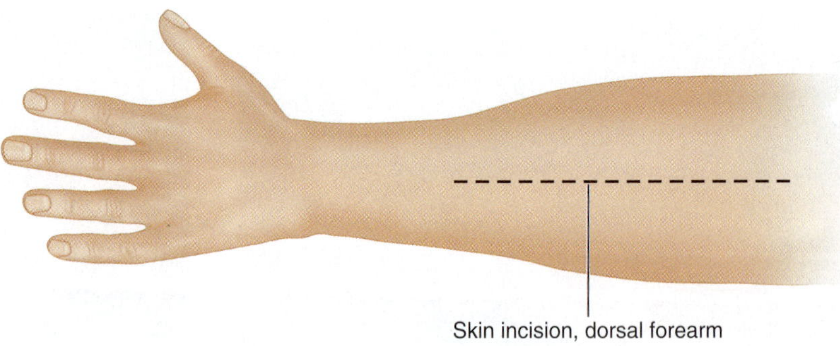

FIGURE 2-13

Forearm

- The standard incision for release of the forearm is a curvilinear incision extending from the medial epicondyle to the proximal wrist crease. It is important to curve this incision over the distal forearm so that a flap of skin can cover the median nerve and the flexor carpi radialis (FCR) tendon (Fig. 2-12).
- A 10- to 15-cm dorsal longitudinal incision beginning 3 to 4 cm distal to the lateral epicondyle toward the Lister tubercle can decompress the dorsal compartment and the mobile wad of muscles (Fig. 2-13). We prefer to use two parallel longitudinal incisions instead of the standard incision.

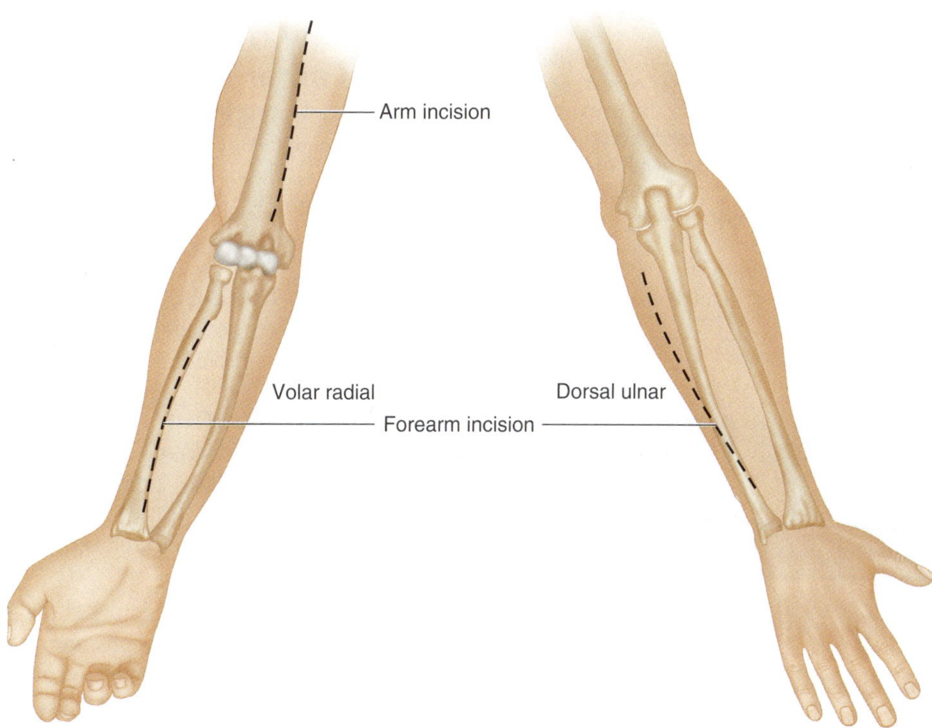

FIGURE 2-14

- One incision is made over the volar radial aspect of the forearm overlying the flexor muscles, and the other is made over the dorsal ulnar aspect over the extensor muscles. This double incision allows decompression of the volar and dorsal compartments and does not expose the median nerve or the tendons at the distal forearm (Fig. 2-14).

Arm

- A medial incision extending from the anterior axillary line to the medial epicondyle can access the anterior and posterior compartments (see Fig. 2-14). The medial incisions can also be used for exposure of the major neurovascular structures in the arm.
- A separate incision over the midportion of the deltoid may be required in rare situations.

PEARLS

One should aim to preserve the cutaneous nerves and veins whenever possible.

The incision for release of the hypothenar compartment should not be over the ulnar border of the hand, but slightly radial to prevent pressure over the scar when the hand is rested (see Fig. 2-9).

When dorsal and volar forearm compartments are involved, it is preferable to release the volar compartment first because the relaxation afforded by the skin and fascia often decompresses the dorsal compartment at the same time.

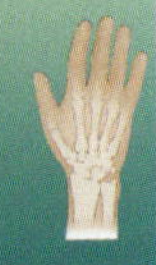

STEP 1 PEARLS

It is important to do the carpal tunnel release through a regular extensile incision that extends to the proximal wrist crease. The limited carpal tunnel release incision used in carpal tunnel syndrome should not be used in this situation because the exposure is poor and fascial release may be inadequate.

STEP 3 PITFALLS

One must take care not to divide the ulnar digital nerve to the small finger.

Procedure

Fasciotomy of the Hand

Step 1: Carpal Tunnel Release

- The incision is deepened, and the palmar aponeurosis is identified. The fibers of the palmar aponeurosis are split longitudinally to expose the transverse carpal ligament (TCL). The distal free edge of the TCL is identified, and the ligament is divided from distal to proximal taking care to protect the median nerve (Fig. 2-15).

Step 2: Thenar Decompression

- The incision is deepened until the abductor pollicis brevis (APB) muscle is visualized. The fascia over the APB is incised (see Fig. 2-15).

Step 3: Hypothenar Decompression

- The incision is deepened until the abductor digiti minimi (ADM) is visualized. The fascia over the ADM is incised (see Fig. 2-15).

Step 4: Decompression of the Dorsal Compartment

- The incision along the radial border of the index metacarpal is used to decompress the first dorsal interosseous and the adductor pollicis (Figs. 2-16 and 2-17). The second dorsal interosseous (between the index and long metacarpals) is also approached via the same incision (see Fig. 2-17).

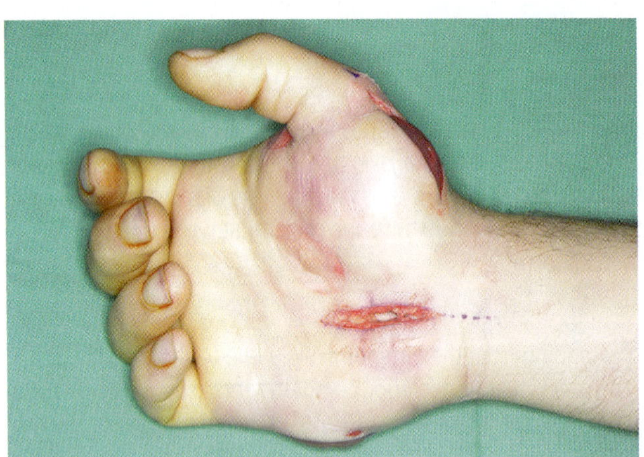

FIGURE 2-15

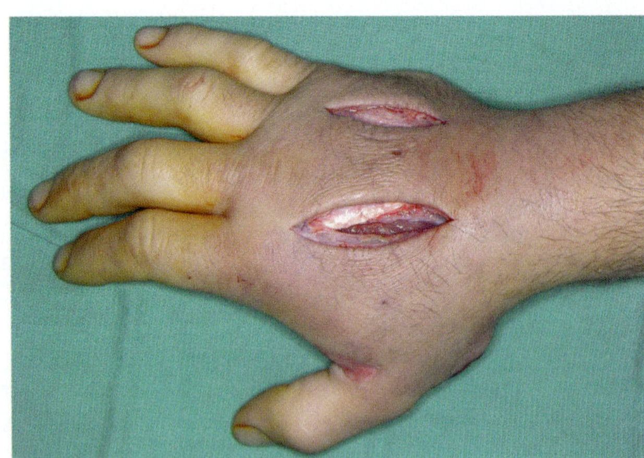

FIGURE 2-16

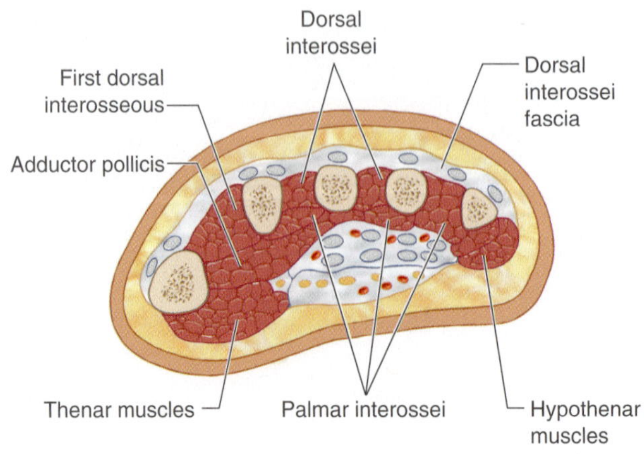

FIGURE 2-17

STEP 4 PEARLS

The release of the skin and superficial fascia is insufficient to decompress the dorsal compartments of the hand. One needs to divide the fascia overlying the interosseous muscle in each intermetacarpal space by retracting the extensor tendons (see Fig. 2-17).

STEP 4 PITFALLS

One must take care to protect branches of the superficial radial nerve and dorsal branch of the ulnar nerve.

STEP 1 PEARLS

If the muscles appear pale, it may be necessary to incise the epimysium to further decompress individual muscles.

It is better to approach the deep muscles after identifying the median nerve and staying ulnar to the median nerve to protect the palmar cutaneous branch of the median nerve. This branch arises from the radial aspect of the median nerve and travels on the ulnar side of the FCR.

- The incision along the radial border of the ring metacarpal is used to decompress the third and fourth dorsal interossei (see Fig. 2-17).

Step 5

- The tourniquet is released and hemostasis secured. One or two tagging sutures may be placed over the carpal tunnel and in other areas to cover any exposed tendons.
- A bulky dressing is applied, and a splint in functional position is provided.

Procedure

Fasciotomy of the Forearm

Step 1: Volar Forearm Release

- The incision is deepened, and the deep fascia of the forearm is divided (Fig. 2-18).
- The deep flexor muscles (pronator quadratus, flexor pollicis longus, and flexor digitorum profundus) may also need to be decompressed. They can be approached by dissecting between the FCR and the palmaris longus (PL).

Step 2: Dorsal Forearm Release

- The incision is deepened, and the deep fascia is divided (Fig. 2-19).
- The mobile wad muscles (brachioradialis, extensor carpi radialis longus and brevis) must be approached via the same incision, and overlying fascia is divided.

Step 3: Two-Incision Release of Forearm

- The two-incision forearm release (volar radial and dorsal ulnar) that we use is depicted in Figures 2-20 and 2-21.

Step 4

- The tourniquet is released and hemostasis secured.
- Any secondary procedures, such as débridement of nonviable muscles and arterial reconstruction, should be done.
- One or two tagging sutures may be placed in the distal volar forearm to cover the median nerve and the FCR.
- A bulky dressing is applied, and a splint in functional position is provided.

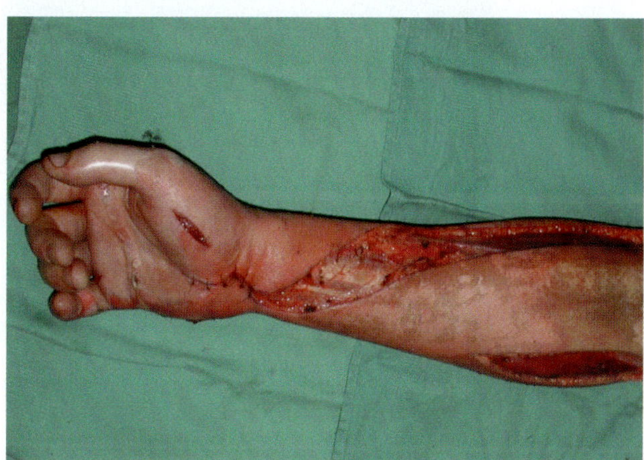

FIGURE 2-18

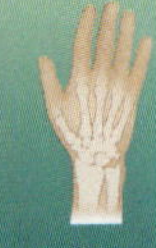

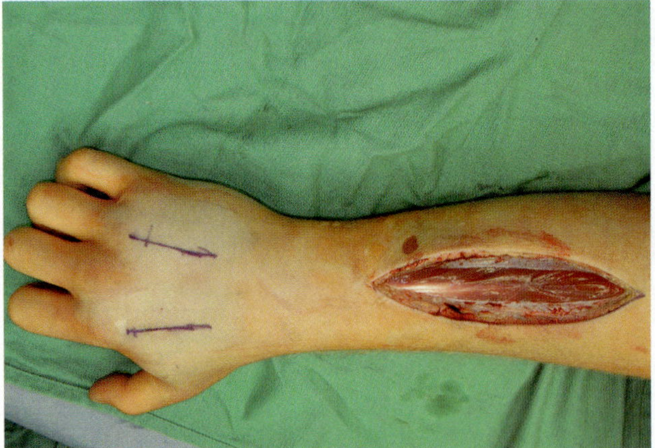

FIGURE 2-19

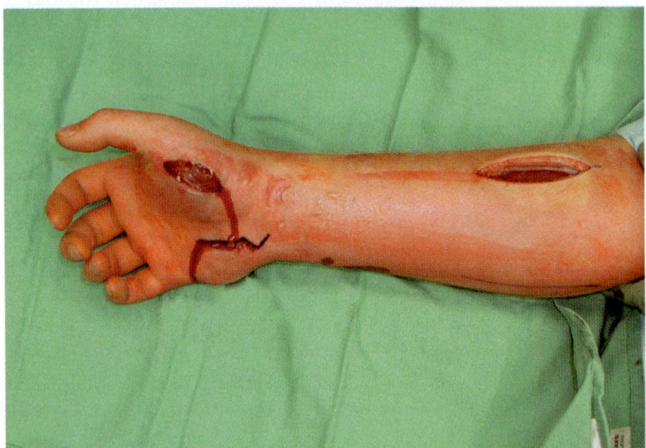

FIGURE 2-20

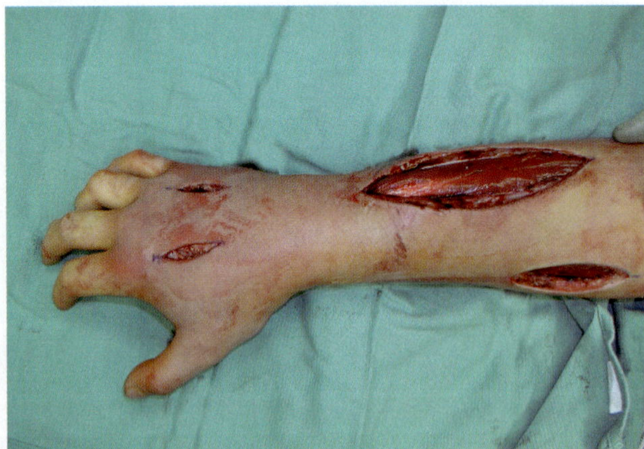

FIGURE 2-21

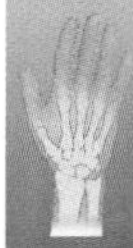

STEP 1 PITFALLS

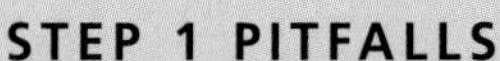

One must take care to protect the medial antebrachial cutaneous nerve.

Procedure

Fasciotomy of the Arm

Step 1: Arm Decompression

- The incision is deepened until the deep fascia. Anterior dissection is carried out initially to decompress the fascia overlying the anterior compartment. Next, the posterior skin flap is mobilized to decompress the posterior compartment.

Step 2

- The tourniquet is released and hemostasis secured. One or two tagging sutures may be placed in the distal arm to cover the ulnar nerve.
- A bulky dressing is applied, and a splint is provided to keep the elbow in 90 degrees of flexion.

Postoperative Care and Expected Outcomes

- The limb should be elevated to decrease swelling and encourage venous return.
- The wound should be reexamined within 24 hours, and, if required, additional débridement is done.
- Wound closure should be planned within 3 to 5 days. Waiting longer makes closure difficult and increases the risk for secondary bacterial colonization. A skin graft may be required occasionally.
- The outcome of fasciotomy depends on how early it is performed. There is usually no morbidity if it is done within 3 to 4 hours. If it is delayed, however, there may be irreversible nerve and muscle injury that will require secondary reconstructive surgery.

Evidence

Bae DS, Kadiyala RK, Waters PM. Acute compartment syndrome in children: contemporary diagnosis, treatment, and outcome. *J Pediatr Orthop*. 2001;21:680-688.

A retrospective study of 33 pediatric patients with compartment syndrome who were treated between 1992 and 1997. Approximately 75% of these patients developed compartment syndrome owing to fracture. Pain, pallor, paresthesia, paralysis, and pulselessness were relatively unreliable signs and symptoms of compartment syndrome in these children. With early diagnosis and expeditious treatment, more than 90% of the patients achieved full restoration of function. (Level IV evidence)

Ouellette EA, Kelly R. Compartment syndromes of the hand. *J Bone Joint Surg [Am]*. 1996;78:1515-1522.

A retrospective review of 19 patients who had been managed with fasciotomy because of compartment syndrome of the hand. All patients had a tense, swollen hand and elevated pressure in at least one interosseous compartment. Carpal tunnel release and decompression of the involved compartments led to a satisfactory result for 13 of the 17 patients who were followed. The remaining 4 patients had a poor result. (Level IV evidence)

Ragland R III, Moukoko D, Ezaki M, et al. Forearm compartment syndrome in the newborn: report of 24 cases. *J Hand Surg [Am]*. 2005;30:997-1003.

A retrospective review of 24 children with compartment syndrome of the forearm at the time of birth. Early treatment was limited to one case, and an emergent fasciotomy was performed with a good outcome. In the other 23 cases, tissue loss, compressive neuropathy, muscle loss, and late skeletal changes were responsible for impaired function. Distal bone growth abnormality was also common. (Level IV evidence)

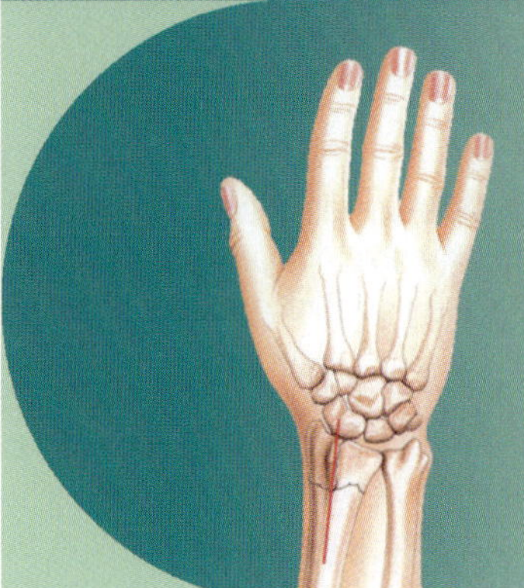

Nail Bed Repair

Pao-Yuan Lin and Sandeep J. Sebastin

Indications

- Open nail bed laceration (Fig. 3-1)
- Closed nail bed laceration with subungual hematoma involving greater than 50% of nail (Fig. 3-2)
- Closed nail bed laceration with displaced distal phalangeal fracture

Examination/Imaging

Clinical Examination

- Complete sensory examination before anesthesia.
- Note pattern of nail bed laceration (simple/stellate), involvement of germinal matrix, and dorsal roof matrix. (Fig. 3-3 shows a crush injury of the right thumb with a stellate laceration involving the sterile and germinal matrices.)
- Look out for associated subtotal pulp amputation (Fig. 3-4).

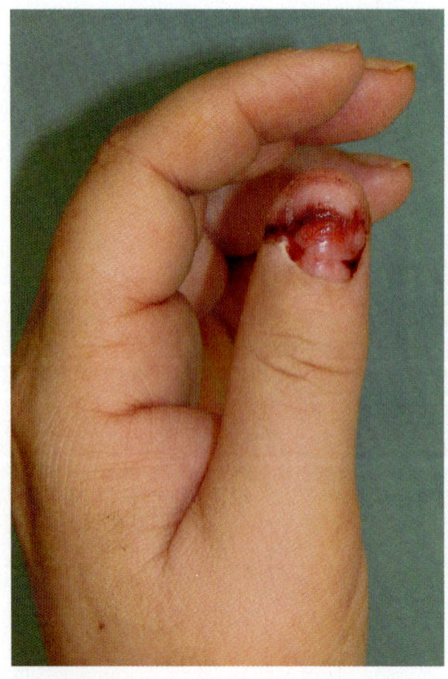

FIGURE 3-1

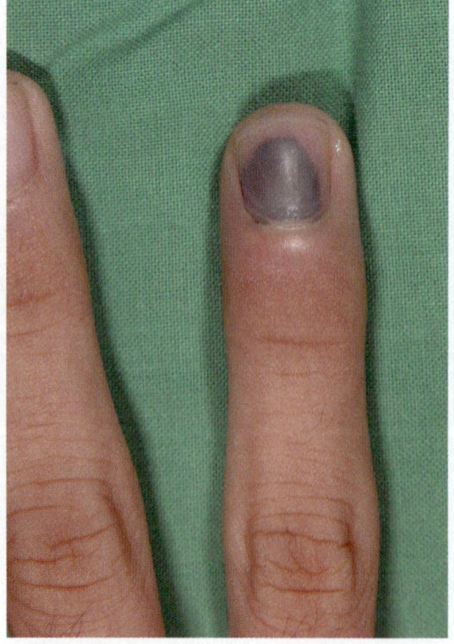

FIGURE 3-2

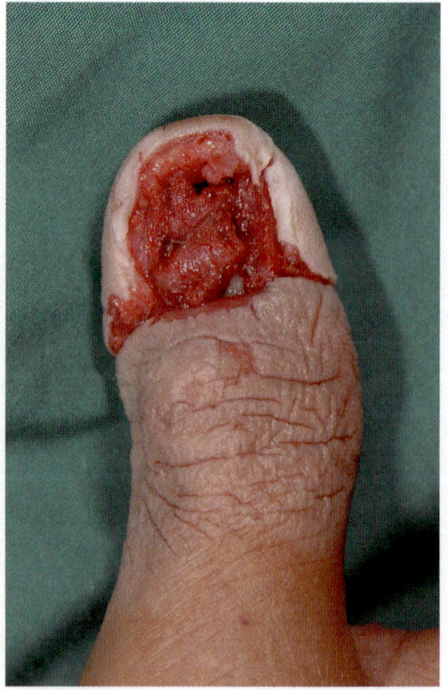

FIGURE 3-3

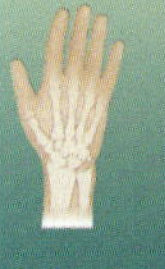

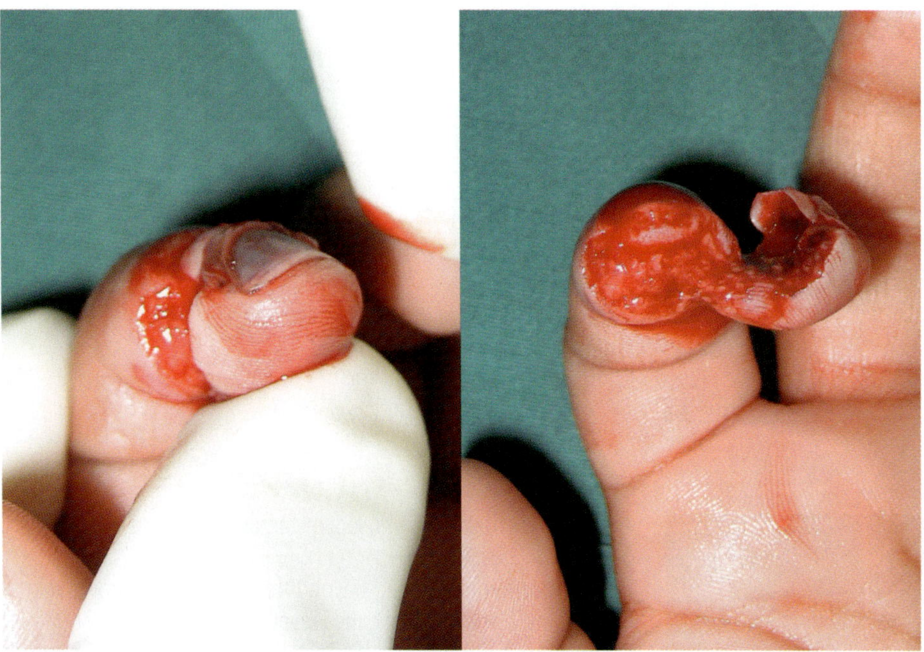

FIGURE 3-4

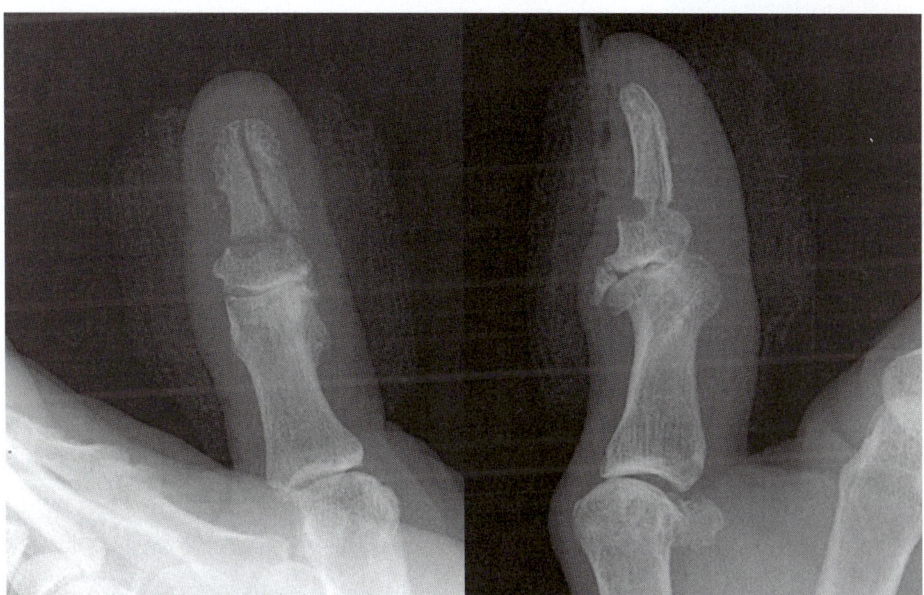

FIGURE 3-5

Imaging

- Radiologic examination should include anteroposterior, lateral, and oblique views of the injured fingers. (Figure 3-5 shows radiographs of the thumb depicted in Figure 3-3.)

Surgical Anatomy

- The nail is a hard structure composed of desiccated, keratinized, squamous cells attached to the nail bed and is the end product of the nail bed's generative efforts. The nail is loosely attached to the germinal matrix but is densely adherent to the underlying sterile matrix and the eponychium.

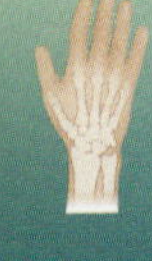

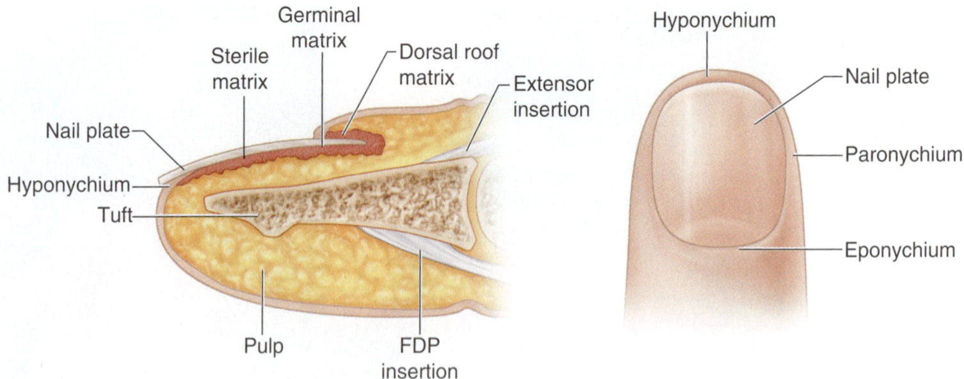

FIGURE 3-6

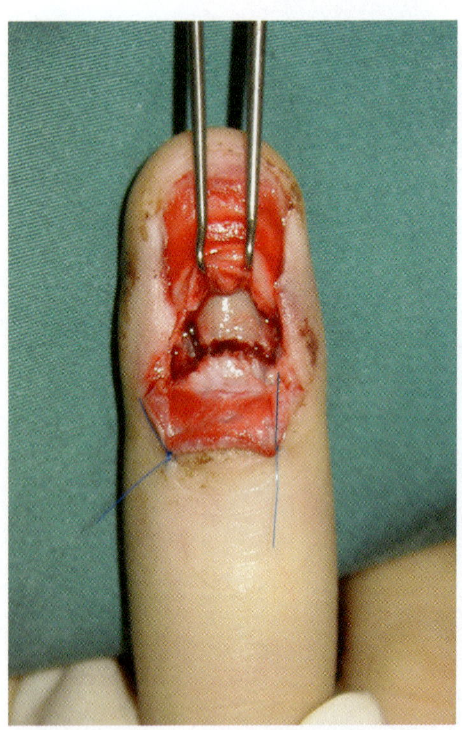

FIGURE 3-7

- The nail bed is composed of sterile matrix, germinal matrix, and dorsal roof matrix (Fig. 3-6).
- The portion of nail bed beyond the lunula is the sterile matrix. The sterile matrix acts as a road bed for the advancing nail. It adds squamous cells to the nail, making it thicker, stronger, and adherent to the bed. Firm adhesion of the nail to the nail bed is essential to the function of the fingertip.
- The germinal matrix is the region of the nail bed proximal to the lunula and responsible for production of the nail plate.
- The dorsal roof matrix is the dorsal portion of the nail bed and is responsible for the luster of the nail plate.

Positioning

- The procedure is performed under tourniquet control. It can be done under local anesthesia. The patient is positioned supine with the affected extremity on a hand table.

Exposures

- A Freer elevator is inserted between the nail plate and the nail bed distally and used to elevate the nail plate off the nail bed from distal to proximal.
- Nail bed lacerations that extend under the nail fold or involve the germinal matrix require elevation of the dorsal roof matrix to expose the laceration and allow a good repair. This is done by making two oblique incisions at the corner of the nail fold and elevating the dorsal roof matrix as a proximally based flap. Two sutures at either corner maintain the flap in position (Fig. 3-7).

PEARLS

In children, general anesthesia is required to facilitate a meticulous repair.

If the laceration involves only the distal portion of sterile matrix, the nail plate needs to be elevated only 1 to 2 mm beyond the laceration.

Examine the undersurface of the nail for any nail bed remnants. They can be used as a free graft.

When the dorsal roof matrix flap is sutured back, it is important to ensure that the suture passes through the full thickness of the tissue.

PITFALLS

The nail bed is adherent to the nail, and occasionally a portion of the nail bed may be elevated along with the nail, especially when the patient has a stellate laceration.

Do not throw the nail away. It can be cleaned and reused as a splint after nail bed repair.

STEP 1 PITFALLS

An aggressive débridement should not be carried out.

STEP 2 PEARLS

A slight gap is preferable to a tight nail bed repair.

A nail bed graft needs to be considered if there is loss of nail bed or there is a gap larger than 4 to 5 mm in the sterile matrix. A split-thickness sterile matrix graft can be harvested from the great toe without much donor morbidity. A gap in or loss of the germinal matrix is difficult to reconstruct. A sterile matrix graft will not replace the function of the germinal matrix. A germinal matrix graft from the toes will cause loss of nail growth in the toes, and the result at the finger may not be successful. It may be reasonable to consider an amputation of the digit proximal to the germinal matrix. An option in patients desiring germinal matrix reconstruction is transfer of toe pulp, using the nail complex as a free flap.

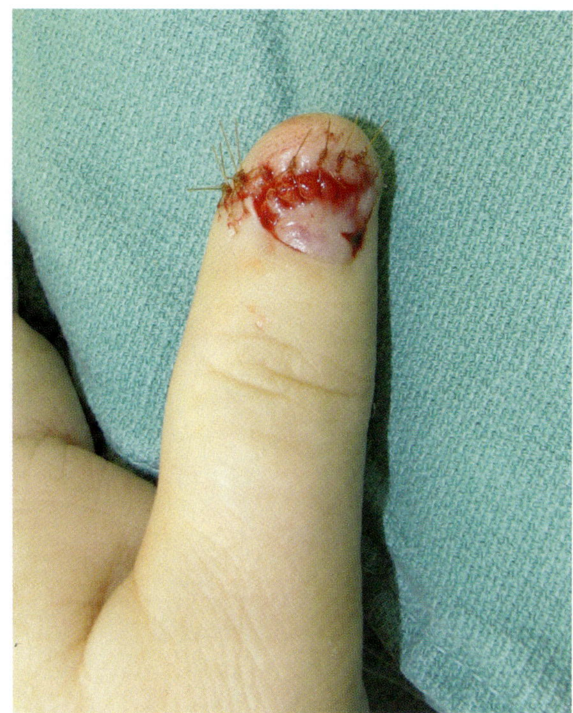

FIGURE 3-8

Procedure

Step 1

- Under loupe magnification, careful minimal débridement of the crushed nail bed is done, and the wound is irrigated.

Step 2

- A tension-free repair of the nail bed is done using 6-0 or 7-0 chromic catgut suture (Fig. 3-8).

Step 3

- The nail is replaced into the nail fold. A figure-of-eight suture or a simple suture from the nail to hyponychium can be used to hold the nail in place.
- This nail serves as a splint for tuft fractures and undisplaced shaft fractures that cannot be or have not been pinned. The nail also prevents the dressing from adhering to the nail bed repair and makes dressing change less painful. Finally, the nail prevents adhesion (synechia) formation between two adjacent injured epithelial surfaces in cases in which the nail bed laceration involves both the germinal matrix and the dorsal roof matrix.

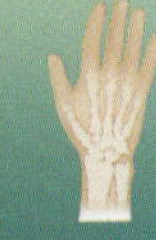

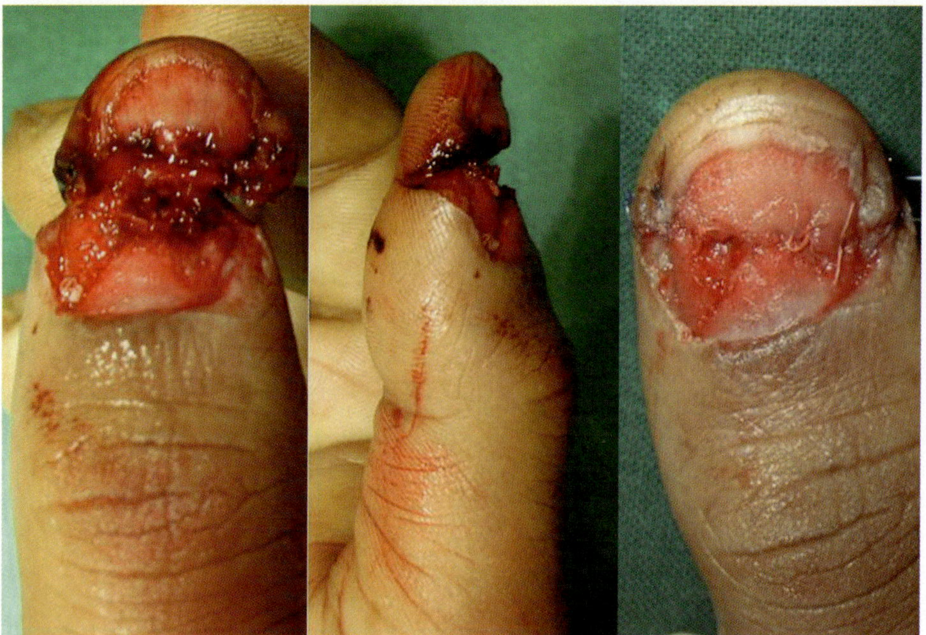

FIGURE 3-9

In severely comminuted stellate nail bed lacerations, it is better to approximate the multiple nail bed flaps with a few strategic sutures instead of attempting an anatomic repair (Fig. 3-9). Good results have been reported with the use of cyanoacrylate glue (Dermabond) in the suturing of such lacerations (Fig. 3-10).

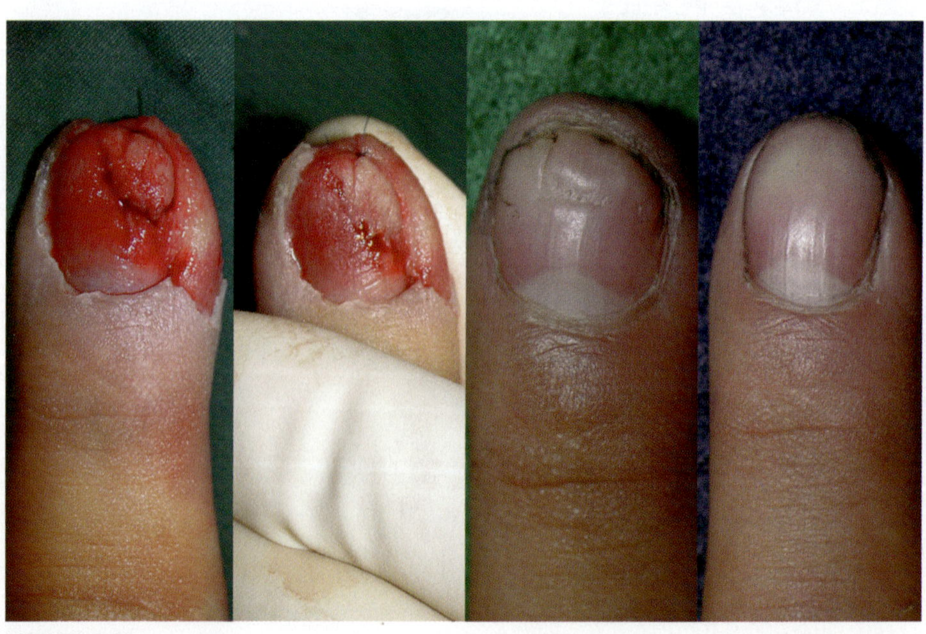

FIGURE 3-10

STEP 3 PEARLS

A couple of holes should be made in the nail using an 18-gauge needle. This provides space for blood to drain (after the tourniquet is released).

If the nail is unavailable or crushed, a sterile artificial silicone nail or a suture package cut in the shape of the nail can be placed within the nail fold (Fig. 3-11). One should remember to make holes for drainage in these nail inserts also.

The nail or an artificial splint should be placed into the nail fold for all lacerations involving the germinal matrix.

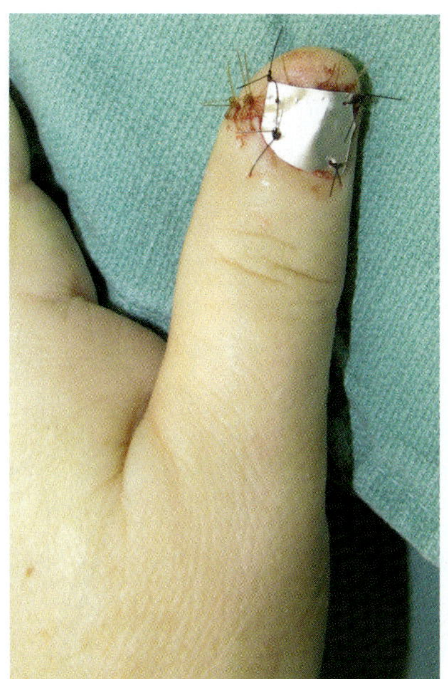

FIGURE 3-11

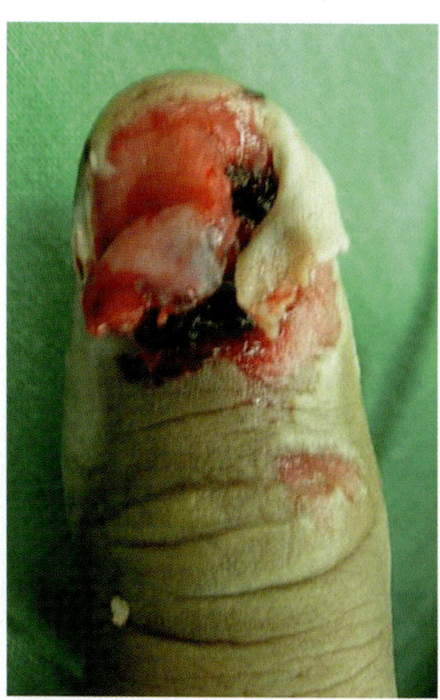

FIGURE 3-12

Procedure

Germinal Matrix Avulsion

Step 1

- A transverse laceration of the germinal matrix at the proximal end of the nail bed (at the junction with the dorsal roof matrix) is referred to as an "avulsion of the germinal matrix." This distally based flap of germinal matrix prolapses out of the nail fold (Fig. 3-12). It is occasionally associated with a displaced fracture of the base of the distal phalanx and prevents closed reduction of the fracture.
- The nail bed flap needs to be reduced back into the nail fold and the reduction maintained with a splint in the nail fold.

Step 2

- A more secure method of maintaining reduction is to elevate the dorsal roof matrix as a flap, as previously described.
- A 5-0 nonabsorbable suture is passed from the dorsum (at the level of the proximal end of the nail bed), a horizontal bite of the nail bed is taken, and the suture is bought back out onto the dorsum. It is then held by a mosquito forceps.

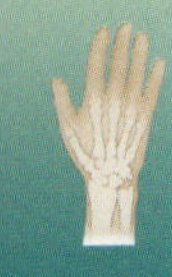

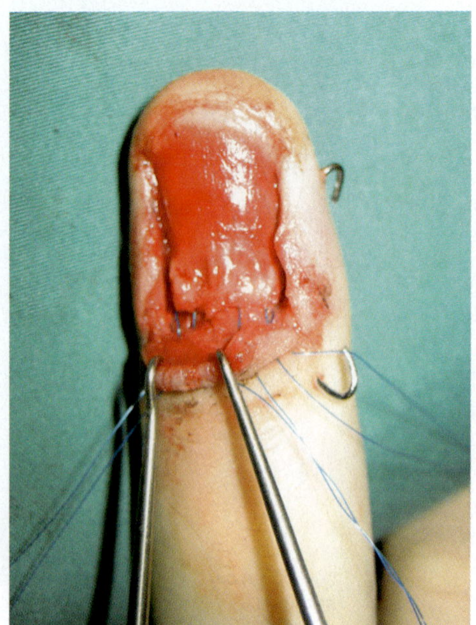

FIGURE 3-13

STEP 3 PITFALLS

The sutures should be tied only after all three or four sutures have been passed. Otherwise, it would become difficult to take a horizontal bite of nail bed after it is reduced under the nail fold.

Step 3

- Two or three more such sutures are passed, so that the entire width of the nail bed is held (Fig. 3-13).
- These sutures are then tied on the dorsum, reducing the nail bed and keeping it in position.

Step 4

- The sutures holding the dorsal roof matrix flap are cut, and the oblique incisions are sutured using 5-0 nonabsorbable suture.

Management of Associated Distal Phalangeal Fracture

- Fractures should be fixated before nail bed repair.
- It is not necessary to fixate distal tuft fractures or very comminuted fractures. The repair of the nail bed and an external split provide adequate stability for most fractures.
- Minimal preliminary shortening of the fracture ends can permit easy nail bed repair in cases in which the nail bed repair is expected to be tight.
- It is better to pin unstable fractures (e.g., transverse fracture between the terminal extensor and flexor insertions). (Figure 3-14 shows intraoperative and late postoperative radiographs of the patient in Figures 3-3 and 3-5.)

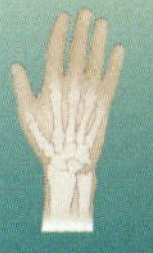

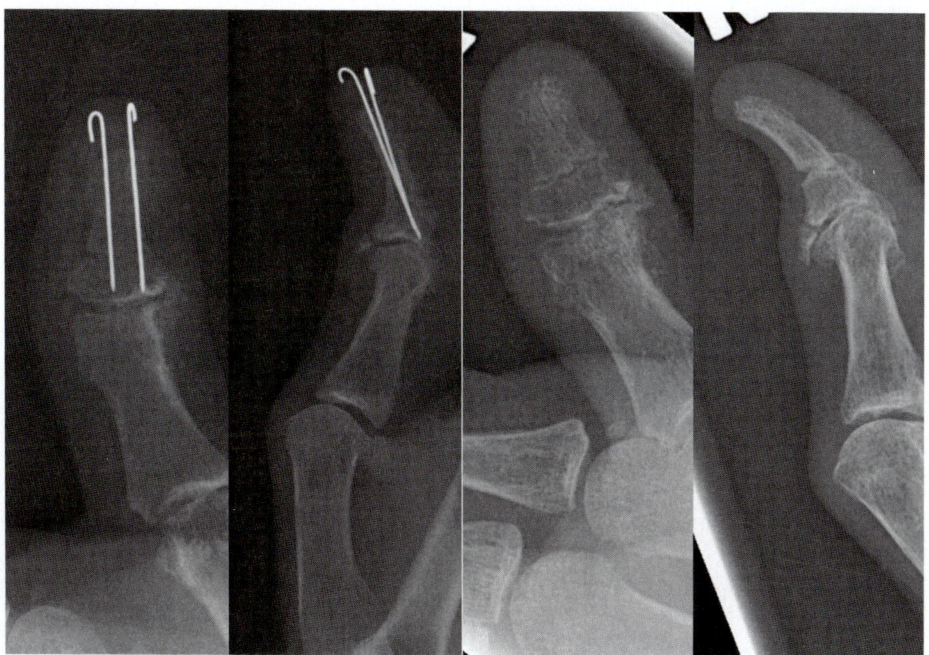

FIGURE 3-14

- Retrograde pinning of the fracture through the fracture site (approached via the nail bed laceration) allows accurate placement of the K-wire.
- A "bamboo split" type of longitudinal fracture can be temporarily stabilized by passing two to three loops of 3-0 or 4-0 absorbable suture (PDS) around the phalanx as a cerclage.
- Trephination of a closed subungual hematoma associated with a fracture should be approached with care. This converts what was initially a closed fracture into an open fracture. It is preferable to drain the hematoma by an open approach by elevation of the nail, irrigation, and nail bed repair.

Postoperative Care and Expected Outcomes

- A nonadherent dressing covered by sterile gauze over a finger dressing is applied.
- A finger splint that immobilizes the distal interphalangeal joint is provided for patients with a tuft or distal phalanx fracture.
- Patients are told that the nail or artificial nail splint may fall out after 2 to 3 weeks as the new nail starts to grow. Complete nail regeneration takes about 4 to 6 months, and the first-generation nail lacks sheen. The second-generation nail, at 9 to 12 months after the injury, is usually of much better quality.
- The quality of the regenerated nail also depends on the initial injury to the sterile and germinal matrix and the age of the patient.

- Figure 3-15 shows the late result of repair of a simple laceration of the sterile matrix after 3 months.
- Figure 3-16 shows the late result of repair of a stellate laceration involving the sterile and germinal matrices of the right index finger after 6 months.
- Figure 3-17 shows the late results of repair of the germinal matrix avulsion shown in Figure 3-12 after 6 months.

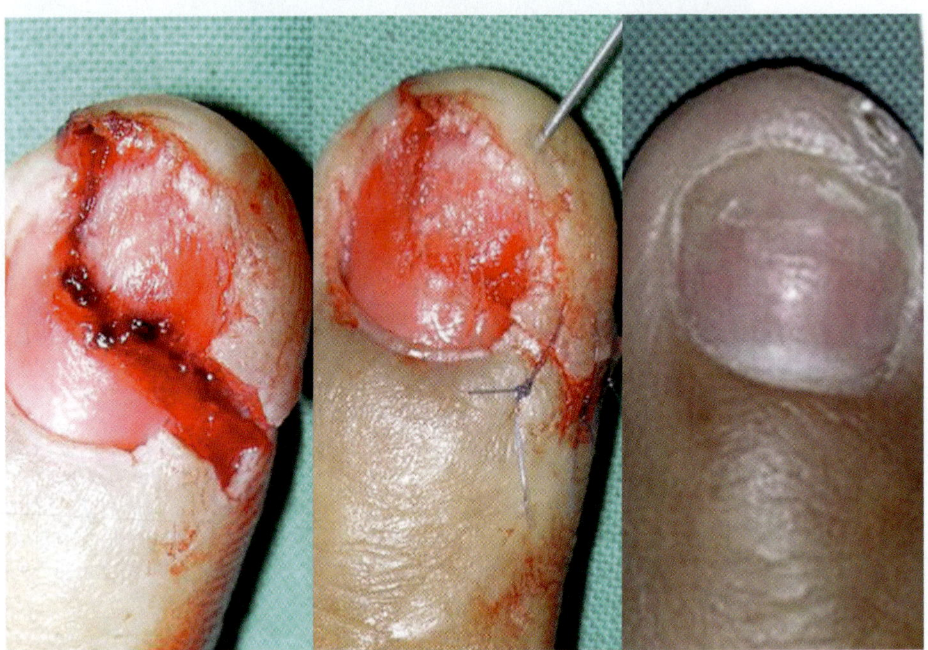

FIGURE 3-15

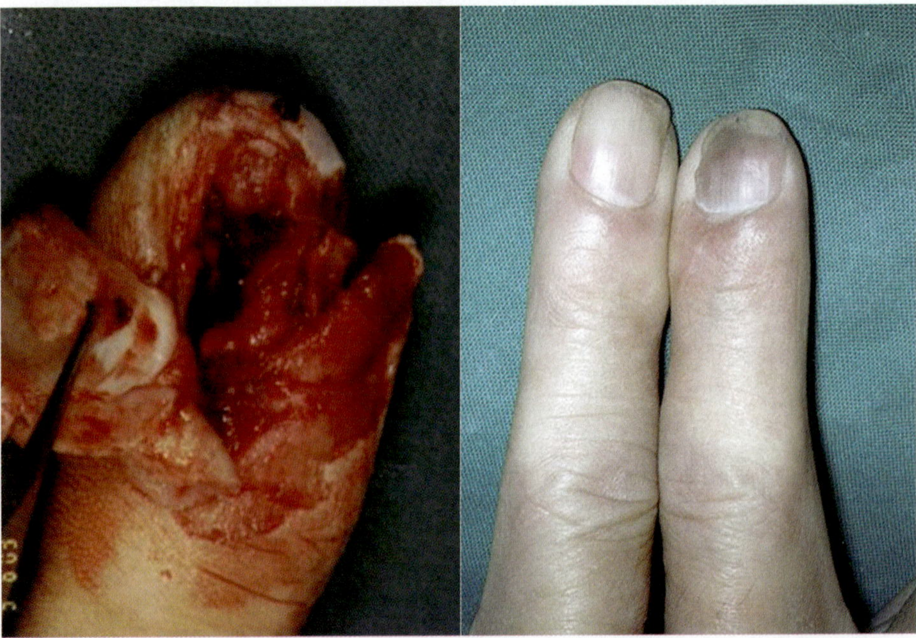

FIGURE 3-16

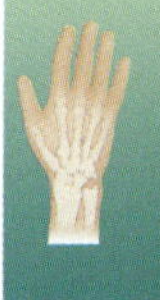

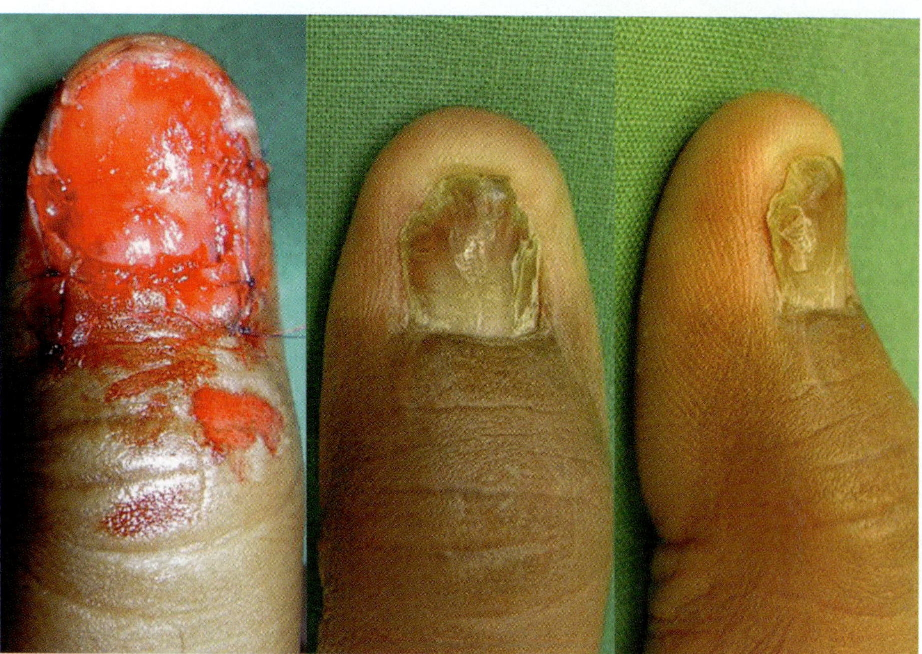

FIGURE 3-17

Evidence

Roser SE, Gellman H. Comparison of nail bed repair versus nail trephination for subungual hematomas in children. *J Hand Surg [Am]*. 1999;24:1166-1170.
Fifty-two children were divided into operative and nonoperative groups. In the operative group, three patients had temporary nail deformity that resolved in 4 months; there were no nail deformities in the nonoperative group. The average cost of treating the operative group was about four times greater than for the nonoperative group ($1263 versus $283). Based on this study, nail removal and nail bed repair are not necessary for children. (Level IV evidence)

Strauss EJ, Weil WM, Jordan C, Paksima N. A prospective, randomized, controlled trial of 2-octylcyanoacrylate versus suture repair for nail bed injuries. *J Hand Surg [Am]*. 2008;33:250-253.
Forty consecutive patients with acute nail bed lacerations were randomly assigned to one of two groups. One group underwent nail bed repair with 6-0 chromic suture, and the nail bed was repaired with Dermabond in the other group. At a mean of 5 months' follow-up, there was no difference in physician-judged cosmetic appearance, patient-perceived cosmetic outcome, pain, or functional ability between the two groups. The average time required for nail bed repair using Dermabond was 9.5 minutes, which was significantly less than that required for suture repair (27.8 minutes). (Level III evidence)

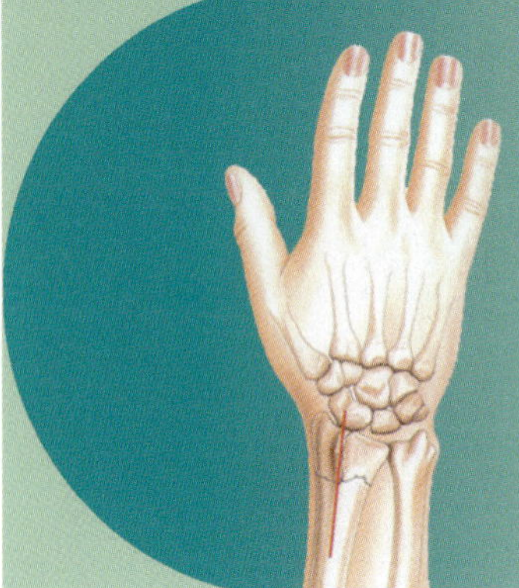

Drainage of Purulent Flexor Tenosynovitis

Brent M. Egeland, Sandeep J. Sebastin, and Kevin C. Chung

Indications

- Clinical diagnosis of acute suppurative tenosynovitis or an infection within the closed space of the fibrous flexor sheath requires early, aggressive treatment.
  - Patients with symptoms lasting longer than 24 to 48 hours
  - Failure of improvement of symptoms with intravenous antibiotics in patients with symptoms for less than 24 hours
  - Diabetic or immunocompromised patient
- Drainage is performed to prevent secondary sequelae of tendon sheath inflammation: stiffness, scarring, or tendon rupture.

Examination/Imaging

Clinical Examination

- Purulent flexor tenosynovitis is a clinical diagnosis.
- Kanavel signs (Fig. 4-1A and B) are as follows:
  - Painful finger held in a slightly flexed position

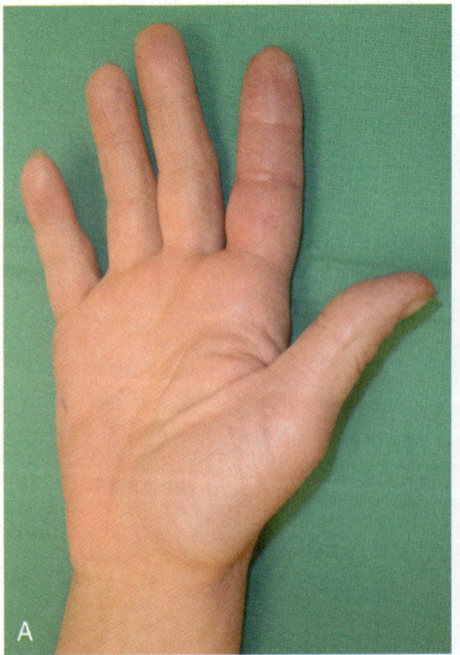

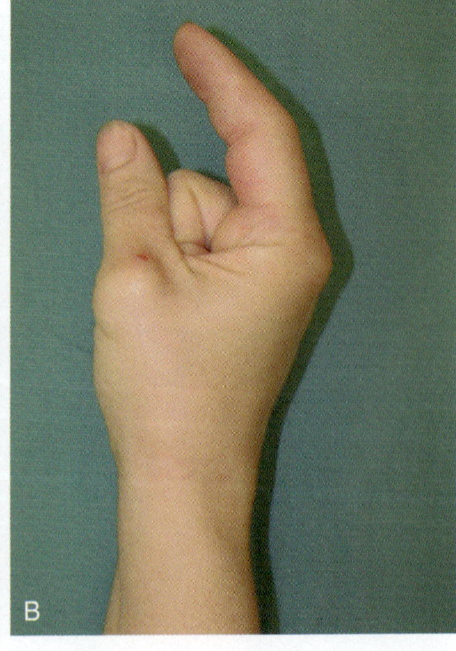

FIGURE 4-1

- Fusiform swelling of the finger, sometimes swelling of the entire hand
- Significant pain with passive extension (or active flexion of the finger)
- Tenderness to palpation along the volar surface of the finger—at the flexor sheath

- Finger erythema is variable.
- Evaluate for possible prior penetrating trauma to the palmar aspect of the digit, which may have seeded bacteria into the tendon sheath.
- Tenosynovitis of the thumb and small finger may be less impressive owing to continuity of the fibrous flexor sheath with larger radial and ulnar bursa that allow spontaneous decompression (Fig. 4-2).
- Infection of the thumb may spread to the small finger and vice versa.
- Examine for signs of gout or other intra-articular processes, which are treated medically.
- Examine for symptoms not confined to one joint. (Gout is typically monoarticular.)
- Without a prior penetrating wound, consider disseminated gonococcal infection or hematogenous spread of bacteria from other sources.

Imaging

- Standard anteroposterior and lateral radiographs of the hand and affected digit should be obtained to rule out a radiopaque foreign body, osteomyelitis, pyoarthrosis, or occult trauma.

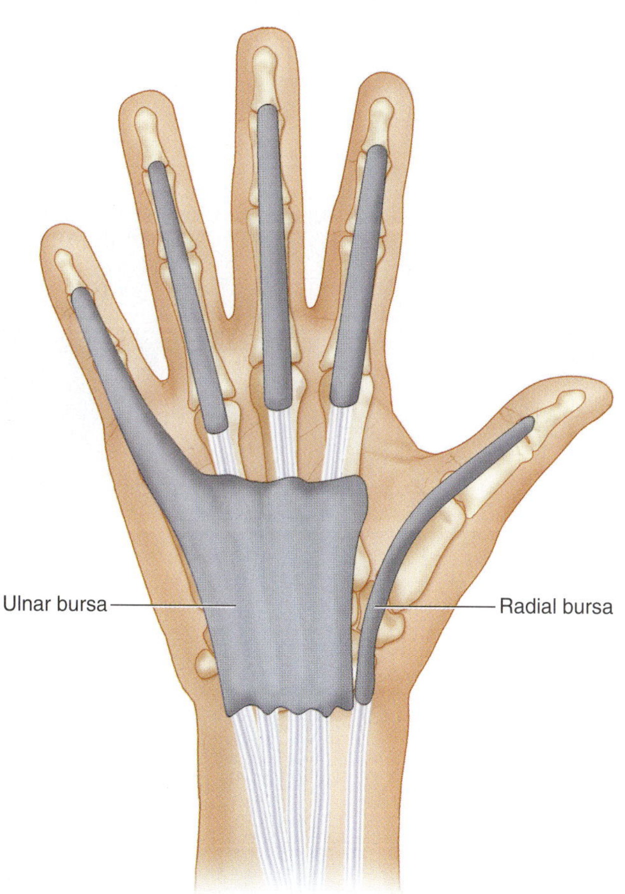

FIGURE 4-2

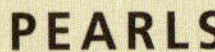

PEARLS

Plan all incisions so that they may be extended distally or proximally as necessary.

Wide exposure of the entire fibrous flexor sheath is reserved for failure of limited exposure. The need for wide exposure is rare and can be associated with exposure of the tendon sheath and neurovascular structures, which leads to desiccation. Most early infections can be treated effectively with antibiotics, hand splinting in intrinsic plus position, and elevation. If the infection does not improve—based on the extent of the erythema and decreased pain—surgical drainage is necessary by the irrigation technique described in this chapter.

Extending the palmar incision proximally may be necessary if the infection has breached the fibrous flexor sheath.

In rare circumstances with ascending infection, a carpal tunnel exposure or volar forearm exposure may be necessary.

PITFALLS

Beware of injury to the neurovascular bundle.

In a midaxial exposure, the incision should be dorsal to the neurovascular bundle.

Inadequate exposure may fail to drain the infection.

Surgical Anatomy

- The fibrous flexor sheath (flexor zone 2) is an enclosed space extending from the metacarpal neck to just proximal to the distal interphalangeal (DIP) joint (see Fig. 4-2).
- The small finger flexor sheath is in continuity with the ulnar bursa, extending to the proximal transverse carpal ligament.
- The thumb flexor sheath is in continuity with the radial bursa, extending to the proximal aspect of the transverse carpal ligament.
- Radial and ulnar bursae may communicate to form a horseshoe abscess via the space of Parona in the volar forearm, between the pronator quadratus and the flexor digitorum profundus.
- The anatomy of the annular pulley system is critical to identifying proximal and distal exposures at A1 and A4, respectively.

Positioning

- The procedure is performed under tourniquet control.
- Use of an Esmarch bandage for exsanguination is risky because it can spread the infection proximally.
- The operation is done under regional or general anesthesia.

Exposures

- Distal exposure is though a longitudinal midaxial incision dorsal to the Cleland ligament, just proximal to the DIP joint on the side opposite the pinch surface, except for the small finger, where the incision is placed radially to avoid the resting ulnar side of the small finger (Fig. 4-3).
- Proximal exposure is via a longitudinal chevron incision at the distal palmar crease just proximal to the A1 pulley.
- In the thumb, a thenar crease incision is used to gain access to the flexor pollicis longus under the distal transverse carpal ligament.

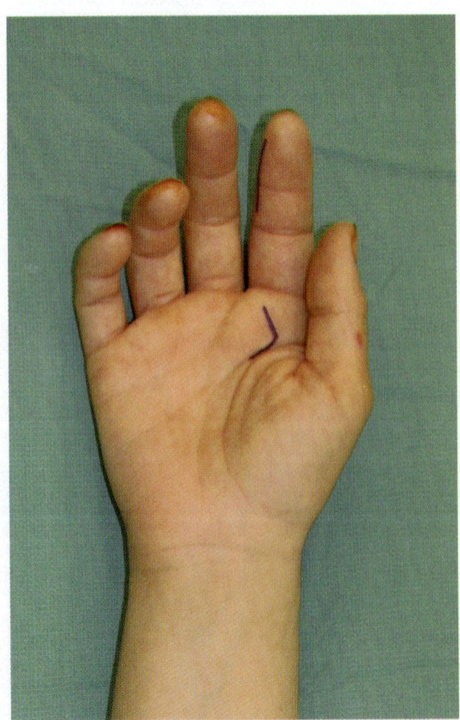

FIGURE 4-3

Procedure

Step 1: Distal Exposure of the Fibrous Flexor Sheath

- Any contaminated puncture wounds should be thoroughly débrided and irrigated.
- A 1-cm midaxial longitudinal incision is made dorsal to the Cleland ligament on the noncontact surface of the finger overlying the A5 pulley (see Fig. 4-3).
- The soft tissues of the finger, including the neurovascular bundles, are elevated in the volar flap of the soft tissue as the incision is carried bluntly down to the lateral aspect of the fibrous flexor sheath at a point overlying the A5 pulley.
- The sheath is entered by sharply dividing the A5 pulley longitudinally over a distance of 5 mm.
- Upon entering the fibrous flexor sheath, purulent material may be encountered; this material should be sent for culture and sensitivity.

Step 2: Proximal Exposure of Fibrous Flexor Sheath

- A longitudinal chevron incision is made over the A1 pulley, corresponding to the proximal aspect of the fibrous flexor sheath (Fig. 4-4).
- Volar soft tissue of the palm can be bluntly dissected and reflected radially and ulnarly to expose the A1 pulley with minimal risk to the neurovascular bundle.
- The A1 pulley does not need to be divided to place the irrigation catheter.

STEP 1 PEARLS

In tenosynovitis, in which an atypical infection is expected, it is important to send the appropriate specimens: Gram stain, culture, sensitivity, acid-fast bacillus stain and culture, nontuberculous mycobacteria culture, fungus stain, and mycotic culture.

If a puncture wound is identified, it is advisable to include this wound in the exposure.

STEP 1 PITFALLS

Too volar an incision places the digital neurovascular bundle at risk.

A small incision in the distal flexor sheath will allow neither adequate decompression nor adequate irrigant egress.

STEP 2 PEARLS

Orientation and placement of incisions should allow for proximal or distal extension in the event of more extensive infection.

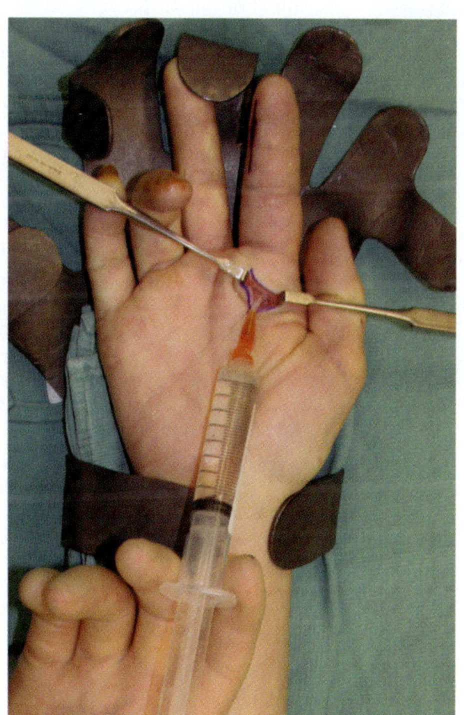

FIGURE 4-4

Step 3: Closed Tendon Sheath Irrigation

- A 16-gauge intravenous catheter is introduced proximally into the fibrous flexor sheath under the A1 pulley (see Fig. 4-4).
- To prevent high-pressure irrigation, a wick or a second irrigation catheter is introduced through the distal incision directed proximally to allow irrigant egress. If the fluid flows easily through the sheath and runs off smoothly over the distal incision, however, a wick is not necessary.
- The tendon sheath should be irrigated with antibiotic-containing saline under gentle pressure until the effluent is clear, typically 500 mL total.
- Drainage wicks should be placed in the proximal and distal incisions, which are left open.
- Continuous irrigation is not used.
- The tourniquet is released, hemostasis is achieved, and the incisions are closed loosely.

STEP 3 PEARLS

An irrigation catheter may be secured in place for continuous or periodic irrigation after the operation, if there is concern about more contamination in the tendon sheath. The need for irrigation of the tendon sheath on the ward is infrequent. It is preferable to irrigate gently through the catheter every 8 hours for 24 hours.

STEP 3 PITFALLS

High-pressure irrigation may spread the infection.

One must be careful not to flush the irrigant into the subcutaneous tissue because this will cause marked swelling in the finger, resulting in finger compartment syndrome.

The fluid should flow readily through the tendon sheath until clear effluent is seen in the distal incision.

Postoperative Care and Expected Outcomes

- The arm and fingers should be immobilized in a bulky splint and elevated.
- If symptoms at presentation do not rapidly improve within 24 to 48 hours, the patient should return to the operating room for additional débridement, irrigation, or wider exposure of infection.
- Intravenous antibiotics for common pathogens, including methicillin-resistant *Staphylococcus aureus*, should be used initially and tailored appropriately.
- Adequate analgesia is necessary to begin early motion.
- The incisions typically heal without specific treatment, but edema may persist for weeks.
- The patient should be informed that scarring along the tendon sheath from the infection might prevent full finger motion.
- Ten to 20% of patients fail to recover full motion.
- About 66% of motion is achieved by 6 weeks, improving to 80% by 30 months.

PITFALLS

Failure to elevate or splint may contribute to difficulty in eradicating infection.

Inadequate intravenous antibiotic therapy may contribute to early recurrence.

Failure to wick the palmar incision open may contribute to recurrence.

Evidence

Abrams RA, Botte MJ. Hand infections: treatment recommendations for specific types. *J Am Acad Orthop Surg*. 1996;4:219-230.
This article presents recommendations for antibiotic treatment of hand infections. The authors clearly discuss treatment options for a variety of infectious conditions in the hand. (Level V evidence)

Lille S, Hayakawa T, Neumeister MW, et al. Continuous postoperative catheter irrigation is not necessary for the treatment of suppurative flexor tenosynovitis. *J Hand Surg [Br]*. 2000;25:304-307.
Retrospective review of 75 patients from two institutions comparing intraoperative débridement alone (20 patients) with postoperative catheter irrigation (55 patients). No statistically significant differences in outcomes were noted. (Level IV evidence)

Neviaser RJ. Closed tendon sheath irrigation for pyogenic flexor tenosynovitis. *J Hand Surg [Am]*. 1978;3:462-466.
The authors describe the use of the catheter irrigation technique presented in this chapter. In this retrospective study, 18 of 20 patients regained full active motion when treated with débridement and 48 hours of continuous irrigation of the sheath. This technique has withstood the test of time and is the recommended technique for the treatment of pyogenic flexor tenosynovitis. (Level IV evidence)

Pang HN, Teoh LC, Yam AKT, et al. Factors affecting the prognosis of pyogenic flexor tenosynovitis. *J Bone Joint Surg [Am]*. 2007;89:1742-1748.
This retrospective review demonstrated poor outcomes in patients who met one or more of five criteria: (1) age more than 43 years; (2) diabetes, vascular disease, or renal failure; (3) subcutaneous purulence; (4) digital ischemia; and (5) polymicrobial question. Patients could be stratified into expected outcome based on the presence or absence of these factors. (Level IV evidence)

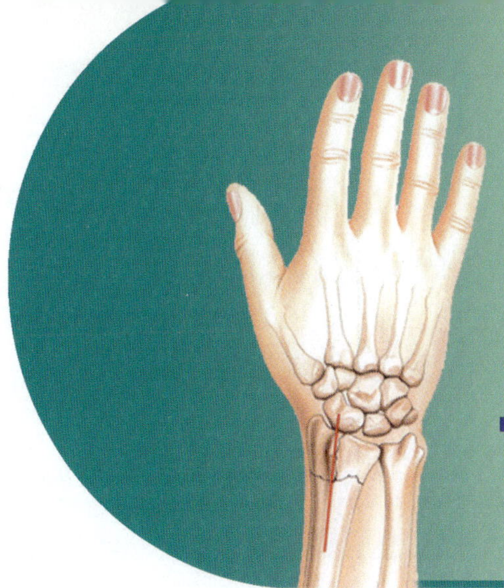

Section II

TENDON CONDITIONS

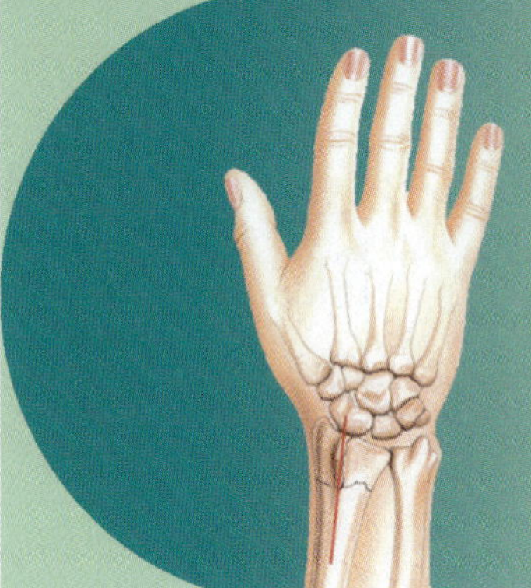

PROCEDURE 5

Surgical Treatment of Trigger Digits

Brent M. Egeland, Sandeep J. Sebastin, and Kevin C. Chung

See Video 2: Surgical Treatment of Trigger Digits

Indications

- Failure of tendon sheath steroid injections
  - Recurrence of triggering after two steroid injections for the thumb, index, long, and ring fingers
  - Recurrence of triggering after one injection in diabetic patients or in patients with long-standing trigger (>6 months), a flexible flexion contracture, or trigger of the small finger. The small finger flexor tendons are narrower compared with the other fingers; therefore, the risk for tendon rupture with repeated steroid injected is much higher.
- A fixed flexion contracture of the proximal interphalangeal (PIP) joint owing to the triggering
- Trigger digits in patients with rheumatoid arthritis
- Congenital trigger finger
- Persistent congenital trigger thumb at 2 years of age

Examination/Imaging

Clinical Examination

- The patient is examined for a palpable nodule at the level of A1 pulley. The patient may be unable to flex the finger or experience a catching when the finger flexes as the enlarged tendon passes through the A1 pulley (Fig. 5-1).
- The grade of triggering should be recorded for follow-up purposes (Table 5-1). One should look for tenderness over the A1 pulley and a palpable nodule. In long-standing triggering, a flexion contracture of the PIP joint may be present, and the degree of contracture should be noted.
- The most frequently involved digit is the ring finger, followed by the thumb and the long, small, and index fingers. Patients who present with primary index finger trigger must be evaluated for associated conditions like diabetes and rheumatoid arthritis.
- In patients with rheumatoid arthritis, one must carefully differentiate between the snapping observed in fingers with early swan-neck deformity and the catching seen in trigger finger. The snapping finger is due to the sudden return of the lateral bands from a dorsal to a palmar location over the condyle of the proximal phalanx as the patient actively corrects the hyperextension deformity. Occasionally triggering may be due to flexor tendon nodules getting caught under the carpal tunnel.

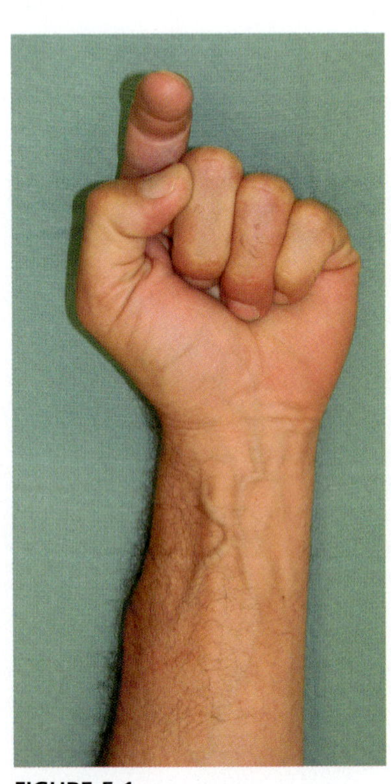

FIGURE 5-1

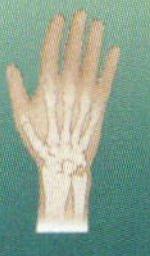

Table 5-1 Grading of Trigger Digits

Grade I	Before triggering	History of triggering, but not demonstrable on examination
Grade II	Active	Demonstrable triggering, but patient can actively overcome the trigger
Grade III	Passive	Demonstrable triggering, but patient cannot actively overcome trigger
• IIIA	• Extension	• Locked in flexion and needs passive extension to overcome trigger
• IIIB	• Flexion	• Locked in extension and needs passive flexion to overcome trigger
Grade IV	Contracture	Demonstrable trigger with flexion contracture of posterior interphalangeal joint

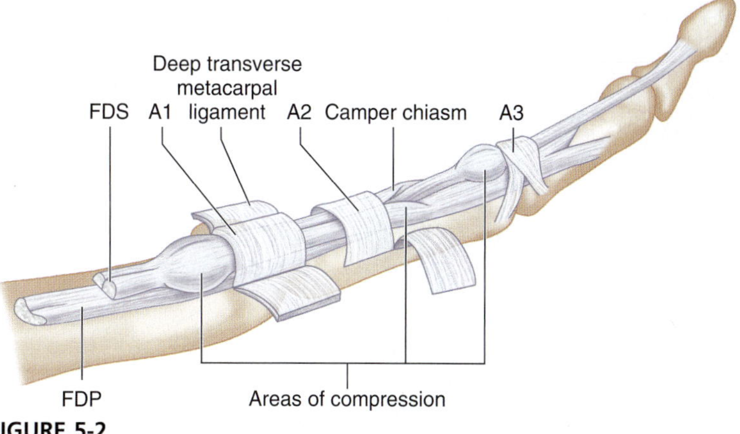

FIGURE 5-2

- Rarely, a locked metacarpophalangeal (MCP) joint can be confused with a trigger finger. A trigger finger primarily affects the interphalangeal joints and is usually gradual in onset, in contrast to the sudden onset of MCP joint locking. MCP joint locking usually results from collateral ligament injury, sesamoid, or osteophyte entrapment.
- Congenital trigger thumb most commonly presents with a fixed flexion deformity, and less commonly with triggering. A characteristic nodule (Notta node) can be palpated on the flexor pollicis longus (FPL) tendon at the region of the A1 pulley. This can help differentiate congenital trigger thumb from other clasped thumb deformities.
- Congenital trigger finger is a distinct entity related to abnormal thickening of the flexor digitorum superficialis (FDS) and flexor digitorum profundus (FDP), calcifications or granulations within the tendons, or abnormal relationship of the tendons at the FDS decussation. The common sites for triggering in a congenital trigger finger are the A1 pulley, the FDS chiasm, and the A3 pulley (Fig. 5-2).

Imaging

- Imaging is most often not necessary. Ultrasound examination can be useful when diagnosis requires confirmation. A radiograph may be useful in a patient with a long-standing flexion contracture to determine the condition of the PIP joint.

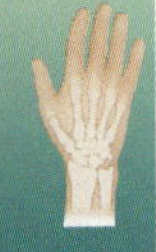

PEARLS

Bruner zigzag incisions are used in patients with rheumatoid arthritis because they may need a wider exposure for tenosynovectomy. Similarly, the zigzag incision is used in pediatric trigger finger to the level of the PIP joint to expose the A2 pulley and FDS decussation.

Surgical Anatomy

- Triggering occurs at the proximal edge of the A1 pulley for the fingers and the thumb.
- The proximal edge of the A1 pulley for the small and ring fingers is in line with the distal palmar crease; for the long finger, it is midway between the distal and proximal palmar creases; and for the index finger, it is in line with the proximal palmar crease. The proximal edge of the A1 pulley of the thumb is at the level of the MCP joint crease.
- Biomechanical studies have shown that the integrity of the A2 and A4 annular pulleys is most important to prevent bowstringing in the fingers. Therefore, it is important to prevent injury to the A2 pulley during division of the A1 pulley. Similarly, the oblique pulley in the thumb prevents bowstringing and should be preserved.

Positioning

- The patient lies supine on the operating table with the affected arm placed on a hand table.
- The procedure is performed under tourniquet control under local anesthesia.

Exposures

- A 1-cm transverse incision is made in line with the distal palmar crease for the long, ring, and small fingers and at the proximal palmar crease for the index finger (Fig. 5-3).

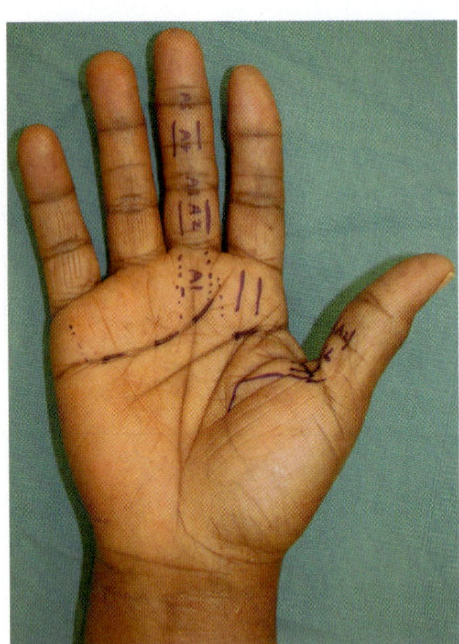

FIGURE 5-3

PITFALLS

The radial digital nerves to the thumb and the index finger are most at risk for injury because they take an oblique course from ulnar to radial close to the A1 pulley. The thumb radial digital nerve is also very subcutaneous and can be accidentally transected with a deep skin incision (Fig. 5-5).

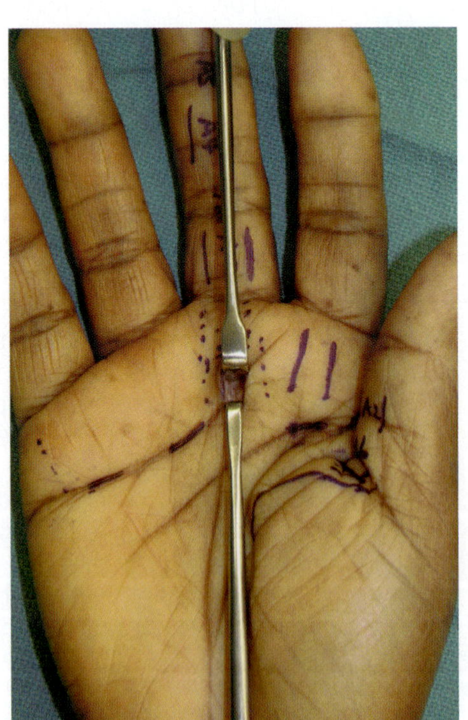

FIGURE 5-4

STEP 1 PEARLS

The scissor tips should be placed parallel to the course of the tendon sheath during soft tissue dissection to avoid injury to the neurovascular bundles.

Patients with rheumatoid arthritis and trigger fingers need flexor tenosynovectomy. A1 pulley release may be done only after tenosynovectomy has failed to relieve the trigger. The release of the A1 pulley may contribute to the MCP joint ulnar drift deformity, especially for the index and long fingers, because of the oblique line of pull of the long flexors for these digits. Because of this tendency, some surgeons recommend resection of one slip of the FDS to provide more space for passage of the FDP, as opposed to an A1 pulley release.

- A 2-cm chevron-shaped apex radial incision is made over the MCP joint crease (a more extensile incision to visualize the digital nerves) for release of thumb trigger.
- The subcutaneous fat is gently spread with scissors to expose the tendon sheath and the A1 pulley. Two Ragnell retractors are held by the assistant to maintain visualization (Fig. 5-4).

Procedure

Primary Trigger Finger Release

Step 1

- The A1 pulley is exposed with gentle traction of the soft tissues and incised with a no. 15 blade (Fig. 5-6).
- Once identified and partially divided, the scissors is used to complete the sheath division (Fig. 5-7).
- Any excessive synovial tissue should also be excised, if encountered.
- A tendon hook is used to provide traction on the FDS, and then the FDP, ensuring that it results in smooth flexion of the PIP joint and distal interphalangeal (DIP) joint, respectively. It is advisable to ask the patient to move the fingers actively to determine whether there is any limitation of tendon excursion.

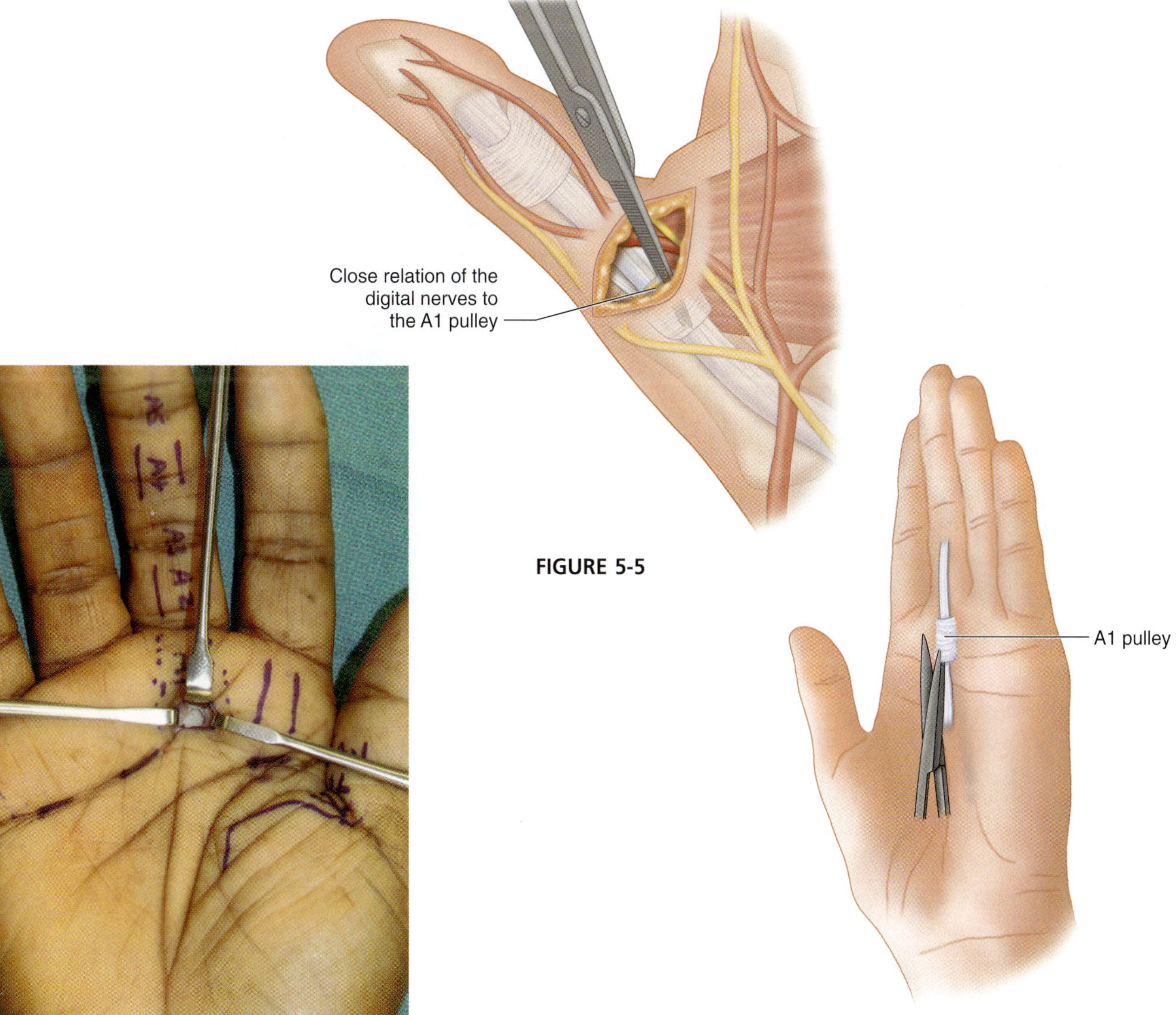

FIGURE 5-5

FIGURE 5-6

FIGURE 5-7

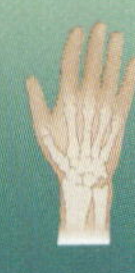

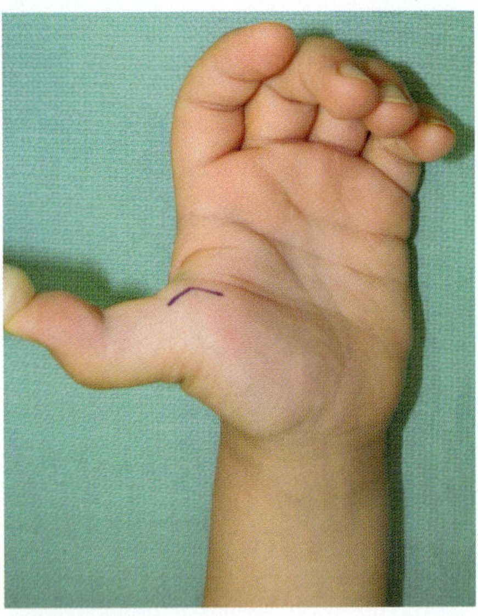

FIGURE 5-8

Step 2

- The tourniquet is released and hemostasis achieved using bipolar electrocautery.
- The skin is closed with interrupted 4-0 nylon sutures.
- A soft, lightly compressive bandage is applied.
- Motion is begun immediately.

Procedure

Congenital Trigger Thumb

Step 1

- A longitudinal chevron incision is designed over the metacarpophalangeal joint crease, corresponding to the A1 pulley (Fig. 5-8).
- The A1 pulley and FPL tendon, often with a focal enlargement called the Notta node, are identified using blunt dissection, with care taken to identify and protect the radial digital nerve (Fig. 5-9).
- The A1 pulley is incised with a no. 15 blade, and the remainder of the division is completed with a tenotomy scissors under direct visualization (Fig. 5-10).

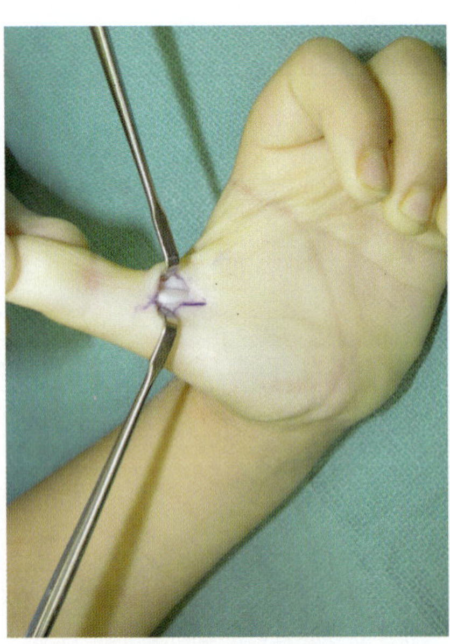

FIGURE 5-9

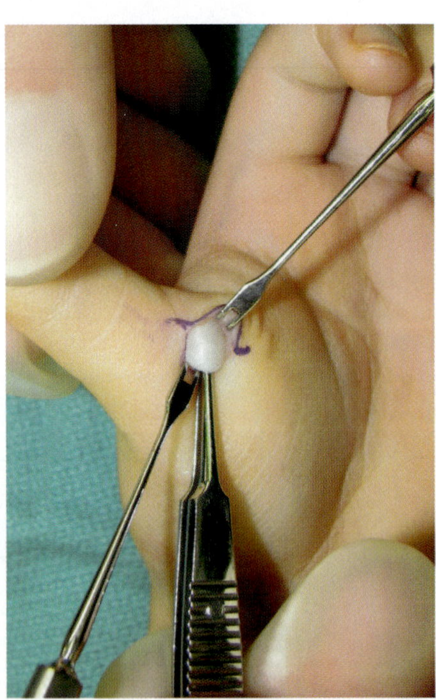

FIGURE 5-10

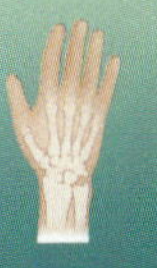

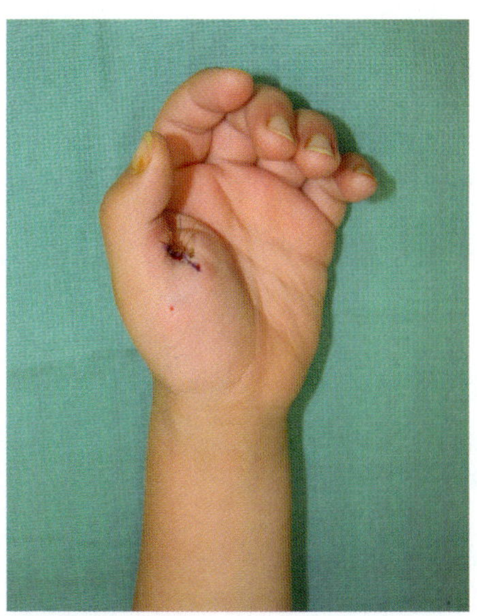

FIGURE 5-11

Step 2

- The tourniquet is released and hemostasis achieved using bipolar electrocautery.
- The incision is closed with 5-0 plain catgut suture (Fig. 5-11).
- A soft, lightly compressive bandage is applied.

Procedure

Congenital Trigger Finger

- Congenital trigger finger is rare. It is usually due to an enlarged tendon or abnormal anatomic relationship of the FDS and FDP at the FDS decussation. Treatment is directed at specific intraoperative findings but may include not only A1 pulley release but also partial resection of the FDP or FDS tendon.

Step 1

- Bruner incisions are made over the A1 and A2 pulleys (Fig. 5-12).
- The A1 pulley is visualized and divided as described previously (Fig. 5-13).

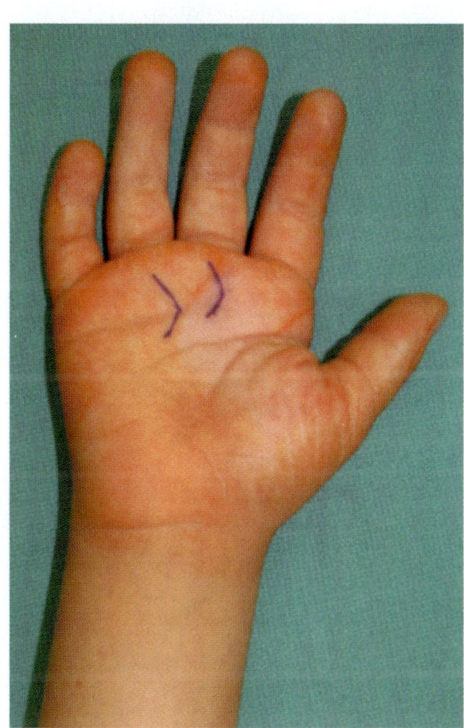

FIGURE 5-12

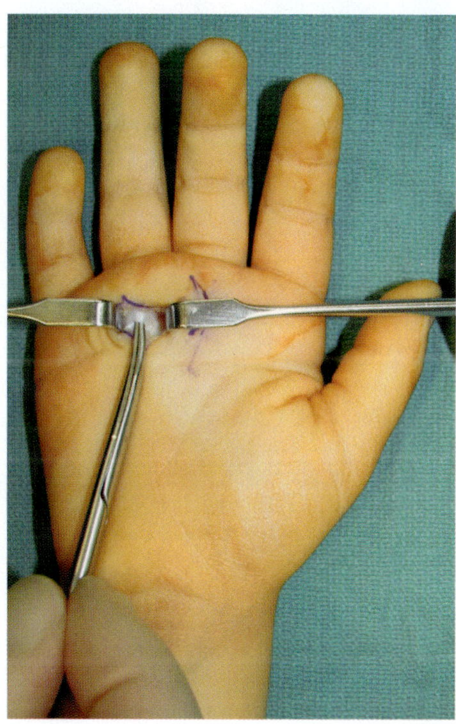

FIGURE 5-13

Step 2

- Intraoperative traction is applied to the flexor tendons, and they are observed for triggering—most commonly at the FDS decussation or under A2 (Fig. 5-14).
- If triggering is observed, the focally thickened tendon is partially shaved to decrease the bulk, and the FDS decussation is opened partially to permit easier movement to the FDP through the decussation.
- If triggering is not yet completely resolved, partial division of A2 may be required (Fig. 5-15).

Step 3

- The tourniquet is released and hemostasis achieved using bipolar electrocautery.
- The incision is closed with 5-0 plain catgut suture.
- A soft, lightly compressive bandage is applied.

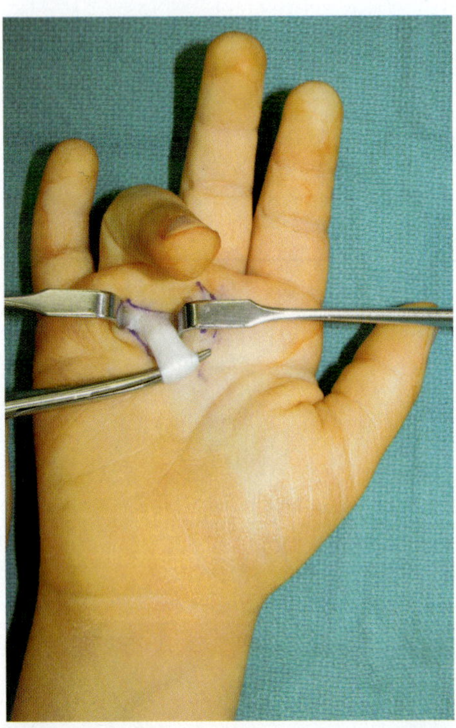

FIGURE 5-14

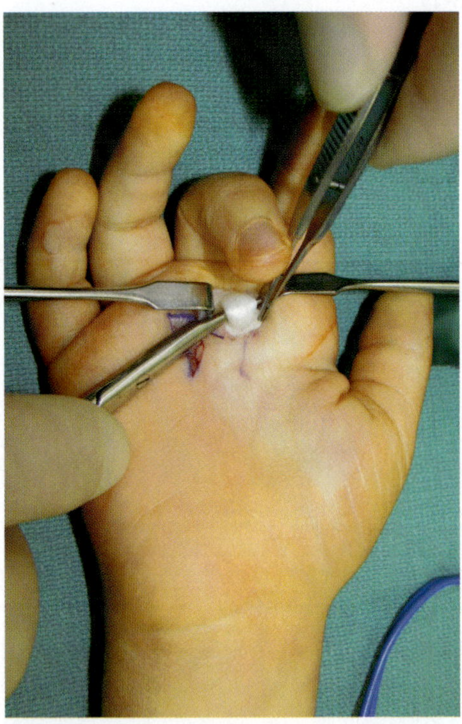

FIGURE 5-15

Evidence

Bae DS, Sodha S, Waters PM. Surgical treatment of the pediatric trigger finger. *J Hand Surg [Am]*. 2007;32:1043-1047.
This retrospective study evaluated 23 pediatric trigger fingers treated over a 10-year period with division of the A1 pulley and resection of a single slip of the flexor digitorum superficialis. Ninety-one percent of fingers had complete resolution of the triggering. There were no complications using the described treatment. (Level IV evidence)

Marks MR, Gunther SF. Efficacy of cortisone injection in treatment of trigger fingers and thumbs. *J Hand Surg [Am]*. 1989;14:722-727.
One hundred consecutive patients with trigger fingers were treated with steroid injection alone. Eighty-four percent of the patients had a favorable response to one injection, and 91% to two injections. This study indicated that steroid injection is quite effective for treating trigger fingers. (Level III evidence)

Wilhelmi BJ, Snyder N, Verbesey JE, et al. Trigger finger release with hand surface landmark ratios: an anatomic and clinical study. *Plast Reconstr Surg*. 2001;108: 908-915.
This study evaluated the anatomic relationships of the A1 pulley to surface landmarks in the hand in 256 fingers. The study demonstrated that the distance from the proximal interphalangeal joint crease to the palmar digital crease is nearly identical to the distance from the palmar digital crease to the proximal edge of A1. (Level V evidence)

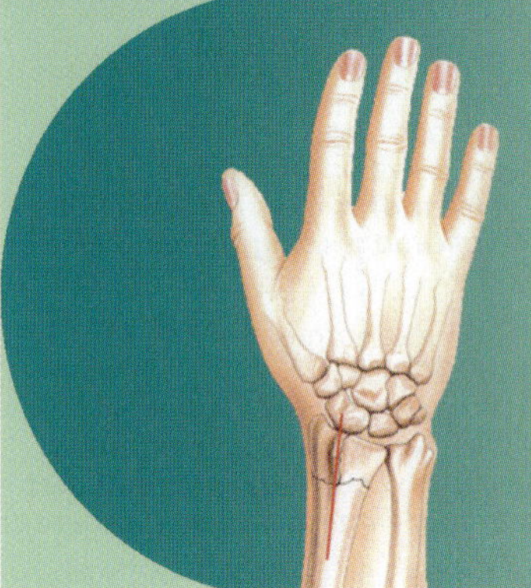

PROCEDURE 6

Surgical Treatment of de Quervain Tendovaginitis

Brent M. Egeland, Sandeep J. Sebastin, and Kevin C. Chung

See Video 3: Release of First Dorsal Compartment for de Quervain Tendovaginitis

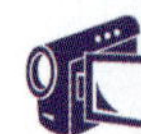

Indications

- Surgery is recommended after failure of conservative treatment measures, including the following:
  - One to two injections of steroids, which should work in up to 70% of patients
  - Wrist splinting for 4 to 6 weeks
  - Avoidance of all inciting activities

Examination/Imaging

Clinical Examination

- The patient has tenderness over the radial styloid and may have triggering of the thumb extensor tendons. The following two tests can be done to confirm the presence of de Quervain disease.
  - *Hitchhiker's sign:* The patient complains of pain localized to the first dorsal compartment when asked to extend and abduct the thumb, as is done when requesting a ride (Fig. 6-1).

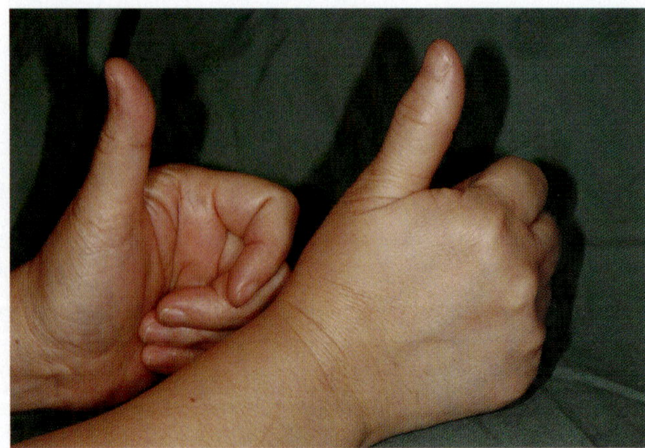

FIGURE 6-1

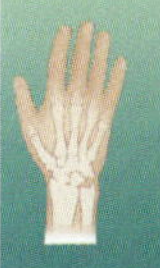

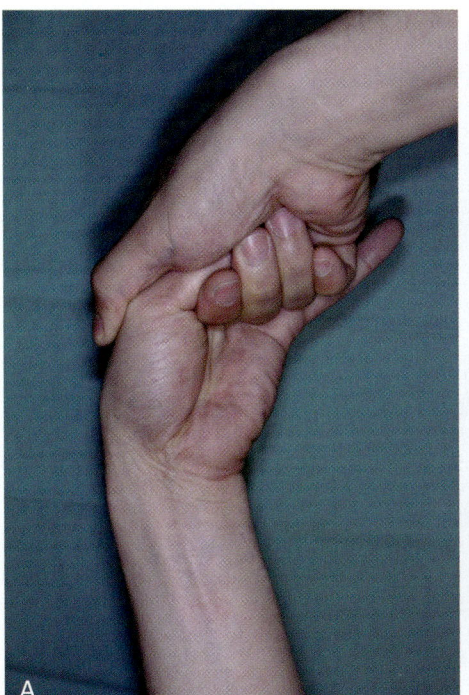

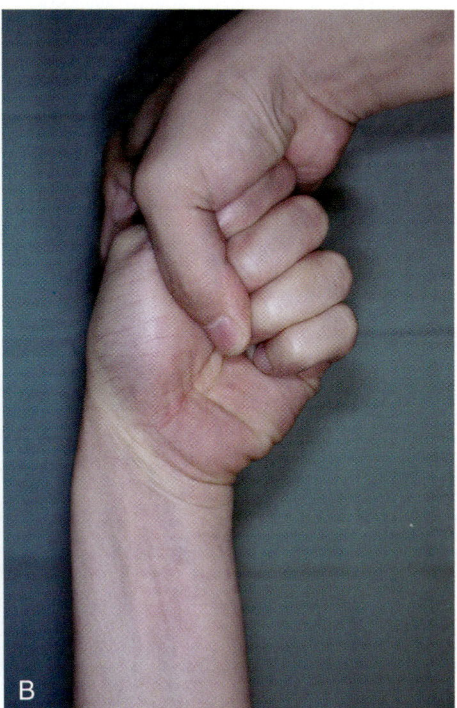

FIGURE 6-2

- *Finkelstein test:* This is done by grasping the patient's thumb and ulnarly deviating the wrist (Fig. 6-2A). This usually results in acute pain over the radial styloid. In the test described by Eichhoff (often misunderstood to be the Finkelstein test), the thumb is placed within the hand and held tightly by the other fingers (Fig. 6-2B). A positive test is when the wrist is painful during ulnar deviation.
- *Extensor pollicis brevis (EPB) entrapment test:* Some patients have separate sheaths for the EPB and abductor pollicis longus (APL), and tendovaginitis may involve either one. This test helps identify pathologic changes involving one or both compartments. The patient is asked to put the palm flat on the table with the wrist in ulnar deviation. First the EPB compartment is tested by asking the patient to lift the thumb directly up (off the table) while the examiner provides resistance over the metacarpal. Next the patient is asked to radially abduct the thumb against resistance, testing the APL. Pain during the first or second maneuvers suggests EPB tendovaginitis and APL tendovaginitis, respectively.

- The examiner must evaluate for and rule out other causes of radial wrist pain. They include thumb basal joint arthritis, scaphoid fracture, Wartenberg syndrome (compression of the superficial sensory branch of the radial nerve between the extensor carpi radialis longus [ECRL] and brachioradialis [BR]), intersection syndrome (tendinitis at the crossing over of the APL and EPB muscle bellies over the ECRL and extensor carpi radialis brevis [ECRB]), scaphotrapeziotrapezoid (STT) arthritis, and Preiser disease (avascular necrosis of the scaphoid).

Imaging

- Plain films should be obtained if the clinical diagnosis is unclear and one needs to consider other differential diagnoses, such as thumb carpometacarpal (CMC) arthritis.

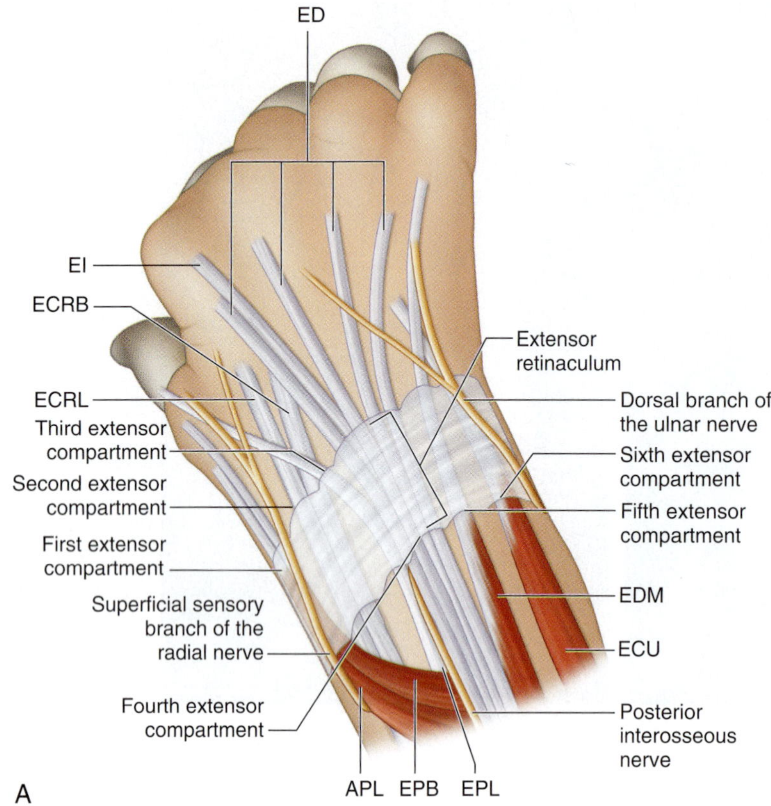

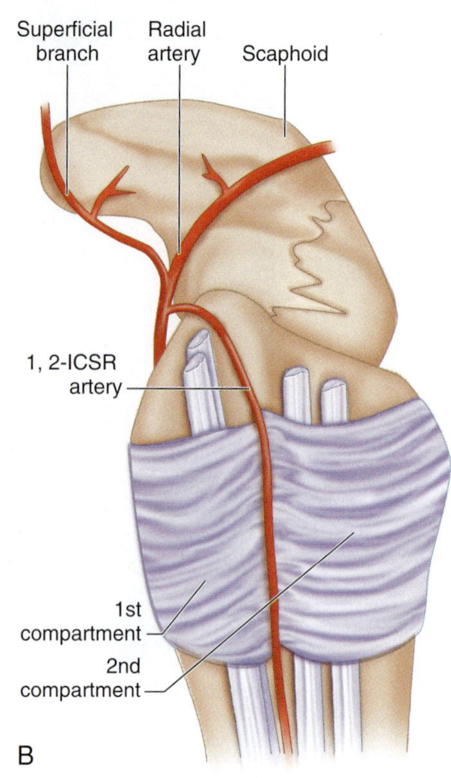

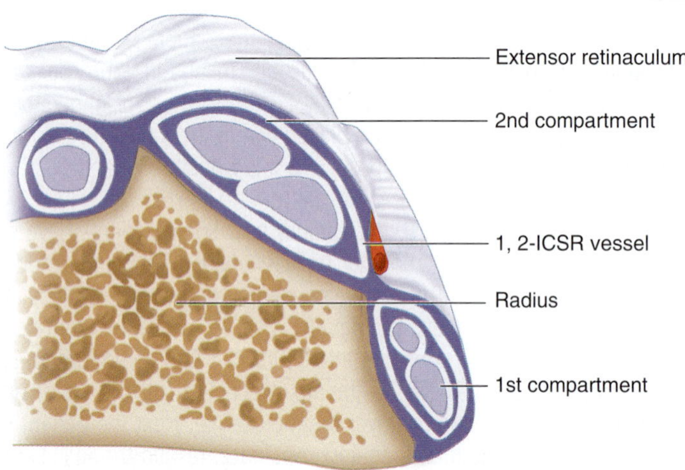

FIGURE 6-3

Surgical Anatomy

- Six extensor compartments have been described over the dorsum of the wrist (Fig. 6-3A).
- The first dorsal compartment is involved in de Quervain tendovaginitis. It contains two tendons, the APL and the EBP (Fig. 6-3B and C). The APL tendon has multiple slips. The APL tendon is more radial and volar, whereas the EPB tendon is ulnar and dorsal. In up to 40% of subjects, there may be a separate subsheath for each of the two tendons.
- The first dorsal compartment is about 2 cm long, with the floor formed by a groove on the radial surface of the radial styloid. The walls are formed by tough intercompartmental connective tissue septa extending from the bony floor to the roof, or extensor retinaculum.

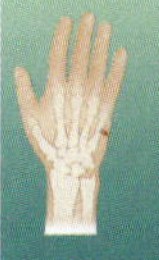

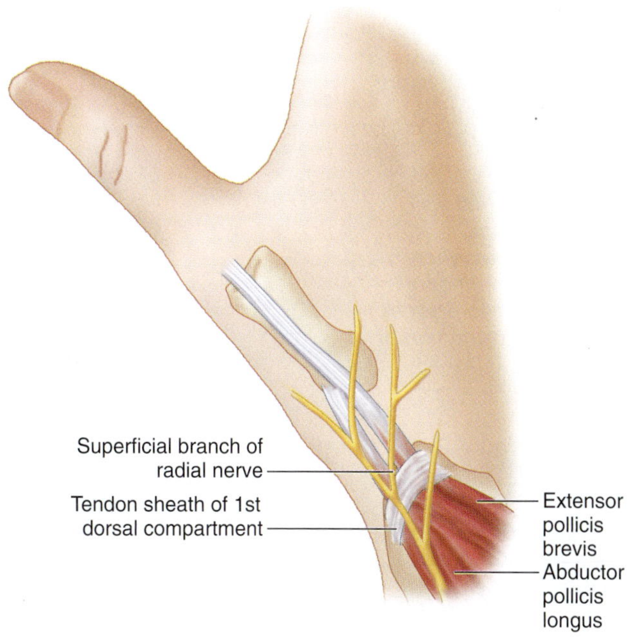

FIGURE 6-4

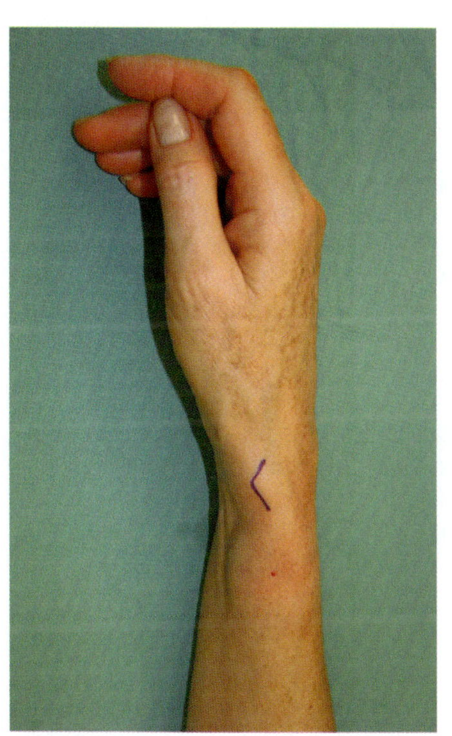

FIGURE 6-5

- The radial artery is volar to the first compartment but is closely related to the floor of the distal end of the first compartment near the radial styloid on its way to the anatomic snuff from a volar to dorsal direction.
- The radial sensory nerve has several branches in the subcutaneous tissue superficial to the extensor retinaculum. Most complications during this operation are a result of traction injury of this nerve, leading to persistent pain at the incision site (Fig. 6-4).

Positioning

- The patient lies supine on the operating table with the affected arm placed on a hand table.
- The procedure is performed under tourniquet control and local anesthesia.

Exposures

- A 3-cm longitudinal chevron incision is made extending proximally from the radial styloid over the first compartment (Fig. 6-5). As soon as the deep portion of the dermis is opened, gentle blunt dissection with a scissors should be used to expose the extensor retinaculum over the first dorsal compartment. The skin flaps can then be gently elevated to fully expose the first compartment.

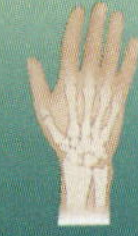

PEARLS

The scissors should be spread in a longitudinal direction to avoid injury to the longitudinally oriented branches of the superficial radial nerve.

The nerve should be identified and protected. It is best to avoid dissection of the nerve, but where required, a thick cuff of perineural fat should be maintained to prevent adhesions of the nerve to the skin or the scar (Fig. 6-6).

PITFALLS

Overzealous retraction of the radial sensory nerve is the major cause of persistence of pain postoperatively.

STEP 1 PEARL

Instead of dividing the first dorsal compartment in the midline, dividing it on the dorsal ulnar border will decompress the compartment, while preventing volar subluxation of the tendons.

STEP 1 PITFALL

One should not mistake the multiple slips of the APL for the EPB (see Fig. 6-8). Traction on the tendons after release should be used to differentiate between the tendons. The EPB subsheath is often hidden under the groove on the radial styloid and easily missed (see Fig. 6-8).

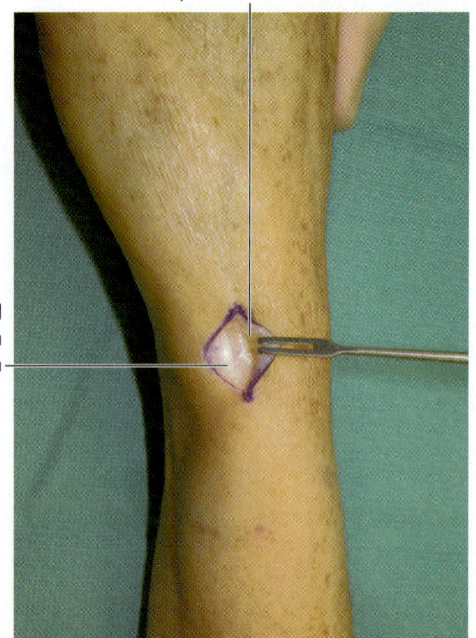

FIGURE 6-6

Procedure

Step 1

- The first dorsal compartment is opened along its entire length with a no. 15 scalpel blade (Fig. 6-7). One should inspect the compartment for presence of any subsheaths, which should be individually released (Fig. 6-8).
- Any hypertrophic synovium should be excised.
- Release is visually confirmed and verified by taking the thumb through a full range of motion (Fig. 6-9).

Step 2

- The tourniquet is released, and careful hemostasis is achieved using bipolar electrocautery, with care taken to avoid cautery injury to the radial sensory nerve.
- The wound is closed with simple cutaneous 4-0 nylon sutures, and a soft dressing is applied.

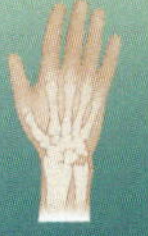

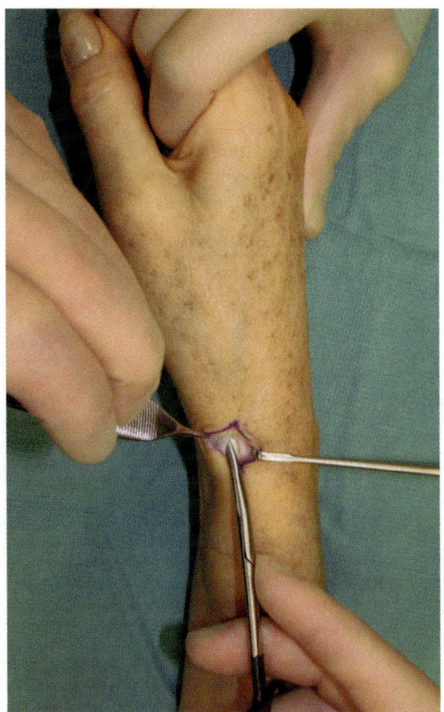

FIGURE 6-7

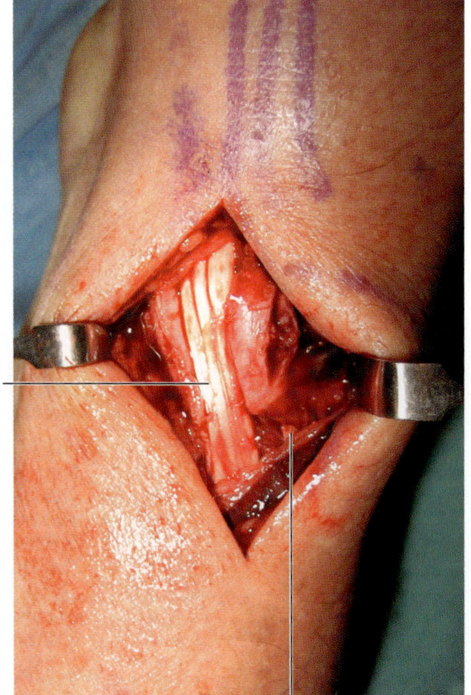

FIGURE 6-8

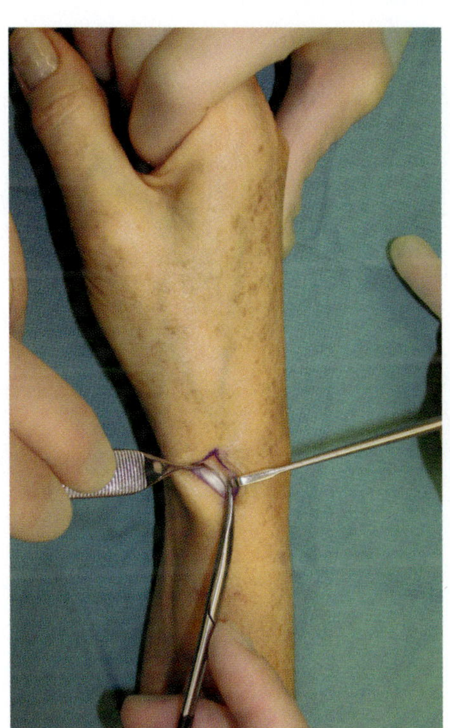

FIGURE 6-9

Postoperative Care and Expected Outcomes

- The patient should wear the gentle compression dressing for several days followed by liberalization of movement as the wound heals.
- The majority of patients (>90%) should have nearly immediate relief of symptoms after release of the first compartment. If symptoms persist, one must consider inadequate release of unrecognized subsheaths within the first compartment.
- Occasionally patients with prolonged symptoms and stiffness may require progressive therapy for active and passive motion and progressive strengthening. This can begin immediately after surgery.
- If a patient develops a sensitive scar, desensitization therapy should be recommended with close clinical follow-up.

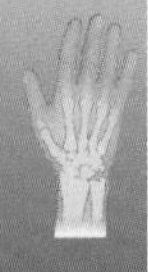

Evidence

Ahuja NK, Chung KC. Fritz de Quervain, MD (1868-1940): stenosing tendovaginitis at the radial styloid process. *J Hand Surg [Am]*. 2004;29:1164-1170.
This is a comprehensive review of the life of Fritz de Quervain, one of the most prominent surgeons of his era. Dr. de Quervain described and proposed surgical treatment for the inflammatory process of the tendon sheath over the first dorsal compartment. This paper also describes other maneuvers to distinguish this condition from associated diseases in this area, including thumb carpometacarpal joint arthritis. (Level V evidence)

Ta KT, Eidelman D, Thomson G. Patient satisfaction and outcomes of surgery for de Quervain's tenosynovitis. *J Hand Surg [Am]*. 1999;23:1071-1077.
This is a three-part retrospective review of 43 patients who underwent surgical treatment for de Quervain tenosynovitis. Follow-up averages 3 years and includes subjective survey data as well as clinical exam data. There was a 5% recurrence rate, one patient (2%) with radial sensory nerve injury, and another with scar tenderness. The cure rate was 88% with a 91% satisfaction rate. (Level IV evidence)

Weiss AC, Akelman E, Tabatabi, M. Treatment of de Quervain's disease. *J Hand Surg [Am]*. 1994;19:595-598.
This longitudinal cohort study of 93 patients with a mean follow-up time of 13 months compared conservative management with splinting versus steroid injection or a combination of the two in treating de Quervain tenosynovitis. This study indicated that any injection had a higher success rate than splinting alone. Ultimately, nearly half of patients underwent surgical release for failure of conservative management. The authors recommend steroid injection without splinting as initial treatment of de Quervain disease. (Level IV evidence)

Witt J, Pess G, Gelberman RH. Treatment of de Quervain tenosynovitis: a prospective study of the results of injection of steroids and immobilization in a splint. *J Bone Joint Surg [Am]*. 1991;73:219-222.
This prospective study evaluated outcomes of lidocaine-steroid injection in 99 wrists with this condition. Satisfactory results occurred in 62% of the wrists, and failure of injection related to potentially missing the abductor pollicis brevis (APB) subcompartment during the injections. The lack of responsiveness with steroid injection may be related to missing the first compartment or missing the separate compartment for the APB tendons. (Level III evidence)

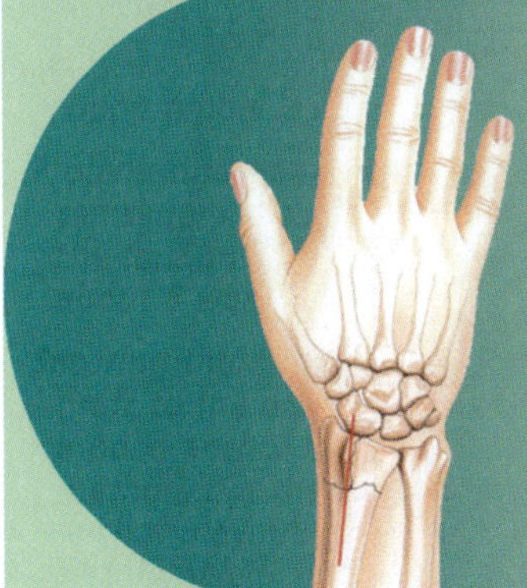

PROCEDURE 7

Acute Repair of Zone 1 Flexor Digitorum Profundus Avulsion

Brent M. Egeland, Sandeep J. Sebastin, and Kevin C. Chung

See Video 4: Acute Repair of Zone 1 Flexor Digitorum Profundus Avulsion

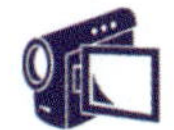

Indications

- Loss of flexion of the distal interphalangeal (DIP) joint may occur owing to avulsion of the flexor digitorum profundus (FDP) from its insertion into the distal phalanx.
- Typical etiology is forced extension of the flexed finger, typically when tackling an opponent in football, which is often called "jersey finger."
- Reattachment is possible if presented 10 to 14 days after injury, or longer if FDP is not retracted proximally because of the restraint provided by the intact vincula.
- If there is a late presentation, the potential need for tendon grafting or other procedures such as DIP fusion or tenodesis must be discussed.
- If tendon grafting is contemplated for late presentation, the patient must have a supple DIP joint. In addition, patient expectations must be appropriate.
  - Patient has a need for DIP joint function.
  - Patient is willing to comply with postoperative precautions and therapy to optimize success.

Examination/Imaging

Clinical Examination

- With the metacarpophalangeal (MCP) and PIP joints in extension, the patient is unable to actively flex the DIP joint (Fig. 7-1).
- A soft tissue mass may be felt, and there may be localized bruising over the volar finger at the location of the retracted stump.

Imaging

- Standard anteroposterior and lateral radiographs are necessary.
- Lateral radiographs may demonstrate an avulsed bony fragment at the DIP or proximally in the finger or palm corresponding to the proximal retraction of the FDP tendon to which the bone fragment is attached (Fig. 7-2).
- Ultrasound may be beneficial in confirming the injury, identifying the location of the retracted tendon preoperatively, and aiding in surgical planning, particularly in late presentations.

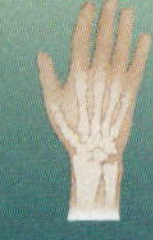

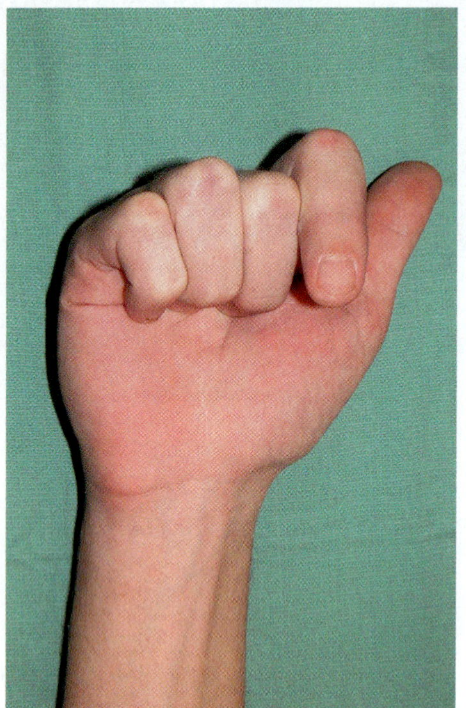

FIGURE 7-1

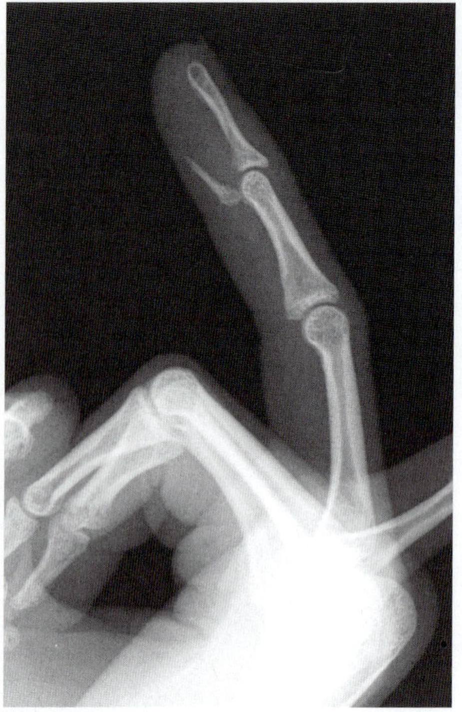

FIGURE 7-2

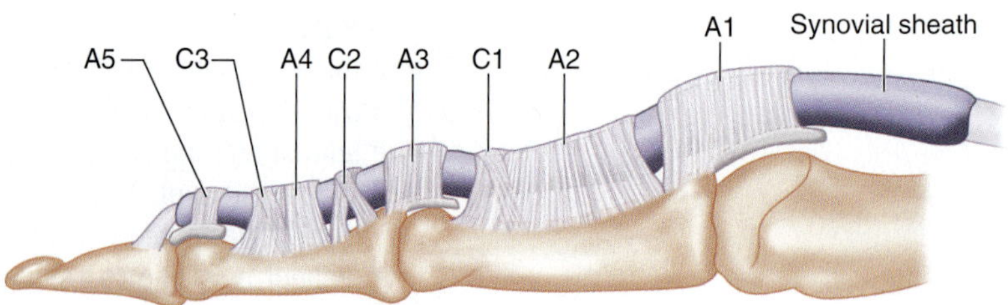

FIGURE 7-3

Surgical Anatomy

- Flexor zone 1 is distal to flexor digitorum superficialis (FDS) insertion over the middle third of the middle phalanx and contains only the FDP, C3, and A5 pulleys (Fig. 7-3).
- Blood supply to the distal FDP is from the vinculum longus profundus (VLP), vinculum brevis profundus (VBP), and distal phalanx at its bony insertion (Fig. 7-4).
- Avulsed tendon can retract proximally in three patterns as defined by Leddy and Packer (1977). Additional types 4 and 5 have been described (Fig. 7-5).
  - *Type 1:* FDP has pulled though zone 2 to lie in the palm or A1 pulley—vincular blood supply is disrupted. The tendon and bone fragment can be passed through the pulley system and repaired with a pullout button.
  - *Type 2:* Most frequent; the FDP retracts to the PIP joint at the FDS chiasma between the A2 and A4 pulleys. Proximal retraction is prevented by intact vincula brevis. Because blood supply is not completely disrupted, delayed repair is possible.

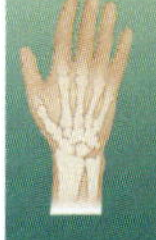

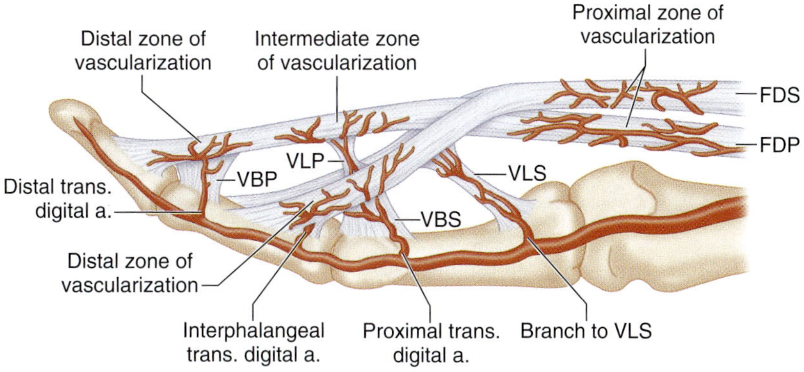

FIGURE 7-4

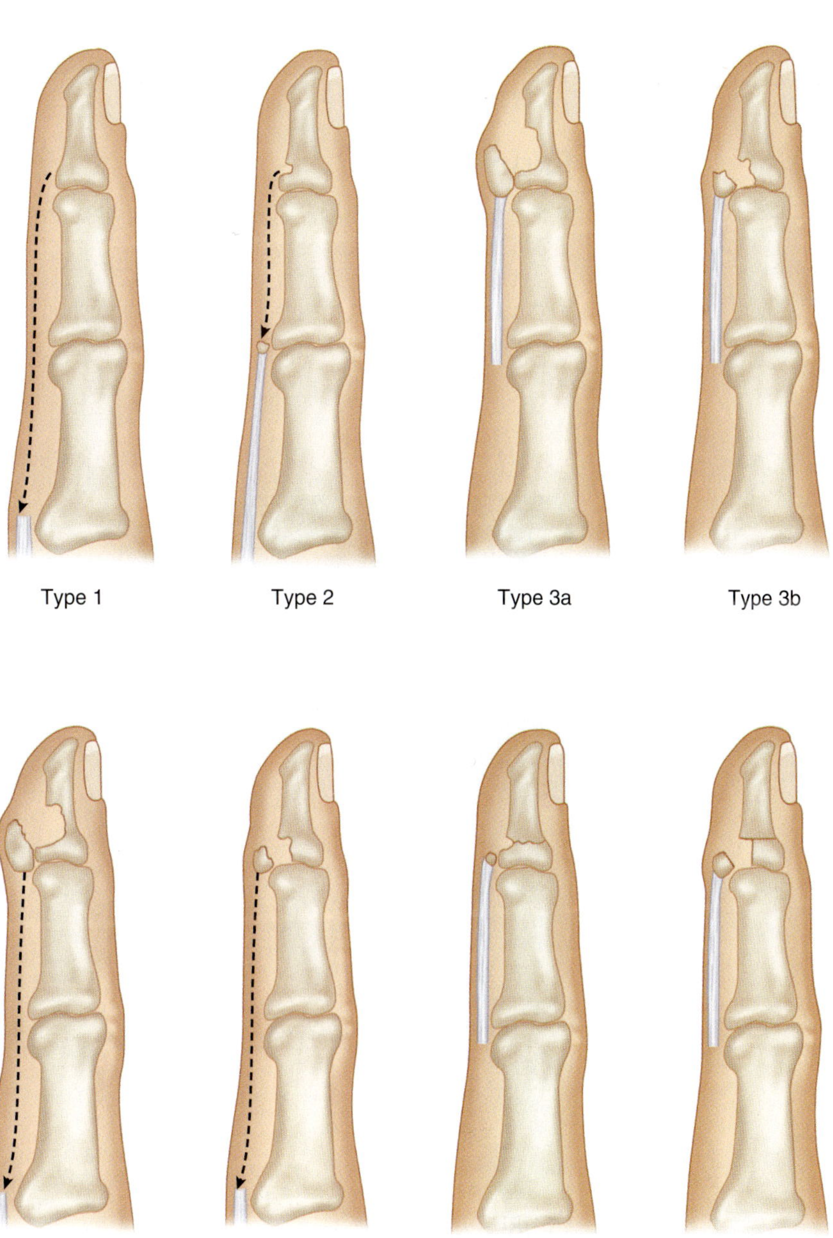

FIGURE 7-5

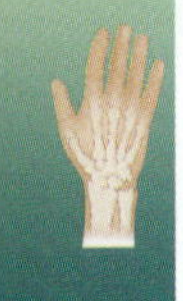

- *Type 3:* A large bone fragment remains attached to the FDP, and tendon does not retract proximal to the A4 pulley.
- *Type 4:* Similar to type 3 except with simultaneous avulsion of the tendon from the bone fragment.
- *Type 5:* Like type 3, but with concomitant fracture of the distal phalanx.

- In most cases, the tendon can be retrieved from the above locations, passed through the pulley system, and reattached to the distal phalanx via pullout button or bone anchor.
- With late presentation of greater than 4 weeks, the myostatic contracture of the avulsed tendon may preclude distal reconstruction, obligating a tendon graft.

Positioning

- The operation is done under local, regional, or general anesthesia under tourniquet control.
- The patient is positioned supine with the affected extremity abducted to 90 degrees onto a radiolucent hand table.
- Access to palmaris and plantaris tendon may be necessary when grafting is needed.

PEARLS

Palmaris tendon may be harvested using transverse incisions spaced every 5 to 7 cm over the volar forearm.

Exposures

- A zigzag Bruner incision will provide the best exposure of the finger. The incision can be extended proximally as needed to retrieve the tendon or provide exposure for repair (Fig. 7-6).
- A palmar incision at the level of the A1 can help in retrieving the tendon to be passed through fibrous flexor sheath to zone 1.

PITFALLS

The neurovascular bundle in the finger must be identified and protected.

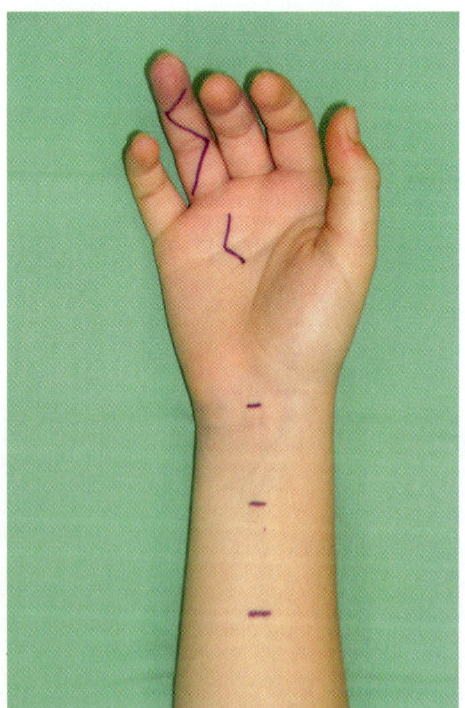

FIGURE 7-6

Procedure

Step 1

- Exploration of the finger with a zigzag incision is used to identify the proximal tendon at one of several classic locations—at A4, between A2 and A4 pulleys, or at A1 (Fig. 7-7).
- The A2 pulley is partially opened to retrieve the proximal tendon (Fig. 7-8).
- At the distal tendon insertion, thin atrophic tendon remains that is not suitable for repair (Fig. 7-9).

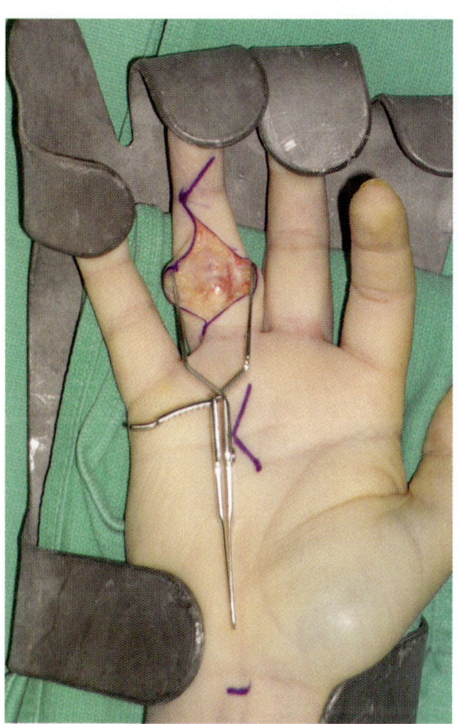

FIGURE 7-7

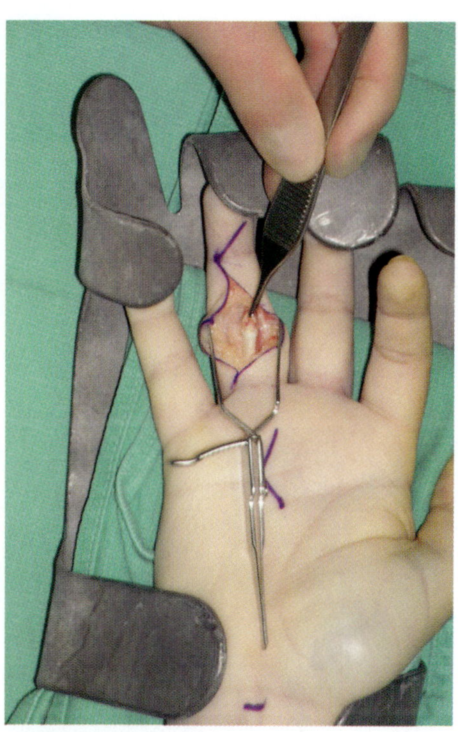

FIGURE 7-8

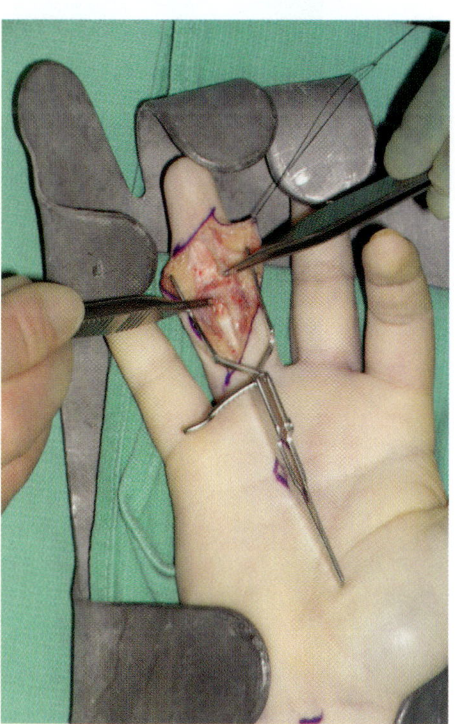

FIGURE 7-9

- Excursion of the proximal tendon is tested and found to be inadequate for tension-free repair (Fig. 7-10).
- The FDP is pulled proximally over the palm and dissected free from the FDS. Scar adhesion is released, which often develops if treatment is delayed.
- This provides additional mobility of tendon to allow primary repair (Fig. 7-11).

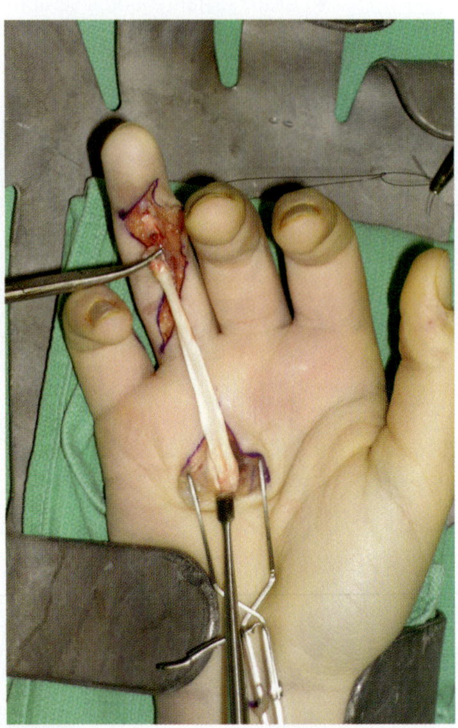

FIGURE 7-10

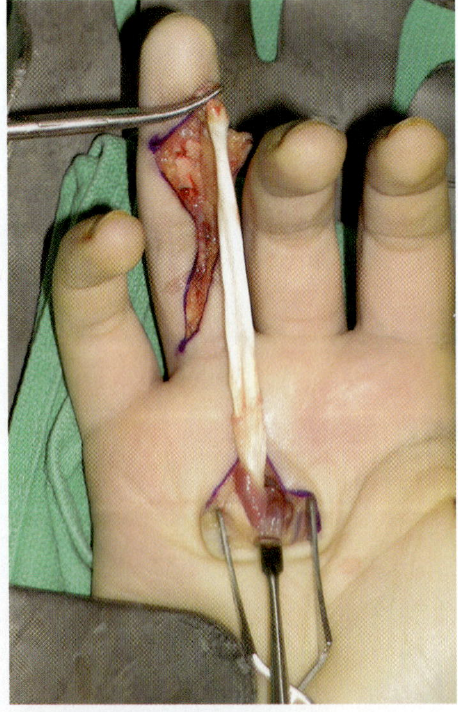

FIGURE 7-11

STEP 1 PEARLS

One should not pull the tendon by the feeding catheter. Rather, the tendon is gently pushed under the A1 pulley. Gentle pulling of the feeding catheter and pushing on the tendon proximally will deliver the tendon through the sheath atraumatically.

STEP 1 PITFALLS

It is important to ensure that the tendon is not twisted as it is manually passed through zone 2 and through the FDS chiasm.

- A small feeding catheter is gently threaded through the A2 pulley into the palmar incision (Fig. 7-12). The feeding catheter is sutured to the proximal profundus tendon using a horizontal mattress suture, and the tendon is gently threaded through the pulley system into the distal incision (Fig. 7-13).
- The wrist is flexed to decrease the tension on the profundus tendon so that more of the tendon can be retrieved into the distal incision. A needle is inserted to hold the tendon in place (Fig. 7-14).

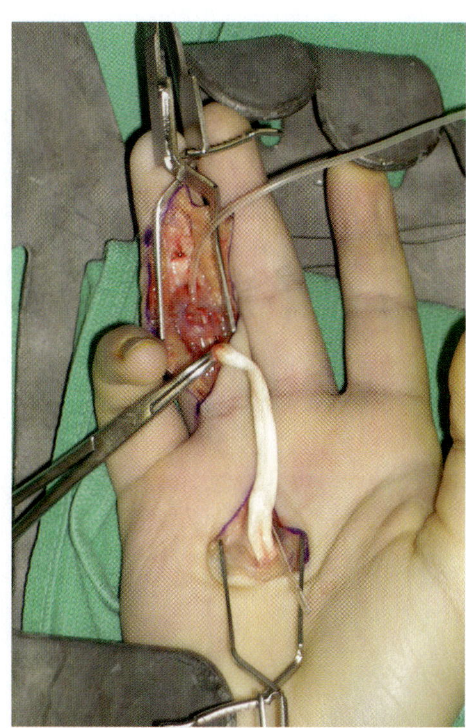

FIGURE 7-12

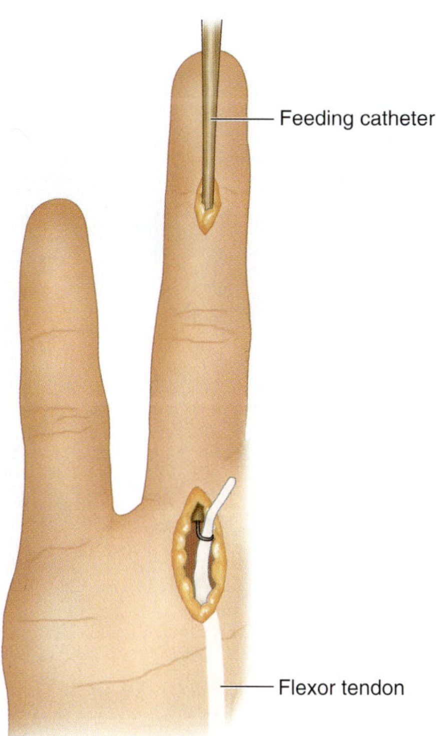

FIGURE 7-13

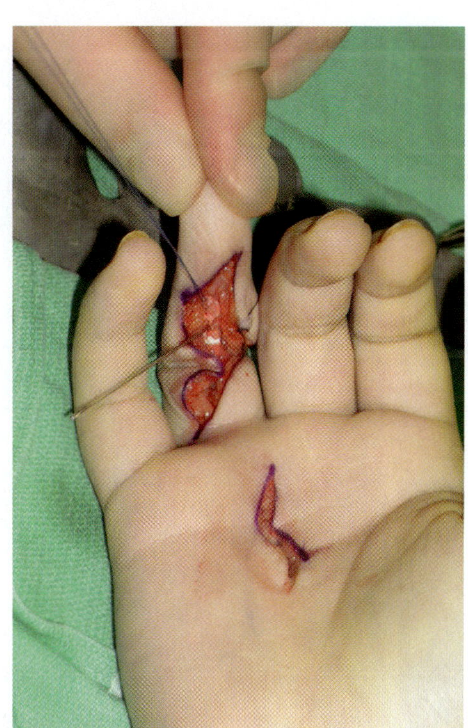

FIGURE 7-14

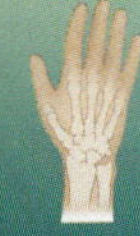

STEP 2 PEARLS

- Prolene sutures are used because they can slide out easily upon healing of the tendon to the bone, which takes about 6 weeks.
- One must be careful when placing the Keith needles through the nail to avoid proximal penetration of the germinal matrix, which may cause nail deformity.
- When tying down the Prolene suture over the nail, the surgeon must observe the tendon sitting securely within the bone trough at the distal phalanx.
- The elevated periosteum can be sutured to the end of the tendon using 4-0 Ethibond braided suture to provide additional support.

Step 2

- In avulsion injuries, direct tenorrhaphy is not possible, and treatment consists of reattaching the proximal tendon to the bone via pullout suture over a button (Fig. 7-15).
- The distal tendon remnant and scar is resected to expose the volar base of the distal phalanx.
- The volar proximal aspect of the distal phalanx is gently débrided until cancellous bone is encountered. A bone tunnel is not necessary (Fig. 7-16).
- Zigzag 3-0 Prolene suture is passed through the distal end of the tendon (Fig. 7-17).
- Keith needle holes are drilled obliquely through the base of the distal phalanx just lateral or distal to the bone through to the dorsum of the finger while avoiding the germinal matrix of the nail.
- The suture ends holding the distal aspect of the FDP tendon are then passed thought the Keith needle holes to be withdrawn over the nail bed.
- The sutures are then secured in place with a bolster, or button, on the dorsal aspect of the finger (Fig. 7-18).

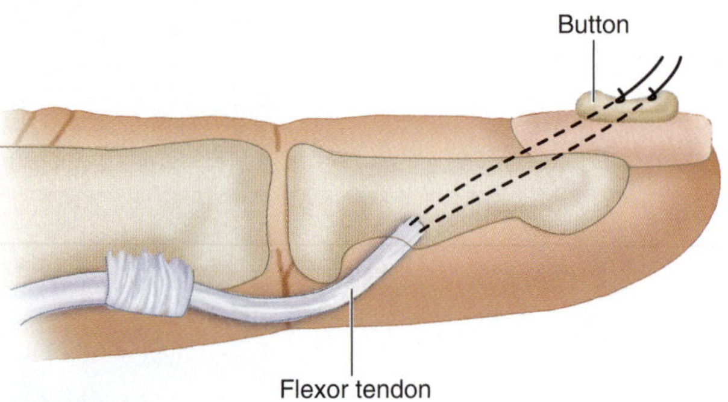

FIGURE 7-15

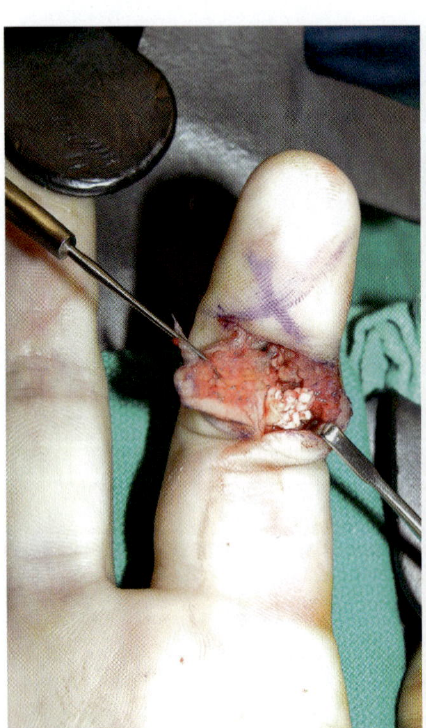

FIGURE 7-16

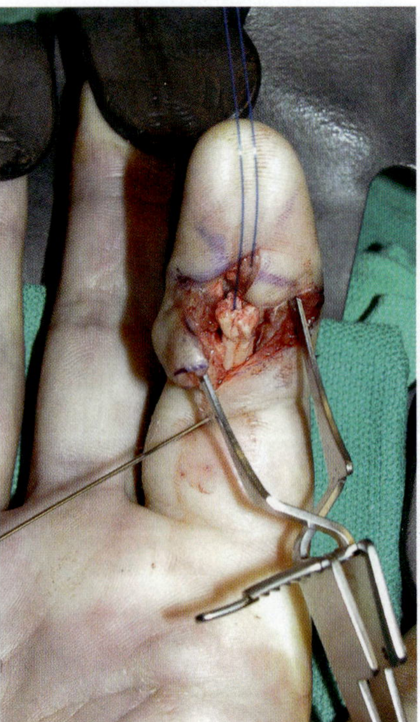

FIGURE 7-17

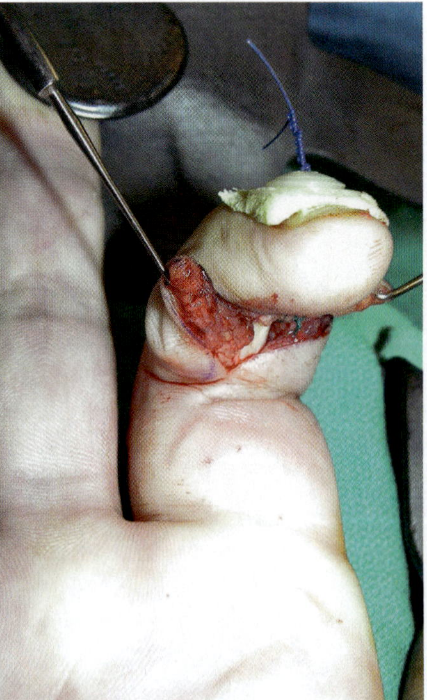

FIGURE 7-18

PITFALLS

Tendon rupture is a distinct possibility if the tendon does not heal to the bone. One should immediately explore the tendon system and place a tendon graft when a rupture is encountered because the tendon sheath will collapse quickly when the sheath is empty. Early exploration is much easier because the tendon sheath is still open, and retrieval and excision of the ruptured tendon within the sheath are relatively easy. However, if the exploration is delayed, the ruptured tendon may be adherent to the pulley system and the tendon sheath may contract, which makes primary tendon grafting difficult.

Postoperative Care and Expected Outcomes

- The patient is placed in a dorsal blocking splint with the wrist flexed at 60 degrees and the MCP joints flexed at 90 degrees to take tension off the tendon repair site (Fig. 7-19).
- The hand is splinted in this posture for about 4 weeks, and passive flexion-extension exercises are initiated for the DIP joint within 1 week.
- After 4 weeks, the splint is gradually extended to provide more tension at the suture line, and the patient is started on gentle active flexion exercises.
- The button and the Prolene suture are removed at 8 weeks after surgery in the clinic.
- Three months after the tendon repair, the patient begins strengthening exercises and continues scar massages to achieve better excursion of the flexor tendon. (Fig. 7-20 demonstrates the early postoperative result of the patient shown in Fig. 7-1.)

Evidence

Leddy JP, Packer JW. Avulsions of the profundus tendon insertion in athletes. *J Hand Surg [Am]*. 1977;2:66-69.

Three types of avulsion injuries of the profundus tendon were proposed. In type 1, the tendon retracts into the palm, whereas in types 2 and 3, the tendon lodges in the tendon sheath in the fingers. The authors provide a comprehensive description of the mechanism of injury and the treatment options. (Level IV evidence)

Sourmelis SG, McGrouther DA. Retrieval of the retracted flexor tendon. *J Hand Surg [Br]*. 1987;12:109-111.

This article proposed the use of a small feeding catheter to retrieve the tendon atraumatically through the tendon sheath. This technique avoids injury to the retracted tendon and the pulley system. This is the technique described in this chapter and is the preferred technique of the author. (Level IV evidence)

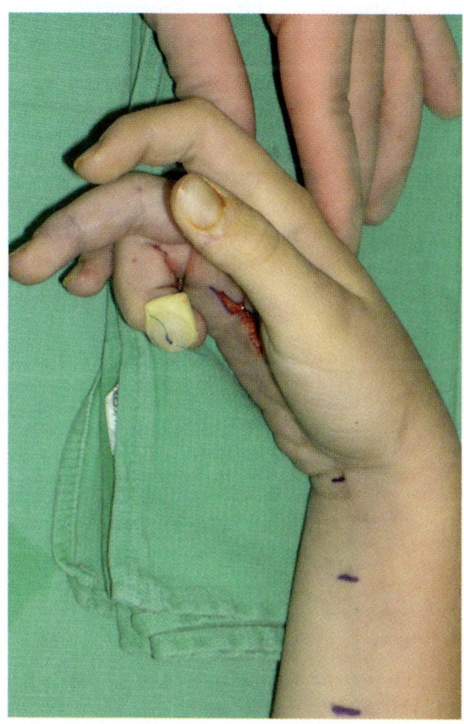

FIGURE 7-19

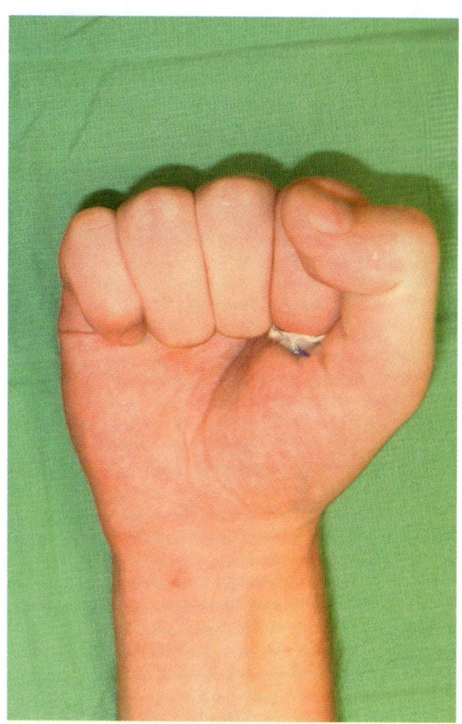

FIGURE 7-20

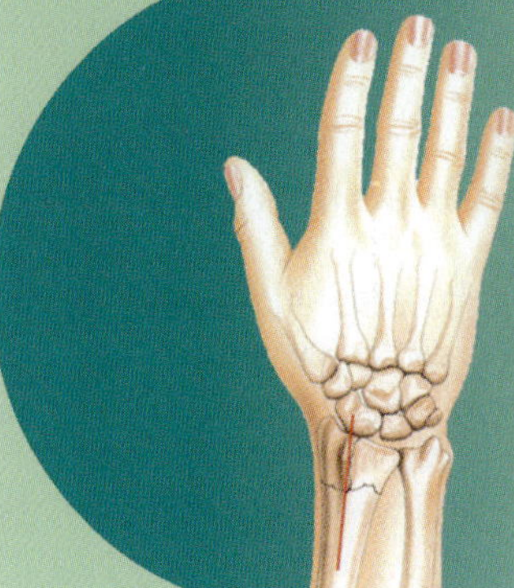

PROCEDURE 8

Acute Repair of Zone 2 Flexor Tendon Injury

Brent M. Egeland, Sandeep J. Sebastin, and Kevin C. Chung

See Video 5: Acute Repair of Zone 2 Flexor Tendon Injury

Indications

- Acute repair of zone 2 flexor tendon injuries is indicated when there is a clean-cut injury with the following findings:
  - Completely divided flexor digitorum profundus (FDP) and/or flexor digitorum superficialis (FDS)
  - Partial flexor tendon injury involving greater than 60% of the tendon substance
  - Minimal wound contamination
- A tendon defect of up to 1 cm can be repaired by end-to-end suturing. Greater losses (up to 2 to 3 cm) may need an intramuscular tendon lengthening via forearm incisions, and larger tendon gaps will need tendon grafting.

Examination/Imaging

Clinical Examination

- Patients present with loss of active distal interphalangeal (DIP) and proximal interphalangeal (PIP) joint flexion if both FDP and FDS are divided, or loss of only DIP joint flexion if only FDP has been injured. On inspection, the normal finger cascade is lost with the affected digit in an extended position.
- The function of the FDP is determined by asking the patient to actively flex the DIP joint of the involved finger.
- Testing for FDS injury is more complex compared with the FDP because the PIP joint is flexed both by the FDS and by the FDP. Therefore, one needs to check the function of the FDS while blocking the action of the FDP.
  - The standard test for the FDS takes advantage of the fact that the FDP tendons to the long, ring, and small fingers share a common muscle belly. The finger being tested is allowed to flex while the action of the FDP tendon is blocked by preventing flexion of the DIP joint of the other two fingers (Fig. 8-1). The standard test is not reliable for the index finger because the index finger FDP has an independent muscle belly (Fig. 8-2). In addition, the action of the FDS of the small finger may be dependent on the FDS to the ring finger, and they may need to be tested together (Fig. 8-3).

Figure 8-7 is adapted from Tang JB. Flexor tendon repair in zone 2C. J Hand Surg [Br]. *1994;19:72-75, with permission from Elsevier. Figure 8-18 is adapted from Strickland JW. Development of flexor tendon surgery: twenty-five years of progress.* J Hand Surg [Am]. *2000;25:214-235, with permission from Elsevier.*

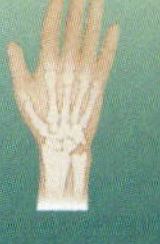

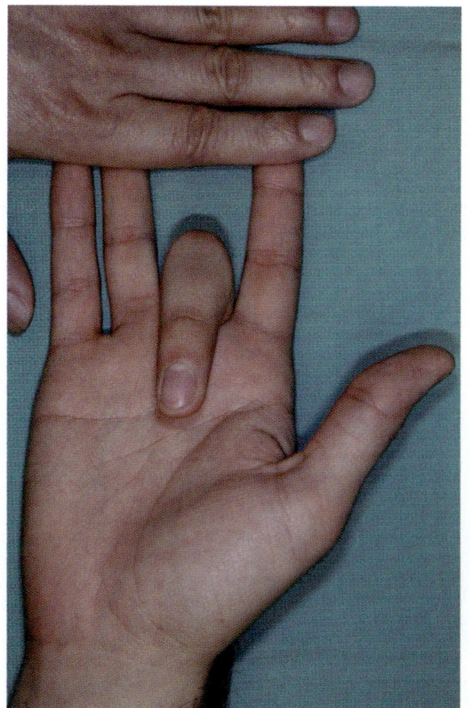

FIGURE 8-1

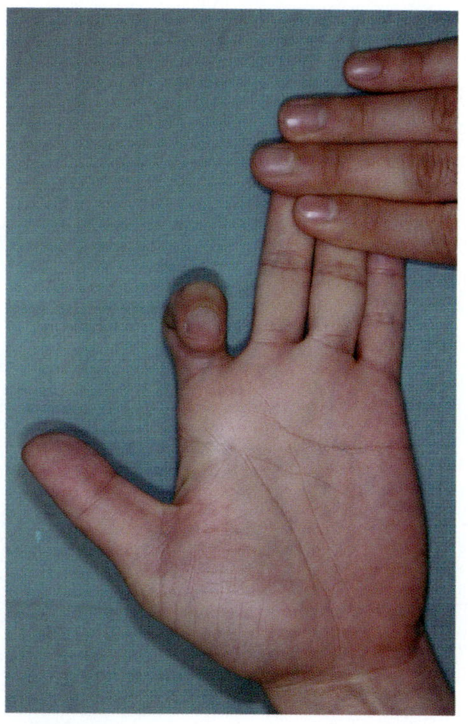

FIGURE 8-2

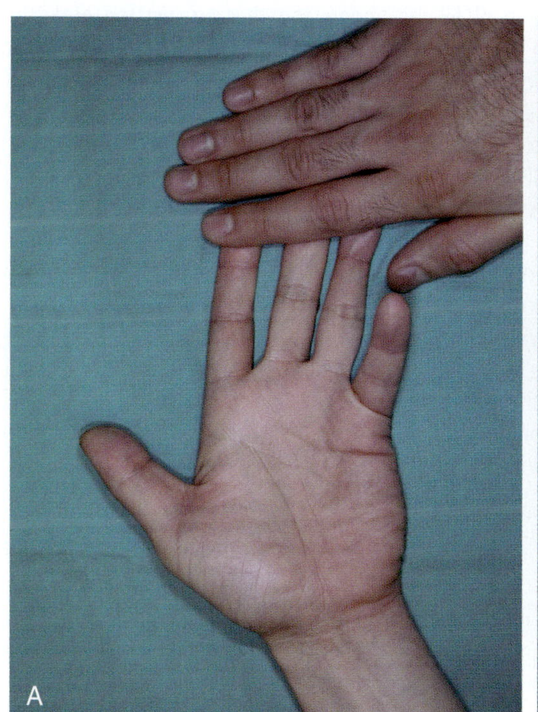

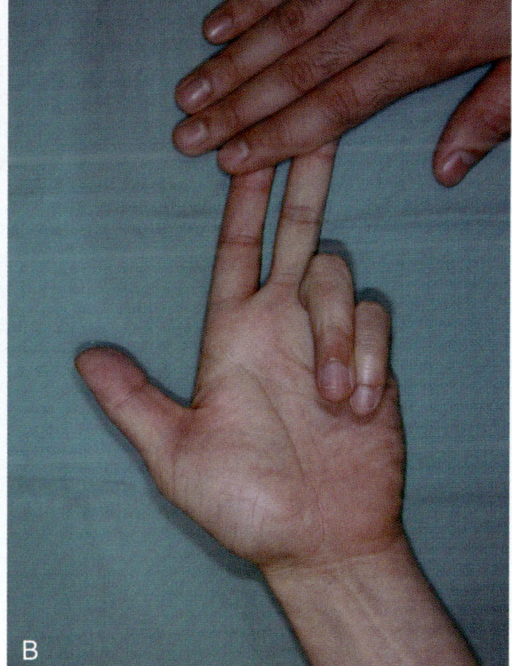

A B

FIGURE 8-3

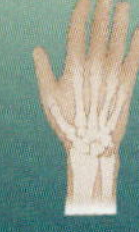

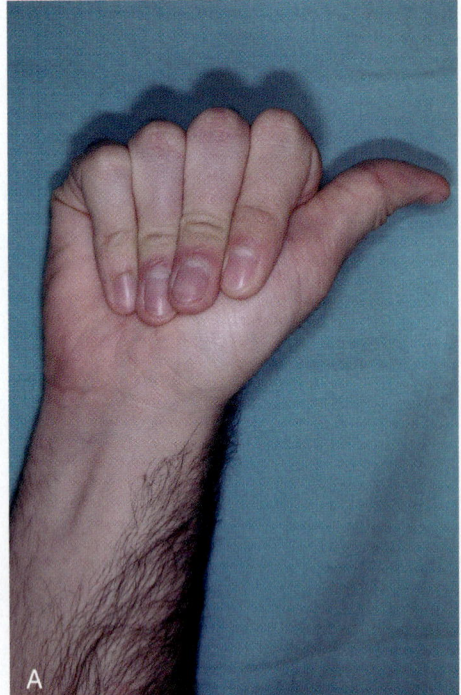

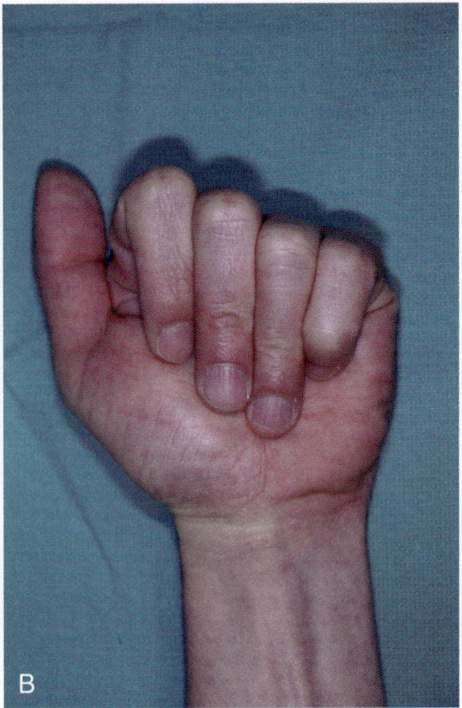

FIGURE 8-4

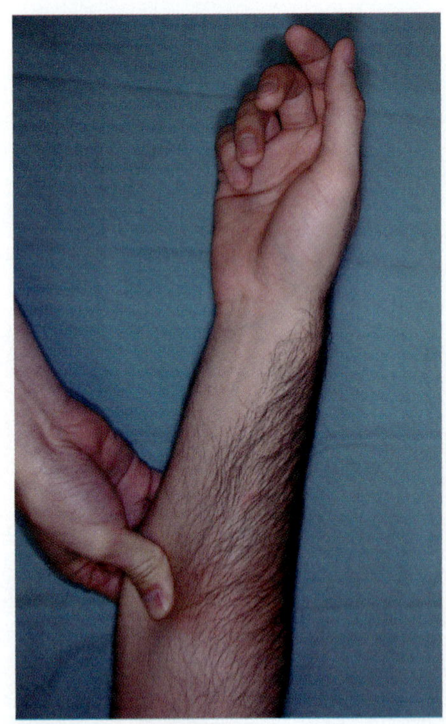

FIGURE 8-5

- Mishra described a modified test whereby the subject is asked to press the fingertip pulp of all the fingers together against the proximal part of the palm, such that the DIP joint is kept extended. If the FDS is acting, the DIP joint remains in a position of extension to hypertension while the MCPJ and PIPJ are fully flexed. If the FDS of any of the fingers is injured or absent, the DIP joint goes into flexion. This test works on the principle that the FDP can flex the PIP joint only after it has flexed the DIP joint. If the DIP joint is maintained in extension, PIP joint flexion is purely a function of the FDS (Fig. 8-4).

- A partial tendon laceration should be suspected in patients in whom active motion is associated with pain or triggering.
- In patients who cannot cooperate (e.g., children or comatose or intoxicated patients), one can look for passive movement of the fingers resulting from the wrist tenodesis effect or by squeezing the forearm muscles (Fig. 8-5). The same maneuvers can be used when trying to differentiate between tendon injury and inability to move as a result of nerve palsy.
- It is important to examine the patient for presence of concomitant injuries to the digital arteries and nerves.

Imaging

- Preoperative imaging studies are not typically necessary, but anteroposterior and lateral x-rays may help identify associated bony injury. When a patient presents with unstable or intra-articular fractures, rigid fixation of the fracture is performed so that judicious tendon mobilization can be performed after tendon repair.

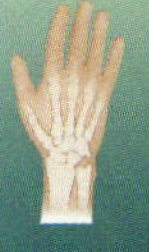

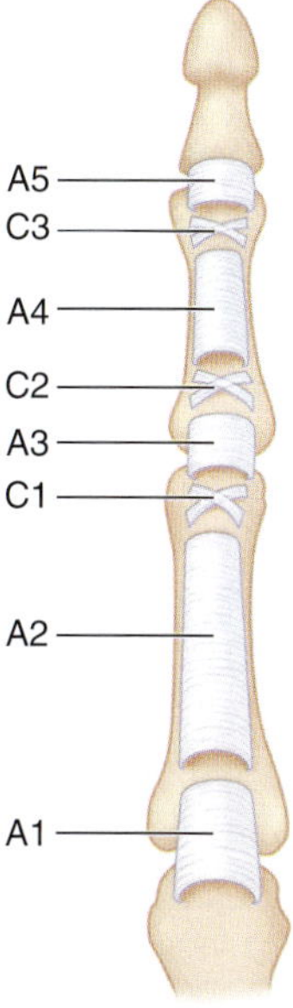

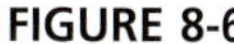

FIGURE 8-6

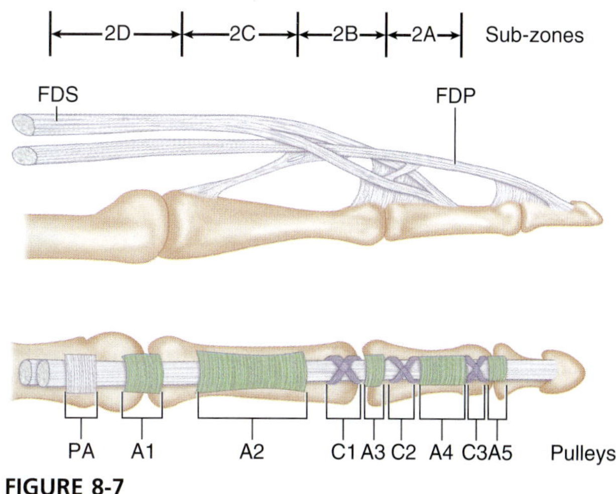

FIGURE 8-7

PEARLS

If the incision needs to be extended to the distal palm, one must avoid placing the incision in the web space to prevent a scar contracture that limits finger extension.

Knowing the mechanism of injury helps in determining the location of the distal cut end of the tendon, and the incision can be planned accordingly. If injury occurred in flexion, the distal cut end will migrate distal to the skin laceration with the finger held in extension. The skin incision will need to be extended distally. If injury occurred in extension, the distal cut end will be at the same level as the skin laceration. Retraction of the proximal cut end depends on the level of injury in relation to the vincular attachment. In zone 2A and 2B injuries, the proximal end may get caught at the A2 pulley. In zone 2C and 2D injuries, the tendon retracts to the distal palm, where the FDP is restricted by the lumbrical muscle attached to the radial side of the FDP.

Surgical Anatomy

- Zone 2 contains both the FDS and FDP tendons and extends from the proximal edge of the A1 pulley in the palm to the insertion of the FDS over the middle phalanx. It includes four annular pulleys (A1, A2, A3, and A4) and two cruciate pulleys (C1 and C2) (Fig. 8-6).
- Zone 2 was subdivided by Tang (1994) into four subzones (Fig. 8-7).
  - *2A:* Includes the C2 and A4 pulleys and has the FDS insertion. Only the FDP tendon glides under the A4 pulley. The A4 pulley is located at the midpoint of the middle phalanx and is 0.5 to 0.8 cm long.
  - *2B:* Includes the C1 and A3 pulleys and has the chiasm portion of the FDS.
  - *2C:* Includes the A2 pulley and represents the narrowest segment of zone 2. The A2 pulley is about 2 cm long and is situated over the proximal two thirds of the proximal phalanx. The middle and distal parts of the A2 pulley are very narrow, and the FDS tendon bifurcates within the midpart of the A2 pulley.
  - *2D:* Includes the A1 pulley and represents the widest portion of zone 2.
- The blood supply to the tendons in this region comes from the vincular system and enters the tendon on the dorsal surface. It is recommended that core sutures be passed in the palmar portion of the tendon.

Positioning

- The patient lies supine on the operating table with the affected arm placed on a hand table.
- A lead hand is used during dissection and tendon repair.

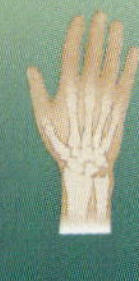

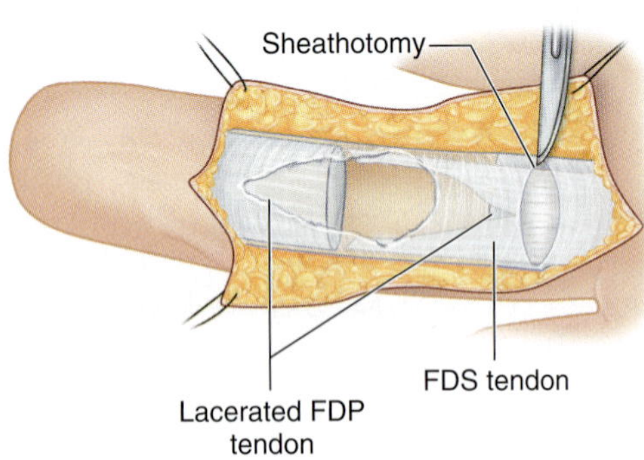

FIGURE 8-8

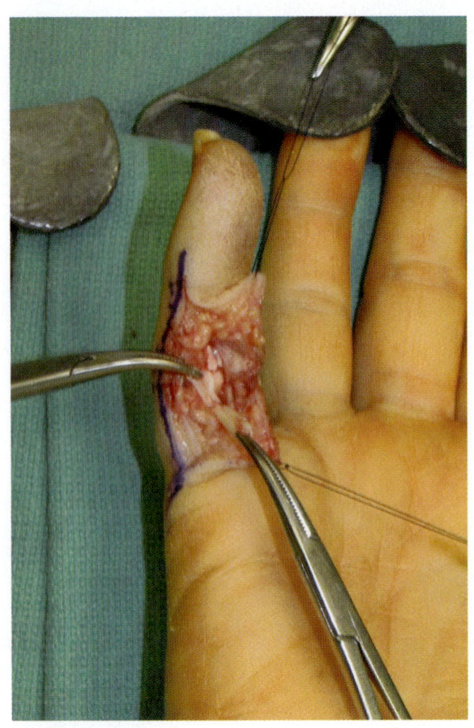

FIGURE 8-9

Exposures

- Bruner incisions or midaxial incisions (by incorporating the transverse lacerations) are designed from the DIP joint to the base of the finger (Fig. 8-8).
- Thick skin flaps are raised in a plane superficial to the tendon sheath to expose the tendon sheath (Fig. 8-9).

Procedure

Step 1: Exposure of Divided Tendons

- The excursion of FDP within zone 2 is approximately 2 cm. To allow this excursion, we divide varying portions of the A2, A3, and A4 pulleys and the flexor sheath, depending on the location of the distal cut end of the tendon with the finger in extension (Fig. 8-10). Selective and limited division of the pulleys allows free movement of the repaired tendon while avoiding clinically significant bowstringing.

Step 2: Retrieval of Proximal Tendon End

- This can be challenging when the tendon has retracted into the palm. The following maneuvers are used in sequence:
  - The first maneuver is to apply gentle pressure in a proximal to distal direction on the forearm with the wrist and metacarpophalangeal (MCP) joint in flexion. This may occasionally coax the tendon through the pulley system, especially for tendons ends that are caught at the A2 pulley.
  - A single attempt with a fine-tipped mosquito forceps passed into the sheath from distal to proximal can be done next.

STEP 2 PEARLS

The tendon should be handled with care to prevent iatrogenic injury and scarring.

STEP 2 PITFALLS

Repeated blind grasps with a hemostat within the fibrous flexor sheath in an attempt to retrieve the proximal tendons should be avoided. Limited incisions in the pulleys will allow atraumatic access to the tendon within zone 2.

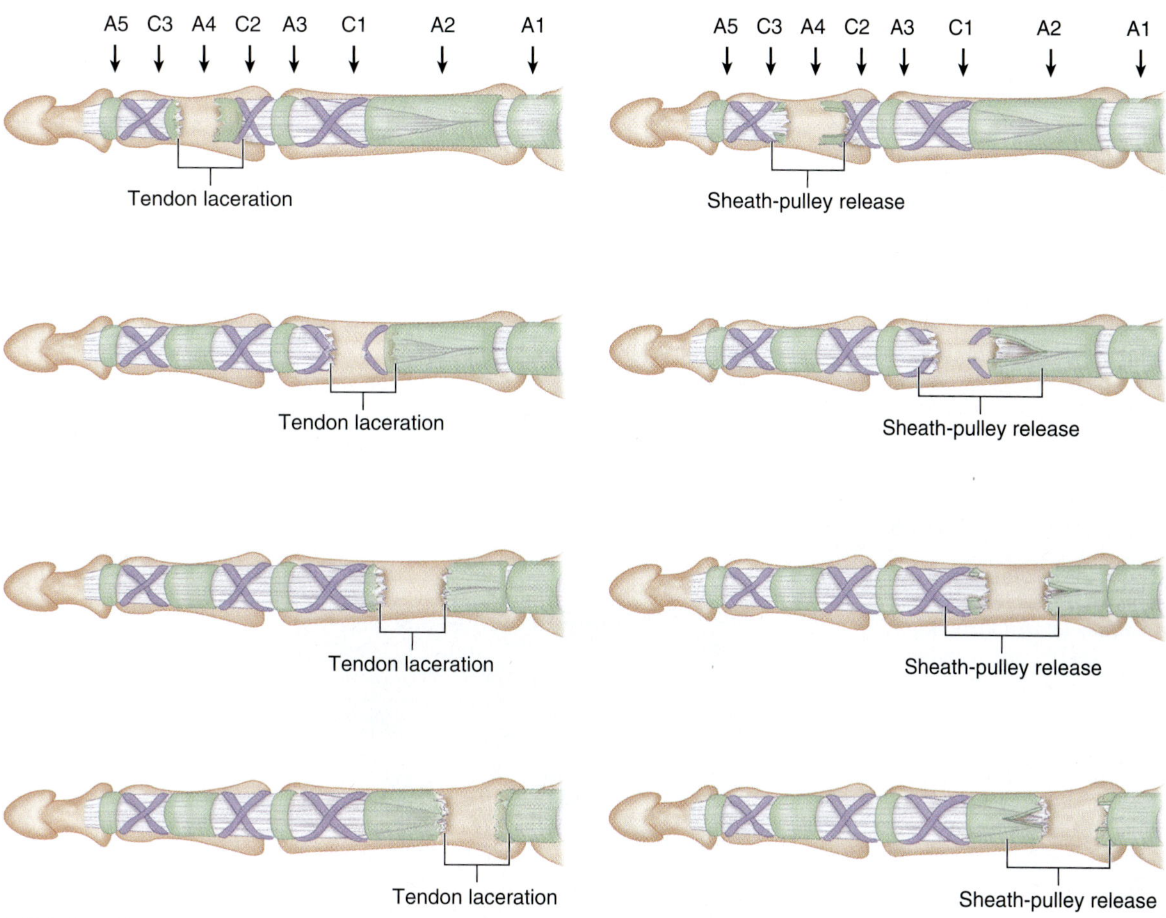

FIGURE 8-10

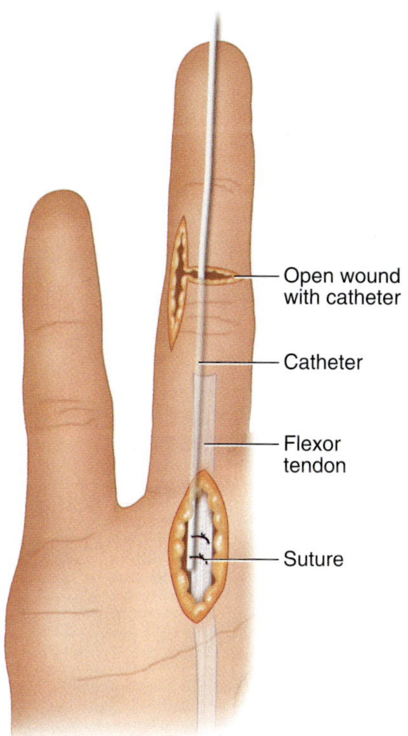

FIGURE 8-11

- If both these maneuvers do not work, the method described by Sourmelis and McGrouther should be tried. A chevron incision is made in the distal palm proximal to the A1 pulley. The flexor tendons are identified. If they are still within the A1/A2 pulley, they are not disturbed. A 5/6 French pediatric feeding tube is passed from retrograde through the flexor sheath to emerge at the proximal incision. The feeding tube is sutured to the palmar surface of the flexor tendon without withdrawing the tendons from the fibrous flexor sheath. If the tendon ends have retracted proximal to the A1 pulley, the feeding tube is sutured to the end of the tendons. Using a combination of pulling the feeding tube at the distal incision and pushing the flexor tendon at the proximal incision, the tendon ends are delivered into laceration (Fig. 8-11).
- After retrieval to the site of repair, the tendon should be secured in place with a hypodermic needle to prevent it from retracting proximally and to allow a tension-free repair.

STEP 3 PEARLS

If the FDS is lacerated at the Camper chiasm, direct mattress repair to the radial and ulnar tendon ends can be performed using 4-0 or 5-0 braided suture.

After tendon repair, the finger should be placed through gentle range of motion to ensure adequate tendon gliding through the pulley system. If the pulleys are restricting free motion, they should be vented by divided them at one edge.

STEP 3 PITFALLS

If a gap is noted during passive mobilization, the repair needs to be done again or strengthened. The gap will heal by scarring, which will be weak and can rupture easily.

It is crucial to orient the FDS and FDP correctly during repair because the tendons may twist in the sheath. Additionally, the lacerated FDP may migrate outside the FDS chiasm, and it should be gently passed through the chiasm. If the vincula is still intact, it must be carefully preserved during the repair.

Step 3: Tendon Repair

- The tendon ends are gently débrided of frayed ends while retaining their length.
- The FDS is repaired before the FDP. An attempt is made to repair both slips of the FDS (Fig. 8-12). This may be difficult, especially in zone 2C, where the A2 pulley is narrowest. In such circumstances, repair of one slip is appropriate. Because of the flatness of the FDS at zone 2, its repair is a simple horizontal mattress suture repair of each slip of the FDS.
- Many methods of tendon repair have been described for the FDP. We use a 6-0 Prolene suture epitendinous repair combined with a 3-0 Ethibond modified double-Kessler core suture (Fig. 8-13).
- First the epitendinous repair of the dorsal half of the tendon is carried out. Sutures bites are taken at 1- to 2-mm intervals approximately 1 to 2 mm from the edge of the tendon. This is a continuous suture repair, and the loops are locked.

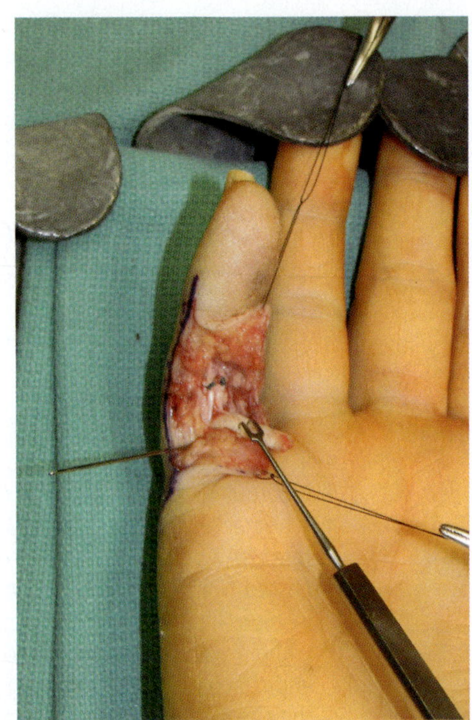

FIGURE 8-12

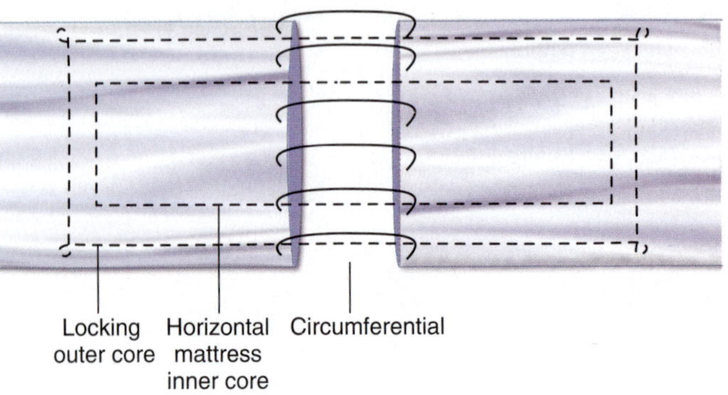

FIGURE 8-13

- Next a modified Kessler core suture is placed in the standard manner (Fig. 8-14). The transverse portion of the suture is locked. It is important to remember that 3-0 Ethibond is a braided suture and does not glide well within the tendon substance. One should therefore pull the required length of the suture through the tendon at first pass. A minimum of 0.7 cm, and most commonly 1 to 1.2 cm, of the tendon is grasped by the longitudinal portion of the suture loop before making the transverse portion.
- A horizontal mattress suture is placed within the previous suture repair using 4-0 Ethibond. Approximately 0.5 to 0.6 cm of the tendon is grapsed by the longitudinal portion of the suture loop before making the transverse portion (Fig. 8-15).
- The palmar half of the epitendonous repair is now completed (Fig. 8-16).

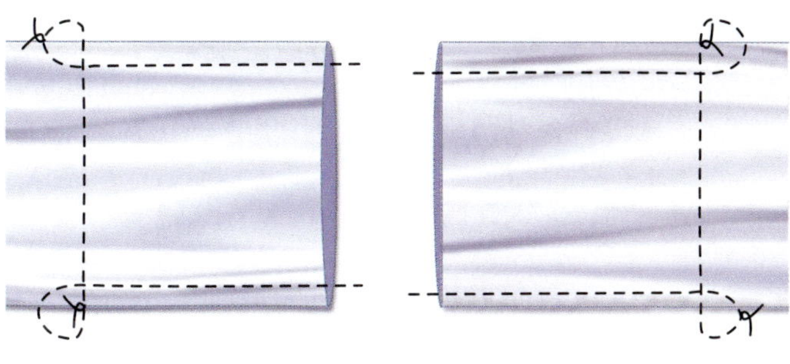

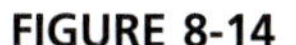
FIGURE 8-14

Horizontal mattress inner-core suture

FIGURE 8-15

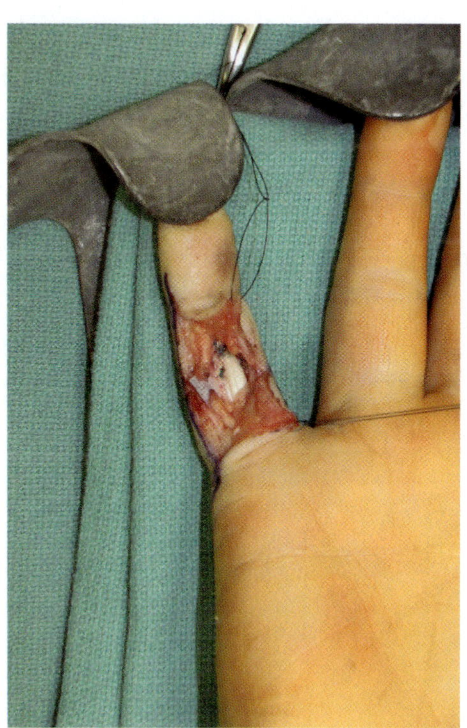

FIGURE 8-16

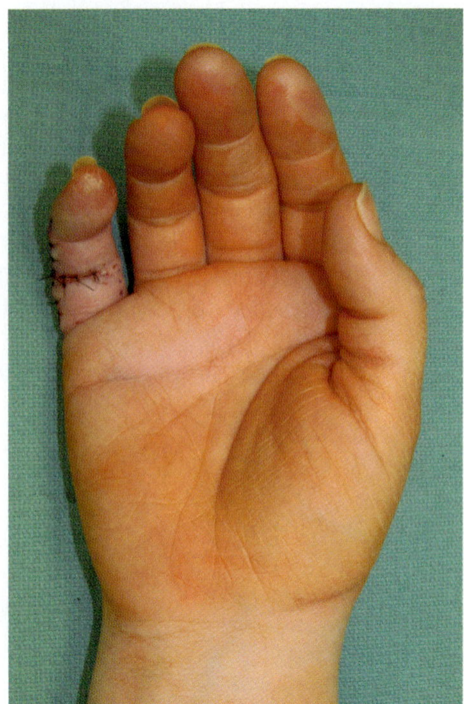

FIGURE 8-17

Step 4: Closure

- The tourniquet is released and hemostasis obtained.
- The skin is loosely closed to accommodate for postoperative edema (Fig. 8-17).

Postoperative Care and Expected Outcomes

- The patient is splinted in 30 degrees of wrist flexion and 60 degrees of metaphalangeal (MP) flexion and with the fingers in slight flexion.
- It is critical for the surgeon and therapist to maintain direct communication during the postoperative period.
- Tendon repair strength declines for the first week after surgery, plateaus for 1 week, and then slowly begins to get stronger. In this initial phase of healing, all strength across the repair is due to the suture and will increase predictably with increasing strand count. During tendon healing, the force applied to the repair should always be below the repair strength, or rupture may occur. Following this logic, and explicitly described later for a four-strand core-suture repair, passive exercises always remain below rupture threshold and are used for the initial 4 weeks following surgery. At 4 weeks, active exercises are safely started. Strengthening is not started until 8 weeks (Fig. 8-18).
- Indiana Early Active Mobilization, or the Tenodesis Program, is initiated on postoperative day 3. This involves both passive exercises using a Modified Duran Program and place-and-hold exercises.
  - The patient's bulky dressing is removed and replaced with a dorsal blocking splint (DBS) to be worn at all times with the wrist in 20 degrees of palmar flexion, MP joints in 70 degrees of flexion, and interphalangeal (IP) joints at neutral. While wearing the DBS, a modified Duran Exercise Program is initiated and continued every 2 hours throughout the day. Specifically, each session involves 25 repetitions of passive flexion and extension of the PIP, then the DIP, and then the entire digit.

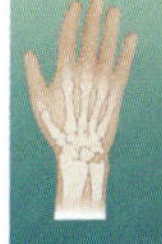

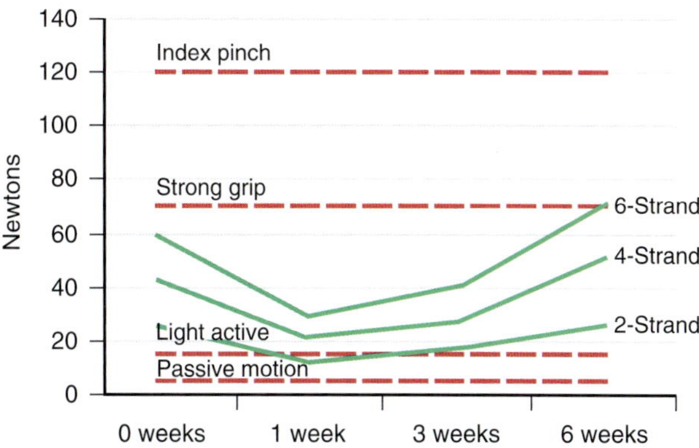

FIGURE 8-18

Table 8-1 Methods of Grading Total Active Motion

Score	ASSH (degrees)	Strickland (%)	Modified Strickland (%)
Excellent	>220	85-100	75-100
Good	200-219	70-84	50-74
Fair	180-199	50-69	25-49
Poor	<180	0-49	0-24

ASSH, American Society for Surgery of the Hand.

  - In addition, a second tenodesis splint is applied. This allows wrist flexion but limits wrist extension to 30 degrees. Within this splint, place-and-hold exercises are performed. This involves composite passive flexion of the digits while simultaneously bringing the wrist from flexion into extension. Once in extension, the patient actively maintains a fist position for 5 seconds and then lets it passively relax, and the wrist drops into flexion.
- At 4 weeks, the tenodesis splint is discontinued, but the place-and-hold exercises continue. Additional active exercises are started, consisting of making a fist while the wrist is in neutral position. Active wrist flexion and extension are allowed. The Modified Duran Program is continued within the DBS.
- At 5 weeks, active extension is allowed.
- At 6 weeks, the DBS is discontinued, and the involved finger is buddy-taped to the adjacent finger. An extension splint is worn at night.
- At 8 weeks, progressive strengthening is started.
- At 10 to 12 weeks, the patient may return to all activities but should not perform heavy lifting until 16 weeks.
- Based on the Total Active Motion (TAM) evaluation system proposed by Kleinert and Verdan, and advocated by the American Society for Surgery of the Hand, most patients should regain good to excellent function after primary repair of flexor tendons (Table 8-1). TAM is calculated by the following formula:
  - TAM = total active flexion (MCP joint + PIP join + DIP joint) – total extension deficit (MCP joint + PIP joint + DIP joint).

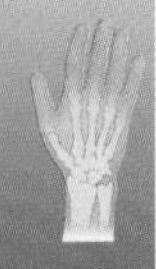

Evidence

Kitis PT, Buker N, Kara IG. Comparison of two methods of controlled mobilisation of repaired flexor tendons in zone 2. *Scand J Plast Reconstr Surg Hand Surg*. 2009;43:160-165.

This study compares active and passive regimens of postoperative motion. Controlled active motion (Kleinert/Washington) was compared with group-controlled passive motion (Duran). The controlled active motion group achieved better results in Total Active Motion (TAM) and Disabilities of the Arm, Shoulder and Hand (DASH) scores. This is the first high-level evidence study demonstrating superiority of early active versus early passive movement. (Level II evidence)

Tang JB. Flexor tendon repair in zone 2C. *J Hand Surg [Br]*. 1994;1:72-75.

This article reports on a randomized prospective clinical study evaluating Total Active Motion (TAM) after repair of both the FDS and FDP, versus the FDP alone, in zone 2B (under the A2 pulley). The results indicated decreased TAM when both FDS and FDP are repaired in this region. Furthermore, there was a higher rate of adhesions or rupture requiring operative management. The author concluded that with a laceration at zone 2C, the FDS should be excised in favor of repairing FDP alone. (Level IV evidence)

Tang JB. Indications, methods, postoperative motion and outcome evaluation of primary flexor tendon repairs in zone 2. *J Hand Surg [Br]*. 2007;32:118-129.

In this expert opinion article, the author presents his practical views on zone 2 flexor tendon repairs. Tang discusses indications, techniques, and postsurgical treatment and outcome measures and further describes methods of sheath-pulley release, tendon repair, postoperative motion, and outcome evaluation. Based on the information in this review, the author notes that predictable outcomes of flexor tendon repair in zone 2 are now routine. (Level V evidence)

Thien TB, Becker JH, Theis JC. Rehabilitation after surgery for flexor tendon injuries in the hand. *Cochrane Database Syst Rev*. 2004;4:CD003979.

This is the only Cochrane review regarding flexor tendon repair, and it specifically reviews postoperative therapy. Six randomized controlled trials were reviewed. Despite widespread use of postoperative therapies, this review found insufficient evidence to define the best mobilization strategy. There was a trend toward early active mobilization strategies. (Level II evidence)

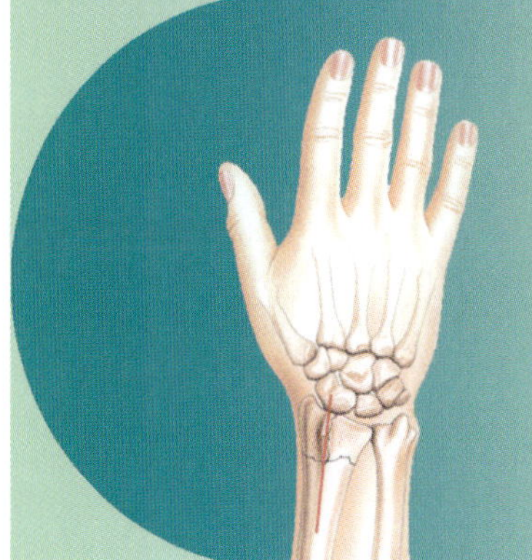

PROCEDURE 9

Staged Flexor Tendon Reconstruction

Brent M. Egeland, Sandeep J. Sebastin, and Kevin C. Chung

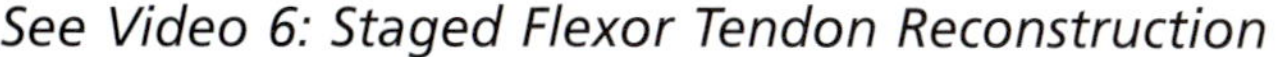

See Video 6: Staged Flexor Tendon Reconstruction

Indications

- Finger that is not amenable to primary or delayed primary repair or a single-stage tendon graft procedure, as in the following cases:
  - Extensive crush injury with underlying unstable fracture or skin loss
  - Soft tissue contractures leading to tissue deficiency (Fig. 9-1)
  - Joint contractures (Fig. 9-2)
  - Inadequate pulley system requiring pulley reconstruction
- Failure of previous treatment
  - Late presentation of ruptured primary or delayed primary tendon repair
  - Failure of single staged tendon graft
- Late presentation (>3 weeks) of a flexor digitorum profundus (FDP) avulsion injury (type 1 and type 4)
- Staged reconstruction of flexor tendons is a technically demanding procedure that should be undertaken cautiously, especially in patients with an intact flexor digitorum superficialis (FDS). Patient selection is key to the success of this procedure. Results are likely to be better in young motivated individuals with good passive range of joint motion and commitment to therapy.

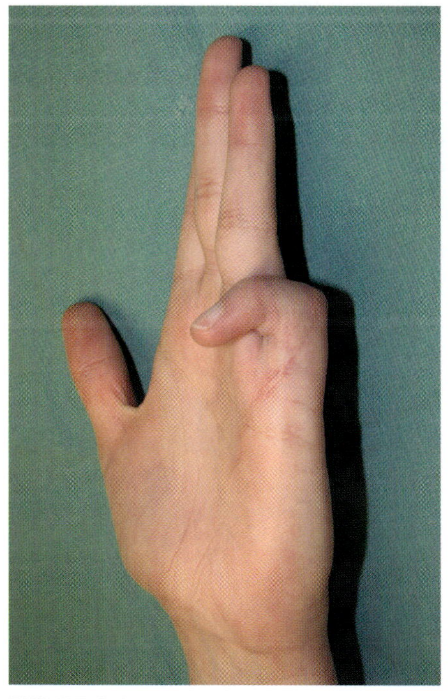

FIGURE 9-1

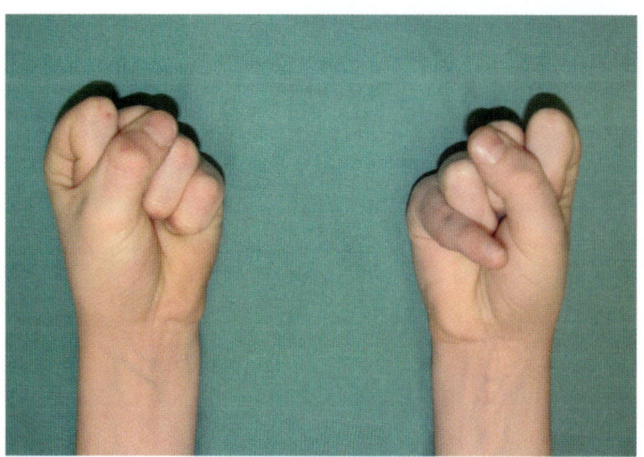

FIGURE 9-2

Examination/Imaging

Clinical Examination

- The patient should be examined to identify specific tendon involvement and reconstructive needs. Patients will present with loss of active distal interphalangeal (DIP) and proximal interphalangeal (PIP) joint flexion if both the FDP and FDS are divided, or loss of only DIP joint flexion if only FDP has been injured. On inspection, the normal finger cascade is lost, with the affected digit in an extended position (see Fig. 9-2).
- The metacarpophalangeal (MCP) and interphalangeal (IP) joints should have full passive range of motion, or they will require capsulotomy before tendon reconstruction (Figs. 9-3 and 9-4).
- The patient must have adequate soft tissue cover, or soft tissue reconstruction may also be necessary.
- The patient must be examined for the presence of the palmaris longus (PL), which is the most frequently used tendon graft. Other options include plantaris, extensor indicis proprius, extensor digiti minimi, and fascia lata. The toe flexors and the proximal FDS from the injured finger are possible sources of intrasynovial tendon grafts.

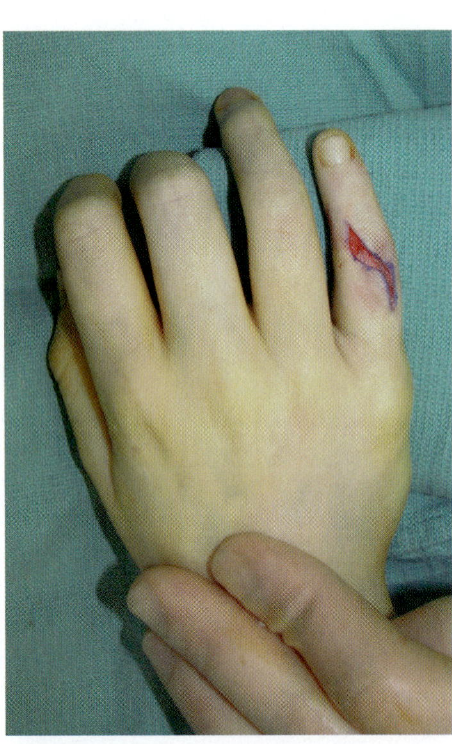

FIGURE 9-3

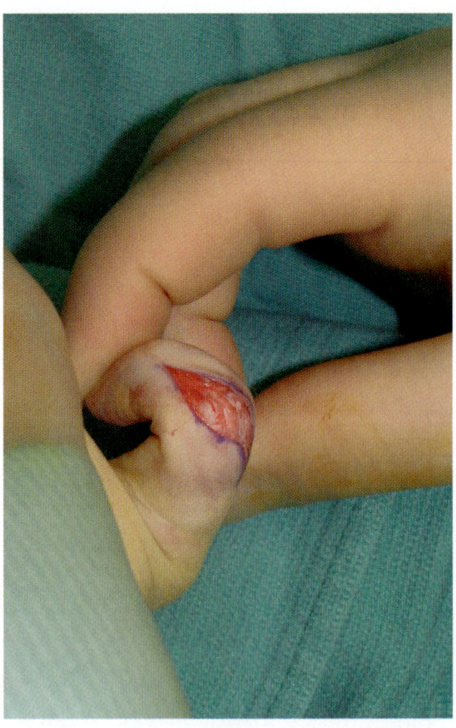

FIGURE 9-4

- *Palmaris longus:* It is absent in 5% to 15% of the population. Many tests have been described for determining the presence of the PL, and we find the Mishra test easy to apply and reliable. The Mishra test is performed by holding the patient's wrist and fingers in hyperextension while asking the patient to flex the wrist. This stretches the palmar aponeurosis and makes the PL taut when the patient attempts wrist flexion (Fig. 9-5).
- *Plantaris:* The absence of plantaris cannot be predicted preoperatively and has been reported in up to 6% to 20% of the population. The distal end of the plantaris is located over the deep medial aspect of the Achilles, midway between the medial malleolus and the posterior margin of the leg.

Imaging

- Preoperative imaging studies are not typically necessary for tendon reconstruction but may be required for commonly associated injuries.

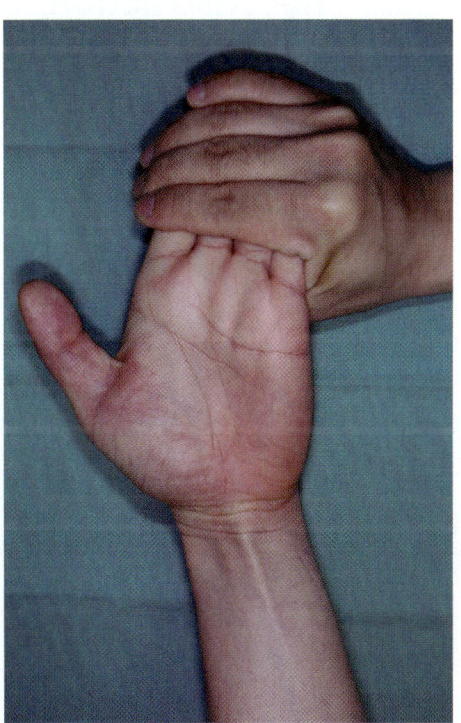

FIGURE 9-5

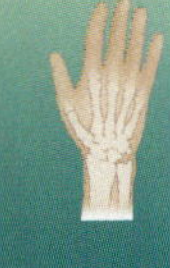

Surgical Anatomy

- The lumbrical muscle prevents further proximal retraction of the FDP tendons. For this reason, the proximal juncture of the tendon graft is usually placed in the palm to the FDP, just distal to the lumbrical origin. The median innervated first and second lumbricals are unipennate and arise from the radial and palmar surface of the FDP tendons to the index and long finger. The ulnar innervated third and fourth lumbricals are bipennate and arise from contiguous surfaces of the long/ring finger FDP tendon and ring/small finger FDP tendon, respectively. If the palm is involved in trauma, the proximal juncture is placed in the forearm.

Positioning

- The patient is placed supine on the operating table with the affected arm placed on a hand table.
- A lead hand is very useful during dissection.
- Access to the plantaris tendon may be necessary during the second stage if the palmaris is absent or a longer tendon graft is required.

PEARLS

If pulley reconstruction is not necessary, two separate incisions may be used: the first for distal palm exposure and the second for exposure of the tendon sheath in the finger.

The neurovascular bundles should be identified outside the zone of injury (related to previous scars) and protected when flaps are raised, as well as for the remainder of the operation.

Stage I: Exploration, Pulley Reconstruction, and Placement of Silicone Rod

Exposures

- Bruner incisions are designed from the mid-distal phalanx to the distal palm. Incisions are planned such that they incorporate any previous scars (Fig. 9-6).
- Thick skin flaps are raised in a plane superficial to the tendon sheath to expose the tendon sheath from the A1 pulley to the DIP joint (Fig. 9-7).

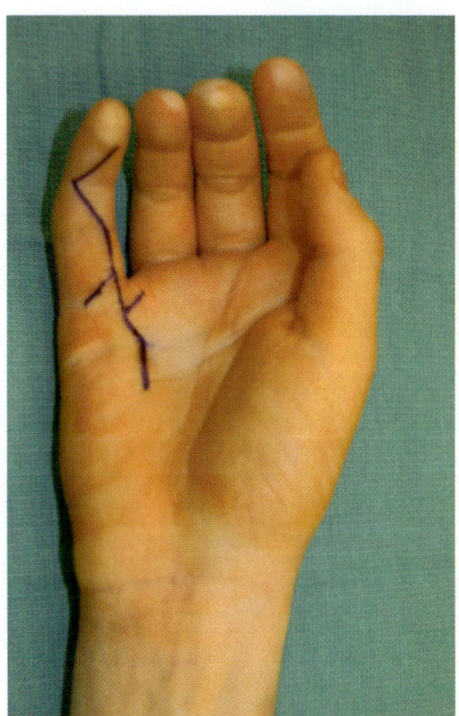

FIGURE 9-6

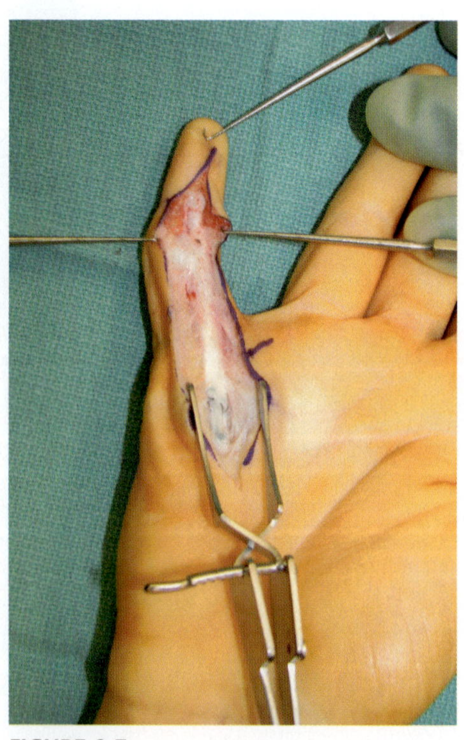

FIGURE 9-7

Procedure

Step 1: Assessment of Pulleys

- The tendon sheath is dissected carefully in an attempt to preserve any remnants of the A2 and A4 pulleys. Usually there is moderate to severe scarring, making it impossible to preserve good-quality pulleys (Fig. 9-8).

STEP 2 PEARLS

Excised good-quality remnants of the FDS or FDP should be saved for later use in pulley reconstruction.

Step 2: Débridement of Scar Sheath and Tendons

- The remnants of the scarred FDS and FDP tendons are excised distal to the lumbrical origin. Approximately 1 cm of the distal FDP insertion (if available) is preserved to provide a distal anchor point for the silicone rod.
- Poor-quality scarred tendon sheath is also excised. An attempt is made to preserve remnants of the A2 and A4 pulleys on the lateral aspect of the phalanges to provide soft tissue for anchoring sutures during pulley reconstruction.
- Joint release via closed capsulotomies or direct release of tight collateral or check-rein ligaments can be performed to achieve full range of motion.

Step 3: Pulley Reconstruction

- We use excised remnants of the FDS and FDP harvested from the finger or from FDS tendon in the palm or forearm to reconstruct the pulley.
- A single pulley is made at the middle phalanx, and two pulleys are made over the proximal phalanx. Pulleys are made by suturing segments of FDS and FDP to the remnants of the pulleys on the lateral aspect of the phalanx and the periosteum using 4-0 Ethibond sutures (Fig. 9-9).

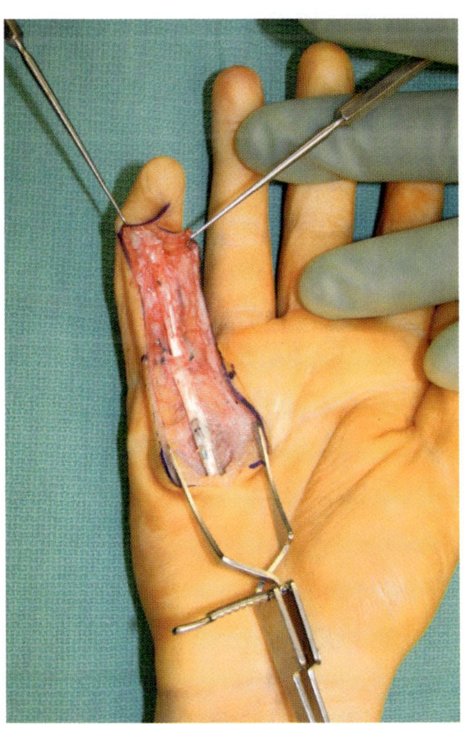

FIGURE 9-8

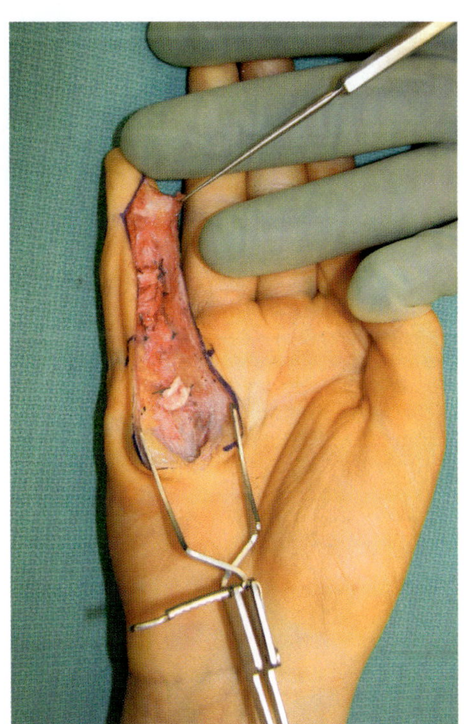

FIGURE 9-9

Step 4: Silicone Rod Placement

- The widest silicone rod that will pass through the pulleys and still glide proximally and distally with passive finger flexion and extension is selected.
- The selected silicone rod is passed from proximal (A1 pulley) to distal until it emerges at the DIP joint. It will need to be gently maneuvered through the remaining or reconstructed pulleys (Fig. 9-10).
- The distal end of the silicone rod is sutured to the remnants of the FDP insertion, the volar plate of the DIP joint, and surrounding soft tissue using 4-0 monofilament suture.
- The proximal end of the silicone rod is left free in the palm or the distal forearm, depending on where the proximal tendon juncture is planned.

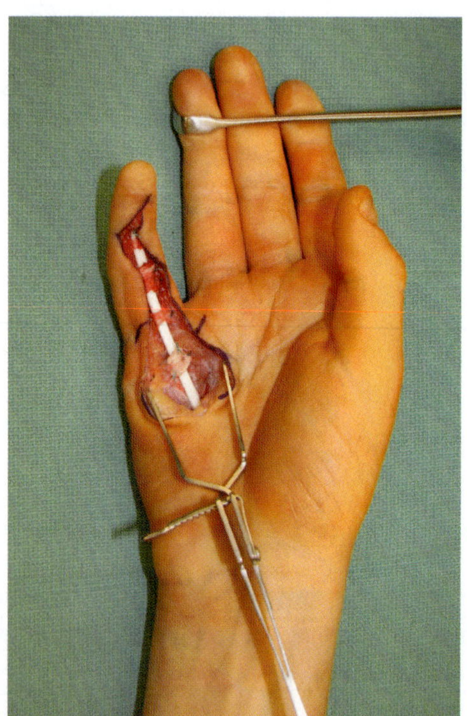

FIGURE 9-10

STEP 4 PEARLS

One must move the finger to ensure that the silicone rod glides freely and that there is no buckling of the silicone rod. The excess length of the silicone rod should be excised proximally. It is important to leave sufficient length such that it does not slip out distal to the A1 pulley with the digit in full extension or hyperextension. It should also not be so long that it gets kinked in the palm or forearm on full flexion of the digits.

If a decision about the proximal juncture has not been made, placing the rod in the forearm allows for the option of grafting either to the palm or to the forearm during the second stage. Typically, tendon grafting to the palm can be facilitated by the palmaris tendon graft, but sometimes the palm is so scarred that the silicone rod must be placed into the distal forearm. In these cases, a plantaris tendon graft is often used to reach the wrist, or, in some situations, a long palmaris longus tendon may reach the distal wrist that requires proximal juncture repair in the carpal tunnel.

The proximal rod should be placed next to the tendon to be used to power the tendon graft. In the palm, the FDP tendon is used, and the tendon repair juncture is at the lumbrical muscle origin. In the wrist, the FDS tendon is preferable because it is superficial and more accessible.

STEP 4 PITFALLS

It is important not to suture the proximal juncture of the silicone rod to the FDP tendon. Although this may seem like a good idea to enable active motion, the juncture between native tendon and silicone rod does not heal and will never be strong enough for active motion. A disruption of the distal juncture will require surgery to prevent proximal migration.

STEP 5 PEARLS

In the event that there is a significant soft tissue defect, local tissue rearrangement, such as the cross-finger flap, may be required for durable coverage of the silicone rod (Figs. 9-12 to 9-15). In heavily injured or contracted fingers, durable soft tissue coverage may even require a separate stage.

Step 5

- The tourniquet is released and hemostasis achieved.
- The skin is closed with interrupted 4-0 nylon sutures (Fig. 9-11).
- A bulky noncompressive volar forearm splint is applied.

Postoperative Care and Expected Outcomes

- Immediately after surgery, the patient is asked to elevate the hand for pain and edema control.
- Within 3 to 5 days, the bulky dressing is replaced with a light compressive dressing. Under the guidance of a therapist, passive range-of-motion exercises begin for the involved digit, and unrestricted active range-of-motion exercises are allowed for the other uninvolved digits.
- Between therapy sessions, the patient is maintained in an extension splint. Pulley tape is placed where pulleys have been reconstructed.
- The extension splint is discontinued by 6 weeks postoperatively and replaced with buddy straps used to link the involved finger with the adjacent finger to enable continuous passive range of motion.
- The second stage of surgery is planned for 3 months after the first stage, or when full passive range of motion is obtained. Furthermore, this time allows for the formation of a retinacular sheath, which will permit gliding of a tendon graft, and for the reconstructed pulleys to become firm and withstand active motion.

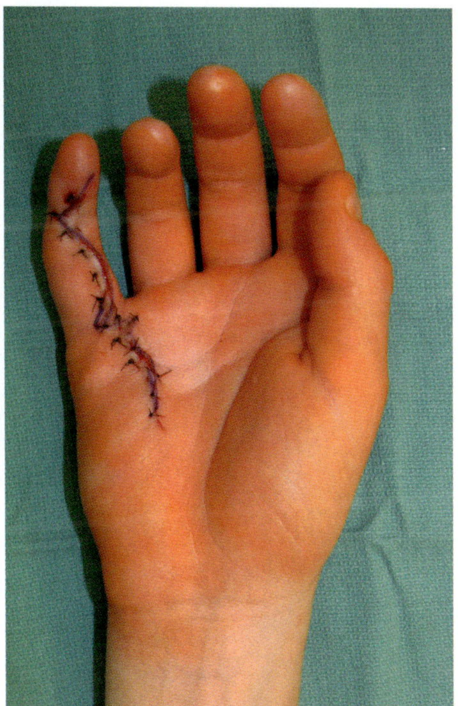

FIGURE 9-11

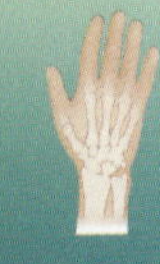

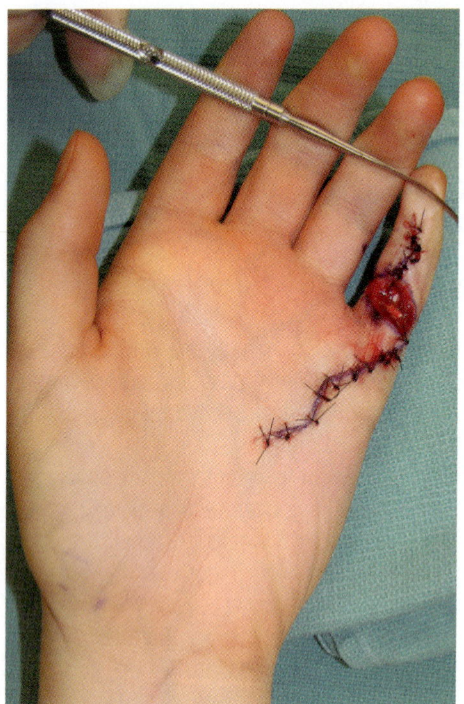

FIGURE 9-12

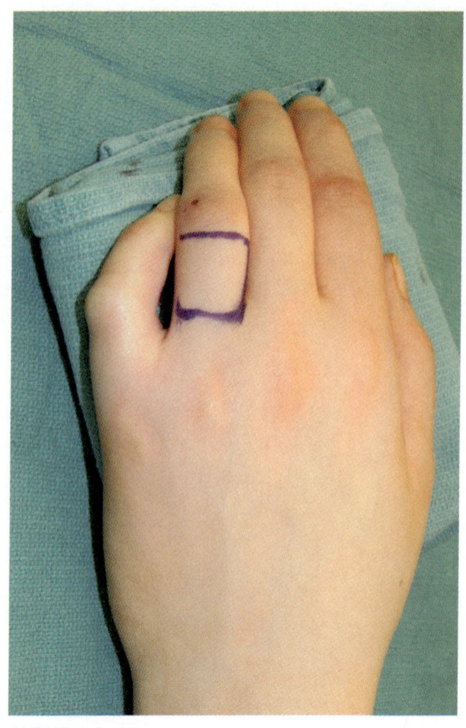

FIGURE 9-13

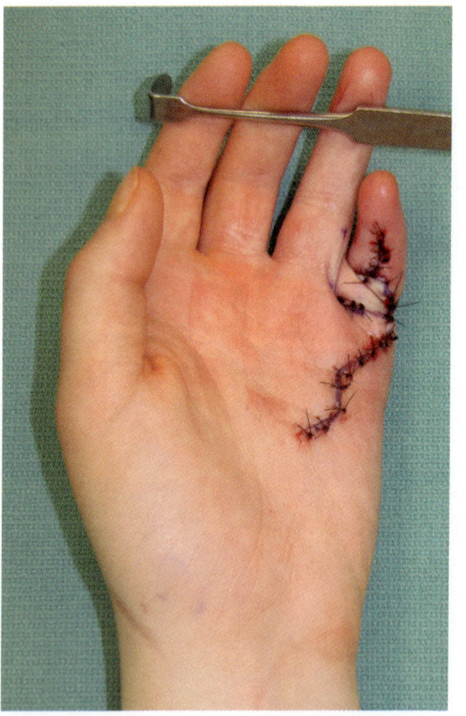

FIGURE 9-14

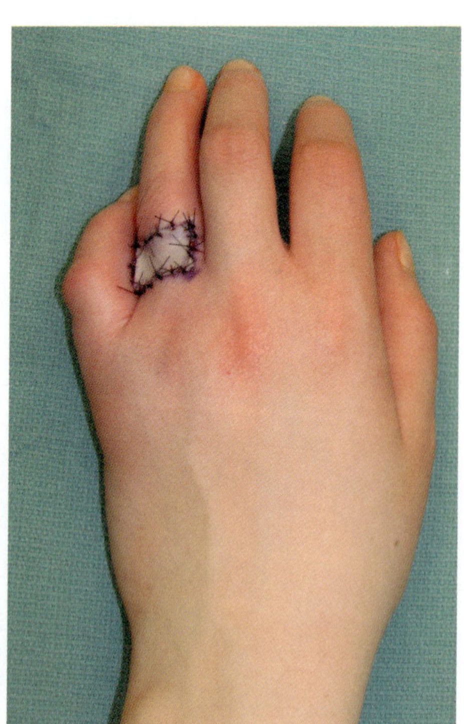

FIGURE 9-15

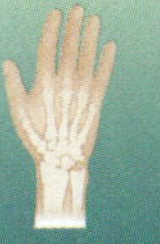

Stage II: Removal of Silicone Rod and Placement of Tendon Graft

Exposures

- Only a limited exposure is required for the second stage. An incision is made at the site of the proposed proximal tendon juncture (distal forearm or distal palm), and the proximal free end of the silicone rod is identified. Another incision is made over the DIP joint, and the distal end of the tendon rod is exposed (Fig. 9-16).

Procedure

Step 1: Harvest of Tendon Graft

- The PL is used if the proximal juncture is in the palm, and the longer plantaris is used if the proximal juncture is in the forearm or if the palmaris is absent.
- The PL tendon is exposed and harvested through a 1-cm transverse incision over the distal tendon at the wrist and three 1-cm transverse incisions in the forearm (Fig. 9-17).

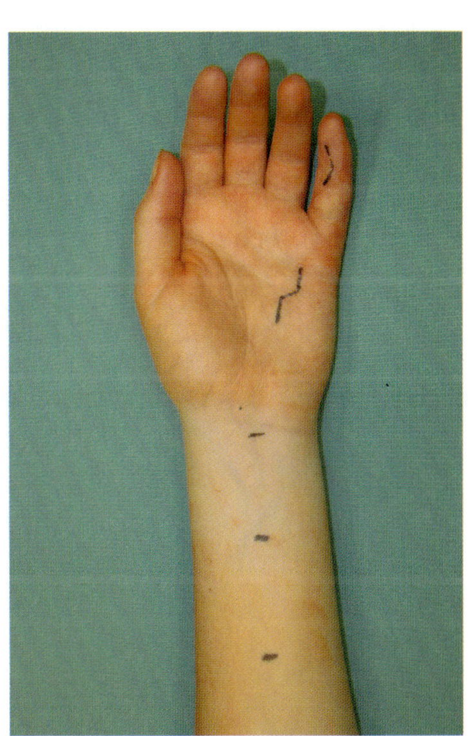

FIGURE 9-16

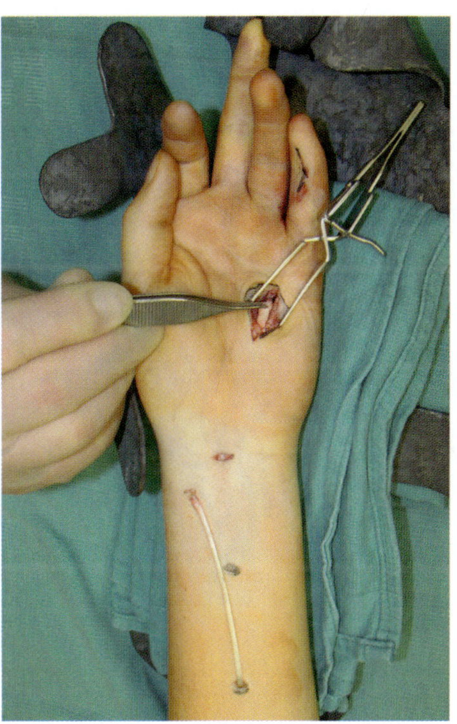

FIGURE 9-17

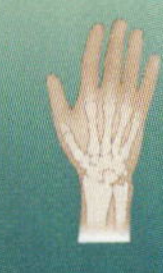

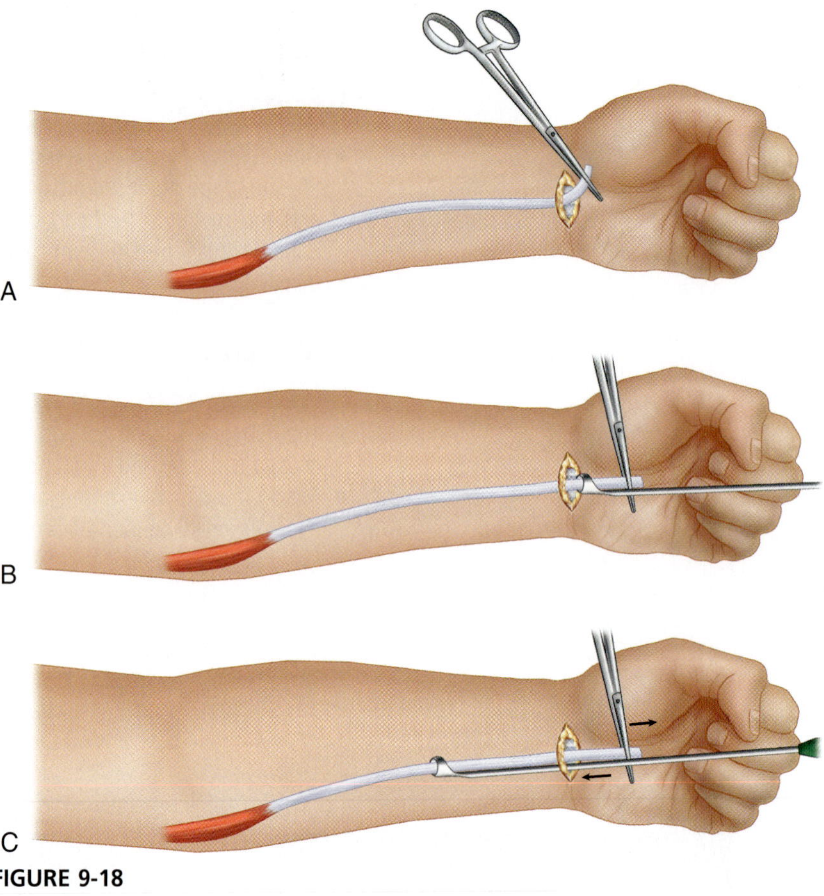

FIGURE 9-18

- The exposed portion of the PL tendon is held with a hemostat, and the tendon is divided distal to the hemostat. The hemostat and tendon are then pulled distally while simultaneously freeing the proximal tendon from the surrounding antebrachial fascia at each incision site. When the musculotendinous junction is encountered, the tendon can be easily extracted with gentle traction at the wrist incision. Alternatively, a Brand tendon stripper can be used (Fig. 9-18A to C).

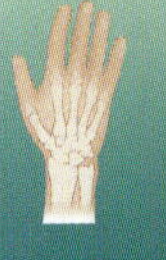

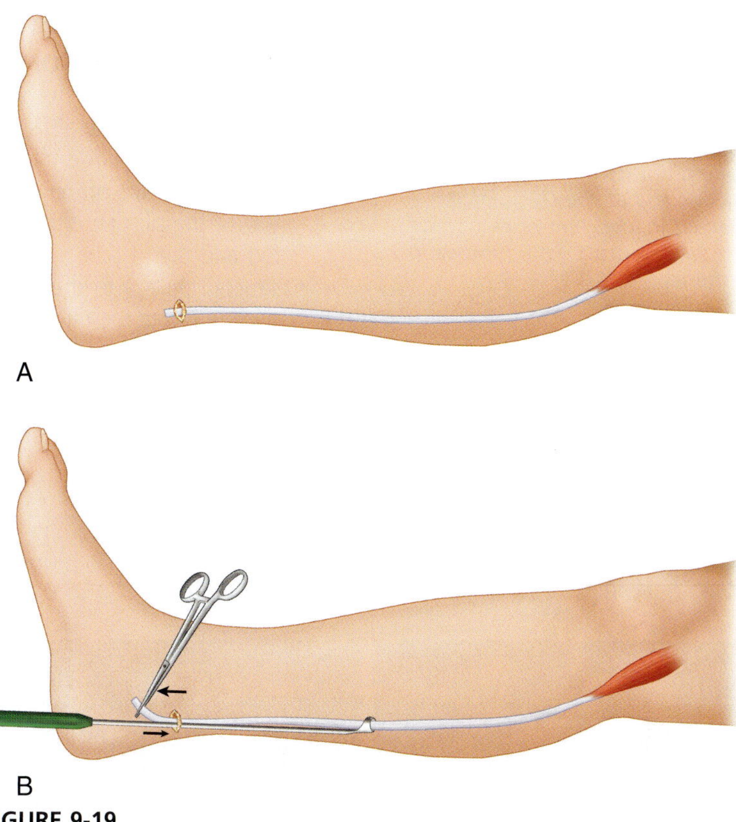

FIGURE 9-19

- The plantaris tendon is exposed by a 2-cm transverse incision just anterior to the Achilles tendon and above the medial calcaneus. The tendon is divided and the distal end passed through a Brand tendon harvester. While maintaining countertraction on the distal end of the tendon, the tendon harvester is advanced proximally to release the tendon at the myotendinous junction. The knee should be kept extended during the harvest to avoid injury to neurovascular structures in the popliteal area (Fig. 9-19A and B).
- The harvested tendon graft is kept in moist gauze to prevent desiccation of the tendon, and all skin incisions are closed using 4-0 nylon.

STEP 2 PEARLS

A mosquito forceps should be attached to the free end of the tendon graft proximally before pulling on the distal end of the silicone rod at the DIP joint to prevent inadvertent retraction of the tendon graft within the palm or finger.

Step 2: Passing the Tendon Graft through the Flexor Tendon Sheath

- The proximal end of the silicone rod is exposed at the palm or wrist, and one end of the tendon graft is sutured to the rod using a horizontal mattress suture with 3-0 Prolene. It is important not to make this juncture bulky (Fig. 9-20).
- The attachments of the silicone rod at the DIP joint are divided, and the distal end of the silicone rod is pulled gradually (Fig. 9-21). This brings the silicone rod and the attached tendon graft through the flexor sheath and the reconstructed pulleys to the DIP joint. The attachment of the proximal end of the silicone rod to the tendon graft is divided, and the silicone rod is discarded.
- One end of the tendon graft is now at the DIP joint and the other at the location of the proximal tendon juncture in the distal palm or distal forearm (Fig. 9-22).

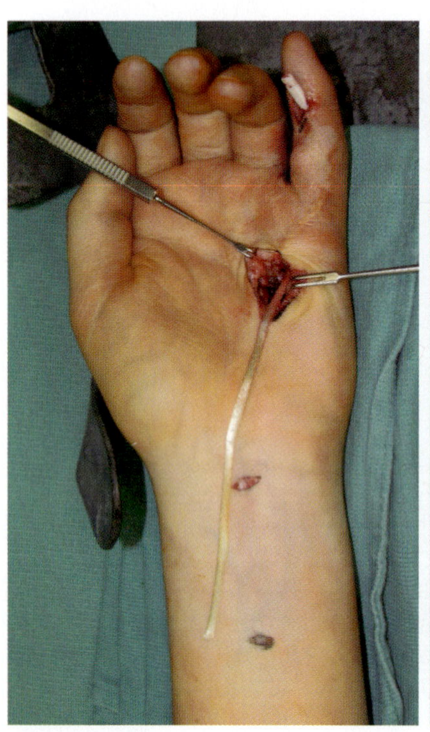
FIGURE 9-20

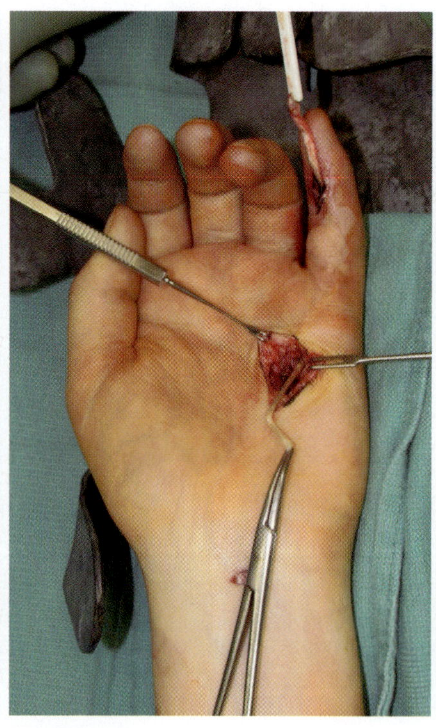
FIGURE 9-21

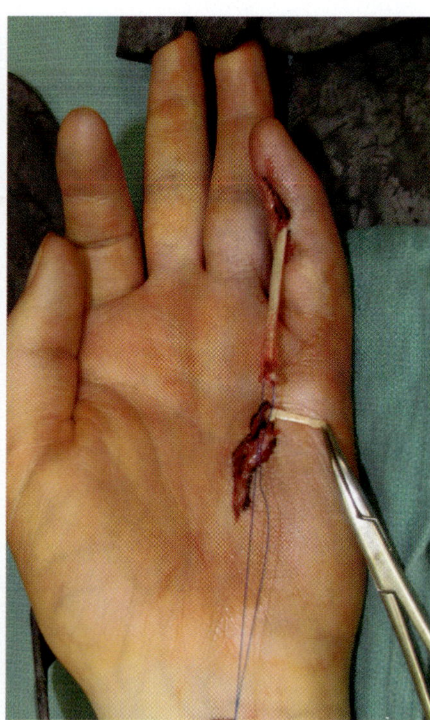
FIGURE 9-22

STEP 3 PEARLS

A bone tunnel is not necessary.

Prolene sutures are used because they can slide out easily after healing of the tendon to the bone, which takes about 6 weeks.

Securing the distal end of the tendon graft to the distal phalanx with a bone anchor is an alternative method, but the prominence of the anchor may protrude through the distal phalanx into the nail bed, which will be most problematic.

STEP 3 PITFALLS

When drilling the Keith needle through the nail, it is important not to drill the needle into the germinal matrix, which will assuredly cause nail deformity. Rather, the Keith needle should initially run parallel to the distal phalanx before perforating through the bone and should exit the nail at the midnail position.

When tying down the Prolene suture over the nail, the surgeon must observe the tendon sitting securely within the bone trough at the distal phalanx.

Step 3: Distal Tendon Repair

- If a sufficient amount of good-quality FDP remnant (>1 cm) is available distally, the distal end of the tendon graft can be sutured directly to the FDP remnant by a double Kessler technique using 4-0 Ethibond sutures. This repair is bolstered by additional sutures to the palmar periosteum of the distal phalanx and the volar plate. This type of repair, however, is usually not strong enough to start passive-motion gliding exercises and should not be entertained in most cases.
- If insufficient distal FDP tendon is available for direct repair, a pull-through suture technique is used to repair the tendon graft to the palmar cortex of the base of the distal phalanx. A Bunnell-type criss-crossing locking suture using 3-0 Prolene is passed through the distal end of the tendon graft. The palmar proximal aspect of the distal phalanx is gently débrided using a fine rongeur until cancellous bone is encountered. Two Keith needles are drilled obliquely through the base of the distal phalanx to the dorsum of the finger and through the nail plate to emerge distal to the lunula (Fig. 9-23). The two ends of the Bunnell suture are passed through the proximal end of the needle, and the needles are withdrawn on the dorsal surface to bring the sutures onto the dorsum. The sutures are then secured in place with a bolster, or button, on the dorsal aspect of the finger (Fig. 9-24). The elevated periosteum and surrounding soft tissue can be sutured to the end of the tendon using 4-0 Ethibond suture to provide additional support.
- The distal skin incision is closed using 4-0 nylon before doing the proximal tendon juncture because the finger will be in a flexed posture after the proximal tendon juncture.

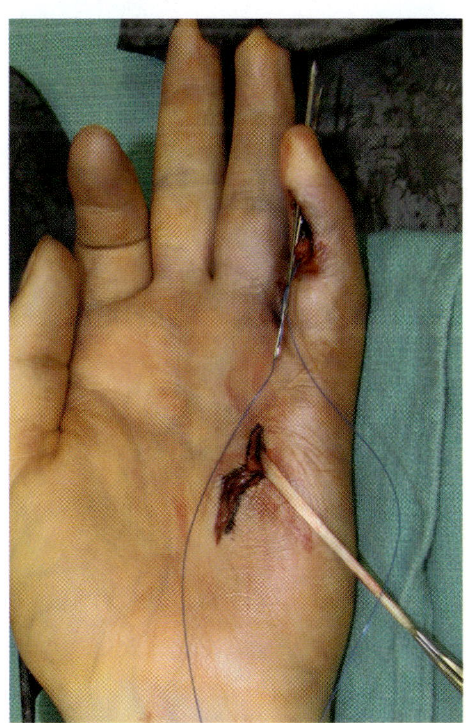

FIGURE 9-23

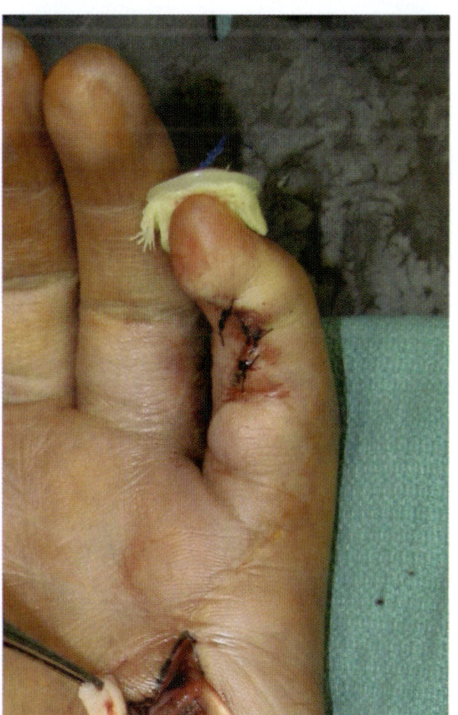

FIGURE 9-24

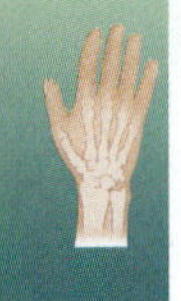

Step 4: Proximal Tendon Repair

- The proximal end of the tendon graft is sutured to the distal end of the selected FDP tendon using a Pulvertaft weave and secured with 4-0 Ethibond sutures (Fig. 9-25). Tension of the graft is adjusted such that the fingers are in a natural cascade with the wrist in neutral position.

Step 5: Wound Closure

- The tourniquet is released and hemostasis secured.
- The remaining skin incisions are closed with 4-0 nylon (Fig. 9-26).
- A dorsal blocking splint is applied with the wrist in 20 degrees of flexion, the MCP joint in 70 degrees of flexion, and the IP joints at neutral.

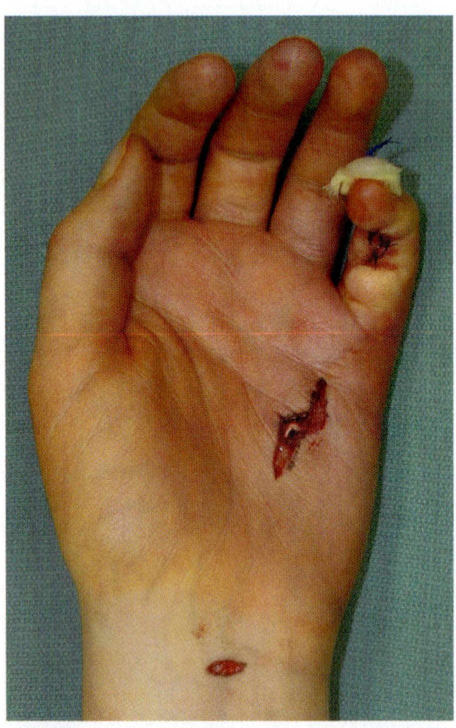

FIGURE 9-25

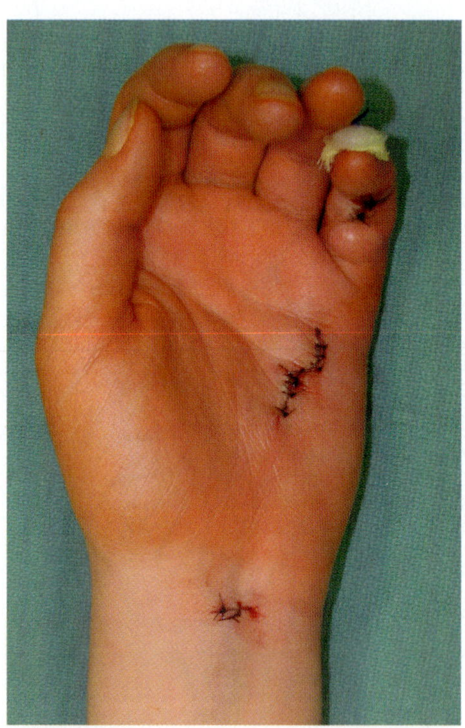

FIGURE 9-26

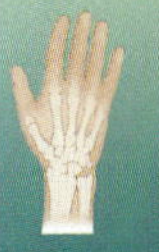

Postoperative Care and Expected Outcomes

- Three days postoperatively, a modified Duran passive range-of-motion exercise program is begun within the confines of the dorsal blocking splint under the close supervision of a hand therapist.
- Three weeks postoperatively, active range of motion is begun within the confines of the splint.
- Four weeks postoperatively, active range of motion is begun with the wrist and fingers outside of the splint.
- Five weeks postoperatively, unrestricted active motion is allowed, with discontinuation of the splint by 6 weeks.
- Strengthening is initiated at 8 weeks with the expectation that the hand can be used in all activities by 12 to 14 weeks postoperatively.
- With this protocol, in the best of hands, about one third of patients achieve good results (greater than 200 degrees of total active motion) (Fig. 9-27A and B). Another one third have fair improvement, and the remainder fail two-stage flexor tendon reconstruction.
- In cases of decreased range of motion despite adequate therapy, flexor tenolysis may be necessary but should be delayed at least 3 to 6 months after tendon grafting.

PEARLS

Care should be taken to avoid interphalangeal joint contractures.

PITFALLS

Because the graft is entirely avascular for several weeks, it is weak and prone to rupture. Therefore, motion must be recovered gradually and cautiously, with only the lightest of active unrestricted flexion and single-joint active and passive extension during the early phases of recovery.

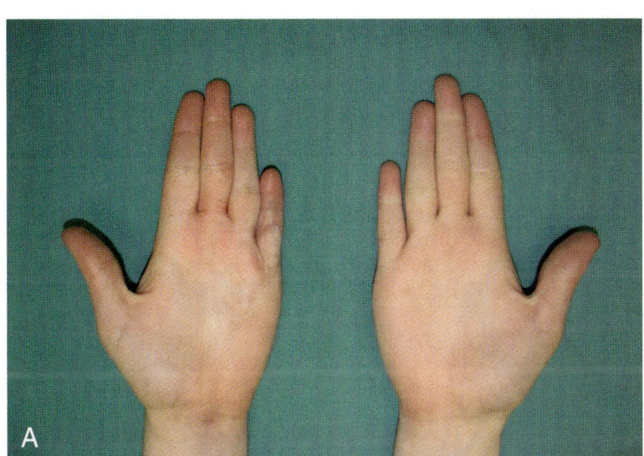

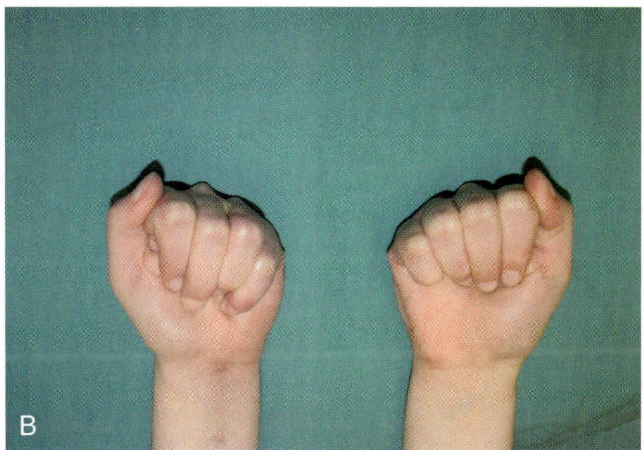

FIGURE 9-27

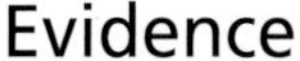

Evidence

Boyes JH, Stark HH. Flexor-tendon grafts in the fingers and thumb: a study of factors influencing results in 1000 cases. *J Bone Joint Surg [Am]*. 1971;53:1332-1342.
This landmark and largest study in the literature reported outcomes of staged tendon reconstruction in 607 fingers and thumbs. (Level IV evidence)

Leversedge FJ, Zelouf D, Williams C, et al. Flexor tendon grafting to the hand: an assessment of the intrasynovial donor tendon—a preliminary single-cohort study. *J Hand Surg [Am]*. 2000;25:721-730.
A small clinical study using intrasynovial donor tendons for flexor tendon reconstruction in 10 patients showed encouraging results compared with the published standard. (Level III evidence)

Thien TB, Becker JH, Theis JC. Rehabilitation after surgery for flexor tendon injuries in the hand. *Cochrane Database Syst Rev* 2004;4:CD003979.
The only Cochrane Database study on flexor tendon reconstruction concluded that there is insufficient evidence from randomized controlled trials to outline the best mobilization strategy after tendon reconstruction. (Level II evidence)

Wehbé MA, Mawr B, Hunter JM, et al. Two-stage flexor-tendon reconstruction: ten-year experience. *J Bone Joint Surg [Am]*. 1986;68:752-763.
Case series of 150 patients who underwent staged tendon reconstruction with interposed Hunter rod followed by immediate protected motion and tendon gliding exercises. Authors demonstrated an increase in Total Active Motion of 74 degrees. Complications were reported. (Level IV evidence)

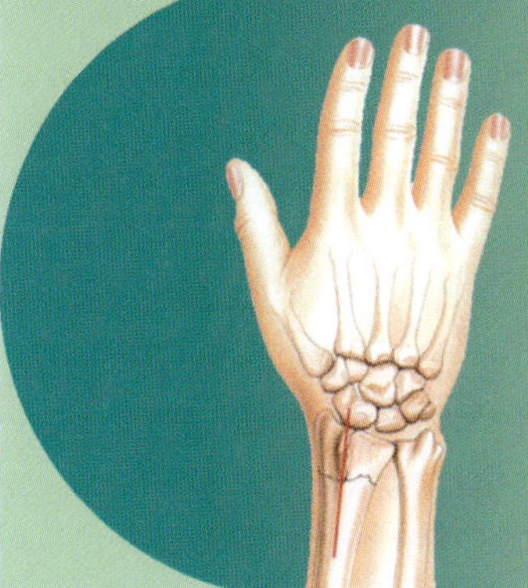

PROCEDURE 10

Extensor Tendon Repair in Zones 1 to 5

Pao-Yuan Lin, Sandeep J. Sebastin, and Kevin C. Chung

See Video 7: Turnover Tendon Flap for PIP Extensor Tendon Injury

Indications

- Open wound with divided extensor tendon involving more than 50% of the width of the tendon

Examination/Imaging

Imaging

- Radiographs of the hand should be obtained to rule out any associated foreign bodies or fractures (Fig. 10-1).

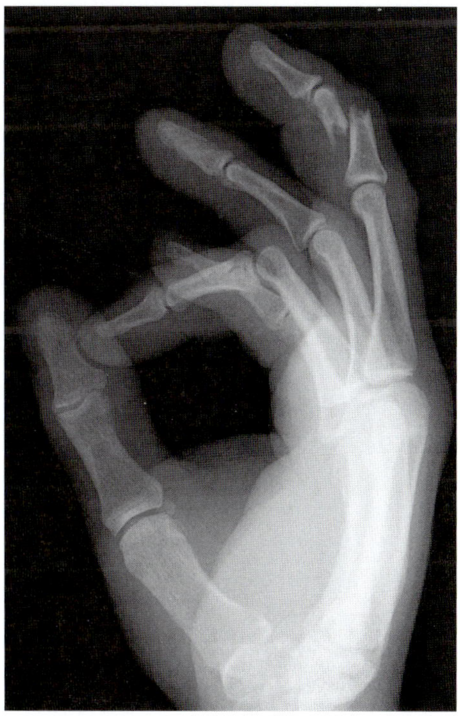

FIGURE 10-1

Surgical Anatomy

- Extensor tendon injuries are divided into nine zones for the fingers and seven zones for the thumb numbered from distal to proximal (Fig. 10-2A). An easy way to remember these zones is to bear in mind that the odd-numbered zones are located over the joints. Therefore zones 1, 3, 5, and 7 are located over the distal interphalangeal (DIP) joint, proximal interphalangeal (PIP) joint, metacarpophalangeal (MCP) joint, and wrist, respectively.
- The extensor tendon is thick over the MCP joint but becomes broad and thin over the dorsum of the proximal phalanx, where it divides into three portions. The central portion becomes the central slip that inserts into the base of the middle phalanx, and the lateral portions join the lateral bands. The tendons of the lumbrical and interosseous muscles form the lateral bands. These lateral bands come together over the middle phalanx and form the most distal part of the extensor tendon that inserts into the base of the distal phalanx (Fig. 10-2B).

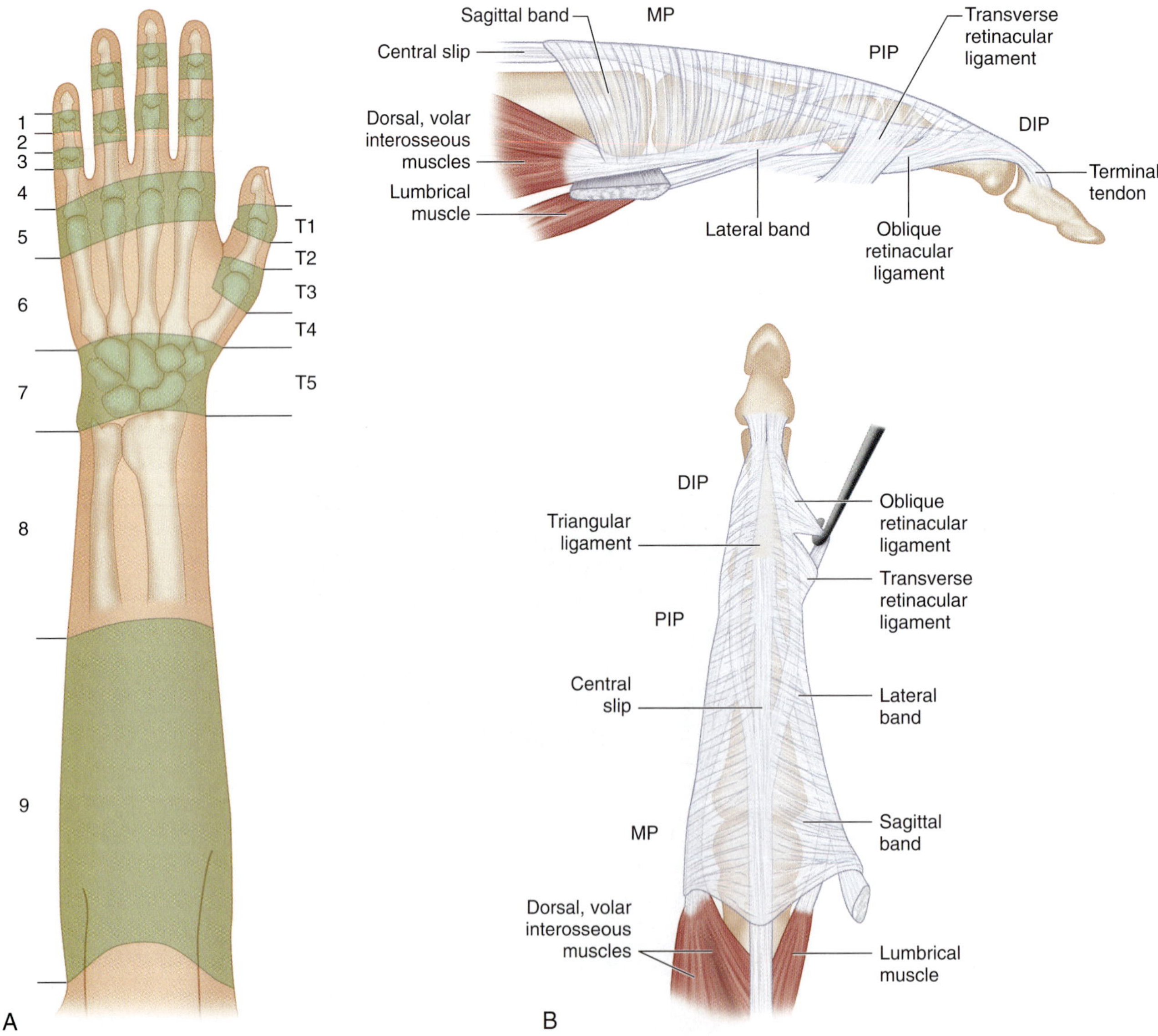

FIGURE 10-2

- At the MCP joint, the extensor tendon is held in position by the sagittal bands, which arise from the volar plate of the MCP joint and the intermetacarpal ligaments, to insert on the extensor hood. Injury to the sagittal bands may result in subluxation of the extensor tendon.
- There is very little excursion of the extensor tendon over the fingers (11 to 17 mm at the MCP joint, 6 to 8 mm at the PIP joint, and 4 to 5 mm at the DIP joint). It is therefore important to do an accurate repair and avoid bunching up the tendon. It is usually possible to pass a core suture through the extensor tendon in the proximal half of zone 4 and in zone 5. However, only a simple suture is possible in zones 1, 2, and 3.
- Lacerations to the extensor pollicis longus (EPL) tendon cannot be tested by simply examining extension of the thumb interphalangeal (IP) joint. The IP joint may be extended by the extensor pollicis brevis (EPB) and the thenar intrinsic muscles via their insertions on the extensor expansion. The EPL is tested by placing the patient's hand flat on a table and asking the patient to lift the thumb off the table (Fig. 10-3).

Positioning

- Extensor tendon repairs can be done under a digital block (zones 1, 2, and 3) or a wrist block (zones 4 and 5). The use of a forearm tourniquet (placed distally over the nonmuscular portion of the forearm) will allow the patient to tolerate the tourniquet for a longer period (30 to 40 minutes) compared with the usual placement over the arm (20 to 30 minutes). The patient is positioned supine with the affected extremity on a hand table.

Exposures

- The existing lacerations are incorporated to raise wide flaps with a broad tip.
- Full-thickness skin flaps are raised superficial to the paratenon.

PITFALLS

Do not raise a flap with a narrow tip. This may lead to tip necrosis and exposure of the repair.

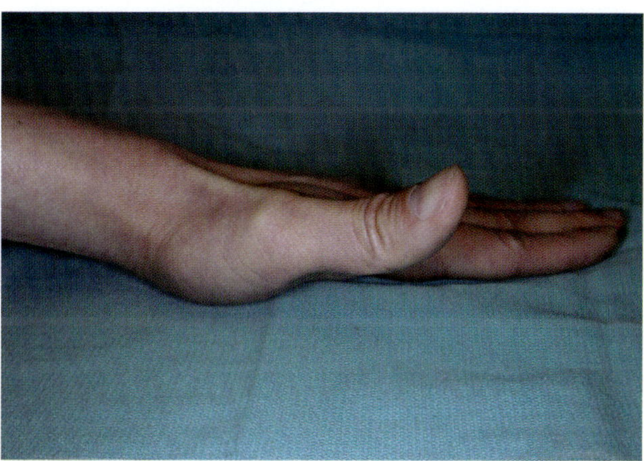

FIGURE 10-3

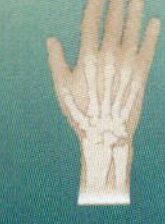

Zone 1 Injury

Clinical Examination

- Patients present with a flexed posture of the DIP joint (mallet finger) and inability to actively extend the DIP joint (Fig. 10-4).
- Patients with an untreated mallet finger, especially those with a preexisting hyperextensible PIP joint, can develop a compensatory swan-neck deformity because of extensor force being directed toward the central slip and leading to hyperextension at the PIP joint.
- Doyle has classified mallet finger into four types (Table 10-1).

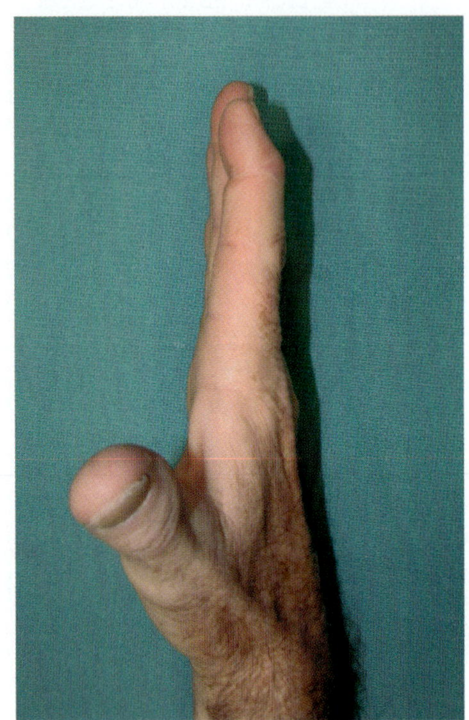

FIGURE 10-4

Table 10-1 Classification of Mallet Finger

Type	Definition
I	Closed injury
II	Associated with overlying skin laceration
III	Associated with tendon and loss of overlying skin (deep abrasion)
IVA	Transphyseal injury in skeletally immature digit
IVB	Associated with avulsion fracture involving 20%-50% of articular surface
IVC	Associated with avulsion fracture involving >50% of articular surface

STEP 1 PEARLS

If there is a gap, a small extensor retinaculum graft can be used to bridge the defect.

If there is not enough distal terminal tendon for suturing, a bone anchor can be used. The bone anchor must be passed before the joint is pinned.

STEP 2 PEARLS

Pinning the joint before tendon repair is optional. It takes the stress off the repair and is valuable in patients who cannot be relied on to wear a splint.

It may be easier to pass the K-wire retrograde by flexing the DIP joint. This will also avoid any bone anchor that has been used for repair.

Procedure

Step 1

- The proximal end of the tendon is mobilized for 5 to 8 mm such that the tendon ends lie close to each other with the joint in neutral position.

Step 2

- The DIP joint is pinned in extension or slight hyperextension using a 0.045-inch K-wire (Fig. 10-5A).

Step 3

- A 4-0 Ethibond horizontal mattress suture is used for tendon repair (Fig. 10-5B).

Step 4

- The tourniquet is released and hemostasis secured. Skin is closed with 5-0 nylon interrupted sutures.
- The K-wire may be cut short and buried under the skin.
- A thermoplastic splint is also provided to immobilize the DIP joint and protect the tip of the K-wire. Additional immobilization of the PIP joint in extension may be required in patients who have an associated swan-neck deformity.

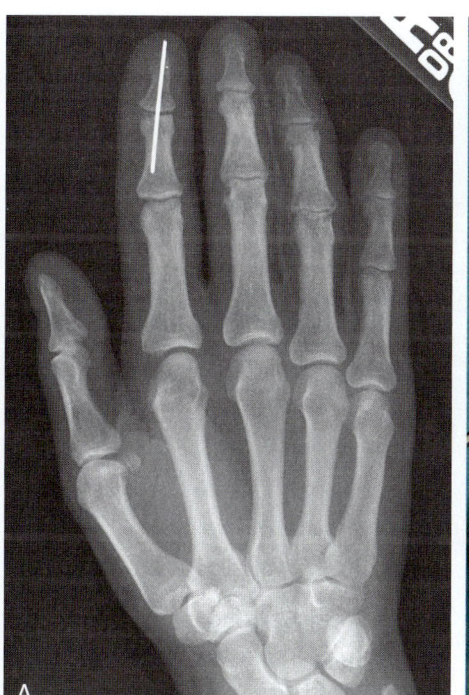

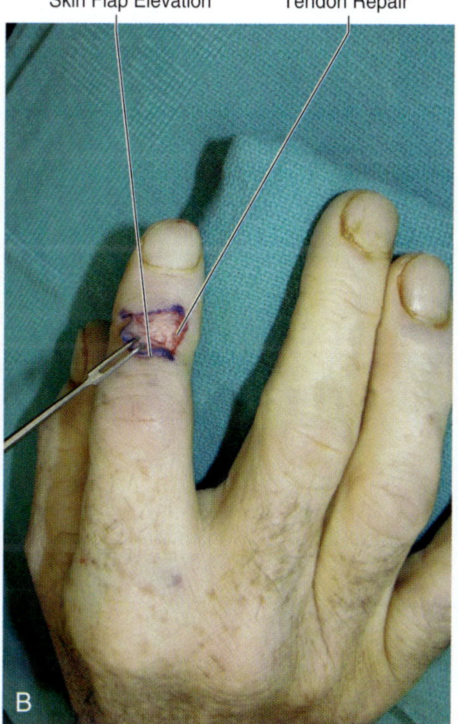

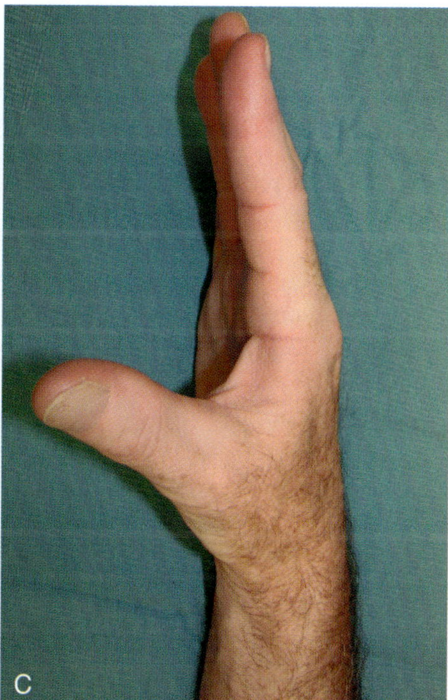

FIGURE 10-5

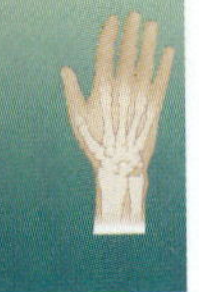

Postoperative Care and Expected Outcomes

- The K-wire should be maintained for 6 weeks, after which time it is removed and the patient is started on gradual mobilization of the DIP joint. The splint is maintained for an additional 4 weeks.
- Patients should be advised to continue mobilizing the PIP joint during the period of DIP joint splintage.
- Seventy percent to 80% of patients with zone 1 extensor tendon injuries have an excellent (no lag) to good (<10-degree lag) outcome (Fig. 10-5C).

Zone 2 Injury

Clinical Examination

- Patients usually do not develop a mallet deformity because one or both of the lateral bands are spared, and the laceration usually involves only the triangular ligament.
- This injury is frequently associated with a fracture of the middle phalanx (see Fig. 10-1).

Procedure

Step 1

- The tendon ends are exposed (Fig. 10-6A).

Step 2

- The DIP joint may be pinned with a 0.045-inch K-wire.

Step 3

- The tendon is repaired using a 4-0 or 5-0 Ethibond horizontal mattress suture (Fig. 10-6B).

Step 4

- The tourniquet is released and hemostasis secured. Skin is closed with 5-0 nylon interrupted sutures.
- The K-wire may be cut short and buried under the skin.
- A thermoplastic splint is also provided to immobilize the DIP joint and protect the tip of the K-wire.

STEP 4 PEARLS

A type III injury with loss of overlying skin will need flap coverage. Available options include a local transposition flap or a reverse dermis cross-finger flap from the adjacent digit.

Postoperative Care and Expected Outcomes

- The K-wire and/or the splint is maintained for 6 weeks. Gradual mobilization is started thereafter, with splintage for an additional 4 weeks (Fig. 10-6C).

Zone 3 Injury

Clinical Examination

- Patients with an injury to the central slip (zone 3) but with intact lateral bands and triangular ligament will be able to extend the PIP joint through the lateral bands that are still dorsal to the axis of the PIP joint. However, if untreated, the triangular ligament is gradually attenuated over a period of 2 to 3 weeks, and the lateral bands sublux volar to the axis of the PIP joint. This results in the lateral bands becoming a flexor of the PIP joint. The patient will now be unable to extend the PIP joint and will present with a boutonnière deformity (flexion of the PIP joint and hyperextension of the DIP joint) (Fig. 10-7).

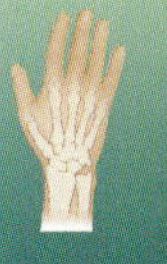

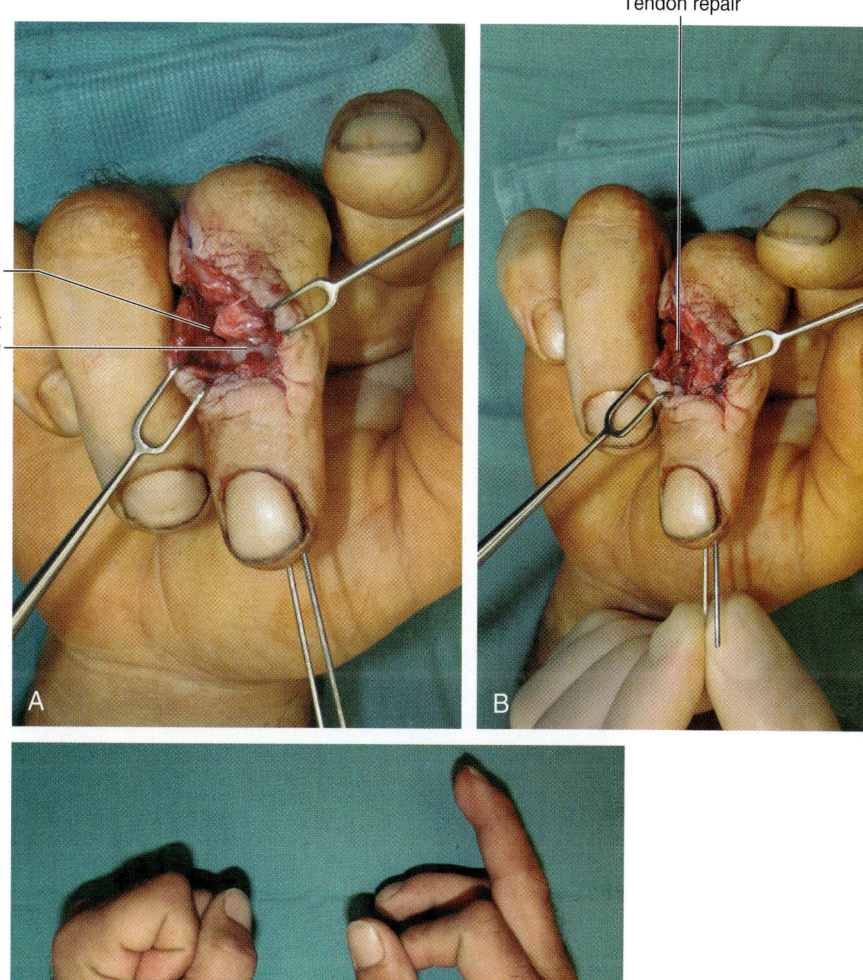

FIGURE 10-6

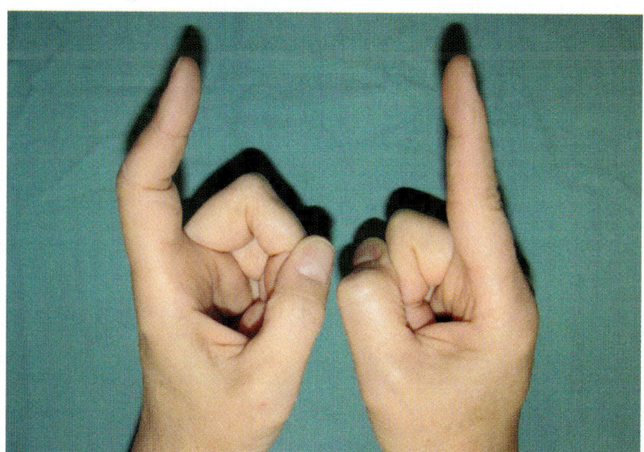

FIGURE 10-7

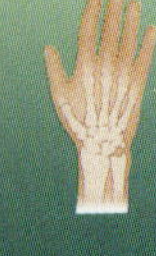

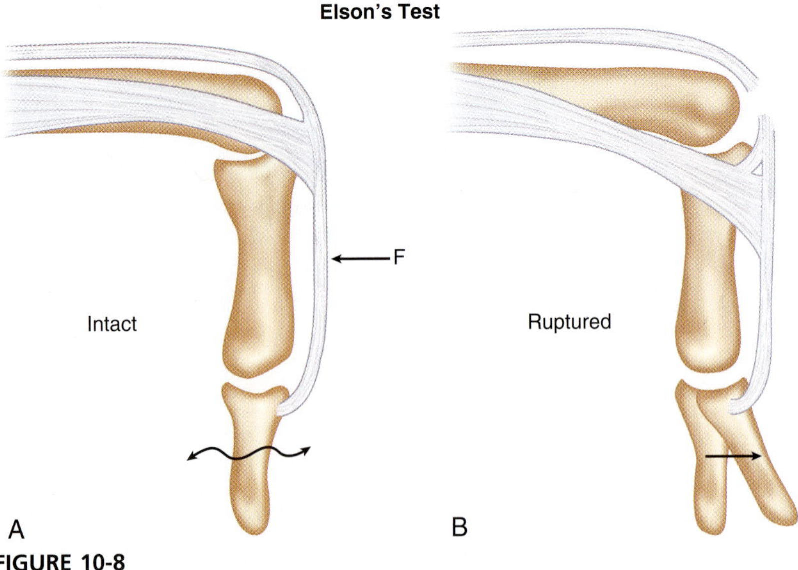

FIGURE 10-8

- The Elson test is useful in diagnosing a central slip injury early (before the development of a boutonnière deformity) and in differentiating a boutonnière deformity from edema of the PIP joint or a PIP joint flexion contracture. The examiner passively flexes the PIP joint to 90 degrees over a tabletop and asks the patient to attempt active extension of the PIP joint while the examiner resists PIP joint extension. Acute rupture of the central slip results in no extension power being felt at the PIP joint and significant extension power, or hyperextension, produced at the DIP joint (Fig. 10-8).

Procedure

Step 1

- The tendon ends are exposed (Fig. 10-9A).

Step 2

- The PIP joint is pinned with a 0.045-inch K-wire.

Step 3

- The tendon is repaired using a 4-0 Ethibond horizontal mattress suture (Fig. 10-9B and C).

STEP 3 PEARLS

If there is a gap, a tendon turndown procedure may be used. Appropriate length of the tendon is raised as a distally based flap from the proximal tendon (Fig. 10-10). Another option would be to use a free tendon graft.

If there is not enough distal terminal tendon for suturing, a bone anchor can be used. The bone anchor must be inserted before the joint is pinned (Fig. 10-11).

Step 4

- The tourniquet is released and hemostasis secured. Skin is closed with 5-0 nylon interrupted sutures.
- A thermoplastic splint is also provided to immobilize the PIP and DIP joints.

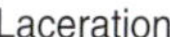

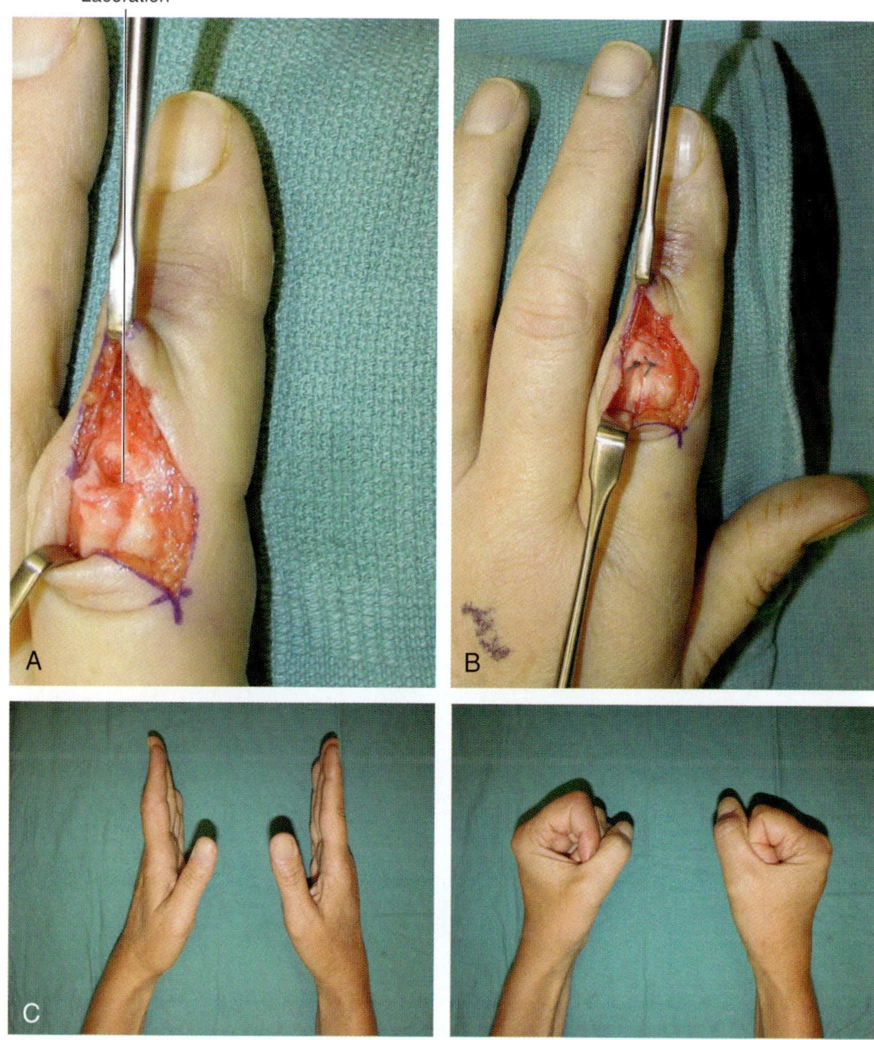

FIGURE 10-9

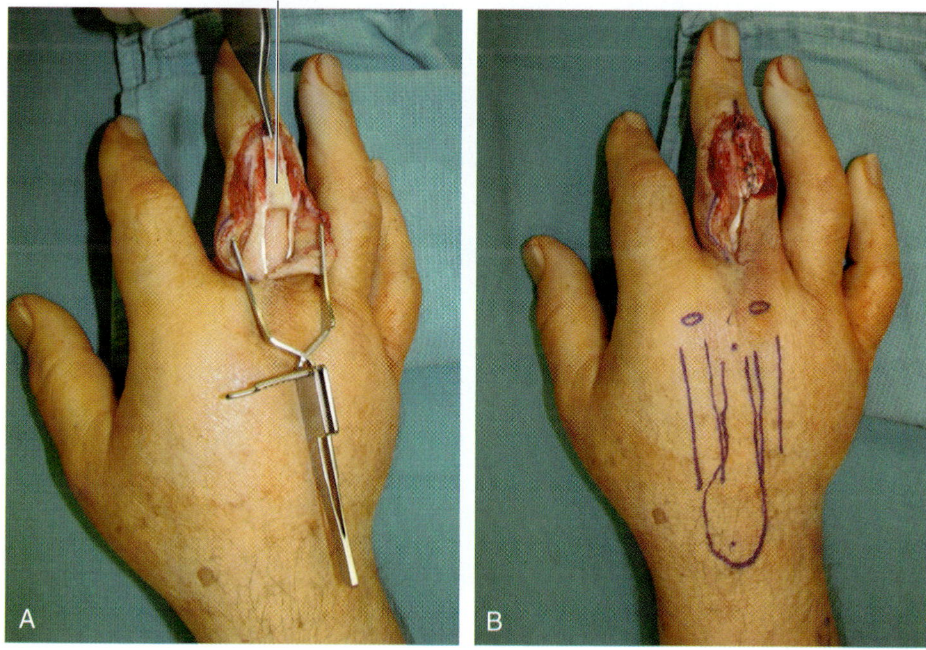

FIGURE 10-10

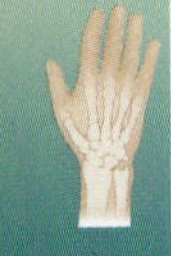

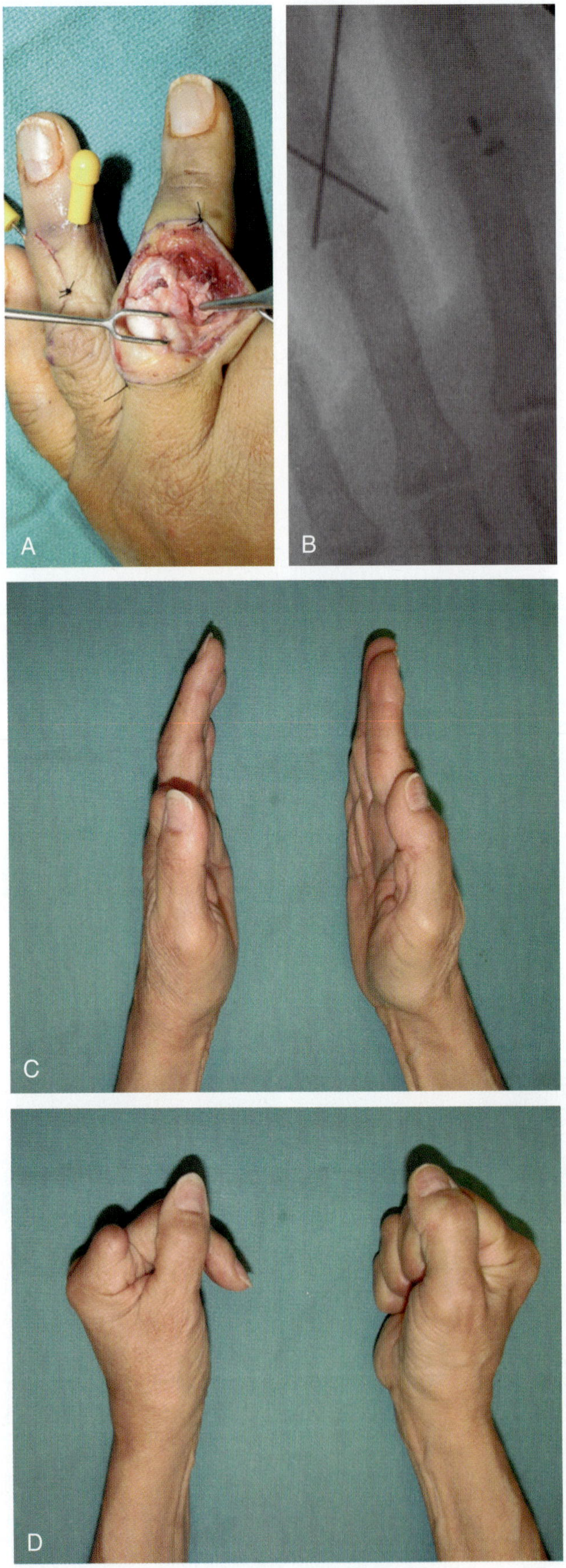

FIGURE 10-11

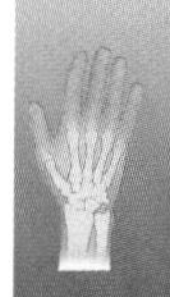

Postoperative Care and Expected Outcomes

- The K-wire and/or splint is maintained for 6 weeks. Intermittent gentle active DIP joint motion is permitted. The PIP joint is mobilized after the K-wire is removed. Gradual mobilization is started with splintage for an additional 4 weeks.

Zone 4 Injury

Clinical Examination

- These are similar to zone 2 injuries and are frequently associated with an underlying fracture.
- There may not be any appreciable extension lag at the PIP joint owing to the continuity of the lateral bands and intrinsic tendons.

Procedure

Step 1

- The divided tendon ends are exposed.
- The PIP and MCP joints are maintained in extension.

Step 2

- If the tendon is thick (proximal half of zone 4), a modified Kessler repair with a 4-0 Ethibond core suture and a 6-0 Prolene epitendinous repair is carried out.
- If the tendon is not thick (distal half of zone 4), a horizontal mattress repair with 4-0 Ethibond suture and a running 6-0 Prolene suture repair is carried out.

Step 3

- The tourniquet is released and hemostasis secured. Skin is closed with 5-0 nylon interrupted sutures.
- A splint to immobilize the wrist in slight extension and the MCP and IP joints in full extension is provided.

Postoperative Care and Expected Outcomes

- The splint is maintained for 4 weeks, and the patient is started on mobilization thereafter. If a core suture repair was possible, the patient can be started on mobilization earlier.

Zone 5 Injury

Clinical Examination

- A human bite injury should always be suspected in an open zone 5 tendon injury. These patients present with a small puncture wound over the knuckle that is associated with extensor tendon dysfunction, pain out of proportion to the presentation (owing to underlying joint infection), and a suspicious history.
- A closed rupture of the sagittal band should be suspected in patients who present with an inability to extend the finger after blunt trauma to the dorsum of the hand. This can be confirmed by passively placing the patient's digit in extension and observing whether the patient can actively maintain the position. If the patient can maintain the position, it indicates a rupture of the sagittal band; if the patient cannot maintain the position, it indicates an extensor tendon rupture (or a nerve palsy).

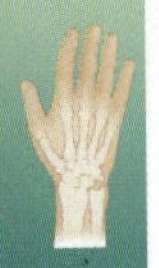

STEP 1 PEARLS

The joint is exposed and inspected by dividing the sagittal band and the joint capsule longitudinally on the lateral aspect of the extensor tendon when a human bite injury is suspected. A wound culture should be obtained before a thorough débridement and washout.

STEP 2 PEARLS

If a human bite injury is suspected, a tendon repair should not be carried out. The wounds should be left open over a drain and a delayed primary closure considered once the infection has been cleared.

- The ability to extend the MCP joint does not necessarily mean that the extensor tendon is in continuity. The patient may still be able to extend the finger using the adjacent extensor tendon via the juncturae tendineae.

Procedure

Step 1

- The skin flaps are mobilized to expose the divided tendon ends (Fig. 10-12A).

Step 2

- The MCP joint is put in full extension with a modified Kessler repair using a 4-0 Ethibond horizontal mattress core suture (Fig. 10-12B).

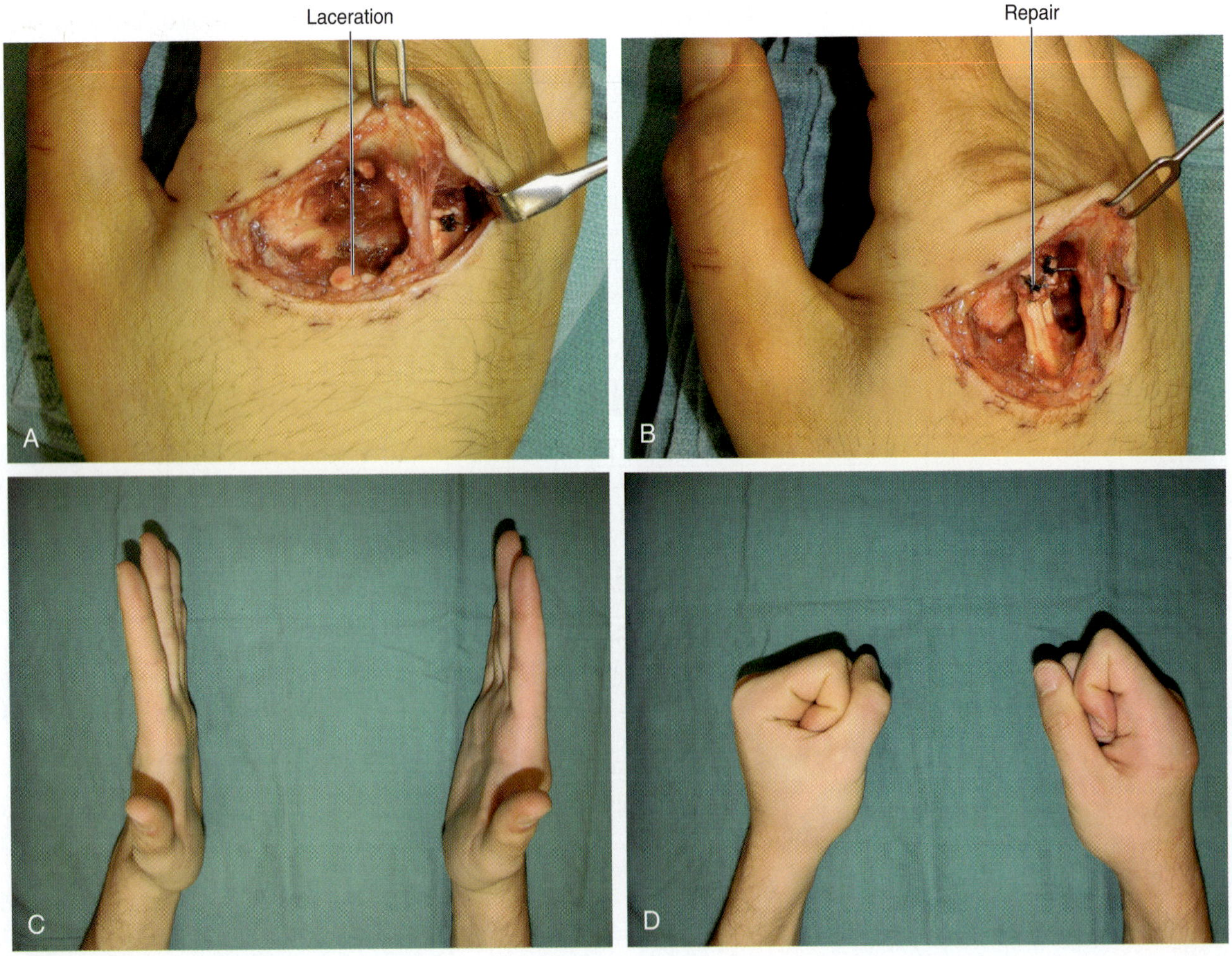

FIGURE 10-12

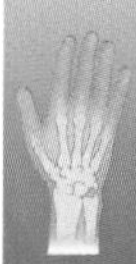

Step 3

- The tourniquet is released and hemostasis secured. Skin is closed with 5-0 nylon interrupted sutures.
- A splint to immobilize the wrist in slight extension and the MCP joint in full extension is provided. The PIP joint is left free.

Postoperative Care and Expected Outcomes

- Patients are started on a graduated therapy protocol 1 week after repair. The splint is maintained for 4 to 6 weeks (Fig. 10-12C and D).

Evidence

Newport ML, Blair WF, Steyers CM Jr. Long-term results of extensor tendon repair. *J Hand Surg [Am]*. 1990;15:961-966.

A retrospective analysis in 62 patients with 101 digits having extensor tendon injury was conducted. Sixty percent of all fingers sustained an associated injury (fracture, dislocation, joint capsule or flexor tendon damage). Patients without associated injuries achieved 64% good/excellent results and Total Active Motion of 212 degrees. Distal zones (1 to 4) had a significantly poorer result than more proximal zones (5 to 8). (Level IV evidence)

Woo SH, Tsai TM, Kleinert HE, et al. A biomechanical comparison of four extensor tendon repair techniques in zone IV. *Plast Reconstr Surg*. 2005;115:1674-1681.

Twelve fresh-frozen cadaver hand-forearm units (48 fingers) were randomly assigned to four suture repair treatments: the double figure-of-eight, the double modified Kessler, the six-strand double-loop, and the modified Becker suturing techniques. The modified Becker suture technique, although not easily performed, proved to be the strongest repair, with a significantly greater resistance to 1-mm and 2-mm gap and the greatest ultimate strength on maximal loading. (Level IV evidence)

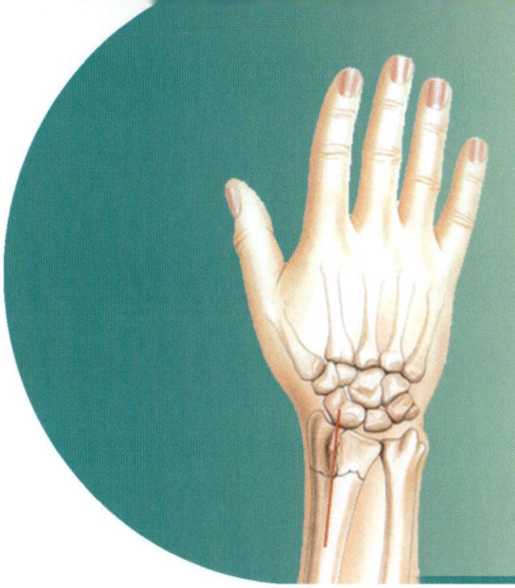

Section III

NERVE INJURY AND NERVE PALSY

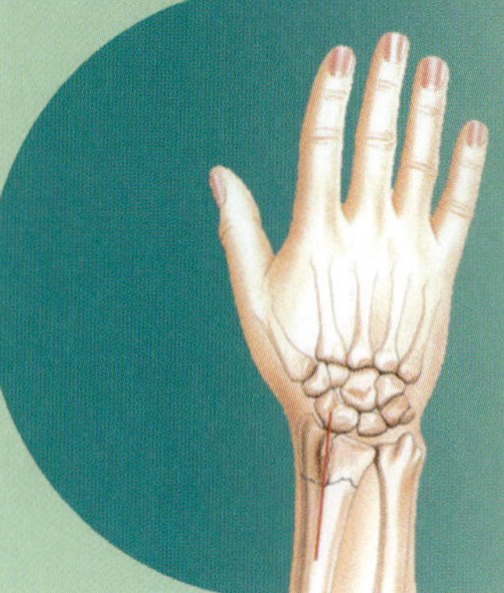

Endoscopic Carpal Tunnel Release

Shimpei Ono, Sandeep J. Sebastin, and Kevin C. Chung

Indications

- Failure of conservative treatment for idiopathic carpal tunnel syndrome (CTS).
- Patient prefers the endoscopic procedure.
- The authors' preferred technique is the limited incision open carpal tunnel release (LOCTR) (see Procedure 12). Studies have not demonstrated significant differences in outcomes between endoscopic carpal tunnel release (ECTR) and LOCTR. ECTR has a steep learning curve, needs a sizeable initial capital investment in video equipment, and incurs the recurring cost of the single-use disposable blade. Although the time taken to perform ECTR is less than for LOCTR, the time expended to set up the equipment mitigates this advantage.
- Occasionally, patients request the endoscopic procedure. They are counseled with regard to the cost and complications. We prefer the single-portal Agee technique to the double-portal Chow technique because the Agee technique avoids a scar in the palm.

Examination/Imaging

Clinical Examination

- The clinical examination for CTS is described in Procedure 12.
- It may be difficult to introduce the scope in patients with a very narrow wrist.

Imaging

- None required

Surgical Anatomy

- The carpal tunnel is a fibro-osseous tunnel that contains the median nerve and the nine flexor tendons to the thumb and the fingers. The roof of the carpal tunnel is formed by the flexor retinaculum, which extends between four bony prominences (proximally: pisiform and tubercle of scaphoid, distally: hook of the hamate and tubercle of trapezium) (Fig. 11-1).
- The flexor retinaculum can be divided into three components (see Fig. 11-1).
  - *Proximal:* Direct continuation of the deep antebrachial fascia
  - *Middle:* Transverse carpal ligament (TCL)
  - *Distal:* Aponeurosis between the thenar and hypothenar muscles
- Some authors consider the flexor retinaculum and the TCL to be synonymous.
- The carpal tunnel is narrowest in both palmar-dorsal and ulnar-radial planes at the level of the hook of the hamate. The other narrow portion of the carpal tunnel is at the proximal edge of the TCL (see Fig. 11-1).
- The important surface landmarks and surrounding neurovascular structures related to the carpal tunnel are as follows (Fig. 11-2):

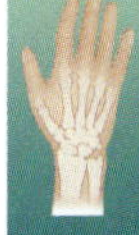

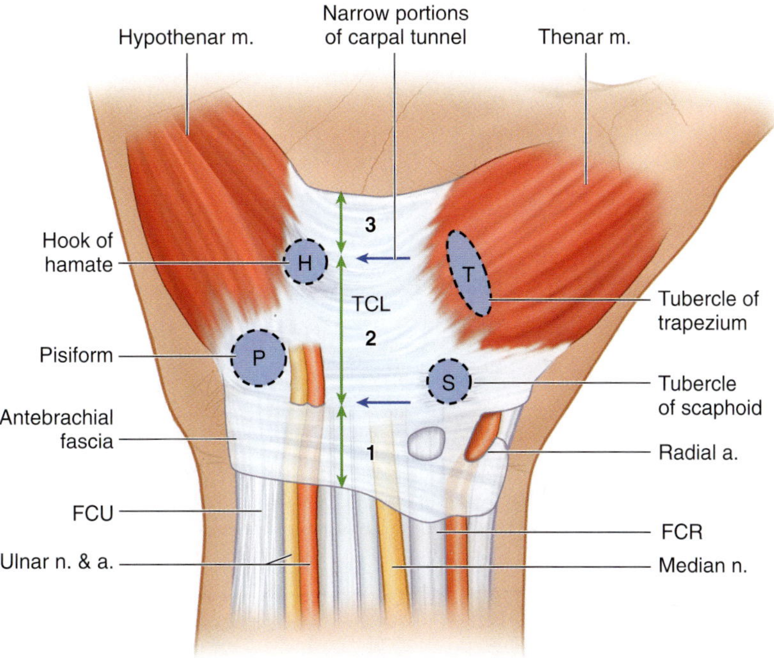

FIGURE 11-1

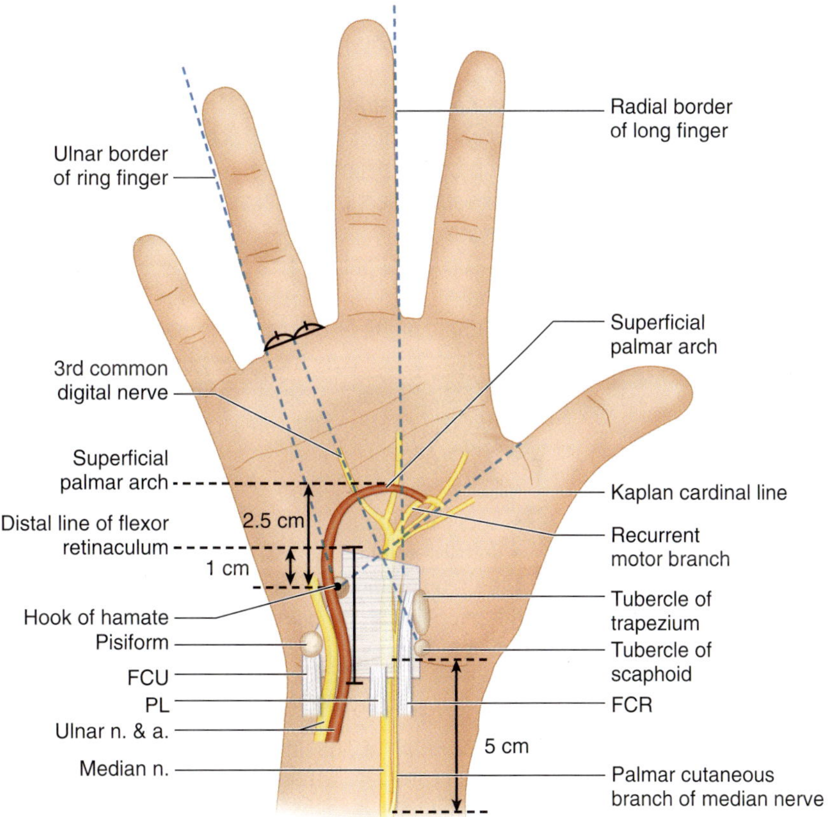

FIGURE 11-2

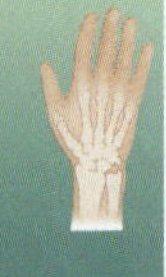

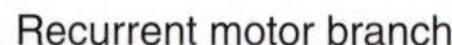

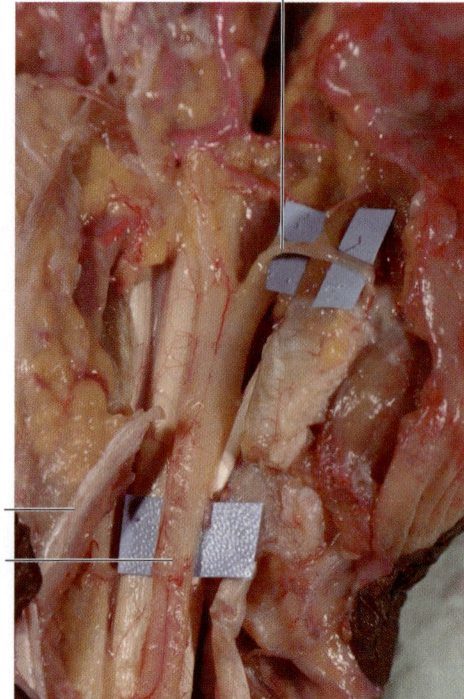

FIGURE 11-3

- The hook of the hamate is palpable 1 cm distal and radial to the pisiform and is in line with the ulnar border of the ring finger.
- The Kaplan cardinal line (KCL) connects the apex of the first web with the thumb in abduction to the hook of hamate. This line is usually parallel to the proximal palmar crease.
- The distal aspect of the flexor retinaculum lies 1 cm distal to the hook of the hamate.
- The superficial palmar arch (SPA) lies about 2.5 cm distal to the hook of the hamate.
- The origin of the recurrent motor branch is surface-marked at the intersection of a vertical line from the radial border of the long finger and KCL. The recurrent motor branch arises from the palmar and ulnar aspect of the median nerve (Fig. 11-3), and three courses of this branch have been described (Fig. 11-4).
  - Extraligamentous (46%)
  - Subligamentous (31%)
  - Transligamentous (23%)
- The third common digital nerve is surface-marked by an oblique line joining the midpoint of the palmar digital crease of the ring finger to the scaphoid tubercle. This nerve is always located distal to the KCL at an average distance of 0.5 cm.
- The palmar cutaneous branch of the median nerve arises from the radial aspect of the median nerve about 5 cm proximal to the wrist crease (see Fig. 11-2). It runs parallel to the median nerve for 1.6 to 2.5 cm and then passes under the antebrachial fascia between the palmaris longus (PL) and the flexor carpi radialis (FCR). About 0.8 cm proximal to the wrist crease, it pierces the antebrachial fascia, becoming superficial to the flexor retinaculum.

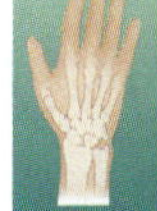

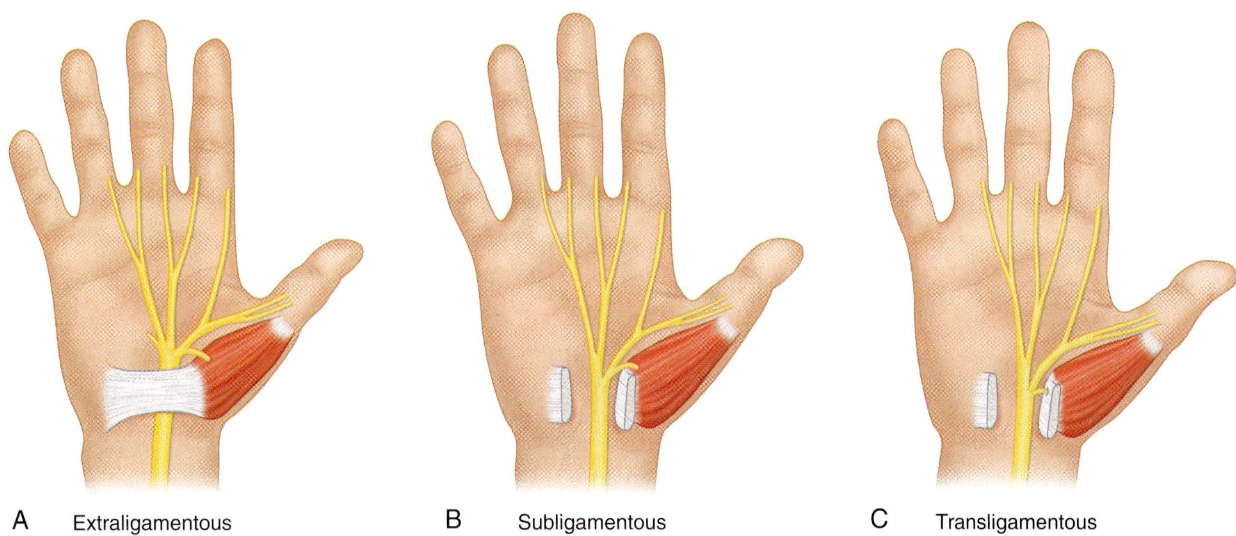

FIGURE 11-4

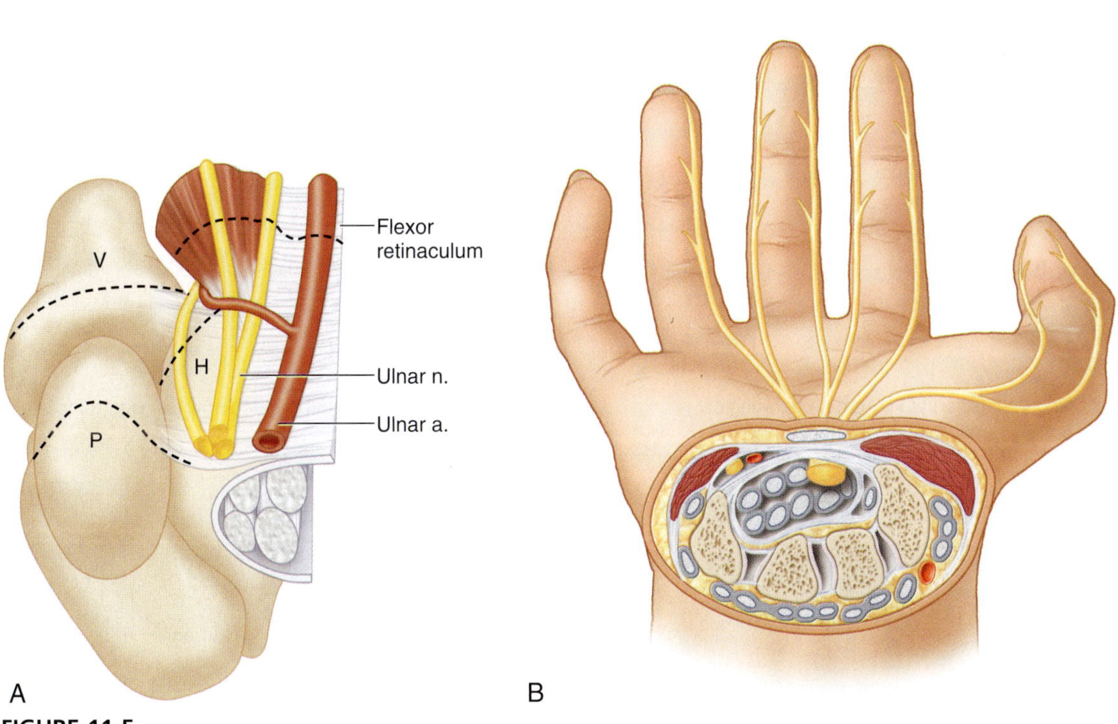

FIGURE 11-5

> **PEARLS**
>
> *The infiltration of local anesthetic within the carpal tunnel can obscure endoscopic viewing and cause fogging of the lens. Care should be taken to infiltrate only the skin and to block the median nerve in the distal forearm rather than under the carpal tunnel.*

- The ulnar nerve and artery overlie the ulnar border of the flexor retinaculum and may be at risk during ECTR. The nerve is generally anterior or ulnar to the hook of the hamate, but the artery is often immediately superficial to the flexor retinaculum lying within a fat-filled space (Fig. 11-5).

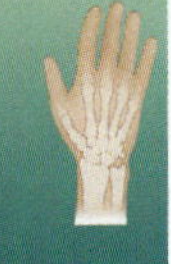

Positioning

- The procedure is performed under tourniquet control with the patient in supine position and the affected extremity on a hand table. The positioning of surgeon, patient, and anesthesiologist is shown in Figure 11-6.
- It can be done under general regional anesthesia, intravenous regional (Bier block) anesthesia, or local anesthesia.

Positioning for right-handed surgeon operating on patient's right hand.

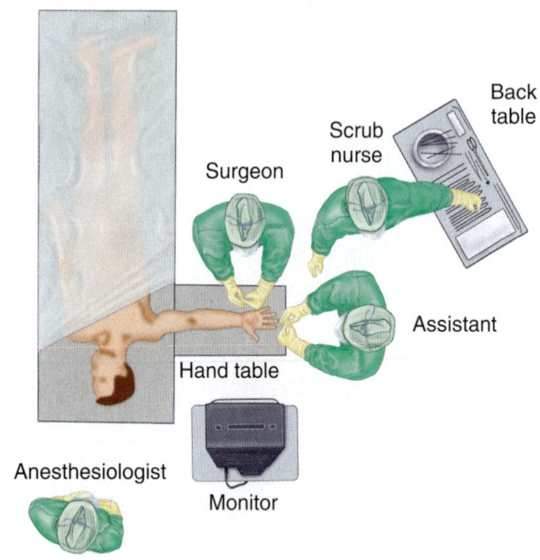

Positioning for right-handed surgeon operating on patient's left hand.

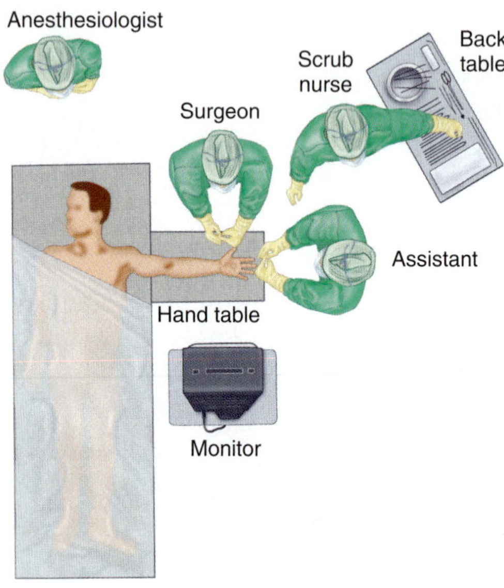

Positioning for left-handed surgeon operating on patient's right hand.

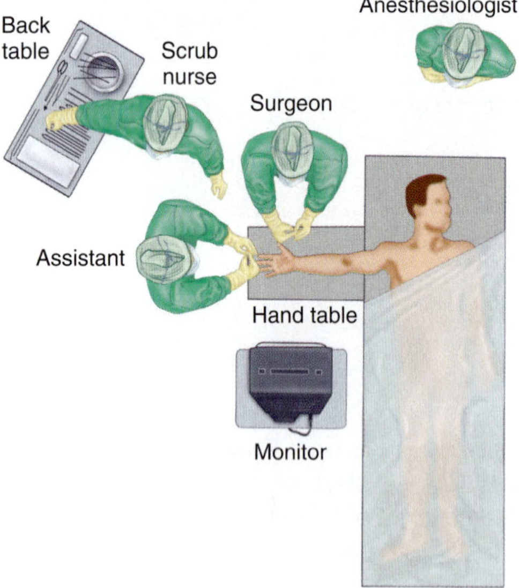

Positioning for left-handed surgeon operating on patient's left hand.

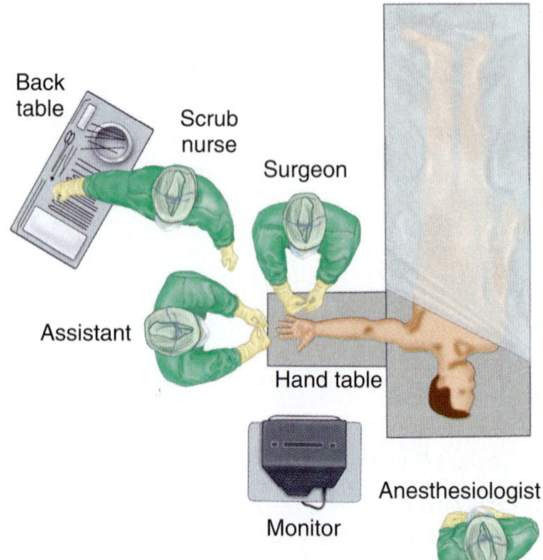

FIGURE 11-6

PEARLS

If more than one wrist flexion crease exists, the most proximal crease is selected because there is less subcutaneous fat.

PITFALLS

Care should be taken not to injure the palmar cutaneous branch of the median nerve and the palmar cutaneous branch of the ulnar nerve.

The median nerve is directly below this flap, so care must be taken during the initial flap incision and elevation, especially in patients who do not have a PL tendon.

Exposures

- We use the 3M Agee Carpal Tunnel Release System for ECTR (Fig. 11-7).
- A 1- to 1.5-cm transverse skin incision is made over the proximal wrist crease, ulnar to the PL tendon and radial to the flexor carpi ulnaris (FCU) tendon (Figs. 11-8 and 11-9).

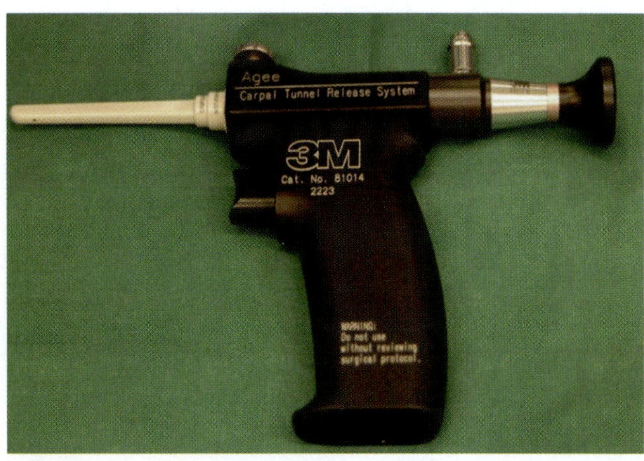

FIGURE 11-7

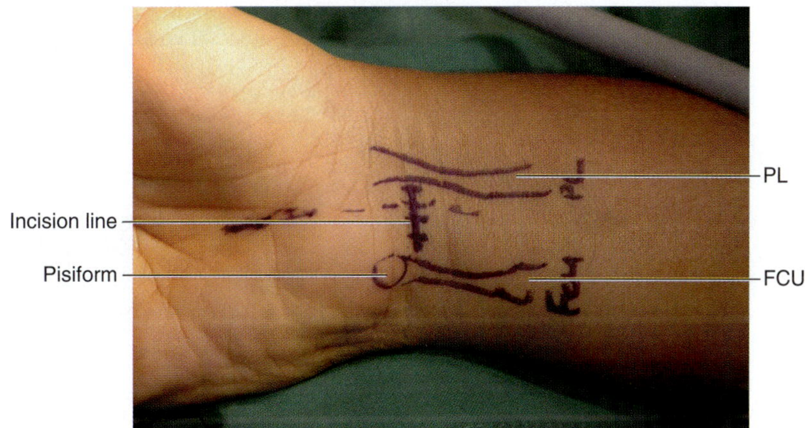

FIGURE 11-8

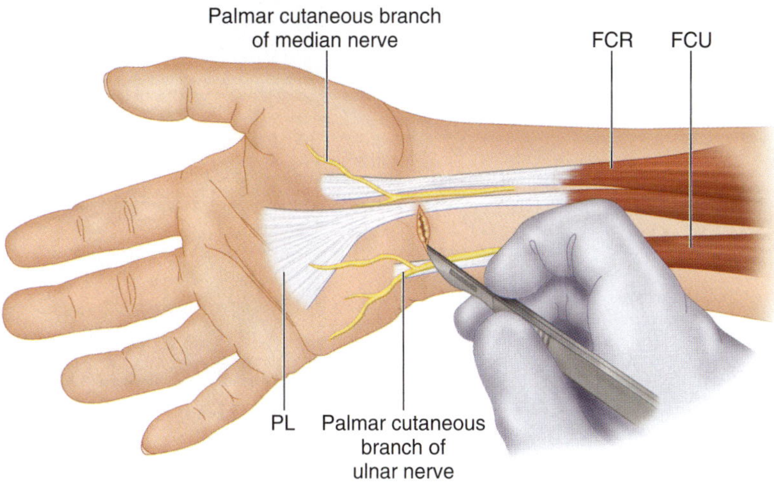

FIGURE 11-9

- Once the incision is made, the underlying loose tissue is dissected by spreading longitudinally to identify and preserve any palmar cutaneous nerves.
- The antebrachial fascia is exposed, and a U-shaped, distally based fascial flap is raised (Fig. 11-10). Elevation of the flap ensures that the endoscope enters the right plane deep to the fascia and not superficial to it.
- The fascial flap is held up using a hemostat to expose the underlying median nerve (Fig. 11-11).

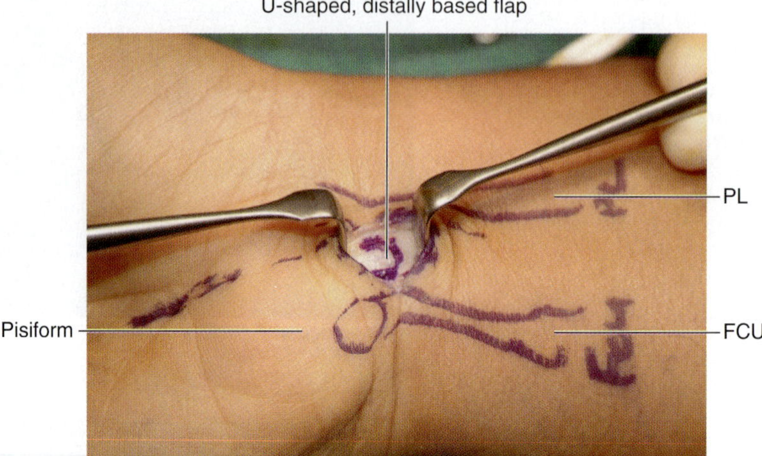

FIGURE 11-10

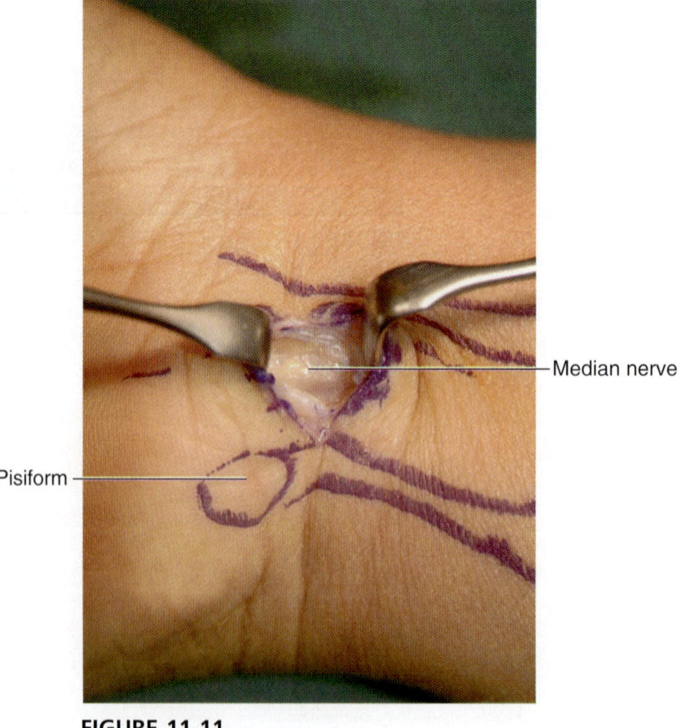

FIGURE 11-11

STEP 1 PITFALLS

Care is taken not to injure the palmar cutaneous branch of the median nerve, which is located on the radial aspect of the PL.

STEP 2 PEARLS

It is good to mark the most proximal point where the tip of the probe can be palpated subcutaneously. This indicates the end of the TCL and provides a visual clue to how far the blade assembly can be advanced safely.

Procedure

Step 1: Release the Forearm Fascia

- Using tenotomy scissors, the antebrachial fascia is released proximally for 1 to 2 cm (Fig. 11-12).

Step 2: Dilate the Carpal Tunnel

- The smallest probe (hamate finder) is inserted under the previously elevated fascial flap. The wrist is held in slight extension, and the probe is gradually advanced in line with the ring finger. The tip of the probe is automatically directed radially by the hamate and should be palpable subcutaneously as it exits the distal free edge of the TCL. The probe is then removed.
- The next-sized probe is inserted (Fig. 11-13), and finally the largest probe is inserted (Fig. 11-14). These probes function both as dilator and to confirm that the probe is within the carpal tunnel and not the Guyon canal.

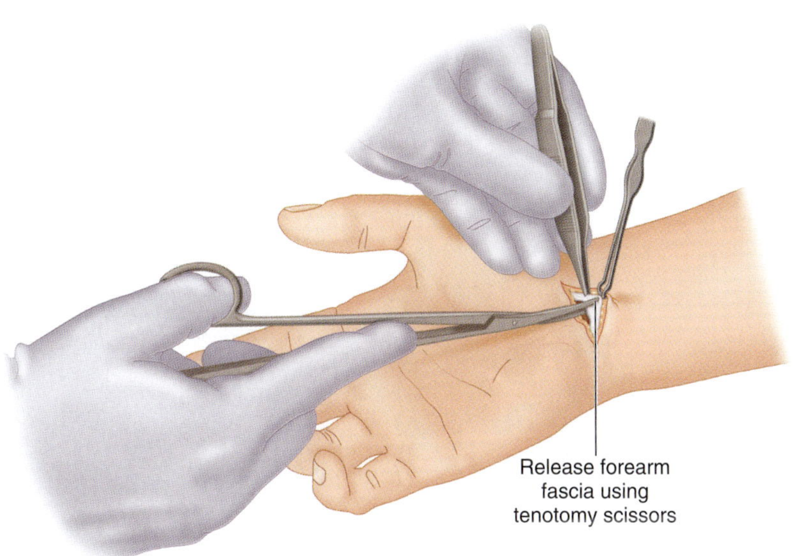

FIGURE 11-12

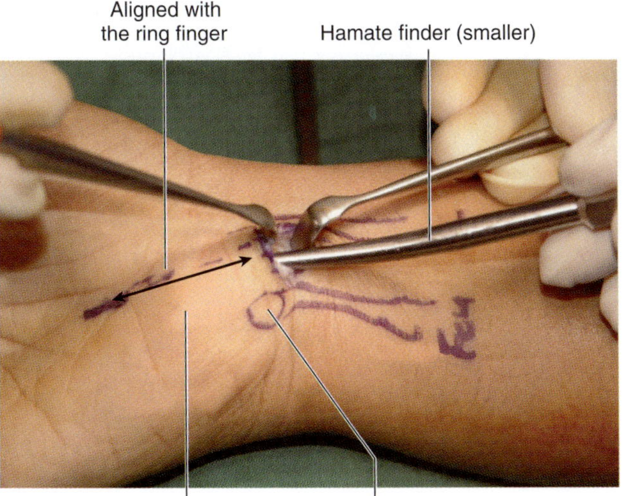

FIGURE 11-13

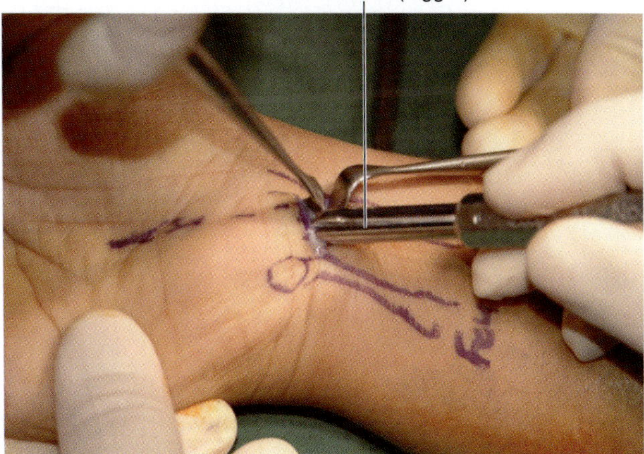

FIGURE 11-14

Step 3: Clear the Synovium

- The synovial separator is then passed into the dilated carpal tunnel. The synovial separator is used to sweep any adherent synovial membranes off the undersurface of the TCL. Adequate clearing of the synovial membrane is indicated by the roughness ("washboard effect") of the transverse fibers of the TCL.

Step 4: Introducing the Blade Assembly into the Carpal Tunnel

- The wrist is placed in slight extension, and the blade assembly is inserted (Figs. 11-15 and 11-16) with the viewing window and blade facing anteriorly (toward the inner aspect of the TCL) (Fig. 11-17).

STEP 4 PEARLS

The device is inserted to a depth of less than 3 cm to avoid injury to the superficial palmar arch or the common digital nerve.

In patients with a narrow carpal tunnel, it may be difficult to insert the blade assembly even after adequate dilation. It is safer in such cases to convert to an open procedure.

STEP 4 PITFALLS

The blade must be kept in a retracted position at all times during insertion of the blade assembly.

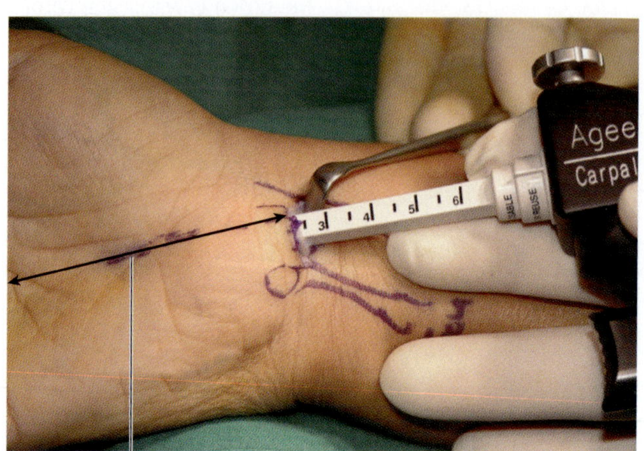

FIGURE 11-15

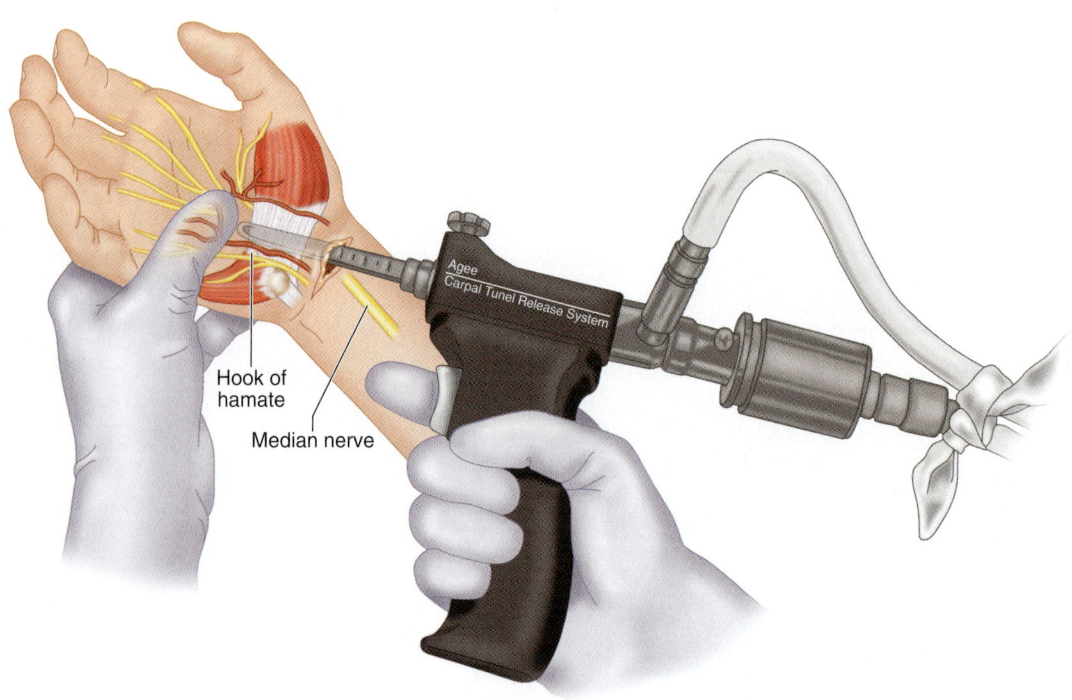

FIGURE 11-16

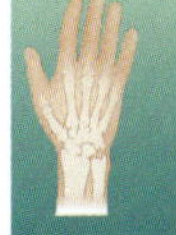

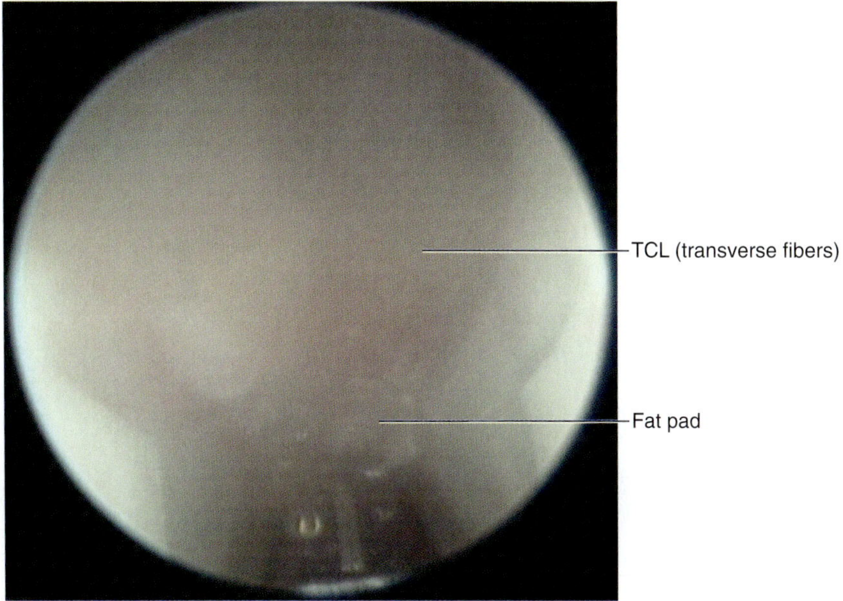

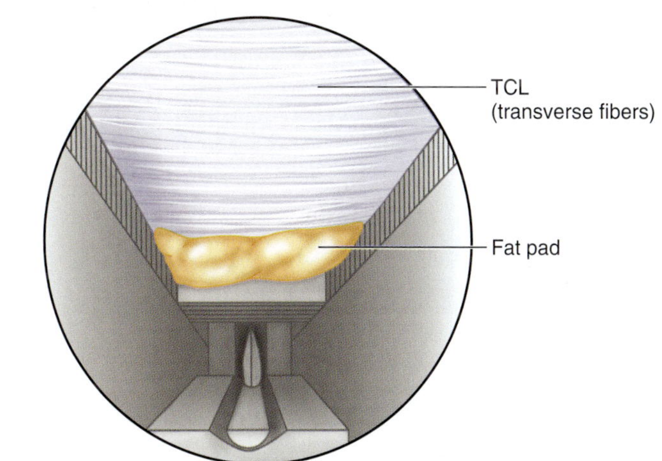

FIGURE 11-17

Step 5: Identifying the Distal End of the TCL

- The following cues can be used to correctly identify the distal end of the TCL:
  - A bundle of fat seen immediately distal to the TCL
  - The loss of the normal transversely running fibers of the TCL
  - The point marked previously using the hamate finder
- The end of the TCL is indicated by transillumination by the light source. Transillumination only occurs distal to the TCL.

STEP 5 PEARLS

If the TCL and its distal free end cannot be clearly defined (because of synovium, flexor tendons, or fogging of endoscope lens), it is safer to convert to an open procedure.

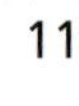

Step 6: Incise the TCL

- Once the distal end of the TCL has been identified, the blade is elevated (Fig. 11-18), and slight pressure is applied on the palmar aspect of the carpal tunnel. The blade is then gradually withdrawn under visual guidance on the monitor to divide the TCL (Fig. 11-19).
- The blade assembly is reinserted (with the blade retracted), and the TCL is inspected to ensure that it has been completely divided. Occasionally, one or two additional passes may be required to complete the cut.
- After division of the ligament, fat will be seen herniating down into the field of vision (Fig. 11-20).

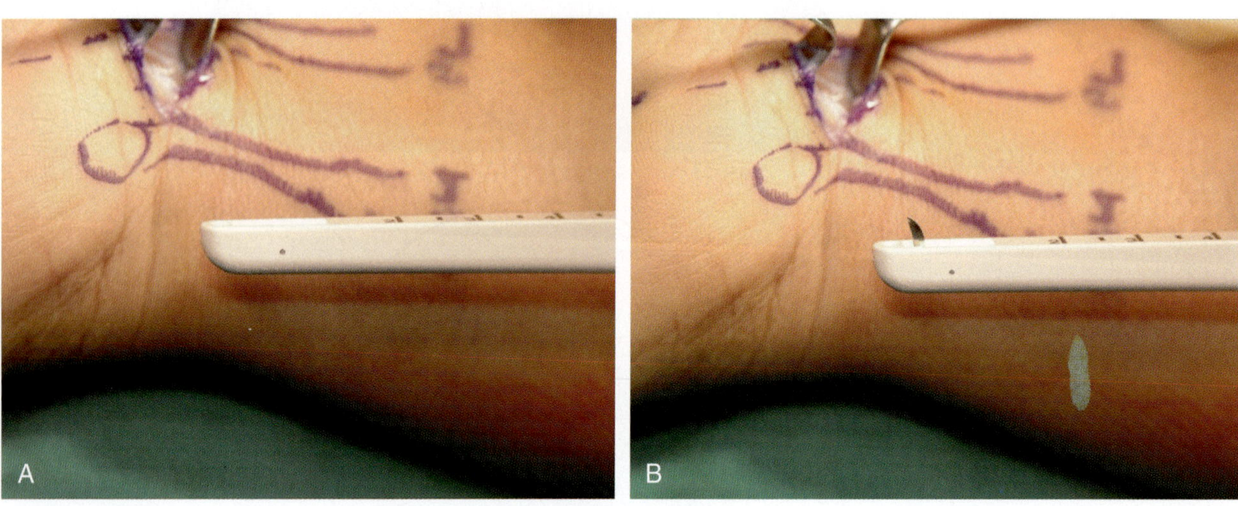

FIGURE 11-18

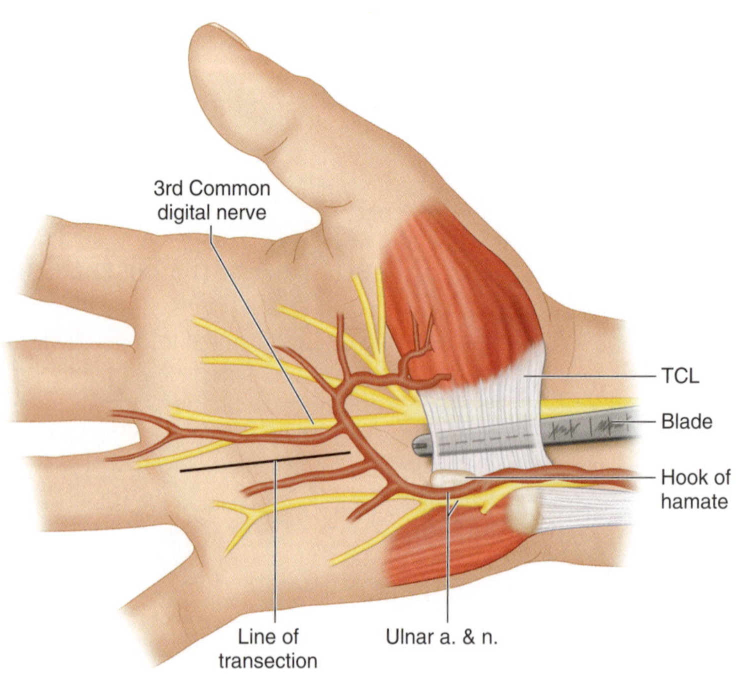

FIGURE 11-19

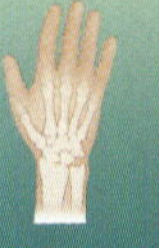

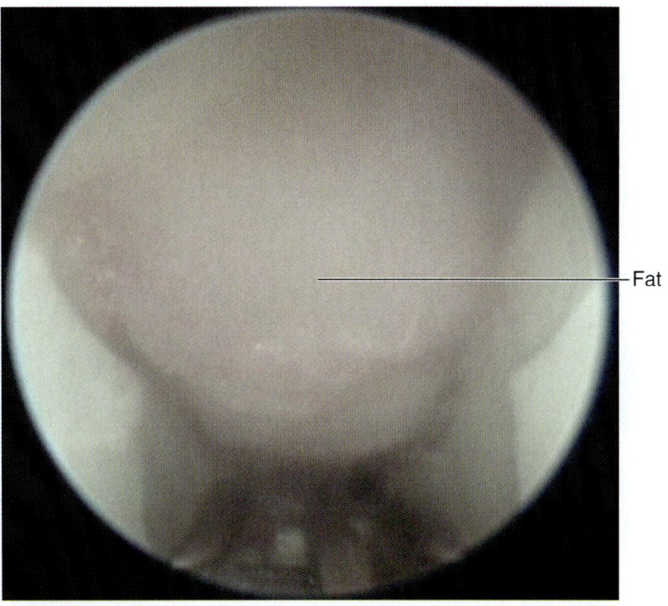

FIGURE 11-20

STEP 6 PEARLS

The presence of a V-shaped cut on the TCL or transverse fibers suggests an incomplete release of the TCL (Fig. 11-21).

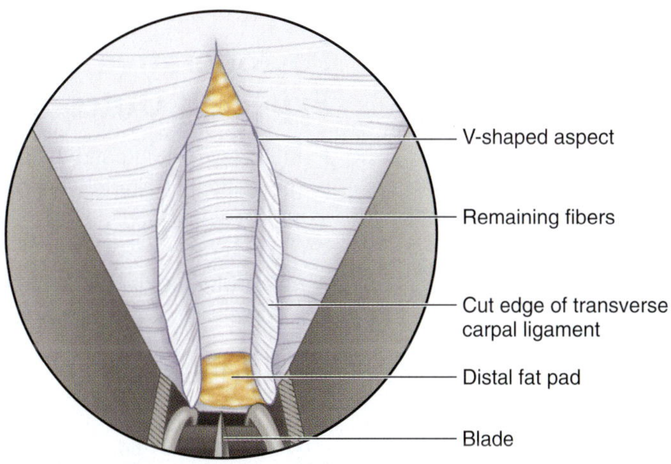

FIGURE 11-21

STEP 6 PITFALLS

The blade assembly must not be inserted beyond the distal edge of the TCL to prevent inadvertent injury to the superficial palmar arterial arch and/or the common digital nerve.

Once the blade is elevated, the assembly must always be withdrawn in a distal to proximal direction. The assembly should never be passed in a proximal to distal direction with the blade elevated. This is especially important when inspecting the TCL for completeness of the division and when additional passes are made to divide an incomplete TCL.

The blade assembly should be withdrawn gently and the blade retracted when nearing the entrance incision to avoid cutting skin.

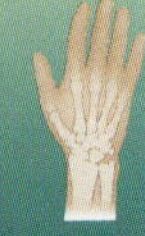

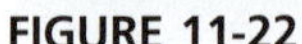

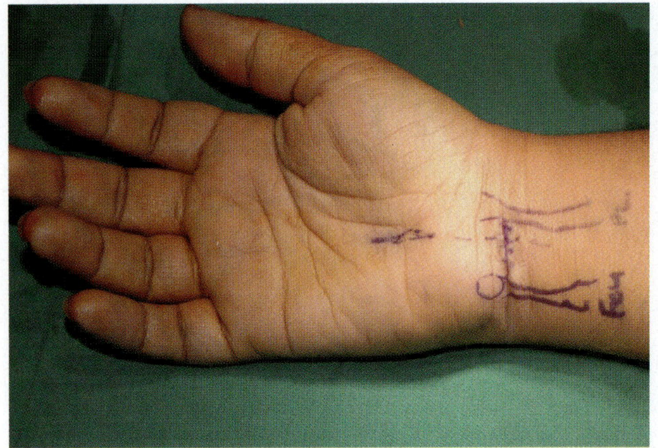

FIGURE 11-22

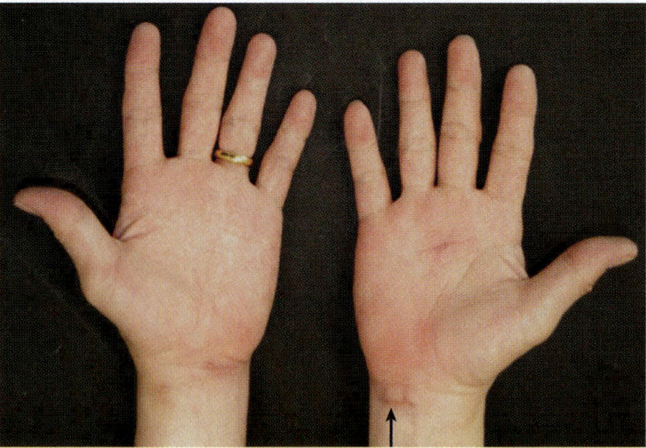

FIGURE 11-23

Step 7: Closure

- The skin incision is closed using 5-0 Monocryl subcuticular suture (Fig. 11-22).
- The hand is wrapped in a bulky compression dressing, and a volar wrist splint is applied.
- Finally, the tourniquet is released.

Postoperative Care and Expected Outcomes

- The bulky dressing and the splint are removed 2 days after surgery.
- The patient is started on range-of-motion and nerve-gliding exercises. The patient is allowed to return to normal activities 3 to 4 weeks after surgery (Fig. 11-23).
- About 95% to 100% of patients obtain relief of their symptoms after ECTR. A complication rate of 1% to 3% has been reported in the literature.

Evidence

Beck JD, Deegan JH, Rhoades D, Klena JC. Results of endoscopic carpal tunnel release relative to surgeon experience with the Agee technique. *J Hand Surg [Am]*. 2011;36:61-64.

A total of 278 patients (358 procedures) underwent ECTR. Twelve patients required conversion to OCTR over a 2-year period. In the first 6 months of practice, 8 of 71 ECTRs were converted to OCTR compared with 1 of 72 in the second 6 months. In year 2, 3 of 215 patients were converted to OCTR. A learning curve for ECTR was present, and the rates of conversion significantly diminished with increased surgeon and anesthesia experience. No patients required repeat surgery for recurrence of carpal tunnel symptoms. The authors reported no major neurovascular complications. (Level IV evidence)

Schmelzer RE, Della Rocca GJ, Caplin DA. Endoscopic carpal tunnel release: a review of 753 cases in 486 patients. *Plast Reconstr Surg*. 2006;117:177-185.

The authors evaluated outcomes of ECTR in a large patient cohort (486 patients, 753 hands). Data included demographics, subjective complaints, prior interventions, preoperative examination findings, and postoperative follow-up. All follow-up data were obtained from a single, independent occupational therapy clinic. Three hundred seventy-seven patients were gainfully employed at presentation, and 206 filed a workers' compensation claim. Four hundred eighty-six patients (100%) obtained symptom relief. Complications included 1 transient median nerve neurapraxia, 6 complaints of residual pain, and 1 complaint of hypersensitivity. Workers' compensation patients and non–workers' compensation patients returned to work full-duty at similar times postoperatively. Ninety percent of employed patients returned to their original occupation. They concluded that ECTR was safe and effective. Patients demonstrated a high return-to-work rate and an extremely low complication rate. The data challenged the belief that endoscopic carpal tunnel release results in higher complication rates. (Level IV evidence)

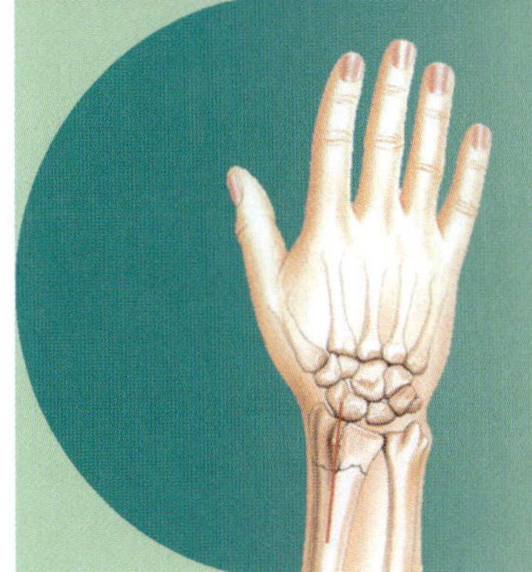

PROCEDURE 12

Open Carpal Tunnel Release

Douglas Sammer

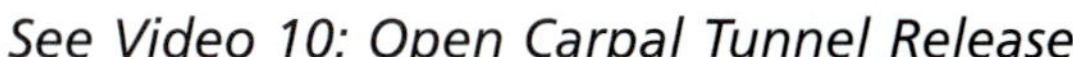

See Video 10: Open Carpal Tunnel Release

Indications

- Diagnosis of carpal tunnel syndrome with one of the following:
  - Mild symptoms unresponsive to conservative management (6 to 12 weeks of nocturnal use of neutral wrist splint)
  - Substantial symptoms, with or without trial of conservative management (continuous symptoms, two-point discrimination changes, or thenar weakness or atrophy)
  - Prolonged duration of symptoms (≥6 months), with or without trial of conservative management

Examination/Imaging

Clinical Examination

- *Phalen test* (Fig. 12-1): The patient's wrist is held in a flexed position for up to 1 minute or until onset of symptoms. A positive test consists of the onset of numbness or paraesthesia in the median nerve distribution. Care must be taken to avoid direct pressure or flexion at the elbow when performing this examination, in order to avoid inducing ulnar nerve symptoms.
- *Carpal tunnel compression test* (Fig. 12-2): The examiner applies direct pressure to the carpal tunnel with his or her thumb for up to 1 minute or until onset of symptoms. A positive test consists of the onset of numbness or paresthesia in the median nerve distribution. As with Phalen test, care is taken to avoid direct pressure or flexion at the elbow when performing this examination.
- *Tinel sign* (Fig. 12-3): The examiner taps directly over the carpal tunnel with his or her long and index fingers. A positive test consists of paresthesia or pain in a median nerve distribution.
- *Two-point discrimination* (tests innervation density; abnormal test is a late finding)
- *Semmes-Weinstein monofilament test* (tests pressure threshold; more sensitive)

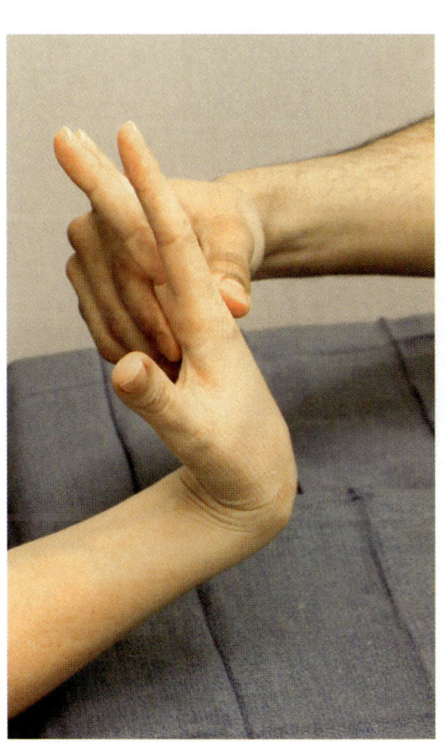

FIGURE 12-1

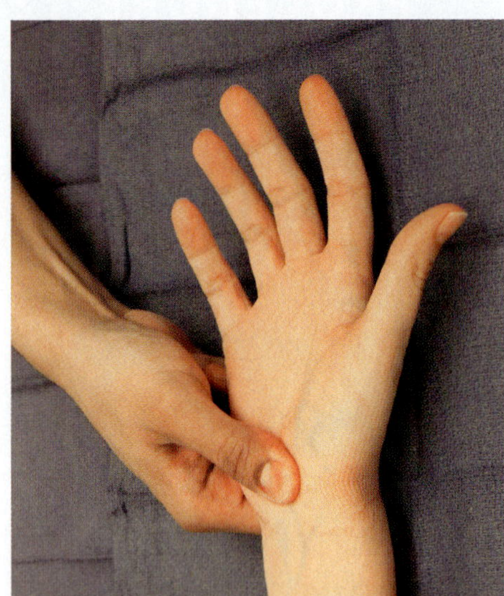

FIGURE 12-2

Imaging/Diagnostic Studies

- Three-view radiographs of the wrist (posteroanterior, lateral, oblique) plus carpal tunnel view: obtained when there is antecedent wrist trauma that may narrow the carpal tunnel. Otherwise, routine wrist x-rays are unnecessary.
- Nerve conduction studies (NCS) and electromyelogram (EMG)
  - Increased distal median nerve sensory latency (>3.5 msec)
  - Increased distal median nerve motor latency (>4.5 msec)
  - Decreased conduction velocity (demyelination) or amplitude (axonal loss)
  - Denervation of thenar muscles on EMG (fibrillation potentials, sharp waves, increased insertional activity)

Surgical Anatomy

- The superficial palmar fascia is a fanlike palmar fascial extension into which the palmaris longus inserts.
- The palmar cutaneous branch of the median nerve (PCN) lies between the flexor carpi radialis and palmaris longus tendons in the distal forearm, but its branches may be found up to 6 mm ulnar to the thenar crease in the palm (Fig. 12-4).
- The transverse carpal ligament (flexor retinaculum) forms the roof of the carpal tunnel.
- The walls of the carpal tunnel are formed by the hamate and triquetrum ulnarly and the scaphoid and trapezium radially.

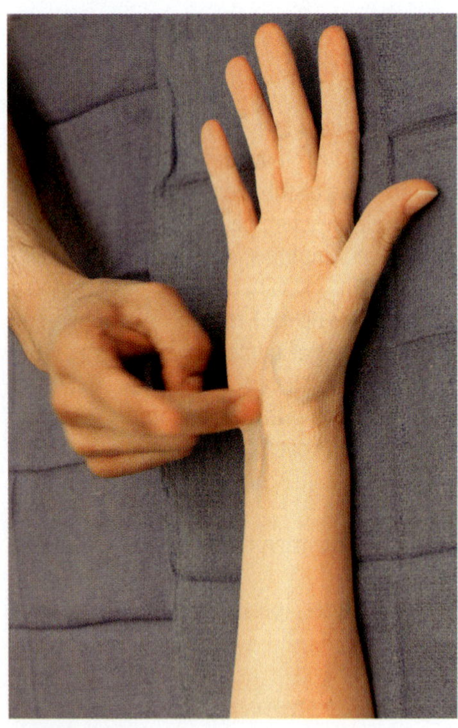

FIGURE 12-3

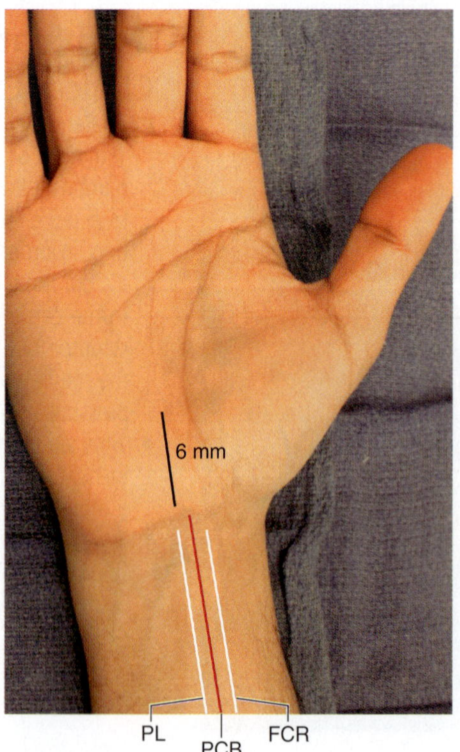

FIGURE 12-4

PEARLS

It is important to keep the incision at least 6 mm ulnar to the thenar crease to prevent injury to the PCN.

The incision should lie ulnar to the longitudinal course of the palmaris longus tendon.

PITFALLS

If the incision is made too ulnar in an effort to avoid the PCN, the dissection becomes more difficult owing to increased palmar fat (hypothenar fat) and the presence of the ulnar neurovascular bundle.

- Nine tendons (four flexor digitorum profundus [FDP] tendons, four flexor digitorum superficialis [FDS] tendons, one flexor pollicis longus [FPL] tendon) travel within the carpal tunnel, along with the median nerve.
- The median nerve lies in the volar and radial quadrant of the carpal tunnel.
- The recurrent motor branch typically arises from the volar-radial aspect of the median nerve at the distal end of the transverse carpal ligament and turns proximally and radially to innervate the thenar muscles. Multiple variations may exist, including a transligamentous course (recurrent motor branch pierces transverse carpal ligament), subligamentous origin, multiple recurrent motor branches, origin of recurrent motor branch from ulnar side of median nerve, recurrent motor branch anterior to transverse carpal ligament, absence of recurrent motor branch (ulnar nerve supplies thenar muscles), and others. Overall, the incidence of an anomalous course is 19%, with a transligamentous recurrent motor branch being the most common anomalous variation.

Exposures

- A 2.5- to 3-cm longitudinal incision is made in the proximal palm.
- The incision does not cross the distal wrist flexion crease.
- The incision should be placed 6 mm ulnar to the thenar crease (Fig. 12-5).

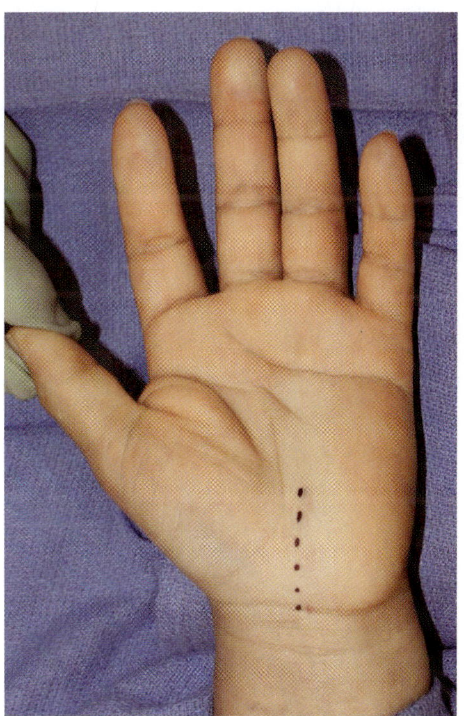

FIGURE 12-5

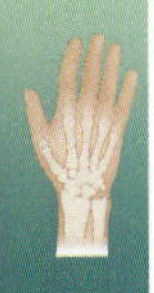

STEP 1 PEARLS

Retraction with skin hooks or blunt Senn retractors aids in dissection through the palmar fat.

Procedure

Step 1

- The incision is made as described earlier (see Fig. 12-5).
- Double skin hooks are used to retract the skin (Fig. 12-6).
- A no. 15 blade is used to incise down to the superficial palmar fascia, which has longitudinal fibers (Fig. 12-7).
- A blunt self-retaining retractor is placed for radial and ulnar retraction, and blunt Senn retractors are used for distal and proximal retraction.

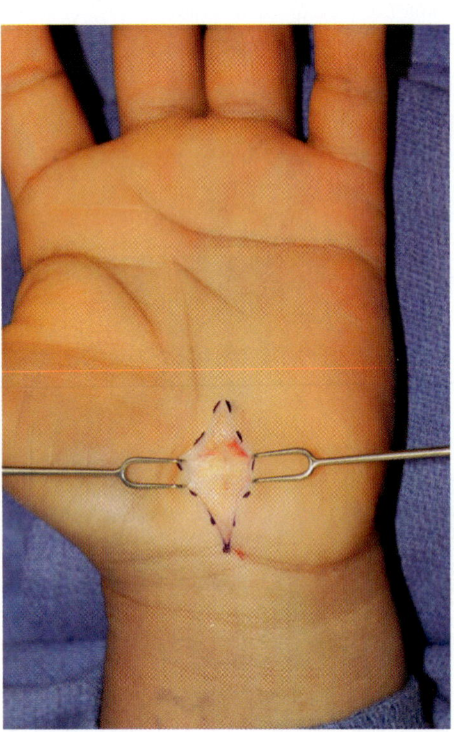

FIGURE 12-6

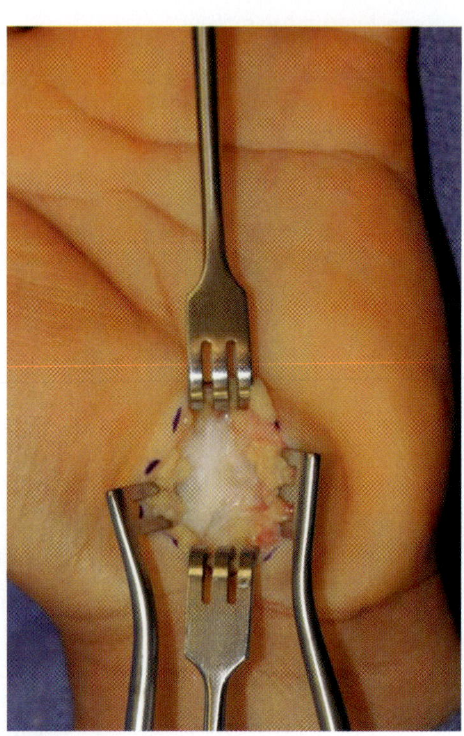

FIGURE 12-7

Step 2

- The superficial palmar fascia is divided longitudinally with a no. 15 blade.
- The transverse carpal ligament is exposed and cleared off with a sponge (Fig. 12-8).

Step 3

- The hook of the hamate is palpated.
- The transverse carpal ligament is divided longitudinally with a no. 15 blade, just radial to the hook of the hamate (Fig. 12-9).

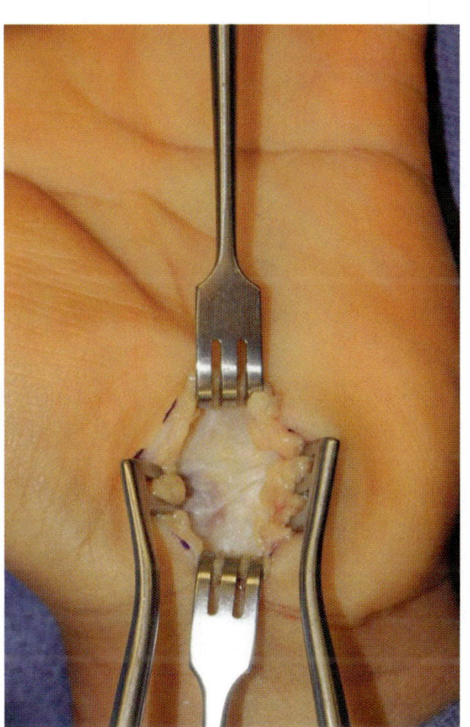

FIGURE 12-8

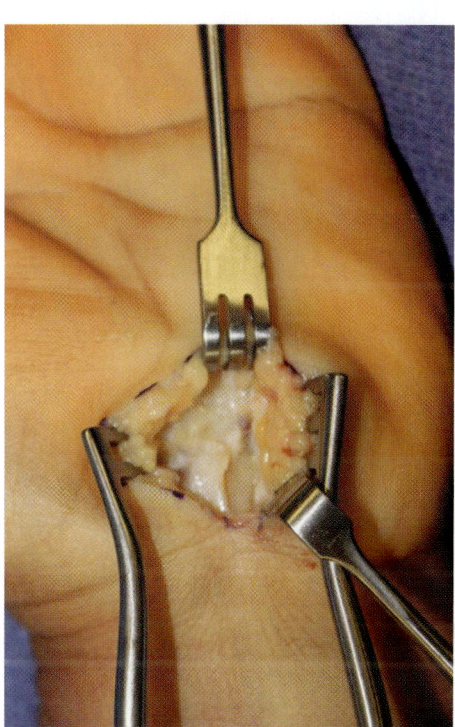

FIGURE 12-9

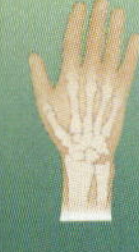

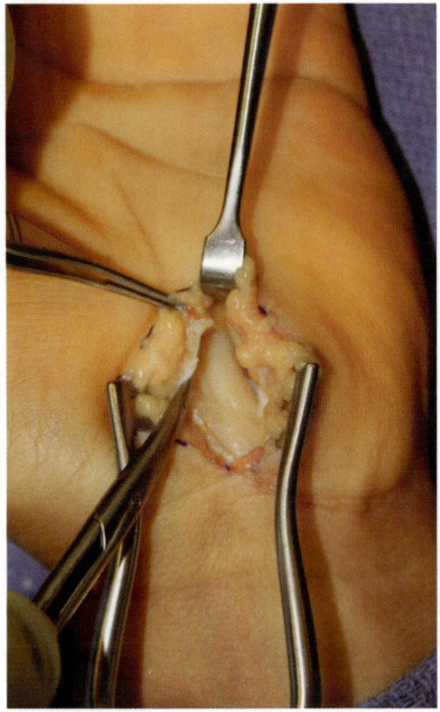

FIGURE 12-10

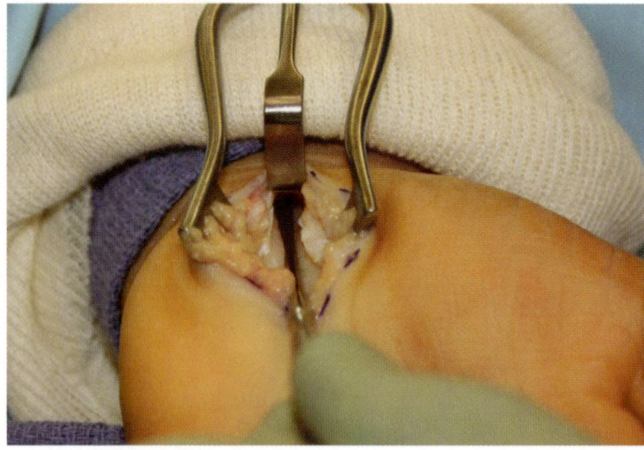

FIGURE 12-11

STEP 4 PEARLS

The presence of perivascular fat indicates proximity to the superficial palmar arch and the distal end of the release.

The surgeon's small finger can be passed distally into the palm; if the release is complete, it should pass easily. Alternatively, the close end of the scissors can be inserted into the wound and, with a pullback motion, can define whether there is residual ligament that has not been divided.

STEP 5 PEARLS

Care is taken not to veer radially or ulnarly, to prevent injury to important structures (PCN and ulnar neurovascular bundle, respectively).

The surgeon's small finger can be passed proximally into the distal forearm.

If tight bands are present, antebrachial fascia may be divided with scissors.

It is important to do this under direct visualization, as opposed to blindly advancing the scissors.

Synovectomy and neurolysis are not necessary unless specifically indicated (e.g., synovectomy in rheumatoid arthritis).

Step 4

- Tenotomy scissors are used to spread distally, just superficial to the transverse carpal ligament.
- Under direct visualization, the distal release is completed with scissors (Fig. 12-10).

Step 5

- Tenotomy scissors are used to spread on top of the ligament proximally.
- A freer elevator is placed under the ligament, and the contents of the carpal tunnel are pressed down and away from the ligament.
- The proximal release is completed under direct visualization with scissors (Fig. 12-11).

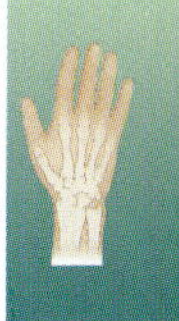

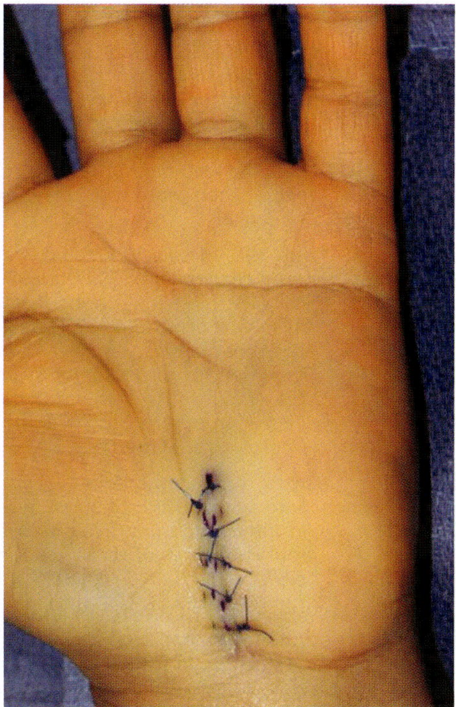

FIGURE 12-12

Step 6

- The skin is closed with 4-0 horizontal mattress Prolene sutures (Fig. 12-12).
- A soft bulky dressing is applied.
- Splinting is unnecessary.

Postoperative Care and Expected Outcomes

- Elevation and finger motion are encouraged.
- Light activity is encouraged when comfortable.
- The dressing can be removed in 3 to 4 days, and handwashing is encouraged.
- Lifting is limited to 5 lb for 6 weeks.
- At 6 weeks the patient can gradually resume full activity.
- With mild and/or intermittent symptoms, relief is often immediate.
- With prolonged or severe symptoms (two-point discrimination changes, thenar weakness), relief of symptoms may occur over many months, and the patient may not experience complete improvement.

Evidence

Freshwater MF, Arons MS. The effect of various adjuncts on the surgical treatment of carpal tunnel syndrome secondary to chronic tenosynovitis. *Plast Reconstr Surg*. 1978;61:93-96.

This classic study demonstrates that routine flexor synovectomy and external neurolysis are unnecessary in patients undergoing carpal tunnel release. In fact, patients who did not receive adjunctive procedures were able to return to work earlier than those who underwent synovectomy and neurolysis. (Level IV evidence)

Keith MW, Masear V, Amadio P, et al. Treatment of carpal tunnel syndrome. *J Am Acad Orthop Surg*. 2009;17:297-405.

Keith MW, Masear V, Chung K, et al. Diagnosis of carpal tunnel syndrome. *J Am Acad Orthop Surg*. 2009;17:389-396.

These two articles represent clinical practice guidelines for the diagnosis and treatment of carpal tunnel syndrome. These guidelines were developed by the American Academy of Orthopaedic Surgeons and subsequently endorsed by the American Association of Neurological Surgeons and the Congress of Neurological Surgeons.

Lanz U. Anatomical variations in the median nerve in the carpal tunnel. *J Hand Surg [Am]*. 1977;2:44-53.

In this classic study, 246 cadaveric hands were examined. The study describes four categories of variations in the anatomy of the median nerve. (Level V evidence)

Watchmaker GP, Weber D, Mackinnon SE. Avoidance of transaction of the palmar cutaneous branch of the median nerve in carpal tunnel release. *J Hand Surg [Am]*. 1996;21:644-650.

This is an excellent anatomic study of the course of the palmar cutaneous branch of the median nerve within the palm and its relationship to proposed carpal tunnel release incisions. (Level V evidence)

PROCEDURE 13

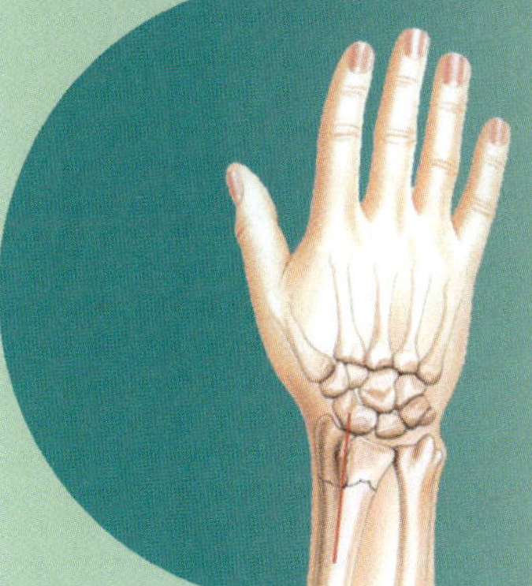

In Situ Cubital Tunnel Decompression

Pao-Yuan Lin, Sandeep J. Sebastin, and Kevin C. Chung

See Video 11: In Situ Cubital Tunnel Decompression

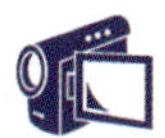

Indications

- In situ decompression of the ulnar nerve is indicated for patients with symptoms that are mild or intermittent (Table 13-1). If there is subluxation or instability of the ulnar nerve and/or ulnar nerve palsy owing to an abnormal osseous architecture of the elbow, in situ decompression is not indicated. In these situations, an anterior transposition is more appropriate to correct the anatomic problem.

Examination/Imaging

Clinical Examination

- *Palpation:* The ulnar nerve is palpated to check for enlargement or subluxation.
- The elbow joint is checked for range of motion.
- Check Tinel sign from the distal forearm to above the elbow along the course of the ulnar nerve. In cubital tunnel syndrome, Tinel sign is present at the medial epicondylar groove or over the proximal end of the flexor carpi ulnaris (FCU) muscle.
- A provocative test for ulnar nerve subluxation is performed by placing the elbow in full flexion with the wrist hyperextended, whereas manual pressure is applied to the nerve for 60 seconds. If the patient's ring and small finger become numb, the ulnar nerve is likely compressed.
- Intrinsic muscle function is tested by asking the patient to cross the long finger over the index finger (i.e., the crossed finger test). Patients with severe ulnar nerve entrapment will not be able to perform this task.

Imaging

- Radiographs of the elbow may be obtained if elbow pathology is suspected, such as valgus cubitus, bone spurs or fragments, a shallow epicondylar groove, osteochondroma, and/or destructive lesions. In most cases of idiopathic ulnar nerve entrapment, however, radiographs are not necessary.
- Electromyography tests and nerve conduction studies are indicated to confirm the area of entrapment and to document the extent of the pathology.
- Nerve conduction studies showing a diminished signal conduction rate of less than 50 meters per second (33% decrease from normal) across the elbow are indicative of nerve compression.

Table 13-1 Ulnar Nerve Entrapment

	Sensory	Motor	Tests
Mild	Paresthesias come and go, vibratory perception increased	Subjective weakness, clumsiness or loss of coordination	Elbow flexion test or Tinel sign may be positive
Moderate	Paresthesias come and go, vibratory perception decreased or normal	Measurable weakness in pinch or grip strength	Elbow flexion test or Tinel sign is positive, finger crossing might be abnormal
Severe	Paresthesias are persistent, vibratory perception decreased, abnormal two-point discrimination	Measurable weakness in pinch and grip strength plus muscle atrophy	Elbow flexion test or Tinel sign may be positive, finger crossing is usually abnormal

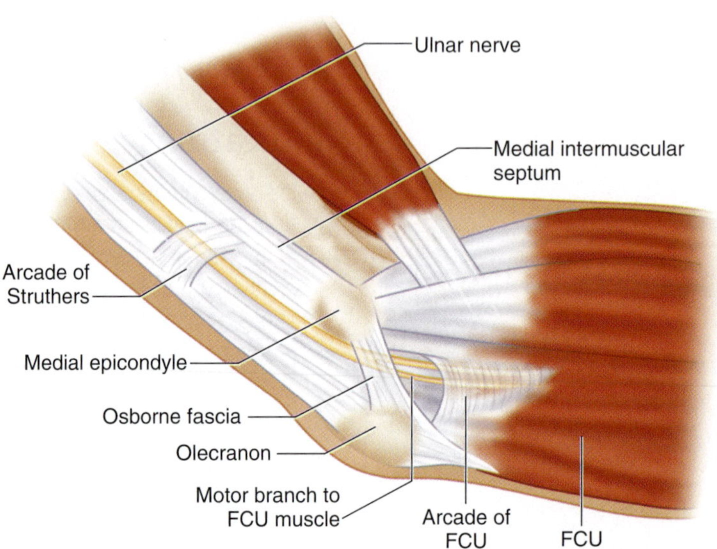

FIGURE 13-1

Surgical Anatomy

- The ulnar nerve is the terminal branch of the medial cord of the brachial plexus. Initially, the ulnar nerve lies medial to the axillary artery. In the upper arm, the ulnar nerve lies posteromedial to the brachial artery, posterior to the intermuscular septum, and anterior to the medial head of the triceps muscle. Approximately 8 cm proximal to the medial epicondyle is the arcade of Struthers, a thin fibrous band. At the elbow, the ulnar nerve travels posterior to the medial epicondyle and medial to the olecranon at the subcutaneous level, then it enters the cubital tunnel. The cubital tunnel is covered by fibroaponeurotic bands and the Osborne fascia (a ligament over the epicondylar groove), which is the fibroaponeurotic tissue between the two heads of the FCU. After passing through the cubital tunnel, the ulnar nerve travels deep into the forearm between the humeral and ulnar heads of the FCU. Distally, the ulnar nerve follows through the FCU to the deep flexor-pronator aponeurosis (Fig. 13-1).

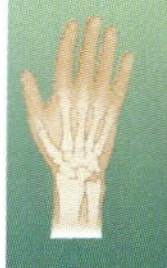

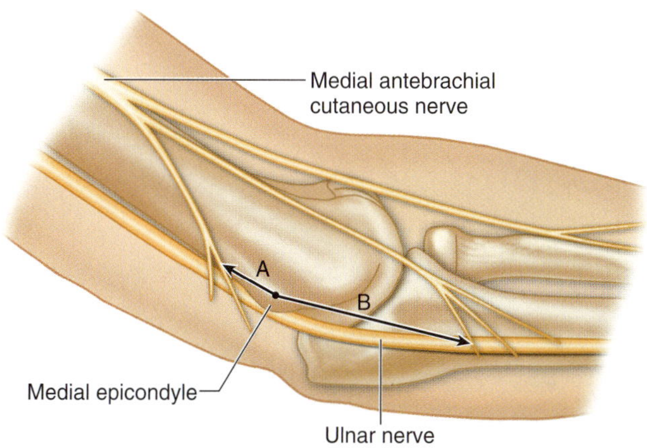

A: The distance (1.8 cm) proximally from the crossing branch to the medial epicondyle
B: The distance (3.1 cm) distally from the crossing branch to the medial epicondyle

FIGURE 13-2

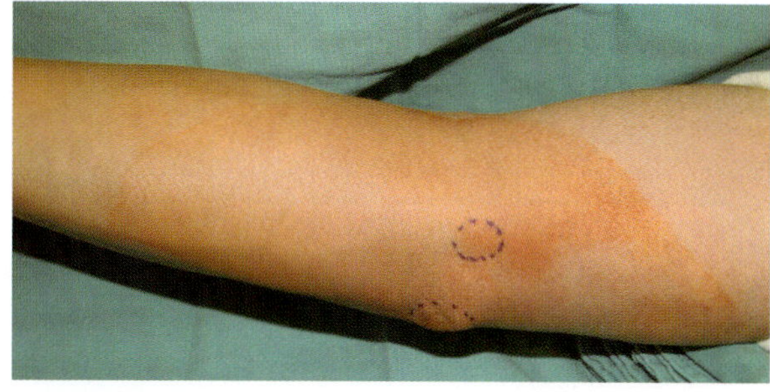

FIGURE 13-3

- The posterior branch of the medial antebrachial cutaneous nerve is at risk of injury during cubital tunnel surgery. The proximal crossing branch lies approximately 1.8 cm proximal to the medial epicondyle, whereas the distal crossing branch is about 3.1 cm distal to the medial epicondyle (Fig. 13-2).
- The ulnar nerve may be easily compressed at five sites (see Fig. 13-1).
  - The arcade of Struthers, a thin aponeurotic band extending from the medial head of the triceps to the medial intermuscular septum. The ulnar nerve passes through the arcade of Struthers in 70% to 80% of patients.
  - The medial epicondyle, where a valgus cubitus deformity caused by malunion or nonunion of a condylar fracture may compress the nerve.
  - The epicondylar groove (proximal part of cubital tunnel), which is a fibro-osseous tunnel bound anteriorly by the medial epicondyle and laterally by the olecranon and ulnohumeral ligament and covered by fibroaponeurotic bands (Osborne fascia).
  - The middle part of the cubital tunnel, where the nerve passes between the two heads of the FCU, which is a continuation of the fibroaponeurotic covering of the epicondylar groove. During elbow flexion, the Osborne fascia is stretched and the tunnel flattened, resulting in a 7- to 20-fold increase in tunnel pressure, ultimately causing pressure on the ulnar nerve. The distal part of the cubital tunnel is formed by the muscle bellies of the FCU.
  - Flexor-pronator aponeurosis. Fascia is located at the point of exit from the FCU.
- The most common sites of ulnar nerve compression are the epicondylar groove and the cubital tunnel.

Positioning

- The procedure is performed under tourniquet control. It can be done under regional or general anesthesia. The patient is positioned supine with the affected extremity on a hand table. The elbow is in 90-degree flexion, with some towels under the elbow to keep the elbow in flexion and supination posture. Placing these towels under the elbow will help in locating the medial epicondyle (Fig. 13-3).

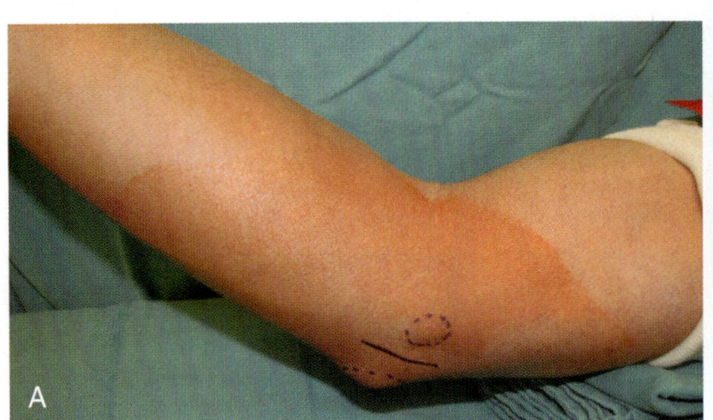

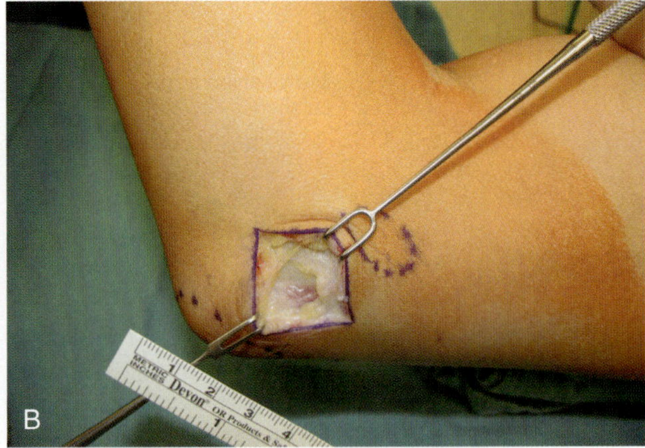

FIGURE 13-4

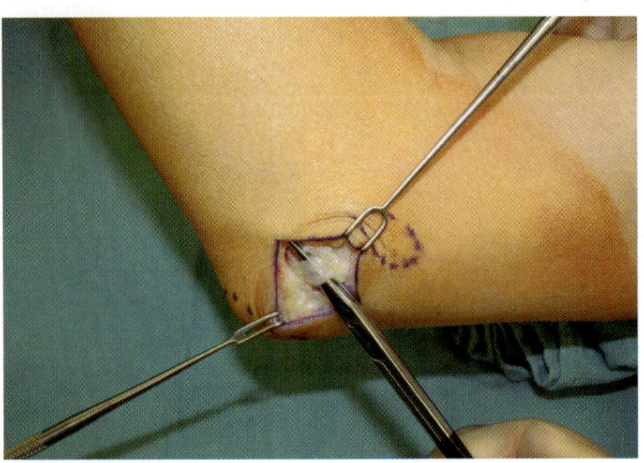

FIGURE 13-5

PEARLS

Using short (3- to 5-cm) skin incisions will help to avoid injury to the medial antebrachial cutaneous nerve (see Fig. 13-2).

STEP 1 PITFALLS

Care should be taken to avoid injury to the medial antebrachial cutaneous nerve. Injury of the cutaneous nerve will result in a painful neuroma (see Fig. 13-2).

Exposures

- The medial epicondyle and olecranon are marked first. A 3-cm skin incision line between the medial epicondyle and olecranon is marked, which is generally drawn a little closer to the medial epicondyle (Fig. 13-4).

Procedure

Step 1

- After tourniquet inflation, the skin and subcutaneous tissue are dissected and divided with a blade, and the Osborne fascia is identified (Fig. 13-5).

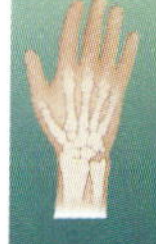

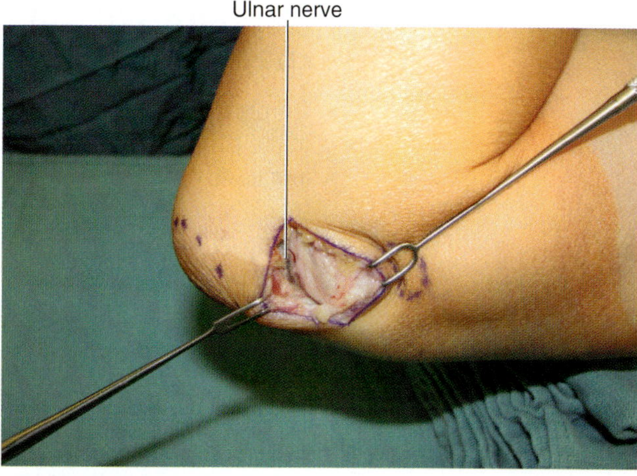

FIGURE 13-6

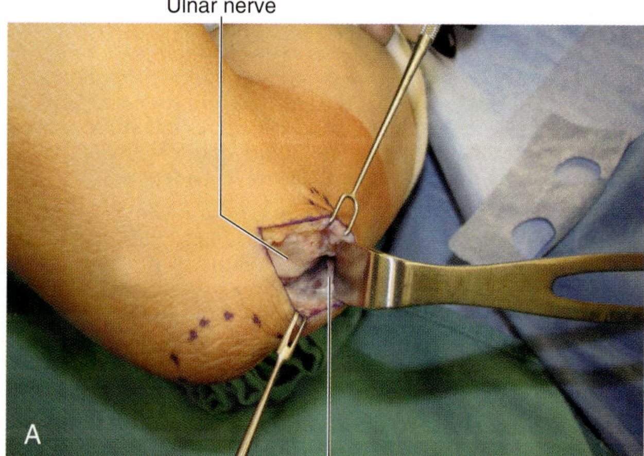

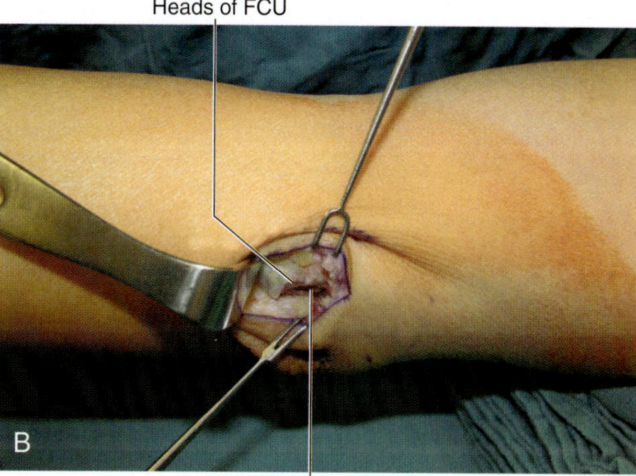

FIGURE 13-7

> **STEP 2 PEARLS**
>
> *The ulnar nerve is secured in its groove with areolar tissue and longitudinal feeding blood vessels. Freeing this areolar tissue will cause ulnar nerve subluxation. Only the compressive fascia band needs to be released, whereas the supporting soft tissue posterior to the ulnar nerve should not be disturbed.*

Step 2

- After Osborne fascia release, the ulnar nerve is identified (Fig. 13-6).
- The skin is retracted proximally and distally at the medial epicondyle. The tightened fascia over the ulnar nerve can be checked using scissors; if the fascia is tight, it may be divided with scissors (Fig. 13-7A and B).
- Distally, the muscle bellies of the FCU should be released if ulnar nerve compression is discovered.

Step 3

- The elbow is moved through a range of movements to check whether the ulnar nerve subluxes.
- If subluxation of the ulnar nerve over the medial epicondyle is noticed, medial epicondylectomy or anterior transposition of the ulnar nerve should be performed to avoid postoperative discomfort from nerve impingement.

Step 4

- Tourniquet is deflated and the wound is compressed for 5 minutes to allow the vessels to retract. In most cases, bleeding will stop spontaneously.
- The skin and subcutaneous tissue are closed with absorbable sutures and then covered with skin strip tapes.
- The patient's elbow is protected in a soft bulky dressing.

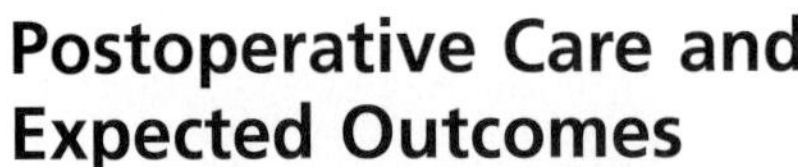

Postoperative Care and Expected Outcomes

- The dressings are removed 2 to 3 days after surgery, and active range of motion of the elbow is started at that time.
- In mild to moderate nerve compression, the in situ decompression procedure should result in marked relief of paresthesias in the ulnar nerve distribution. The motor weakness may take a much longer time to recover.

Evidence

Miller RG, Hummel EE. The cubital tunnel syndrome: treatment with simple decompression. *Ann Neurol.* 1980;7:567-569.
A retrospective review of 12 patients with progressive cubital tunnel syndrome treated with simple decompression of the ulnar nerve. Eleven of the 12 patients had clinical and electrophysiologic evidence of improvement. Patients with the best outcomes had (1) mild weakness, (2) recent onset of symptoms, and (3) a mild abnormality of the sensory action potential preoperatively. (Level IV evidence)

Nathan PA, Istvan JA, Meadows KD. Intermediate and long-term outcomes following simple decompression of the ulnar nerve at the elbow. *Chir Main.* 2005;24:29-34.
A retrospective review of 102 cases of cubital tunnel syndrome in 74 patients treated with simple decompression of the ulnar nerve. Overall, 82% of patients were regarded as having 75% or more improvement in range of motion at the elbow following the surgery. Most patients (61%) were found to have improved ulnar nerve conduction velocities at follow-up. In this study, simple decompression resulted in excellent intermediate and long-term relief of symptoms in a substantial majority of patients. (Level IV evidence)

Tanigughi Y, Takami M, Tamake T, et al. Simple decompression with small skin incision for cubital tunnel syndrome. *J Hand Surg [Br].* 2002;27:559-562.
A retrospective review of 18 elbows in 17 patients treated by simple decompression using only a 1.5- to 2.5-cm skin incision with no endoscopic assistance. Clinical results were evaluated as "excellent" for 4 elbows, "good" for 10, and "fair" for 4. The 4 patients with a "fair" outcome had diabetes mellitus, with marked atrophy of the interosseous muscle and unmeasurable nerve conduction velocities. (Level IV evidence)

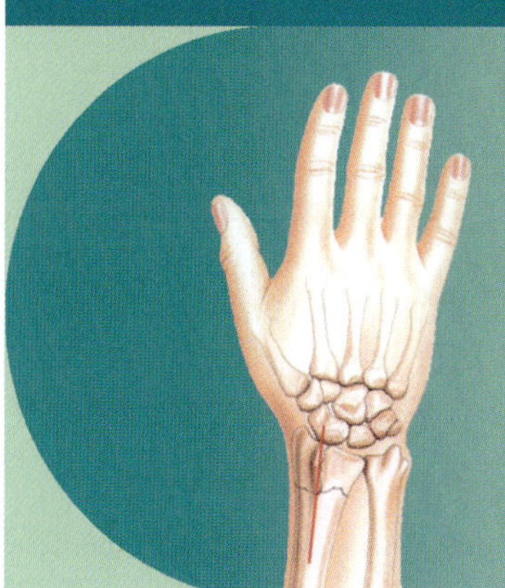

PROCEDURE 14

Distal Anterior Interosseous Nerve Transfer to Motor Branch of Ulnar Nerve

Pao-Yuan Lin, Sandeep J. Sebastin, and Kevin C. Chung

See Video 12: Distal Anterior Interosseous Nerve Transfer to Motor Branch of Ulnar Nerve

Indications

- For recovery of intrinsic muscle function in a patient with a high ulnar nerve injury (near or above the elbow) to shorten the distance between the donor nerve and the recipient muscles
  - In patients with ulnar nerve injuries at the mid-distal forearm, direct nerve repair or nerve grafts are more suitable options than nerve transfers.
  - In patients with demyelinating neuropathy such as leprosy, nerve transfer procedures are not indicated.

Examination/Imaging

Clinical Examination

- Check motor function of the anterior interosseous nerve (AIN).
  - The patient is examined to ensure that the function of the flexor pollicis longus (FPL) (flexion of thumb interphalangeal joint) and the flexor digitorum profundus (FDP) of the index finger (flexion of index finger distal interphalangeal joint) is preserved. These two muscles are innervated by the AIN and can be checked by asking the patient to make the OK sign.
  - The other muscle that is innervated by the AIN is the pronator quadratus (PQ). This is done by testing pronation of the forearm with the elbow in full flexion (to eliminate the contribution of the pronator teres).
- Check the joints of the ring and small fingers. The joints of the hand should be supple. If mild contractures of the joints are discovered, the patient will require hand therapy before any nerve transfer procedures are performed.

Imaging

- Electromyography of the ulnar and median nerves should be performed if the nerve-muscle function is not clear.

Surgical Anatomy

- The ulnar nerve enters the anterior (flexor) compartment of the forearm between the two heads of flexor carpi ulnaris (FCU) and innervates one and a half muscles (FCU and medial half of FDP to the ring and small fingers). It runs along the ulna with the ulnar artery, and the two travel distally under the FCU. Proximal to the wrist, the fascicles of the motor branch lie ulnar to the sensory fascicles. The ulnar nerve and artery pass superficial to the flexor retinaculum into the Guyon canal. In the Guyon canal, the ulnar artery is radial to the ulnar nerve. At the radial side of the pisiform bone, the ulnar nerve is divided into the superficial and deep branches. The deep branch of the ulnar nerve curves laterally to supply the hypothenar muscles and runs across the palm with the deep palmar arch; it terminates by supplying the first dorsal interosseous and the deep head of the flexor pollicis brevis (Fig. 14-1).
- The AIN is a branch of the median nerve that supplies the deep muscles on the front of the forearm. It accompanies the anterior interosseous artery and runs on the anterior surface of the interosseous membrane in the interval between the FPL and FDP, supplying the whole of the former and the radial half of the latter. The AIN terminates in the volar capsule of the wrist joint after it innervates the PQ (see Fig. 14-1).

PEARLS

The facial bands of the hypothenar muscle should be released to visualize the motor branch of the ulnar nerve.

PITFALLS

It is easy to injure the palmar cutaneous branch of the median nerve if the incision is too close to the thenar crease (see Fig. 14-1).

Positioning

- The procedure is performed under general anesthesia under tourniquet control. Regional anesthesia is not used so that nerve stimulation can be performed. The patient is positioned supine with the affected extremity on a hand table.

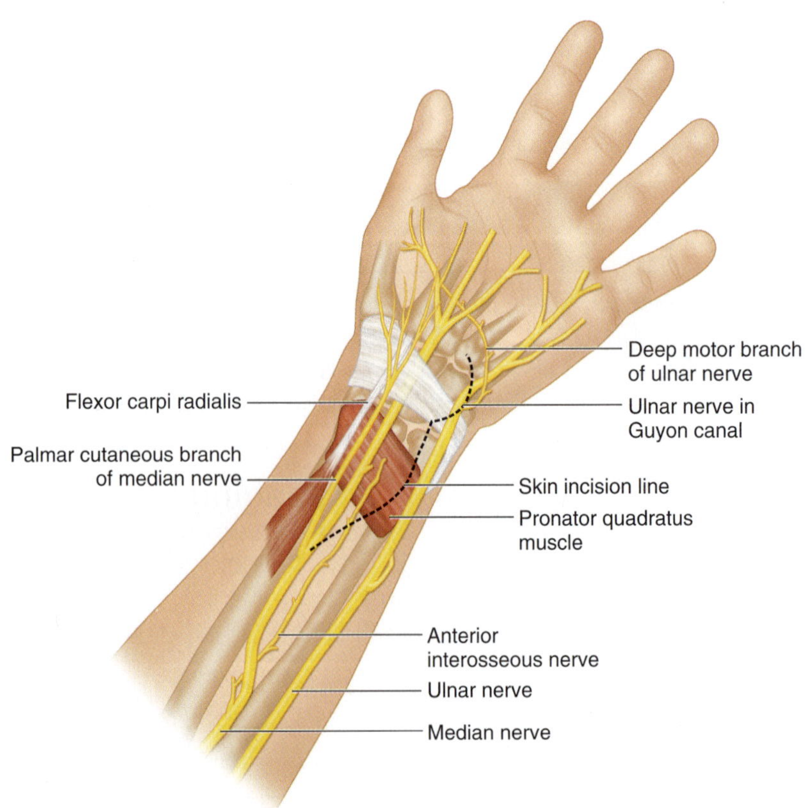

FIGURE 14-1

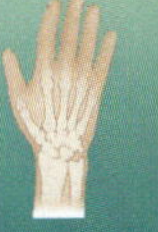

Exposures

- A 10-cm curvilinear incision begins at the pisiform and curves gently radially and proximally. This incision will expose the ulnar nerve in Guyon canal and the AIN in the distal forearm (Fig. 14-2). The skin and subcutaneous fat are dissected in the distal half of the incision to expose the ulnar nerve in Guyon canal. In the proximal half of the incision, the antebrachial fascia is divided ulnar to the palmaris longus. The median nerve is identified below the palmaris longus to expose the flexor tendons. The palmaris longus, median nerve, and flexor tendons to the radial two fingers are retracted radially, and the flexor tendons to the ulnar fingers are retracted ulnarly to expose the PQ.

Procedure

Step 1

- The Guyon canal is opened, and the deep motor branch of the ulnar nerve is identified at the level of the hook of the hamate (Fig. 14-3).

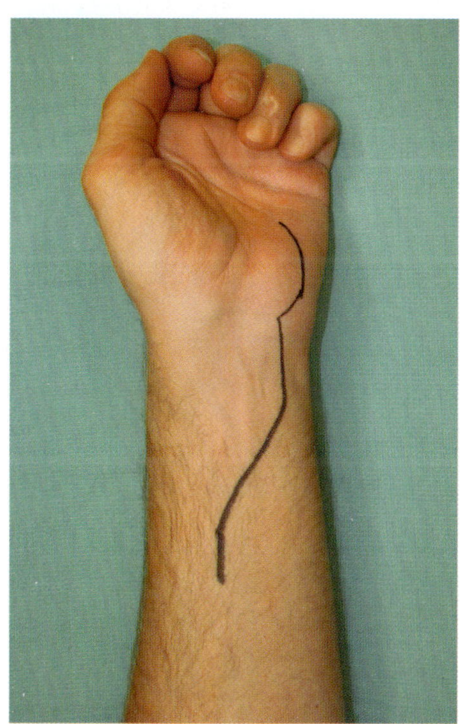

FIGURE 14-2

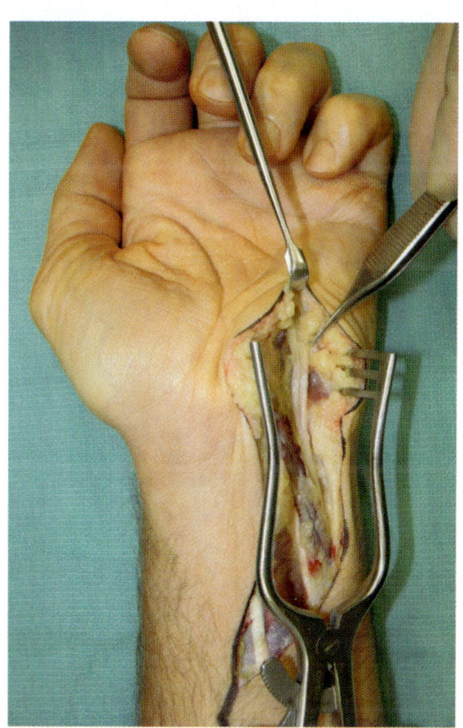

FIGURE 14-3

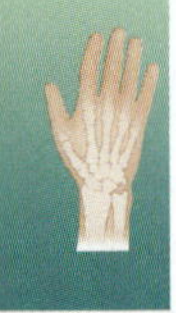

Step 2

- The motor branch of the ulnar nerve in the hand is dissected proximally into the forearm for about 10 cm from the hook of the hamate (Fig. 14-4) to a point that is proximal to the AIN (Fig. 14-5).

Step 3

- The AIN is identified proximal to the PQ. This is confirmed using a nerve stimulator and should show marked contraction of the PQ. Intramuscular dissection of the AIN within the PQ is performed.
- At about the midportion of the PQ, the AIN begins to branch. The AIN is divided proximal to this branching point.

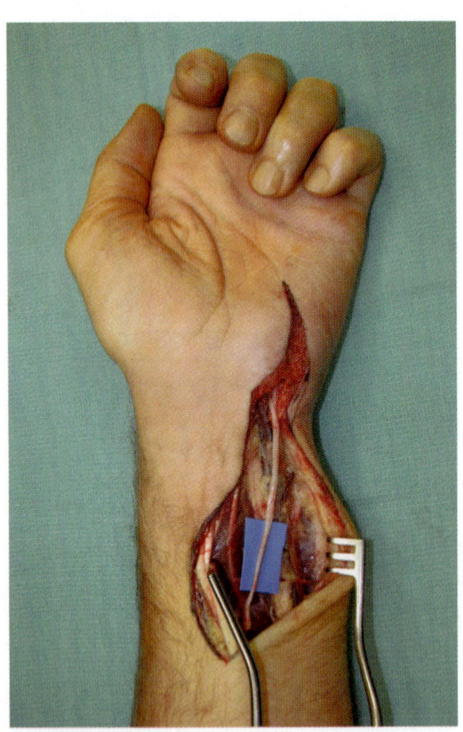

FIGURE 14-4

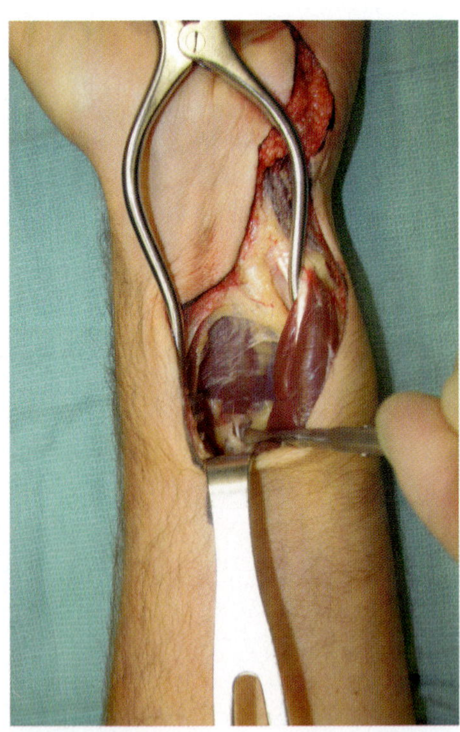

FIGURE 14-5

STEP 4 PEARLS

The motor branch of the ulnar nerve is divided at an adequate distance proximally so that a nerve graft is not necessary to reach the distal end of the AIN. The use of nerve graft will markedly decrease the axon count reaching the muscles and hamper muscle recovery.

The motor branch of the ulnar nerve should be passed underneath the flexor tendons to keep it on the same plane as the AIN to avoid compression of nerve while the flexor tendons glide during movement.

STEP 4 PITFALLS

Isolation of the wrong fascicular group will result in a nonfunctional result.

Step 4

- The motor branch of the ulnar nerve is divided in the forearm using microscissors and passed under the flexor tendons to reach the divided AIN within the PQ (Fig. 14-6).

Step 5

- Direct epineural repair of the motor branch of the ulnar nerve to the PQ branch of the AIN in end-to-end fashion is achieved using 9-0 nylon sutures under microscope magnification (Fig. 14-7).
- The wrist and digits are taken through a full range of motion to make sure that there is no tension at the nerve repair site.

Step 6

- The tourniquet is deflated and careful hemostasis achieved by micro-bipolar cauterization.
- A dorsal short-arm splint is applied to maintain the wrist in neutral position.

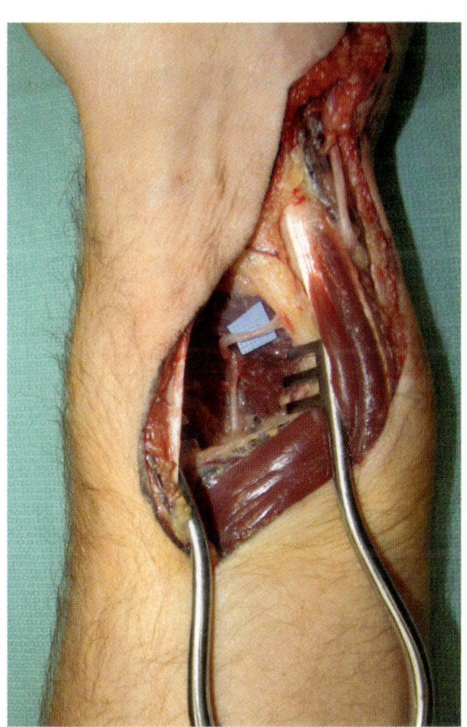

FIGURE 14-6

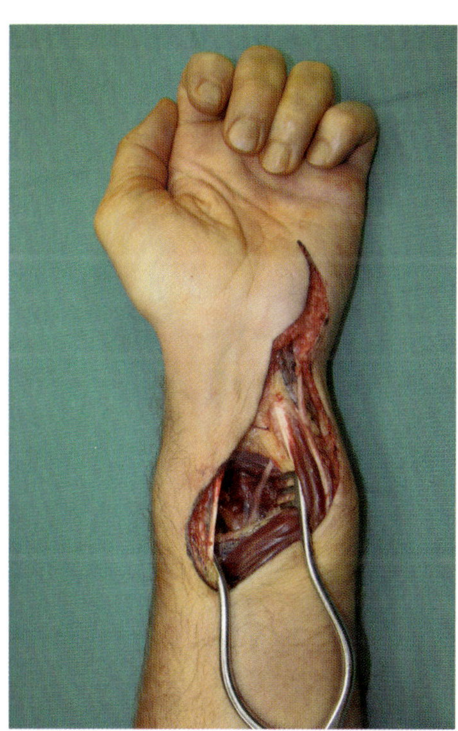

FIGURE 14-7

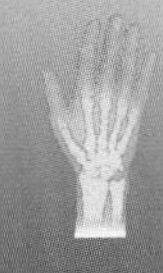

Postoperative Care and Expected Outcomes

- A splint is used to maintain the wrist in neutral position for 3 weeks. The patient is instructed in range-of-motion exercise of the fingers, elbow, and shoulder to maintain movement and nerve gliding proximal and distal to the repair site.
- Postoperative rehabilitation includes motor rehabilitation. The patient is initially instructed in resisted forearm pronation exercises. With evidence of reinnervation of the intrinsic muscles, the patient is then instructed in pinching exercises in resisted forearm pronated positions.
- Although the distal anterior interosseous nerve is not a powerful donor, one can at least expect to prevent clawing, improve pinch strength, and avoid tendon transfers.

Evidence

Haase SC, Chung KC. Anterior interosseous nerve transfer to the motor branch of the ulnar nerve for high ulnar nerve injuries. *Ann Plast Surg*. 2002;49:285-290.
This paper presented two cases of high ulnar nerve injuries that received anterior interosseous nerve transfers to the motor branch of the ulnar nerve. The intrinsic muscles functioned normally at 1-year follow-up. (Level V evidence)

Novak CB, Mackinnon SE. Distal anterior interosseous nerve transfer to the deep motor branch of the ulnar nerve for reconstruction of high ulnar nerve injuries. *J Reconstruct Microsurg*. 2002;18:459-463.
Retrospective chart review of eight patients who sustained high ulnar nerve injury received anterior interosseous nerve transfer to the deep motor branch of the ulnar nerve. All patients had reinnervation of the ulnar nerve intrinsic muscles of the hand. Lateral pinch and grip strength were improved, and all patients were able to fully flex the metacarpophalangeal joints of the ring and small fingers and to make a complete fist. (Level IV evidence)

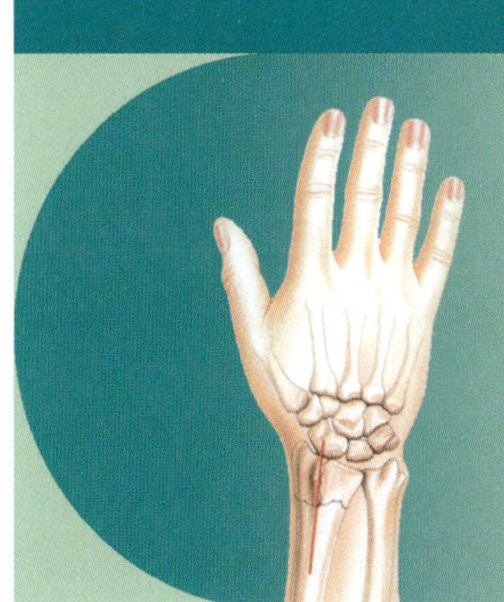

PROCEDURE 15

Nerve Transfer Techniques for Elbow Flexion in Brachial Plexus Palsy

Lynda J. Yang

See Video 13: Nerve Transfers for Elbow Flexion in Brachial Plexus Palsy (Ulnar Fascicle to Musculocutaneous Nerve)

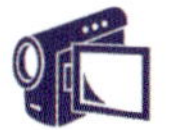

Indications

- Lack of elbow flexion/supination
- Available functional donor nerve with a lesser-valued function (e.g., ulnar fascicle to flexor carpi ulnaris with normal muscle power) in close proximity with recipient nerve/muscle
- Available recipient nerve without distal injury (e.g., intact musculocutaneous nerve branch to biceps in patients with supraclavicular brachial plexus injury)
- Donor and recipient nerves ideally with agonistic functions (e.g., flexion of elbow, wrist)

Examination/Imaging

Clinical Examination

- Examine the involvement of all muscles that contribute to elbow flexion—biceps, brachialis, and brachioradialis—to determine the site of injury (e.g., nerve root versus peripheral nerve).
- Examine the active and passive range of motion at the elbow.
- Examine the integrity of the vascular supply to the arm.
- Examine the integrity of the donor nerve/muscle (e.g., flexor carpi ulnaris).
- Determine whether the biceps muscle is ruptured, because end-organ injury would preclude nerve transfer.

Surgical Anatomy

- Pertinent surgical anatomy includes the neurovascular anatomy in the medial aspect of the arm.

Positioning

- Position the patient supine with the arm extended onto a surgical arm board.
- In patients with decreased shoulder range of motion, an external positioning device can be used to place the arm in abduction and external rotation to reveal the medial aspect of the upper arm (Fig. 15-1).

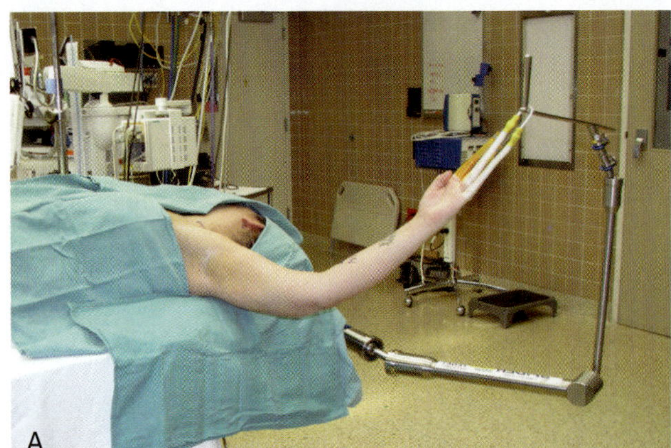

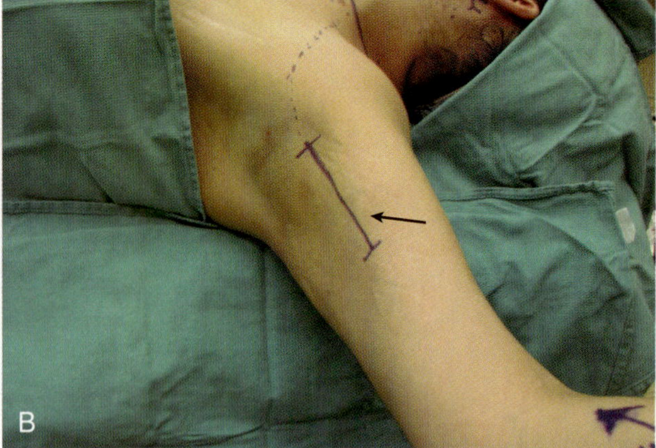

FIGURE 15-1

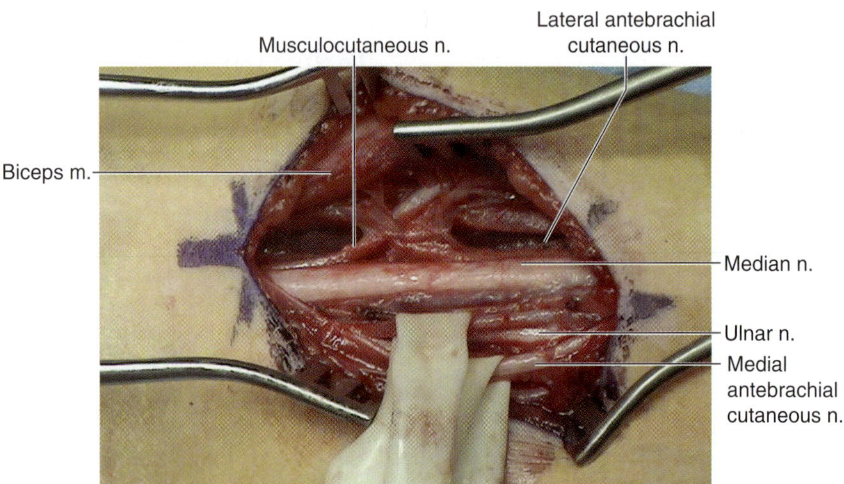

FIGURE 15-2

PEARLS

The ulnar nerve is more medial than the median nerve. The brachial artery is adjacent to the median nerve (Fig. 15-2).

The first nerve exposed is usually the medial antebrachial cutaneous nerve that can be traced proximally to the medial cord and ulnar nerve.

The musculocutaneous nerve and its branches can be found under the biceps muscle; identifying the lateral antebrachial cutaneous nerve and tracing it proximally to expose the main trunk of the musculocutaneous nerve may facilitate exposure.

The fascicle of the ulnar nerve to the flexor carpi ulnaris usually lies in the volar radial position within the ulnar nerve.

Exposures

- *Ulnar fascicle to musculocutaneous nerve:* An incision is made along the medial arm from the pectoralis muscle insertion site to distally, with the incision overlying the path of the neurovascular bundle that lies between the biceps and triceps (see Fig. 15-1).
- *Double fascicular nerve transfer for elbow flexion:* The double fascicular nerve transfer for elbow flexion employs (1) the ulnar nerve fascicles innervating the flexor carpi ulnaris to the musculocutaneous branch innervating the biceps; and (2) the median nerve fascicles innervating the flexor carpi radialis to the musculocutaneous branch innervating the brachialis.

STEP 1 PEARLS

Ensure careful identification and protection of the median nerve, ulnar nerve, and brachial artery (Fig. 15-3).

The branches of the musculocutaneous nerve to the biceps can be dissected proximally by opening the epineurium until its fascicles become physically inseparable from the parent nerve, then transected sharply to serve as the recipient nerve (Fig. 15-4).

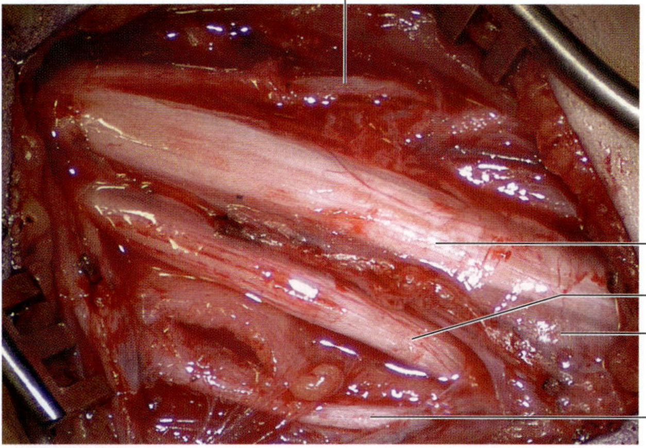

FIGURE 15-3

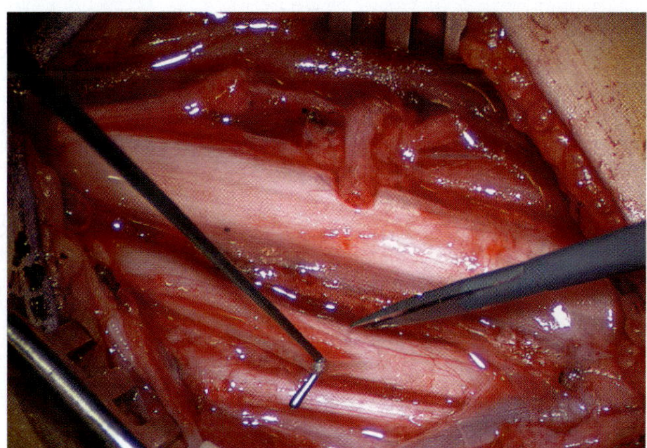

FIGURE 15-4

Procedure

Step 1

- Open the biceps fascia to reveal the branch of the musculocutaneous nerve innervating the biceps muscle and transect it proximally.

STEP 2 PEARLS

Careful intraneural dissection will reveal one or two fascicles with diffuse innervation of the distal muscles with emphasis on the flexor carpi ulnaris (usually found superficially in the ulnar nerve) using intraoperative nerve stimulation; avoid those fascicles with primary innervation to the hand intrinsic muscles.

Step 2

- Isolate the appropriate ulnar nerve fascicles for use as the donor by opening the epineurium of the ulnar nerve (see Fig. 15-4).
- The desired fascicles can be dissected proximally and distally until they are of adequate length for a tension-free coaptation with the musculocutaneous nerve. The fascicles are then transected sharply as distally as possible and coapted with the appropriate recipient nerve (see Fig. 15-4).

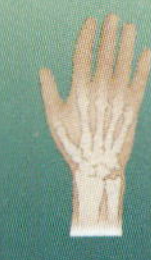

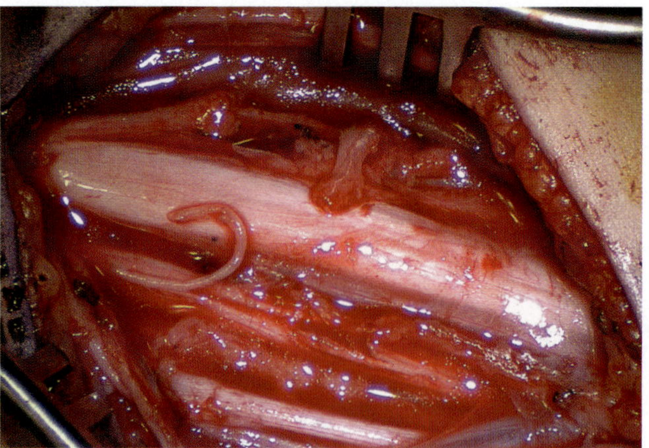

FIGURE 15-5

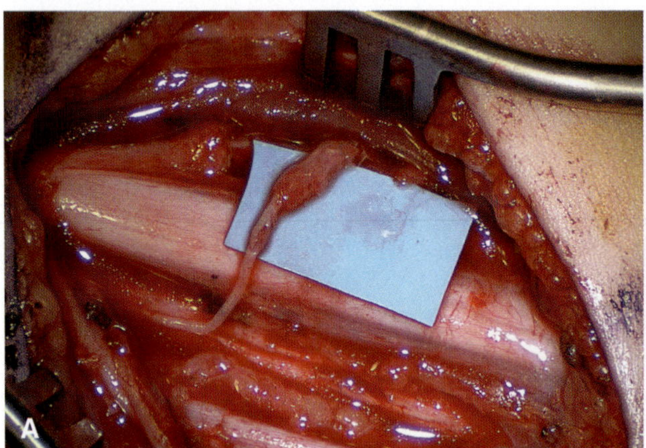

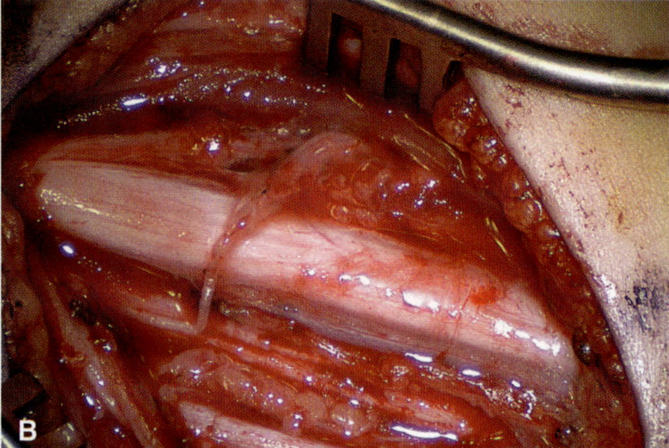

FIGURE 15-6

STEP 2 PITFALLS

Transecting the donor too proximally or the recipient too distally may necessitate the use of a nerve graft, which is not desirable for optimal outcome (Fig. 15-5).

STEP 3 PEARLS

The fascicles that primarily serve to innervate the flexor carpi radialis (confirm function of fascicles with intraoperative nerve stimulation) are optimal for use as donor nerve.

Tension-free coaptation is desirable (Fig. 15-6).

Step 3

- If both the musculocutaneous branches to the biceps and brachialis are desired, in addition to the dissection for the ulnar nerve fascicles, an intraneural dissection of the median nerve is undertaken.
- Locate the branch of the musculocutaneous nerve innervating the brachialis distal to the branch to the biceps.

Postoperative Care and Expected Outcomes

- A soft wrap or sling can be used with care to avoid pressure on the medial aspect of the arm.
- Physical therapy for range of motion can start 4 to 6 weeks postoperatively.
- Recovery of reinnervated muscle function occurs from 6 months to 3 years postoperatively.
- The expected outcome of the surgery is improved active elbow flexion.

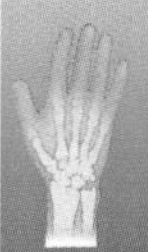

Evidence

Bertelli JA, Florianopolis SC, Ghizoni MF, Tubarao SC. Reconstruction of C5 and C6 brachial plexus avulsion injury by multiple nerve transfers: spinal accessory to suprascapular, ulnar fascicles to biceps branch, and triceps long or lateral head branch to axillary nerve. *J Hand Surg [Am]*. 2004;29:131-139.
This retrospective study reports the results of nerve transfer surgery on 10 adult patients at a mean of 2 years after surgery. All patients who underwent ulnar fascicle to musculocutaneous nerve transfer had recovered elbow flexion ≥ MRC 3 (with 70% ≥ MRC 4). (Level IV evidence)

Carlsen BT, Kircher MF, Spinner RJ, et al. Comparison of single versus double nerve transfers for elbow flexion after brachial plexus injury. *Plast Reconstr Surg*. 2011;127:269-276.
This retrospective review of patients who underwent single versus double nerve transfer for elbow flexion comprised 55 patients (23 single, 32 double). Fourteen of 21 single- and 24 of 30 double-nerve transfer patients showed MRC ≥4 after at least 1 year of follow-up. Outcomes were similar between the two groups for elbow flexion and supination strength. (Level IV evidence)

Goulet B, Boretto JG, Lazerges C, Chammas M. A comparison of intercostal and partial ulnar nerve transfers in restoring elbow flexion following upper brachial plexus injury (C5-C6 ± C7). *J Hand Surg [Am]*. 2010;35:1297-1303.
This retrospective study reports the results of nerve transfer surgery on 23 adult patients at a mean of 32 months after surgery. Twenty of 23 patients who underwent ulnar fascicle to musculocutaneous nerve transfer had recovered elbow flexion ≥ MRC 3. (Level IV evidence)

Mackinnon SE, Novak CB, Myckatyn TM, Tung TH. Results of reinnervation of the biceps and brachialis muscles with a double fascicular transfer for elbow flexion. *J Hand Surg [Am]*. 2005;30:978-985.
This retrospective study reports the results of nerve transfer surgery on six adult patients at mean of 20.5 months after surgery. The patients who underwent ulnar fascicle to musculocutaneous nerve (biceps) transfer coupled with median fascicle to musculocutaneous nerve (brachialis) transfer had recovered mean elbow flexion (MRC 4+). (Level IV evidence)

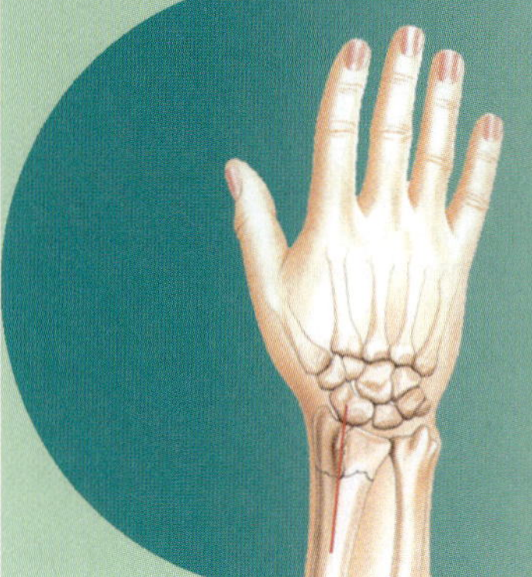

Treatment of a Nerve Gap in the Hand

Sandeep J. Sebastin and Kevin C. Chung

Indications

- A segmental defect in a nerve can result from the following:
  - Trauma (Fig. 16-1)
  - Excision of a tumor (Fig. 16-2)
  - Excision of a neuroma-in-continuity (Fig. 16-3)
  - Iatrogenic (e.g., excision of Dupuytren cord)

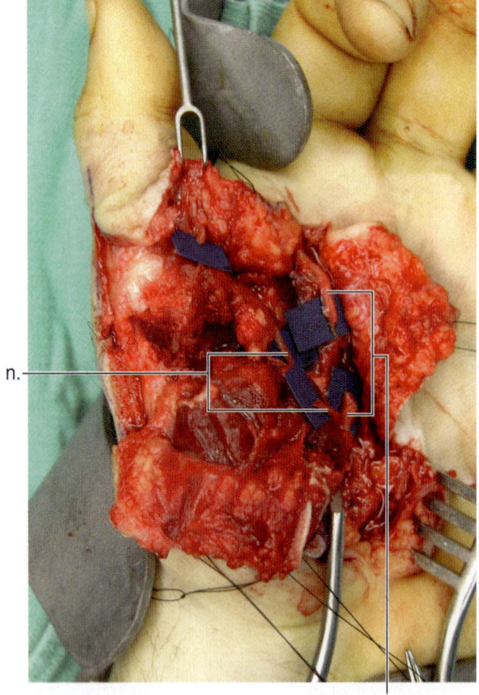

FIGURE 16-1

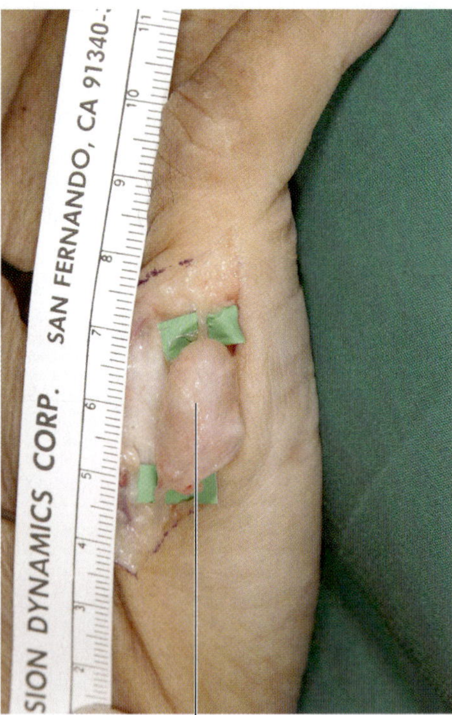

FIGURE 16-2

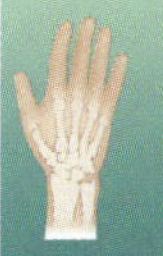

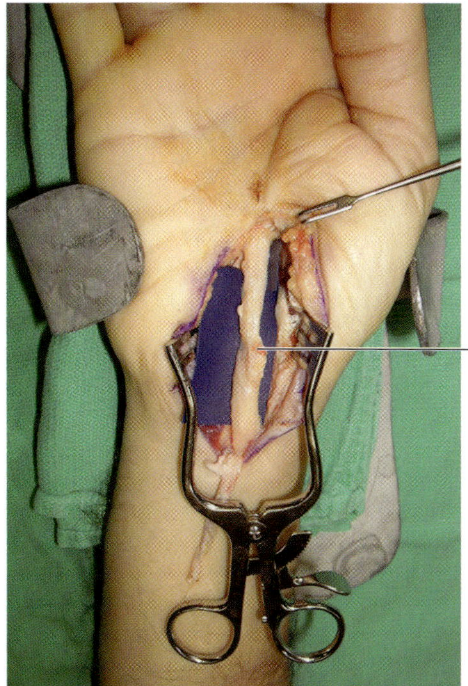

FIGURE 16-3

- Nerve grafting should be considered in the following cases:
  - A single 8-0 suture is unable to keep the nerve ends together.
  - Greater than 30-degree flexion of the interphalangeal (IP) joint is required to bridge the gap.
  - Greater than 10% elongation of the exposed portion of the nerve is required. Depending on the level of injury, each end of a proper digital nerve can be mobilized for 3 to 4 cm at most. Therefore, the maximal elongation that is permissible without risking nerve ischemia is approximately 6 to 8 mm.

Examination/Imaging

Clinical Examination

- The possibility of nerve grafting should be discussed for all patients in whom a digital nerve injury is suspected. Potential nerve graft sources and their morbidity should also be discussed (detailed later). It is better to avoid harvesting a nerve graft from the same limb in patients who have preexisting nerve-related pain/paresthesia because it adds another nociceptive focus.
- It may be difficult to establish sensory loss in children. The absence of wrinkling following immersion of the child's hand in warm water for 5 to 7 minutes indicates loss of sympathetic innervation and can help with diagnosis.

Imaging

- No imaging is required.

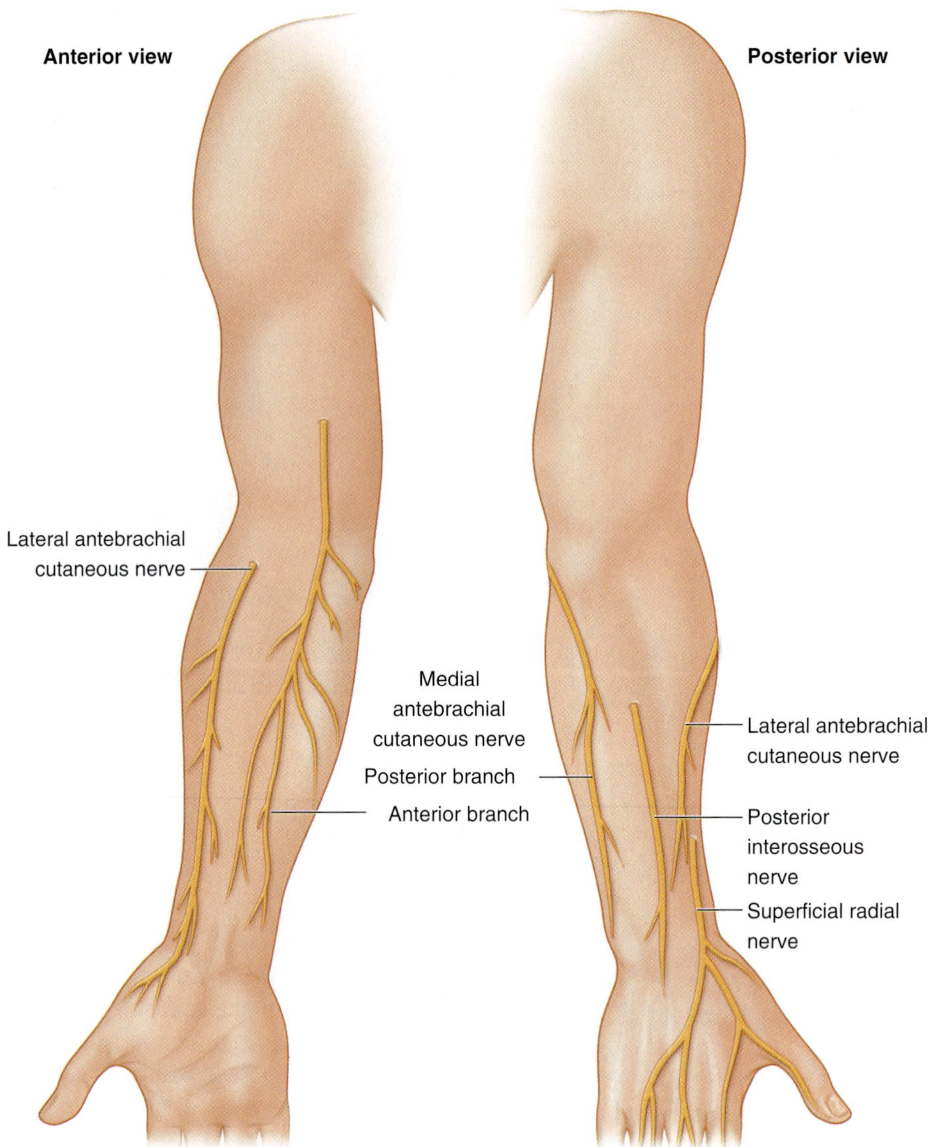

FIGURE 16-4

Surgical Anatomy

- A variety of substitutes have been described for reconstituting nerve defects. They include nerve (autograft/allograft), biological conduits (e.g., vein, muscle), and artificial conduits (e.g., polyglycolic acid, nanofiber).
- The available nerve autografts include the posterior interosseous nerve (PIN), superficial radial nerve, medial and lateral antebrachial cutaneous nerves, and sural nerve (Fig. 16-4). We do not use the superficial radial nerve or the lateral antebrachial cutaneous nerves because they provide innervation to potentially valuable areas of skin.
- *PIN:* The distal portion of the PIN is a purely sensory nerve that innervates the wrist joint. It is identified in the radial aspect of the floor of the fourth extensor compartment deep to the tendons of the extensor digitorum communis (EDC) and the extensor indicis proprius (EIP). It can then be followed proximally for a distance of 5 to 7 cm adjacent to the posterior interosseous artery on the dorsal aspect of the interosseous membrane. It has a cross-sectional area of approximately 0.5 to 0.8 mm^2 and contains one to two fascicles.

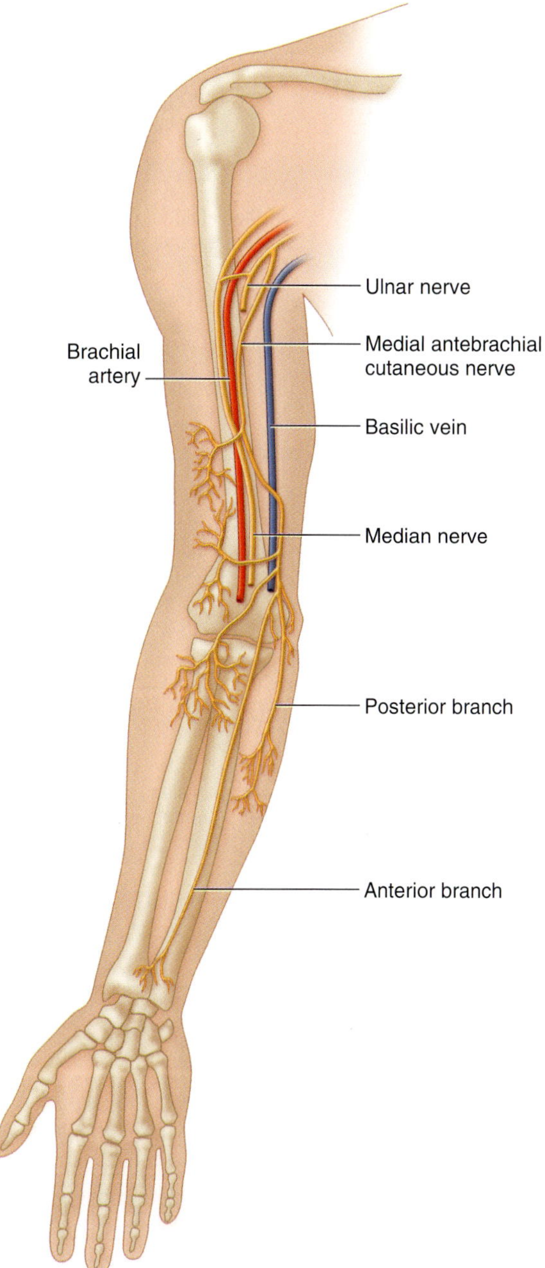

FIGURE 16-5

- *Medial antebrachial cutaneous nerve (MABCN):* This is a purely sensory nerve that arises directly from the medial cord of the brachial plexus (C8, T1) and runs along the axillary vein. It then accompanies the basilic vein in the proximal half of the arm and pierces the deep fascia in the midarm. It splits into anterior and posterior branches in the distal third of the arm. The anterior branch innervates the anteromedial surface of the forearm, whereas the posterior branch innervates the posterior and ulnar aspect of the elbow and forearm (Fig. 16-5). The anterior branch of MABCN is used for nerve graft harvest to avoid sensory loss over the elbow. The anterior branch crosses the elbow between the medial epicondyle and the biceps tendon, usually in front of the antecubital vein, and courses superficial to the flexor carpi ulnaris muscle, ending 10 cm from the wrist. A 20-cm long graft can be harvested based on the anterior branch. It has a cross-sectional area of approximately 0.6 to 1 mm^2 and contains three to four fascicles.

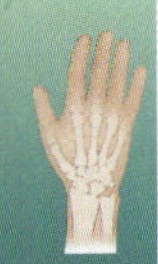

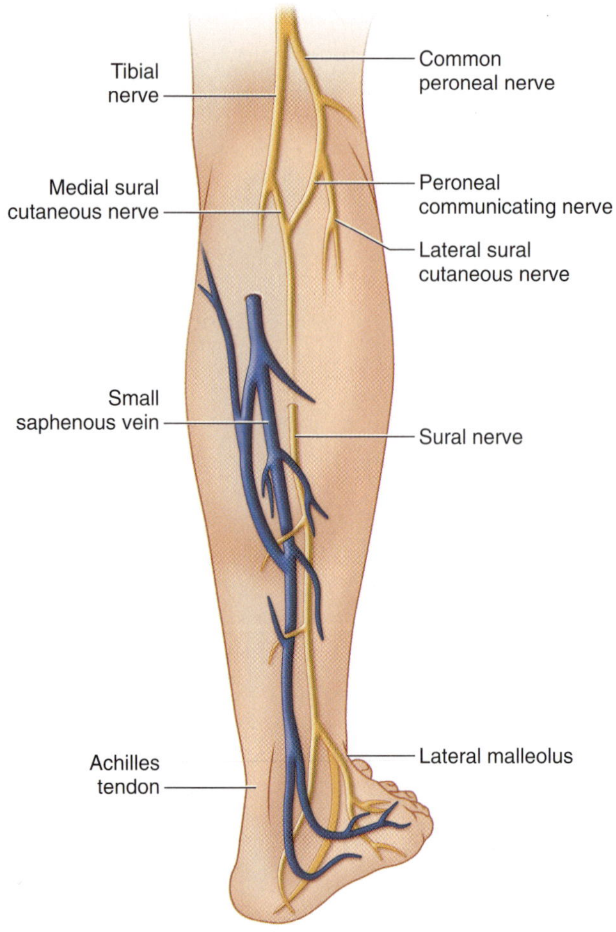

FIGURE 16-6

- *Sural nerve:* The sural nerve is a purely sensory nerve formed by the union of the medial and lateral sural cutaneous nerves (sural communicating nerve). The medial sural cutaneous nerve arises from the tibial nerve and pierces the deep fascia of the leg between the heads of the gastrocnemius in the upper third of the leg. It is then joined by the lateral sural cutaneous nerve branch of the peroneal nerve to form the sural nerve. The sural nerve descends along the lateral margin of the Achilles tendon with the small saphenous vein between the lateral malleolus and the calcaneus (Fig. 16-6). It innervates the lateral aspect of the lower third of the leg and the lateral aspect of the ankle, heel, and foot. A 40-cm–long graft can be harvested based on the sural nerve and medial sural cutaneous nerves. The sural nerve has a cross-sectional area of approximately 2.5 to 3.0 mm^2 and contains six to eight fascicles.

Positioning

- The procedure is performed under tourniquet control using 3.0× to 3.5× loupe magnification for the initial dissection and an operating microscope for the nerve repairs.
- The patient is positioned supine with the affected extremity on a hand table.
- The leg must be prepared and a thigh tourniquet applied, if a sural nerve graft is anticipated.

PEARLS

Positioning the patient in a semi-lateral position (chest facing the involved limb) will make it easier to harvest the contralateral sural nerve, especially when a sturdy assistant is not available to hold the leg.

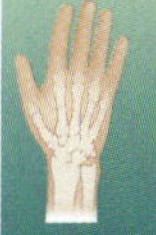

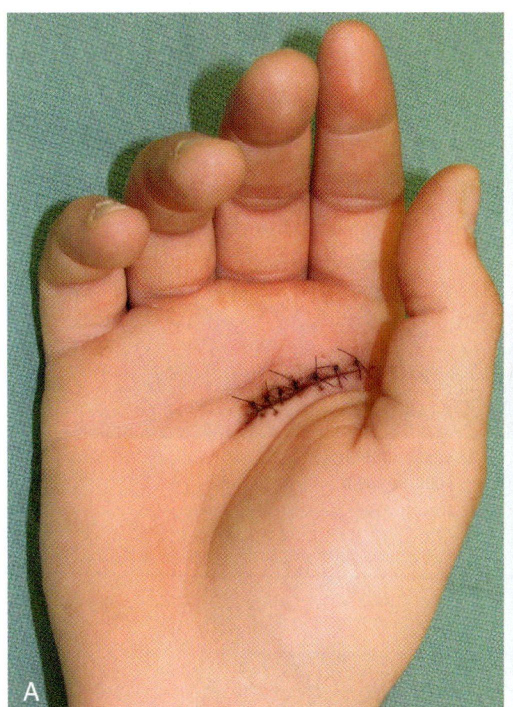

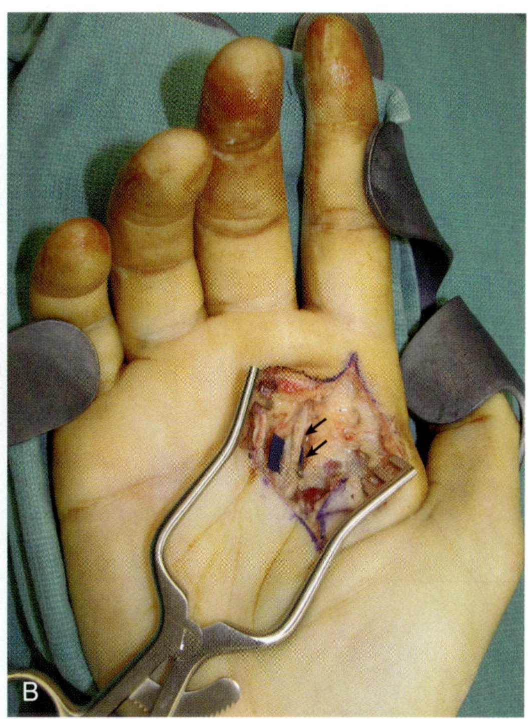

FIGURE 16-7

PEARLS

It is preferable not to cross the web space by the Bruner incision to prevent the development of a contracture band. If an incision needs to extend from the palm to the digit, it is better to leave a small bridge of intact skin at the web and tunnel the nerve graft.

It is important to identify the nerve in normal (uninjured) tissue planes proximal and distal to any existing laceration. These nerves are then followed to find the divided ends that may be encased in scar tissue.

PITFALLS

Avoid injury to branches of the superficial radial nerve when exposing the PIN.

Exposures

- A Bruner zigzag incision that incorporates any previous lacerations is made. Thick skin flaps are raised in a plane superficial to the tendon sheath (Fig. 16-7B).
- Nerve grafts should not be harvested until the divided nerve ends have been exposed, the ends have been débrided, and the required length of nerve graft has been calculated.
- The PIN is exposed by a longitudinal incision ulnar to the Lister tubercle. The extensor retinaculum over the fourth compartment is incised, and the tendons of the EDC and EIP are retracted. The PIN is found on the radial aspect of the floor of fourth compartment. Depending on the length of the nerve required, the skin incision can be extended proximally. There is often a bulbous dilation at the distal termination of the PIN. This should be excised. The average length of a PIN graft is usually 4 to 5 cm.
- The MABCN is exposed by a longitudinal incision on the anteromedial aspect of the forearm at the junction of the proximal and middle third of the forearm. This incision begins 2 cm anterior and 2 to 3 cm distal to the medial epicondyle. The anterior branch of the MABCN can be found within the subcutaneous tissue (Fig. 16-8). If more than one branch is found, the branch that better matches the recipient nerve diameter is selected. Depending on the length of nerve required, the skin incision can be extended proximally.
- The sural nerve is exposed by a 2-cm longitudinal incision midway between the lateral malleolus and the calcaneus. It is close to the lateral margin of the Achilles tendon and lies lateral to the small saphenous vein. The required length of the nerve is then dissected proximally. The use of multiple transverse 1-cm stepladder incisions gives a more aesthetic result compared with a single longitudinal incision.

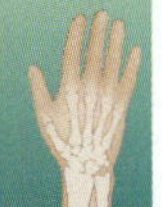

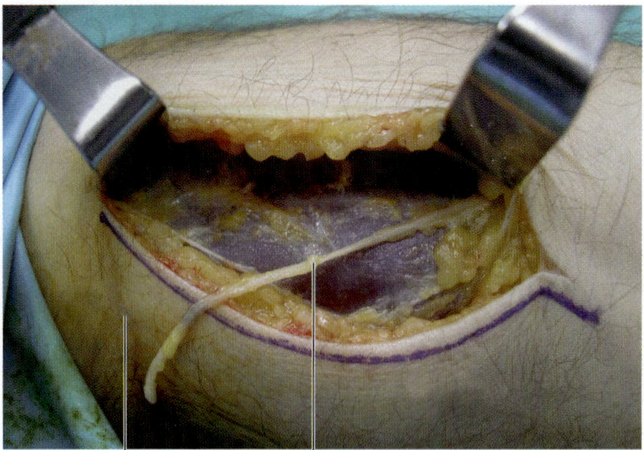

FIGURE 16-8

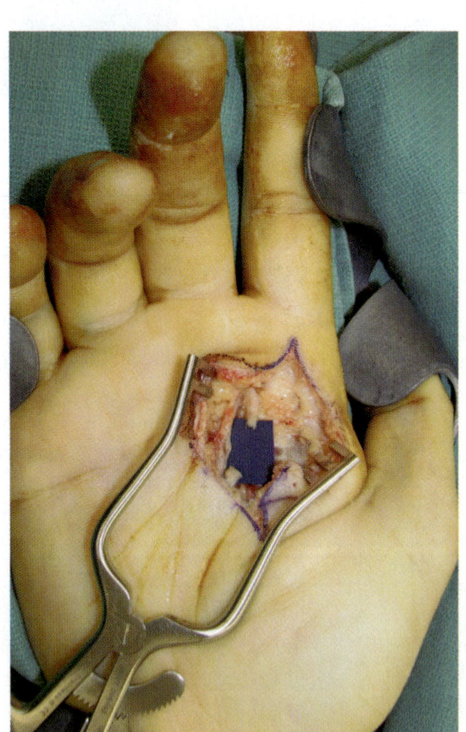

FIGURE 16-9

STEP 1 PEARLS

Trimming of the nerve ends should be done conservatively in a graduated fashion to avoid cutting off too much nerve.

It is important to use a sharp microscissors reserved for this purpose. The use of a blunt scissors can lead to a crushed cut with unevenly cut fascicles. A fresh no. 15 blade can also be used for this purpose, provided that the nerve can be placed on a firm, nonslippery surface. We have found that a sterile razor blade and a gauze-wrapped wooden spatula are ideal in preparing the ends of the divided nerve as well as the nerve graft (Fig. 16-10).

Procedure

Step 1: Preparation of Nerve Ends

- The divided nerve ends are mobilized for 1 to 2 cm depending on the location of injury.
- The nerve ends are then trimmed until healthy fascicles are visualized (Fig. 16-9).

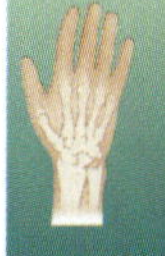

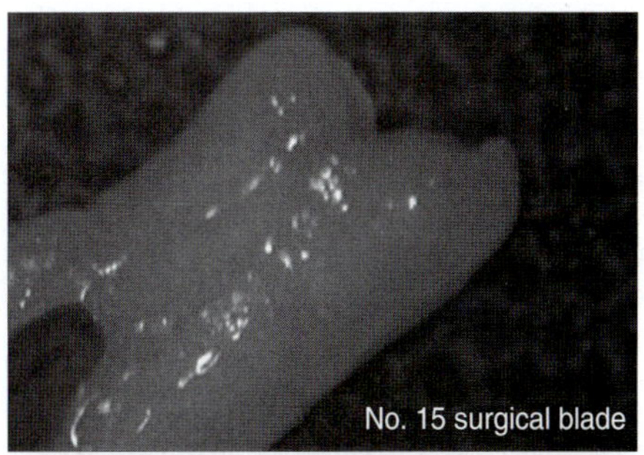

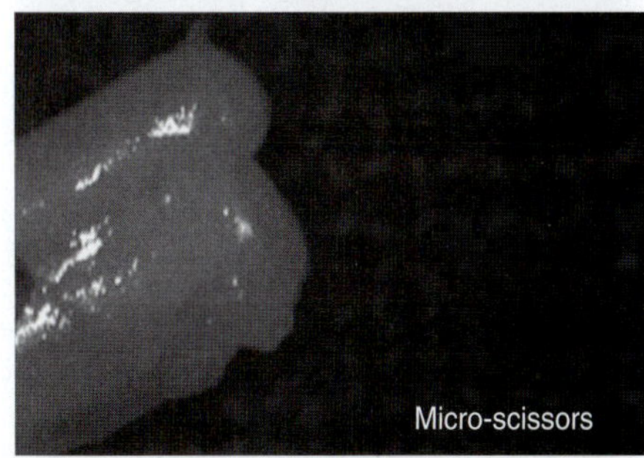

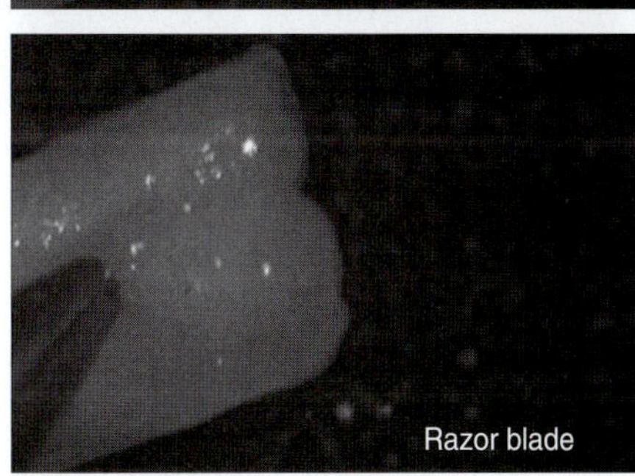

FIGURE 16-10

STEP 2 PEARLS

In a patient with an associated tendon injury, it is preferable to graft a nerve defect rather than suture it, even under slight tension, because the nerve repair is likely to rupture during early mobilization for the tendon injury.

In a traumatic situation with skin loss associated with segmental loss of a digital artery and nerve (up to 10 mm), it may be possible to use a homodigital neurovascular island flap based on the proximal end of divided artery and nerve. This flap can be advanced 10 mm, allowing closure of the skin as well as primary repairs of the digital nerve and artery.

STEP 3 PEARLS

We prefer to use a conduit (vein conduit/PGA conduit) for a digital nerve gap that is less than 3 cm (Fig. 16-11).

For digital nerve gaps that are 3 cm or larger, we use a nerve autograft (Figs. 16-12 and 16-13).

We use a vein graft for nondigital nerve defects (dorsal cutaneous nerves and superficial radial nerve) because the vein grafts are available locally and an additional incision is not usually required (Fig. 16-14).

We also prefer the use of vein conduit in elderly patients (>65 years) because the results of nerve grafting are poor in this population. The use of vein conduit minimizes the risk for neuroma formation and avoids the morbidity associated with harvest of nerve grafts.

Step 2: Assessment of Nerve Gap and Possibility of Primary Repair

- The gap between the nerve ends is measured with the IP joint and metacarpophalangeal (MCP) joint in full extension.
- One should proceed with nerve grafting if the gap is greater than 10 mm. Additional mobilization and slight flexion of the IP joint will allow tension-free repair of gaps smaller than 5 mm. For gaps that are 5- to 10-mm wide, a single 8-0 nylon suture can be used to assess tension of the repair with the joint in 30-degree flexion. If the suture can hold the nerve ends together, a primary repair is attempted.

Step 3: Selection of Nerve Graft

- A nerve graft should be 10% to 15% longer than the measured gap to account for shrinking of the graft as a result of elastic recoil.
- The selection of nerve autografts for digital nerve defects depends on the number, length, and location of the nerve gap.
  - Single, short (about 3 cm), and distal nerve gap: PIN graft
  - Single, long (4 to 8 cm) nerve gap: MABCN graft
  - Multiple, short nerve gaps: MABCN graft
  - Multiple, long nerve gaps: sural nerve graft

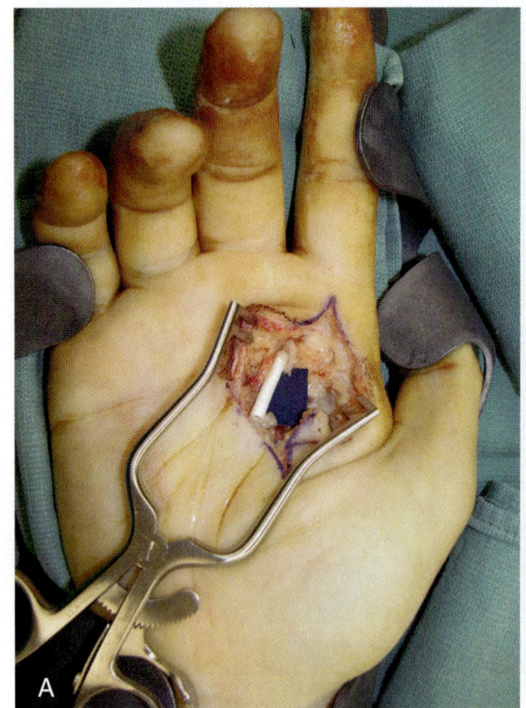

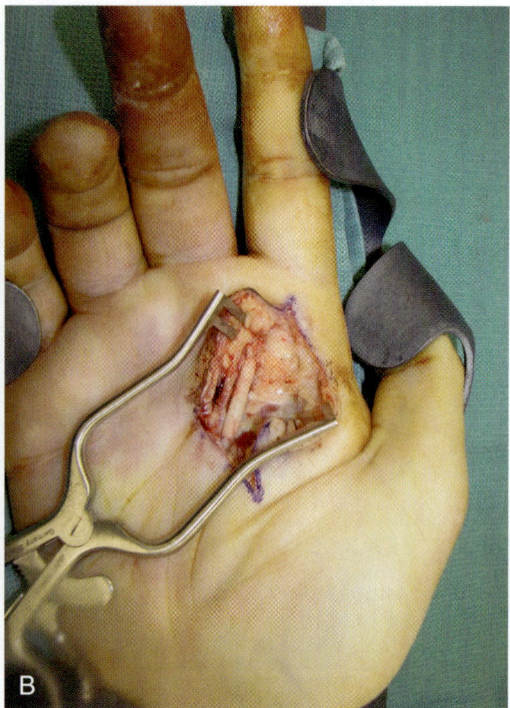

FIGURE 16-11

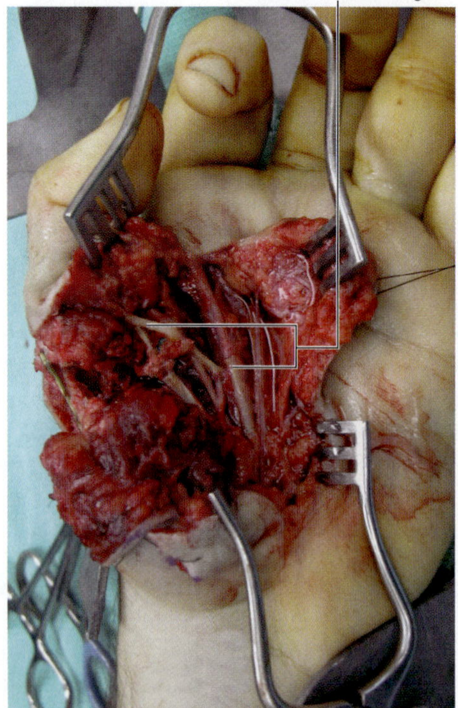

FIGURE 16-12

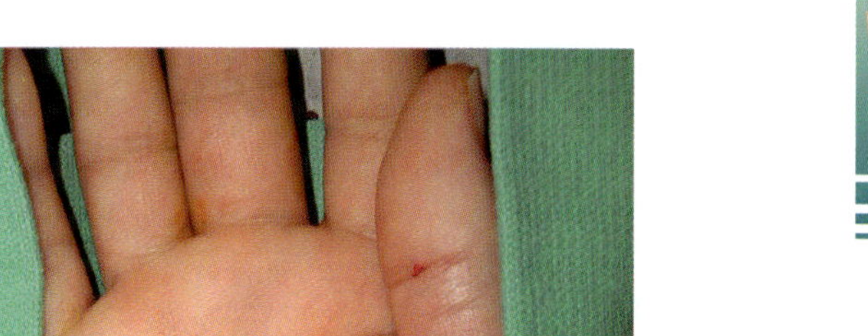

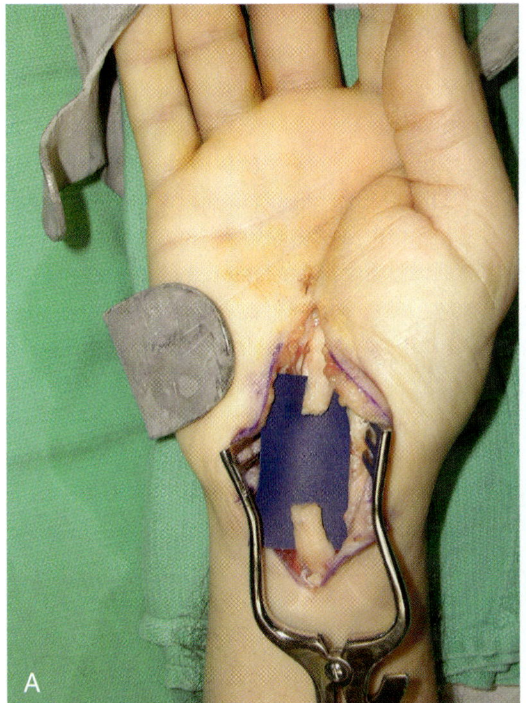

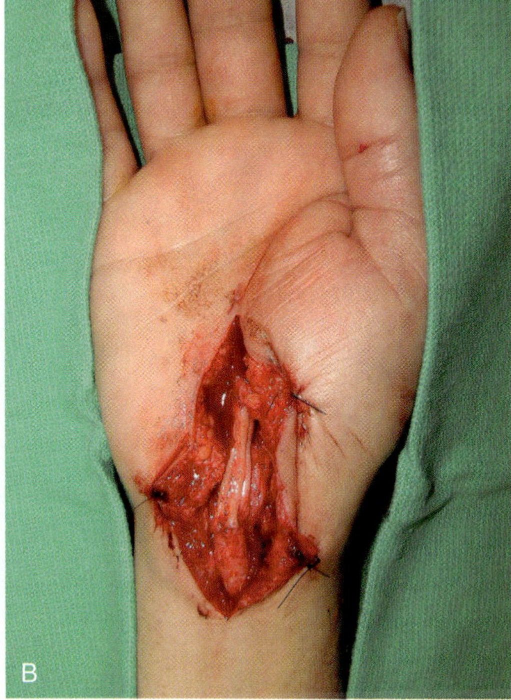

FIGURE 16-13

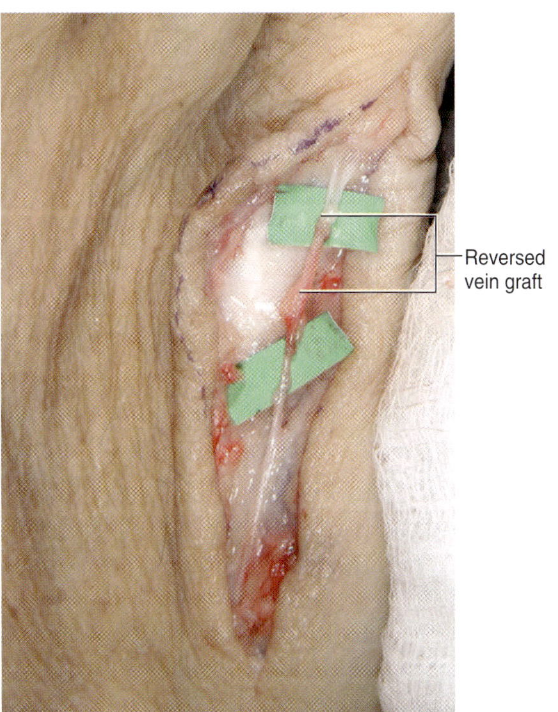

FIGURE 16-14

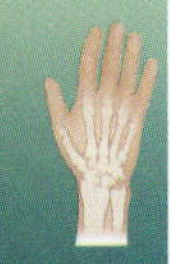

STEP 4 PEARLS

The nerve graft should be handled with care using fine-tipped micro-instruments.

The graft should be 10% to 15% longer than the measured defect.

It is important to mark any one end of the nerve graft (proximal or distal). We feel that it is better to reverse the nerve graft when bridging the defect. This may prevent outgrowth of axons from the branches.

If a vein conduit is being used, it should also be reversed so that the valves do not obstruct axonal growth.

STEP 4 PITFALLS

The graft must be placed in a moist gauze and separated from other gauze pieces so that it is not inadvertently discarded.

STEP 5 PEARLS

The tourniquet time should be minimized and nerve repair done after release of the tourniquet.

We pass a suture in the midline of the back wall first, followed by the far lateral wall, the near lateral wall, and finally the midline anterior wall.

Step 4: Harvest of Nerve Graft

- An appropriate length of nerve graft is harvested from the selected site.
- The tourniquet is released and hemostasis secured at the nerve graft donor site and the recipient site.

Step 5: Suture of Nerve Graft

- Suturing the nerve grafts is done under a microscope.
- A group fascicular repair is done by placing three or four sutures circumferentially. We use 9-0 Ethilon in the fingers and 8.0 Ethilon in the palm.

Step 6: Wound Closure

- The wound is closed with intermittent 5-0 nylon sutures.
- A dorsal splint is provided to maintain the IP joint in neutral position and the MCP joint in 50 to 60 degrees of flexion.

Postoperative Care and Expected Outcomes

- The patient is started on early mobilization within the splint. There should be no tension at the repair site in a nerve graft, and patients can be mobilized early, as opposed to after a primary repair, which would require a longer period of immobilization. The splint can be discontinued after 2 to 3 weeks, and patients are advised to avoid hyperextension for another 2 to 3 weeks.
- More than 90% of patients (<65 years) get S3 or greater sensory recovery after a nerve graft (Fig. 16-15—late postoperative result of patient in Figs. 16-1 and 16-12). This equates to recovery of pain and touch sensation, disappearance of hyperesthesia, and ability to localize stimulus. However, there is imperfect recovery of two-point discrimination.

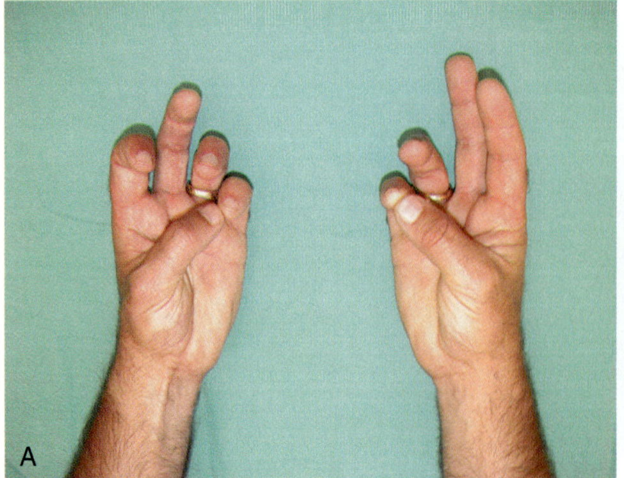

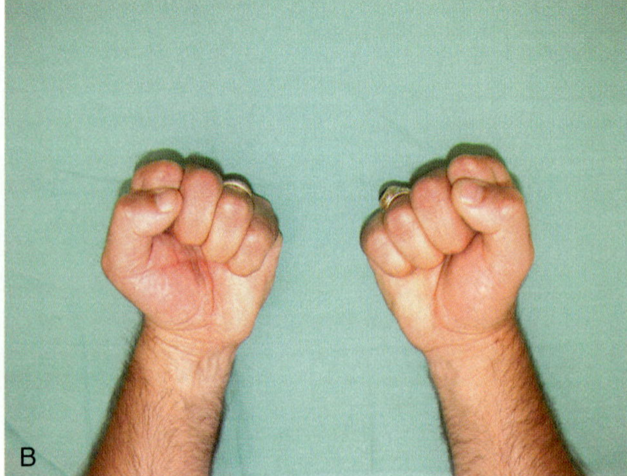

FIGURE 16-15

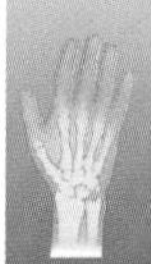

Evidence

Higgins JP, Fisher S, Serletti JM, Orlando GS. Assessment of nerve graft donor sites used for reconstruction of traumatic digital nerve defects. *J Hand Surg [Am]*. 2002;27:286-292.

The authors harvested nerve segments from 10 fresh cadavers. They included the lateral and medial antebrachial cutaneous nerves (LABCN, MABCN), posterior and anterior interosseous nerves (PIN, AIN), and sural nerves. They also harvested segments of the proper and common digital nerves. They analyzed these nerves with regard to the cross-sectional area and the number of fascicles to match the anatomic characteristic of the graft with the recipient digital nerve. According to their analysis, the PIN is best matched by cross-sectional area to the distal proper digital nerve. The LABCN and MABCN are best matched to the proximal proper digital nerve, and the sural nerve is most anatomically similar to the common digital nerve. (Level IV evidence)

Rinker B, Liau JY. A prospective randomized study comparing woven polyglycolic acid and autogenous vein conduits for reconstruction of digital nerve gaps. *J Hand Surg [Am]*. 2011;36:775-781.

The authors performed a randomized controlled study comparing a PGA conduit to a vein graft for digital nerve defects ranging from 4 to 25 mm. They enrolled 42 patients with 76 nerve repairs, and 37 patients with 68 nerve repairs were valuable for follow-up at 6 months and 1 year. They found no statistically significant difference between the two groups with regard to static and moving two-point discrimination. Smoking and workers' compensation patients had a worse sensory recovery. There was no difference in cost between the two procedures. The savings produced by not having a commercial implant in the vein group was almost exactly offset by the expense of the extra operating time necessary for vein harvest. There were two extrusions in the PGA conduit group requiring reoperation. (Level II evidence)

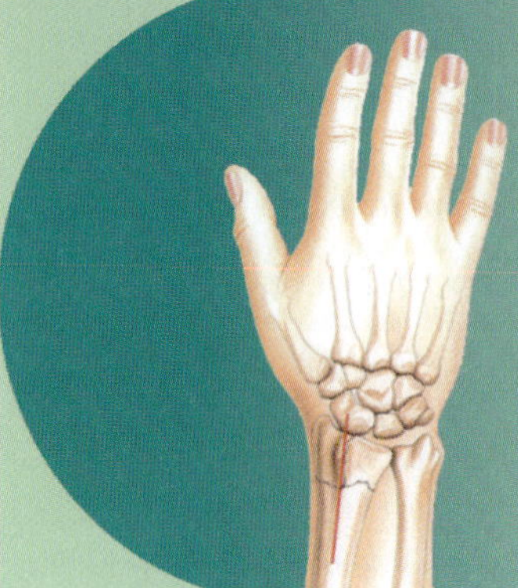

PROCEDURE 17

Surgical Treatment of Neuromas in the Hand

Sandeep J. Sebastin and Kevin C. Chung

Indications

- Neuroma with the following characteristics:
  - Identifiable cause of nerve injury
  - Painful (localized area of tenderness with pain radiating in the distribution of the involved nerve)
  - Associated with functional limitation
  - No improvement with initial conservative treatment (desensitization, taping, massage, ultrasound, transcutaneous electrical nerve stimulation [TENS])
- A neuroma can result from the following:
  - Trauma (unrepaired nerve laceration, blunt crush, and amputation)
  - Iatrogenic (de Quervain release, trigger release, percutaneous pinning of distal radius fractures, poor repair of nerve, and carpal tunnel release)
  - Chronic irritation (bowler's thumb)

Examination/Imaging

Clinical Examination

- Patients may present with pain associated with scar and altered sensation (hypoesthesia, hyperalgesia, or anesthesia). The pain may be spontaneous or result from pressure over the neuroma, movement of adjacent joints, or light touch in the vicinity of the neuroma.
- A painful neuroma by itself is not an indication for surgery. Information regarding the cause of injury, contributing factors (e.g., bowling, method of holding equipment), workers' compensation and litigation issues, and functional status of the patient must be obtained. Patients must also be evaluated for the presence of complex regional pain syndrome.
- The location of the neuroma in relation to any overlying scar and the presence of a Tinel sign must be noted (Fig. 17-1).

Imaging

- No imaging is required.

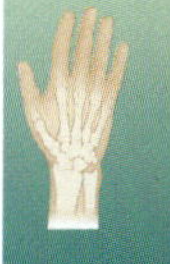

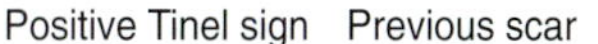

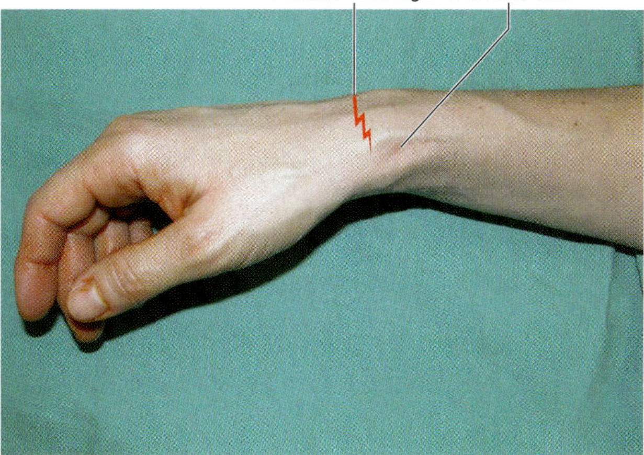

FIGURE 17-1

Surgical Anatomy

- A neuroma of the hand can be an end neuroma or an in-continuity neuroma. End neuromas are frequently associated with digital amputation and involve the proper digital nerves. In-continuity neuromas most often result from poor surgical repair and involve the median and ulnar nerves at the wrist. Both end neuromas and in-continuity neuromas can also result from unrecognized iatrogenic injury (e.g., superficial radial nerve, palmar cutaneous branch of median nerve) or delayed presentation of a partially or completely divided nerve.
- The hand and wrist have been classified into three zones based on the location of the neuroma (Fig. 17-2). Zone I represents the digits and includes neuromas arising from the digital nerves, their dorsal branches, and the terminal branches of the nerves innervating the dorsum of the hand. Zone II represents the body of the hand and includes the common digital nerves, the palmar cutaneous branches of the median nerve, and the palmar and dorsal cutaneous branches of the ulnar nerve. Zone III represents the radial border of the wrist and forearm and includes the superficial radial nerve, the lateral antebrachial cutaneous nerve, the medial antebrachial cutaneous nerve, and the posterior cutaneous nerve of the forearm.
- Although a neuroma can involve any sensory nerve in the hand, the superficial radial nerve is particularly prone to developing a neuroma, and these neuromas are difficult to manage. The nerve becomes subcutaneous about 7 cm proximal to the radial styloid by piercing the fascia between the brachioradialis (BR) and the extensor carpi radialis longus (ECRL) (Fig. 17-3). It is believed that the nerve may be compressed between the tendons of the ECRL and BR. In 3% to 10% of the population, it passes through the tendon of the brachioradialis, tethering it proximally. These factors, combined with its superficial location, may explain the predisposition to iatrogenic injury and neuroma formation.

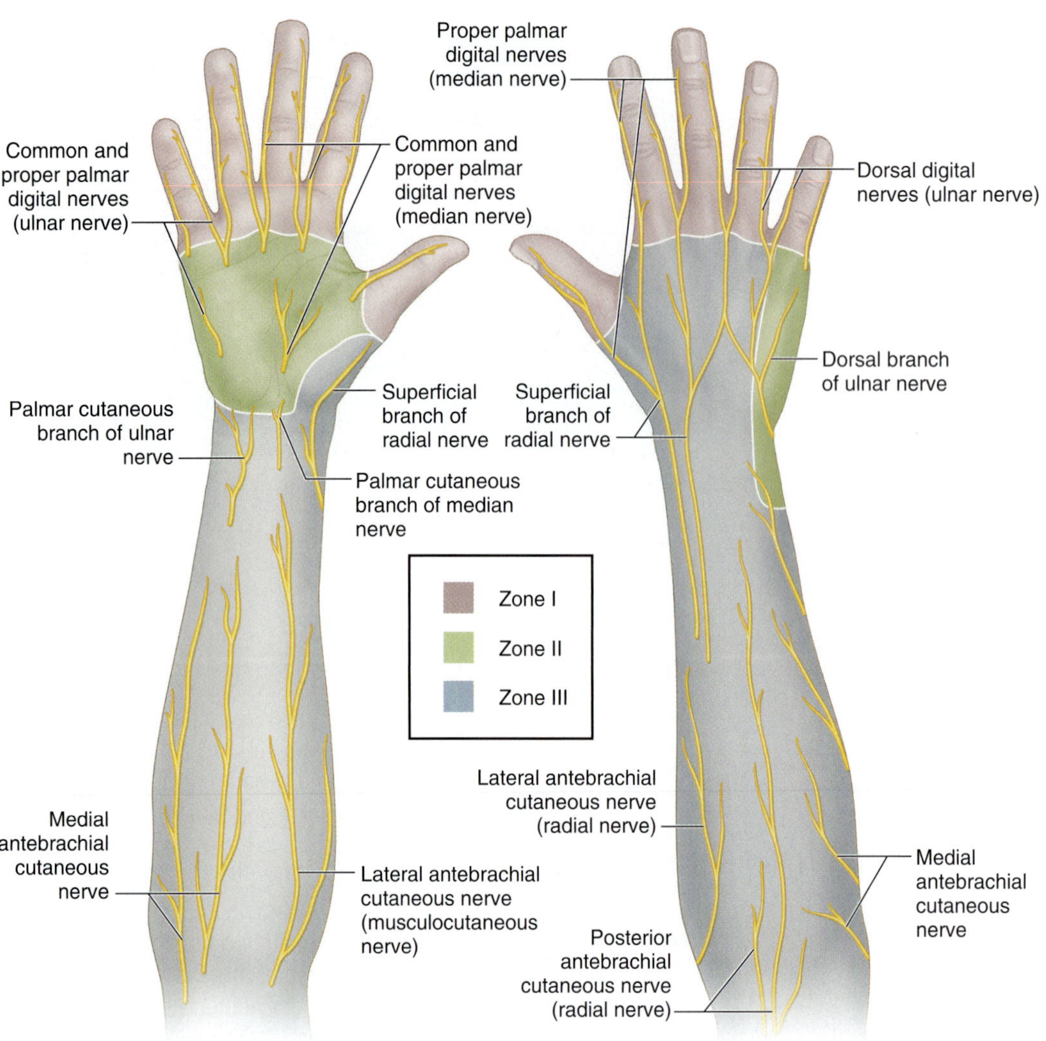
Proper palmar digital nerves (median nerve)
Common and proper palmar digital nerves (ulnar nerve)
Common and proper palmar digital nerves (median nerve)
Dorsal digital nerves (ulnar nerve)
Dorsal branch of ulnar nerve
Palmar cutaneous branch of ulnar nerve
Superficial branch of radial nerve
Superficial branch of radial nerve
Palmar cutaneous branch of median nerve
Zone I
Zone II
Zone III
Lateral antebrachial cutaneous nerve (radial nerve)
Medial antebrachial cutaneous nerve
Lateral antebrachial cutaneous nerve (musculocutaneous nerve)
Medial antebrachial cutaneous nerve
Posterior antebrachial cutaneous nerve (radial nerve)

FIGURE 17-2

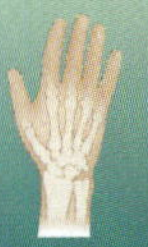

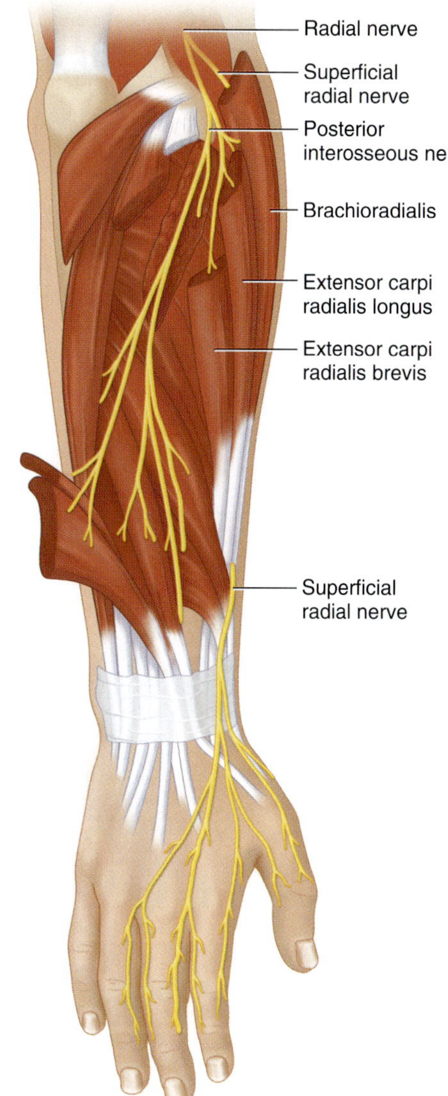

FIGURE 17-3

TREATMENT OPTIONS

- Our surgical treatment of neuromas is based on the availability of an appropriate distal nerve, the local tissue environment, and the anatomic zone of the neuroma.
- If an appropriate distal target is available, we use a nerve graft to bridge the defect caused by resection of the neuroma. If the local tissue environment is not suitable for a nerve graft, we wrap the nerve graft in a vein, an artificial nerve conduit, or a locally transposed fat flap.
- If an appropriate target is not available, we resect the neuroma and relocate the proximal end. The relocation of the proximal end depends on the anatomic zone.
  - In a distal zone I neuroma (distal and middle phalanx), we allow the proximal end to retract proximally into unscarred tissue. In a proximal zone I neuroma (proximal phalanx and distal metacarpal shaft), we bury the neuroma into the metacarpal.
  - In a zone II neuroma, we transpose the end into the pronator quadratus.
  - In a zone III neuroma, we transpose the end into the brachioradialis.
- We have occasionally used the technique of centro-centralization for a digital nerve neuroma. This involves resection of the neuroma and suturing of the digital nerves to each other. Gorkisch and colleagues (1984) suggested dividing one of the digital nerves 5 to 10 mm proximal to the repair site and performing an additional repair. This creates a nerve graft segment and prevents the development of a neuroma at the original nerve repair site (Fig. 17-4).

Positioning

- The procedure is performed under tourniquet control using a 3.0× to 3.5× loupe magnification.
- The patient is positioned supine with the affected extremity on a hand table.
- If a cable nerve graft is anticipated, the leg should be prepped for harvest of a sural nerve graft. It is better to avoid harvesting a nerve graft from the same limb in patients with complex regional pain syndrome, who have preexisting nerve-related pain/paresthesia, because it adds another nociceptive focus.

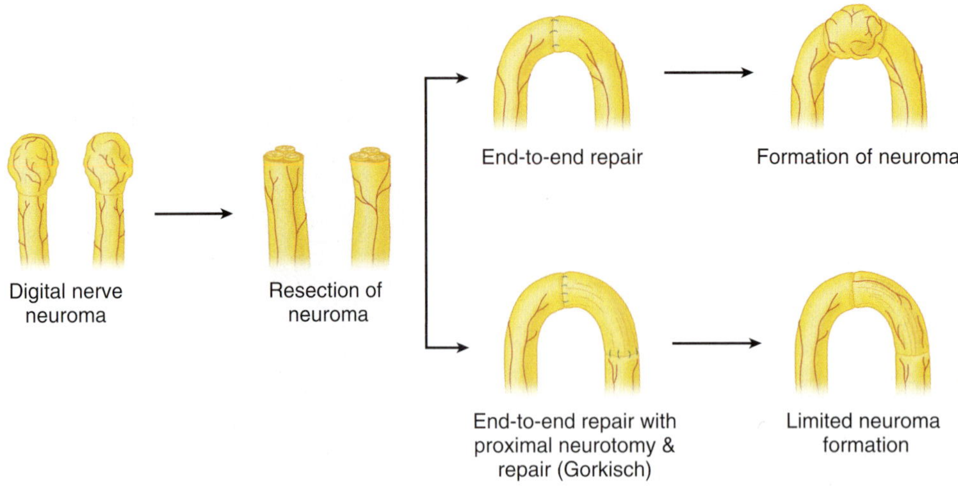

FIGURE 17-4

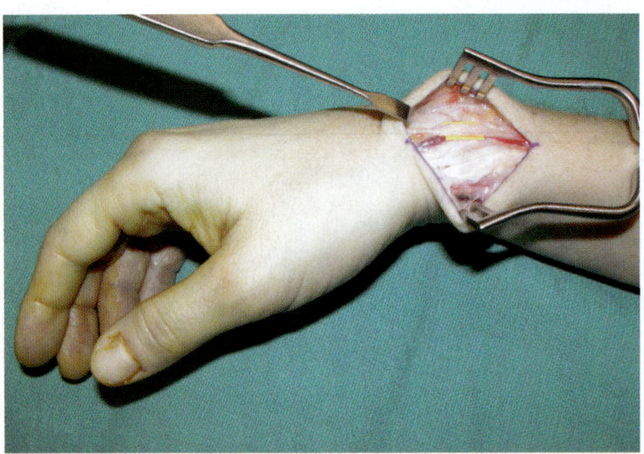

FIGURE 17-5

> **STEP 1 PEARLS**
>
> *The nerve should be identified in normal tissue planes first. Dissecting the nerve through the scar tissue is dangerous and can lead to inadvertent additional nerve injury.*

Procedure

Available Distal Nerve

Step 1

- A 38-year-old woman presented with tenderness over the superficial radial nerve after release of the first dorsal compartment for de Quervain tendovaginitis. The sensory function of the nerve was intact. She had a Tinel sign in the distribution of the superficial radial nerve on percussion of the scar (see Fig. 17-1).
- An incision in line with the previous scar was made and extended proximally and distally (Fig. 17-5).

STEP 2 PEARLS

The nerve should be handled carefully with micro-instruments to prevent further foci of nerve injury.

An internal neurolysis of the superficial radial nerve is not recommended.

STEP 3 PEARLS

We use the adventitial side of the vein graft to cover the nerve. This is believed to bring the adventitial Schwann cells, collagen, and laminin in contact with regenerating axons and provide a better microenvironment for axonal regeneration.

STEP 3 PITFALLS

Care should be taken to ensure that the sutures do not catch the nerve and strangulate some fascicles.

Step 2

- The nerve was dissected free from all surrounding scar tissue (Fig. 17-6). A decision was made to maintain the nerve in continuity because the patient had intact sensory function. It was decided to cover the nerve with a vein graft to improve the local tissue environment and prevent further scarring around the nerve.

Step 3

- A 3- to 4-cm–long vein graft is harvested locally. The graft is split open and wrapped around the scarred area of the nerve using a few interrupted 8-0 Ethilon sutures (Fig. 17-7).

Step 4

- The tourniquet is released and hemostasis secured.
- The nerve is positioned so that it is not directly under the skin incision.
- A local anesthetic agent is infiltrated around the nerve.
- The skin incision is closed in a single layer using 4-0 nylon.
- A bulky dressing is applied.

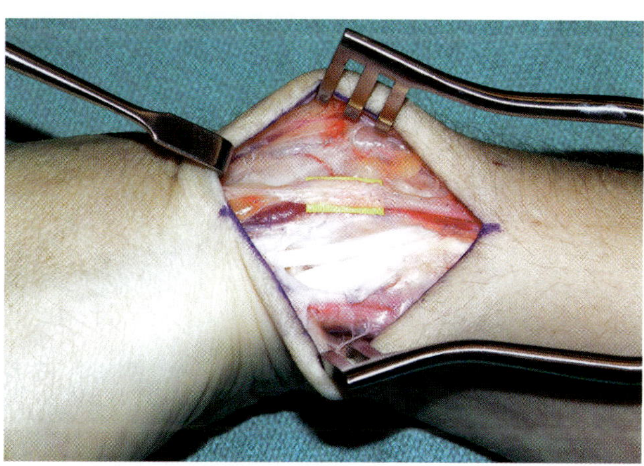

FIGURE 17-6

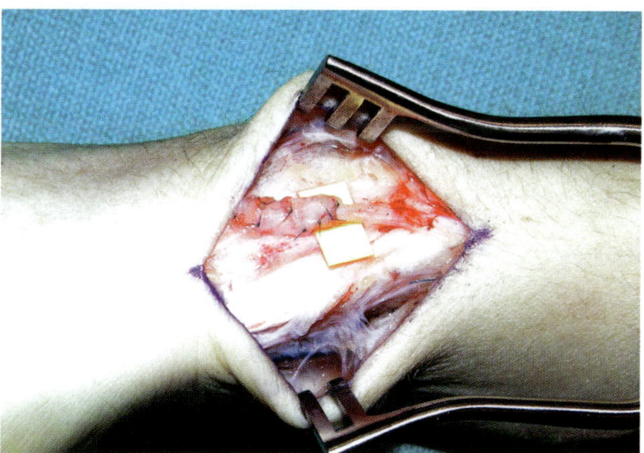

FIGURE 17-7

Procedure

No Distal Nerve Available

Step 1

- A 46-year-old woman presented late with severe burning pain over the superficial radial nerve 3 months after a forearm laceration. The laceration was sutured in the emergency department. On examination, the patient had diminished sensation in the first web, and a Tinel sign was localized to the scar.
- An incision was made over the area of tenderness, and the neuroma of the superficial radial nerve was identified and mobilized (Figs. 17-8 and 17-9).

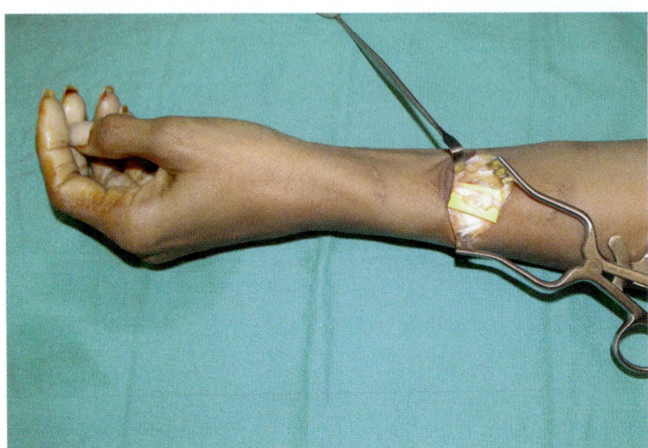

FIGURE 17-8

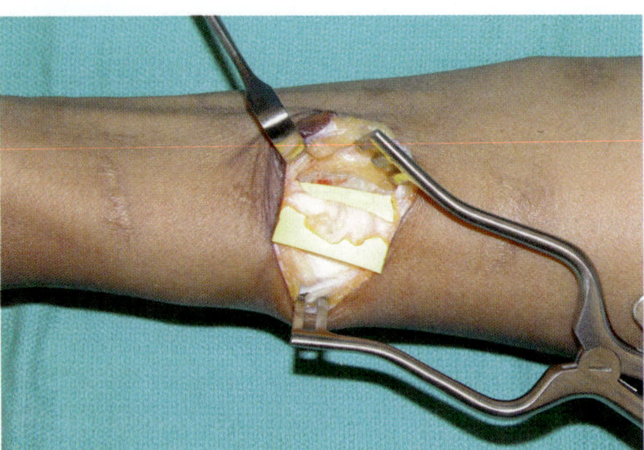

FIGURE 17-9

Step 2

- The neuroma was resected. A decision was made to bury the proximal end under the flexor carpi radialis (FCR). The brachioradialis was not used because it was still tendinous at that location and would have required extension of the incision and more proximal mobilization of the nerve.

Step 3

- The fascicles of the superficial radial nerve were gently separated and sutured to the undersurface of the FCR with a few interrupted 8-0 nylon sutures (Fig. 17-10).
- A single 5-0 Prolene suture was used to suture the nerve to the muscle sheath proximally to reduce the tension on the distal nerve fascicle-muscle suture (Fig. 17-11).

Step 4

- The tourniquet is released and hemostasis secured.
- A local anesthetic agent is infiltrated around the nerve.
- The skin incision is closed in a single layer using 4-0 nylon.
- A bulky dressing is applied.

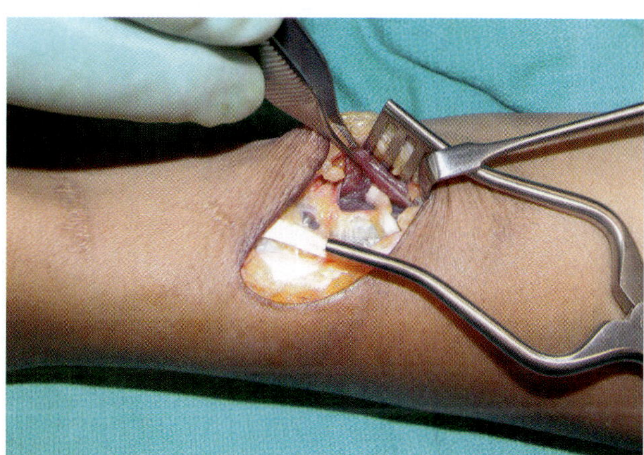

FIGURE 17-10

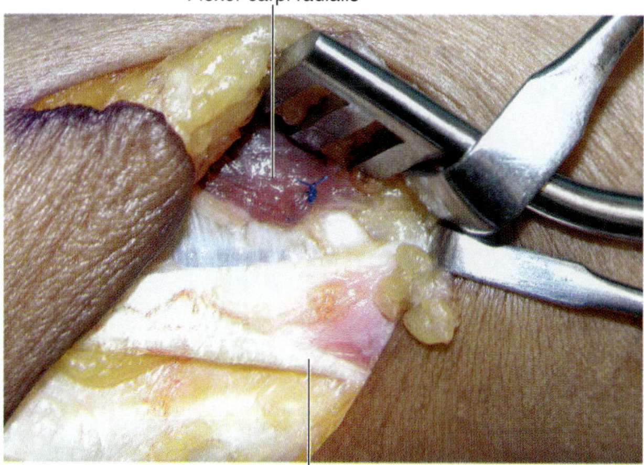

FIGURE 17-11

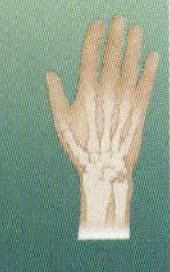

Procedure

Centro-Centralization of a Digital Nerve

Step 1

- A 43-year-old woman presented with pain at the tip of an index finger amputation stump. She had undergone an amputation of the index finger through the middle phalanx following a table saw injury 6 months previously, and her symptoms had not resolved with conservative measures.
- Bilateral midaxial incisions were made and a palmar skin flap elevated (Fig. 17-12).
- The digital nerves were identified in the proximal part of the incision and followed distally to a large neuroma of the radial digital nerve and a smaller neuroma of the ulnar digital nerve (Fig. 17-13).

Step 2

- The ends of the neuroma were resected, and they were sutured to each other using a few 8-0 interrupted Ethilon sutures (Fig. 17-14).

STEP 2 PEARLS

In this case, a proximal division of one of the digital nerves and repair as suggested by Gorkisch and colleagues (1984) was not done because the overlying skin flap was quite thick.

Step 3

- The tourniquet is released and hemostasis secured.
- A local anesthetic agent is infiltrated around the nerve.
- The skin incision is closed in a single layer using 4-0 nylon.
- A bulky dressing is applied.

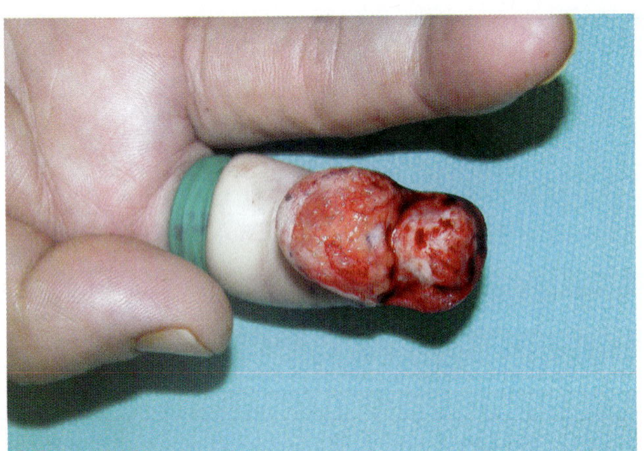

FIGURE 17-12

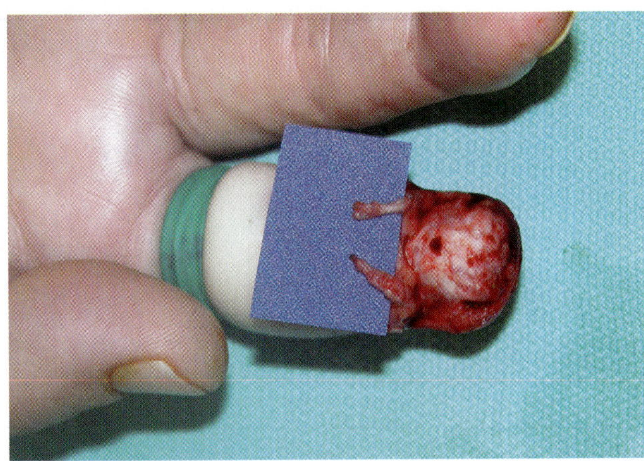

FIGURE 17-13

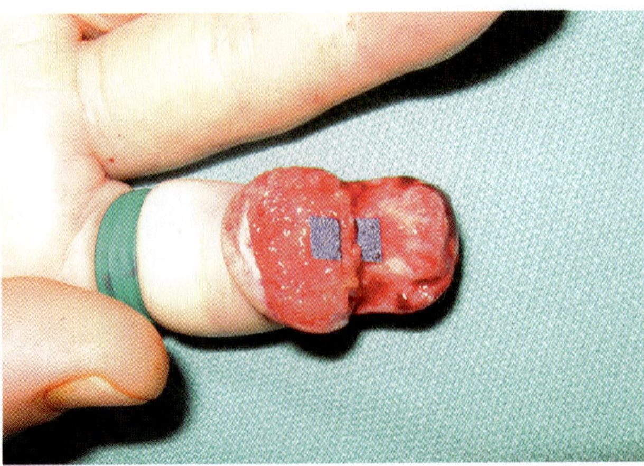

FIGURE 17-14

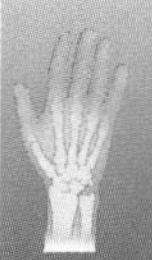

Postoperative Care and Expected Outcomes

- A splint is not applied, and patients are started on early mobilization to allow the nerve to glide within the tissue planes and decrease adhesions. Prevention is the best treatment of neuromas. One should be especially careful when operating in the vicinity of the superficial radial nerve.
- The relocation of neuromas into muscle has given better results compared with burial in bone. Greater than 90% of patients have an improvement in their symptoms.

Evidence

Dellon AL, Mackinnon SE. Treatment of the painful neuroma by neuroma resection and muscle implantation. *Plast Reconstr Surg*. 1986;77:427-438.
The authors describe the procedure of neuroma excision and placement of the proximal end into a muscle. They operated on 78 neuromas in 60 patients and demonstrated good to excellent results in 82% of the patients. The transposition of the nerve into small superficial muscles with significant excursion (abductor pollicis longus and extensor pollicis brevis) resulted in treatment failure. (Level IV evidence)

Gorkisch K, Boese-Landgraf J, Vaubel E. Treatment and prevention of amputation neuromas in hand surgery. *Plast Reconstr Surg*. 1984;73:293-299.
The authors describe the technique of centro-central nerve union with autologous transplantation. They suture the ends of two nerves (or split one nerve into two) after resecting the neuroma. One of the nerves is then divided 5 to 10 mm proximal to the repair site and repaired again creating a nerve segment skin to a nerve graft. The creation of this graft segment prevents the regenerating axons from both nerves meeting at the suture area. Instead they meet in the graft segment. The intact frame of the graft segment prevents the axons growing outward. They conducted studies in an animal model and did electron microscopic studies to prove this. Subsequently they did this procedure on 30 patients, and only one developed a neuroma. (Level IV evidence)

Sood MK, Elliot D. Treatment of painful neuromas of the hand and wrist by relocation into the pronator quadratus. *J Hand Surg [Br]*. 1998;23:214-219.
The authors classified neuromas based on their anatomic location into zones I, II, and III. They reported on 13 neuromas in 10 patients. These neuromas were present in the palm and dorsum of the hand (zone II). They were resected and relocated into the pronator quadratus muscle. All 10 patients had marked improvement in pain. (Level IV evidence)

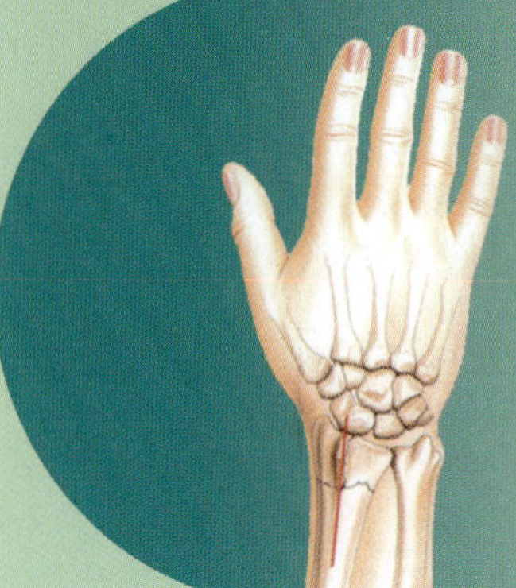

Tendon Transfers for Carpal Tunnel Syndrome

Sandeep J. Sebastin and Kevin C. Chung

See Video 14: Tendon Transfer for Anterior Interosseous Nerve Palsy (FDS to FPL)

Indications

- Severe carpal tunnel syndrome (CTS) with thenar atrophy and inability to abduct or oppose the thumb
- Failed nerve recovery after repair/reconstruction of the median nerve
- Hansen disease (leprosy)
- Neurologic disorders (for example, Charcot-Marie-Tooth disease, syringomyelia)
- Congenital differences

Examination/Imaging

Clinical Examination

- *Sensation:* It is important to document the level of sensation in the thumb and fingers preoperatively. Patients may also have diminished sensation in the ulnar nerve distribution. The potential functional benefit of a tendon transfer will be diminished in a patient with sensory loss, and these patients must be counseled about the likely poorer outcome after surgery.
- *Joints:* To get a good result from the tendon transfer, patients must have good passive range of motion at the thumb metacarpophalangeal (MCP) joint and the thumb carpometacarpal (CMC) joint. It is not uncommon for patients to have basal joint arthritis with a supination and adduction deformity of the thumb and first web-space contracture. This should be addressed before a tendon transfer is considered.
- *Motor:* Many motors have been described for opponensplasty. Our first preference is the palmaris longus (PL) followed by the extensor indicis proprius (EIP), if the PL is absent. We rarely use the flexor digitorum superficialis (FDS) of the ring finger because of the greater morbidity (weakening the power grip, risk for proximal interphalangeal [PIP] joint flexion contracture, swan-neck deformity) and because the soft tissue pulley attenuates over time. Although the tension fraction of PL (1.2%) and EIP (1%) is theoretically less than the combined tension fraction of abductor pollicis brevis (APB) (1.1%) and opponens pollicis (OP) (1.9%), the transfer only needs enough strength to position the thumb in abduction.

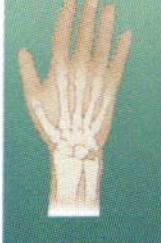

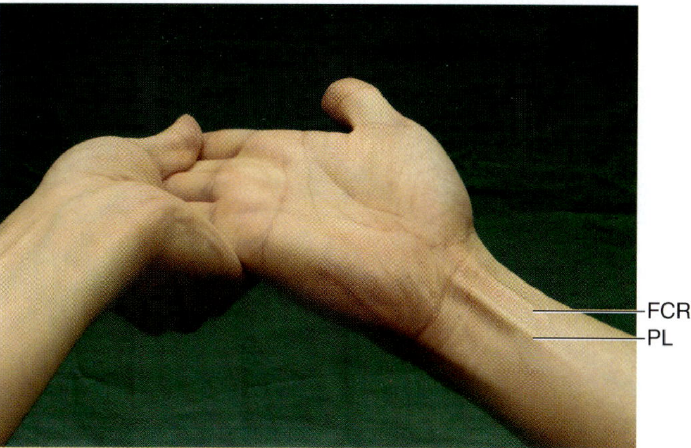

FIGURE 18-1

- The transfer of the PL (Camitz transfer) is typically performed for an elderly patient with CTS and severe thenar atrophy. The Camitz transfer is considered a "freebie" procedure because the incision used for CTS can be extended to the wrist in a zigzag fashion to obtain the PL augmented by the palmar fascia to attach into the ABP insertion at the radial MCP joint. As with any freebie procedure, however, the direction of tendon pull is not in line with the APB muscle but rather is more parallel to the forearm, which does diminish the biomechanical construct of this tendon transfer procedure. For an elderly patient with modest functional requirements, this transfer does serve the purpose of restoring some abduction and will permit the patient to recover acceptable thumb function.
- We use the test described by Mishra to determine the presence of the PL. The traditional test described by Schaeffer requires the patient to abduct and oppose the thumb to the small finger and flex the wrist. A patient with thenar atrophy will find it difficult to do so. The Mishra test is performed by holding the patient's wrist and fingers in hyperextension, while asking the patient to flex the wrist. This stretches the palmar aponeurosis and makes the PL taut when the patient attempts wrist flexion (Fig. 18-1).

Imaging

- X-ray of the hand to look for basal joint arthritis
- Nerve conduction studies

Surgical Anatomy

- Thumb opposition is a complex movement produced by a combination of flexion, palmar abduction, and pronation and requires participation of both the MCP and CMC joints. The prime muscle of thumb opposition is believed to be the APB with contributions from the OP and flexor pollicis brevis (FPB).
- The muscles affected after low median nerve palsy are the APB, OP, superficial head (radial head) of the FPB, and the radial two lumbricals (first and second). The first three muscles are innervated by the recurrent motor branch of the median nerve, whereas the latter two are innervated by the first and second common palmar digital nerve branch of the median nerve.

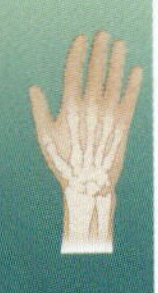

PEARLS

The palmar portion of the incision can follow the interthenar crease for a more aesthetic scar.

The zigzag at the wrist crease should have its apex directed ulnarly to prevent injury to the palmar cutaneous branch of the median nerve.

PITFALLS

The palmar cutaneous branch of the median nerve should be identified immediately ulnar to the flexor carpi radialis and radial to the PL tendon in the distal forearm.

- Reasonable thumb abduction and opposition may be retained after isolated median nerve injury or severe carpal tunnel syndrome as a result of preserved ulnar nerve function (retained innervation of the deep head of the FPB and variability in thenar muscle innervation by connection between the ulnar and median nerves). Figure 18-2 shows the preoperative appearance of the hand with severe CST on the right. Note the thenar atrophy and inability to palmarly abduct the right thumb.
- The midpalmar portion of the palmar aponeurosis has three layers: superficial longitudinal fibers, deeper transverse fibers, and deepest vertical fibers. Only the superficial longitudinal fascia is obtained in continuity with the PL to maximize the length of this tendon to reach the APB insertion.

Positioning

- The procedure is performed under tourniquet control. It is usually performed under sedation and local anesthesia because this procedure is rather expedient and there is no need to take unnecessary anesthetic risk in elderly patients. The patient is positioned supine with the affected extremity on a hand table.

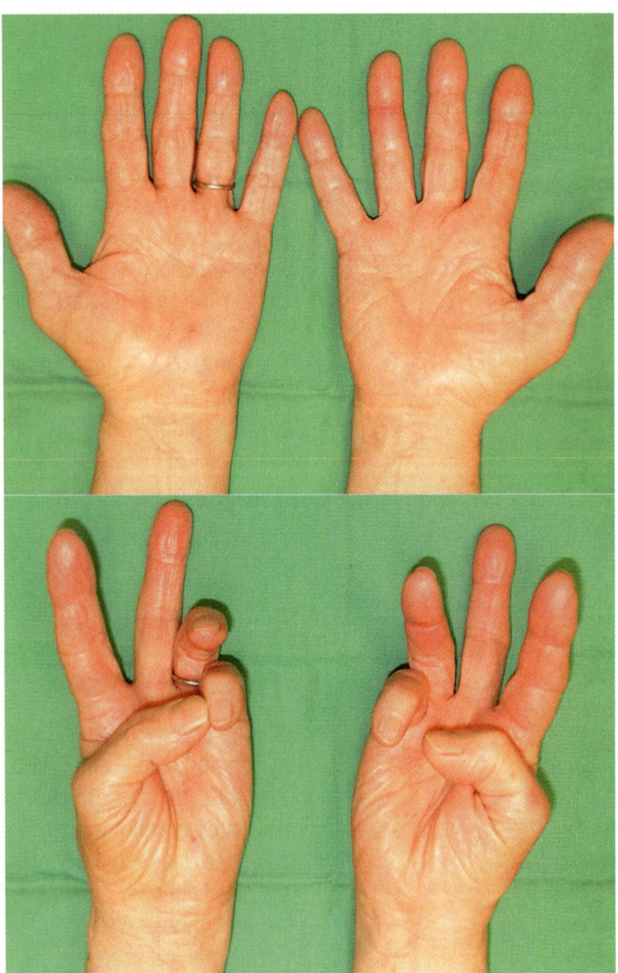

FIGURE 18-2

Exposures

- An incision is made in line with the third web space extending from 1 cm proximal to the proximal palmar crease to a point 2 cm proximal to the wrist crease (Fig. 18-3).
- The incision is extended in a zigzag fashion at the wrist crease.
- The skin and subcutaneous tissue are dissected sharply with a no. 15 knife blade to expose the tendon of the PL in the distal forearm and the palmar aponeurosis in the palm (Fig. 18-4).
- A second 2-cm longitudinal chevron-shaped incision is made over the dorsoradial aspect of the thumb MCP joint.
- The skin and subcutaneous tissue are dissected free to expose the tendon of the APB.

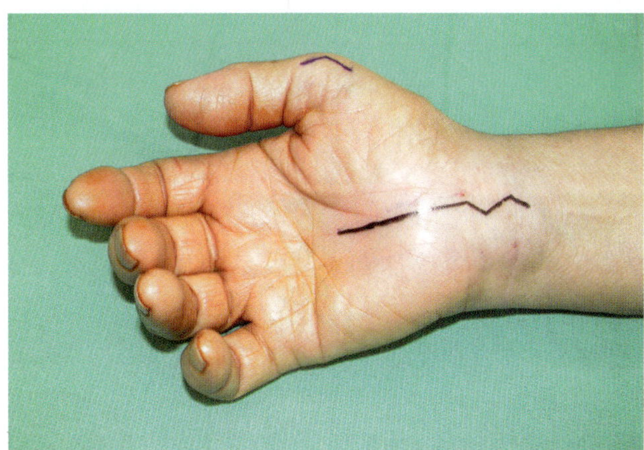

FIGURE 18-3

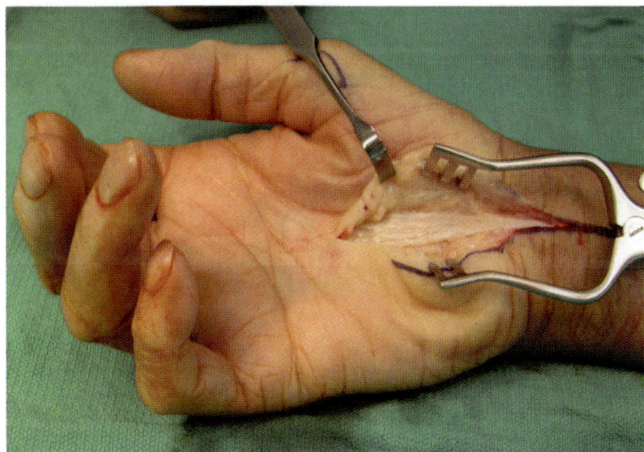

FIGURE 18-4

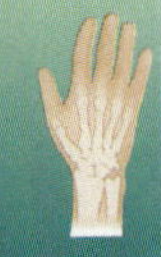

STEP 1 PEARLS

Identify the digital neurovascular bundles in the palm distal to the superficial transverse palmar ligament (thickening of the transverse fibers of the palmar aponeurosis between the proximal and distal palmar creases).

The previously marked segment of the palmar aponeurosis can be elevated in the plane superficial to the neurovascular bundle. This plane lies between the deeper vertical fibers of the palmar aponeurosis and the superficial transverse and longitudinal fibers.

It is better to elevate a longer and wider strip of palmar aponeurosis than what is required.

STEP 1 PITFALLS

Elevating a structurally intact strip of palmar aponeurosis is the most challenging aspect of this procedure, and attention must be paid to maintaining the integrity of the palmar aponeurosis while protecting the underlying neurovascular structures.

Many small perforating vessels pass through the aponeurosis to supply the overlying soft tissue. They must be carefully cauterized to prevent postoperative hematoma.

STEP 2 PEARLS

The distal tendon of the PL lies superficial to the antebrachial fascia, whereas the proximal tendon and muscle are deep to the antebrachial fascia. The attachments of the tendon to the antebrachial fascia must be released to permit free movement of the tendon (Fig. 18-7).

STEP 2 PITFALLS

One must be aware of the palmar cutaneous branch of the median nerve that lies radial to the PL and the median nerve deep to the PL.

Procedure

Step 1

- A 1- to 1.5-cm–wide strip of palmar aponeurosis is marked out and elevated from distal to proximal by maintaining continuity with the palmaris longus tendon over the carpal tunnel (Fig. 18-5).

Step 2

- The strip of palmar aponeurosis and contiguous PL tendon are pulled distally and freed from any tissue in the forearm that restricts movement of the PL (Fig. 18-6).

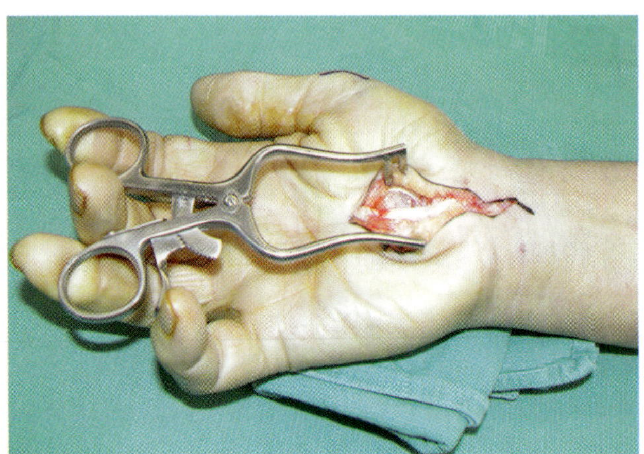

FIGURE 18-5

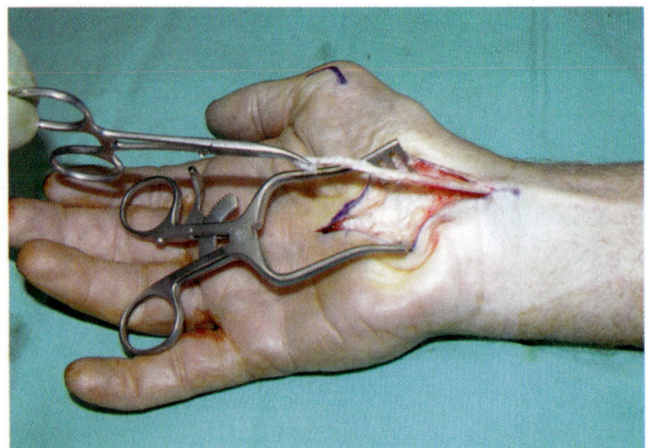

FIGURE 18-6

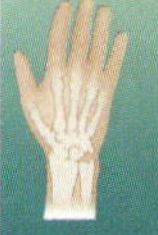

STEP 4 PEARLS

It is better to have the proximal end of the tunnel in the distal forearm rather than the wrist crease to obtain a straight line of pull.

STEP 4 PITFALLS

The palmar cutaneous branch of the median nerve should be protected when the tunnel is created. The tunnel should be made in a plane deeper to the nerve in the distal forearm.

STEP 5 PEARLS

A grasping suture can be passed through the distal end of the palmar aponeurosis and left long before tunneling. The hemostat can hold the suture instead of the aponeurosis to minimize injury to the aponeurosis. The length of the suture will also allow retrieval of the tendon, should it inadvertently slip back into the tunnel.

Maintain the tendon hemostat until the aponeurosis is sutured to the APB.

STEP 5 PITFALLS

The length of the palmar aponeurosis extension is usually just enough to reach the thumb MCP joint (see Fig. 18-7). The aponeurosis is easily frayed, and one should handle it with care to make a strong repair possible.

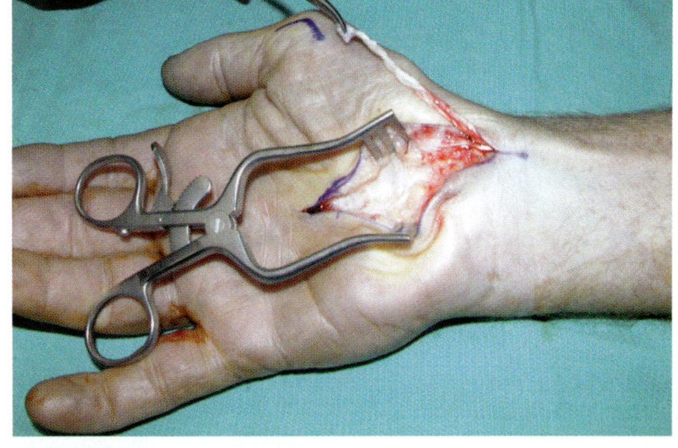

FIGURE 18-7

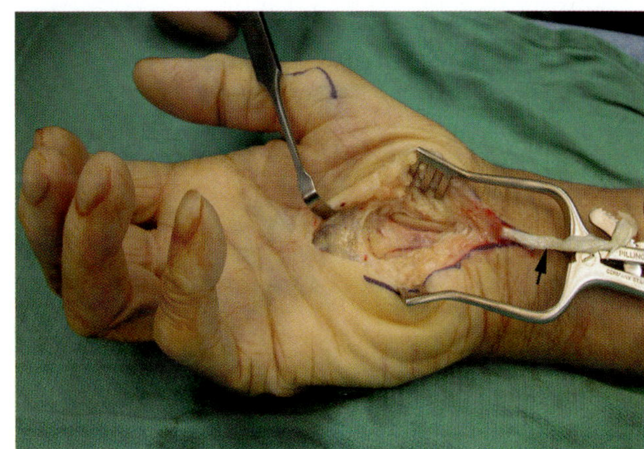

FIGURE 18-8

Step 3

- A complete release of the carpal tunnel is carried out by dividing the transverse carpal ligament (Fig. 18-8).

Step 4

- A wide subcutaneous tunnel is created between the thumb MCP joint incision and the distal forearm incision.

Step 5

- A hemostat passed from the thumb MCP joint through the subcutaneous tunnel is used to grasp the palmar aponeurosis extension of the PL and to bring it out from the thumb incision.

Step 6

- The tourniquet is released, hemostasis is secured, and the wound is closed with nylon sutures.

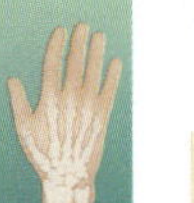

STEP 7 PEARLS

Alternate insertion sites for opponensplasty include (1) a dual insertion on the APB and the dorsal capsule to stabilize the MCP joint passively in addition to providing opposition and (2) an insertion on the dorsoulnar aspect of the MCP joint to provide pronation by an insertion onto the extensor pollicis brevis (EPB). We believe that a dual insertion may not serve a dual function and that the transfer will predominantly act on the tighter insertion. Also, pronation occurs passively with thumb abduction. We therefore prefer a simple APB insertion in isolated low median nerve palsy.

It should be sutured with enough tension so that the thumb can be maintained in full palmar abduction with the wrist in neutral position after the assistant is no longer maintaining the position (Fig. 18-9). A single preliminary suture can be placed to determine whether the tension is appropriate.

Check the effect of wrist tenodesis on thumb abduction with the single suture in situ to determine whether the repair is too tight or too loose. When the tension has been set correctly, one should be able to place the thumb in the plane of the hand with the wrist flexed, and the thumb should be in full palmar abduction with slight flexion of the wrist. Setting of tension is an admirable goal, but the length of this tendon is barely sufficient to reach the ABP insertion. This situation is similar to EIP transfer in that it is unnecessary to be precise in setting the tension because the tension is already set by the just-enough length of the transferred tendon to reach the ABP insertion.

STEP 7 PITFALLS

Do not lift the tendons toward you when doing the first suture. This will result in a lax repair once the tendon drops into its natural position.

STEP 8 PITFALLS

Ensure that the branches of the superficial radial nerve are not caught in the tendon repair or the skin closure.

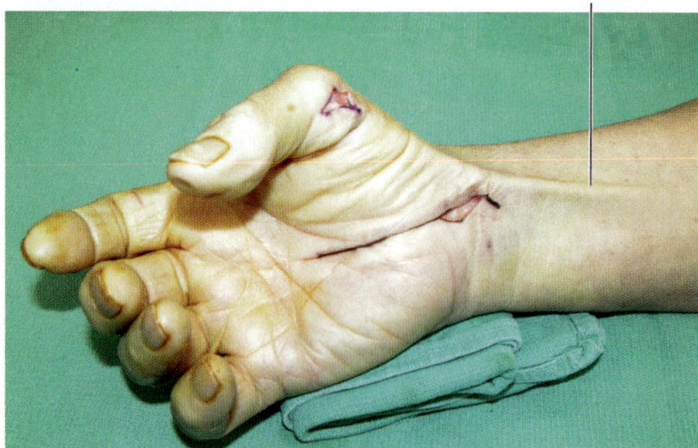

FIGURE 18-9

Step 7

- With an assistant holding the wrist in neutral position and the thumb in full palmar abduction, the palmar aponeurosis is weaved through the tendon of the APB and sutured to itself and the APB using 4-0 Ethibond sutures.

Step 8

- The incisions over the distal forearm and thumb MCP joint are closed, with the assistant maintaining the wrist in neutral position and the thumb in full palmar abduction.

Postoperative Care and Expected Outcomes

- A thumb spica splint that maintains the thumb in full palmar abduction and the wrist in flexion is applied postoperatively. Ten days after surgery, the wound is inspected, sutures are removed, and the position is maintained using a removable thumb spica splint that the patient will wear for another 3 weeks (provided that the patient is reliable in keeping the splint on at all times, except in the daily cleaning of the hand). Thereafter, the patient is encouraged to move the thumb and is started on gradual strengthening exercises. A protective removable splint is also provided for night wear and general protection for the next 4 weeks. The protective splint is discontinued 2 months after surgery, and the patient is allowed unrestricted activity.
- The PL transfer (Camitz transfer) restores palmar abduction and is not a true opponensplasty. It gives good results in severe CTS because the patients may regain some opposition over time as a result of carpal tunnel release. It is usually not recommended for traumatic median nerve palsy when the PL is divided or scarred. Most authors have reported more than 90% restoration of thumb abduction with a Camitz transfer in severe CTS.

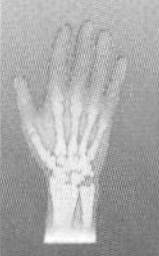

Evidence

Braun RM. Palmaris longus tendon transfer for augmentation of the thenar musculature in low median palsy. *J Hand Surg [Am]*. 1978;3:488-491.
A retrospective review of 28 cases of palmaris longus transfer for restoring thumb abduction in patients with carpal tunnel syndrome, thenar muscle injury, and median nerve injury. The author reported good function in all 28 cases. (Level IV evidence)

Foucher G, Malizos C, Sammut D, et al. Primary palmaris longus transfer as an opponensplasty in carpal tunnel release: a series of 73 cases. *J Hand Surg [Br]*. 1991;16:56-60.
A retrospective review of 73 cases of Camitz transfers performed for severe carpal tunnel syndrome. The authors reported good results in 93% of PL transfers inserted into the APB tendon and in 87% inserted into the dorsal capsule or EPB tendon. However, there was a greater loss of thumb MCP extension when the insertion was into the dorsal capsule or EPB tendon. Eight percent of APB insertions lost 10 to 15 degrees of thumb MCP extension, whereas 20% of capsule/EPB insertions lost 15 to 25 degrees of extension. Other complications included dystrophic reactions in 3 of 73 cases and 1 case of radial translation of the transfer that led to a loss of thumb abduction. (Level IV evidence)

Terrono AL, Rose JH, Mulroy J, Millender LH. Camitz palmaris longus abductorplasty for severe thenar atrophy secondary to carpal tunnel syndrome. *J Hand Surg [Am]*. 1993;18:204-206.
A retrospective review of 29 cases of Camitz transfer for severe carpal tunnel syndrome. The authors reported a 94% satisfaction rate after PL abductorplasty. Thumb function improved in 27 of 29 cases, and the authors stated that formal hand therapy was unnecessary. (Level IV evidence)

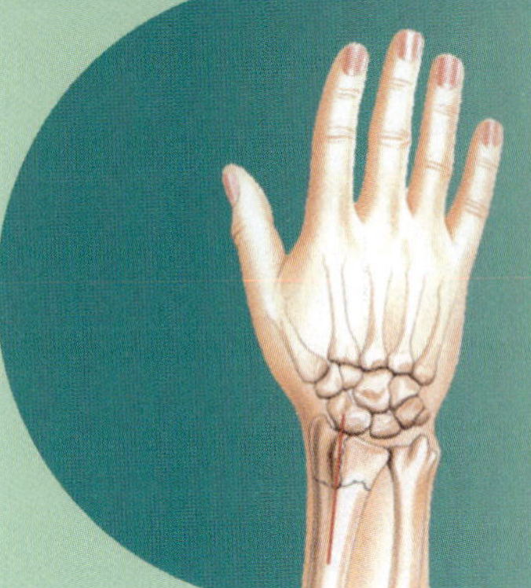

PROCEDURE 19

Tendon Transfers for Ulnar Nerve Palsy

Sandeep J. Sebastin and Kevin C. Chung

See Video 15: Tendon Transfers for High Median and Ulnar Nerve Palsy

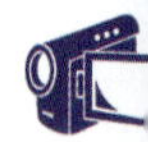

Indications

- Delayed presentation (>1 year) of an ulnar nerve laceration
- Failed motor recovery after repair/reconstruction of the ulnar nerve
- Failed motor recovery after release of ulnar nerve compression at Guyon canal or cubital tunnel
- Persistent motor weakness after completion of drug therapy in Hansen disease (leprosy)
- Neurologic disorders (for example, Charcot-Marie-Tooth disease, syringomyelia)

Examination/Imaging

Clinical Examination

- *Functional deficit:* The loss of function in ulnar nerve palsy results from the claw deformity, which causes an abnormal pattern of finger flexion, weak thumb key pinch, small finger abduction deformity, and loss of ring and small finger distal interphalangeal (DIP) joint flexion (Fig. 19-1). However, these problems may not be functionally disabling in all patients, and some may require correction of only

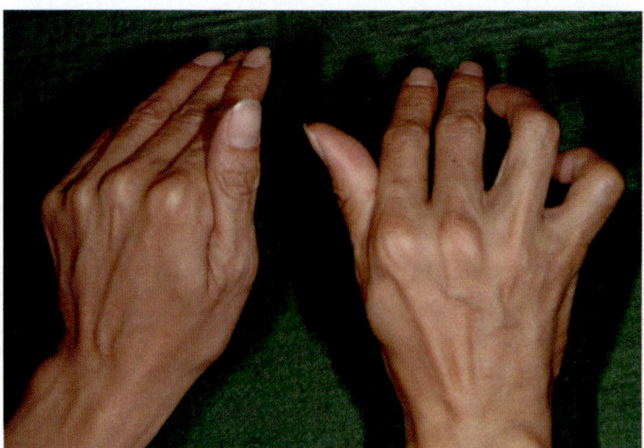

FIGURE 19-1

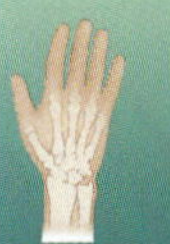

one aspect. It is important to determine this and then to set a sequence for the appropriate corrective procedures. It is better to correct the lack of DIP joint flexion first, followed by transfers for restoring thumb key pinch, and finally correction of the claw deformity because it is difficult to establish appropriate intrinsic plus posture of the hand.

- *Claw deformity (Duchenne sign):* This is the characteristic resting posture of the ring and small fingers with hyperextension of the metacarpophalangeal (MCP) joints and flexion of the interphalangeal (IP) joint. It results from the unopposed action of the radial nerve–innervated long extensors at the MCP joint (hyperextension) and median nerve–innervated flexor digitorum superficialis at the proximal interphalangeal (PIP) joint (flexion) in the presence of paralyzed ulnar nerve–innervated interosseous muscles and the third and fourth lumbricals that normally flex the MCP joint and extend the PIP joint. The MCP joint hyperextension deformity may not appear immediately after an ulnar nerve injury and depends on the laxity of the MCP joint volar plate. The deformity is more pronounced in patients with a lax volar plate and develops over time in patients with a taut volar plate.
  - In a high ulnar palsy, the deformity appears less severe because the flexor digitorum profundus to the ring and small fingers (innervated by the ulnar nerve) is paralyzed and the patient has no claw at the DIP joint (ulnar nerve paradox). Therefore, the increase in severity of a claw deformity after repair of a high ulnar nerve injury is a good prognostic sign and indicates reinnervation of the ring and small finger flexor digitorum profundus (FDP) (Fig. 19-2).
  - A claw deformity results in an abnormal pattern of finger flexion because the IP joint flexes before the MCP joint. In a normal hand trying to grasp an object, the MCP joint flexes first (intrinsic action), followed by the long flexors (IP joint) to wrap the hand around the object. In ulnar nerve paralysis, the IP joint flexes before the MCP joint, which pushes the object out of the hand (Fig. 19-3).

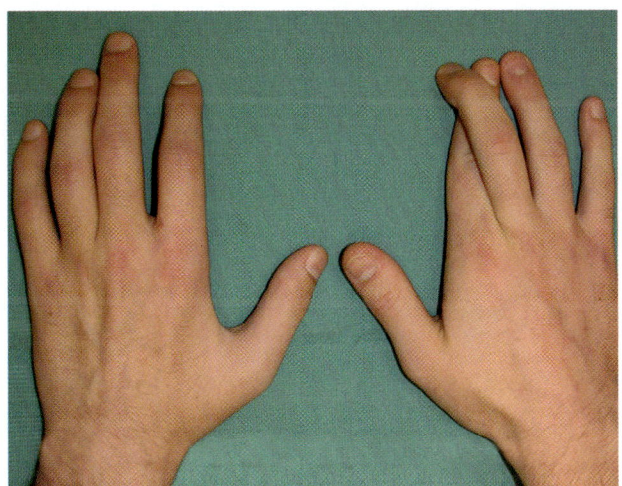

Appearance 3 months after repair of ulnar and median nerve lacerations in the midarm. Note absence of claw deformity

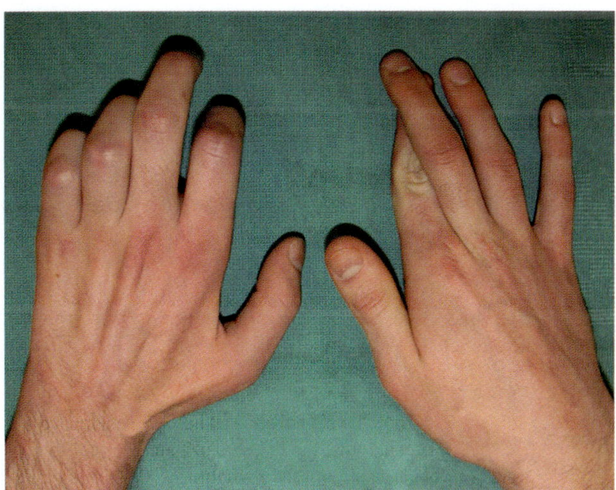

Appearance at 9 months showing deformity following recovery of long flexors. Note guttering in intermetacarpal space due to interosseous muscle wasting

FIGURE 19-2

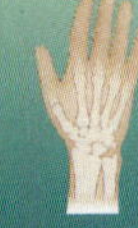

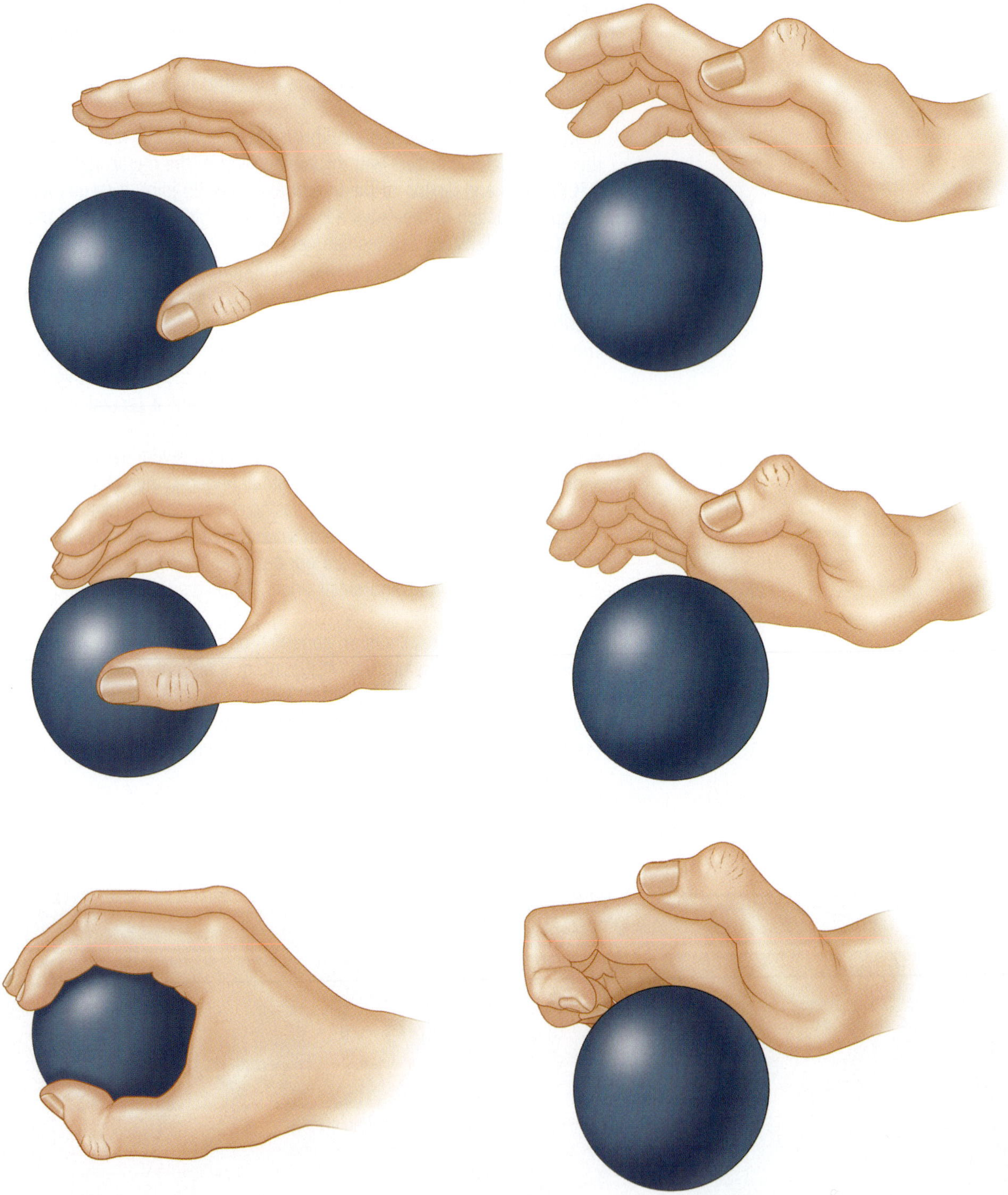

FIGURE 19-3

- In an ulnar nerve palsy, the claw deformity usually involves only the ring and small fingers because the median nerve–innervated first and second lumbricals retain their function. In Hansen disease (leprosy) and lacerated wounds involving both nerves, the patient may have clawing of all four fingers.

- *Weak thumb key pinch:* This results from paralysis of the ulnar nerve–innervated adductor pollicis and first dorsal interosseous. In addition to the obvious muscle wasting in the first web space, a positive Froment sign demonstrates the muscle deficit. The patient is asked to pinch sheets of paper between the thumb and index finger of both hands. A positive Froment sign is indicated by marked thumb IP joint flexion in the affected hand as a result of the patient using the median nerve–innervated flexor pollicis longus to hold the sheet of paper, rather than using the adductor pollicis (Fig. 19-4).
- *Small finger abduction deformity (Wartenberg sign):* The small finger is abducted at rest, and putting the hand into a pocket can become difficult. This deformity results from unopposed action of the radial nerve–innervated extensor digitorum minimi (EDM) in the presence of the paralyzed ulnar nerve–innervated third palmar interosseous muscle that normally adducts the small finger. EDM causes abduction of the small finger in addition to extension because it has an insertion on the ulnar aspect of the base of the proximal phalanx (Fig. 19-5).

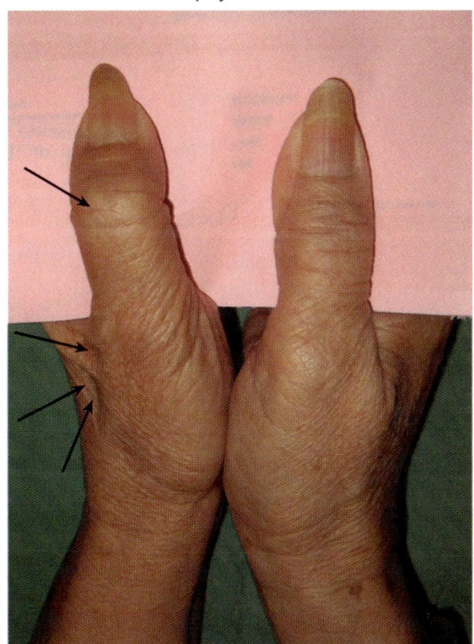

FIGURE 19-4

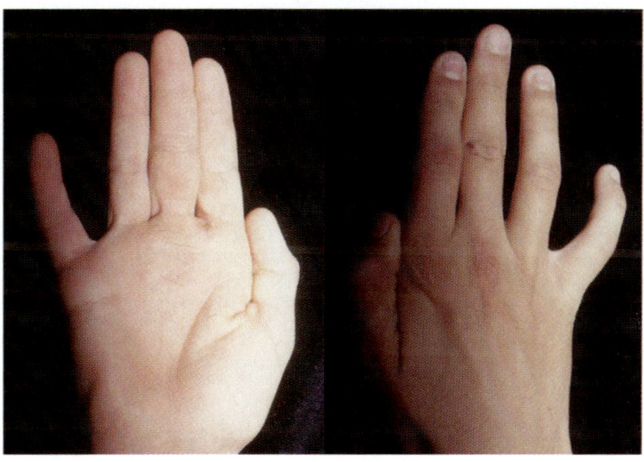

FIGURE 19-5

- *Loss of small and ring finger DIP joint flexion (Pollock sign):* This is seen in high ulnar nerve palsy with loss of innervation to the FDP of the ring and small fingers. The flexor digitorum superficialis (FDS) and the FDP of the index and long fingers are innervated by the median nerve (Fig. 19-6).
- *Sensation:* It is important to document the level of sensation in the thumb and the fingers preoperatively. Loss of sensation on the dorsoulnar aspect of the hand, which is innervated by the dorsal branch of ulnar nerve, can help differentiate a high ulnar nerve lesion (e.g., cubital tunnel compression) from a low ulnar nerve lesion (e.g., Guyon canal compression), which should have preserved sensation over the dorsal-ulnar hand (Fig. 19-7).

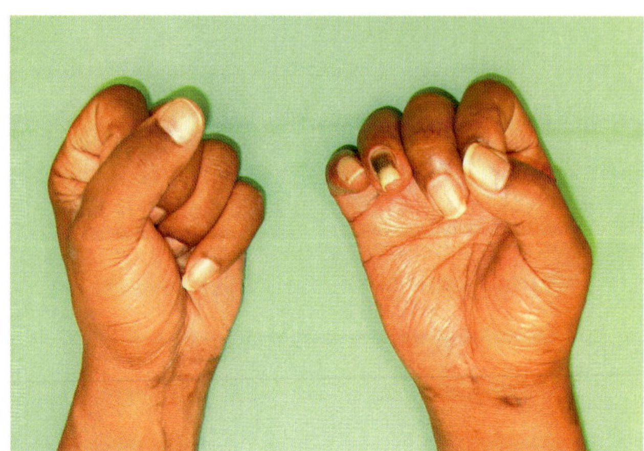

FIGURE 19-6

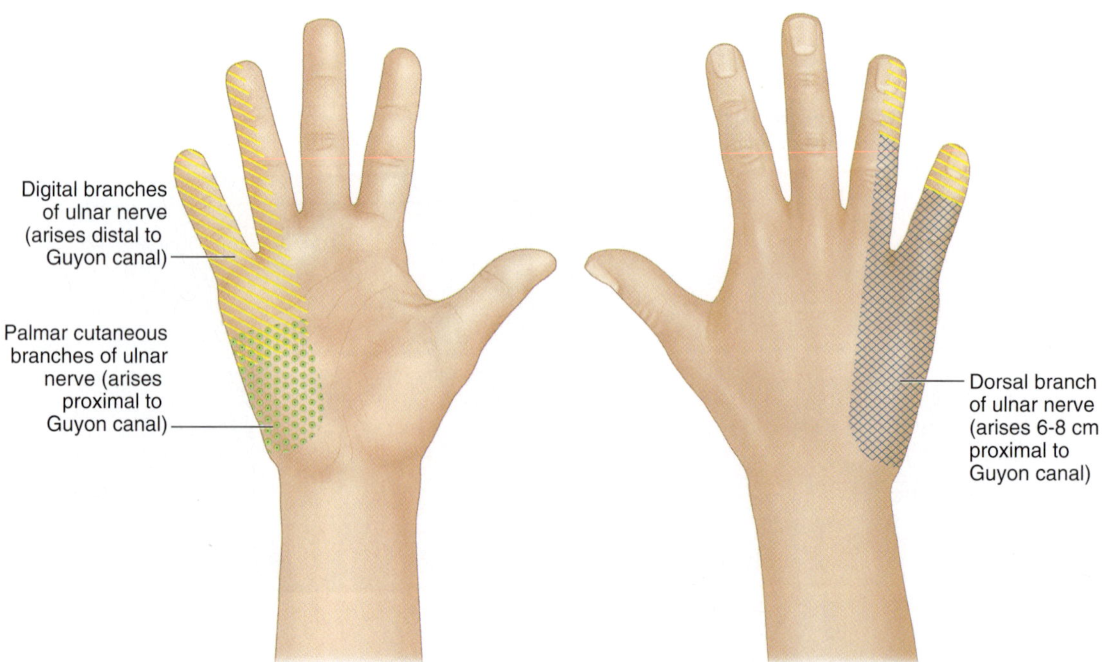

FIGURE 19-7

- *Joints:* To achieve a good result from the tendon transfer, patients must have good passive range of motion at the IP and the MCP joints. The most important aspect of assessment of an ulnar nerve palsy is determining whether the patient can extend the PIP joint with the examiner correcting the MCP joint hyperextension (Bouvier maneuver) (Fig. 19-8).
  - *Full active PIP joint extension:* This indicates that the extensor mechanism is competent (Fig. 19-8A). This patient only needs correction of the MCP joint hyperextension and can use the intact extensor mechanism to obtain PIP joint extension. A static or a dynamic procedure will suffice for this patient. A static procedure is preferred because it is simpler.
  - *Incomplete active PIP joint extension with full passive extension:* This indicates that the PIP joint is competent but that the extensor mechanism is incompetent (Fig. 19-8B and C). This patient will need a dynamic transfer, which is described later, to extend the PIP joint through the lateral band.
  - *Incomplete active and passive PIP joint extension:* This indicates that there is a flexion contracture of the PIP joint (e.g., palmar skin shortage, stiff PIP joint) that needs to be addressed before any tendon transfers are considered (Fig. 19-8D).

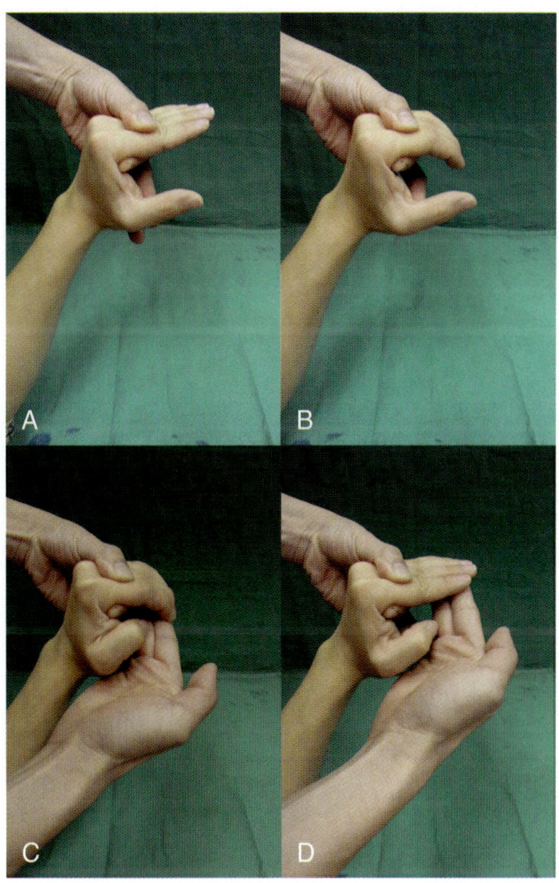

FIGURE 19-8

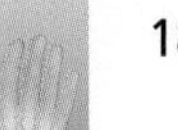

- *Selection of motor:* We use a static procedure (MCP joint volar plate advancement) for correction of the claw deformity in patients who are able to achieve full active extension of the PIP joint. In patients unable to achieve full PIP joint extension, we use a dynamic transfer and prefer the long or ring finger FDS as a motor. We prefer to use the ring finger FDS in low ulnar nerve palsy because the FDS is important for chuck grip, which is predominantly a function of the thumb and index and long fingers. In patients with high ulnar nerve palsy with a weak or absent FDP to the ring finger, the FDS remains the only flexor of the ring finger, and it is prudent to use the long finger FDS. Other motors that have been described include the extensor indicis proprius (EIP) and EDM (both have insufficient length, resulting in excessive tension of the extensor apparatus), wrist flexors (flexor carpi radialis [FCR], palmaris longus [PL]), and wrist extensors (extensor carpi radialis longus [ECRL], extensor carpi radialis brevis [ECRB]). (All need a tendon graft.) We use the ECRB lengthened with a PL tendon graft as the motor for restoring thumb pinch. Other motors that have been described include the brachioradialis, ECRL, extensor carpi ulnaris (ECU), EIP, and FDS.

Imaging

- X-ray of the hand to examine the MCP and PIP joints
- X-ray of the elbow (Fig. 19-9)
- Nerve conduction studies

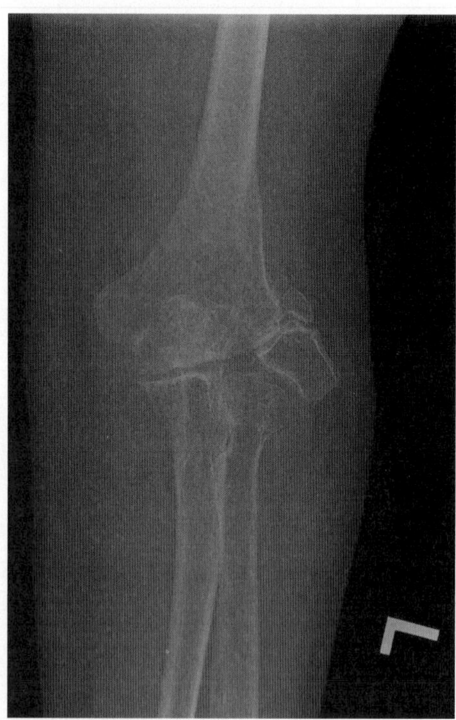

FIGURE 19-9

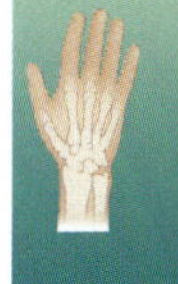

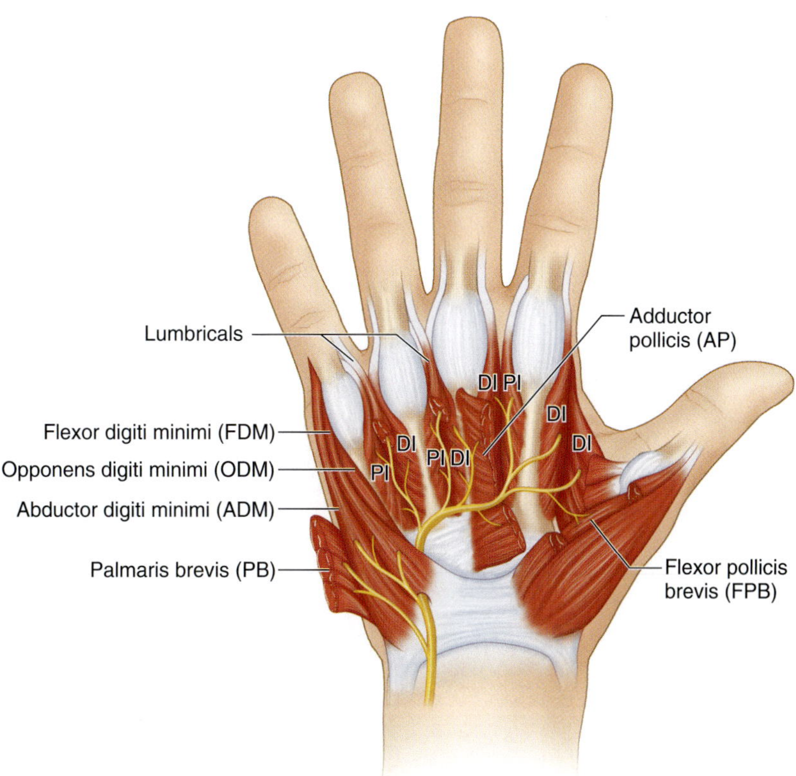

FIGURE 19-10

Surgical Anatomy

- The muscles affected after low ulnar nerve palsy are the four hypothenar muscles (abductor digitorum minimus [ADM], flexor digitorum minimus [FDM], opponens digitorum minimus [ODM], and palmaris brevis [PB]), seven interossei muscles (four dorsal and three palmar), third and fourth lumbricals, and two thenar muscles (adductor pollicis [AP] and the deep head of the flexor pollicis brevis [FPB]). All these muscles are innervated by the deep motor branch of the ulnar nerve (Fig. 19-10).
- In high ulnar nerve palsy, the flexor carpi ulnaris (FCU) and the ulnar half of the FDP (ring and small fingers) are affected in addition to the muscles listed earlier.

Positioning

- The procedure is performed under tourniquet control.
- The patient is positioned supine with the affected extremity on a hand table.

PEARLS

Two longitudinal incisions in line with the ring and small fingers will give better exposure, whereas a transverse incision is more aesthetic.

PITFALLS

Keeping the soft tissue dissection in line with the metacarpal shaft will avoid injury to the neurovascular bundles.

Procedure 1—Static Correction of Claw Deformity with an MCP Joint Volar Plate Advancement

Exposures

- A 3-cm transverse incision is made in line with the distal palmar crease overlying the ring and small finger MCP joints (Fig.19-11A and B).
- The skin and subcutaneous fat are dissected, and common digital neurovascular bundles are identified and protected.
- The flexor tendon sheaths of the ring and small fingers are identified, and the A1 pulley is exposed (Fig. 19-12).

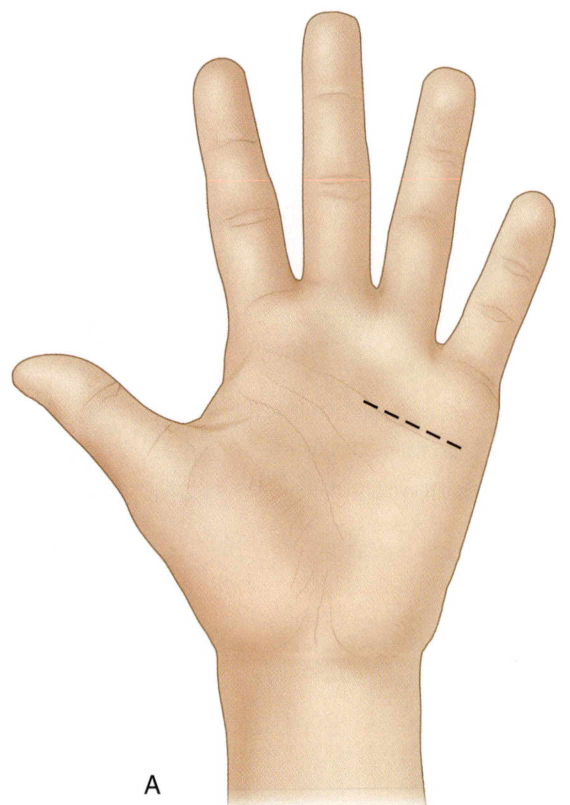

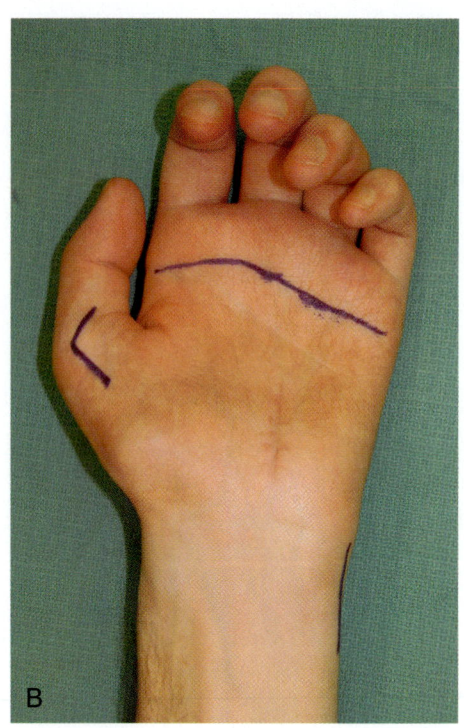

FIGURE 19-11

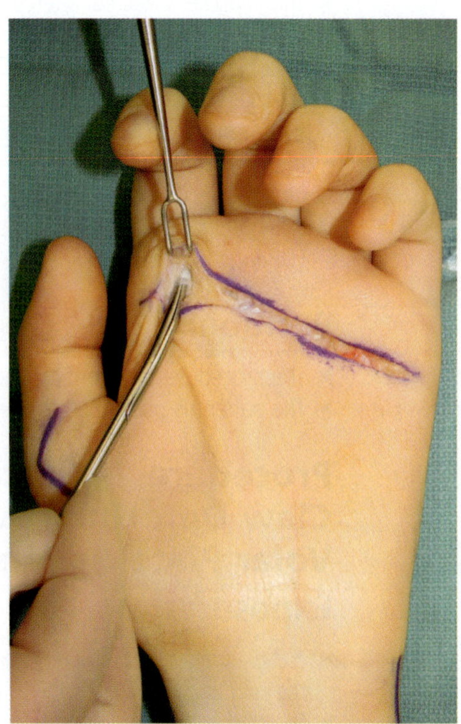

FIGURE 19-12

STEP 1 PITFALLS

Take care not to extend the pulley division to the A2 pulley.

Procedure

Step 1

- The A1 pulley of each finger is completely divided and the flexor tendons retracted to expose the volar plate of the MCP joint (Fig. 19-13).

Step 2

- The neck of the metacarpal (immediately proximal to the volar plate) is cleared of soft tissue, including periosteum.

Step 3

- A distally based flap of the volar plate is created by making two parallel longitudinal incisions and releasing the proximal attachment over the head of the metacarpal (Fig. 19-14A and B).

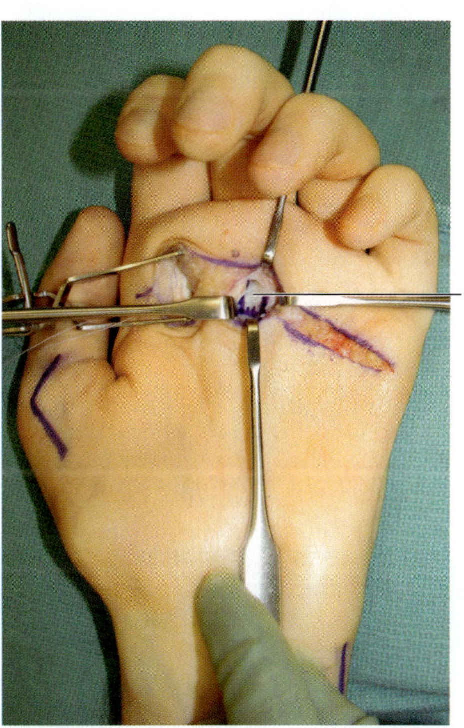

FIGURE 19-13

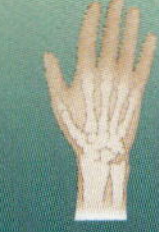

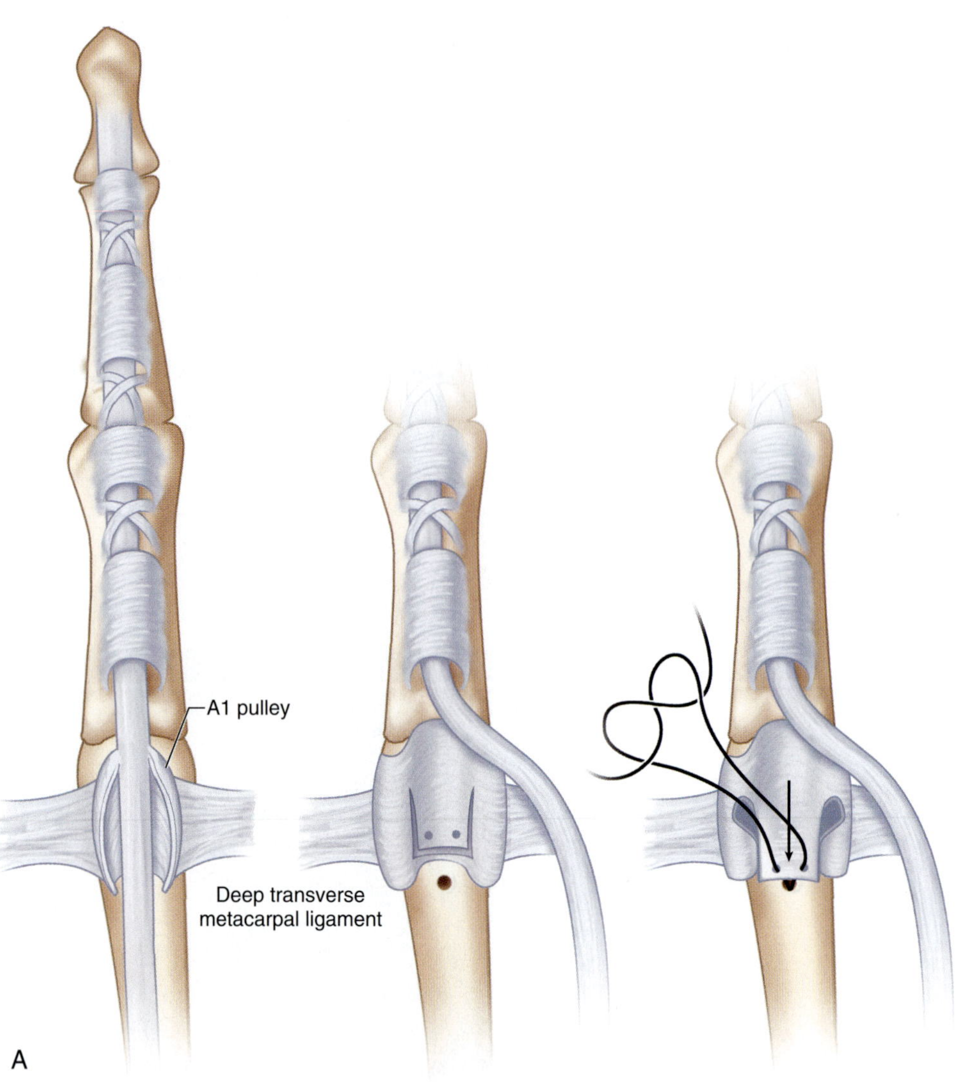
A1 pulley
Deep transverse metacarpal ligament
A

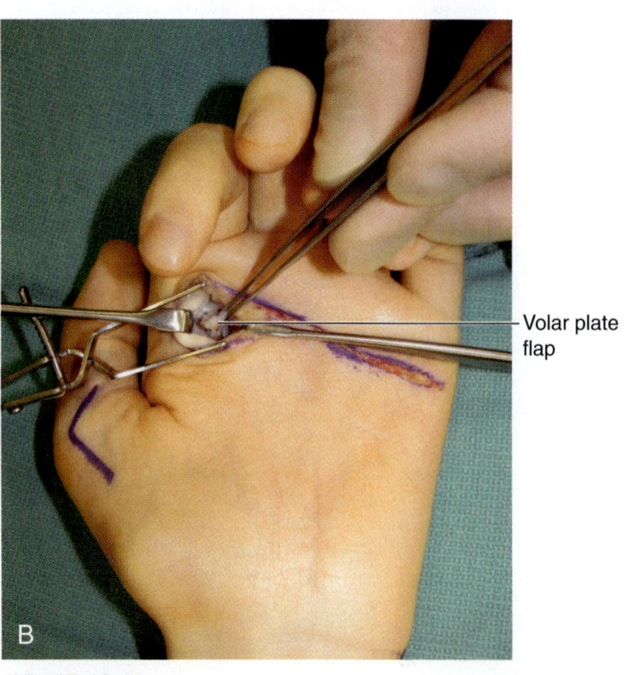
Volar plate flap
B

FIGURE 19-14

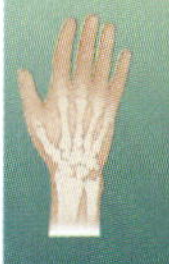

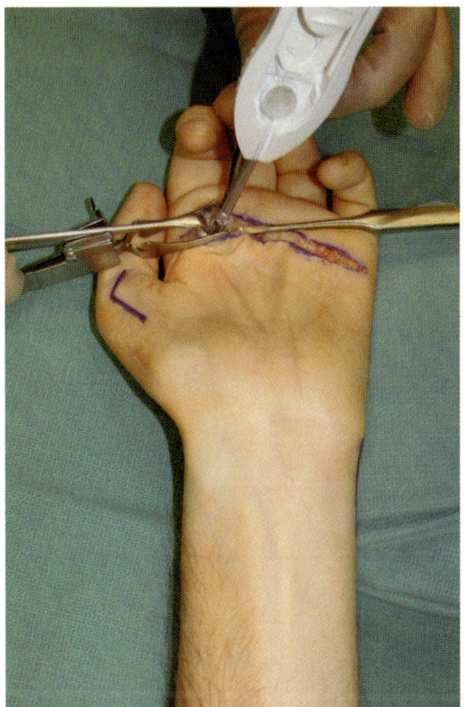

FIGURE 19-15

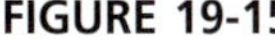

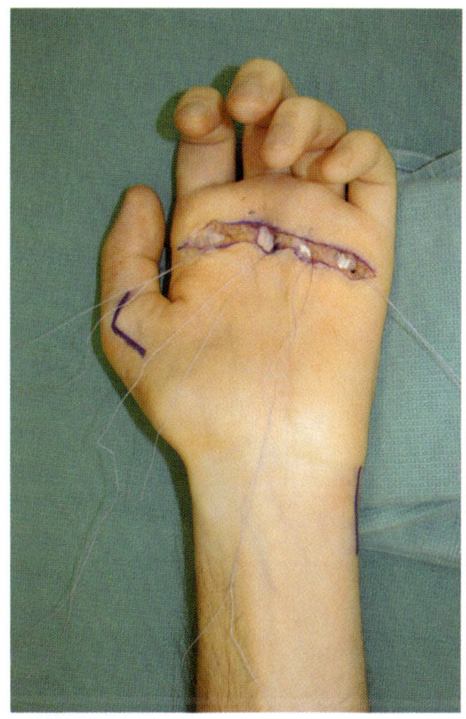

FIGURE 19-16

STEP 4 PEARLS

It is better to create a wide flap.

STEP 4 PITFALLS

Care must be taken not to detach the base of the volar plate flap from the base of the proximal phalanx.

STEP 5 PEARLS

It is better to pass the sutures for all the fingers through the volar plate and tie them at the end instead of completing one finger and then proceeding to the next (Fig. 19-16). Passing the suture through the volar plate requires significant retraction, and an adjacent flexed finger will hinder this.

The suture must hold a good bite of the thick portion of the volar plate.

Step 4

- A mini-Mitek bone anchor suture is inserted on the palmar surface of the neck of the metacarpal (Fig. 19-15).

Step 5

- The bone anchor sutures are passed through the proximal end of the flap and tied down.

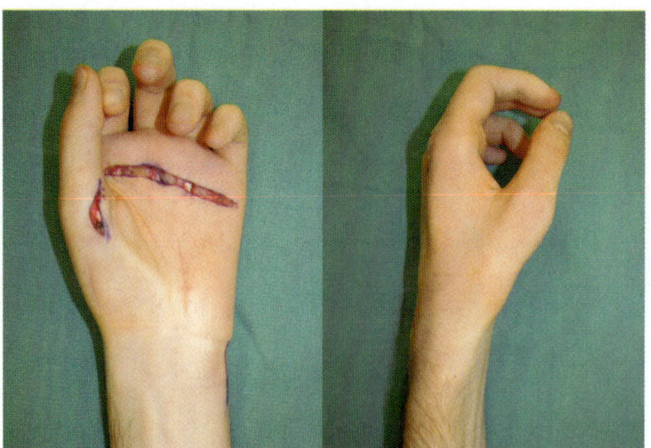

FIGURE 19-17

Step 6

- The wrist is maintained in a neutral position, and the ring finger capsular flap is sutured down to the neck of the metacarpal using the bone anchor sutures such that the MCP joint is flexed to about 45 to 50 degrees. The ring finger MCP joint should have slightly greater flexion compared with the long finger (Fig. 19-17).
- The small finger flap is sutured next to obtain 50 to 55 degrees of MCP joint flexion and should be slightly more in comparison to the ring finger.

STEP 6 PEARLS

The amount of MCP joint flexion required to produce full PIP joint extension preoperatively can guide the surgeon regarding the degree of MCP joint flexion required intraoperatively.

Some authors recommend excising a 1.5-cm ellipse of skin (dermodesis) to prevent stretching the volar plate and overcorrecting the deformity.

Postoperative Care and Expected Outcomes

- The hand is splinted with the wrist in neutral and the MCP joint in 50 to 60 degrees of flexion. The IP joints are left free to move.
- Ten days after surgery, the wound is inspected, sutures are removed, and the position is maintained using a removable splint that the patient will wear for another 4 weeks, provided that the patient is reliable in keeping the splint on at all times, except in the daily cleaning of the hand. Thereafter, the patient is encouraged to move the MCP joint, and a knuckle-bender splint is provided. One should avoid passive stretching of the MCP joint. A protective removable splint is also provided for night wear and general protection for the next 4 weeks. The knuckle-bender and protective splints are discontinued 2 months after surgery, and the patient is allowed unrestricted activity.
- Volar plate advancement is a simple procedure that gives good results in patients who can fully extend the PIP joint when the MCP joint is held in flexion. A bone anchor fixation of the volar plate reduces the incidence of loss of correction over time as a result of stretching. This procedure is not recommended for patients engaged in heavy manual labor who will certainly stretch the volar plate. A dynamic transfer may be more appropriate.

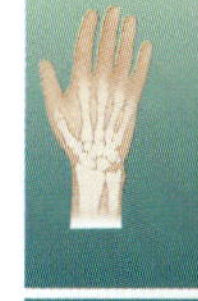

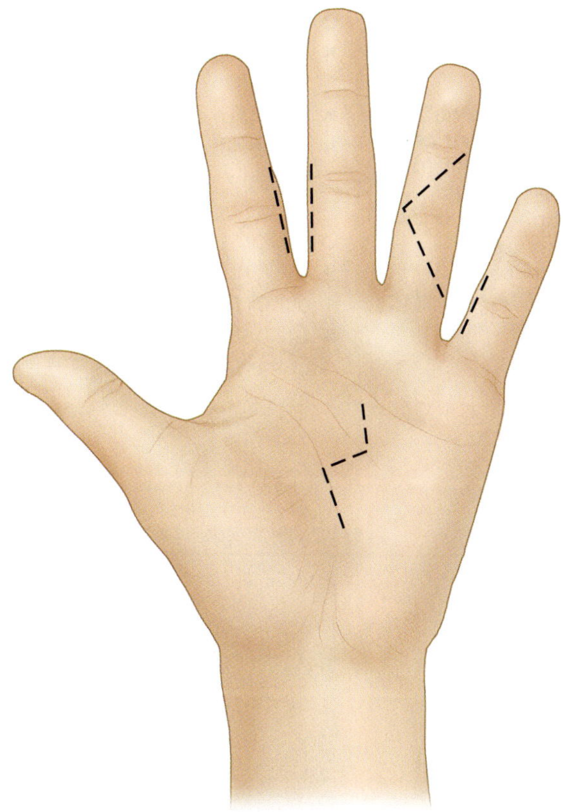

FIGURE 19-18

PEARLS

Additional lateral incisions can be made on the ulnar aspect of the index finger and radial aspect of the long finger if a claw correction of all four fingers is required.

The ulnar lateral band of the index and the radial lateral bands of the long, ring, and small fingers are chosen so that the tendon transfer can produce some adduction of these digits in addition to flexion at the MCP joint and extension at the PIP joint.

The long finger FDS should be used in patients with a high ulnar nerve palsy.

Procedure 2—Dynamic Correction of Claw Deformity with Transfer of Ring Finger FDS

Exposures

- A Bruner-type incision centered over the PIP joint is made over the ring finger. Both neurovascular bundles are identified and retracted laterally to expose the flexor tendon sheath. Subsequently, the radial neurovascular bundle is retracted ulnarly, and a tissue plane is developed deep to it to expose the radial lateral band, which will receive the tendon transfer.
- A second 3-cm longitudinal zigzag incision is made in the midpalm proximal to the proximal palmar crease. The skin and subcutaneous fat are dissected, and the common digital neurovascular bundles and the superficial arch are identified and protected. The flexor tendons are exposed.
- A third 2-cm longitudinal incision is made on the radial aspect of the small finger proximal phalanx. The soft tissue is dissected to expose the radial lateral band (Fig. 19-18).

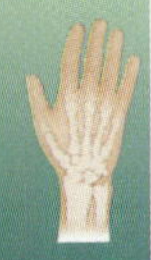

Step 1

- The A3 pulley of the ring finger is opened, and both slips of the FDS are identified.
- Both slips of the FDS are divided as distally as possible.
- The divided ends are held with a hemostat and pulled distally to identify the chiasma, which is then divided.

STEP 1 PEARLS

In patients who have a hyperextensible PIP joint, dividing the FDS proximal to the PIP joint can prevent the development of a swan neck deformity because the distal FDS insertion may be adherent to the volar plate and serve as a restraint. In patients who have a stiff PIP joint, the FDS should be divided distal to the PIP joint to prevent development of a flexion contracture.

STEP 1 PITFALLS

Incomplete division of the chiasma will make it impossible to retract the FDS out of the palmar incision.

Step 2

- The ring finger FDS tendon is identified at the midpalmar incision and withdrawn out of the incision.
- The distal split in the FDS tendon is completed all the way in the visible portion of the tendon (Fig. 19-19).

STEP 2 PEARLS

It is easy to split the FDS tendon into two as one can follow the natural split in the tendon. A knife is more suitable for this purpose. If claw correction of four fingers is required, the tendon has to be split into four parts. This needs to be done carefully (Fig. 19-20).

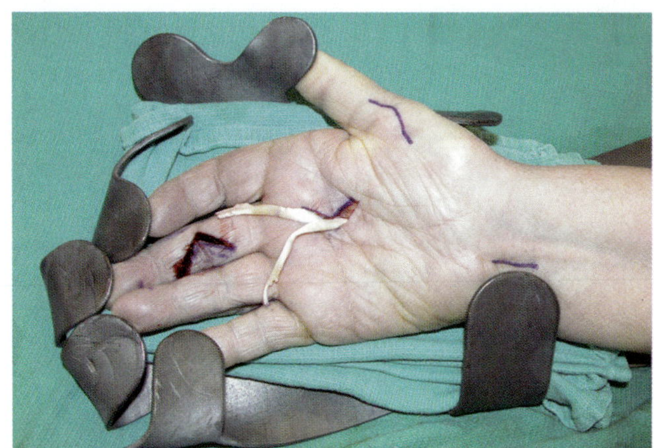

FIGURE 19-19

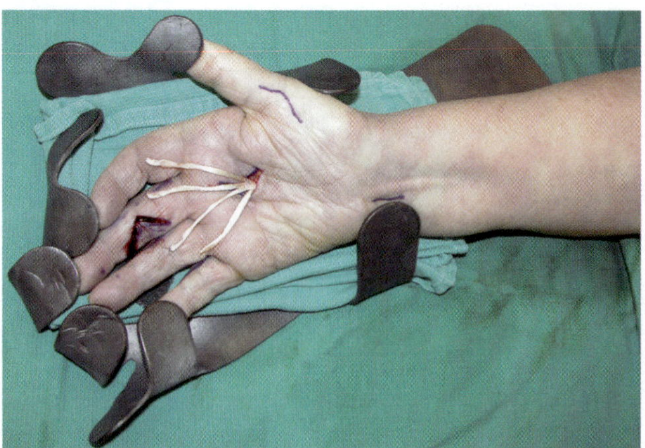

FIGURE 19-20

Step 3

- The origin of the lumbrical muscle from the FDP is identified. A mosquito forceps or a tendon passer is passed from the palmar incision along the lumbrical through the lumbrical canal (remaining superficial/palmar to the deep transverse metacarpal ligament) to exit on the incision made on the radial side of the small finger (Fig. 19-21).
- The jaws of the mosquito forceps are used to hold another mosquito forceps, which is brought into the palmar wound by withdrawing the first forceps. The tip of the mosquito forceps holds the distal end of the ulnar slip of the FDS and brings it out of the radial aspect of the small finger. The mosquito forceps is not removed and continues to hold the tendon.

STEP 2 PITFALLS

Ensure that the tendon is retracted out of the A1 pulley and is not looped around the superficial palmar arch or any of the neurovascular structures.

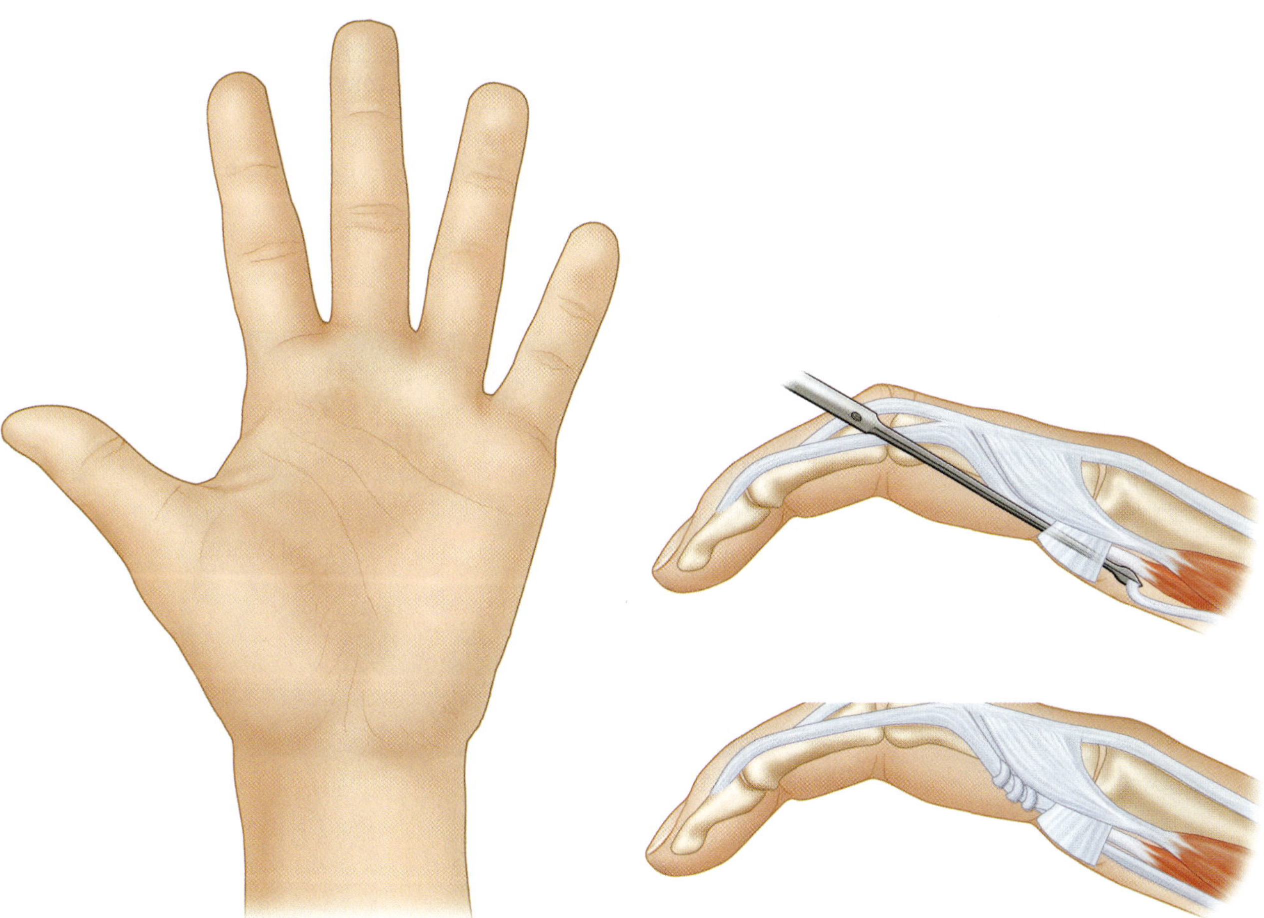

FIGURE 19-21

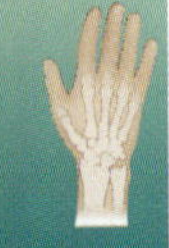

STEP 3 PITFALLS

The key step in this surgery is to remain volar to the axis of the MCP joint by passing the tendon through the lumbrical canal, remaining palmar to the deep transverse metacarpal ligament. This direction of pull will ensure MCP flexion after the tendon is attached to the lateral band.

STEP 5 PEARLS

The MCP joint cascade can be corrected by tightening or loosening the FDS attachment to the lateral band.

The desired tension is to keep the MCP joint in about 60 to 70 degrees of flexion and the IP joint in full extension, with the wrist at about 20 degrees of extension. In most cases, the ideal tension cannot be established because of the large amount of excursion of the FDS, which reaches 70 mm. Therefore, getting close to this posture is acceptable because the FDS, which is considered a smart tendon because of its excursion, can modulate the tension to reach an acceptable posture (Fig. 19-23).

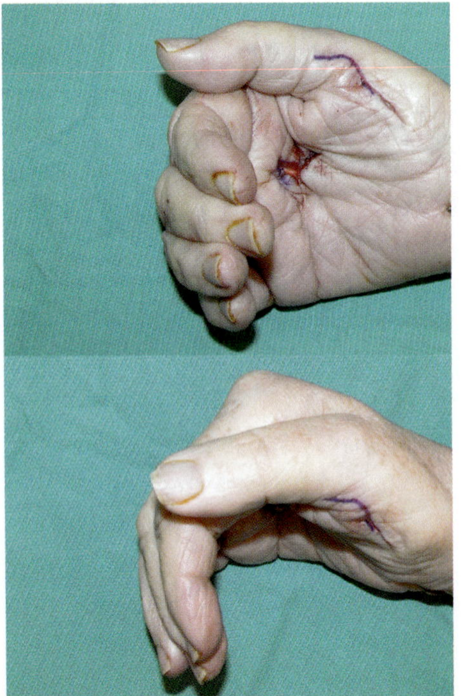

FIGURE 19-23

- The same procedure is repeated to bring the radial slip of the FDS through the lumbrical canal on the radial aspect of the ring finger (Fig. 19-22).

Step 4

- The tourniquet is released and hemostasis secured. The midpalmar incision and the distal half of the ring finger incision are closed.

Step 5

- The forearm is pronated, and a rolled-up towel is placed in the palm so that the wrist is in neutral position and the MCP joints are flexed beyond the rolled towel.
- The hemostat holding the FDS slip on the radial side of the ring finger is pulled to bring the MCP joint into about 60 degrees of flexion. (Aim to get slightly greater flexion than the adjacent long finger so that the normal cascade can be obtained.) The PIP joint is held in full extension by the assistant, and a single preliminary suture of the FDS to the lateral band is made.
- The tension and the finger cascade are confirmed by taking the wrist through a gentle range of motion. If the tension is correct, two or three nonabsorbable horizontal mattress sutures are placed between the FDS and the lateral bands.

Step 6

- The remainder of the skin incisions are closed with 5-0 nylon.

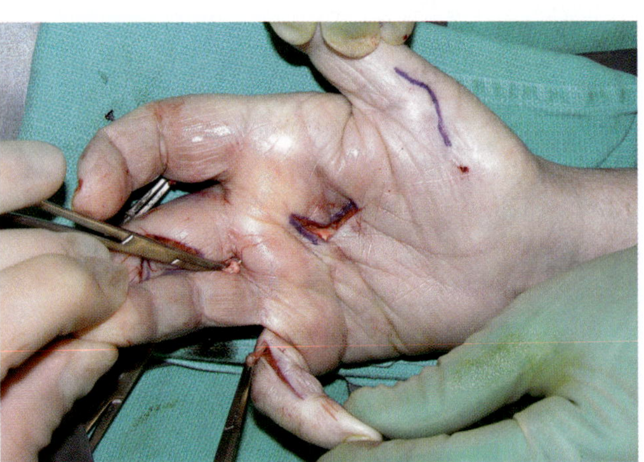

FIGURE 19-22

Postoperative Care and Expected Outcomes

- The hand is splinted with the wrist in neutral position, the MCP joint in 60 to 70 degrees of flexion, and the IP joints in full extension.
- Ten days after surgery, the wound is inspected, sutures are removed, and the position is maintained using a removable splint that the patient will wear for another 4 weeks, provided that the patient is reliable in keeping the splint on at all times, except in the daily cleaning of the hand. Thereafter, the patient is given a dorsal blocking splint that keeps the MCP joint flexed but allows full extension and flexion of the IP joint for another 4 weeks. The splint is discontinued 2 months after surgery, and the patient is allowed unrestricted activity.
- The transfer of FDS reliably corrects MCP joint hyperextension but does not improve grip strength and may not fully correct the loss of PIP joint extension. This procedure gives good results in supple joints, although the patient may develop a swan neck deformity from loss of volar restraint provided by the FDS.

PEARLS

If the PL is determined to be absent preoperatively, half of the tendon of the ECRB can be used as a tendon graft. Approximately 10 cm of tendon graft will be required to bridge the gap between the distal end of the ECRB and the adductor tendon. Another option is to consider the plantaris tendon.

PITFALLS

One should look out for the branches of the superficial radial nerve in the dorsal incisions and the palmar cutaneous branch of the median nerve radial to the PL in the volar incision.

STEP 1 PEARLS

The ECRB may have a portion of its insertion on the base of the index metacarpal. Care should be taken to protect the ECRL insertion.

Procedure 3—Restoration of Thumb Adduction with an ECRB Tendon Transfer

Exposures

- A 3-cm longitudinal incision is made starting at the base of the ulnar aspect of the long finger metacarpal and extending distally. The soft tissue is dissected, and the ECRB is exposed at its insertion onto the base of the long metacarpal. Distally, the dorsal interosseous fascia overlying the interspace between the long and ring metacarpals is divided, and interosseous muscles are exposed (Fig. 19-24).
- Through this incision, the ECRB tendon is identified immediately proximal to the extensor retinaculum.
- A 1-cm longitudinal incision is made on the ulnar aspect of the thumb MCP joint, and the soft tissue is dissected to expose the insertion of the adductor pollicis.
- A 1-cm incision is made at the proximal wrist crease, and the tendon of the palmaris longus is identified and exposed.

Step 1

- The ECRB is divided at its insertion.

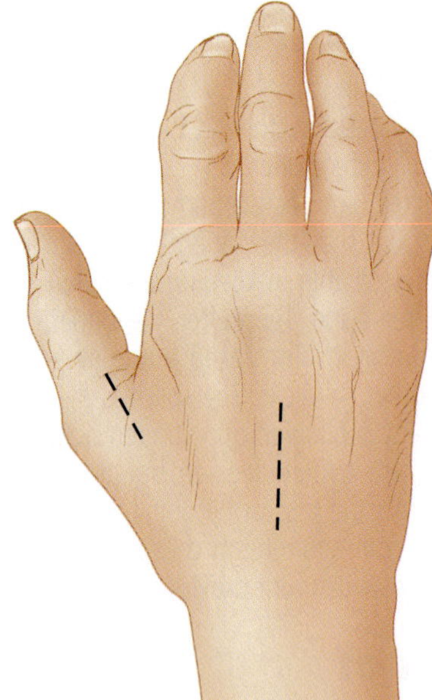

FIGURE 19-24

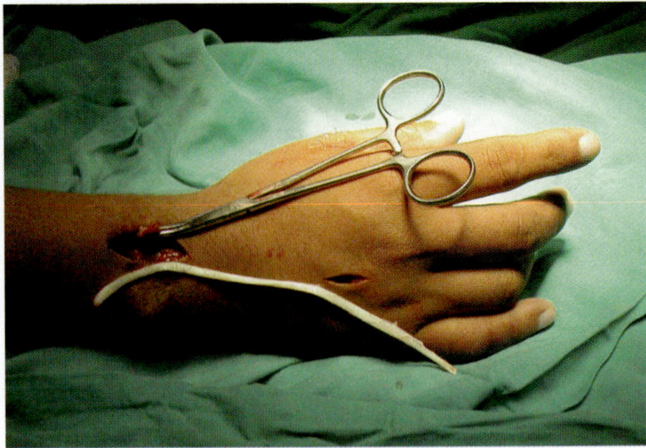

FIGURE 19-25

Step 2

- The ECRB tendon is withdrawn proximal to the extensor retinaculum (Fig. 19-25).

Step 3

- The exposed portion of the PL tendon is held with a hemostat, and the tendon is divided distal to the hemostat.
- The hemostat is used to pull the tendon distally and free it from the surrounding antebrachial fascia.
- The PL is harvested using three 1-cm transverse incisions in the forearm.

STEP 3 PITFALLS

Confirm that it is the PL that you are dividing. There have been reports of inadvertent harvest of the median nerve.

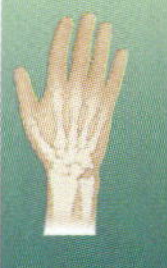

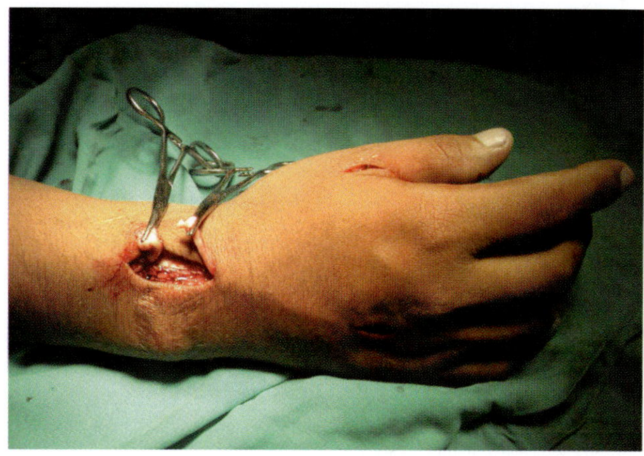

FIGURE 19-26

STEP 4 PEARLS

This tendon juncture should be planned so that it does not lie at the middle and ring metacarpal interspace. The bulky weave may not glide well in this narrow interspace.

Step 4

- The PL tendon graft is sutured to the distal cut end of the ECRB using a Pulvertaft weave (Fig. 19-26).

Step 5

- A subcutaneous tunnel is made superficial to the extensor retinaculum to pass the tendon.

Step 6

- A curved hemostat is used to make a subcutaneous tunnel from the ulnar aspect of the thumb MCP joint to the third to fourth intermetacarpal space. This tunnel is made superficial (palmar) to the adductor pollicis but deep (dorsal) to the flexor tendons (Fig. 19-27).
- The hemostat then grabs the ECRB extended by the PL graft and brings it out to the thumb.

STEP 7 PEARLS

Tension adjustment is checked by wrist tenodesis. When the wrist is extended, the thumb should fall into abduction, and with the wrist in flexion, the thumb should lie firmly against the palm (Fig. 19-28).

Step 7

- The tendon is sutured to the tendon of the adductor pollicis with the wrist in neutral position. Tension is adjusted so that the thumb lies just palmar to the index finger.

Step 8

- The tourniquet is released, and all skin incisions are closed with 5-0 nylon.

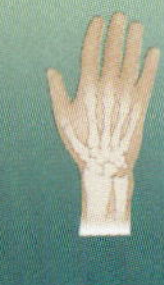

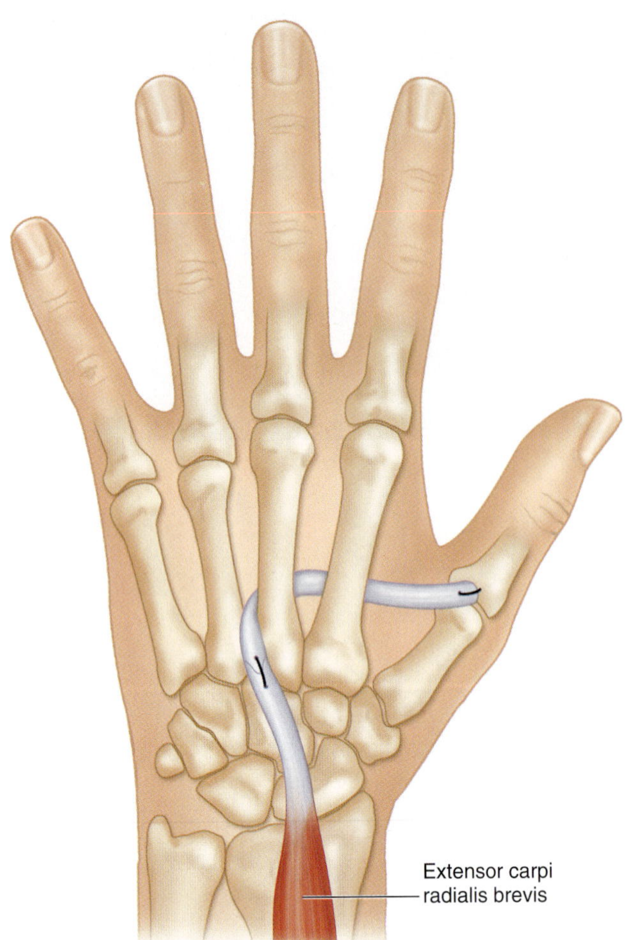

FIGURE 19-27

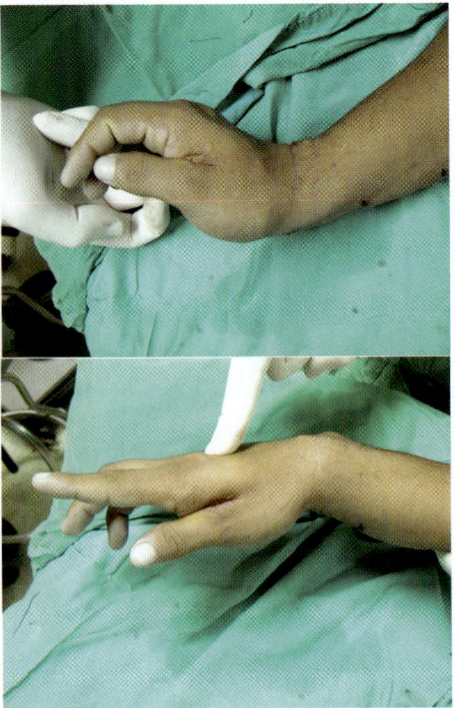

FIGURE 19-28

Postoperative Care and Expected Outcomes

- The hand is splinted with the wrist and thumb in neutral position.
- Ten days after surgery, the wound is inspected, sutures are removed, and the position is maintained using a removable splint that the patient will wear for another 4 weeks, provided that the patient is reliable in keeping the splint on at all times, except in the daily cleaning of the hand. Thereafter, the patient is given a protective splint and encouraged to move the thumb and wrist.
- The transfer of ECRB restores thumb pinch and improves the ability to perform activities of daily living. Patients recover about 50% of the pinch strength of the contralateral thumb. This transfer may restrict thumb opposition and palmar abduction.

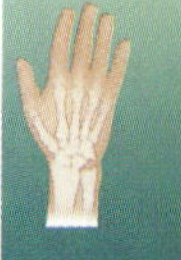

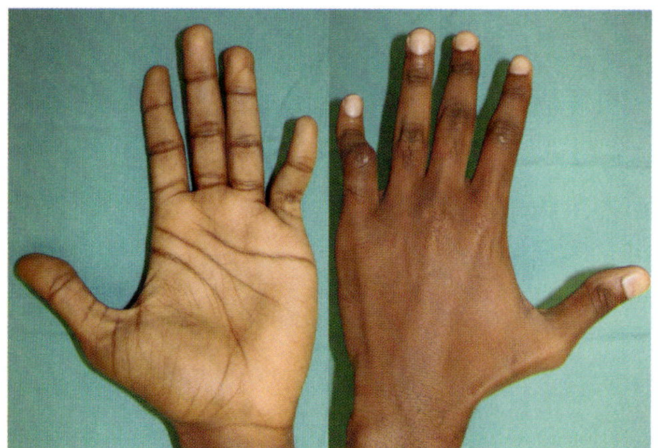

FIGURE 19-29

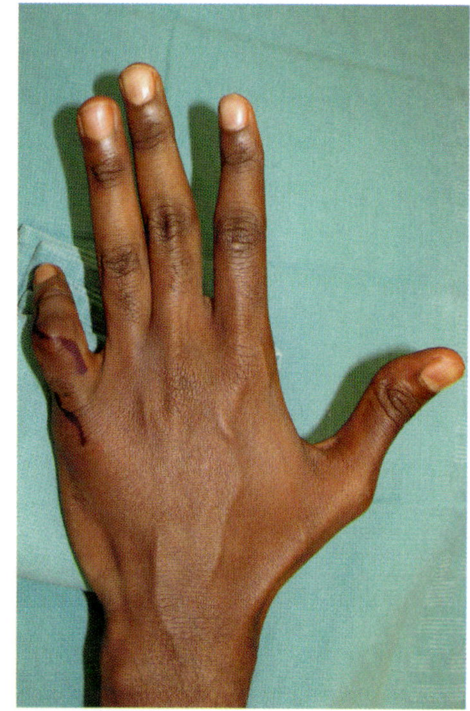

FIGURE 19-30

PITFALLS

Care should be taken to protect branches from the dorsal branch of the ulnar nerve.

Procedure 4—Correction of Abduction Deformity (Wartenberg Sign) of Small Finger

Exposures

- A 3-cm chevron-shaped incision with the apex directed ulnarly is made over the dorsal aspect of the small finger MCP joint. The skin and soft tissue are dissected to expose the tendon of the EDM (Figs. 19-29 and 19-30).
- The radial collateral ligament of the small finger MCP joint is exposed by making a longitudinal incision in the proximal portion of the extensor hood overlying the radial aspect of the small finger MCP joint.

Step 1

- The ulnar insertion of the EDM is detached from the extensor hood and dissected proximally from the remainder of the EDM for about 2 to 3 cm proximal to the MCP joint.
- This tendon is now passed radially under the EDM and the extensor digitorum communis (EDC) to the small finger to reach the radial side of the small finger MCP joint.

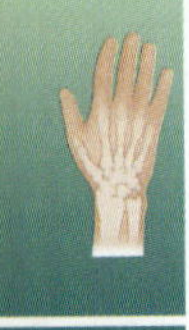

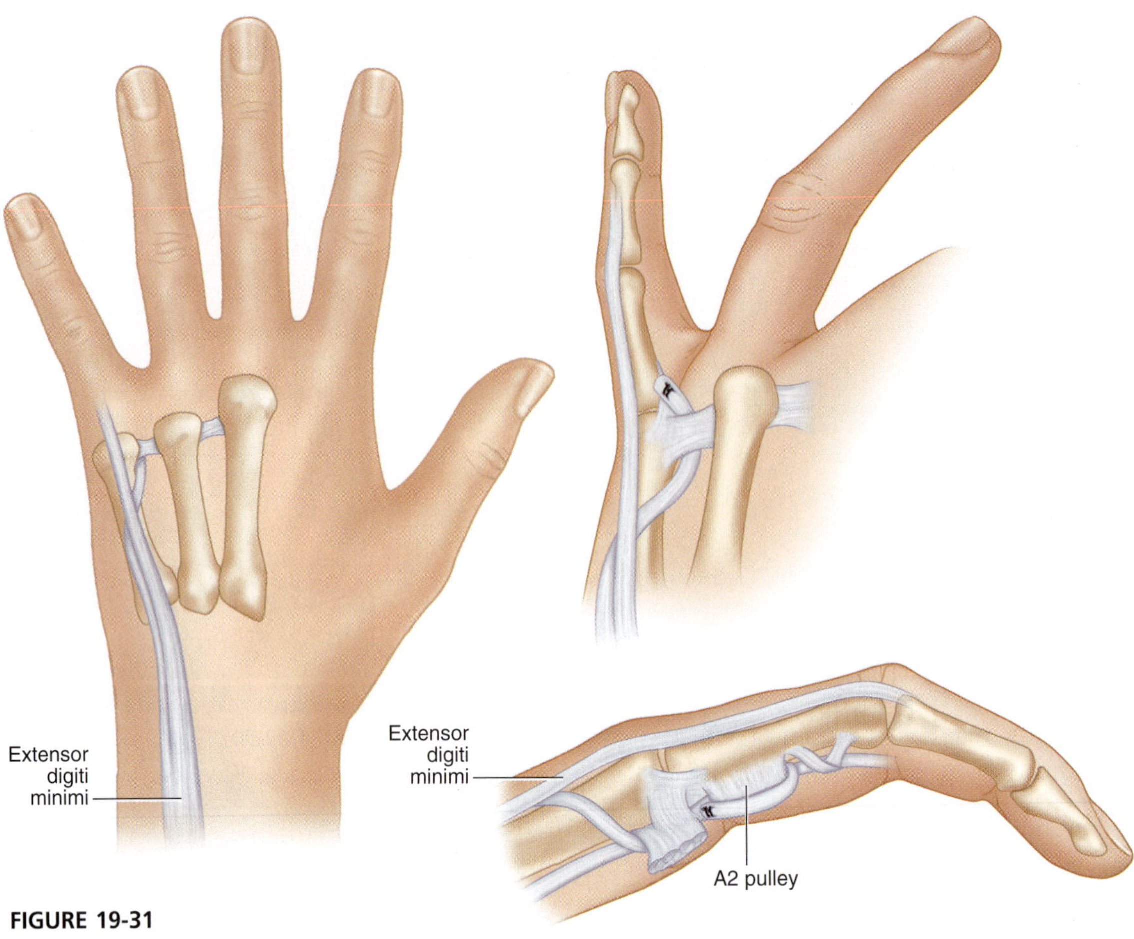

FIGURE 19-31

STEP 2 PEARLS

The transfer of the ulnar half of the EDM tendon to the radial collateral ligament is useful in patients with low ulnar nerve palsy who have an abduction deformity but do not have clawing or have clawing that has been corrected by a previous transfer.

In patients who have clawing, an additional 2.5-cm oblique palmar incision is made between the distal palmar crease and the proximal digital crease of the small finger. The common digital neurovascular bundle is identified and retracted radially to expose the deep transverse metacarpal ligament. The EDM tendon is retrieved using a hemostat and passed from dorsum to palmar between the fourth and fifth metacarpals, remaining palmar to the deep transverse metacarpal ligament. It is passed through a slit made in the proximal half of the A2 pulley and sutured to itself with the assistant holding the wrist in neutral position, the MCP joint in 20 degrees of flexion, and the small finger adducted (see Fig. 19-31).

Step 2

- The tendon is sutured to the phalangeal attachment of the radial collateral ligament with the wrist in neutral position with the assistant holding the small finger adducted (Fig. 19-31).

Step 3

- The tourniquet is released, hemostasis is secured, and the skin is closed with 5-0 nylon.

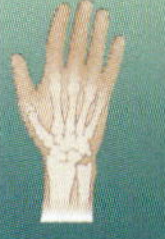

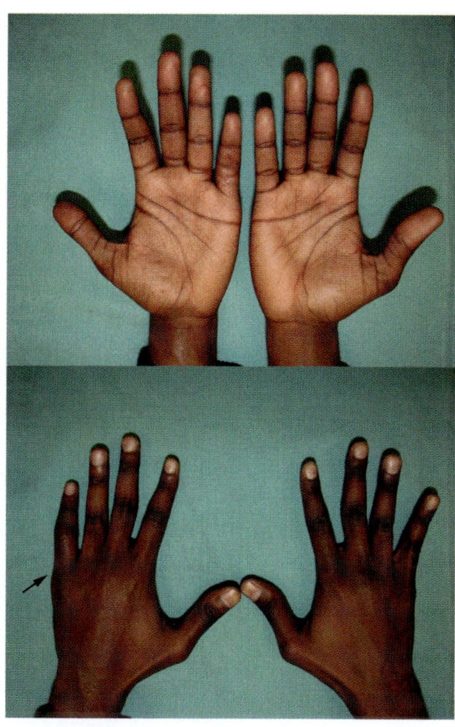

FIGURE 19-32

Postoperative Care and Expected Outcomes

- A splint is applied that keeps the small and ring fingers MCP joints in 60 to 70 degrees of flexion and the wrist in neutral position. The IP joints are left free.
- Ten days after surgery, the wound is inspected, sutures are removed, and the position is maintained using a removable splint that the patient will wear for another 4 weeks, provided that the patient is reliable in keeping the splint on at all times, except in the daily cleaning of the hand. Thereafter, the patient is encouraged to move the MCP joint, and a protective removable splint is also provided for night wear and general protection for the next 4 weeks. The protective splint is discontinued 2 months after surgery, and the patient is allowed unrestricted activity (Fig. 19-32).
- This is a simple procedure to correct an annoying disability.

Procedure 5—Side-to-Side FDP Transfer for Restoration of Ring and Small Finger DIP Joint Flexion Strength (High Ulnar Palsy)

Exposures

- A 4-cm longitudinal incision is made 2 cm proximal to the wrist crease ulnar and parallel to the tendon of the palmaris longus. The antebrachial fascia is divided, and the PL tendon is retracted radially. The median nerve is identified and retracted radially. Next, the FDS tendons to the ring and long finger are identified and retracted radially. Immediately below are the FDS tendons to the small and index fingers. The index FDS is retracted radially, and the small FDS is retracted ulnarly. This exposes the four FDP tendons.

PITFALLS

The palmar cutaneous branch of the median nerve runs on the radial aspect of the PL.

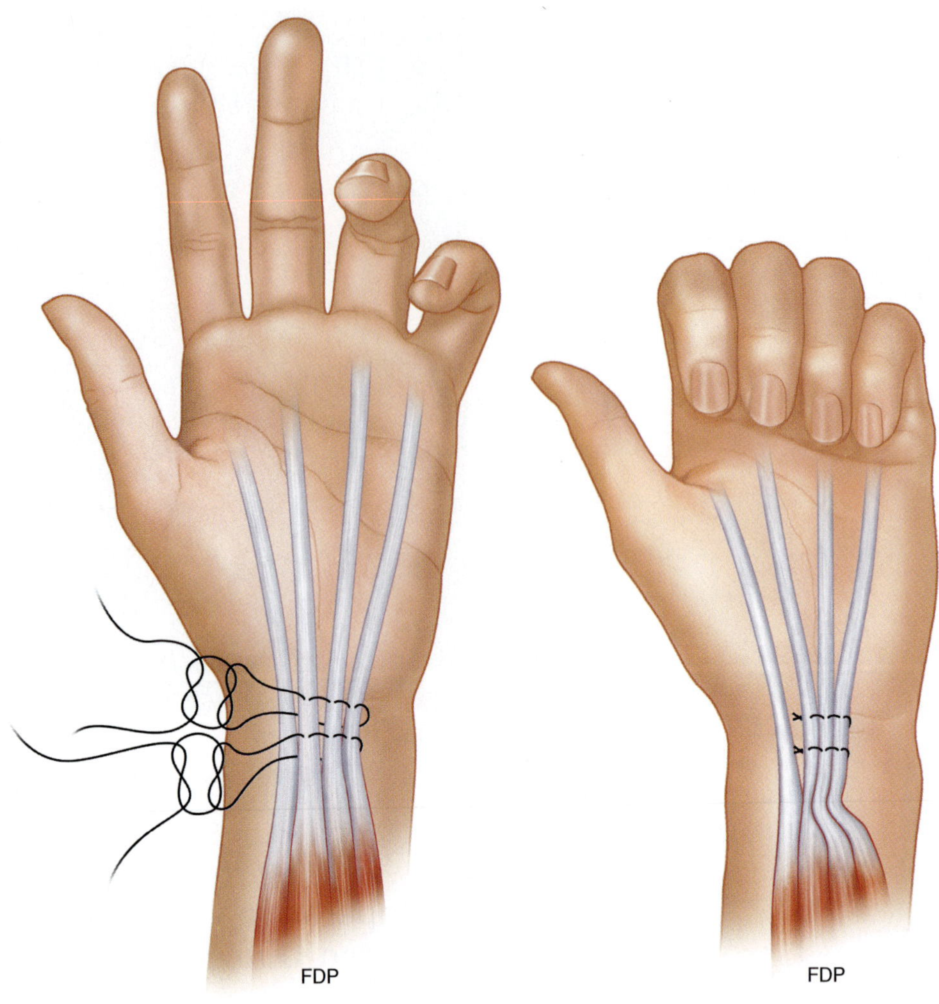

FIGURE 19-33

> **STEP 1 PEARLS**
>
> *The FDP of the index finger is not included in the transfer to allow some independent function of the index finger.*

Step 1

- An assistant holds the wrist in neutral position and maintains the MCP and IP joints to obtain a normal finger cascade.
- The FDP tendons of the small and ring fingers are then sutured to the FDP of the long finger using two or three horizontal mattress sutures (Fig. 19-33).

Step 2

- The tourniquet is released, hemostasis is secured, and the skin is closed with 5-0 nylon.

Postoperative Care and Expected Outcomes

- A protective dorsal blocking splint is provided that keeps the MCP joint in 60 to 70 degrees of flexion and the wrist in neutral position. The patient is allowed to actively move the IP joints.
- Ten days after surgery, the wound is inspected, sutures are removed, and the protective splint is maintained for another 4 weeks. Thereafter, the splint is removed, and the patient is allowed unrestricted activity.
- This procedure should be performed before claw correction, and patients should be warned that the surgery will exaggerate the claw deformity.

Evidence

Hastings H, McCollam SM. Flexor digitorum superficialis lasso tendon transfer in isolated ulnar nerve palsy: a functional evaluation. *J Hand Surg [Am]*. 1994;19:275-280.
This prospective outcome study demonstrated no significant improvement in grip strength after surgery for patients who returned for late follow-up an average of 40 months after Zancolli FDS lasso procedure. (Level II evidence)

Ozkan T, Ozer K, Gulgonen A. Three tendon transfer methods in reconstruction of ulnar nerve palsy. *J Hand Surg [Am]*. 2003;28:35-43.
This prospective clinical series compared the FDS four-tail procedure, the ECRL four-tail procedure, and the Zancolli lasso procedure. The ECRL four-tail procedure and the Zancolli lasso procedure were found to provide greater grip strength. The FDS four-tail procedure was found to result in greater improvements in correcting the claw deformity. (Level II evidence)

Smith RJ. Extensor carpi radialis brevis tendon transfer for thumb adduction: a study of power pinch. *J Hand Surg [Am]*. 1983;8:4-15.
Smith performed this operation on 15 patients with paralysis or loss of the adductor muscle. In 8 patients, he simultaneously performed a tendon transfer to the first dorsal interosseous tendon, using the extensor indicis proprius in 4 patients and an accessory slip of the abductor pollicis longus in the other 4. He reported one episode of synovitis at the index-long interspace, but 14 of his 15 patients reported significant improvement. Overall thumb pinch strength was doubled by the procedure, rising from 25% (preoperatively) to 50% (postoperatively) of the strength of the contralateral thumb. (Level IV evidence)

Trevett MC, Tuson C, de Jager LT, Juon JM. The functional results of ulnar nerve repair: defining the indications for tendon transfer. *J Hand Surg [Br]*. 1995;20:444-446.
This clinical series provided follow-up on patients with ulnar nerve palsies and reported patient functional impairment. Manual laborers with ulnar nerve palsy had difficulty coping at work, whereas sedentary workers tended to be able to cope. The authors suggest early tendon transfers in patients involved in manual labor to avoid an unnecessarily long waiting period. (Level IV evidence)

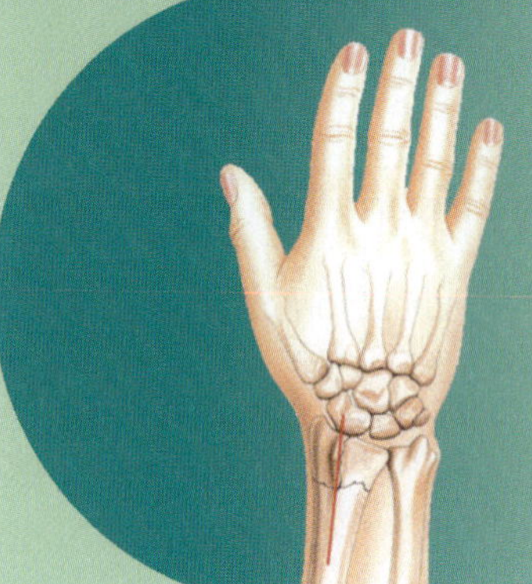

Tendon Transfers for Radial Nerve Palsy

Sandeep J. Sebastin and Kevin C. Chung

See Video 16: Standard Tendon Transfer Sequence for Radial Nerve Palsy

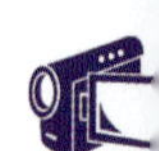

See Video 17: Alternate Tendon Transfer Sequence for Radial Nerve Palsy When PL Is Absent

Indications

- Delayed presentation (>1 year) of a radial nerve injury
- Failed motor recovery after repair/reconstruction of the radial nerve
- Failed motor recovery after decompression of the radial/posterior interosseous nerve

Examination/Imaging

Clinical Examination

- *Functional deficit:* The loss of function in radial nerve palsy results from the wrist drop deformity, which causes an inability to extend the wrist and the finger metacarpophalangeal (MCP) joints and to extend and abduct the thumb (Fig. 20-1). The loss of wrist extension weakens power grip, and the loss of finger and thumb extension makes it difficult to grasp objects. It is important to differentiate radial nerve palsy (above the elbow) from posterior interosseous nerve (PIN) palsy (below the elbow). The extensor carpi radialis longus (ECRL) receives its innervation by a branch of the radial nerve that arises above the elbow. It is therefore spared in a lesion of the PIN, and patients can extend the wrist, although with radial deviation (Fig. 20-2).
- *Sensation:* Sensory loss in the areas innervated by the superficial radial nerve (anatomic snuffbox and dorsum of first web) can help differentiate a radial nerve lesion from a lesion of the PIN, which should have preserved sensation over the dorsum of the first web (Fig. 20-3).
- *Joints:* To get a good result from the tendon transfer, patients must have good passive range of motion at the wrist and the MCP joint. One of the common transfers uses wrist flexors for obtaining finger and thumb MCP joint extension. The excursion of wrist flexors is approximately 33 mm, whereas finger extension requires a tendon excursion of 50 mm. This difference in excursion is obtained by the natural tenodesis effect, and patients are able to obtain full finger extension when the wrist is flexed.

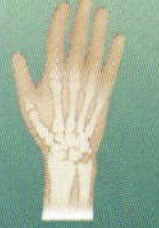

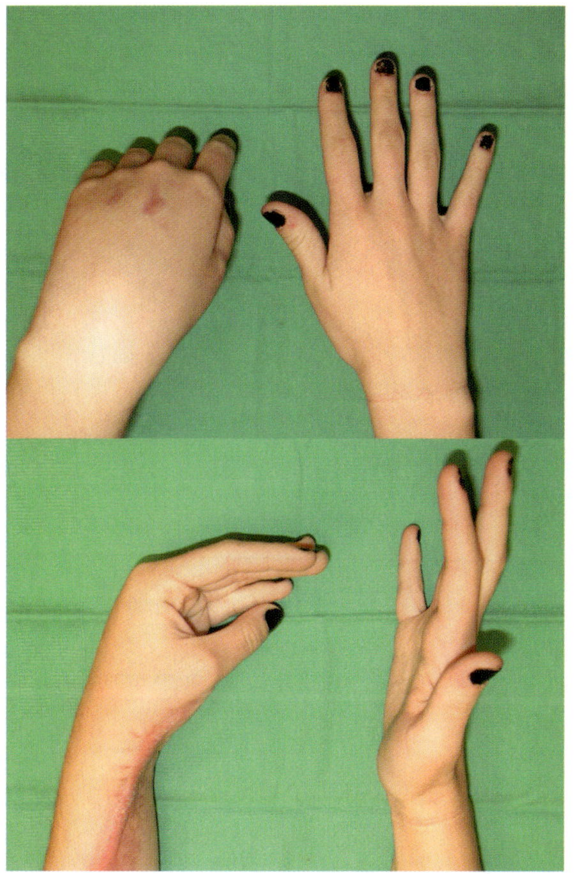

FIGURE 20-1

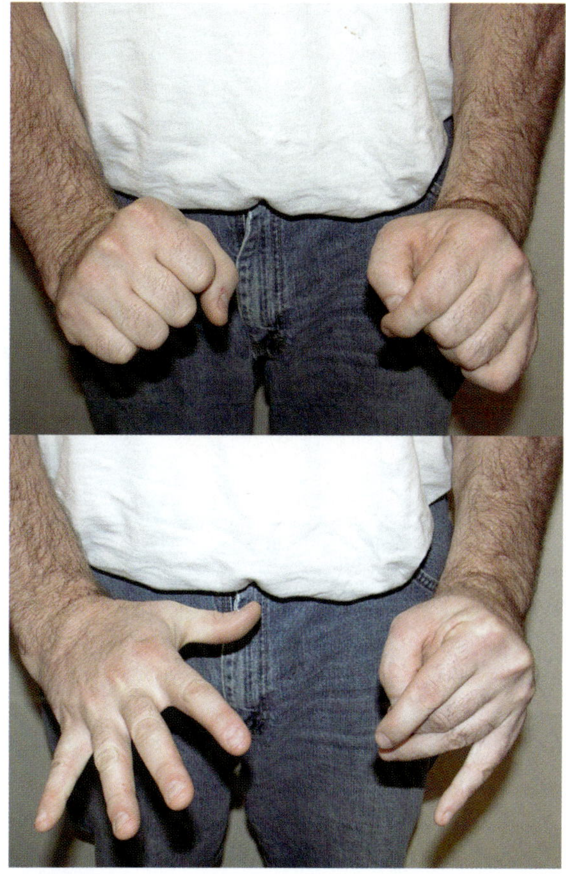

FIGURE 20-2

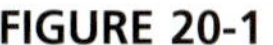

- *Selection of motor:* Our preferred motors are as follows. Patients with PIN palsy do not require a transfer for wrist extension because the ECRL is functional.
  - *Wrist extension:* We transfer the pronator teres (PT) to the extensor carpi radialis brevis (ECRB).
  - *Finger extension:* We transfer the flexor carpi radialis (FCR) to the extensor digitorum communis (EDC). We prefer the FCR to the flexor carpi ulnaris (FCU) because the FCR is simpler to harvest without many proximal attachments. The FCU requires a bit more dissection to free up the muscle from its attachment along the ulna, and the FCU has an additional function of stabilizing the ulnar side of the wrist. Also, in patients with a PIN palsy (with an intact ECRL), the FCU remains the only ulnar deviator of the wrist, and its transfer may lead to excessive radial deviation.
  - *Thumb extension:* We transfer the palmaris longus (PL) to the extensor pollicis longus (EPL). In patients who do not have the PL, we use the flexor digitorum superficialis (FDS) from the long finger for motor. In these cases, we transfer the FDS of the long finger to the EPL and extensor indicis proprius (EIP) and the FCR to the EDC of the long, ring, and small fingers. This allows extension of the thumb and index fingers independent of the other digits to improve pinch.

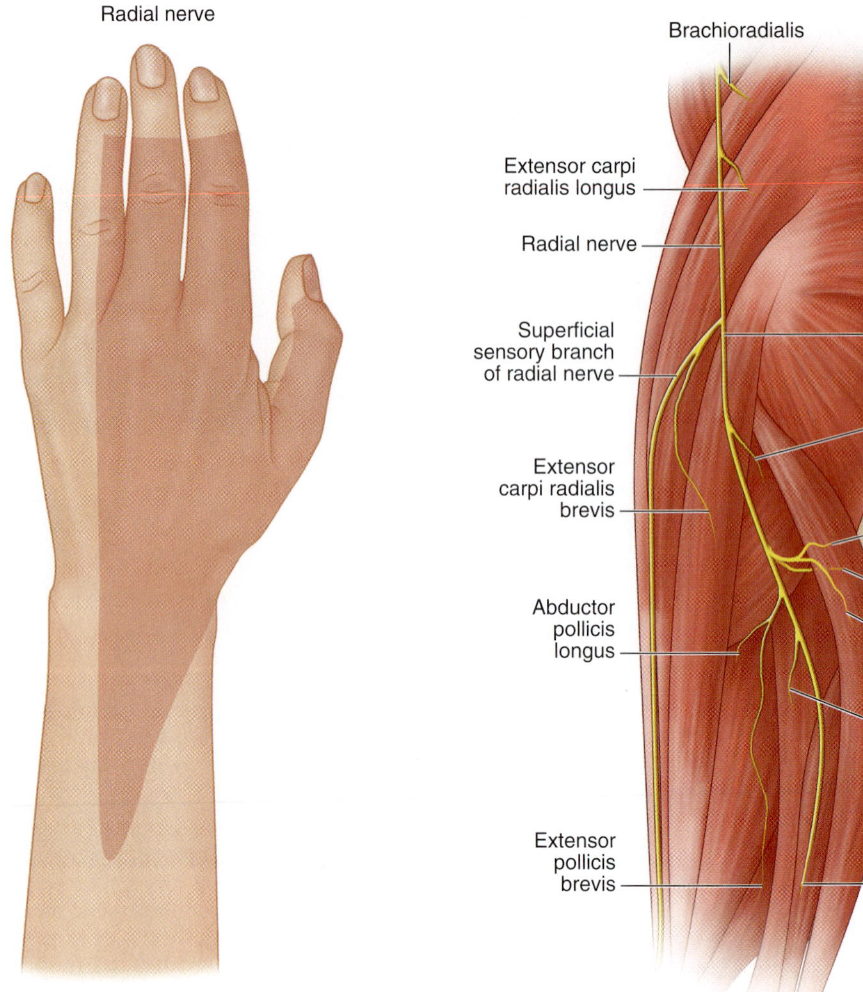

FIGURE 20-3

FIGURE 20-4

Imaging

- Electrodiagnostic studies are often used to confirm the diagnosis of a nerve problem. For radial nerve palsy, these nerve studies are not particularly useful because muscle testing and careful examination should be able to identify the functional deficits and the available tendons that can be transferred.

Surgical Anatomy

- The radial nerve divides into the superficial radial nerve and the posterior interosseous nerve at the level of the lateral epicondyle (about 1 to 2 cm above the elbow joint). It gives off branches that innervate the brachioradialis (BR) and the ECRL before this division. The ECRB has variable innervation that can arise from the radial nerve, superficial radial nerve, or PIN. The remaining extensor compartment muscles are innervated in the following order by the PIN: supinator, EDC, extensor carpi ulnaris (ECU), extensor digiti quinti minimi (EDQM), abductor pollicis longus (APL), extensor pollicis longus (EPL), extensor pollicis brevis (EPB), and extensor EIP (Fig. 20-4).

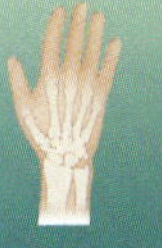

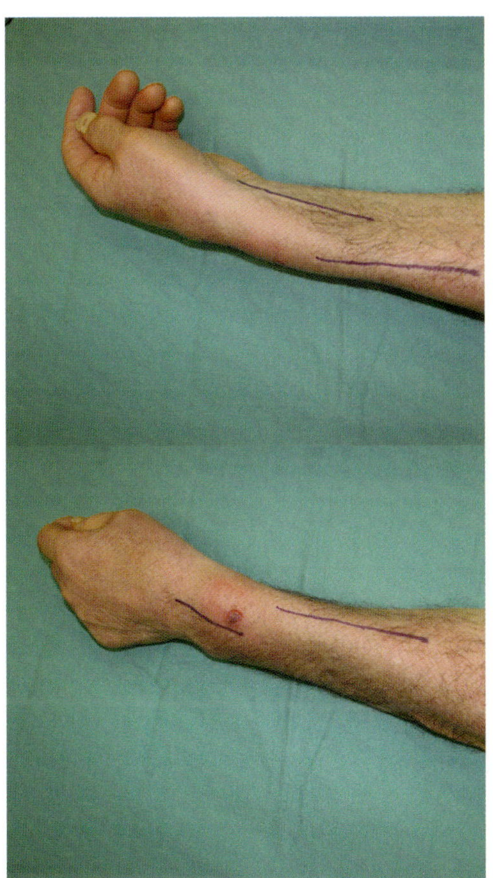

FIGURE 20-5

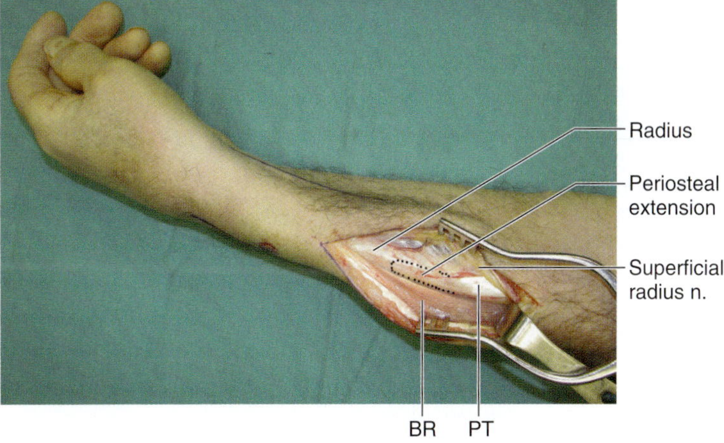

FIGURE 20-6

Positioning

- The procedure is performed under tourniquet control.
- The patient is positioned supine with the affected extremity on a hand table.

Exposures

- A 6-cm longitudinal incision is made over the volar radial aspect of the mid-forearm (Fig. 20-5). This incision is centered over the palpable musculotendinous junction of the ECRB and ECRL. The forearm fascia is divided, and the tendons of ECRB and ECRL are identified. The BR is identified radial to the ECRL and retracted ulnarly along with the ECRL. The superficial branch of the radial nerve should be identified under the BR and protected. This will bring into view the insertion of the PT (Fig. 20-6).
- A 4-cm longitudinal incision is made over the Lister tubercle (see Fig. 20-5). The extensor retinaculum is exposed and the third compartment opened to free the EPL. The EIP, EDC, and EDQM tendons are identified proximal to the extensor retinaculum.
- A 6-cm longitudinal incision is made over the volar aspect of the distal forearm beginning at the proximal wrist crease in line with the FCR (see Fig. 20-5). The tendons of the FCR and the PL are identified, taking care to protect the radial artery, the palmar cutaneous branch of the median nerve, and the median nerve. If the PL is absent, the FDS to the long finger is identified by deeper dissection through the same incision. The long finger is used instead of the ring finger to preserve the strength of the power grip by the ring finger. The FDS tendons to the long and ring fingers lie in a plane superficial to the FDS tendons to the index and small fingers.

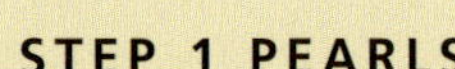

Procedure

Step 1

- The PT is detached from its insertion on the radius (see Fig. 20-6).

Step 2

- The PT muscle-tendon unit must be mobilized proximally to free it from any attachments that will limit subsequent excursion.

Step 3

- The PT is rerouted superficial to the BR and the ECRL around the radial border of the forearm to reach the musculotendinous junction of the ECRB.

Step 4

- The PT is sutured end to side to the ECRB using a Pulvertaft weave with multiple 4-0 nonabsorbable sutures (Fig. 20-7). During this suture, the wrist is maintained in 45 degrees of extension by the assistant. A single preliminary suture is placed first, and the tension is confirmed by determining whether the position is maintained without being held by the assistant.

Step 5

- The FCR tendon (Fig. 20-8A) is divided at the wrist crease and mobilized up to the mid-forearm. A subcutaneous tunnel is made around the radial border of the forearm using a blunt-tipped mosquito forceps that will redirect the FCR tendon in a straight line to the previously exposed EDC tendons (Fig. 20-8B).

STEP 1 PEARLS

A 3- to 4-cm strip of periosteum distal to the insertion of the PT should be harvested in continuity with the PT (see Fig. 20-6). The length of the PT is usually just enough to reach the ECRB, and harvesting this additional periosteal extension makes a strong repair of the PT to the ECRB possible.

A portion of the ECRL tendon can also be used as a tendon graft to strengthen the repair site, given that the ECRL is redundant.

STEP 2 PITFALLS

Care should be taken to prevent injury to the superficial branch of the radial nerve, the radial artery, and the innervation to the PT during the proximal dissection.

STEP 4 PEARLS

Although dividing the ECRB and doing an end-to-end repair will allow a straighter line of pull, we prefer to do an end-to-side repair. The length of the PT is usually just enough to reach the ECRB, and we feel it is safer to do an end-to-side repair to avoid excessive tension in the tendon repair juncture. An end-to-side repair is also better in patients whose recovery of the radial nerve is expected and in whom the transfer has been done as an internal splint to provide wrist extension in the intervening period.

It is better to err on the side of suturing the extensor tendon transfers too tightly rather than too loosely because the extensors tend to stretch out with time.

STEP 4 PITFALLS

Do not lift the tendons toward you when doing the first suture because this will result in a lax repair once the tendon drops into its natural position.

STEP 5 PEARLS

The innervation of the FCR should be protected during proximal mobilization of the muscle.

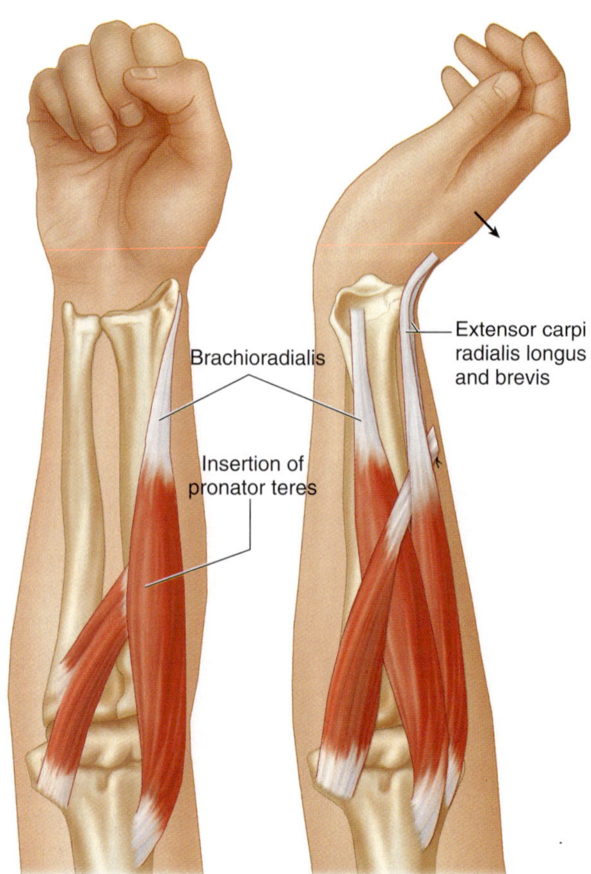

FIGURE 20-7

Step 6

- With an assistant holding the wrist in 45 degrees of extension and the finger MCP joint in full extension, the FCR tendon is weaved in an end-to-side fashion to the EDC tendons to the index, long, ring, and small fingers using 4-0 nonabsorbable suture (Fig. 20-9).

Step 7

- The PL tendon is divided at the distal wrist crease and mobilized proximally up to the mid-forearm.

STEP 5 PITFALLS

The radial artery, palmar cutaneous branch of the median nerve, and superficial radial nerve should be protected during mobilization of the FCR and creation of the tunnel.

STEP 6 PEARLS

The EDQM needs to be included in the transfer only if traction of the EDC does not result in adequate extension of the small finger MCP joint.

The FCR tendon should be sutured to each EDC slip separately, and the tension must be adjusted for each slip individually.

Correct tension can be confirmed by the wrist tenodesis. The fingers should extend fully with the wrist in flexion, and passive flexion of the fingers should be possible with the wrist in full extension (Fig. 20-9).

Some authors have suggested dividing the EDC proximal to the extensor retinaculum, withdrawing it, rerouting it superficial to the retinaculum, and doing an end-to-end repair to allow a straighter line of pull. We do not feel this step is necessary, and our results have been consistently acceptable with our suggested approach.

STEP 6 PITFALLS

Ensure that the tunnel is wide and allows a straight line of pull.

STEP 7 PITFALLS

The palmar cutaneous branch of the median nerve and the median nerve should be identified and protected.

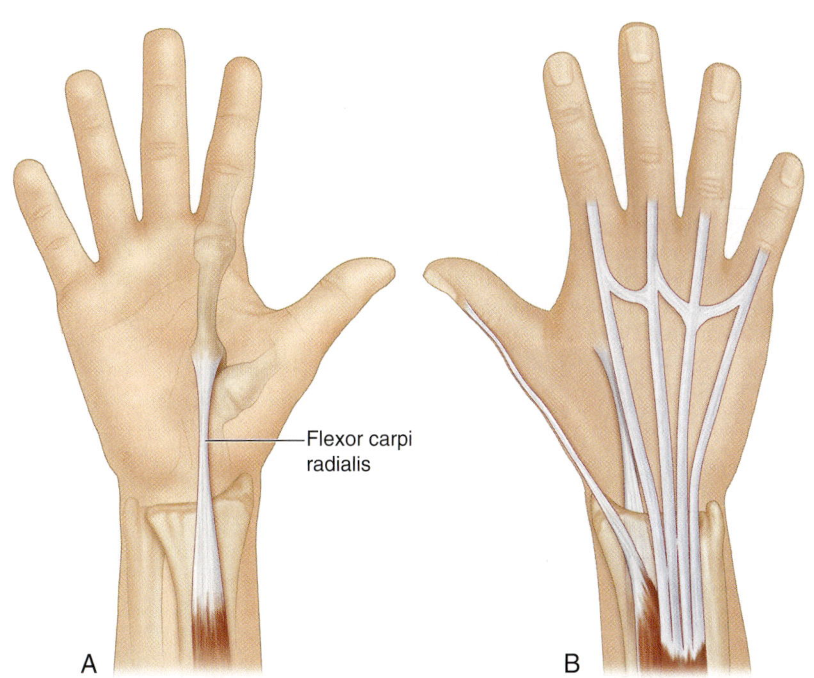

FIGURE 20-8

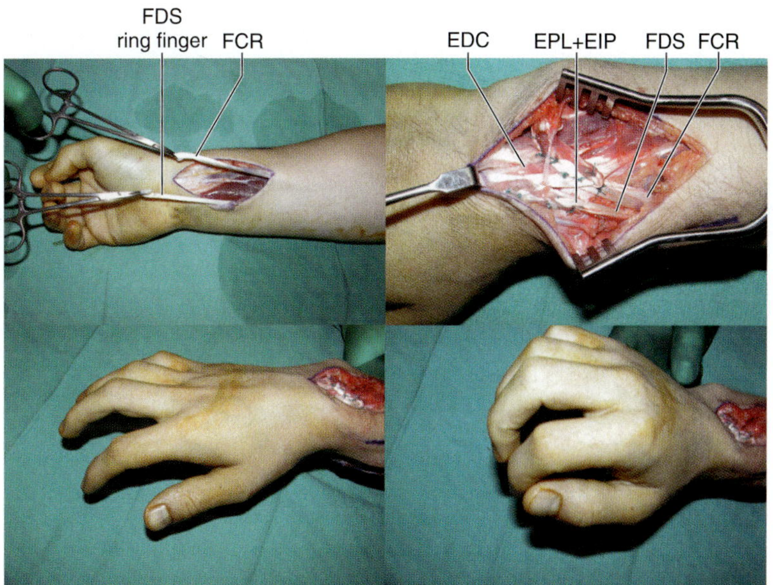

FIGURE 20-9

Step 8

- The EPL tendon is divided at the musculotendinous junction proximal to Lister tubercle. It is then withdrawn distally out of the retinaculum and rerouted superficial to it, to reach the region of the anatomic snuffbox.

Step 9

- A subcutaneous tunnel is created to redirect the PL tendon toward the rerouted EPL tendon in the anatomic snuffbox.

Step 10

- An end-to-end Pulvertaft weave of the EPL and PL tendons is done with an assistant maintaining the wrist in 45 degrees of extension and the thumb in full extension and abduction (Fig. 20-10).

Step 11

- The tourniquet is released, hemostasis is secured, and all incisions are closed.

STEP 9 PEARLS

It is important to divide the EPL and reroute it superficial to the extensor retinaculum for the transfer to provide some thumb abduction in addition to extension.

STEP 10 PEARLS

Correct tension can be confirmed by wrist tenodesis. The thumb should abduct and extend fully with the wrist in flexion, and passive flexion and adduction of the thumb should be possible with the wrist in full extension (Fig. 20-11; see Fig. 20-9).

If the PL is absent, we transfer the FDS of the long finger to the EIP and EPL (both divided proximal to the extensor retinaculum, withdrawn out, and rerouted superficially). In these cases, the FCR is transferred only to the EDC (including the index finger) and the EDQM (if indicated) (see Fig. 20-9).

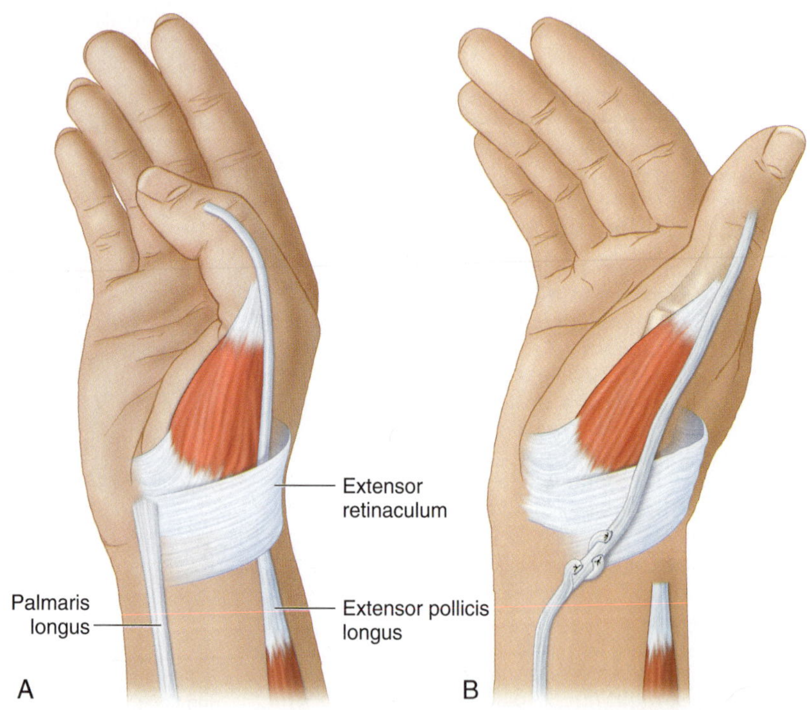

FIGURE 20-10

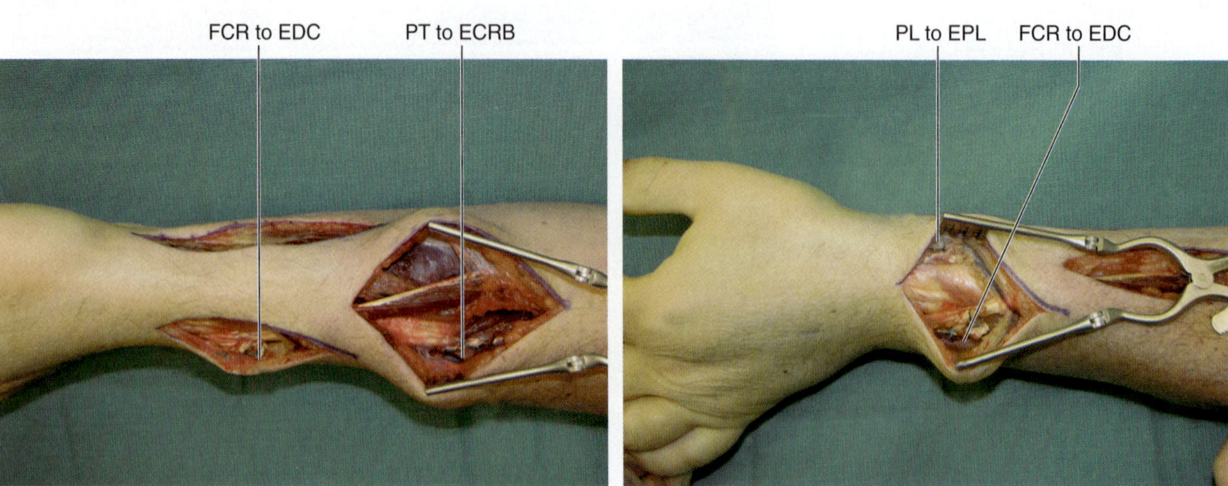

FIGURE 20-11

Postoperative Care and Expected Outcomes

- A long-arm plaster of Paris splint is applied that keeps the wrist in 45 degrees of extension, the finger MCP joint in full extension, and the thumb in maximum abduction and extension. The finger interphalangeal joints are left free.
- Ten days after surgery, the wound is inspected, sutures are removed, and the position previously described is maintained using a removable splint for 4 weeks. After this time, the splint can be worn as needed and the patient is started on tenodesis exercises under the guidance of a therapist. (Figures 20-12 and 20-13 show the late results of patients shown in Figures 20-1 and 20-2, respectively.)
- Most reports suggest that tendon transfer procedures for radial nerve palsy are rewarding, with patients demonstrating improved thumb, wrist, and finger extension. On average, patients regained 50% of the power grip and pinch of the normal side. The limitations included difficulty in grasping or releasing large objects and early fatigue.

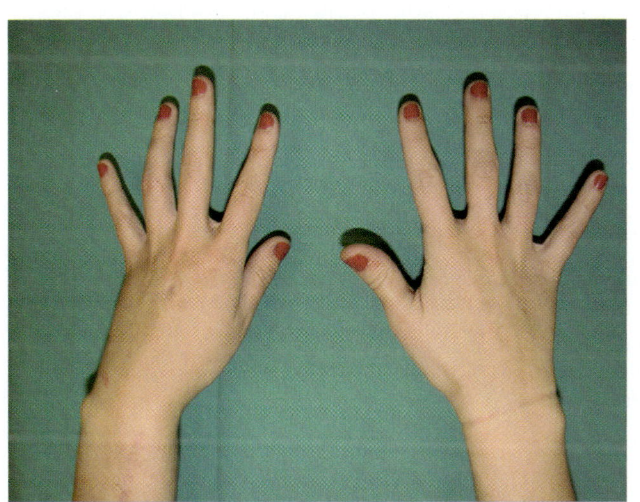

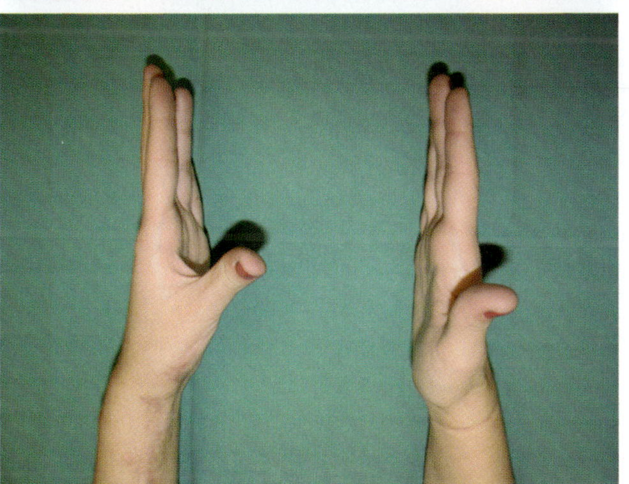

FIGURE 20-12

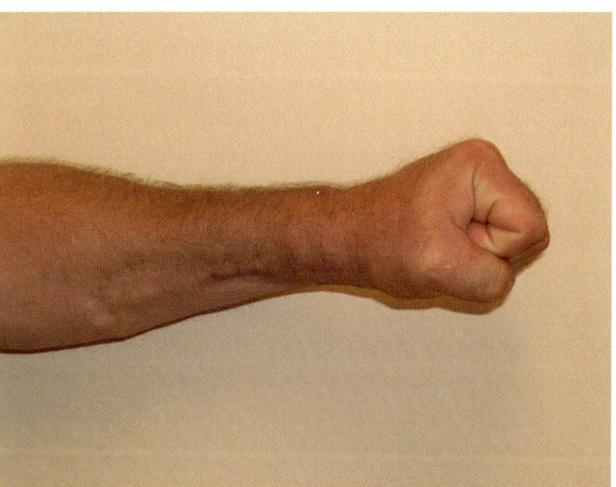

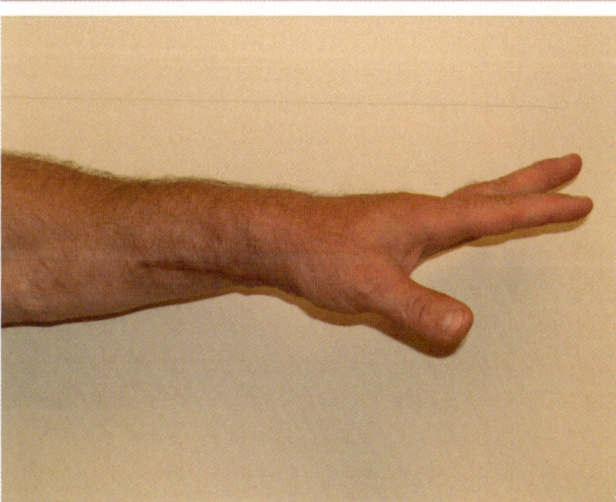

FIGURE 20-13

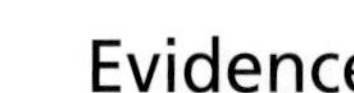

Evidence

Chotigavanich C. Tendon transfer for radial nerve palsy. *Bull Hosp Joint Dis Orthop Inst*. 1990;50:1-10.

The author reviewed 50 patients (43 with high radial nerve palsies and 7 with low palsies) who underwent FCU or long finger FDS transfer to the EDC. In all patients, the PL was transferred to the EPL, and, in 40 patients, the PT was transferred to the ECRL and ECRB. All regained useful hand function. Manual muscle testing demonstrated grade 4 or 5 wrist extension strength in 82%, finger MCP joint extension in 90%, and thumb extension in 92%. Good or excellent results were achieved by Tajima's finger, thumb, and wrist motion criteria in 43 patients. Five cases with FCU transfer had radial wrist deviation. No problems with grip weakness were noted in patients in whom the FDS was used as a donor, but the author stressed the use of only one FDS. (Level IV evidence)

Chuinard RG, Boyes JH, Stark HH, et al. Tendon transfers for radial nerve palsy: use of superficialis tendons for digital extension. *J Hand Surg [Am]*. 1978;3:560-570.

The authors reviewed 22 patients who had the FDS of the long finger transferred to the EDC slips and the FDS of the ring finger transferred to the EPL and EIP. PT was transferred to the ECRL and ECRB. The FCR was inserted into the APL. They also developed a method to objectify results based on flexion and extension of the fingers and the wrist and abduction and extension of the thumb. By their assessment criteria, 16 patients (73%) achieved a good or excellent result. (Level IV evidence)

Skoll PJ, Hudson DA, de Jager W, et al. Long term results of tendon transfers for radial nerve palsy in patients with limited rehabilitation. *Ann Plast Surg*. 2000;45:122-126.

The authors retrospectively reviewed 22 patients who were treated for high radial nerve palsy with transfers of the FCU to the EDC, the PT to the ECRB, and the PL to the rerouted EPL. They used the FCR instead of the FCU in patients with PIN palsy. Using Chuinard's criteria, the authors reported 19 good to excellent results for wrist extension, 20 for finger extension, 20 for thumb extension, and 21 for thumb abduction. Power grip was approximately one half that of the contralateral side. Ten of the 15 patients with the FCU transfer and 2 of the 7 patients with the FCR transfer had a wrist radial deviation posture at rest. All but 1 patient were able to perform activities of daily living. The Jebson test took an average of 1.46 times longer than was expected. Patient satisfaction was graded at 6.5 out of 10, with the most common complaints being stiffness and lack of dexterity and power. Thirteen of 17 patients who were employed before injury were able to return to their previous work. However, only 1 of the 7 heavy manual laborers returned to his preinjury occupation. (Level IV evidence)

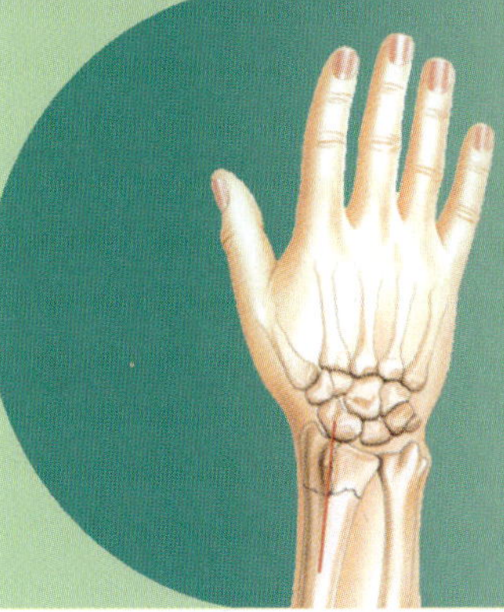

Steindler Flexorplasty

Pao-Yuan Lin, Sandeep J. Sebastin, and Kevin C. Chung

Indications

- Late presentation of upper trunk brachial plexus palsy (C5-C6; C5-C6-C7) without recovery of elbow flexion.
  - Steindler procedure is preferred to a pedicled latissimus dorsi (LD) transfer or free functioning muscle transfer, if the patient has good function of the wrist and finger flexors.
  - A pedicled LD transfer or free functioning muscle transfer can be considered if the wrist flexors are weak.
  - A pectoralis major–biceps transfer can be considered in patients who have a weak biceps (partial recovery). The pectoralis major cannot replace the function of the biceps but can augment it.
- Arthrogryposis patients lacking elbow flexion.

Examination/Imaging

Clinical Examination

- The patients should have adequate strength in the flexor pronator mass, especially the wrist flexors [flexor carpi radialis (FCR) and flexor carpi ulnaris (FCU)]. This can be assessed by asking the patient to flex the wrist against resistance.
- The patient should have good wrist extension to counteract the possible development of a wrist flexion contracture.
- The patients should have adequate passive flexion of the elbow. If passive flexion of the elbow is limited owing to a tight triceps, then triceps lengthening may be necessary to increase passive range of motion.

Imaging

- Plain radiograph of the elbow should reveal normal elbow articulation.

Surgical Anatomy

- The common flexor-pronator muscles originate from the medial epicondyle. The following muscles are elevated during this procedure: pronator teres, FCR, palmaris longus, FCU, and flexor digitorum superficialis (Fig. 21-1). The flexor digitorum profundus is left in situ (see Fig. 21-1).
- The ulnar nerve must be protected during elevation of the flexor-pronator mass. It may be transposed anteriorly in the submuscular plane.

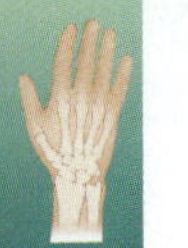

- The medial (ulnar) collateral ligament of the elbow should be protected during elevation of the flexor-pronator mass. It originates at the posterior distal aspect of the medial epicondyle and inserts into the base of the coronoid process of ulna. It is composed of three bands: anterior, posterior, and transverse (Fig. 21-2).

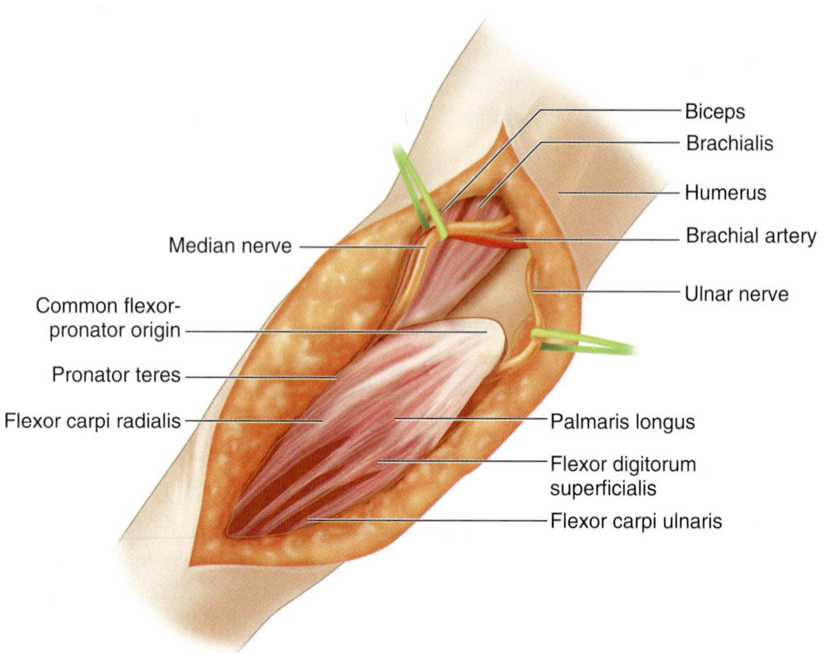

FIGURE 21-1

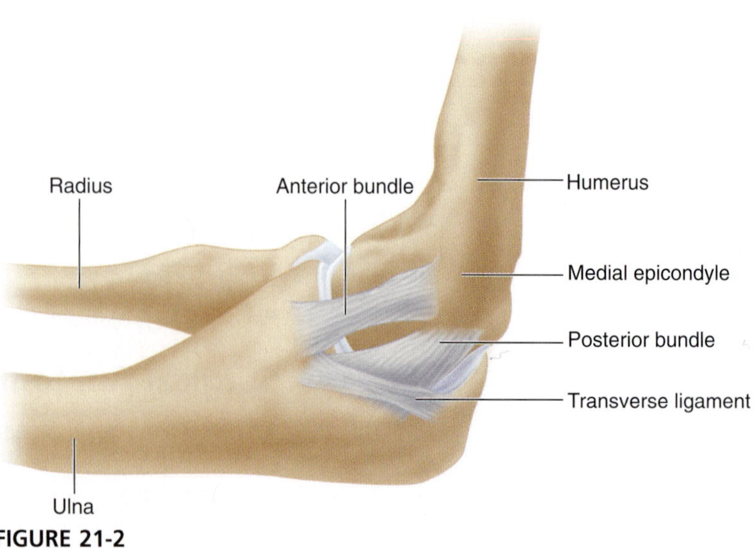

FIGURE 21-2

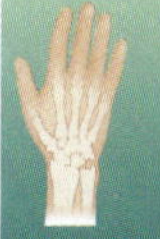

Positioning

- The patient is positioned supine with the affected extremity on a hand table. The procedure is performed under general or regional anesthesia, and a sterile tourniquet is placed as high up the arm as possible.

Exposures

- A 10-cm longitudinal curvilinear incision centered over the medial epicondyle is made (Fig. 21-3).
- A skin flap is elevated while protecting the medial antebrachial cutaneous nerve. After elevation of the skin flap, one will see the flexor-pronator mass attaching to the medial epicondyle (Fig. 21-4).

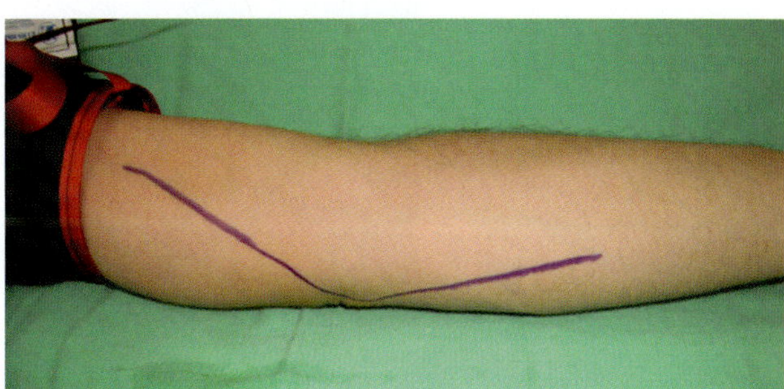

FIGURE 21-3

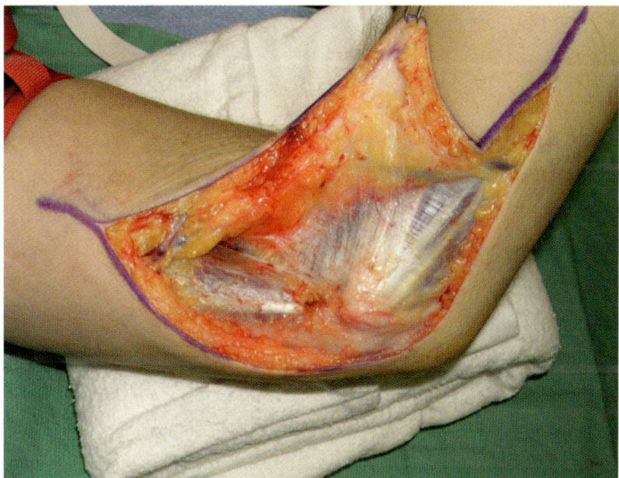

FIGURE 21-4

- The ulnar nerve is protected, and a vessel loop is placed around the nerve for identification and gentle traction (Fig. 21-5).
- Lateral to the flexor-pronator mass, the brachial artery and median nerve are seen entering the arch over the superficialis muscles (Fig. 21-6).

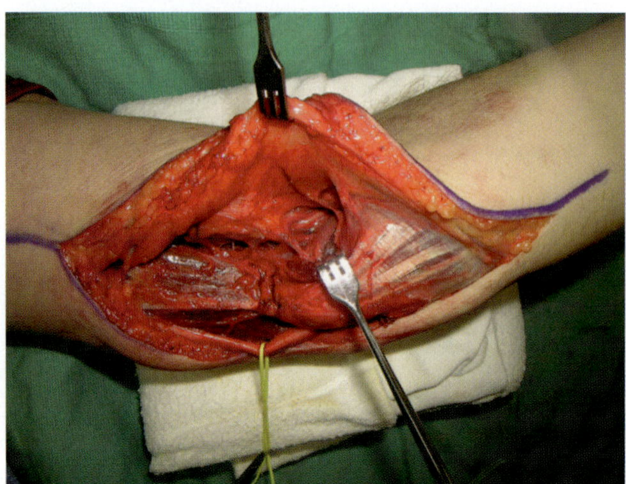

FIGURE 21-5

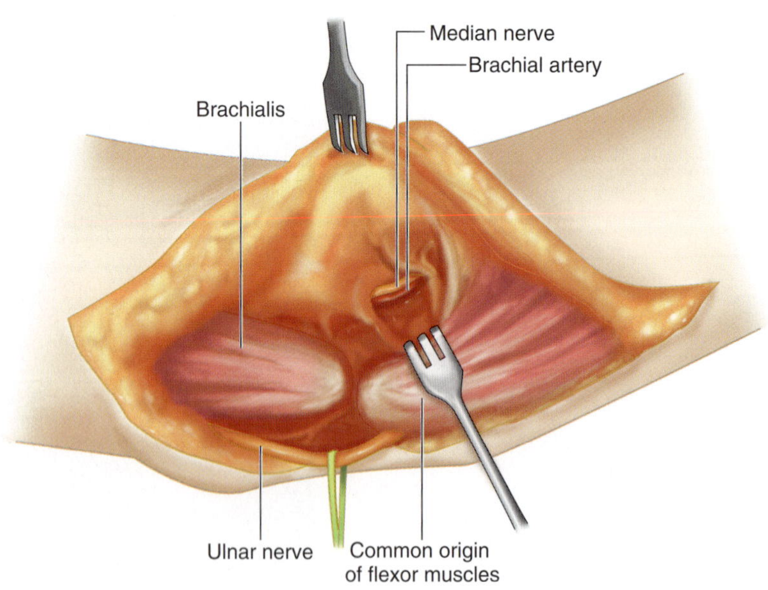

FIGURE 21-6

Procedure

Step 1

- The index finger is placed under the flexor-pronator mass to develop an interval plane between the median nerve and the entire flexor-pronator mass (Fig. 21-7). The ulnar head of FCU is dissected from the ulna.

Step 2

- An osteotome is used to elevate the common pronator-flexor origin along with a segment of bone measuring about 2 × 2 × 1 cm (Fig. 21-8).

Step 3

- The common flexor-pronator origin is separated from the anterior surface of the joint.

STEP 1 PEARLS

Passing a finger around the flexor-pronator mass will define the dissection plane and make harvesting of the osteomuscular flap easier (see Fig. 21-7).

STEP 1 PITFALLS

One must be careful to preserve the small nerve branches from the median nerve and ulnar nerve that innervate the flexor muscles.

STEP 2 PITFALLS

The ulnar collateral ligament of the elbow must be protected while performing the osteotomy of the medial epicondyle.

STEP 3 PITFALLS

The ulnar nerve must be fully mobilized before elevation of the flexor-pronator mass to prevent traction and injury to the nerve (Fig. 21-9).

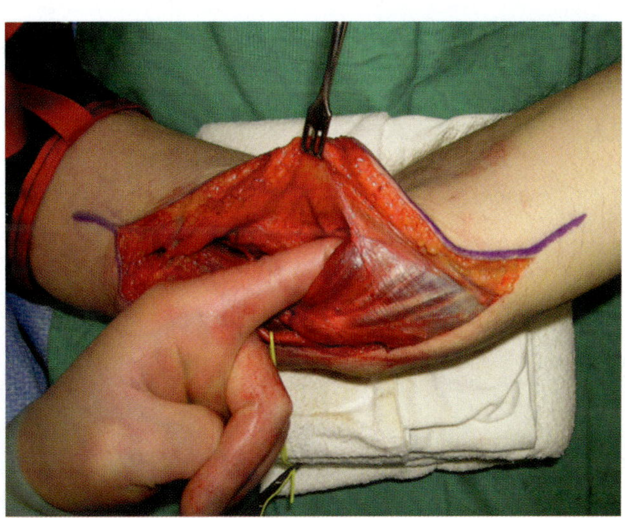

FIGURE 21-7

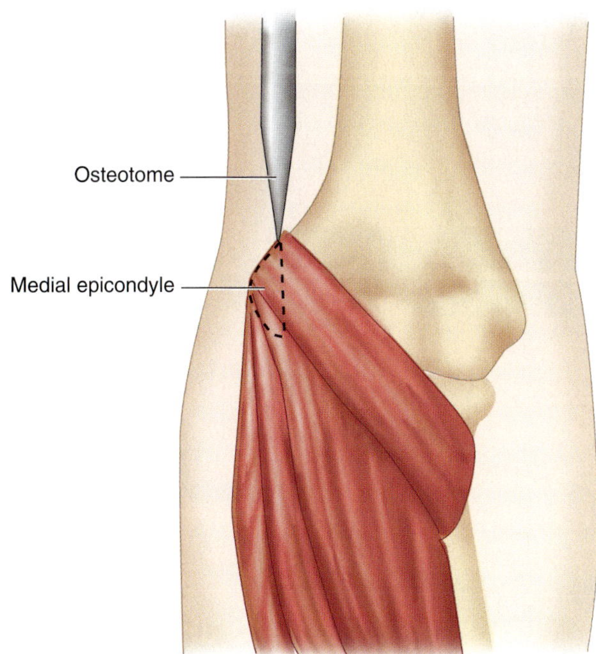

FIGURE 21-8

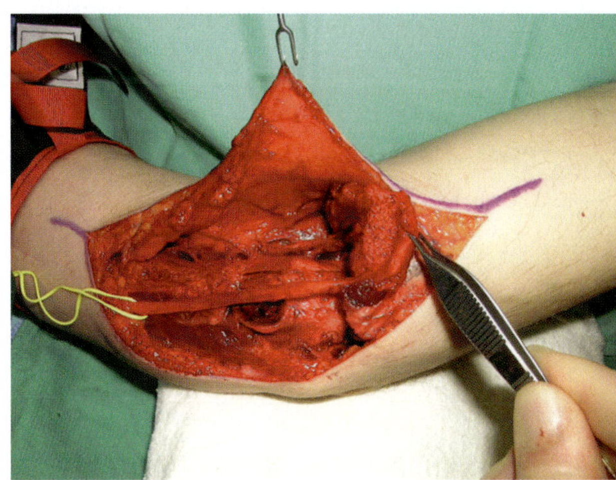

FIGURE 21-9

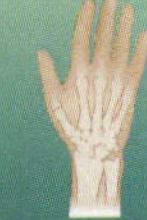

Step 4

- A cortical window is developed between the biceps and brachialis muscles to provide a bone attachment site for the osteotomized medial epicondyle. The fixation site of the new common pronator-flexor origin is about 5 to 7 cm proximal on the humerus, creating 130 degrees of elbow flexion.

STEP 4 PEARLS

- A bur is used to core out a trough on the humerus so that the medial epicondyle can be seated within the trough (Fig. 21-10).

Step 5

- The medial epicondyle can be provisionally fixed to the trough created in the distal humerus and secured using a towel clip.
- Secure fixation to the humerus is achieved by passing a 3.5-mm cortical screw over a washer through the medial epicondyle. A 2.5-mm drill bit and a 3.5-mm tap are used for this purpose (Fig. 21-11).
- After securing the bone, the ulnar nerve is then transposed anteriorly under the flexor-pronator mass. The muscle is then closed over the native medial epicondyle using 2-0 Vicryl sutures.

STEP 5 PITFALLS

- The median nerve and brachial artery should be inspected carefully after fixation to ensure that there is compression, or entrapment.

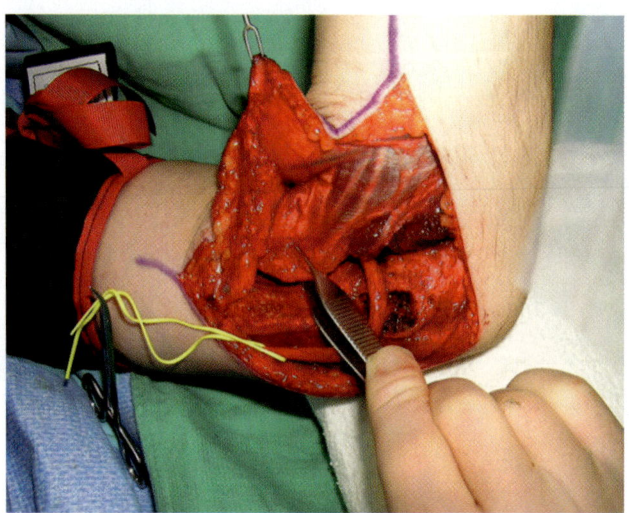

FIGURE 21-10

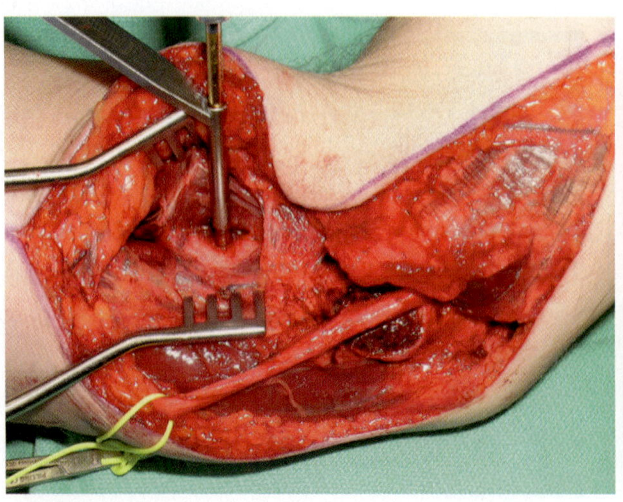

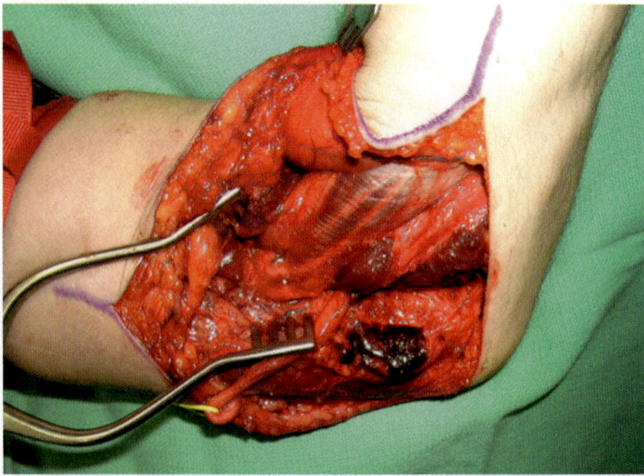

FIGURE 21-11

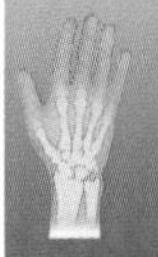

Postoperative Care and Expected Outcomes

- The elbow is splinted at 90 degrees for 6 weeks to allow fusion of the osteotomized medial epicondyle to the humerus. After 2 weeks, the sutures are removed, and a thermoplastic splint is made to immobilize the elbow at 90 degrees of flexion for another 4 weeks. During the first 6 weeks, the patient should move the fingers to prevent contracture. After 6 weeks, the patient is started on gentle gravity-assisted extension of the elbow while initiating elbow flexion exercises. After 12 weeks, resisted flexion is started.
- It is not advisable for the patient to stretch to achieve full extension of the elbow because the purpose of this operation is to achieve sufficient elbow flexion, which is more beneficial to the patients. The patient can be expected to achieve an arc of flexion of 30 to 100 degrees that will reach to the mouth.

Evidence

Chen WS. Restoration of elbow flexion by modified Steindler flexorplasty. *Int Orthop*. 2000;24:43-46.
A retrospective review of eight patients who underwent modified Steindler flexorplasty was conducted. Union between the humerus and transferred bone block was achieved at 3 months. The maximum flexion achieved ranged from 110 to 130 degrees. (Level IV evidence)

Dutton RO, Dawson EG. Elbow flexorplasty: an analysis of long-term results. *J Bone Joint Surg [Am]*. 1981;63:1064-1069.
A retrospective review of 25 patients who underwent Steindler elbow flexorplasty between 1952 and 1976 was conducted. The mean length of the follow-up was 9.3 years. The mean arc of active flexion after flexorplasty was 95 degrees. The postoperative loss of elbow extension averaged 36 degrees. The mean postoperative active pronation and supination were 79 degrees and 51 degrees, respectively. At final evaluation, 14 patients were judged to have excellent; 6, good; 4, fair; and 1, poor function. (Level IV evidence)

Goldfarb CA, Burke MS, Manske PR, et al. The Steindler flexorplasty for the arthrogrypotic elbow. *J Hand Surg [Am]*. 2004;29:462-469.
A retrospective review of 17 elbows in 10 patients with an average age of 7 years being treated surgically with the Steindler flexorplasty procedure was conducted. The mean follow-up period was 5 years. All patients obtained active elbow flexion against gravity averaging 85 degrees (range, 30 to 120 degrees); patients were able to lift an average of 1 kg through their entire arc of elbow flexion postoperatively. Subjectively, 9 of the 10 patients were satisfied with the outcome of the surgery. (Level IV evidence)

Liu TK, Yang RS, Sun JS. Long-term results of the Steindler flexorplasty. *Clin Orthop Relat Res*. 1993;296:104-108.
A retrospective review of 71 consecutive patients who were treated with a modified Steindler flexorplasty from 1970 to 1987 was conducted. The average clinical follow-up was 8.2 years. The outcome was excellent in 32%, good in 47%, fair in 13%, and poor in 8%. The mean arc of active elbow flexion was 114 degrees; the average elbow extension loss, 28 degrees; the mean active pronation, 74 degrees; and supination, 30 degrees, postoperatively. (Level IV evidence)

Monreal R. Steindler flexorplasty to restore elbow flexion in C5-C6-C7 brachial plexus palsy type. *J Brachial Plex Peripher Nerve Inj*. 2007;2:15.
A retrospective follow-up study of 12 patients who had undergone surgical reconstruction of the flail upper limb by Steindler flexorplasty and wrist arthrodesis to restore elbow flexion was conducted. The etiology of elbow weakness was in all patients brachial plexus palsy (C5-C6-C7 deficit). The average duration of clinical follow-up was 28 months. Eleven patients were found to have very good or good function of the transferred muscles. (Level IV evidence)

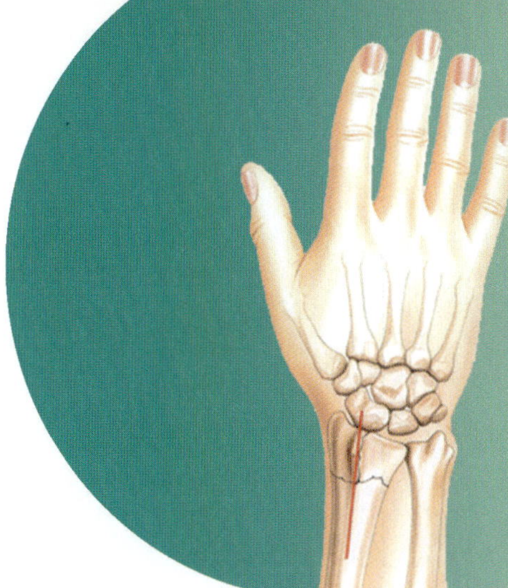

Section IV

MUSCULOTENDINOUS UNIT LENGTHENING AND TENDON TRANSFERS FOR SPASTIC CONDITIONS

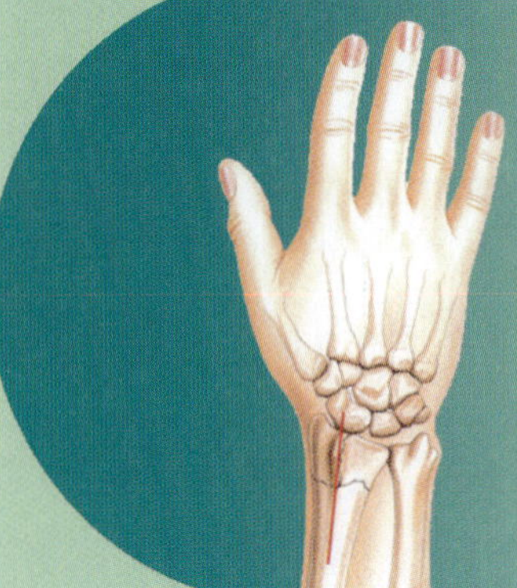

Intrinsic Muscle Release for Thumb-in-Palm Deformity

Harry A. Hoyen and Patrick J. Messerschmitt

See Video 19: Intrinsic Muscle Release for Thumb-in-Palm Deformity and Adductor Release Using a Thenar Incision

Indications

- Spastic contracture of the thumb adductor muscle results in excessive thumb metacarpal adduction and thumb-in-palm deformity.
- In mild or moderate degrees, grasp and pinch are affected when other intrinsic and extrinsic contractures result in compromise of skin care and hygiene.
- This procedure is often combined with other surgical release procedures for the thumb, fingers, and wrist.

Examination/Imaging

Clinical Examination

- Examination of the hand demonstrates an adducted position of the thumb metacarpal across the palm of the hand (Figs. 22-1 and 22-2).
- Additional deformities of the wrist and hand frequently can coexist with the thumb-in-palm deformity (Fig. 22-3).
- Evaluate for flexion deformities of the thumb metacarpophalangeal joint and/or thumb interphalangeal joint, which would require concomitant releases of the flexor pollicis brevis or flexor pollicis longus, respectively.

Surgical Anatomy

- Thenar muscles, flexor pollicis longus, adductor pollicis, lumbricals, and interosseous muscles
- Recurrent motor branch of the medial nerve and the common digital nerves
- Superficial and deep palmar arterial arches

Positioning

- The patient is positioned supine with the arm extended onto a surgical arm board.
- A nonsterile tourniquet is placed high on the arm before surgical preparation to allow better visualization during the procedure.

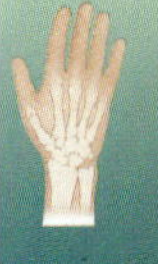

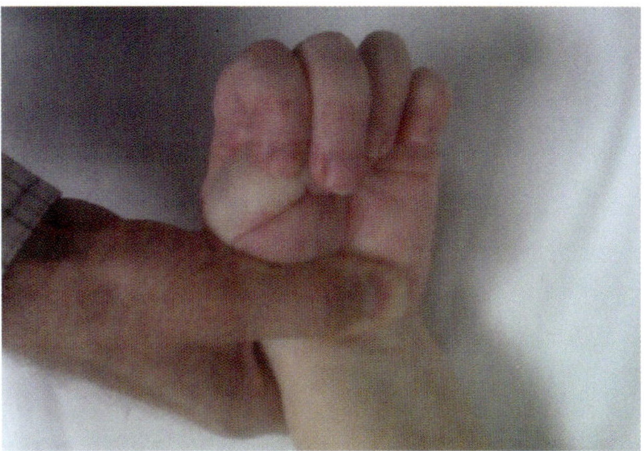

FIGURE 22-1

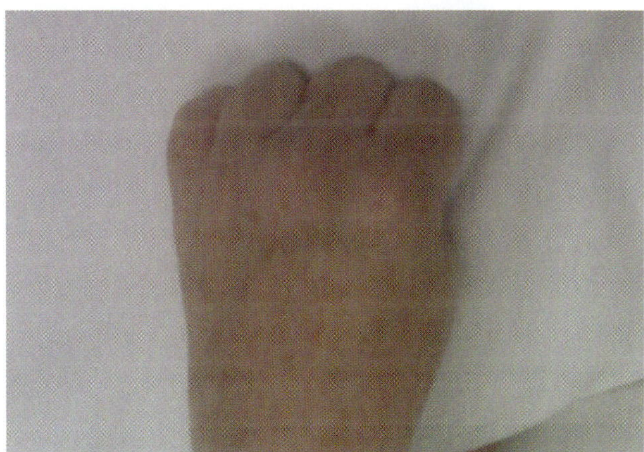

FIGURE 22-2

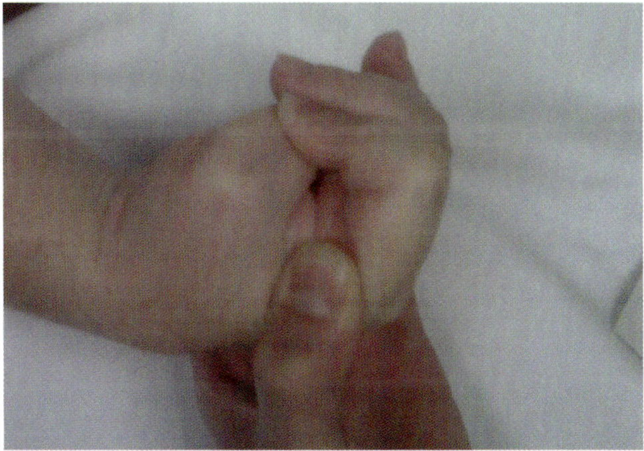

FIGURE 22-3

PEARLS

Severe adduction contractures may require Z-plasty exposure of the first web space, which facilitates release of both skin contracture and involved spastic muscles.

Exposures

- A palmar incision is made paralleling the thenar crease (Fig. 22-4).
- The long finger flexor tendons are the next most dorsal structure after the palmar fascia has been divided. Retract the flexor tendons ulnarly.
- Identify the lumbrical muscle and common digital artery and nerve.
- Gently retract the lumbrical muscle and the neurovascular bundle ulnarly to visualize the enveloping thumb adductor muscle fascia. The thumb adductor muscle, with transverse muscle fibers beneath, originates on the radial side of the long finger metacarpal (Fig. 22-5).

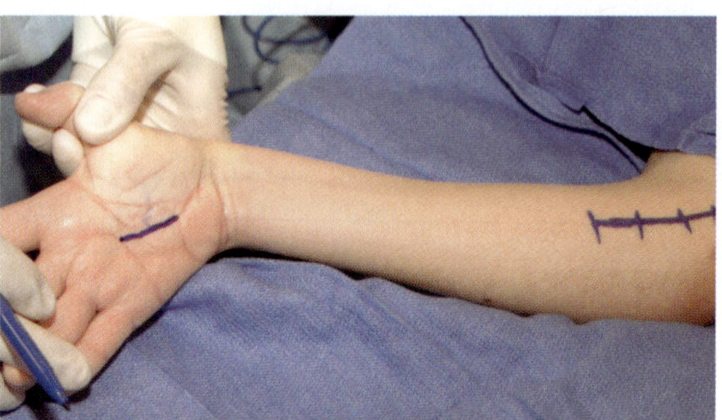

FIGURE 22-4

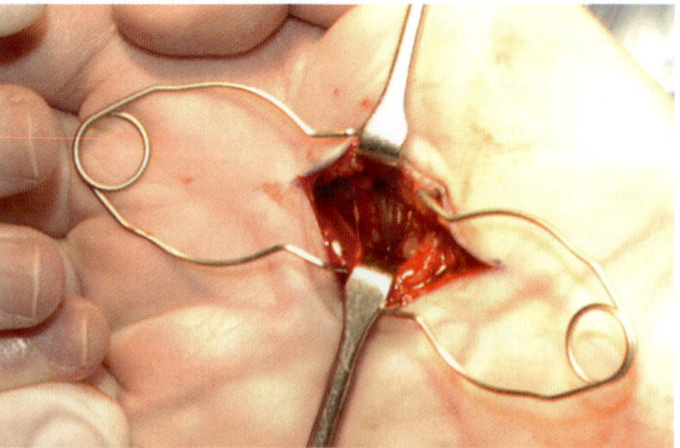

FIGURE 22-5

STEP 1 PEARLS

Preserve the deep ulnar nerve branch to the adductor pollicis.

Preserve the deep palmar vascular arch.

STEP 2 PEARLS

Preserve the motor branch of the median nerve to the thenar muscles.

The first dorsal interosseous muscle can be released from the thumb metacarpal base if residual contracture remains; however, this is usually not necessary.

Pin the thumb metacarpal in abduction with smooth K-wires if tightness persists.

STEP 2 PITFALLS

Avoid injury to the perforating branch of the radial artery.

Obtain meticulous hemostasis after tourniquet deflation before wound closure.

Procedure

Step 1

- Sharply release the origin of the thumb adductor muscle from the long finger metacarpal.
- Passively abduct the thumb, allowing the thumb adductor musculature to pull radially and ensure complete release (Fig. 22-6).

Step 2

- If necessary, proceed to release of thenar muscle contracture.
- Origins of both heads of flexor pollicis brevis, opponens pollicis, and abductor pollicis brevis muscles are identified on the volar carpal ligament and sharply sectioned with care (Fig. 22-7).
- Again, passively abduct and extend the thumb, allowing the muscles to retract.

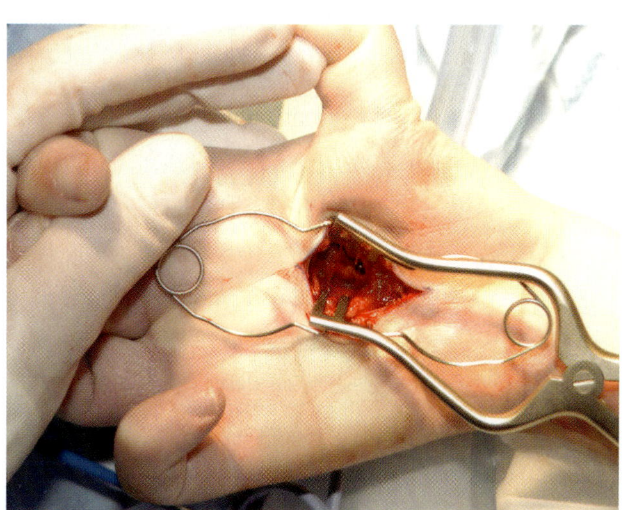

FIGURE 22-6

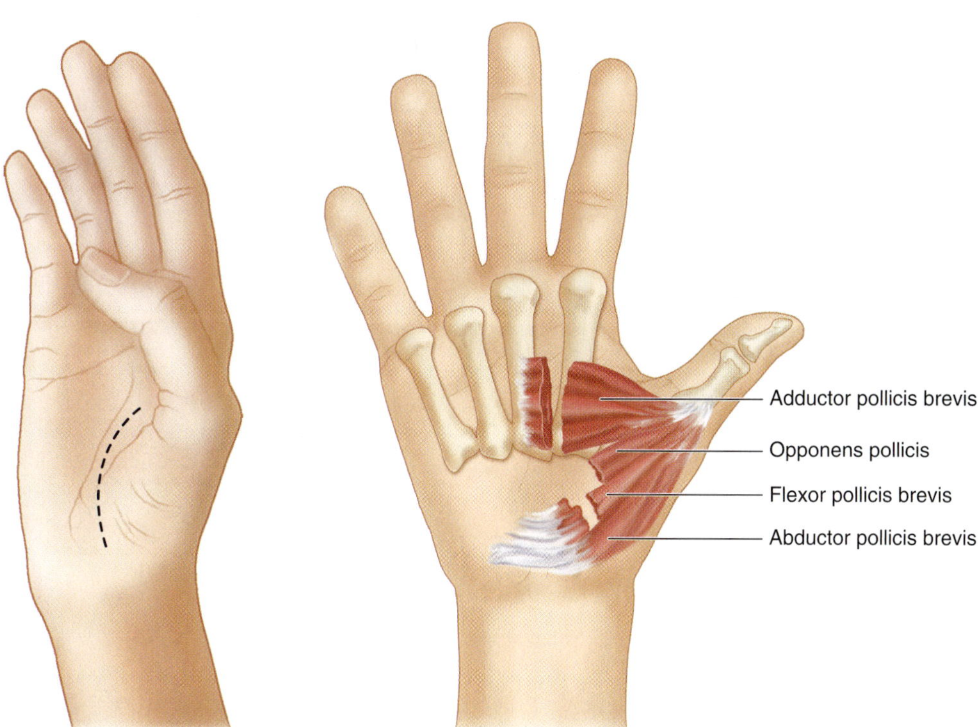

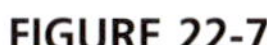

FIGURE 22-7

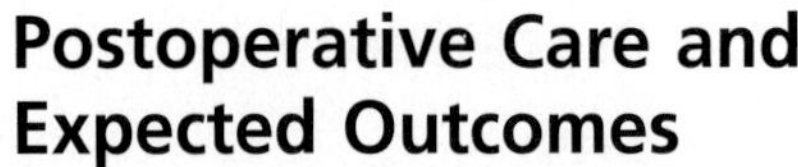

Postoperative Care and Expected Outcomes

- The postoperative thumb-spica splint is applied with the thumb metacarpal positioned in extension and abduction. This permits the fibrosis that bridges the muscle defect to incorporate in a better anatomic position. Avoid thumb metaphalangeal hyperextension.
- After 4 weeks, the patient is converted to a full-time fabricated C-splint between the index metaphalangeal joint and the thumb proximal phalanx. This holds the thumb in extension and abduction and maintains opening of the first web space. The splint is removed for bathing and exercises.
- Eight to 10 weeks postoperatively, the patient is advanced to wearing the splint at night only. If the patient is skeletally mature, the splint can be discontinued 3 to 6 months postoperatively.

Acknowledgment

We would like to give a special thanks to the author of this chapter in the previous edition, Ann E. Van Heest, as her work served as an excellent foundation for and contribution to this chapter.

Evidence

House J, Gwathmey F, Fidler M. A dynamic approach to the thumb-in-palm deformity in cerebral palsy. *J Bone Joint Surg [Am]*. 1981;63:216-225.
This classic article described the spastic thumb-in-palm deformity secondary to cerebral palsy. It also highlighted the Upper Extremity Functional Use Classification as an outcome tool to use after surgery. (Level IV evidence)

Inglis AE, Cooper W, Bruton W. Surgical correction of thumb deformities in spastic paralysis. *J Bone Joint Surg [Am]*. 1970;52:253-268.
This classic article described the spastic thumb-in-palm deformity secondary to cerebral palsy. Surgical methods and outcomes are presented. (Level IV evidence)

PROCEDURE 23

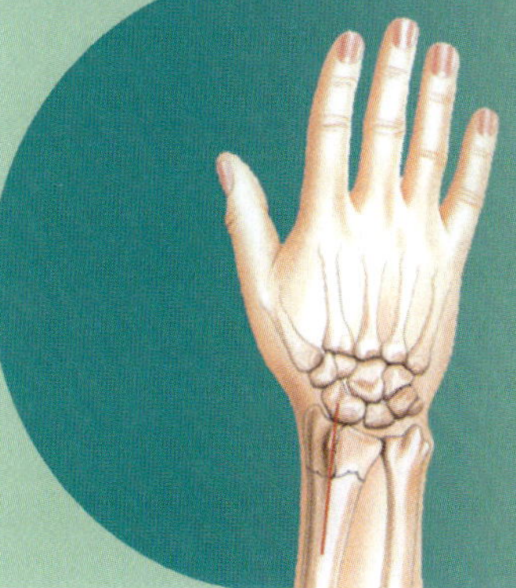

Fractional Lengthening of the Flexor Tendons

Harry A. Hoyen and Patrick J. Messerschmitt

See Video 20: Fractional Lengthening of the Flexor Tendons

Indications

- Wrist and finger flexion deformity due to spastic muscle contracture in which the fingers cannot be passively extended fully despite positioning the wrist in flexion.
- Situation in which flexor lengthening up to 15% to 20% of the muscle is required; otherwise, superficialis-to-profundus tendon transfer is necessary.
- Conditions in which finger and hand flexion is to be preserved for functional purposes. The preoperative condition is functionally limiting, especially with activities of daily living.

Examination/Imaging

Clinical Examination

- Preoperative examination is helpful in determing the contribution of the finger and wrist contracture from the spastic properties of the finger flexor tendons.
- Examine the involvement of all muscles that contribute to wrist flexion: palmaris longus, flexor carpi radialis, and flexor carpi ulnaris (FCU), and those primarily responsible for finger flexion: flexor digitorum sublimis and flexor digitorum profundus (FDP).
- Excessive flexion of distal interphalangeal (DIP) joints indicates FDP involvement.
- Excessive flexion of proximal interphalangeal (PIP) joints without significant contracture of DIP joints suggests flexor digitorum sublimis involvement.
- Examining the wrist in flexion may aid in delineating the effect of the flexor digitorum sublimis from the FDP on the contracture.
- It is also necessary to examine the small hand articulations to determine the effect of fixed joint contractures. This may represent an articular arthrofibrosis and would not improve with a muscle/tendon procedure.

Surgical Anatomy

- Pertinent surgical anatomy includes the volar forearm muscles (palmaris longus, flexor carpi radialis, flexor carpi ulnaris, flexor digitorum superficialis, FDP, pronator teres, pronator quadratus), median nerve, ulnar nerve and artery, and radial artery. Cross-sectional anatomy should be reviewed before intervention.

PEARLS

The ulnar nerve is more volar and ulnar than the ulnar artery. The FDP tendons are supplied by segmental arterioles from the ulnar artery. Hemostasis of these vessels is important in preventing postoperative hematoma.

Identify the median nerve before any musculotendinous recessions. It can be difficult to differentiate the median nerve from the finger flexor tendons, especially under tourniquet application. The vascularity of the nerve is different from the tendon. The nerve is typically supplied by longitudinal vessels. One cannot rely on the tension of the structures in these severe contracture situations.

Positioning

- Position the patient supine with the arm extended onto a surgical arm board.
- A nonsterile tourniquet is placed high on the arm before surgical preparation to allow better visualization during the procedure.

Exposures

- A longitudinal volar incision over the junction of the mid to distal third of the forearm is used. This corresponds to the myotendinous junction of the volar flexor musculature.
- Division of the volar forearm fascia exposes the underlying musculotendinous junctions (Fig. 23-1).
- Cutaneous volar veins should be mobilized and ligated as necessary.

Procedure

Step 1

- The tendinous portion of the myotendinous structure is identified, carefully verifying that the muscular portion is in continuity. The tendon is then identified into the distal muscle belly, without disturbing the muscle fibers (Fig. 23-2).

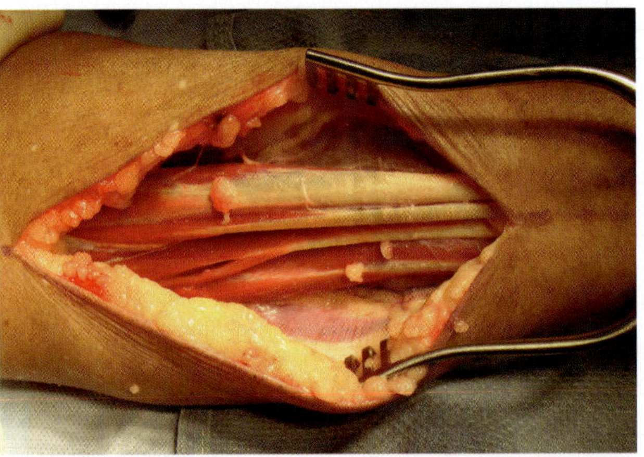

FIGURE 23-1

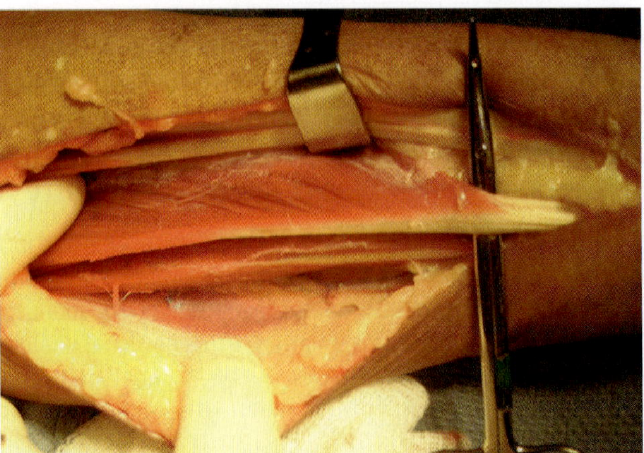

FIGURE 23-2

STEP 1 PEARLS

Ensure careful identification and protection of the median nerve, ulnar nerve, and ulnar artery.

STEP 1 PITFALLS

The flexor tendons need to be divided at a location within the muscle. A division too distal will result in a simple tenotomy.

STEP 2 PEARLS

Incise the tendinous portion only, leaving the underlying muscle belly intact. The muscle will provide structural and nutritional support for tendon reconstitution.

- The tendon will be divided at the transition from muscle to tendon. Some of the superficial muscle fibers may need dissection to adequately identify this location.
- With a wrist flexion contracture, the tendons for the FCR and FCU are first divided. A proximal and distal division of the FCU tendon may be necessary because the myotendinous portion of the FCU extends very distally and over a wide range.

Step 2

- A sharp tendon division is made at the musculotendinous junction in each flexor digitorum superficialis tendon (Fig. 23-3).
- Each digit is passively stretched into extension, allowing the tendon and muscle fibers to slide distally. A 2- to 3-cm gap between the two ends of the tendon will be visualized (Fig. 23-4).

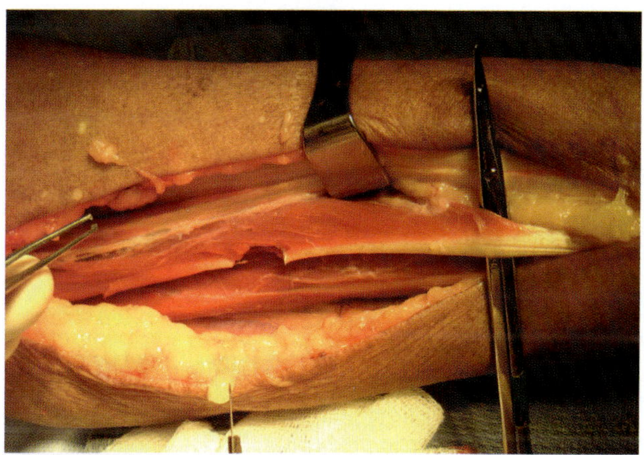

FIGURE 23-3

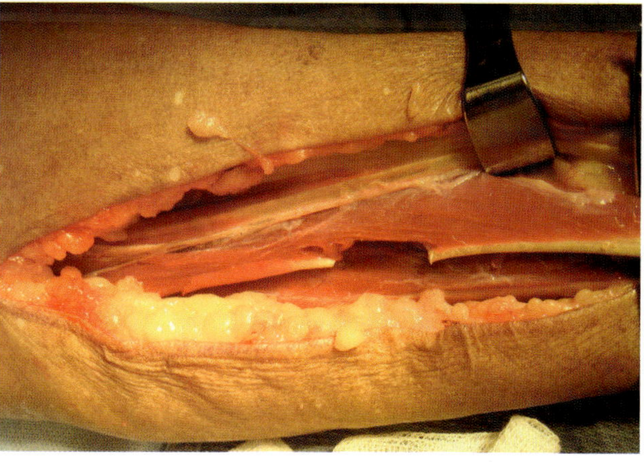

FIGURE 23-4

STEP 3 PEARLS

The posture of the fingers needs to be inspected. A second recession may be necessary if correction of the finger posture is not adequate.

All of the finger flexor recessions (FDP and FDS) should be performed before proceeding with second recessions.

Step 3

- Once all flexor digitorum superficialis tendons are lengthened appropriately, lengthening of the FDP tendons is usually necessary to obtain better digital extension. The examination under anesthesia is helpful in determining the preoperative need to lengthen the FDS and FDP.
- Meticulous dissection deep to the FDP tendons includes hemostasis of segmental arterioles from the ulnar artery (Fig. 23-5).
- The FDP tendons are completely visualized and isolated for lengthening (Fig. 23-6).
- A similar tendon division is made at the musculotendinous junction of each FDP tendon (Fig. 23-7).

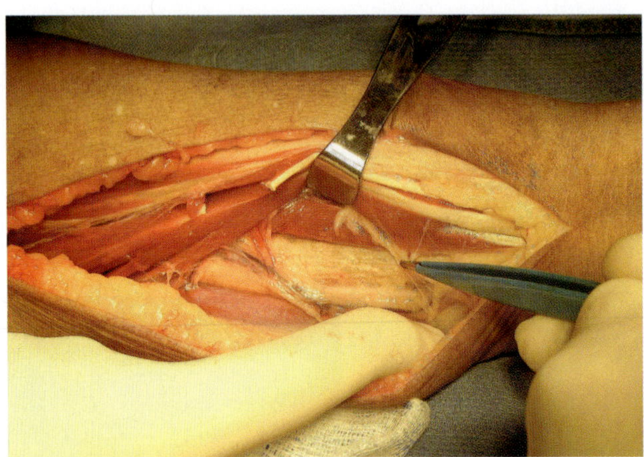

FIGURE 23-5

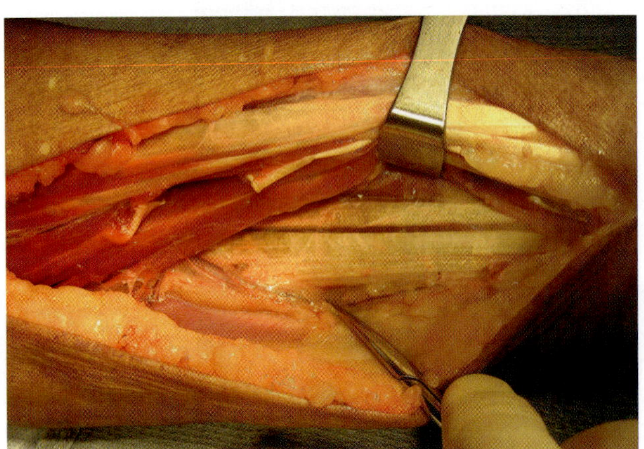

FIGURE 23-6

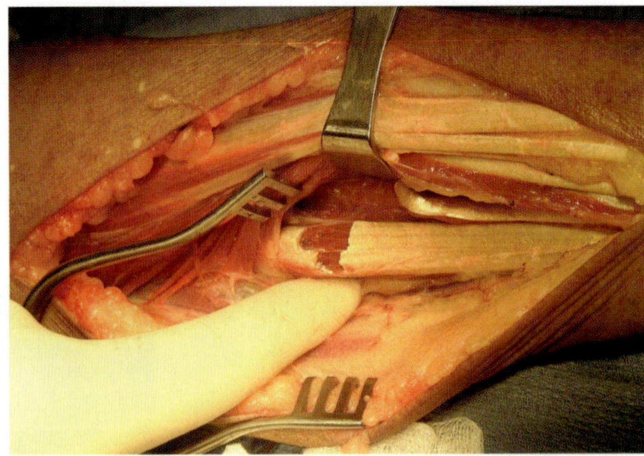

FIGURE 23-7

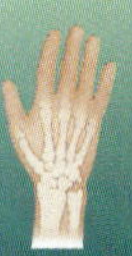

STEP 4 PEARLS

The tension on the median and ulnar nerves should be noted with the wrist in a neutral to 15-degree extension position. This may limit the postoperative positioning of the fingers and wrist during the immobilization period.

Step 4

- The tourniquet is deflated, and meticulous hemostasis is obtained. Postoperative hematoma may occur owing to the muscle dissection and lengthening.

Postoperative Care and Expected Outcomes

- The patient is positioned with the wrist and fingers in extension, as determined by the stretch on the neurovascular structures. A dorsal and volar plaster splint is applied intraoperatively.
- After the postoperative swelling has subsided (7 to 10 days), the wound is inspected. A fiberglass cast is applied to maintain the finger and wrist position. The cast is maintained for an additional 4 weeks to allow the muscle and tendon structures to heal in a lengthened position.
- After the cast is removed, a custom wrist-hand orthosis is fabricated to maintain the passive extension achieved intraoperatively. The orthosis is worn for an additional month on a full-time basis, then advanced to night wear only for an additional 3 to 6 months.
- The expected outcome of the surgery is improved passive wrist and finger extension.

Evidence

Keenan MAE, Abrams RA, Garland DE, et al. Results of fractional lengthening of the finger flexors in adults with upper extremity spasticity. *J Hand Surg [Am].* 1987;12:575-581.

This classic article describes the technique for fractional lengthening of the finger flexors. Surgical indications and treatment outcomes are outlined. (Level IV evidence)

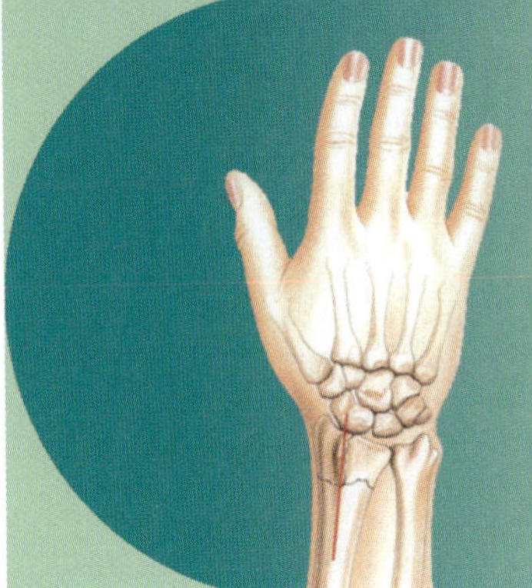

Superficialis-to-Profundus Tendon Transfer

Harry A. Hoyen and Patrick J. Messerschmitt

Indications

- This procedure is indicated for fixed finger deformities secondary to flexor digitorum superficialis and flexor digitorum profundus tendon spasticity. The muscle properties have been permanently altered owing to the contracture severity and chronicity.
- These patients have marked functional impairment and have expected limited upper extremity use. The procedure is often used for facilitating skin care and hand hygiene problems.
- The determination between this type of transfer and a fractional lengthening needs to be evaluated by preoperative assessment. Comanagement with the family and caregivers is essential for identifying the preoperative needs.
- It should be explained that finger stiffness is common after surgery and that a different type of contracture may be present. The position of the contracture is changed to a posture that aids in maintaining hygiene and overall care.

Examination/Imaging

Clinical Examination

- Preoperative evaluation is important to determine the contribution of the different volar flexor muscles to the finger contracture. Examine finger extension at both maximum wrist flexion and maximum wrist extension.
- The finger flexion deformity will be worse with maximum wrist extension than with maximum wrist flexion if the deformity is secondary to contracture of the flexor digitorum superficialis and flexor digitorum profundus tendons. In different neurologic conditions, the wrist flexor musculature may also be spastic.
- Assess the metacarpophalangeal, proximal interphalangeal, and distal interphalangeal joints of each digit because fixed contractures may require concomitant treatment (closed manipulation, open capsulotomies, or joint fusions).

Surgical Anatomy

- Pertinent surgical structures include all volar forearm muscles (palmaris longus, flexor carpi radialis [FCR], flexor carpi ulnaris [FCU], flexor digitorum superficialis [FDS], flexor digitorum profundus [FDP], pronator teres, pronator quadratus), median nerve, ulnar nerve and artery, and radial artery.

Positioning

- The patient is positioned supine with the arm extended onto a surgical arm board.

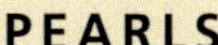

PEARLS

If a concomitant anterior elbow release is to be undertaken, perform the elbow release first to facilitate positioning of the forearm.

PITFALLS

Ensure careful identification and protection of the median nerve and the ulnar nerve and artery. Avoid excessive retraction or distraction of these neurovascular structures during the lengthening procedure.

- A nonsterile tourniquet is placed high on the arm to permit better manipulation of the elbow during the procedure. If an elbow procedure is also necessary, a sterile tourniquet is used. Visualization of the volar forearm can be difficult if there is elbow flexion and forearm pronation contracture. In these instances, sterile bumps are necessary under the dorsal forearm. General anesthesia with muscle relaxation is also helpful to overcome the deforming force of the pronator teres.

Exposures

- A longitudinal volar forearm approach from the mid-forearm to the proximal wrist crease is used.
- The FDS and FDP need to be visualized from the level of the musculotendinous junction to the level of the entrance into the carpal tunnel. The incision should be extended as necessary to identify the flexor tendons and median nerve (Fig. 24-1).
- Meticulous hemostasis is necessary with ligation of the small perforating vessels (Fig. 24-2).

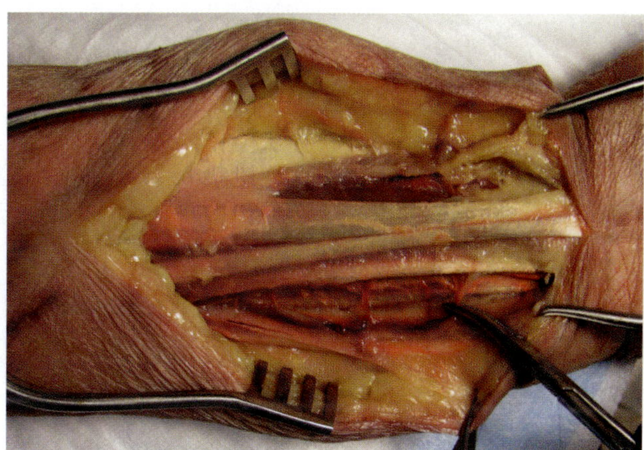

FIGURE 24-1

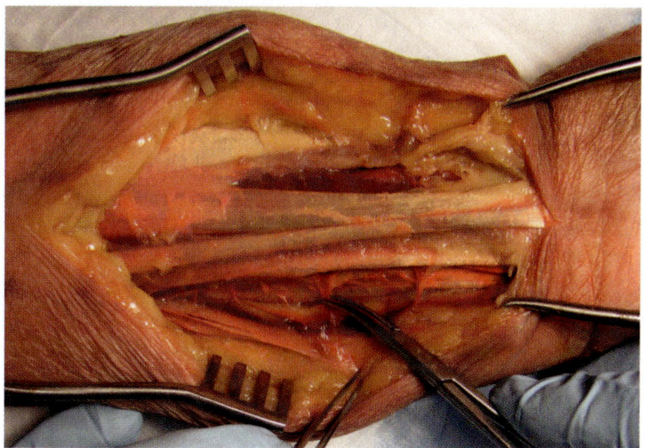

FIGURE 24-2

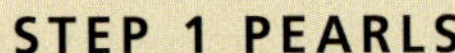

STEP 1 PEARLS

Maintain the superficialis tendons in the position of a normal cascade when placing the stay stitch.

Maximum finger flexion delivers the tendons into the surgical field and takes advantage of the full accessible tendon length.

A myotendinous recession or fractional lengthening may be necessary for the FCR and FCU when there is excessive wrist flexion (similar to fractional lengthening of finger flexors described in previous section). Likewise, if there is an excessive forearm pronation contracture, a release of the pronator teres insertion from the radius can be performed.

STEP 1 PITFALLS

The median nerve can resemble a flexor tendon, especially under tourniquet control. A limited exsanguination preserves the longitudinal vascular supply of the median nerve and may aid in identification.

Procedure

Step 1

- The palmaris longus is identified, and a tenotomy is performed proximally within the incision. Identify the FDS and FDP tendons, the median nerve as it courses between the FDS and FDP muscle bellies, and the ulnar neurovascular bundle adjacent to the deep FDP muscle belly. Protect these neurovascular structures throughout the tenotomy procedures (Figs. 24-3 and 24-4).
- Just proximal to the transverse carpal ligament, a nonabsorbable suture is placed across the FDS tendons of the index, long, ring, and small fingers in a running, locking manner. This creates a single tendon unit (Fig. 24-5).
- Wrist flexion facilitates the exposure of the distal FDS tendons.
- The FDS tendons are then sharply transected as distally as possible (Fig. 24-6).

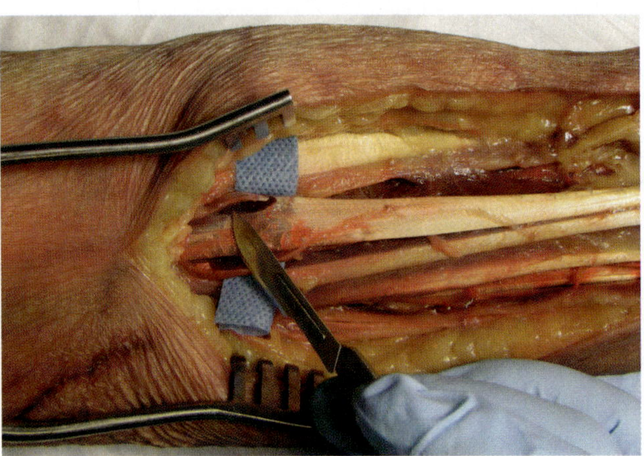

FIGURE 24-3

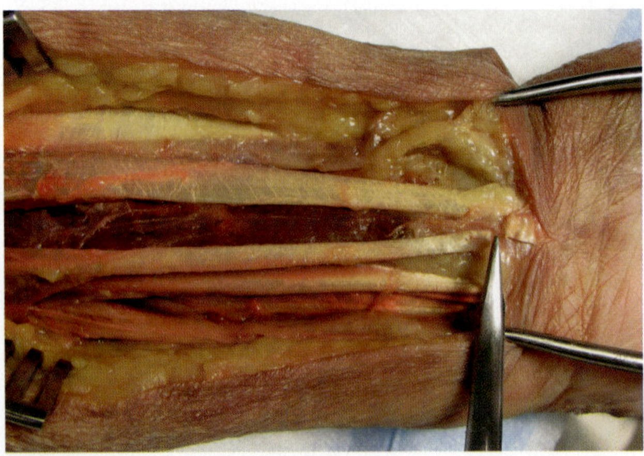

FIGURE 24-4

Step 2

- Retract the FDS tendon unit proximally to expose the underlying FDP tendons (Fig. 24-7).
- A similar nonabsorbable suture is then placed across the FDP tendons to the index, long, ring, and small fingers at their most proximal convergence, again creating a single myotendinous unit (Fig. 24-8).

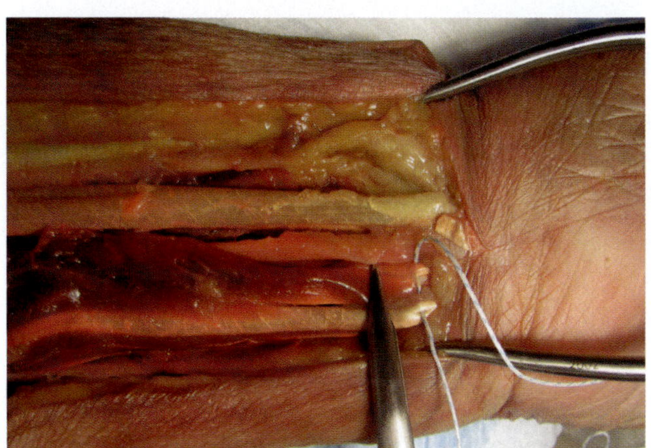

FIGURE 24-5

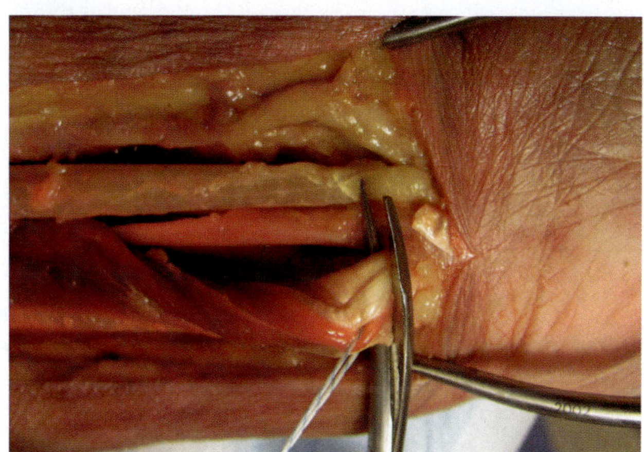

FIGURE 24-6

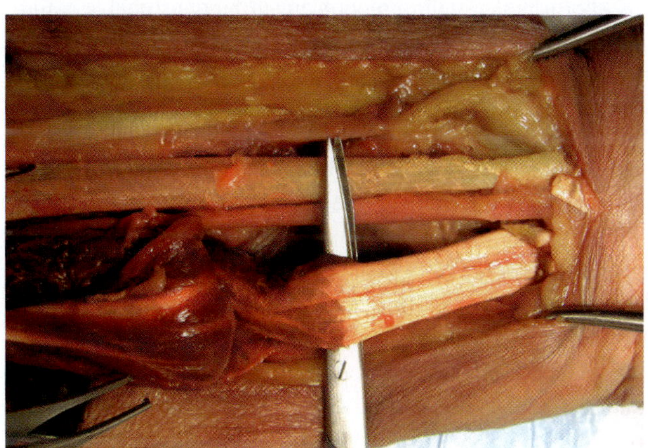

FIGURE 24-7

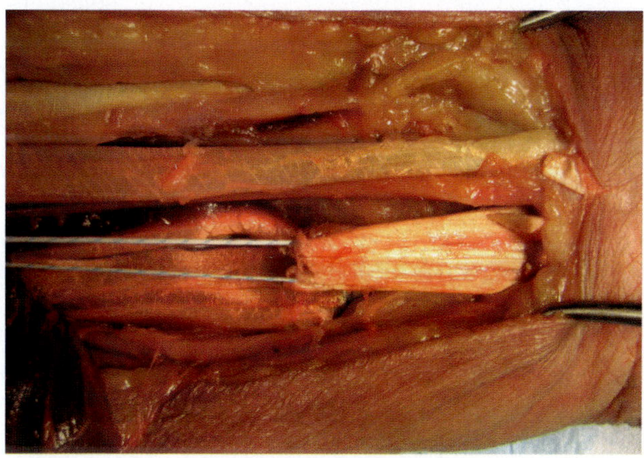

FIGURE 24-8

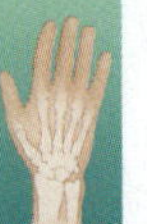

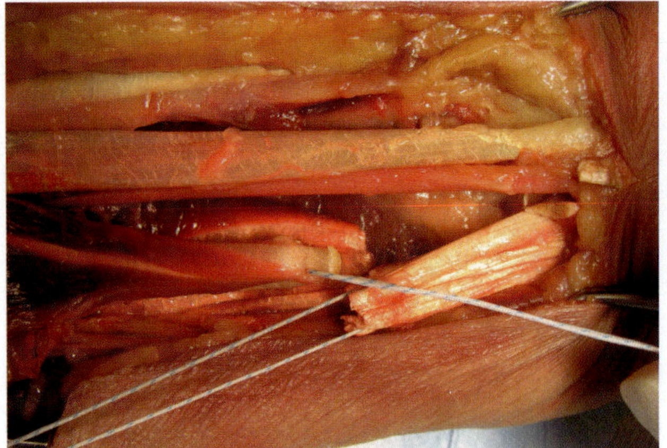

FIGURE 24-9

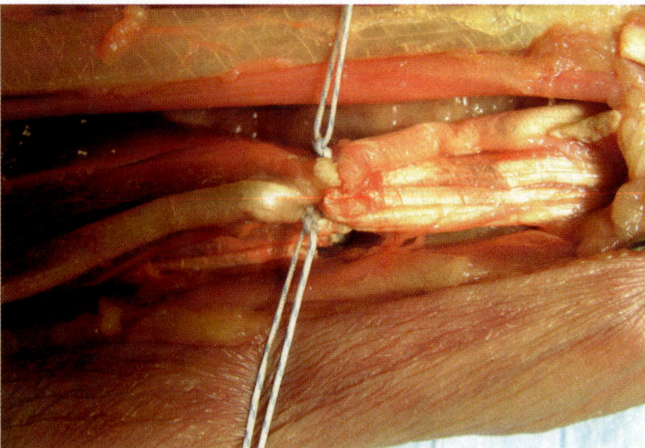

FIGURE 24-10

Step 3

- The FDP tendons are then sharply transected as proximally as possible so that the FDS tendons proximally can be transferred to the FDP tendons distally. The muscle of the FDP will now provide the force for the tendons of the FDS.
- Suture the distal ends of the superficialis tendons to the proximal ends of the profundus tendons while holding the fingers and wrist in a position of maximum extension. Check finger position and evaluate for corrected finger extension and maintenance of normal finger cascade before wound closure (Fig. 24-9).
- A nonabsorbable, braided suture is used to secure the transfer. Multiple horizontal mattress sutures or a running, locking technique is used (Fig. 24-10).
- A layered closure of the subcutaneous tissue with absorbable sutures is performed. The skin is approximated with a monofilament, nonabsorbable suture.

STEP 3 PEARLS

The tourniquet should be deflated and meticulous hemostasis obtained before wound closure. There are multiple segmental arteries from the ulnar artery to the FDP. These vessels require coagulation.

STEP 3 PITFALLS

Ensure that there is not excessive distraction placed on the neurovascular structures. The excursion of the median nerve may be a limiting factor in severe contractures.

Postoperative Care and Expected Outcomes

- Postoperative immobilization is achieved with dorsal and volar splints that hold the fingers and wrist in near-full extension. After swelling subsides (7 to 10 days), the wound is inspected and sutures are removed. Cast immobilization is used for a further 4 weeks.
- The patient is then placed into a full-time fabricated forearm-based splint to keep the wrist and fingers in extension. The splint is removed for bathing and hand therapy exercises. Active finger flexion and extension are permitted.
- After 1 month of full-time wear, the patient is advanced to wearing the splint at night only. If the patient is skeletally mature, the splint can be discontinued 3 to 6 months postoperatively.

PITFALLS

Postoperative finger motion limitation is typically present. The position of the fingers is better for hygiene and assistive care. It is important to counsel the care providers that the contracture has been transferred to a better position.

Evidence

Braun RM, Vise GT, Roper B. Preliminary experience with superficialis to profundus tendon transfer in the hemiplegic upper extremity. *J Bone Joint Surg [Am].* 1974;56:466-472.
This classic article provides background regarding the use of superficialis-to-profundus tendon transfer in treatment of spastic hand contractures. Improvement in hygiene and cosmetic appearance is described. (Level IV evidence)

Keenan MAE, Korchek JI, Botte MJ, et al. Results of transfer of the flexor digitorum superficialis tendons to the flexor digitorum profundus tendons in adults with acquired spasticity of the hand. *J Bone Joint Surg [Am].* 1987;69:1127-1132.
This article describes the technique for superficialis-to-profundus tendon transfer and discusses both the surgical indications and clinical outcomes. (Level IV evidence)

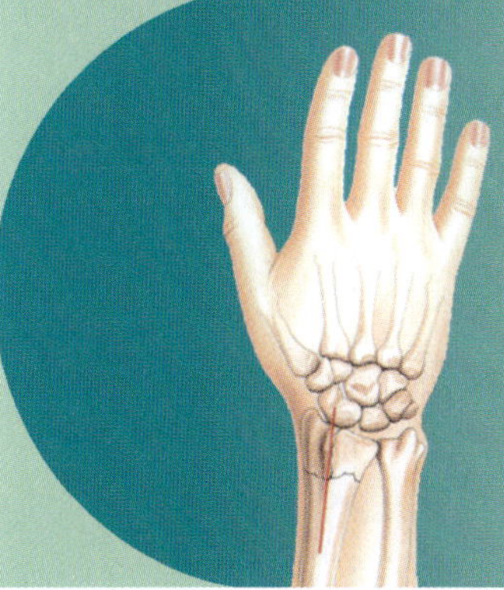

Flexor Pronator Slide

Harry A. Hoyen and Patrick J. Messerschmitt

Indications

- A sustained functional impairment of the spastic upper extremity with a fixed forearm pronation, wrist flexion, and finger flexion deformity.
- Some retained voluntary motor control of forearm supination, wrist extension, and finger extension must be present.
- This is more commonly recommended in an established Volkmann forearm contracture.

Examination/Imaging

Clinical Examination

- Preoperative examination of the upper limb reveals a fixed contracture of the forearm in pronation with contracture of the wrist and fingers. Grasp and release motions of the hand are impaired owing to the fixed wrist position.
- In a forearm Volkmann contracture, there is volar deep soft-tissue adhesions and fibrosis. There is often some retained finger and thumb flexion.

Surgical Anatomy

- Pertinent surgical structures include the volar forearm musculature, ulnar nerve, median nerve, brachial artery, and neurovascular structures adjacent to the interosseous membrane.
- Unlike other contracture release procedures, the proximal anatomy is more relevant in this surgical procedure. The location of the median and ulnar nerves in the proximal forearm is vitally important.

Positioning

- The patient is positioned supine with the arm extended onto a surgical arm board.
- A nonsterile tourniquet is placed high on the arm before surgical preparation to allow better visualization during the procedure. Dissection in the proximal forearm and elbow may be necessary.

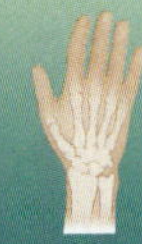

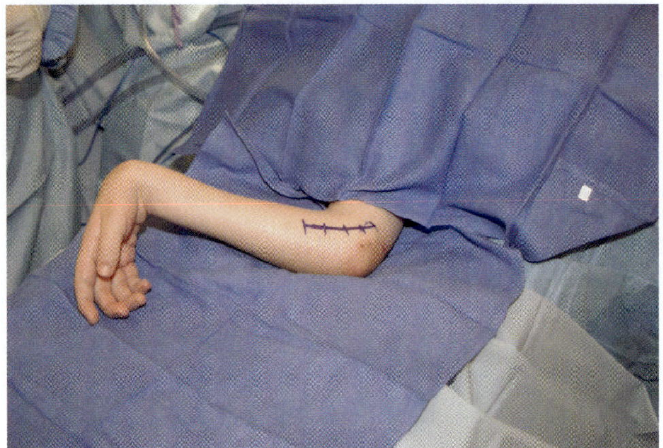

FIGURE 25-1

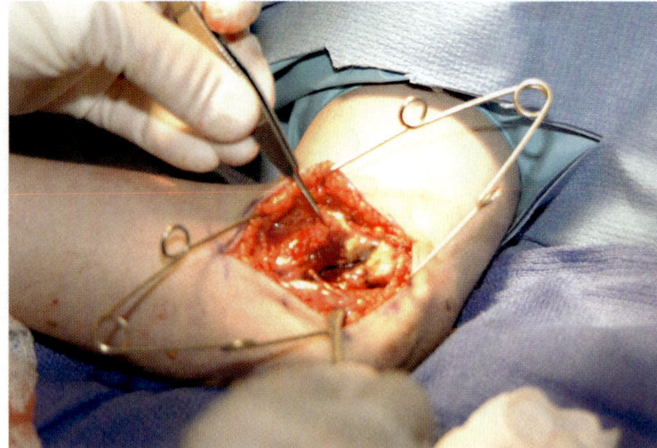

FIGURE 25-2

Exposures

- An anteromedial, longitudinal incision at the elbow situated over the medial epicondyle (Fig. 25-1) is made.
- Superficial dissection includes identification and protection of the medial antebrachial cutaneous nerve. Wide subcutaneous flaps are necessary from the cubital tunnel region to the anterior forearm.

PEARLS

It may be difficult to establish a plane between the flexor-pronator fascia and the subcutaneous tissue. There are multiple perforating vessels to the dermal layer that will require coagulation.

The dissection needs to extend to the median nerve as it enters between the deep and superficial heads of the pronator teres. This is similar to the exposure for a submuscular ulnar nerve transposition.

Procedure

Step 1

- The ulnar nerve is identified proximal to the medial epicondyle, and a decompression is performed through to the deep flexor carpi ulnaris muscle fibers.
- The anterior dissection involves a similar decompression of the median nerve as it enters the flexor musculature. The nerve needs to be completely free of adhesions to the flexor-pronator muscles such that the entire muscle group can slide distally after it is released.
- A plane should be established between the posterior and anterior exposures. This plane is just anterior to the elbow capsule and the anterior band of the medial collateral ligament.
- The entire flexor-pronator mass is then dissected from the medial epicondyle origin. It is elevated from the anterior elbow capsule and proximal portion of the intraosseous membrane (Fig. 25-2).
- The lateral border of the flexor digitorum superficialis, palmaris longus, and flexor carpi radialis is elevated from the intraosseous membrane. The median nerve has terminal motor branches in this region and requires careful dissection. The deep portion of the entire muscle group is then elevated.
- Dissection extends to the deep portion of the muscle origin.

STEP 1 PEARLS

Identify the ulnar nerve proximally and release the cubital tunnel in a distal direction.

The deep dissection will permit identification of the medial collateral ligament. In cases of an elbow contracture, it may be difficult to separate the structure.

The flexor-pronator muscle group needs to be sufficiently mobilized from the elbow capsule and ligament such that the ulnar nerve can be transposed.

STEP 1 PITFALLS

The median nerve motor branches are directly within the deep exposure of the pronator. The distal motor branches are at risk during the more anterior exposure.

Step 2

- At the conclusion of the release, the entire flexor-pronator muscle origin will migrate distally (Fig. 25-3A and B).
- This slide effectively translates the muscle origin distally to lengthen the muscles and allow greater supination, wrist extension, and finger extension (Fig. 25-4).
- A submuscular transposition of the ulnar nerve is usually necessary. The ulnar nerve is placed adjacent to the median nerve in the anterior forearm.

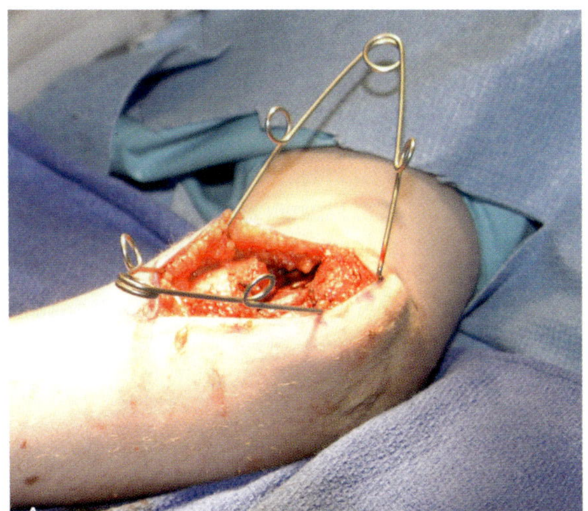

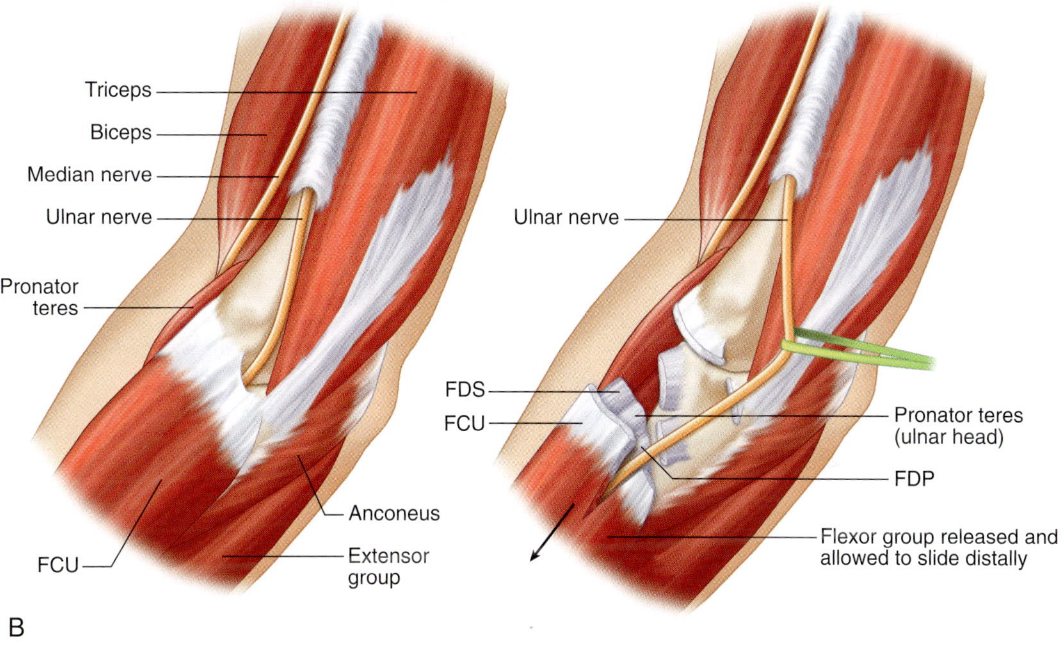

FIGURE 25-3

STEP 2 PEARLS

The tourniquet should be deflated and meticulous hemostasis obtained before wound closure.

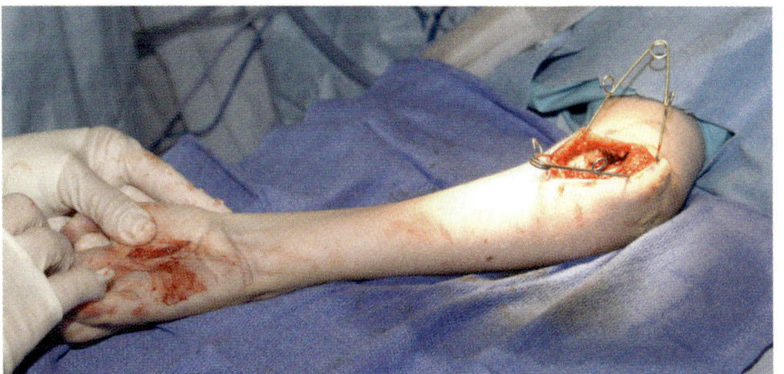

FIGURE 25-4

Postoperative Care and Expected Outcomes

- The forearm and hand are immobilized with long-arm dorsal and volar splints that hold the fingers and wrist in near full extension, with concomitant elbow extension and forearm supination.
- After the swelling subsides, the splint can be changed into a cast.
- The immobilization is continued for 1 month and then advanced to a full-time splint that is forearm based to keep the wrist and fingers in extension. The splint is removed for hygiene purposes and for daily exercises.
- There is gradual transition of the splint to a night-time splint over the next several months.
- Unrestricted activities usually resume 3 to 4 months postoperatively, although in more chronic cases, a splint is worn during rest periods for several additional months.

Acknowledgment

We would like to give special thanks to the author of this chapter in the previous edition, Ann E. Van Heest, whose work served as an excellent foundation for and contribution to this chapter.

Evidence

Inglis AE, Cooper W. Release of the flexor-pronator origin for flexion deformities of the hand and wrist in spastic paralysis. *J Bone Joint Surg [Am]*. 1966;48: 847-857.

White WF. Flexor muscle slide in the spastic hand: the Max Page operation. *J Bone Joint Surg [Am]*. 1972;54:453-459.

These classic articles describe the release of the flexor-pronator origin to effectively lengthen the muscles that originate from the medial epicondyle. Treatment options and outcomes are outlined. (Level IV evidence)

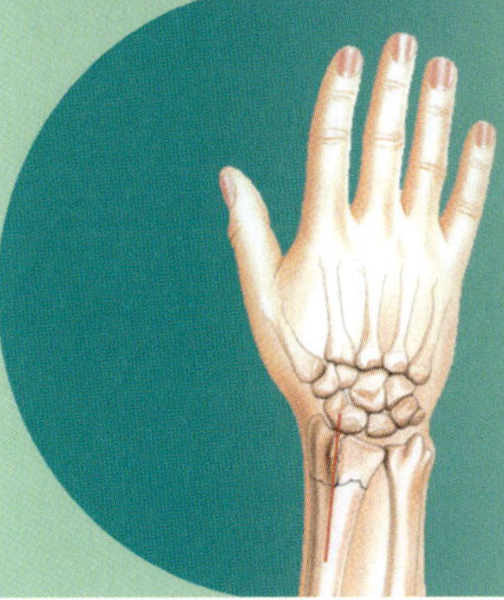

PROCEDURE 26

Reconstruction of Key Pinch in Tetraplegia Patients

Pao-Yuan Lin, Sandeep J. Sebastin, and Kevin C. Chung

See Video 21: Tendon Transfer for Lateral Pinch in Tetraplegic Patients (BR to FPL, FPL to EPL, ECRL to FDP)

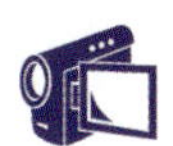

Indications

- Procedure is used in patients with cervical spine injury with partial upper limb paralysis (spinal cord injury at or below C5 cervical segment) with at least grade 4 strength of the brachioradialis (BR).
- General considerations
  - More than 12 months have passed after the injury with stabilized motor recovery.
  - Patient is medically stable and motivated.
  - Patients with poor sensation of the hand may not be candidates for tendon reconstruction because the lack of sensory feedback may present difficulties in use of the reconstructed hand.
- Specific considerations for key pinch
  - Patients with intact wrist extensors (extensor carpi radialis longus [ECRL]) (group 2) are the best candidates for key pinch reconstruction because the BR can be transferred to the flexor pollicis longus (FPL) to get an active key pinch.
  - Only a passive key pinch can be achieved in group 1 patients because they lack wrist extension, and the priority is to get wrist extension. The BR is transferred to the extensor carpi radialis brevis (ECRB) to restore wrist extension, and a passive key pinch is obtained by tenodesis of the FPL, extensor pollicis longus (EPL), and abductor pollicis longus (APL) to the distal radius.

Examination/Imaging

Clinical Examination

- Tetraplegia patients are classified based on the number of functional muscles with grade 4/5 Medical Research Council (MRC) strength below the elbow (Table 26-1). Based on what the patient has, the patient's needs are matched by using a combination of tendon transfers, tenodesis, and arthrodesis to optimize surgical reconstruction.

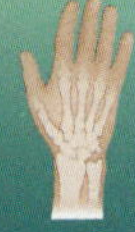

Table 26-1 International Classification for Surgery of the Hand in Tetraplegia

Motor Group	Functioning Muscles (Grade 4 or Greater)
0	No available muscles
1	BR
2	BR and ECRL
3	BR, ECRL, and ECRB
4	BR, ECRL, ECRB, and PT
5	BR, ECRL, ECRB, PT, and FCR
6	BR, ECRL, ECRB, PT, FCR, and finger extensors
7	BR, ECRL, ECRB, PT, FCR, finger and thumb extensors
8	Lacks only intrinsics

BR, brachioradialis; ECRL, extensor carpi radialis longus; ECRB, extensor carpi radialis brevis; FCR, flexor carpi radialis; PT, pronator teres.

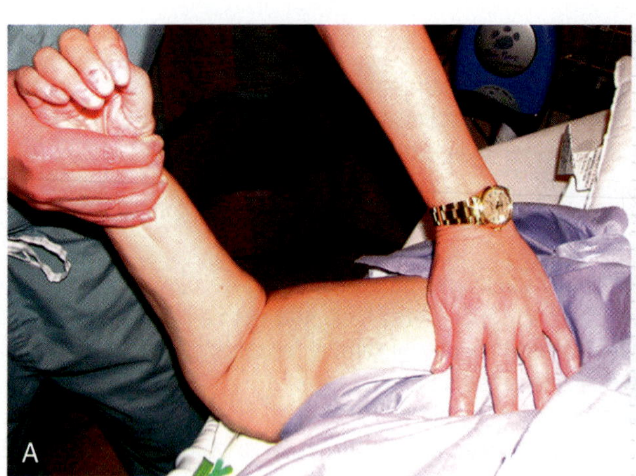

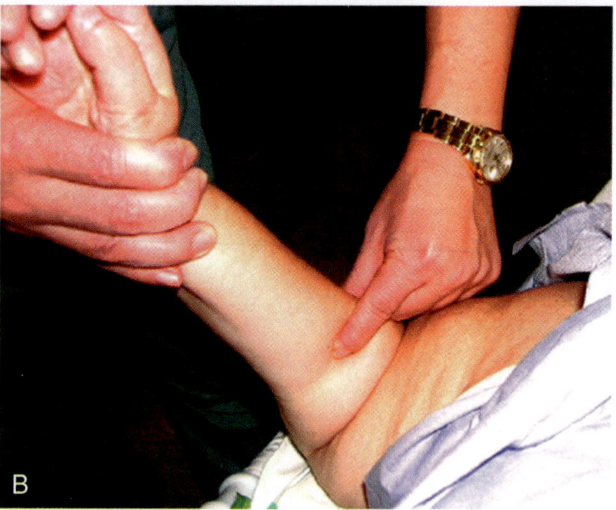

FIGURE 26-1

- The purpose of the key pinch reconstruction is to allow the patient to produce a tenodesis effect to firmly pinch an object between the tip of the thumb and the radial border of the index finger. The differential excursion between the extrinsic flexor and extensor tendon system results in the tenodesis effect. When the wrist is extended, the flexor tendon becomes tight, resulting in finger flexion. With the wrist flexed, the fingers extend secondary to tightening of the extrinsic extensor tendons. Patients with tetraplegia use the tenodesis effect to help develop patterns of pinch function to assist in activities of daily living.
- It is important to assess the strength of the BR. Muscles chosen for transfer should be at least MRC grade 4 because they lose one grade after transfer. This is done by holding the patient's elbow in midprone position and asking the patient to flex the elbow against resistance (Fig. 26-1). This will contract the

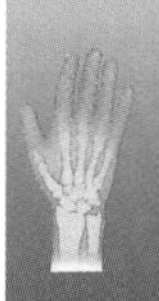

BR. The examiner tries to move the contracted BR. If the BR cannot be moved easily with BR contraction, it is suitable for transfer. On the other hand, if the BR is flaccid and can move easily during contraction, the muscle may not be strong enough for transfer.

- The index finger should also be assessed. If the index finger is flaccid, it may not provide a strong post for the thumb. The flexor digitorum superficialis (FDS) of the index finger can be sutured to the A1 pulley or the volar plate in a lasso procedure so that the index finger can be flexed to act as a post for the reconstructed thumb.
- The procedures required to achieve key pinch in group 1 and group 2 tetraplegia patients are as follows:
  - Group 1 (only BR)
    - Split FPL-to-EPL transfer (to stabilize thumb interphalangeal [IP] joint)
    - FPL tenodesis to volar radius (to provide passive key pinch during wrist extension)
    - EPL and APL tenodesis to dorsal radius and lateral radius, respectively (to allow thumb to abduct and extend during wrist flexion for the release phase of key pinch)
    - BR to ECRB (to provide active wrist extension and passive key pinch by tenodesis)
    - FDS lasso procedure (if index finger metacarpophalangeal [MCP] joint flexion is deemed inadequate for key pinch)
  - Group 2 (BR and ECRL)
    - Split FPL-to-EPL transfer (to stabilize thumb IP joint)
    - BR to FPL (to provide active thumb pinch)
    - EPL and APL tenodesis to dorsal radius and lateral radius, respectively (to allow thumb to abduct and extend during wrist flexion for the release phase of key pinch)
    - FDS lasso procedure (if index finger flexion is deemed inadequate for key pinch)

Surgical Anatomy

- Figure 26-2 presents the segmental innervation (C5 to T1) of muscles of the elbow, forearm, and hand, and Figure 26-3 shows the relevant anatomy of the procedure.

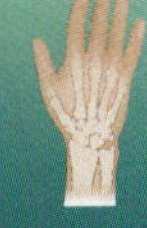

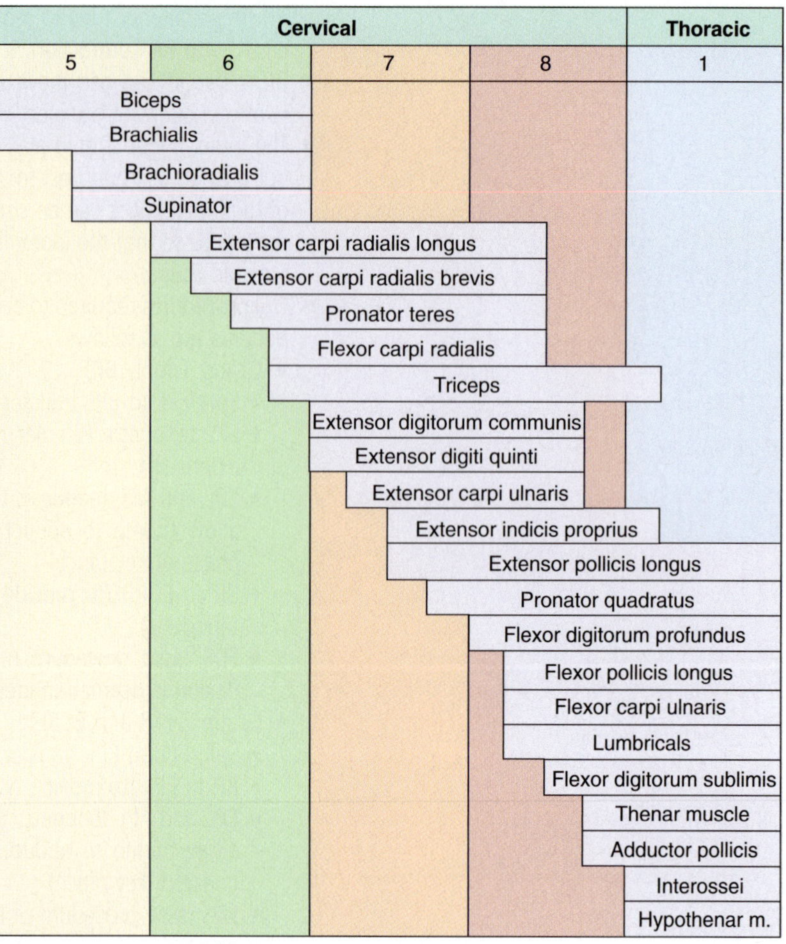

FIGURE 26-2

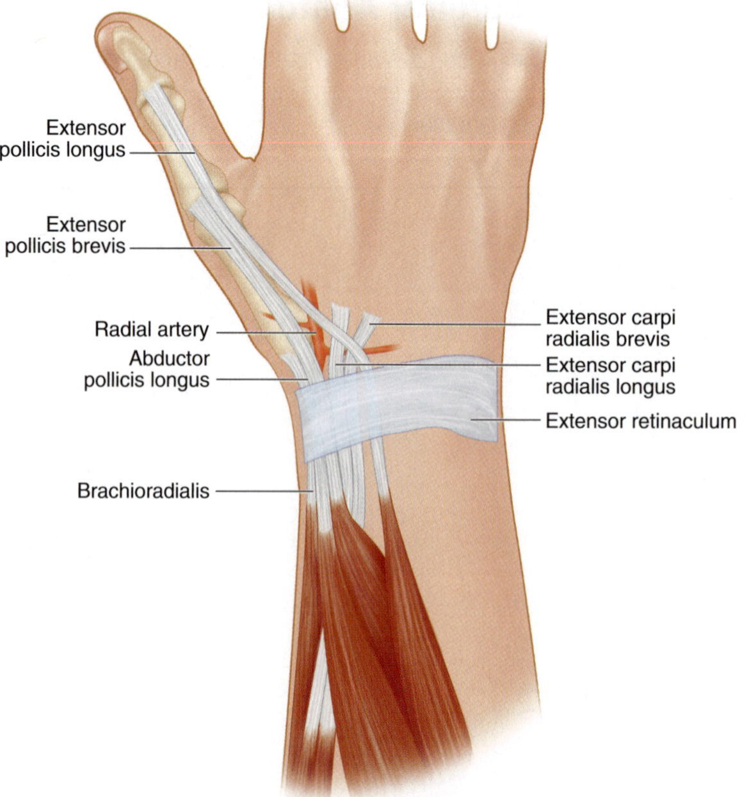

FIGURE 26-3

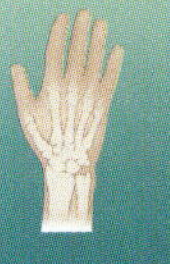

Positioning

- The procedure is performed under general or regional anesthesia and tourniquet control. The patient is positioned supine with the affected extremity on a hand table.

PITFALLS

Care should be taken to avoid injury to the radial digital nerve of the thumb, superficial sensory branches of the radial nerve, and palmar cutaneous branch of the median nerve during these exposures.

Exposures

- A 3-cm longitudinal incision is centered over the IP joint on the radial side of the thumb (Fig. 26-4). This incision is used for the split FPL-to-EPL transfer. The A2 pulley is identified and released to expose the FPL tendon. The FPL tendon must be dissected quite proximally to obtain a sufficiently long tendon that can reach the EPL over the dorsum of the thumb IP joint.
- A 6-cm longitudinal incision is made on the dorsoradial aspect of the wrist extending proximally from the radial styloid. This incision is used to expose the APL tendon and the BR insertion.
- A 6-cm longitudinal incision is made on the dorsum of distal forearm extending 2 cm beyond the Lister tubercle and 4 cm proximal to it. This incision is used to expose the ECRB and EPL tendons.
- A 6-cm longitudinal incision is made on the volar aspect of the distal forearm over the flexor carpi radialis (FCR) tendon. This incision is used to expose the FPL tendon.
- A 3-cm longitudinal chevron-shaped incision is made over the palmar aspect of the index finger MCP joint. This incision will be required only if a lasso procedure of the index finger FDS is planned.

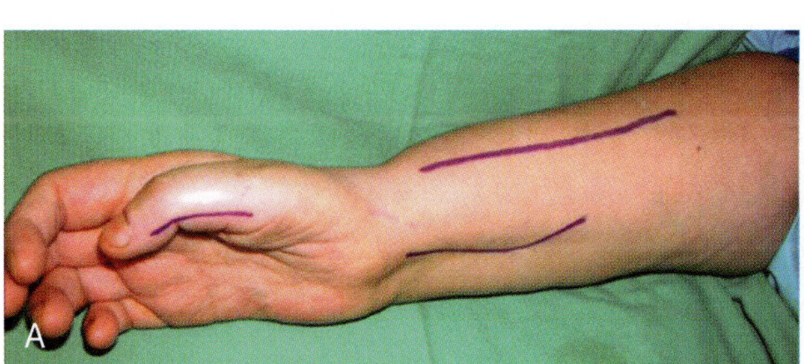

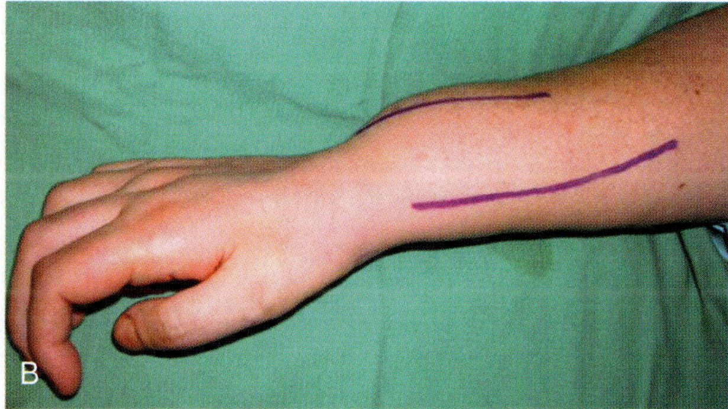

FIGURE 26-4

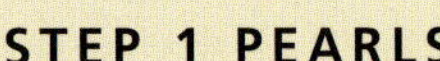

STEP 1 PEARLS

The FPL-to-EPL tenodesis procedure is performed first. This is particularly important because the reconstructed FPL tendon for the key pinch procedure will result in maximum flexion at the MCP joint level and not at the IP level. Extensive flexion of the thumb IP joint will cause a mallet deformity that is not the optimal posture to pinch between the thumb and the index finger (Fig. 26-6).

Procedure

Step 1: Split FPL-to-EPL Transfer

- One half of the FPL tendon is transected distally, and this half is then sutured to the EPL tendon to achieve extension of the IP joint to neutral position. The tendons are sutured using 3-0 horizontal mattress sutures (Fig. 26-5).

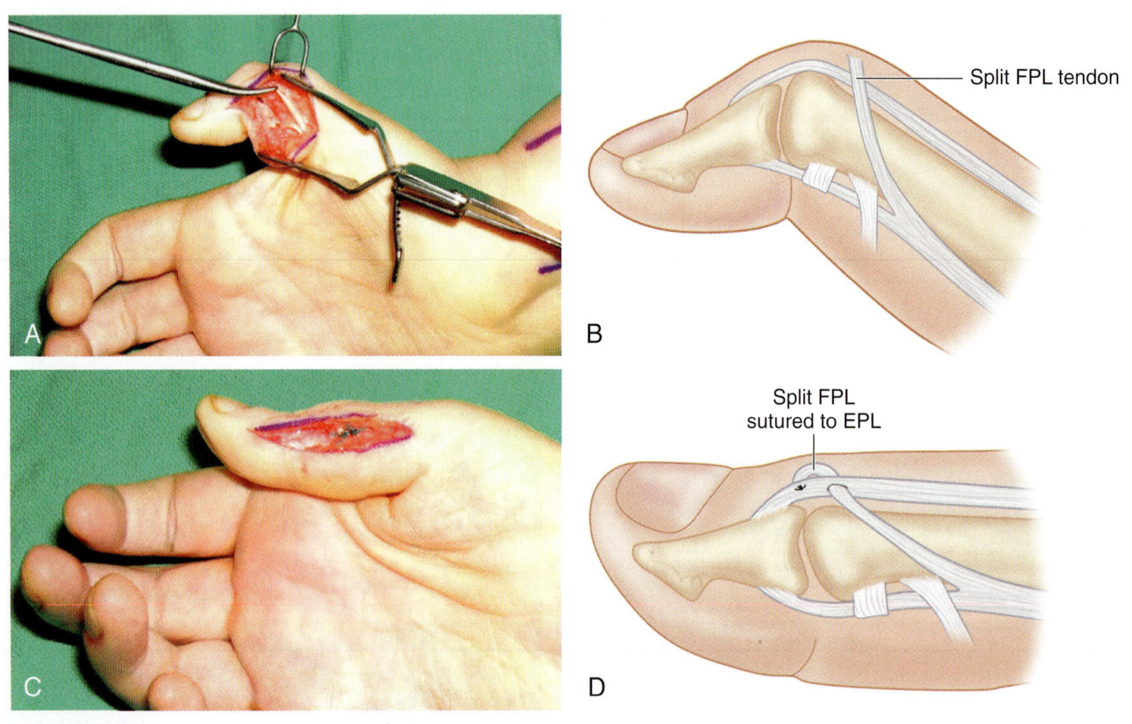

FIGURE 26-5

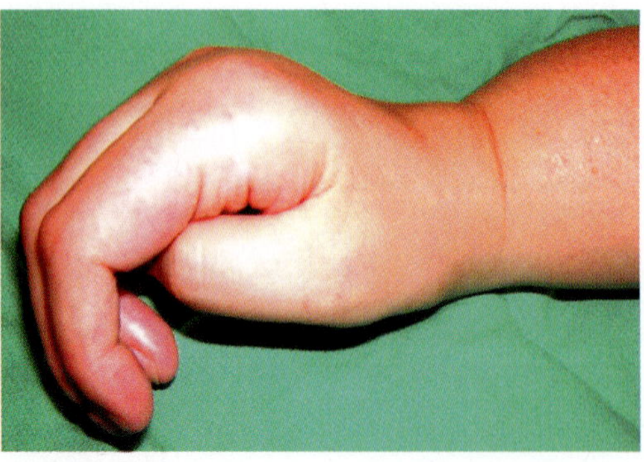

FIGURE 26-6

Step 2: APL Tenodesis

- The APL tendon is identified in the first dorsal compartment and divided proximal to the first dorsal compartment.
- The distally based APL tendon is brought out of the first dorsal compartment distally and secured to the radius using a Mitek Mini bone anchor. It should be secured to the dorsal surface of the radius so that the direction of pull during wrist flexion will result in maximal thumb abduction (Fig. 26-7).

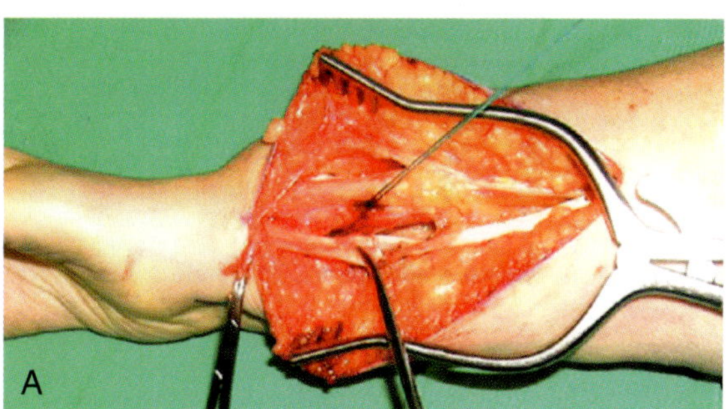

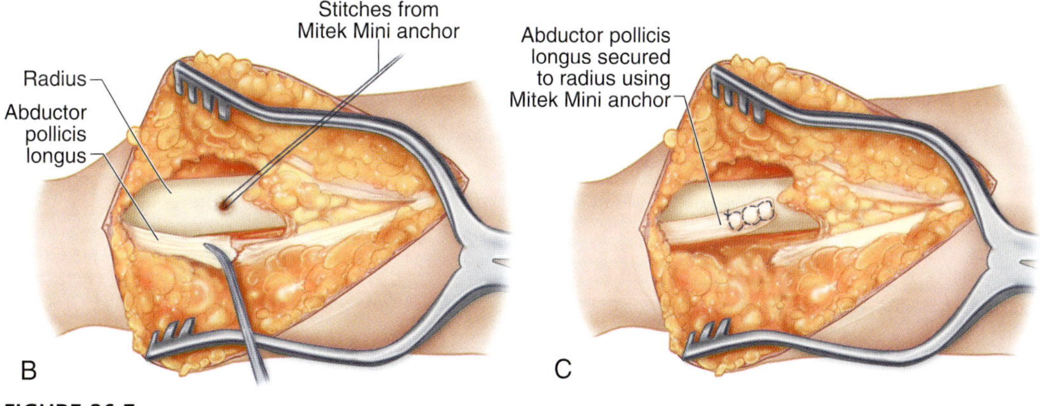

FIGURE 26-7

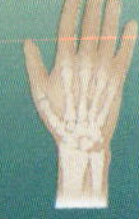

STEP 3 PEARLS

When the tendons are secured to the bone, the result is more predictable, and loosening should not be a problem. Loosening with attachment to the extensor retinaculum may be an issue. The tendon inset in Figure 26-8C shows a method of EPL tenodesis to the extensor retinaculum by making a loop around Lister tubercle. By this method, one can also suture the EPL to Lister tubercle to strengthen the attachment.

Step 3: EPL Tenodesis

- The EPL tendon is then isolated from the dorsal incision and divided proximal to the extensor retinaculum. It can be secured to either the radius or the extensor retinaculum (Fig. 26-8).

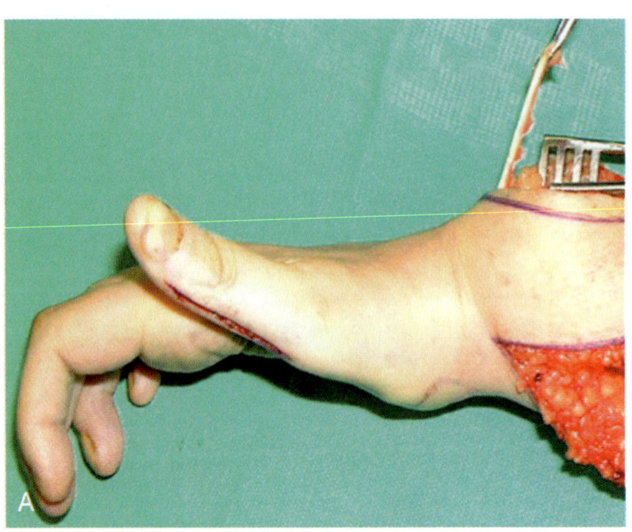

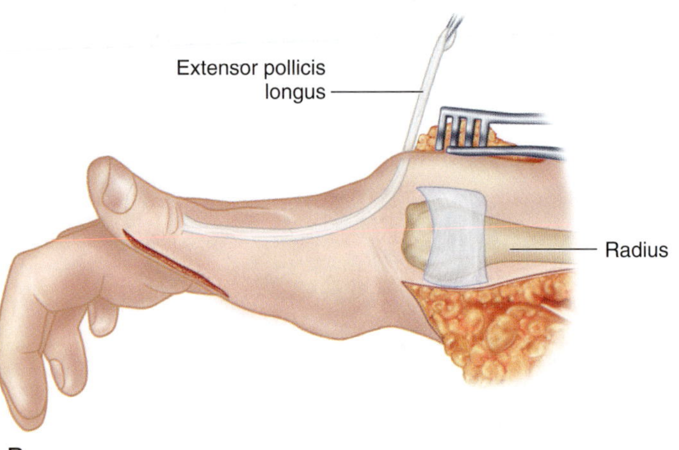

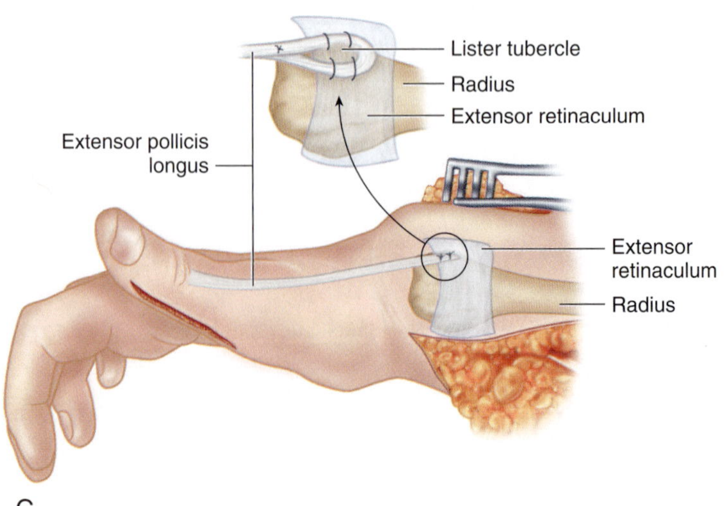

FIGURE 26-8

Step 4: Tenodesis of FPL

- This is done in patients who do not have a strong wrist extensor, and the BR is used for wrist extension rather than transferred to the FPL. The FPL is identified below the FCR in the same plane as the flexor digitorum profundus, but radial to it.
- The FPL is divided 1 cm proximal to the proximal edge of the pronator quadratus (PQ) and anchored to the volar surface of the distal radius proximal to the PQ using a Mitek Mini bone anchor (Fig. 26-9).

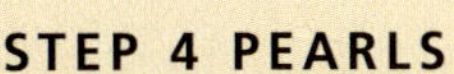

STEP 4 PEARLS

A tenodesis of the extensor pollicis brevis (EPB) to the dorsum of the thumb metacarpal has been described to avoid excessive flexion at the MCP joint.

Step 5: BR-to-ECRB Transfer

- The BR tendon is dissected off its insertion and mobilized proximally.
- A short subcutaneous tunnel is made so that the BR tendon can reach the ECRB.
- The ECRB is identified ulnar to the ECRL, and an end-to-side Pulvertaft weave repair is performed between the BR and ECRB using 2-0 Ethibond (Fig. 26-10). The end-to-side repair is more secure, and the direction of pull will still be straight.
- The tension is set such that the repair is able to hold the wrist in neutral position with the elbow in 45 degrees of flexion. With the elbow flexed, the wrist should passively flex, and with the elbow extended, the transfer should tighten.

STEP 5 PEARLS

Care must be taken to protect the superficial radial nerve as it passes below the BR and becomes superficial by passing between the BR and ECRL about 5 to 9 cm proximal to the radial styloid.

The BR is invested in fascia along its course in the forearm and must be mobilized from the distal radius and forearm fascia to provide adequate excursion.

Step 6: BR-to-FPL Transfer

- This is done in patients who have strong wrist extension. Here the BR is used to provide active pinch by transferring it to the FPL.
- The FPL and BR are divided as described previously. A short subcutaneous tunnel allows the BR to reach the FPL.
- A repair of the FPL and BR is done using a Pulvertaft weave with 2-0 Ethibond sutures (Fig. 26-11).
- Tension is set so that with wrist flexion, the patient's thumb will abduct and extend in this release phase of the operation (Fig. 26-12A). With the wrist extended, sufficient tension on the FPL tendon must achieve a strong enough flexion of the thumb metacarpophalangeal joint so that the pulp of the thumb will press firmly against the radial side of the middle phalanx of the index finger (Fig. 26-12B).

STEP 6 PEARLS

The BR is passed deep (dorsal) to the radial artery.

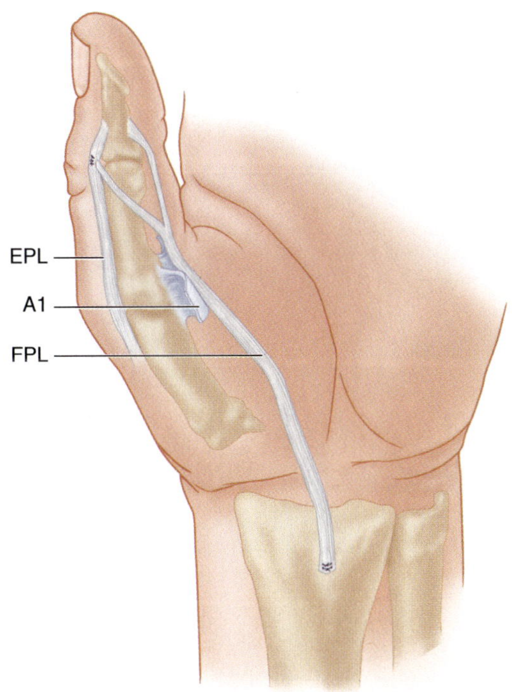

FIGURE 26-9

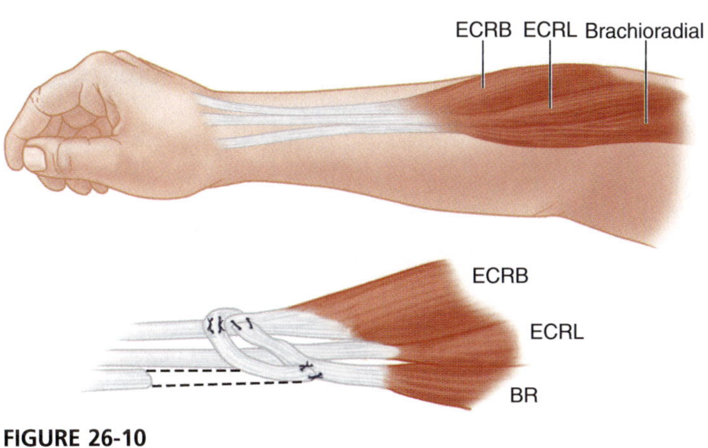

FIGURE 26-10

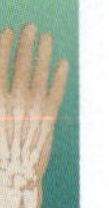

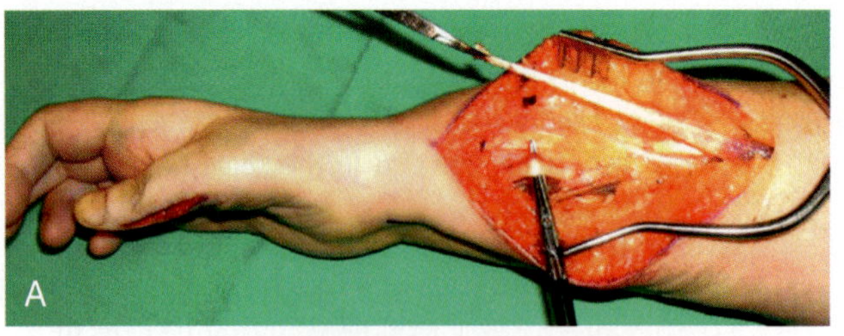
A

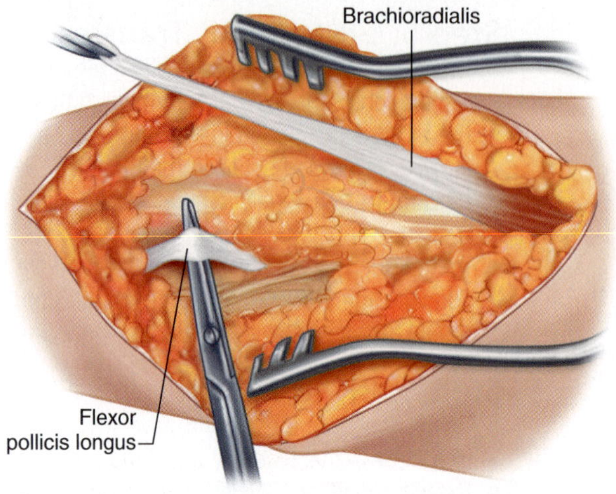
Brachioradialis
Flexor pollicis longus
B

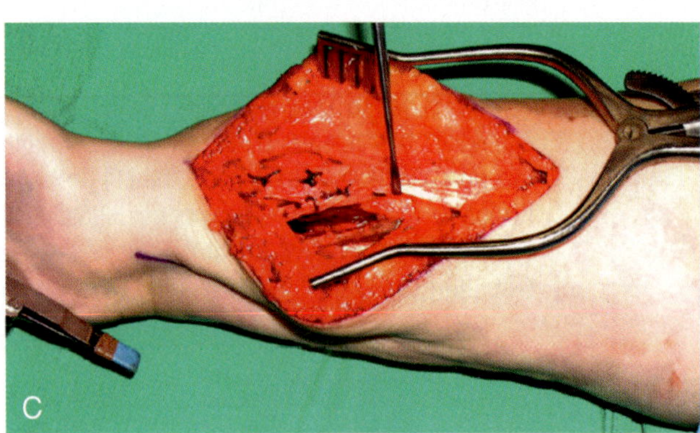
C

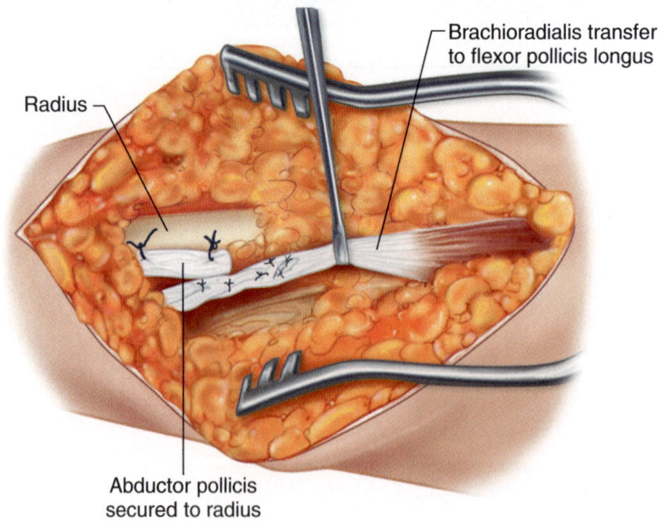
Brachioradialis transfer to flexor pollicis longus
Radius
Abductor pollicis secured to radius
D

FIGURE 26-11

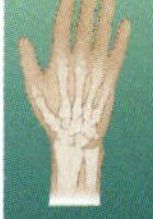

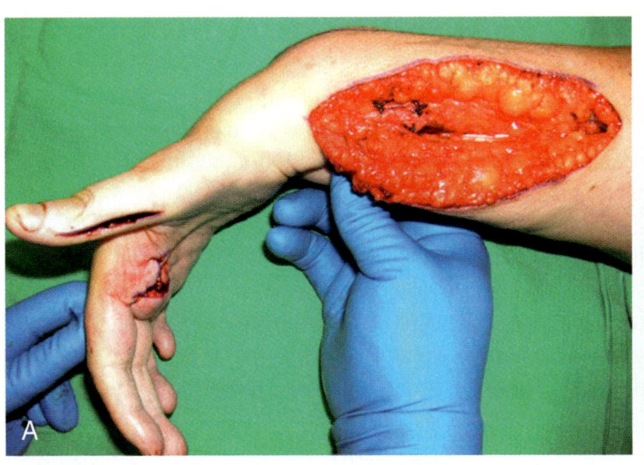

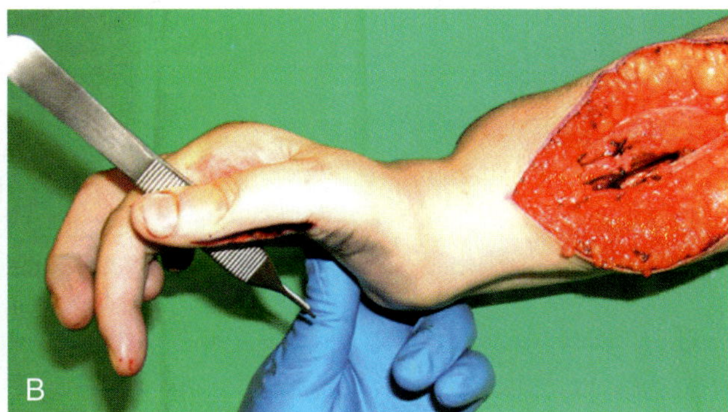

FIGURE 26-12

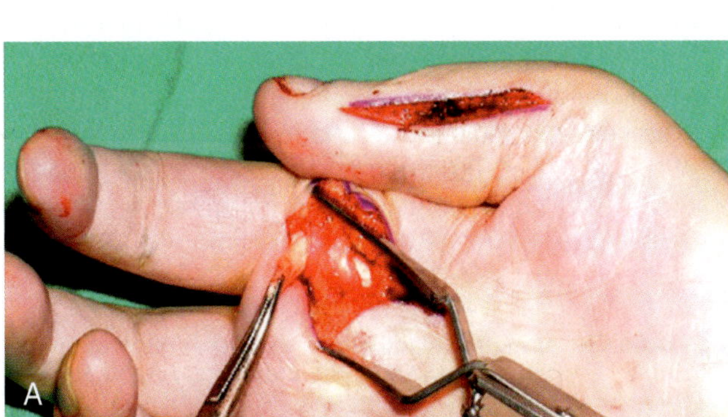

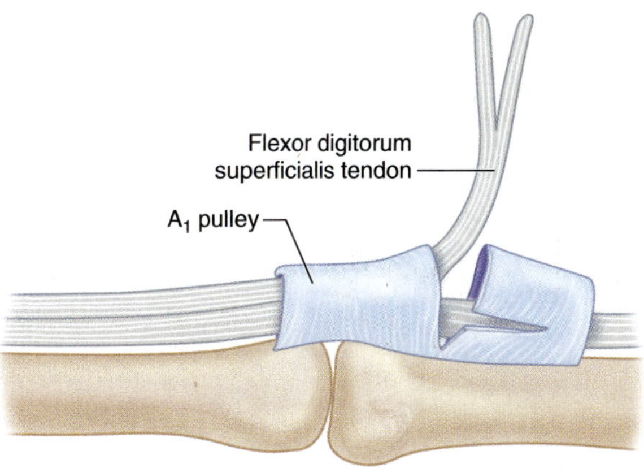

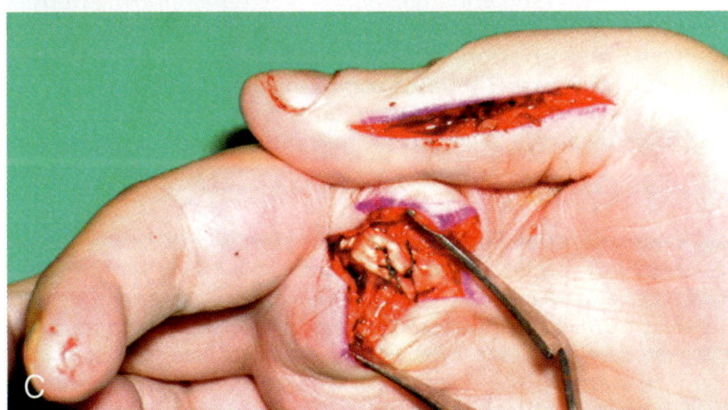

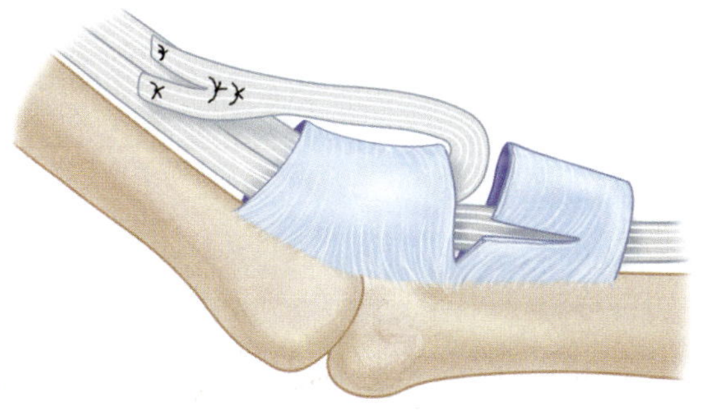

FIGURE 26-13

STEP 7 PEARLS

Check the tenodesis effect to ensure that with flexion of the wrist, the thumb abducts and extends in the release phase of the operation, and with the wrist extended, the pulp of the thumb pinches strongly against the radial border of the index finger.

Step 7: Index Finger MCP Joint Flexion Using an FDS Lasso

- If the index finger MCP joint is flaccid and not sufficiently flexed to meet the thumb, the Zancolli lasso procedure will flex and stabilize the index MCP joint so that the thumb pulp will meet the radial border of middle phalanx of the index finger during key pinch.
- The A1 and A2 pulleys are defined clearly, and a space is developed between them by dissection.
- Both slips of the FDS are divided distal to the A1 pulley (Fig. 26-13A and B).
- The distal ends of the tendon slips are folded over the A1 pulley and sutured to the proximal tendon and the A1 pulley using horizontal 2-0 Ethibond mattress sutures (Fig. 26-13C and D).
- Tension is adjusted to maintain the index finger MCP joint in 50 to 60 degrees of flexion.

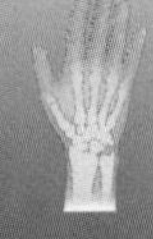

Postoperative Care and Expected Outcomes

- A long-arm cast that immobilizes the elbow in midprone position and 90 degrees of flexion, the wrist in extension, and the thumb in abduction is given to patients who undergo a BR-to-ECRB transfer (group 1).
- A long-arm cast that immobilizes the elbow in midprone position and 90 degrees of flexion, the wrist in 10 to 20 degrees of flexion, and the thumb in abduction is given to patients who undergo a BR-to-FPL transfer (group 2).
- Patients wear a splint for 4 weeks to allow healing of the tendon junctures. This is followed by mobilization, when the patient learns to adapt to the tenodesis effect and achieve sufficiently strong key pinch to perform activities of daily living.
- In selected patients with sufficient muscle function and sensibility, effective lateral pinch can be predictably restored by use of appropriate tendon transfer and tenodesis to provide flexion and extension of the digits and maintain intrinsic balance.
- If a postoperative key pinch strength can reach 2 kg, the patient is able to perform a large range of activities of daily living, such as pushing a button on a remote control, manipulating a key in and out of an entrance lock, opening and closing a vertical or horizontal zipper, inserting a standard card into an automated teller machine and retrieving it, and even manipulating a three-prong plug out of a wall socket. The mean postoperative strength was 1 kg higher for procedures using an active motor than for procedures applying a tenodesis.

Evidence

Hamou C, Shah NR, Curtin CM, et al. Pinch and elbow extension restoration in people with tetraplegia: a systematic review of the literature. *J Hand Surg [Am]*. 2011;34:692-699.

A systematic review between 1966 and 2007 about pinch and elbow extension was addressed. Results from 377 pinch reconstructions in 23 studies were summarized. The overall mean postoperative strength measured after surgery for pinch reconstruction was 2 kg. The most common complications were flexion contracture of the elbow or of the thumb (25% of the complications), stretching or rupture of repair (22% of the complications), and loosening of pins across the thumb interphalangeal joint (21% of the complications). (Level III evidence)

Paul SD, Gellman H, Waters R, et al. Single-stage reconstruction of key pinch and extension of the elbow in tetraplegic patients. *J Bone Joint Surg [Am]*. 1994;76:1451-1456.

A retrospective review of BR-to-FPL transfer to restore key pinch and deltoid-to-triceps transfer to restore elbow extension in nine patients was conducted. The average time from the injury to the operation was 5 years, and the average duration of follow-up was 31 months. Key pinch improved from essentially none preoperatively to an average of 0.9 kg postoperatively: an average of 1.4 kg for the patients who had tetraplegia at the C6 level and an average of 0.4 kg for those who had tetraplegia at the C5 level. (Level IV evidence)

Vastamäki M. Short-term versus long-term comparative results after reconstructive upper-limb surgery in tetraplegic patients. *J Hand Surg [Am]*. 2006;31:1490-1494.

A retrospective review of short-term and long-term comparative studies was conducted. The surgical procedures of key pinch reconstruction included FPL tenodesis to radius, release A1 pulley of the thumb, and fixation of the IP joint of the thumb with a K-wire. Twenty-nine key pinch procedures in 27 patients were evaluated at 4-year follow-up (short-term), and 10 key pinch procedures were evaluated at 21-year follow-up (long-term). In the 21 years between surgery and evaluation, the strength of key pinch had diminished by 21%, from a mean of 1.4 kg (range, 0.6 to 3.0 kg) to 1.1 kg (range, 0.3 to 3.0 kg), a 1% strength loss each year. (Level IV evidence)

PROCEDURE 27

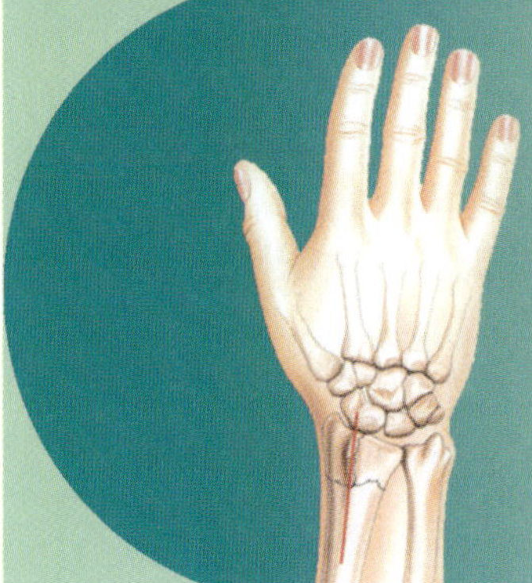

Flexor Carpi Ulnaris–to–Extensor Carpi Radialis Brevis Transfer

Sandeep J. Sebastin and Kevin C. Chung

Indications

- Cerebral palsy patient with a hyperactive flexor carpi ulnaris (FCU) and weak or absent wrist extension
- Late presentation of neonatal brachial plexus palsy with an ulnar deviation deformity and absent wrist extension

Examination/Imaging

Clinical Examination

- *Cerebral palsy:* The flexion deformity in cerebral palsy can be due to spasticity of the wrist flexors, weak wrist extensors, and/or a volar wrist capsular contracture. It is important to differentiate among these causes. An attempt at overcoming muscle spasticity should be done by applying gentle sustained resistance to the spastic force. If the wrist can be extended passively, it rules out capsular contracture. If the wrist cannot be extended passively, but the wrist flexors do not feel spastic, it suggests a wrist capsular contracture. If the spasticity cannot be overcome, a median and ulnar nerve block at the elbow can temporarily eliminate the flexor spasticity and allow an assessment of active and passive wrist extension. An FCU-to–extensor carpi radialis brevis (ECRB) transfer is indicated in patients who have a spastic FCU and good passive wrist extension (no capsular contracture) but lack active wrist extension. Before considering an FCU-to-ECRB transfer, one must ensure that the patient has the following:
  - A functioning FCR, or the transfer will result in a wrist extension deformity
  - Active digital extension with the wrist held in slight extension. If there is some active digital extension, but it is limited by the tight digit flexors owing to the wrist extension, a concomitant lengthening of the digital flexors will be required (Fig. 27-1). If there is no active digital extension, the patient will need lengthening of the digital flexors and augmentation of digital extension with a long finger FDS-to-EDC transfer.
- *Neonatal brachial plexus palsy (NBPP):* The ulnar deviation deformity in this group of patients can be due to the FCU or the extensor carpi ulnaris (ECU). Either one of these tendons can be used for obtaining wrist extension depending on the predominant cause of the ulnar deviation deformity. In NBPP, the FCU is passed around the radius to the extensor carpi radialis longus (ECRL) to get some radial balance to the hand at the wrist. In cerebral palsy, the transfer is made around the ulna to the ECRB. This chapter describes the procedure in cerebral palsy.

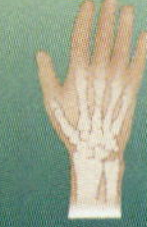

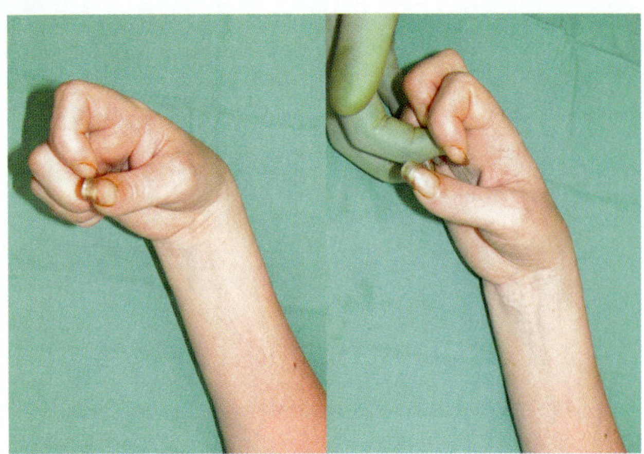

FIGURE 27-1

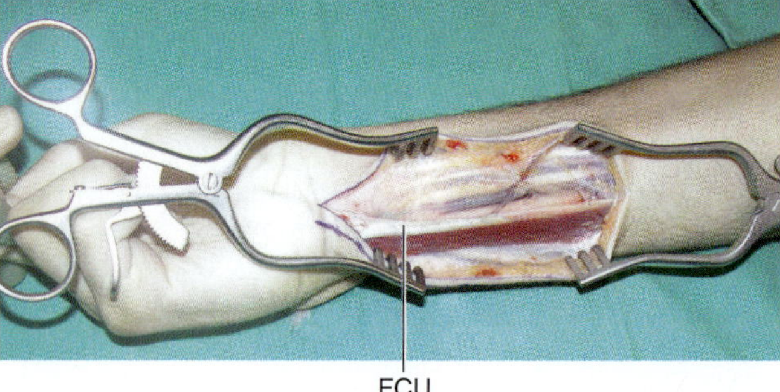

FIGURE 27-2

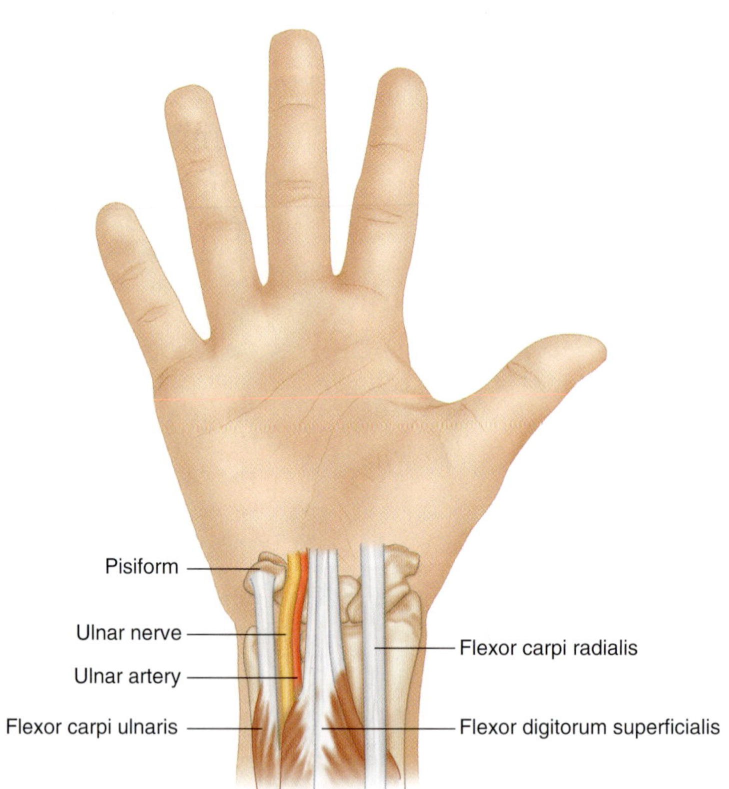

FIGURE 27-3

Surgical Anatomy

- The purely tendinous portion of the FCU is quite short as the muscle extends distally along the tendon. In addition, the muscle is attached along the ulna over a long distance. The muscle must be detached quite proximally to have adequate excursion of the transferred FCU (Fig. 27-2).
- The ulnar artery and nerve are very closely related to the undersurface of the FCU and must be protected during mobilization of the FCU (Fig. 27-3).

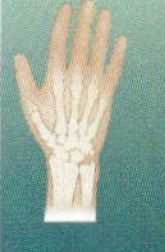

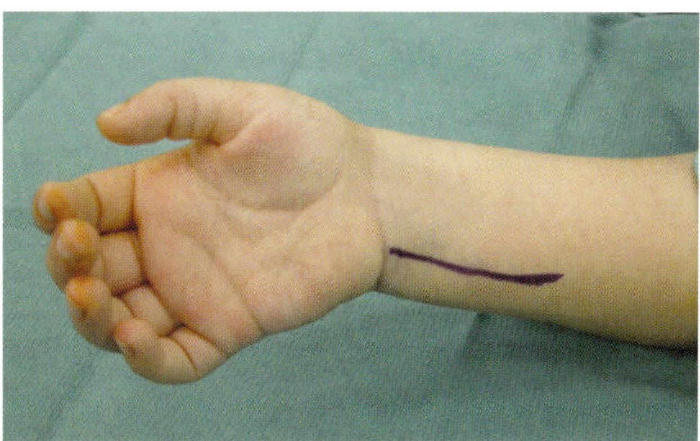

FIGURE 27-4

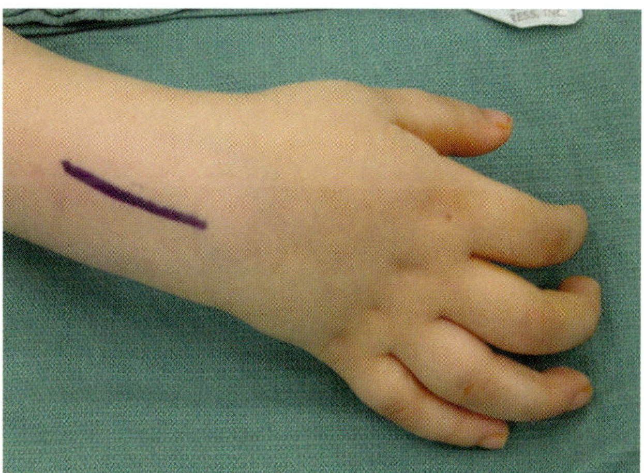

FIGURE 27-5

Positioning

- The patient is placed in the supine position, and the operation is performed under tourniquet control.

Exposures

- A 4-cm longitudinal incision over the volar forearm extending proximally from the pisiform is made, in line with the palpable FCU tendon (Fig. 27-4). Skin and subcutaneous tissue are dissected, and the FCU tendon is exposed.
- A 6-cm longitudinal incision over the dorsal forearm extending proximally from the base of the long finger metacarpal is made (Fig. 27-5). Skin and subcutaneous tissue are dissected to expose the extensor retinaculum. The second dorsal extensor compartment is opened, and the tendons of the ECRL and ECRB are identified.

PITFALLS

One must watch out for branches of the superficial radial sensory nerve during exposure of the ECRB.

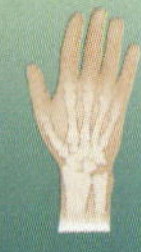

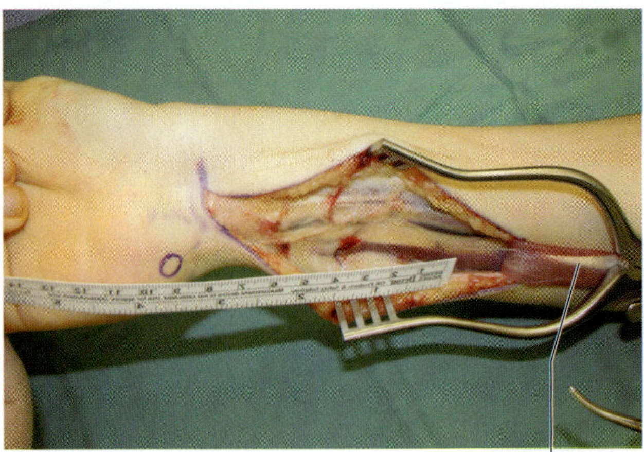

FIGURE 27-6

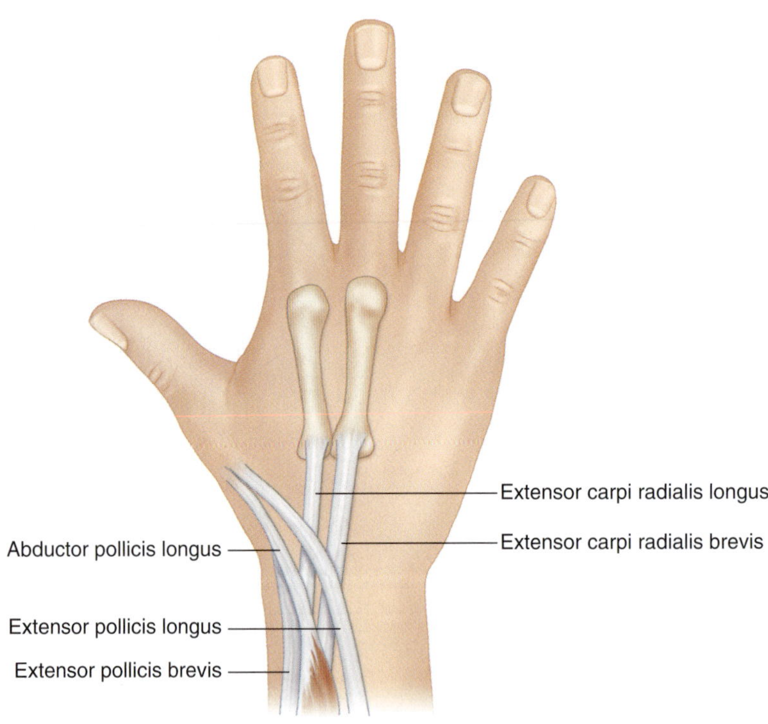

FIGURE 27-7

STEP 1 PEARLS

The ulnar neurovascular bundle, which is under the FCU, must be preserved. Typically, there is a fascial layer covering the neurovascular bundle that should not be disturbed.

STEP 2 PEARLS

It is important to make the subcutaneous tunnel along the shortest, most direct route between these two tendons. Otherwise, the transferred tendon will move over time into the shortest route. This will make the transferred tendon lax and less effective.

The tendon is passed superficial to the extensor tendons of the first and third compartments (adductor pollicis longus [APL], extensor pollicis brevis [EPB], and extensor pollicis longus [EPL]) (Fig. 27-7).

Procedure

Step 1

- The FCU is detached from its insertion on the pisiform and dissected as proximally as possible to release all the fascia attachments to the ulna so that the muscle has adequate excursion (Fig. 27-6).

Step 2

- The FCU tendon is passed around the ulnar aspect of the forearm, over the skin, to the point where it intersects with the ECRB. The route of the FCU tendon is marked.
- A wide subcutaneous tunnel is made along the route from the dorsal incision to the volar incision, and the FCU tendon is delivered in the dorsal wound.

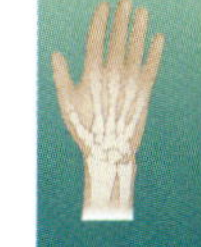

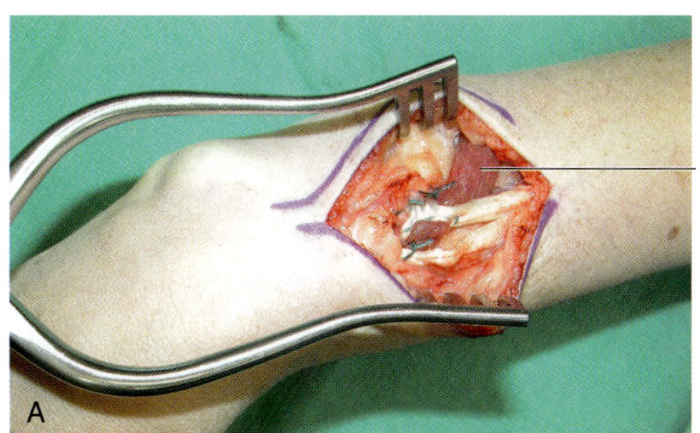

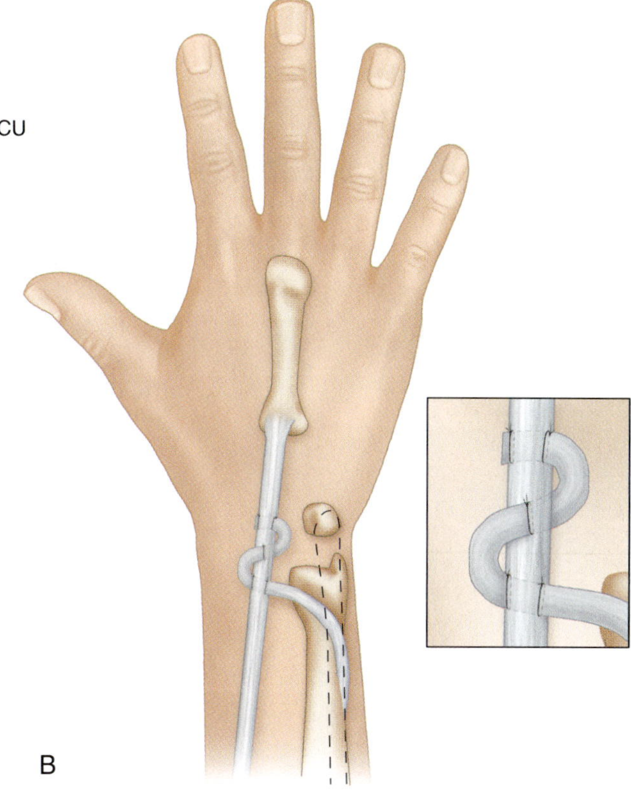

FIGURE 27-8

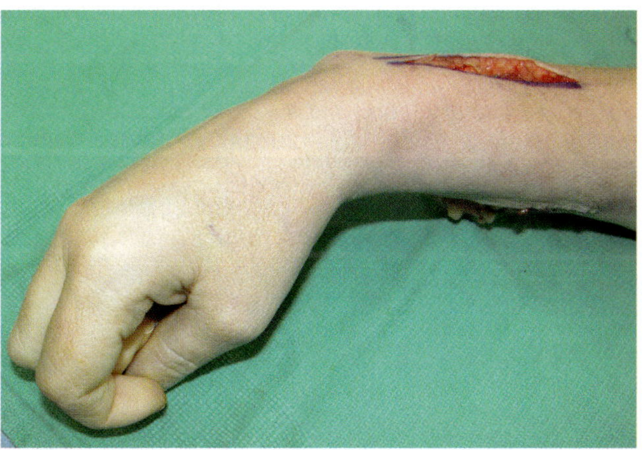

FIGURE 27-9

STEP 3 PEARLS

It is not necessary to divide the ECRB tendon, given that this tendon may still be innervated and partially functional.

The tendon weave should be done such that the weave does not encroach on the intersection with the APL and EPB during wrist extension.

Step 3

- The FCU tendon is weaved into the ECRB tendon using the Pulvertaft weave with 3-0 Ethibond suture (Fig. 27-8A and B).
- The tension is set with the wrist in neutral or 30 degrees of flexion. One must not overtighten the transfer to achieve wrist extension beyond neutral because the patient typically does not have sufficiently strong finger extensors to extend the fingers and will rely on tenodesis effect with the wrist in flexion to extend the fingers (Fig. 27-9).

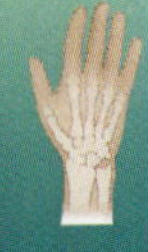

STEP 3 PITFALLS

If passive flexion of the wrist to 20 degrees is not possible, the tendon repair is too tight and should be loosened.

Step 4

- The tourniquet is released, hemostasis is secured, and the incisions are closed in layers.

Postoperative Care and Expected Outcomes

- The patient's wrist is splinted in neutral position for 4 weeks, followed by range-of-motion exercises. The patient wears a removable splint for an additional 4 weeks. Most patients can extend the wrist actively, but if spasticity is not controlled, they may develop recurrent wrist contracture. These patients are advised to wear a volar wrist extension splint at night.
- This transfer has shown good results with improvements in resting wrist posture and arc of wrist motion. However, it is associated with a loss in wrist flexion, and the range of motion usually remains unchanged.

Evidence

Thometz JG, Tachdjian M. Long-term follow-up of the flexor carpi ulnaris transfer in spastic hemiplegic children. *J Pediatr Orthop*. 1988;8:407-412.

This report is a retrospective study of 25 cerebral palsy patients who underwent FCU transfer to the wrist extensors. The mean follow-up period was 8 years and 1 month. The mean active wrist extension was 44.2 degrees, and the mean flexion was 19.0 degrees. The patients had an effective result except for loss of flexion of the wrist after the operation. (Level IV evidence)

Tonkin M, Gschwind C. Surgery for cerebral palsy. Part 2: flexion deformity of the wrist and fingers. *J Hand Surg [Am]*. 1992;17:396-400.

The authors performed flexor aponeurotic release, FCU tenotomy, FCU-to–extensor carpi radialis transfer, flexor pronator slide, and proximal row carpectomy in 34 patients with cerebral palsy. They reported that 30 patients were improved functionally and cosmetically. (Level IV evidence)

Wolf TM, Clinkscales CM, Hamlin C. Flexor carpi ulnaris tendon transfer in cerebral palsy. *J Hand Surg [Am]*. 1998;23:340-343.

In this retrospective study, 16 patients participated in comparison of wrist position, analysis of outcome predictors, and subjective and objective assessment of function after FCU transfer to relieve flexion contracture of the wrist in cerebral palsy. The average follow-up was 4 years; the patients showed improvement in the general resting position, and the center of the arc of motion averaged 6 degrees of pronation and 9 degrees of extension. The authors noted that the most important factor determining the outcome of the operation was the ability of the patient to achieve finger extension. (Level IV evidence)

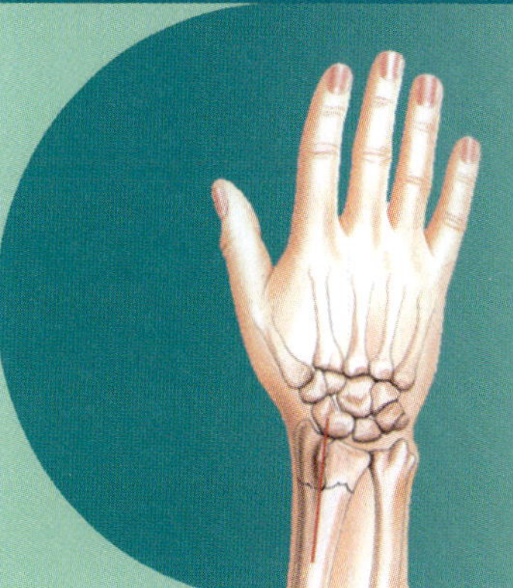

PROCEDURE 28

Pronator Teres Rerouting

Sandeep J. Sebastin and Kevin C. Chung

Indications

- Moderate pronation deformity with no active supination but good passive supination
- Cerebral palsy
- Neonatal brachial plexus palsy

Examination/Imaging

Clinical Examination

- The pronation deformity can be classified into mild (forearm is in partially prone position with preserved active and/or passive motion), moderate (forearm is fully pronated with preserved active and/or passive motion), or severe (forearm is fully pronated with no active and/or passive motion—fixed pronation contracture). A mild deformity does not need surgery because the posture puts the hand in a functional position. No surgery is required for patients with moderate pronation deformity that can actively supinate the hand to neutral. If the patient can actively supinate the arm but cannot bring it to neutral, a release of the pronator quadratus (PQ) and a flexor-pronator slide can be considered. Pronator teres (PT) rerouting is useful in patients who have no active supination but full passive supination. Patients with a fixed pronation contracture may need release of the PQ, a flexor-pronator slide, release of the interosseous membrane, and occasionally a corrective osteotomy to place the forearm in neutral position.
- Before considering PT rerouting, one must ensure that the patient has the following:
  - Good passive supination of the forearm
  - A functional PQ. One of the pronators should be preserved to avoid a supination deformity. The PQ is tested by checking the ability of the patient to pronate the forearm with the elbow in full flexion. Maintaining the elbow in flexion takes the tension off the PT.

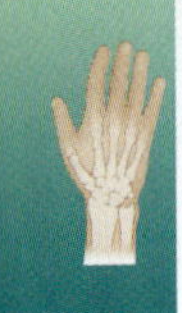

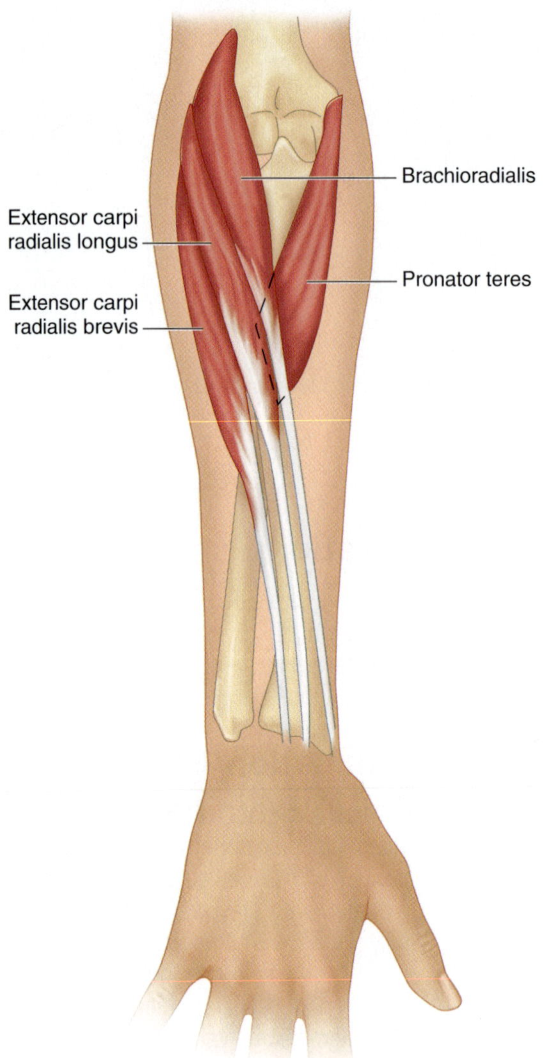

FIGURE 28-1

Surgical Anatomy

- The PT originates at the medial epicondyle and inserts over the volar surface of the radius via a wide fascial attachment.
- The insertion of the PT is found at the mid-forearm under the brachioradialis (Fig. 28-1).
- The superficial radial nerve, which is under the brachioradialis, should be isolated and protected.

Positioning

- The patient is placed in the supine position.

Exposures

- A 6-cm longitudinal incision is made over the volar radial aspect of the mid-forearm (Fig. 28-2). This incision is centered over the palpable musculotendinous junction of the extensor carpi radialis brevis (ECRB) and extensor carpi radialis longus (ECRL). The forearm fascia is divided, and the tendons of the ECRB and ECRL are identified (Fig. 28-3A and B). The brachioradialis is identified radial to

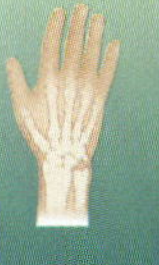

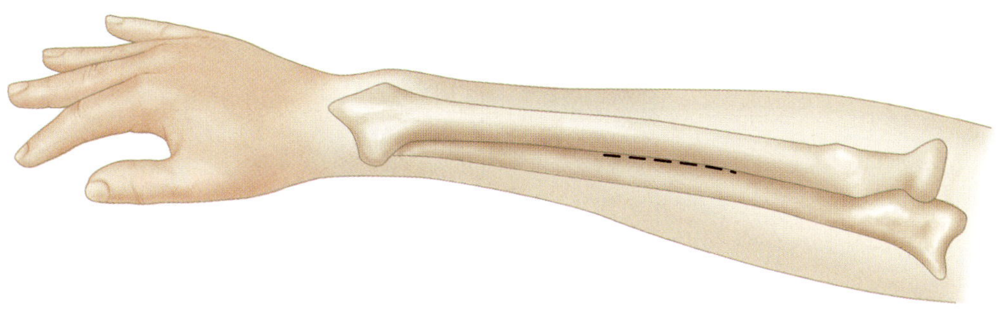

FIGURE 28-2

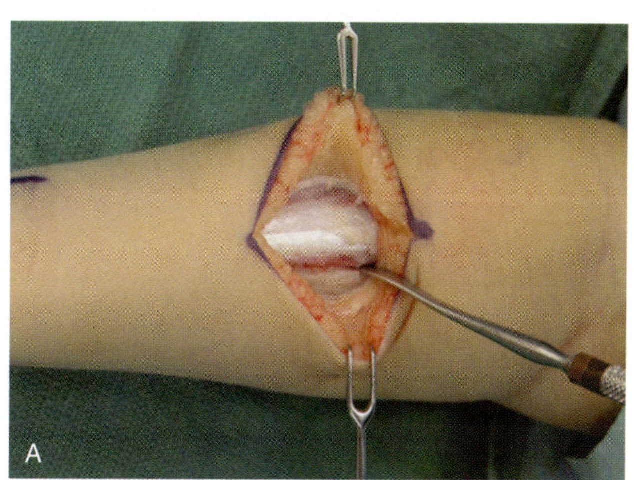

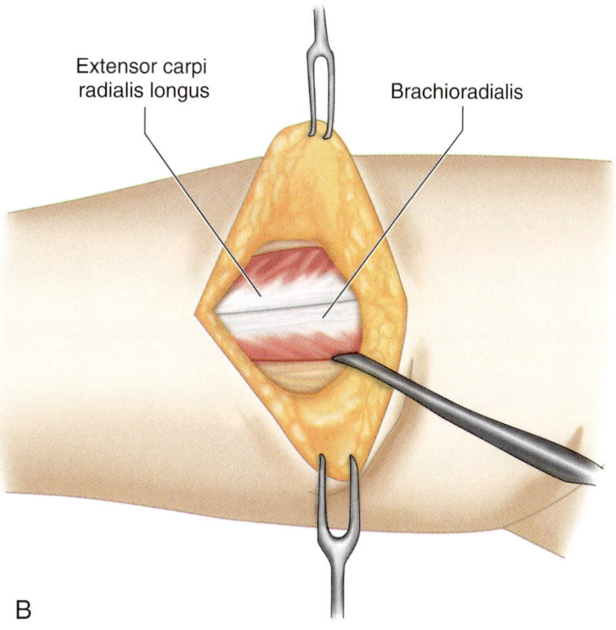

FIGURE 28-3

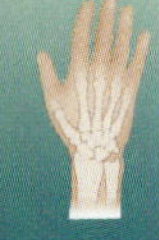

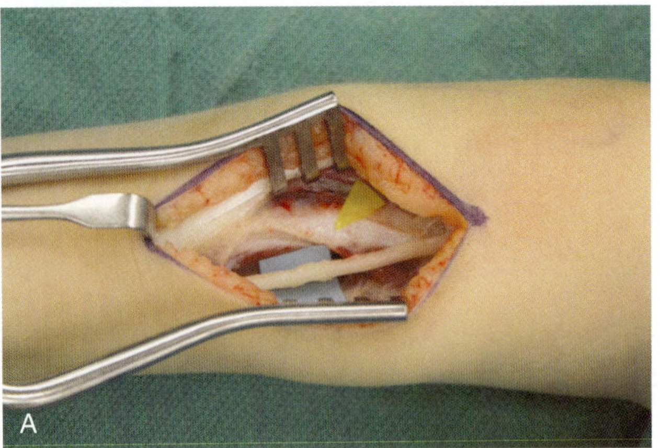

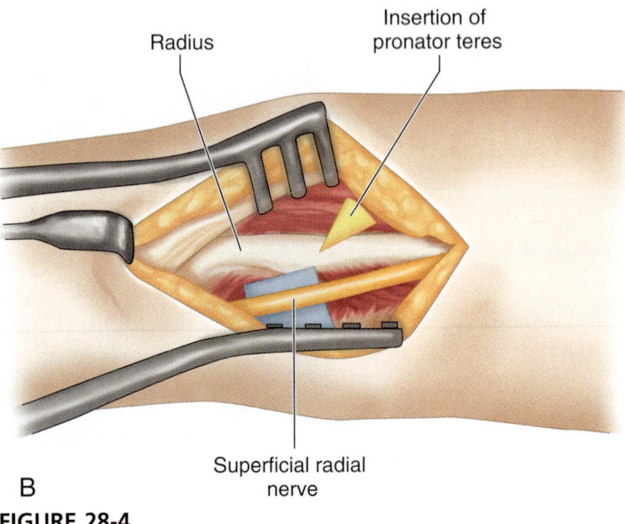

FIGURE 28-4

the ECRL, and it is retracted ulnarly along with the ECRL. The superficial branch of the radial nerve should be identified under the brachioradialis and protected. This will bring into view the insertion of the PT (Fig. 28-4A and B).

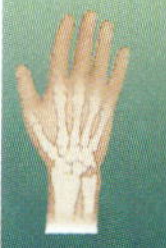

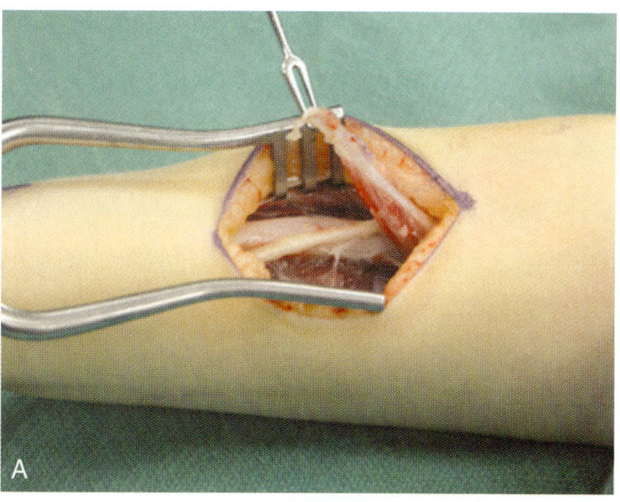

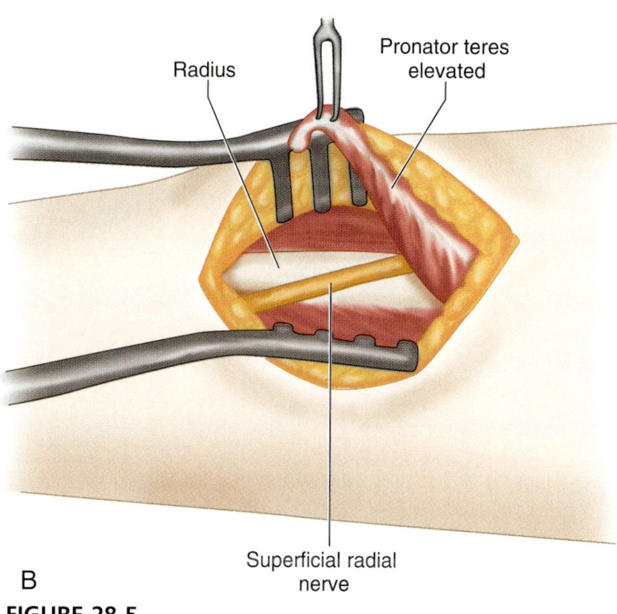

FIGURE 28-5

> **STEP 1 PEARLS**
>
> *A 3- to 4-cm strip of periosteum distal to the insertion of the PT should be harvested in continuity with the PT.*

> **STEP 2 PITFALLS**
>
> *Care should be taken to prevent injury to the superficial branch of the radial nerve, the radial artery, and the innervation to the PT during the proximal dissection.*

Procedure

Step 1

- The PT is detached from its insertion on the radius (Fig. 28-5A and B).

Step 2

- The PT muscle-tendon unit must be mobilized proximally to free it from any attachments that will limit subsequent excursion.
- The PT should have easy excursion with traction.

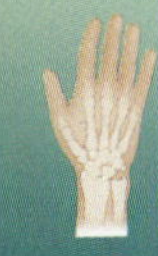

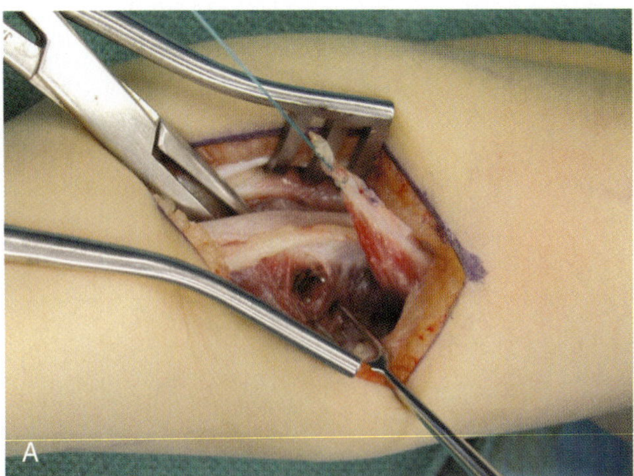

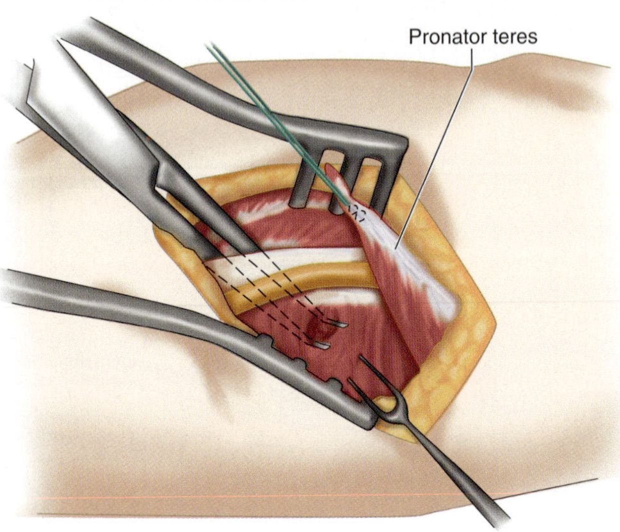

B

FIGURE 28-6

Step 3

- A 3-0 Ethibond suture is weaved to the fascia and tendon structure using the Bunnell stitch. The Bunnell stitch is a crisscrossing, weaving stitching pattern of the tendon to prevent pullout of the sutures (Fig. 28-6A and B).

Step 4

- The attachments of the interosseous membrane are divided over a 3-cm distance at the level of the pronator insertion (see Fig. 28-6B).

Step 5

- A right-angle clamp is introduced from the dorsal aspect of the radius through the opening in the interosseous membrane made previously to emerge on the volar side of the radius (see Fig. 28-6B).

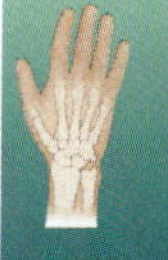

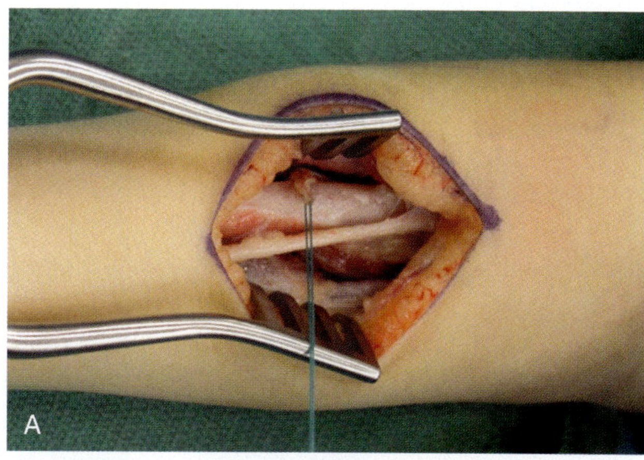

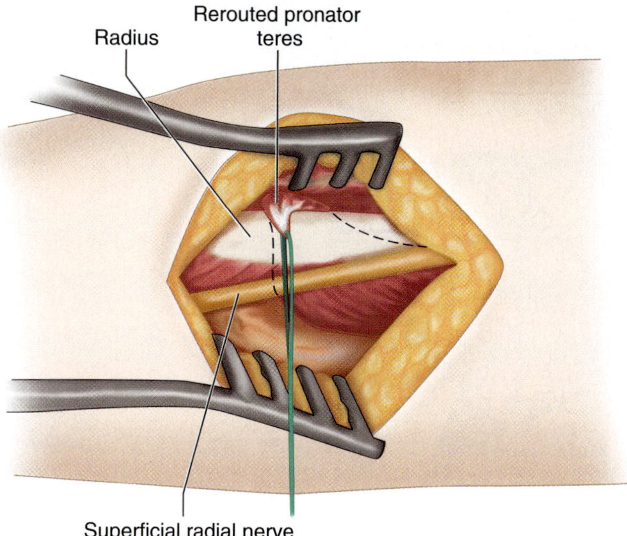

FIGURE 28-7

Step 6

- The detached PT tendon with the Bunnell stitch is held by the right-angle clamp and delivered onto the dorsal aspect of the radius. This rerouting of the PT insertion from the volar to the dorsal side converts it into a supinator of the forearm (Fig. 28-7A and B).

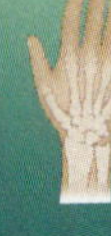

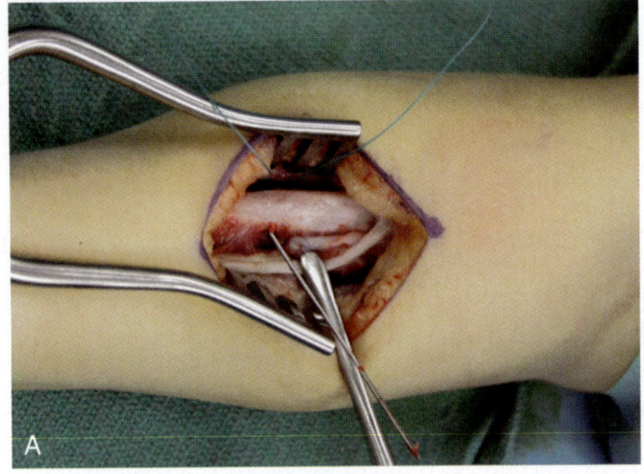

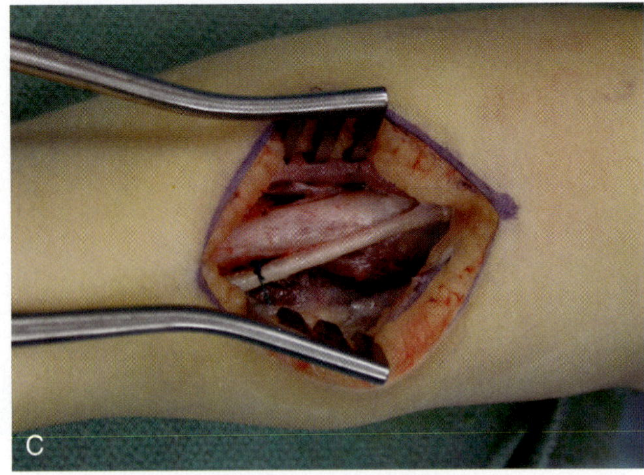

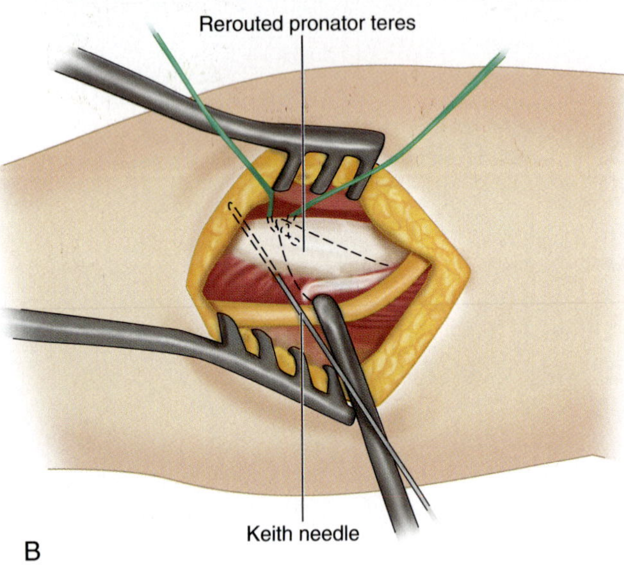

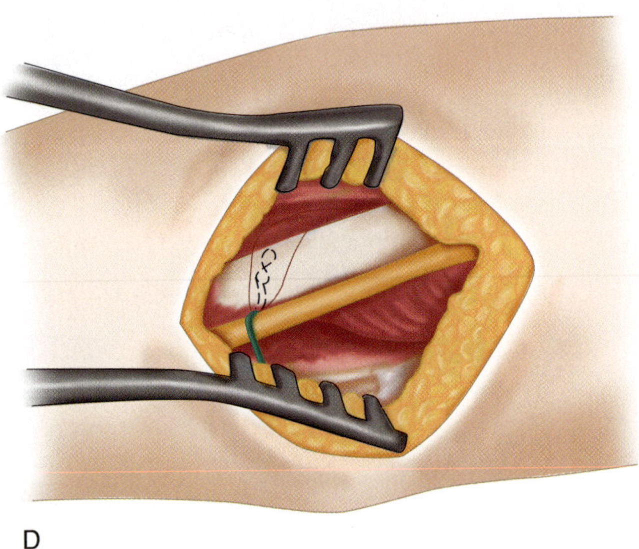

FIGURE 28-8

Step 7

- The PT is now attached to the radius. The attachment of the PT to the bone can be achieved in several ways. A Mitek Mini bone anchor can be inserted over the dorsal radius to provide attachment of the sutures.
- Our preference is to use a Keith needle to drill two holes through the radius, and then to pass the sutures through the radius and tie them over the opposite cortex. This form of attachment is quite strong (Fig. 28-8A to D).
- Tension is set to keep the forearm in the neutral position.

Step 8

- The tourniquet is released, hemostasis is secured, and the incision is closed in layers.

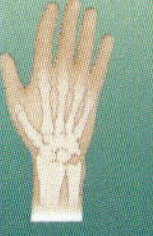

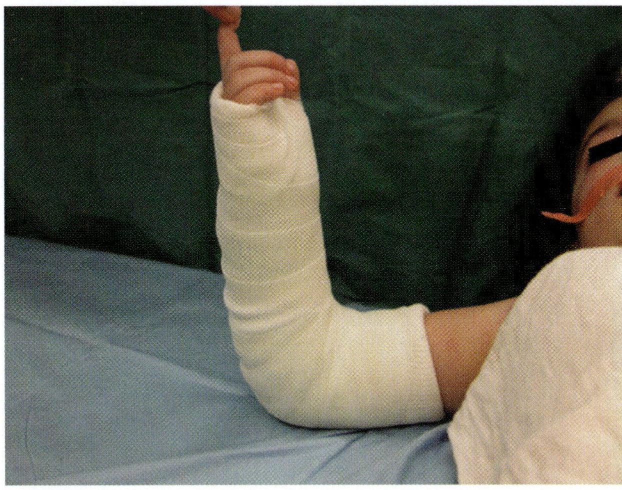

FIGURE 28-9

Postoperative Care and Expected Outcomes

- The forearm is splinted in the fully supinated position above the elbow for the next 6 weeks to allow reattachment of the fascia and tendon to the radius (Fig. 28-9). After 6 weeks of splinting, the patient is allowed unrestricted motion. Therapy typically is not necessary because the patient should automatically be able to learn how to use the tendon transfer for supination. Another advantage of the rerouting procedure is to take tension off the PT (a weak elbow flexor) to enable the patient to extend the elbow.
- The patient can expect an improvement in active supination ranging from 45 to 90 degrees. However, there will be some loss of pronation. The results are less satisfactory in patients who do not have active pronation before the procedure.

Evidence

Gschwind C, Tonkin M. Surgery for cerebral palsy. Part 1: classification and operative procedures for pronation deformity. *J Hand Surg [Am]*. 1992;17:391-395.

This paper discusses the correction of pronation deformity in cerebral palsy patients. The authors note that patients who have active supination beyond neutral position do not need correction. For patients who can only supinate to neutral position, the authors recommend PQ release with or without a flexor aponeurotic release. A flexor aponeurotic release involves a 2-cm transverse strip excision of the forearm fascia 6 cm distal to the medial epicondyle. The purpose of this excision is to remove and release the contracted forearm fascia. For a patient who has no active but full passive supination, the authors recommended a PT rerouting procedure. In a patient with no active supination and tight passive supination, they recommended a PQ release with a flexor aponeurosis release. (Level IV evidence)

Sakellarides HT, Mital MA, Lenzi WD. Treatment of pronation contractures of the forearm in cerebral palsy by changing the insertion of the pronator radii teres. *J Bone Joint Surg [Am]*. 1981;63:645-652.

The authors reported the results of 22 cerebral palsy patients with pronation contracture treated with a PT rerouting procedure. Eighty-two percent of the patients had good to excellent results and gained 46 degrees of active supination when compared with preoperative measurements. (Level IV evidence).

Strecker WB, Emanuel JP, Daily L, Manske PR. Comparison of pronator tenotomy and pronator re-routing in children with spastic cerebral palsy. *J Hand Surg [Am]*. 1988;13:540-543.

This study compared the results of 41 cerebral palsy patients who had a PT rerouting procedure with those of 16 patients who had PT tenotomy. The average gains in supination were 78 degrees for the rerouting and 54 degrees for the tenotomy procedure. (Level III evidence)

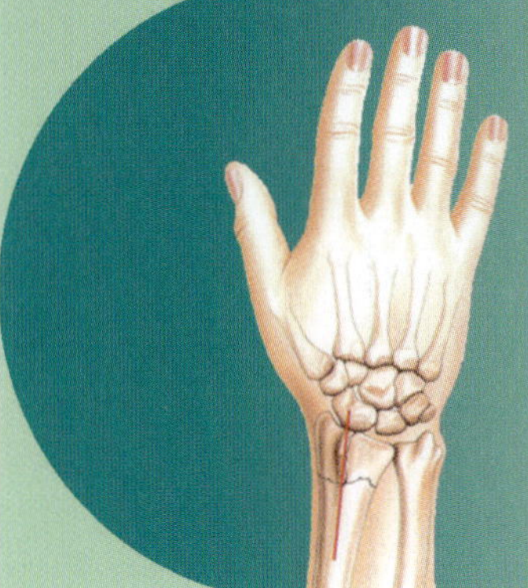

PROCEDURE 29

Release of a Spastic Elbow Flexion Contracture

Sandeep J. Sebastin and Kevin C. Chung

See Video 22: Biceps and Brachialis Lengthening

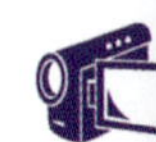

Indications

- Fixed elbow flexion contracture as a result of long-standing muscle spasticity as seen in cerebral palsy, stroke, or traumatic brain injury
  - More than 40 degrees in patients with volitional control of the elbow and hand
  - More than 100 degrees in patients without volitional control (for hygiene)

Examination/Imaging

Clinical Examination

- The three major causes of an elbow flexion contracture resulting from spasticity are cerebral palsy, stroke, and traumatic brain injury. There are some differences in the approach to treatment among these three causes.
  - *Cerebral palsy:* The functional use of the hand and upper limb should be evaluated before surgery is considered. This is usually possible only in late childhood (6 to 12 years) and requires multiple visits. The patient should be asked to perform activities with both hands, and videotaping the child is helpful. Reconstruction in older patients should be undertaken carefully because they may have learned to compensate for their disabilities. The aim is to differentiate between spastic muscle, muscle contracture, and joint contracture. This requires the patient to relax and can be difficult. Patients with muscle spasticity demonstrate full range of motion of an affected joint, whereas those with muscle contracture and joint contracture do not. Children do not usually present with joint contractures. It is also important to determine voluntary use of the hand, sensibility, intelligence quotient, and the presence of athetosis because these factors affect the functional result that may be achieved with surgery. Wheelchair-bound patients (with lower limb involvement) are less troubled by elbow spasticity than ambulatory patients because most of their upper limb use is limited to height of the wheelchair.

- *Stroke:* Surgery for correcting spastic contractures in stroke patients should be considered after they are neurologically stable. Spontaneous neurologic recovery occurs in the first 6 months, and stroke patients are considered to be neurologically stable at 12 months. Hemiplegia with a nonfunctional upper extremity and a less involved lower extremity is the most common presentation in stroke. The degree of spasticity seen in stroke is less because the patients are usually older with weaker muscles and the period of spontaneous recovery is shorter. For the same reasons, the recovery of motor function in stroke is also poor. Therefore, surgical procedures in stroke patients help more in correction of the contracture than in improving function.
- *Traumatic brain injury:* Spontaneous neurologic recovery can occur for up to 18 months after injury, and surgery should be deferred until this period. In contrast to patients with stroke, patients with traumatic brain injury are likely to be younger with quadriplegic involvement and may have concomitant peripheral nerve injuries, deformities from fractures, and heterotopic ossification. The degree of spasticity is much greater, and the recovery of motor function is also better. However, the degree of cognition and patient cooperation may be lower.

- *Extent of release:* The spastic muscles that contribute to an elbow flexion contracture are the biceps brachii, the brachialis, and the brachioradialis. Depending on the degree of contracture and amount of volitional control, they can be either lengthened or divided sequentially. The lacertus fibrosis is always divided, and an anterior capsulectomy of elbow joint or a Z-lengthening of the antecubital skin may be rarely required.

Imaging

- *X-ray of the elbow joint:* Radiography can help differentiate muscle contracture from joint contracture. It is especially useful in traumatic brain injury, in which heterotopic ossification around the elbow is common and can be associated with compression of the ulnar nerve.
- *Nerve block:* A local anesthetic nerve block can be used to differentiate between muscle spasticity and muscle contracture.
- *Dynamic electromyography:* This helps in identifying spastic and flaccid muscles and can help with the surgical decision-making process. It can show the muscles under volitional control and determine phasic activity.

Surgical Anatomy

- The cubital fossa, bounded medially by the pronator teres and laterally by the brachioradialis, contains the lateral cutaneous nerve of the forearm, the tendon of the biceps brachii, the brachial artery, and median nerve. The brachial artery and median nerve are located medial to the biceps brachii, and the lateral cutaneous nerve of the forearm is lateral to the biceps brachii. The lacertus fibrosus, also known as the bicipital aponeurosis, continues distally as deep fascia of the forearm (Fig. 29-1).

Positioning

- The patient is placed in the supine position.
- A pneumatic tourniquet is placed as high as possible toward the axilla so that it does not interfere with the operative field (Fig. 29-2).

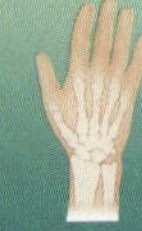

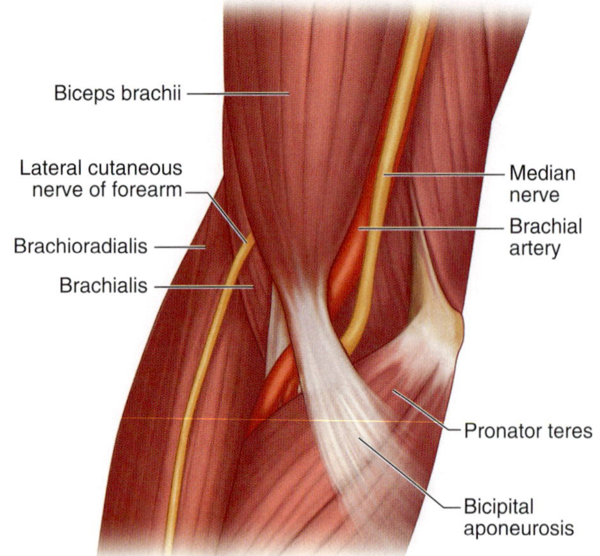

FIGURE 29-1

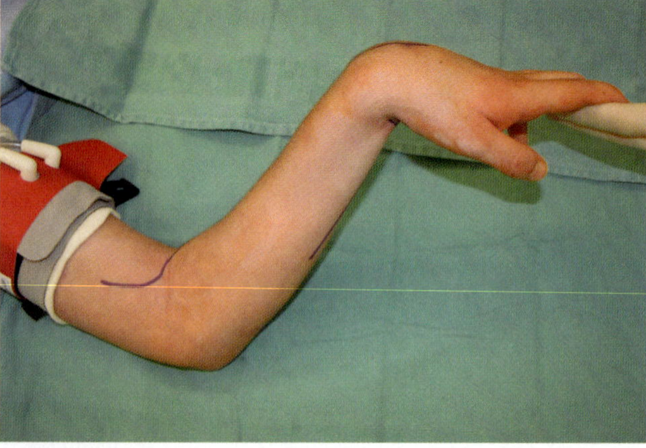

FIGURE 29-2

PEARLS

A longitudinal incision on the lateral aspect of the elbow should be considered in patients who have more than 100 degrees of flexion contracture. This will allow design of multiple Z-plasties during wound closure.

Exposures

- A 15-cm long "lazy S"–shaped incision is made over the antecubital fossa. The incision begins on the lateral aspect of the arm over the origin of the brachioradialis muscle and gently curves over the antecubital crease distally toward the anteromedial aspect of the forearm (see Fig. 29-2).
- The subcutaneous dissection is continued from medial to lateral, to expose the cubital fossa. The lacertus fibrosus and the biceps brachii tendon are identified (Fig. 29-3A and B). The median nerve and brachial artery are identified medial to the biceps tendon, and the lateral antebrachial cutaneous nerve is identified lateral to the biceps tendon emerging from the interval between the biceps and brachialis.

Procedure

Step 1

- The bicipital aponeurosis, located medial to the biceps brachii tendon, is elevated and should be resected completely (Fig. 29-4).

Step 2

- The contracted biceps brachii is exposed and dissected distal to its insertion. The decision regarding the degree of biceps lengthening should be made at this time. A fractional lengthening is performed for mild contractures, and a Z-lengthening is performed for more severe contractures.
- A fractional lengthening is performed by making two transverse and slightly oblique cuts, 1 to 2 cm apart, halfway through the tendinous portion of the musculotendinous junction, with care taken to leave the muscle fibers intact. One cut is made on the lateral side of the tendon, and the other cut is made on the medial side. Passive extension of the elbow allows separation of these tenotomy sites, keeping the muscle in continuity.
- A Z-lengthening (step-cut) is performed over as much length of the tendon as possible because this gives more tendon substance to do a strong repair (see Fig. 29-4).

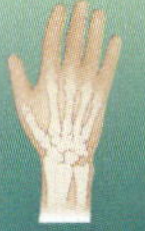

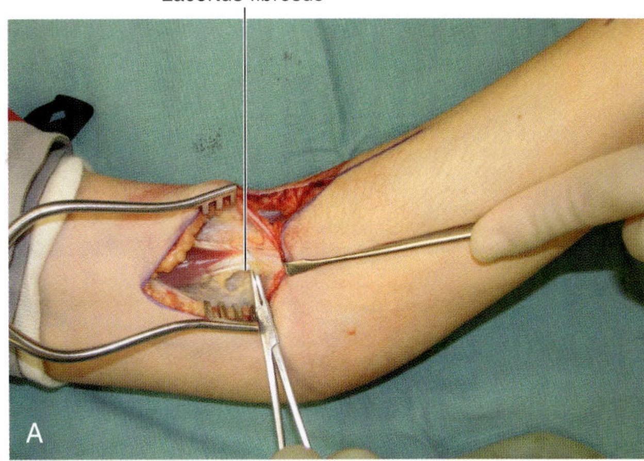

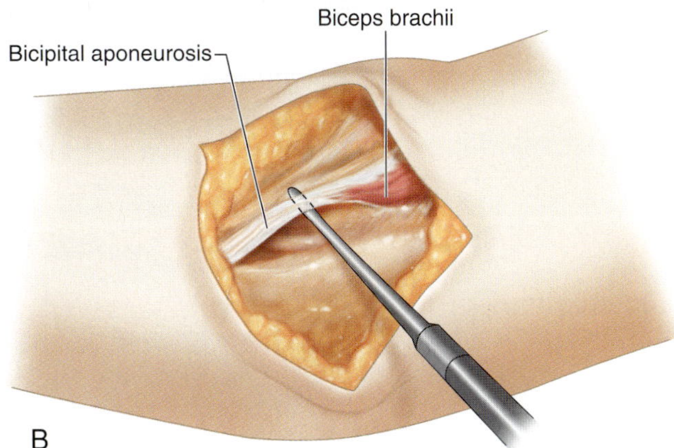

FIGURE 29-3

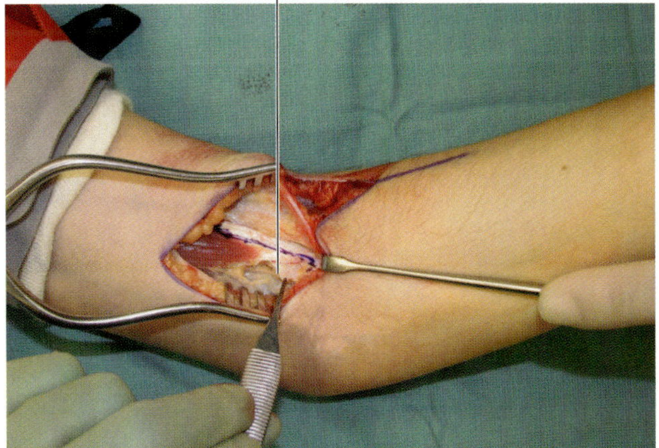

FIGURE 29-4

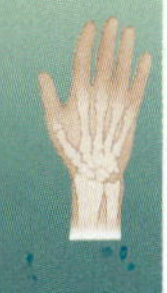

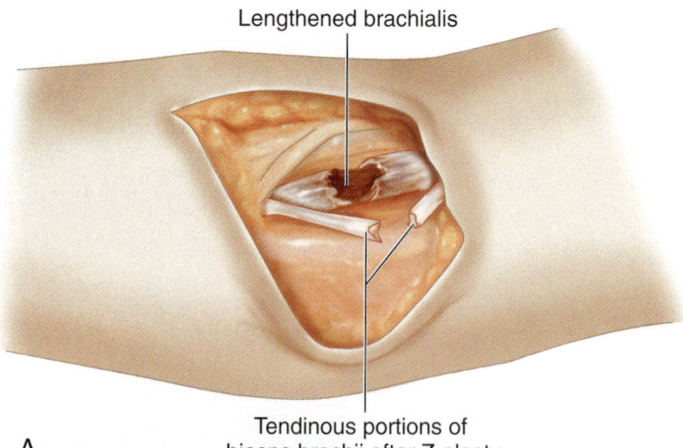

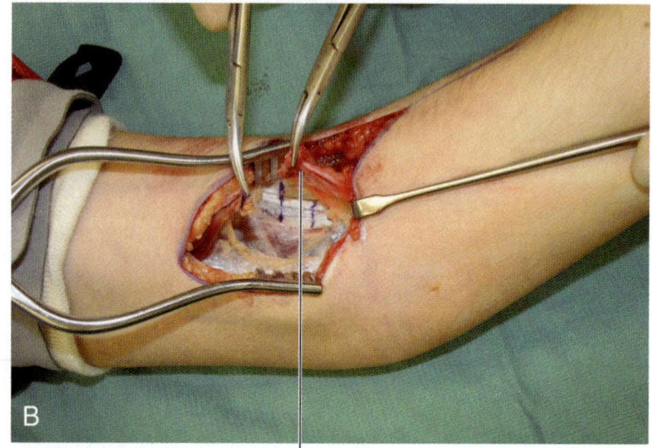

FIGURE 29-5

STEP 3 PEARLS

If a double-incision release of the brachialis is planned, the proximal incision should be made first. If the distal incision is made first, the proximal migration of the brachialis will make it difficult to make the second incision (Fig. 29-6).

Step 3

- The release of the biceps brings the brachialis into view. Depending on the degree of contracture and the volitional control of the patient, a partial or complete release of the brachialis can be done.
- A partial release can be done using one or two incisions (Fig. 29-5A). A double incision gives more release. A transverse incision is made over the aponeurotic portion on the anterior aspect of the muscle, leaving the muscle intact. If two incisions are used, they are spaced about 1 to 2 cm apart (Fig. 29-5B).
- In patients who have severe contractures without volitional control, the brachialis can be completely transected using electrocautery.

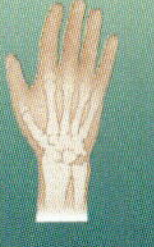

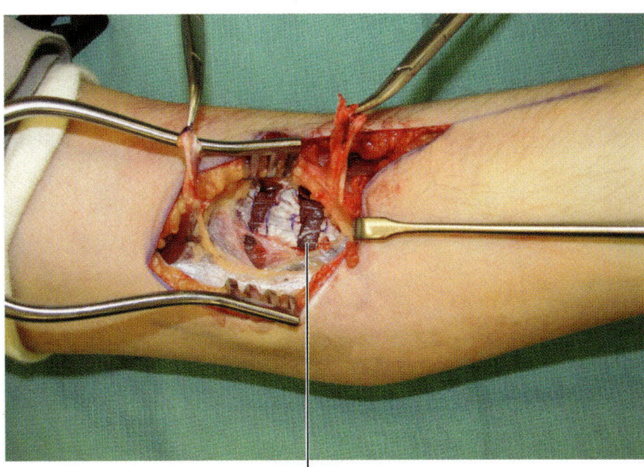

FIGURE 29-6

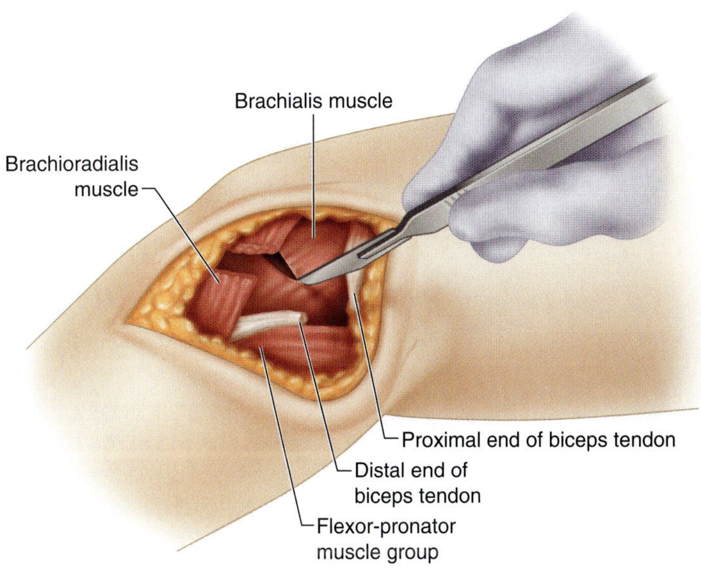

FIGURE 29-7

Step 4

- At this point, assessment of the brachioradialis is done. A partial or complete release of the brachioradialis can be performed, depending on the degree of spasticity and the volitional control of the patient. Dissection is carried out between the brachialis and the brachioradialis.
  - A partial release is done by detaching the origin of the brachioradialis by a combination of blunt dissection and electrocautery. This allows the origin of the brachioradialis to slide distally.
  - A complete release is done by dividing the brachioradialis through its muscle belly using electrocautery (Fig. 29-7).

Step 5

- An anterior capsulectomy of the elbow joint or a Z-plasty of the antecubital skin is required only in the rare very severe contracture.

STEP 4 PEARLS

If the brachioradialis has volitional control and the elbow contracture is not very severe, a partial release can be done through a separate 3-cm longitudinal incision made on the dorsoradial aspect of the mid-forearm. The tendinous portion of the brachioradialis is on its deeper surface; the muscle needs to be reflected to visualize this portion. A transverse incision is used to divide only the tendon, keeping the muscle in continuity.

STEP 4 PITFALLS

The radial nerve needs to be identified and protected during any procedure on the brachioradialis.

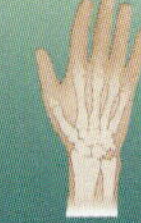

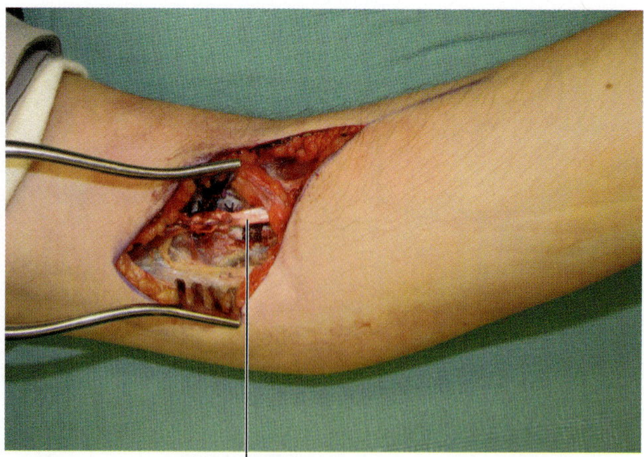

FIGURE 29-8

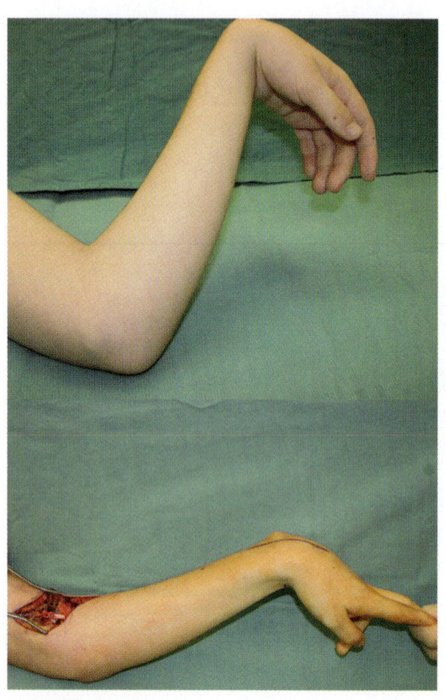

FIGURE 29-9

Step 6

- The biceps tendon is sutured with a Pulvertaft type weave using 3-0 Ethibond sutures with the elbow in 30 degrees of flexion (Fig. 29-8).

Step 7

- The tourniquet is released, hemostasis is secured, and all incisions are closed.
- Tension over the wound closure is relieved by advancing the lateral skin by the S-shaped incision.

Postoperative Care and Expected Outcomes

- A long-arm plaster of Paris splint that keeps the elbow at 30 degrees of flexion is applied.
- Ten days after surgery, the wound is inspected, and sutures are removed. If a Z-lengthening of the biceps was done, the elbow is splinted for an additional 4 weeks in 30 degrees of flexion. Active and passive range of motion is initiated thereafter. Night splints are used for an additional 3 weeks to protect the biceps tendon repair. If only a fractional lengthening of the biceps was done and there was no repair of the biceps tendon, the patient can be started on mobilization immediately.
- Patients who undergo fractional lengthening of the biceps can expect a 10- to 30-degree improvement in the flexion contracture without appreciable loss of flexion power. Patients who undergo Z-lengthening can expect up to a 45- to 60-degree improvement in flexion contracture, but they do lose elbow flexion power. It is important to avoid full extension of the elbow in patients with volitional control because difficulty with elbow flexion after a full release may become a greater problem for the patient (Fig. 29-9).

Evidence

Mital MA. Lengthening of the elbow flexors in the cerebral palsy. *J Bone Joint Surg [Am]*. 1979;61:515-522.

This report describes the correction of elbow flexion contracture in 32 elbows of 26 children with cerebral palsy using Z-plasty of the biceps brachii and transverse tenotomy of the brachialis. The average extension gain after surgery is 40 degrees. (Level IV evidence)

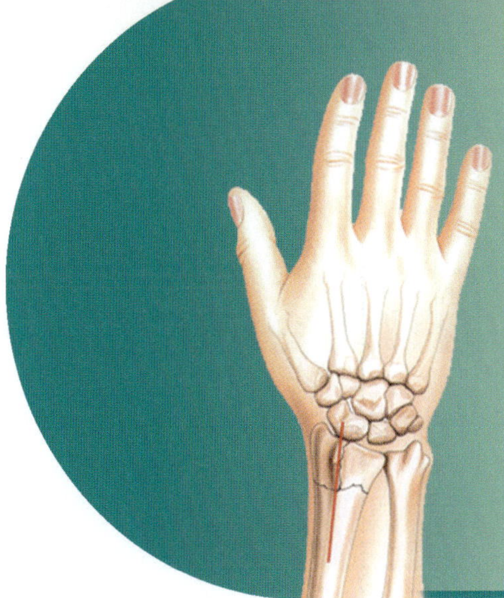

Section V

RECONSTRUCTION OF RHEUMATOID HAND DEFORMITIES

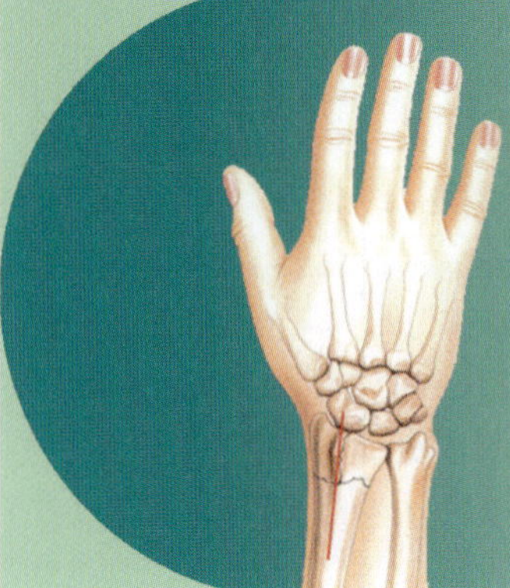

Synovectomy

Shimpei Ono, Sandeep J. Sebastin, and Kevin C. Chung

Indications

- Asymptomatic persistent synovitis despite 3 to 4 months of systemic therapy
- Symptomatic synovitis associated with the following:
  - Restricted range of motion
  - Trigger finger
  - Tendon rupture
  - Nerve compression (carpal tunnel syndrome; rarely, posterior interosseous nerve at the elbow)
  - Joint instability

Examination/Imaging

Clinical Examination

- *Dorsal wrist:* Extensor tendon synovitis can clearly be seen and palpated as a soft swelling on the dorsum of the wrist. Isolated dorsal tenosynovitis is painless. When patients with dorsal tenosynovitis complain of pain, one must look for involvement of the radiocarpal or radioulnar joints. Wrist mobility may be limited in this situation. It is also important to assess for the presence of ruptured extensor tendon and differentiate it from subluxation of the extensor tendons over the dorsum of the metacarpophalangeal (MCP) joints.
- *Palmar aspect of hand:* The presence of synovitis over the palmar aspect of the hand is indicated by the presence of (1) swelling (Fig. 30-1), (2) discrepancy between active and passive range of motion (Fig. 30-2), and (3) palpable crepitus along the course of the flexor tendon on active and passive flexion of the digit. This crepitus is best felt by asking the patient to flex the interphalangeal (IP) joints while applying some pressure over the tendon proximal to the A1 pulley of the flexor tendon sheath. The patient may also have triggering of the fingers. Flexor tendon ruptures occur infrequently compared with extensor tendon ruptures. One must also look for carpal tunnel syndrome as a result of proliferative synovitis within the carpal tunnel.

Imaging

- Radiographic examination should always be done before surgery. Surgery to address joint pathology may be required along with tenosynovectomy.

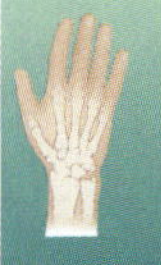

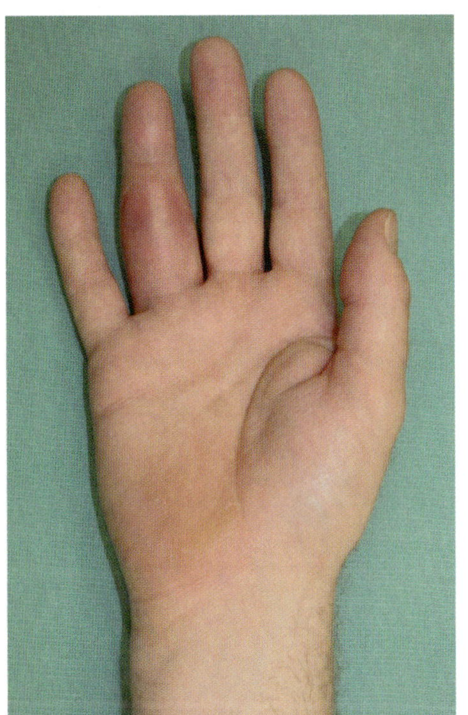

FIGURE 30-1

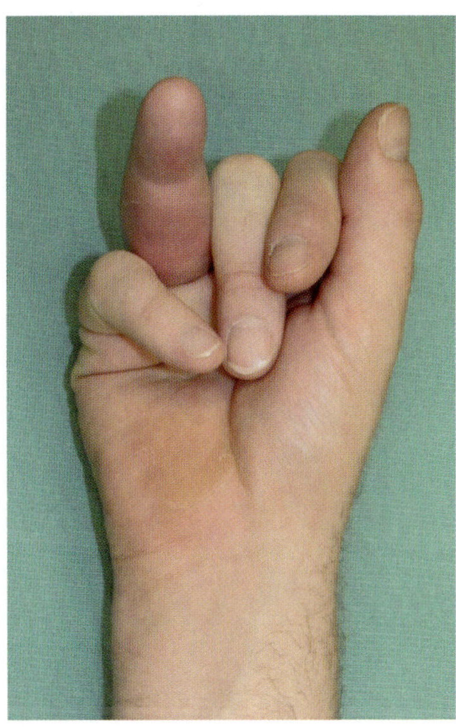

FIGURE 30-2

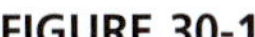

Surgical Anatomy

- Synovitis is the hallmark of rheumatoid arthritis (RA), and, in the hand, it involves the synovial lining of the tendon sheath (tenosynovium) and the joint. Flexor tendons are covered by the tenosynovium under the carpal tunnel and in the digital flexor sheath, whereas extensor tendons are covered by tenosynovium only under the extensor retinaculum. Synovitis of the hand involves the extensor tendons more frequently than the flexor tendons.
- Extensor tendon involvement is frequently seen over the dorsum of the wrist and results from synovitis progressing from the distal radioulnar joint and tenosynovitis under the extensor retinaculum. In contrast, the changes in the extensor tendon seen at the interphalangeal joints are caused by the underlying joint synovitis and not tenosynovitis.
- Three main groups of flexor tenosynovitis can be distinguished: isolated carpal tenosynovitis (20%), palmodigital tenosynovitis (50%), and diffuse tenosynovitis (30%). The index, long, and small fingers are most frequently involved. A flexor tendon rupture in the digital flexor sheath is almost always secondary to infiltrative synovitis and usually involves the flexor digitorum superficialis (FDS) at the proximal interphalangeal (PIP) joint. This is probably because the FDS splits into two slips in the distal third of the proximal phalanx. This decreases the thickness of the tendon and increases the surface area in contact with the invading synovium.

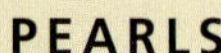

PEARLS

An extended carpal tunnel incision can be made if access is required more proximally.

PITFALLS

The skin must be handled with great care because vascularity and quality of skin are often impaired by rheumatoid disease and/or rheumatoid medications.

The skin incisions must be planned carefully to allow complete access to the diseased area without forceful retraction.

The neurovascular bundles must be identified and protected.

Tenosynovectomy

1. Digital Flexor Synovectomy

Exposures

- A Bruner type incision is made in the fingers extending onto the distal palm (Fig. 30-3).
- The skin flaps are raised in a plane superficial to the flexor tendon sheath. This brings into view the sausage-shaped mass of distended synovium (Fig. 30-4).

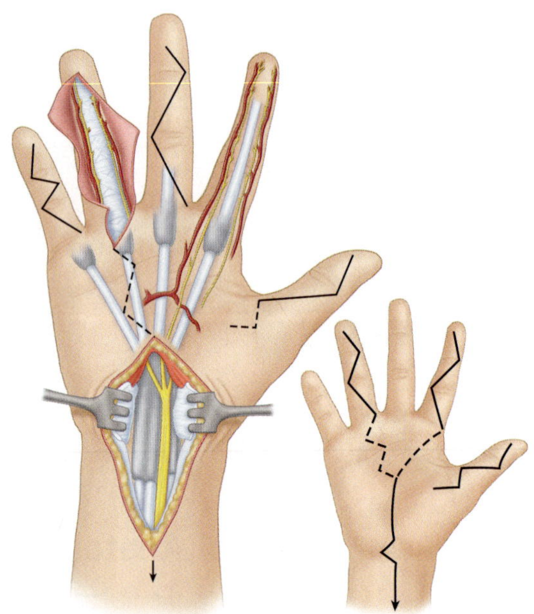

FIGURE 30-3

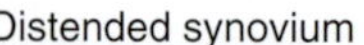

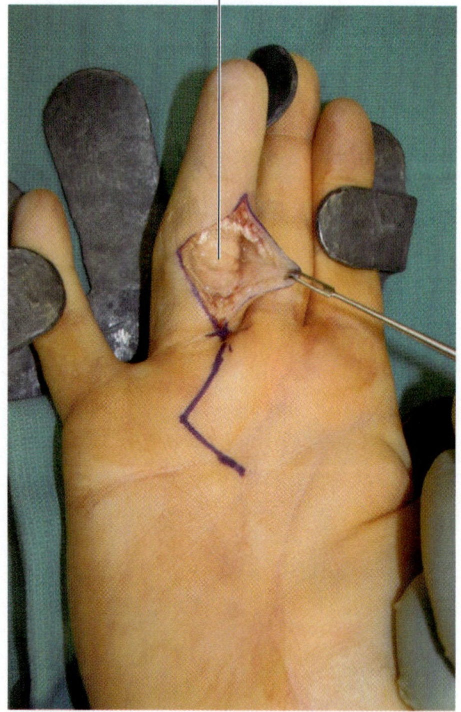

FIGURE 30-4

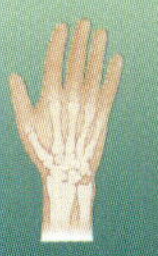

STEP 1 PEARLS

Occasionally, the tenosynovitis infiltrates into the tendon substance, resulting in a frayed tendon surface. In such cases, the frayed surface should be trimmed.

A tendon defect resulting from the excision of a nodule can be closed with a horizontal mattress suture.

STEP 1 PITFALLS

The slips of the FDS may be infiltrated with tenosynovitis, and the surgeon may be tempted to excise the FDS tendon, which should be avoided because of the progressive nature of the disease. The FDS is the prime flexor of the PIP joint, and excising it may result in a swan neck deformity.

Care is taken not to injure the neurovascular bundles and resect the tendon pulleys accidentally.

STEP 2 PEARLS

If surgery is performed with the patient under local anesthesia or a Bier block, active range of motion can be visualized and any residual diseased areas addressed.

If "catching" is found when testing for tendon excursion after tenosynovectomy, check for flexor tendon nodules in digits and/or palm.

If triggering of finger persists after tenosynovectomy, an A1 pulley release is performed.

STEP 2 PITFALLS

The release of the A1 pulley may contribute to the MCP joint ulnar drift deformity, especially for the index and long fingers, because of the oblique line of pull of the long flexors for these digits. Some investigators recommend resection of one slip of the FDS to provide greater space for passage of the FDP instead of A1 pulley release.

Procedure

Step 1: Synovectomy

- Flexor tendon synovectomy is performed by pulling the FDS and flexor digitorum profundus (FDP) tendons alternatively through the openings in the tendon sheath. The area of tenosynovitis can then be excised from each tendon using a combination of sharp and blunt dissections (Fig. 30-5).

Step 2: Checking Passive Range of Motion

- After the tenosynovectomy, the smooth gliding of tendons (FDS and FDP) is confirmed by flexion and extension of the fingers (Fig. 30-6).

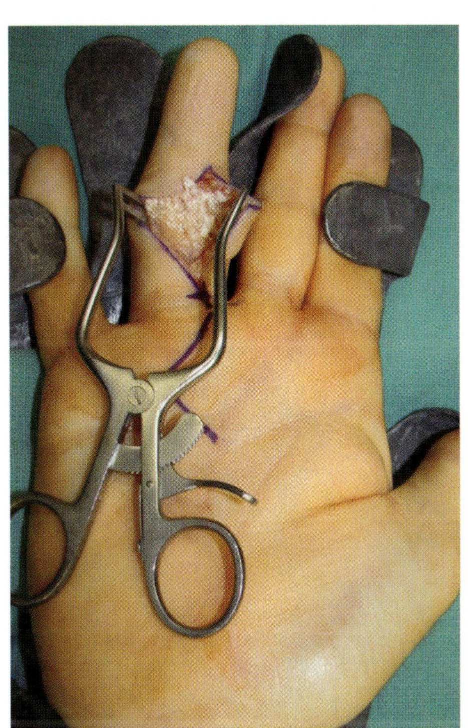

FIGURE 30-5

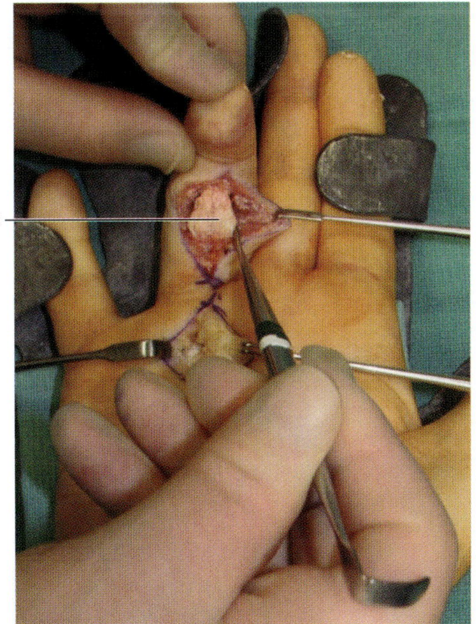

FIGURE 30-6

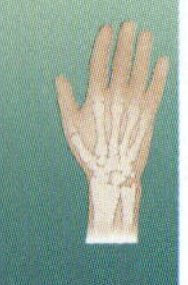

Step 3: Checking for Intrinsic Tightness

- In the presence of intrinsic muscle contracture, the lateral bands should be divided. While maintaining the MCP joint in extension, the lateral bands are divided from volar to dorsal until the PIP joint can be passively flexed.

Step 4: Skin Closure

- The tourniquet is released, and hemostasis is obtained.
- The skin is closed loosely using 4-0 interrupted nylon sutures.

Postoperative Care and Expected Outcomes

- A generously padded volar plaster of Paris slab extending to the fingertips is applied while maintaining the fingers in an intrinsic-plus posture and the wrist in moderate extension. The hand is kept elevated, and gentle mobilization is started in 4 to 7 days.
- Digital flexor tenosynovectomy is a safe and effective method for restoring function to rheumatoid patients with flexor tenosynovitis to prevent further complications such as the flexor tendon rupture.

2. Flexor Synovectomy in the Carpal Tunnel and Distal Forearm

Exposures

- An extended carpal tunnel incision is made (see Fig. 30-3). This longitudinal incision extends 2 cm distal to the wrist crease and 4 cm proximal to it. The distal limb of the incision is required only if a carpal tunnel release is indicated and is made parallel to the thenar crease. The proximal limb of the incision is made over the palmaris longus (PL). The limbs are connected by a transverse incision over the wrist crease.
- The forearm fascia is divided ulnar to the PL to expose the median nerve and flexor tendons in the proximal portion of the incision. The subcutaneous fat is bluntly dissected to expose the transverse carpal ligament in the distal portion. The transverse carpal ligament is divided along its entire length (Fig. 30-7).

PEARLS

Care is taken to protect the palmar cutaneous branch of the median nerve that runs radial to the PL (Fig. 30-8).

The distal limb of the incision must not be too radial (indicated by muscle fibers of the abductor pollicis brevis) or too ulnar (indicated by larger fat globules of Guyon canal).

Procedure

Step 1: Synovectomy

- The hypertrophic tenosynovium surrounding the flexor tendons is excised (Fig. 30-9).

Step 2: Checking for Free Tendon Excision

- Traction is applied to the flexor tendons to check finger motion. Smooth motion of the fingers and thumb should be present.

STEP 2 PITFALLS

"Catching" signals the presence of tendon nodules in the palm or digits. If smooth motion of the tendons is not present, the involved tendon must be explored as far distally as necessary to remove the nodules.

Step 3: Skin Closure

- The tourniquet is released, and hemostasis is obtained.
- The skin is closed using 4-0 nylon.

Postoperative Care and Expected Outcomes

- Postoperative immobilization is supported by a volar wrist splint in neutral position followed by immediate active finger motion.
- Flexor tenosynovectomy with decompression of the nerve prevents permanent pain, numbness, thenar muscle loss, and spontaneous rupture, as well as preserving independent tendon gliding function.

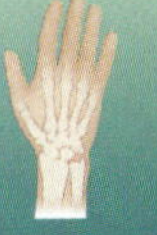

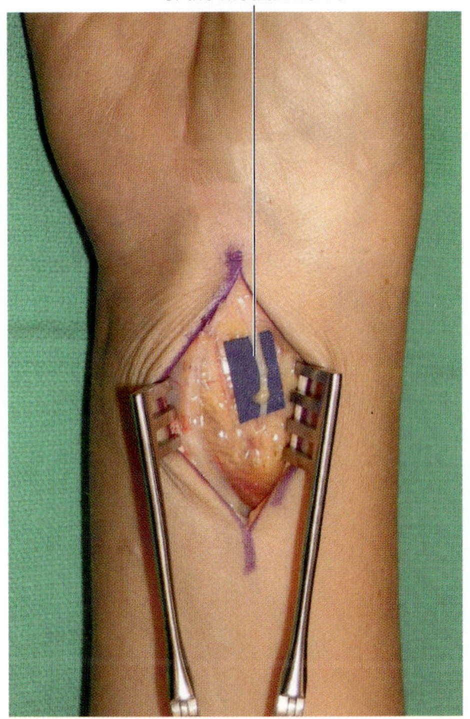

FIGURE 30-7

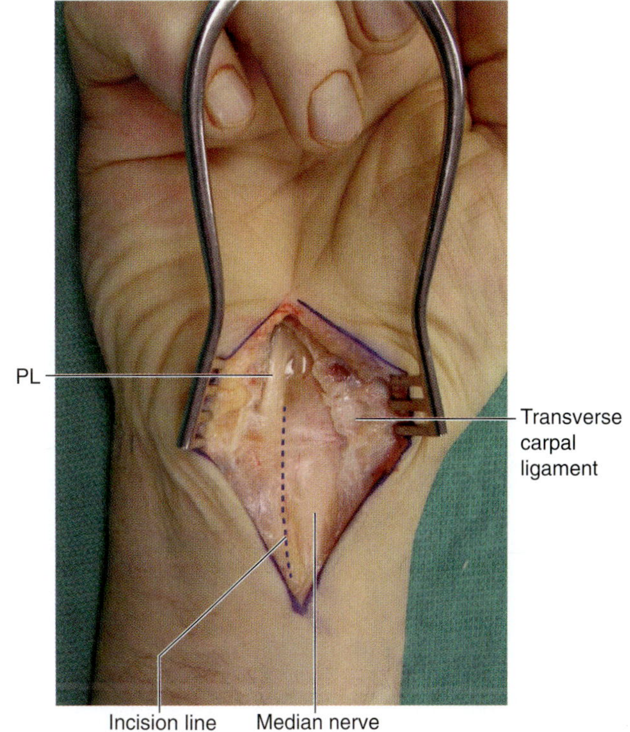

FIGURE 30-8

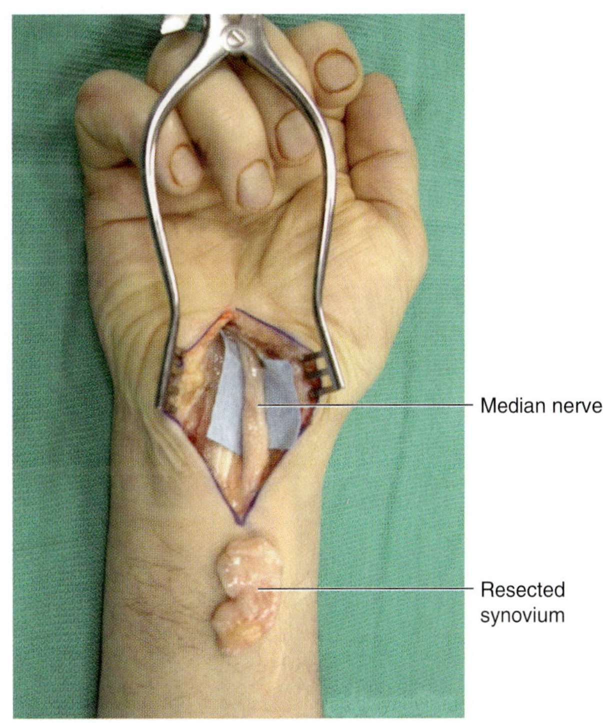

FIGURE 30-9

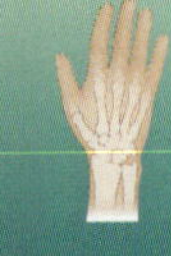

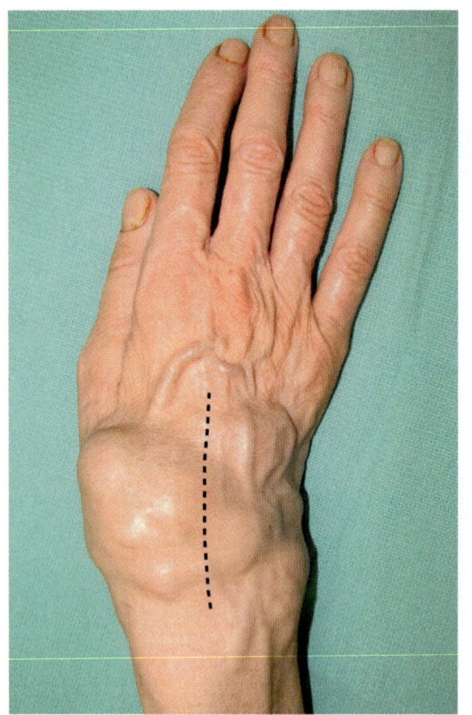

FIGURE 30-10

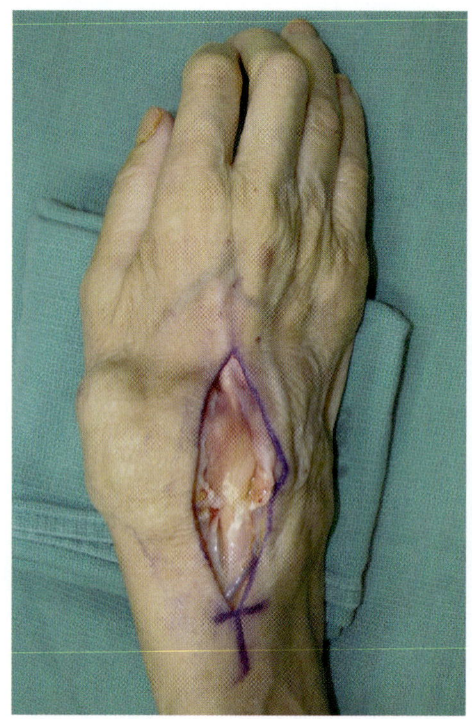

FIGURE 30-11

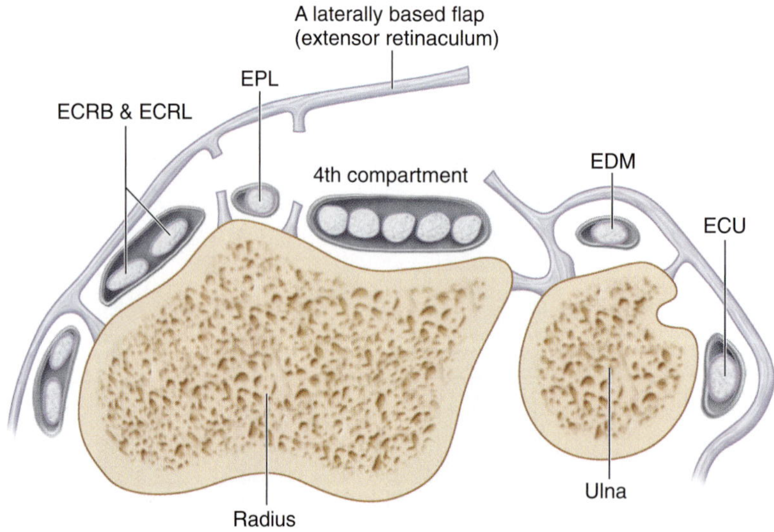

FIGURE 30-12

3. Dorsal Wrist Synovectomy

Exposures

- An 8-cm dorsal longitudinal incision centered over the radiocarpal joint is made (Fig. 30-10).
- Sharp dissection is carried down to the extensor retinaculum over the fourth compartment in this case.
- The extensor retinaculum is incised longitudinally over the fourth compartment (Fig. 30-11). The vertical septae between the extensor compartments are divided, thus raising the retinaculum as a laterally based flap (Fig. 30-12). This exposes the extensor tendons and the hypertrophic synovium.

PEARLS

Care is taken to preserve the main longitudinal veins and not to injure branches of the radial sensory nerve.

When the retinaculum flaps are elevated, the first dorsal compartment is not opened unless it is involved significantly.

An alternative exposure involves elevating the extensor retinaculum as a radially based flap by opening it over the fourth or fifth compartment. This flap is divided into two flaps by splitting it transversely (Fig. 30-13). During closure, one flap is passed below the extensor tendons and the other above the tendons (Fig. 30-14). This approach provides a gliding bed for the tendons and creates a barrier between the tendons and the underlying bone and wrist joint.

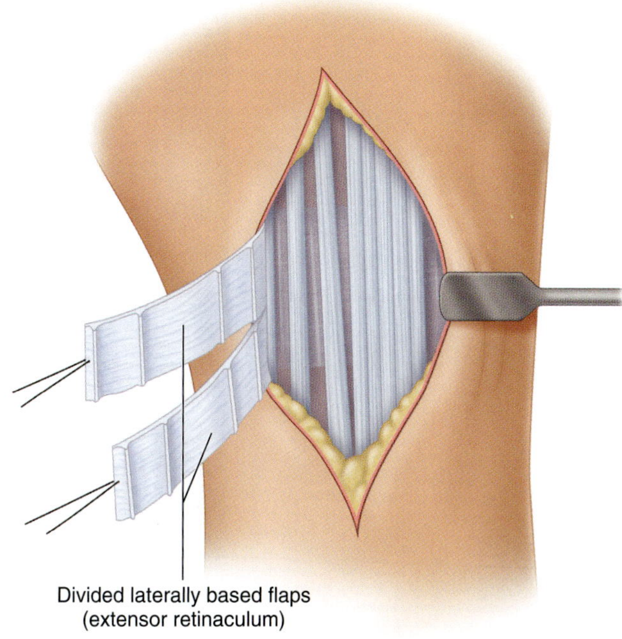

FIGURE 30-13

STEP 1 PEARLS

As much of the diseased synovium is removed as possible, although it is sometimes necessary to leave material that is densely adherent to the extensor tendon surface to avoid disrupting the tendon substance.

Frayed areas of the tendons are repaired with interrupted 5-0 Ethibond braided sutures.

After a complete tenosynovectomy has been performed, the wrist joint is evaluated. If synovitis is present, the joint is opened, and a wrist synovectomy is performed.

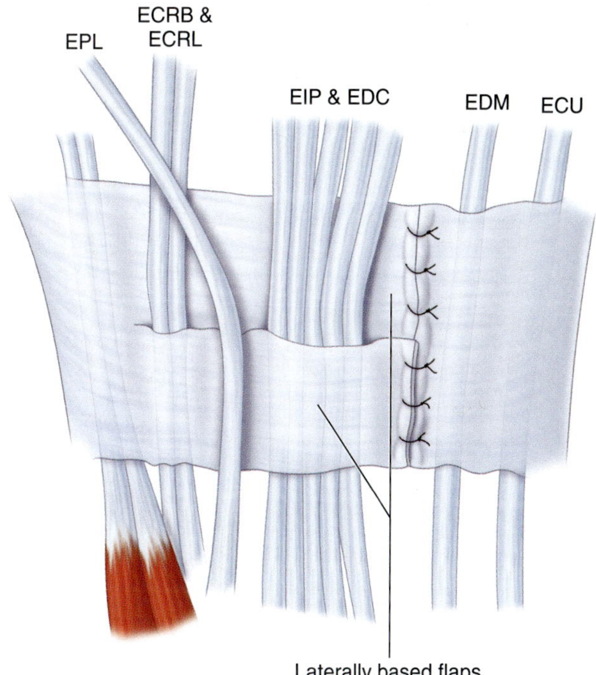

FIGURE 30-14

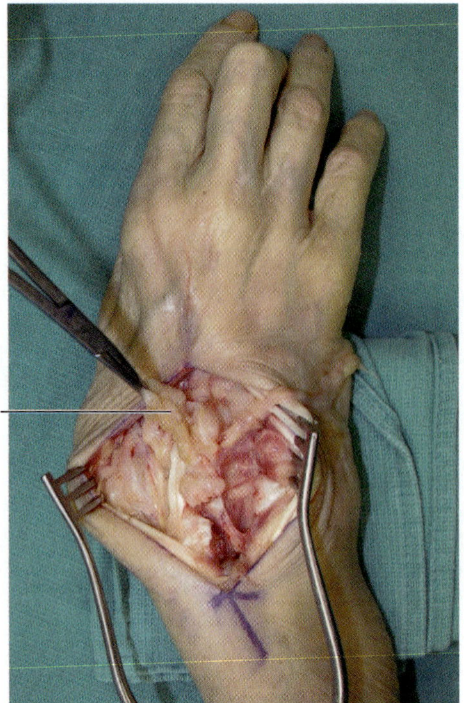

FIGURE 30-15

Procedure

Step 1: Synovectomy

- Hypertrophic synovium is removed from the extensor tendons sharply with a no. 15 blade and occasionally with small scissors (Fig. 30-15).

Step 2: Repair of the Extensor Retinaculum

- The extensor retinaculum flap is repaired using 4-0 Vicryl.

Step 3: Skin Closure

- The tourniquet is released, and hemostasis is obtained.
- The skin is closed using 4-0 nylon.

Postoperative Care and Expected Outcomes

- The hand and wrist are immobilized in a bulky conforming dressing and volar plaster splint. The wrist is held in neutral and the MCP joint in extension to prevent extensor lag until active extension is possible. The IP joints are left free.
- Hand motion is started 24 to 48 hours after surgery. Active extension and flexion exercises are emphasized. The wrist is supported with a volar splint for 2 weeks after the procedure.
- Although the appearance of the tendons within the compartments affected by tenosynovitis may be poor (as evidenced by fraying), tendon rupture rarely occurs after dorsal tenosynovectomy is performed.

Joints Synovectomy

1. *Wrist Synovectomy*

Exposures

- The first part is the same as for dorsal wrist synovectomy. After a complete tenosynovectomy has been performed, the wrist joint is evaluated. If synovitis is present, the joint is opened, and a wrist synovectomy is performed.
- If one needs to access the radiocarpal joint, the floor of third compartment is incised longitudinally, and if access to the distal radioulnar joint is required, the floor of the fifth compartment is opened.

Procedure

Step 1: Synovectomy

- The synovium in the joints is removed with a small, curved rongeur.
- The dorsal aspects of the ulna and radius are examined, and any bony spicules, which might cause attrition ruptures, are removed with a rongeur.
- The distal ulna is resected at the same time if it is dislocated and prominent dorsally (see Procedure 83).

Step 2: Closure

- The tourniquet is released, and hemostasis is obtained.
- The dorsal wrist capsule is repaired with 3-0 Ethibond sutures.
- The extensor retinaculum is repaired as described previously.
- The skin is closed using 4-0 nylon.

Postoperative Care and Expected Outcomes

- A resting volar wrist splint should be provided to immobilize the wrist for 4 weeks while permitting finger motion.

PEARLS

Traction sutures are placed on the skin flaps to provide gentle retraction of the skin.

The longitudinal dorsal veins are preserved.

PITFALLS

It is important to remember that the anatomy is not normal, and usually the extensor tendons are ulnarly subluxed in the valley between the heads of the metacarpals.

2. *Metacarpophalangeal Joint Synovectomy*

Exposures

- A transverse incision is made over the head of the metacarpals for multiple MCP joint synovectomy and a longitudinal "lazy S"–shaped incision is used when a single joint is being addressed. The skin flaps are retracted to expose the extensor mechanism over the MCP joint.
- The radial sagittal band is divided 1 to 2 mm lateral to the extensor tendon, and the extensor mechanism is retracted. The dorsal capsules are incised transversely to expose the MCP joint.

Procedure

Step 1

- The synovium in the MCP joint is removed with a small, curved rongeur.

STEP 1 PEARLS

Traction applied to the finger allows easier access to the joints.

Step 2: Soft Tissue Reconstruction (Extensor Tendon Centralization)

- The attenuated radial sagittal band and joint capsule of the affected finger is tightened to centralize its extensor tendon with 3-0 Ethibond mattress sutures.

STEP 2 PEARLS

MCP joint synovectomy is sometimes combined with the crossed intrinsic transfer or MCP joint arthroplasty.

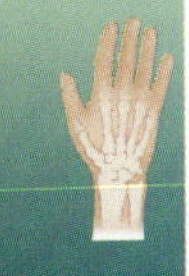

Step 3: Closure

- The tourniquet is released, and hemostasis is obtained.
- The skin is closed using 4-0 nylon.

Postoperative Care and Expected Outcomes

- Active motion is begun 1 to 2 days postoperatively, and a program of dynamic splinting similar to that after MCP joint arthroplasty is used for 4 weeks.

3. Proximal Interphalangeal Joint Synovectomy

Exposures

- A curvilinear longitudinal skin incision on the dorsum of the PIP joint is used. If synovial bulging is limited to one side, a lateral incision can be used. Skin flaps are elevated to expose the extensor mechanism.
- The joint can be approached either between the central slip and the lateral band or palmar to the lateral band, depending on the location of the disease. The joint is approached dorsal to the collateral ligament.

Procedure

STEP 1 PEARLS

Traction applied to the finger allows easier access to the joints.

Step 1: PIP Joint Synovectomy

- A small rongeur is used to excise the synovium (Fig. 30-16).
- A small curette is useful to clear the synovial recesses on the palmar and dorsal aspects of the head of the proximal phalanx.

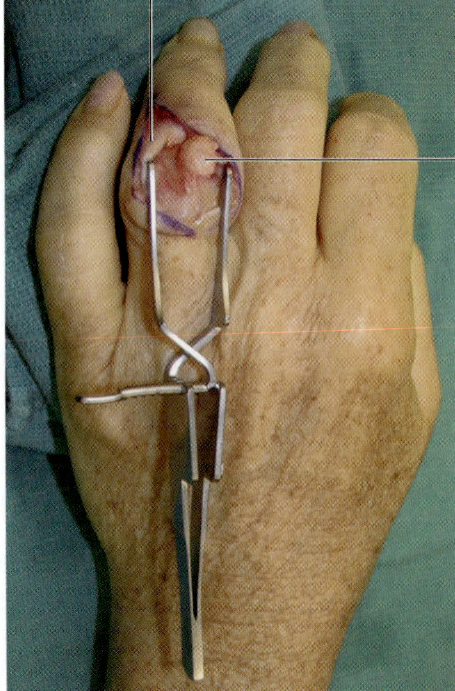

FIGURE 30-16

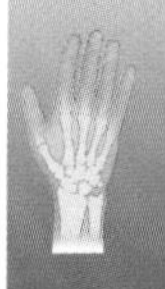

Step 2: Closure

- The tourniquet is released, and hemostasis is obtained.
- The incision in the extensor mechanism is repaired with 4-0 Ethibond sutures.
- The skin is closed using 4-0 nylon.

Postoperative Care and Expected Outcomes

- The joint is splinted in extension until the patient is able to perform active extension, and gentle mobilization is started after 4 to 7 days.

Evidence

Tolat AR, Stanley JK, Evans RA. Flexor tenosynovectomy and tenolysis in longstanding rheumatoid arthritis. *J Hand Surg [Br]*. 1996;21:538-543.

The authors presented a total of 43 patients (49 hands; 424 flexor tendons) who had rheumatoid arthritis of more than 15 years' duration at the time of surgery. The cases were clinically assessed at a mean follow-up of 5.7 years (range, 1.2 to 12 years). The results suggest that the patients had excellent sustained pain relief (mean score = 0.9) and were highly satisfied with the outcome of the procedure (mean score = 2.2). Eighty-one percent had adequate pulp-to-pulp and key pinch. Range of finger motion (total active motion, TAM) was excellent to good in 45% and fair in 22%. In 33%, TAM was graded as poor, and these cases were found to be multifactorial in origin, with associated significant joint disease, preoperative tendon ruptures, extensive digital surgery, readhesions, and combinations of operative procedures that adversely affect the rehabilitation program. The authors concluded that flexor tenosynovectomy with tenolysis is a useful procedure with a low rate of recurrence. (Level IV evidence)

Wheen DJ, Tonkin MA, Green J, Bronkhorst M. Long-term results following digital flexor tenosynovectomy in rheumatoid arthritis. *J Hand Surg [Am]*. 1995;20: 790-794.

The authors reviewed retrospectively the results of patients who underwent flexor tenosynovectomy for rheumatoid flexor tenosynovitis in the palm and digit. Fifteen patients (61 fingers) were reviewed for at least 1 year (average, 4 years) after surgery. An average of 2.2-cm improvement in active flexion (pulp to distal palmar crease) was observed. A significant difference in preoperative and postoperative results was found. Sixty-seven percent of digits were classified as having excellent or good results, 21% as fair results, and 12% as poor results. The clinical recurrence rate was 31%, and the reoperation rate was 15%. Only minimal complications from the extended surgical approach were observed. Debulking the fibro-osseous canal by excising a slip of flexor digitorum superficialis was associated with a reduction in the recurrence and reoperation rates. (Level IV evidence)

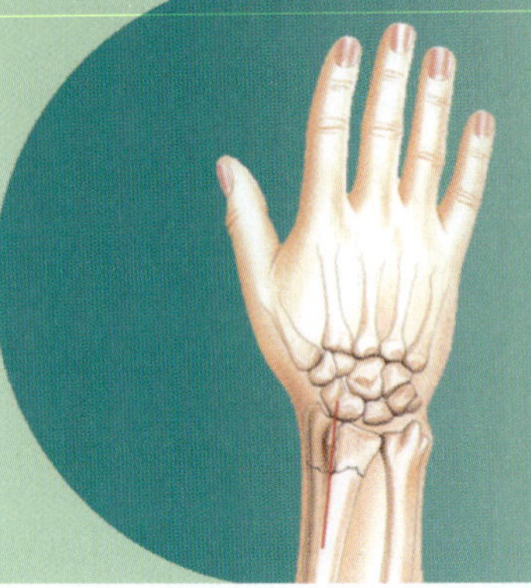

Tendon Transfers for Extensor and Flexor Tendon Ruptures

Shimpei Ono, Sandeep J. Sebastin, and Kevin C. Chung

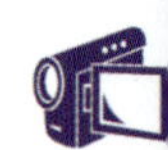

See Video 23: Tendon Transfers for the Ruptured Flexor and Extensor Tendons

Indications

- Rupture of long digital flexor and extensor tendons

Examination/Imaging

Clinical Examination

- The most frequently ruptured tendons in rheumatoid arthritis (RA) are the extensor digiti minimi (EDM), followed by the extensor digitorum communis (EDC) tendons to the small, ring, long, and index fingers, in that order; the extensor pollicis longus (EPL); the flexor pollicis longus (FPL); and, rarely, the flexor digitorum superficialis (FDS) and the flexor digitorum profundus (FDP).
- Patients with isolated small finger extensor tendon (EDM) rupture may still be able to extend the small fingers through the EDC or through the juncturae connecting it to the ring finger (Fig. 31-1). However, these patients will not be able to perform independent extension of the small finger with the other fingers flexed.

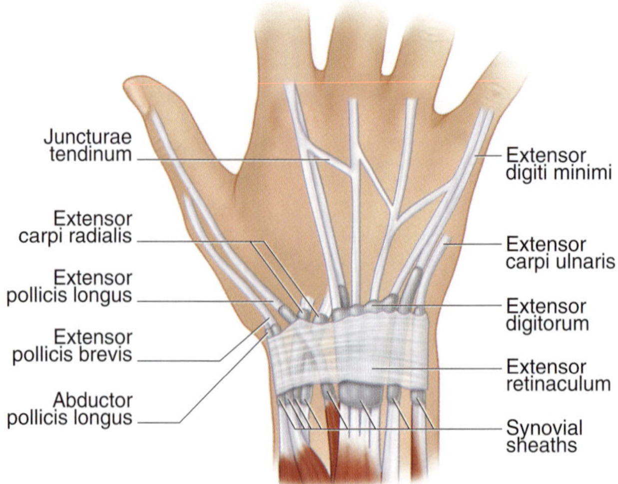

FIGURE 31-1

- Patients with rupture of the EDC to one finger may still be able to extend the finger owing to the juncturae connecting it to intact adjoining fingers. However, patients are usually unable to extend the finger when they have ruptured more than one EDC (Fig. 31-2). The inability to extend the finger in RA may also be caused by ulnar subluxation of the extensor tendons over the head of the metacarpal (Fig. 31-3) and rarely is due to posterior interosseous nerve palsy resulting from elbow synovitis. To differentiate between these causes, it is useful to passively extend the finger and ask the patient to hold it there. Patients with tendon rupture or nerve palsy will be unable to maintain the finger in extension, whereas patients with subluxation will be able to do so as the tendon relocates over the metacarpophalangeal (MCP) joint with finger extension. Patients with tendon rupture will also lose the tenodesis effect of finger extension with wrist flexion, whereas the tenodesis effect will be preserved in nerve palsy.
- The function of the EPL is tested by asking the patient to lay the palm of the hand flat on the table and then asking the patient to lift the thumb away from the table (retropulsion).

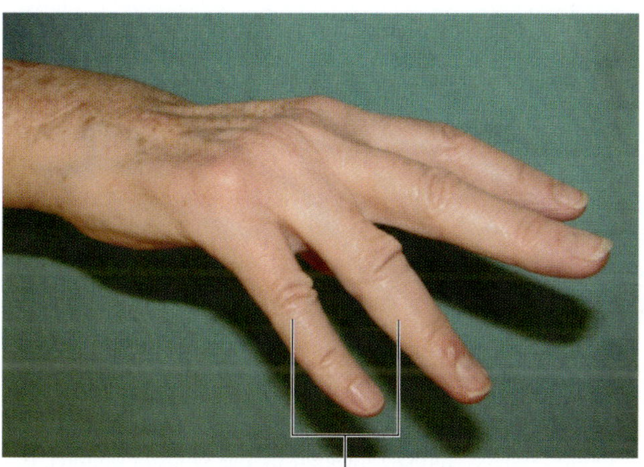

FIGURE 31-2

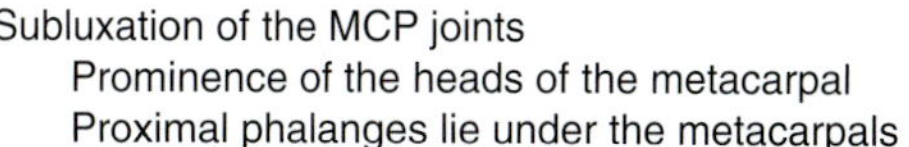

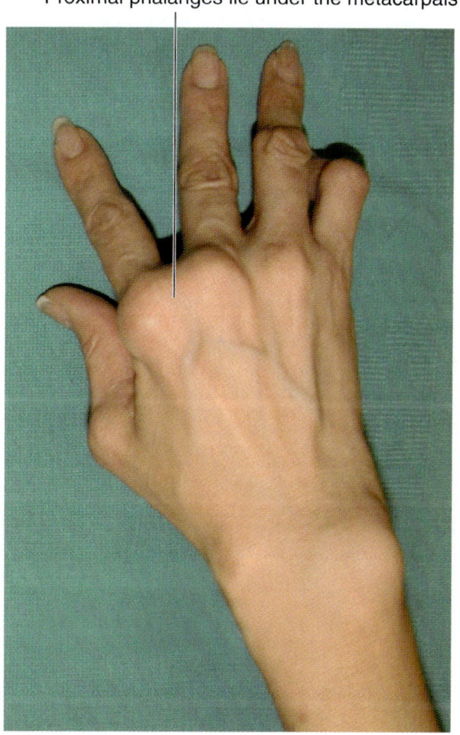

FIGURE 31-3

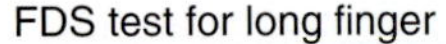
FDS test for long finger

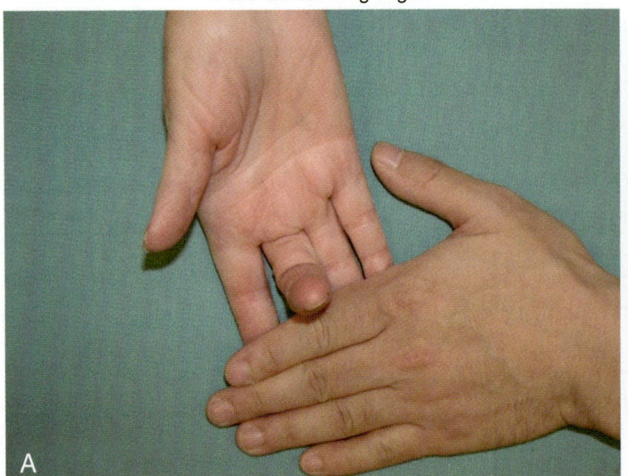

FDS test for ring finger

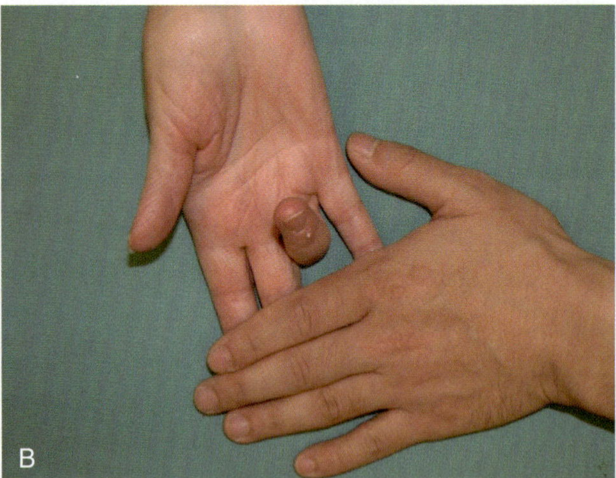

FIGURE 31-4

- One must also examine the integrity of the EIP by testing for independent extension of the index finger with the other fingers held in flexion. The function of the FDS and FDP is also checked. The EIP and FDS to the ring and long fingers are often used as motors for tendon transfers in patients with rupture of multiple extensor tendons. Figure 31-4 shows testing for FDS function of the long and ring fingers.

Imaging

- It is important to obtain radiographs of the wrist to evaluate the distal radioulnar (DRU), midcarpal, and radiocarpal joints. Pathology involving these joints will also need to be addressed at the time of tendon reconstruction to prevent progressive deformity and rerupture of the reconstructed tendons.

Surgical Anatomy

- Tendon rupture in RA occurs as a result of either synovitis or attrition over an eroded bone. The tendon may be directly invaded by the synovial pannus. This occurs in regions where the tendon is covered by tenosynovium (extensor retinaculum, carpal tunnel, and digital flexor sheath). Rupture may also result from ischemia caused by pressure from underlying proliferative synovitis. This occurs in regions where the tendon is in close relation to joints (DRU, radiocarpal, proximal interphalangeal [PIP] joints). Attritional rupture frequently involves the EDM at the ulnar head (Fig. 31-5), EPL at the Lister tubercle, and FPL in the carpal tunnel caused by a flexed scaphoid (see Fig. 31-5). Synovitis between the scaphoid and lunate leads to rupture of the scapholunate ligament and collapse of the scaphoid (scaphoid becomes horizontal with the distal pole protruding into the carpal tunnel).

Treatment Considerations

- Direct repair of ruptured tendons is usually not possible because the ruptured ends are of very poor quality. Additionally, these patients frequently present late, and a tendon graft is also not a reliable option owing to proximal myostatic contraction. A tendon transfer is the preferred option for reconstruction. Depending on the number of ruptured tendons, this may involve a simple end-to-side repair to an intact adjacent tendon or may require transfer of a new motor from the extensor or flexor side (Table 31-1; Fig. 31-6).

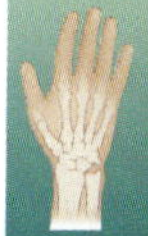

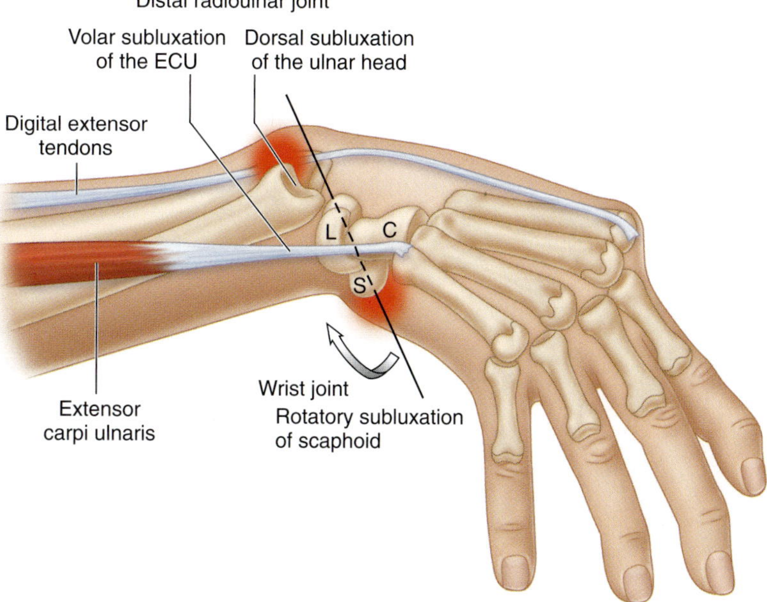

FIGURE 31-5

Table 31-1 Number of Ruptured Tendons and Treatment Considerations

No.	Impairment	Diagnosis	Preferred Option	Alternative Option
1.	Inability to extend small finger	Rupture of EDM at ulnar head	End-to-side repair of EDM to EDC to ring finger	
2.	Inability to extend small and ring fingers	Rupture of EDC to ring and small under extensor retinaculum and EDM at ulnar head	EIP transfer to EDC to ring and EDM	
3.	Inability to extend small, ring, and long fingers	Rupture of EDC to long, ring, and small under extensor retinaculum and EDM at ulnar head	EIP transfer to EDC to ring and EDM End-to-side repair of EDC to index and long	
4.	Inability to extend small, ring, long, and index fingers	Rupture of EIP, EDC to index, long, ring, and small under extensor retinaculum, and EDM at ulnar head	FDS long to EDC to index and long FDS ring to EDC to ring, small and EDM	
5.	Inability to extend thumb	Rupture of EPL at Lister tubercle	EIP to EPL	ECRL to EPL EDM to EPL
6.	Inability to extend thumb and small, ring, long, and index fingers	Rupture of EPL at Lister tubercle, EIP, EDC to index, long, ring, and small under extensor retinaculum, and EDM at ulnar head	FDS long to EPL and EDC to index FDS ring to EDC long, ring, small, and EDM	
7.	Inability to flex thumb	Rupture of FPL in carpal tunnel	BR to FPL	ECRL to FPL FDS long to FPL Thumb IP joint fusion
8.	Inability to achieve independent flexion of PIP joint	Rupture of FDS	PIP joint synovectomy to prevent rupture of FDP	
9.	Inability to flex DIP joint	Rupture of FDP	DIP joint arthrodesis	Tenodesis of DIP joint
10.	Inability to flex IP joint	Rupture of FDS and FDP	Staged flexor tendon reconstruction	

BR, brachioradialis; DIP, distal interphalangeal; ECRL, extensor carpi radialis longus; EDC, extensor digitorum communis; EDM, extensor digiti minimi; EIP, extensor indicis proprius; EPL, extensor pollicis longus; FDP, flexor digitorum profundus; FDS, flexor digitorum superficialis; FPL, flexor pollicis longus; IP, interphalangeal; PIP, proximal interphalangeal.

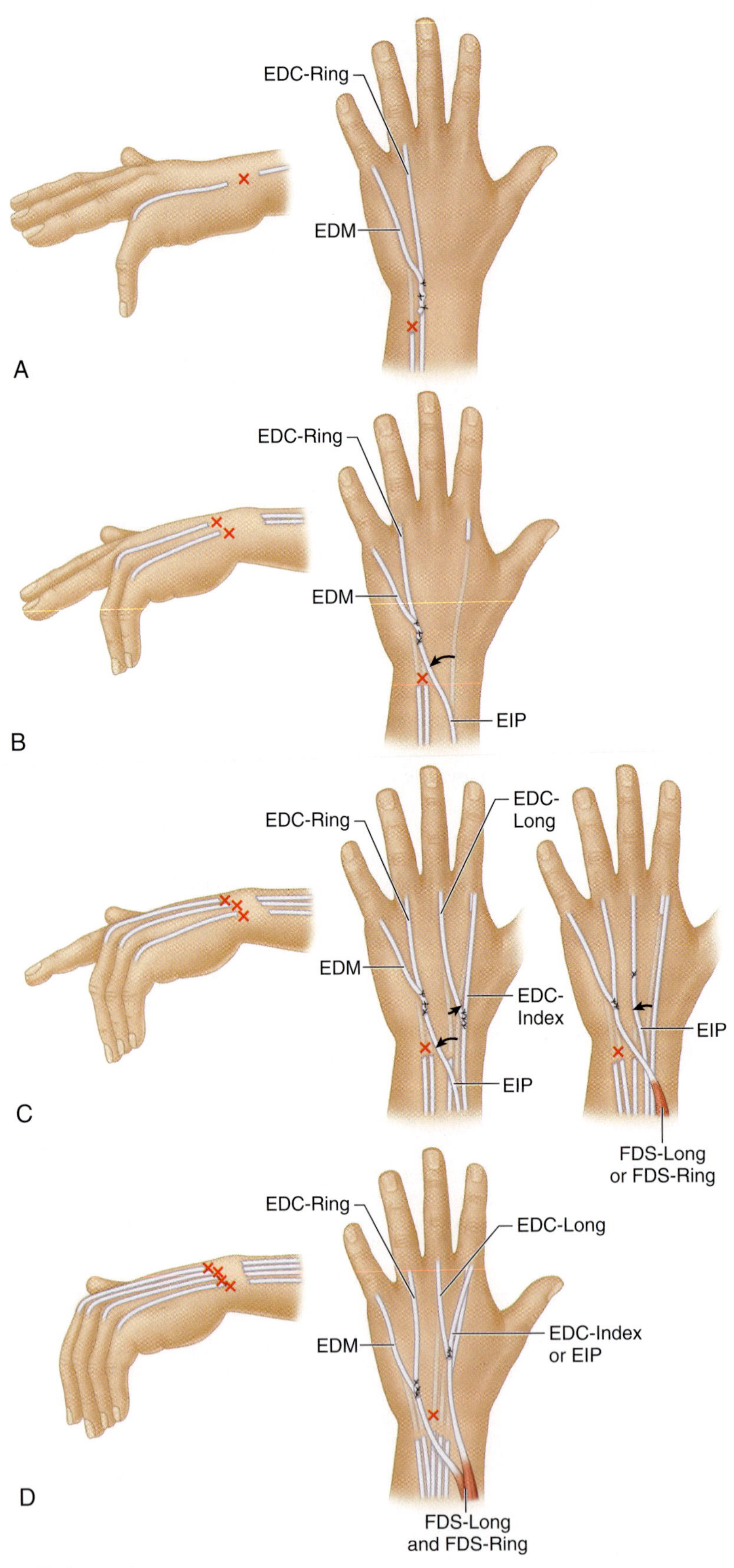

EDC-Ring
EDM
A
EDC-Ring
EDM
EIP
B
EDC-Ring
EDC-Long
EDM
EDC-Index
EIP
EIP
FDS-Long or FDS-Ring
C
EDC-Ring
EDC-Long
EDM
EDC-Index or EIP
FDS-Long and FDS-Ring
D

FIGURE 31-6

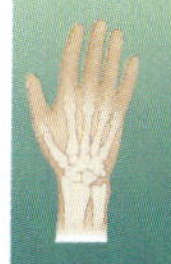

- It is important to address the cause of the tendon rupture at the time of tendon reconstruction. This may require tendon and joint synovectomy and procedures to address any joint instability and bony erosions. For example, if the patient has small-finger extensor tendon rupture, it is highly likely that the ring finger extensor tendon will rupture subsequently, and this process will progress, resulting in ruptures of all the extensor tendons to the fingers. Therefore, when a patient has an extensor tendon rupture of the small finger, tendon reconstruction and either tenosynovectomy or distal ulna excision, or a combination of both, must be performed to prevent progressive ruptures of the other tendons.

Exposures

PEARLS

The skin flaps are raised superficial to the extensor retinaculum, and care is taken to preserve the longitudinal dorsal veins to limit postoperative swelling and the superficial sensory nerve branches.

- A 6-cm longitudinal incision is made over the dorsum of the wrist in line with the long finger metacarpal (Fig. 31-7). Skin flaps are raised to expose the extensor retinaculum (Fig. 31-8). The extensor retinaculum is elevated using a stair-step design (Fig. 31-9). The stair-step incision is used to permit easier closure of the extensor retinaculum in a side-to-side fashion, rather than a straight line closure, which may be difficult because of the swelling under the retinaculum that puts pressure over the retinacular closure. Furthermore, if there is

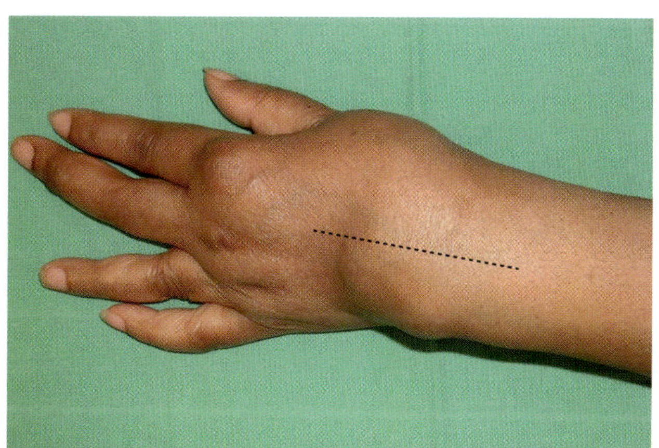

FIGURE 31-7

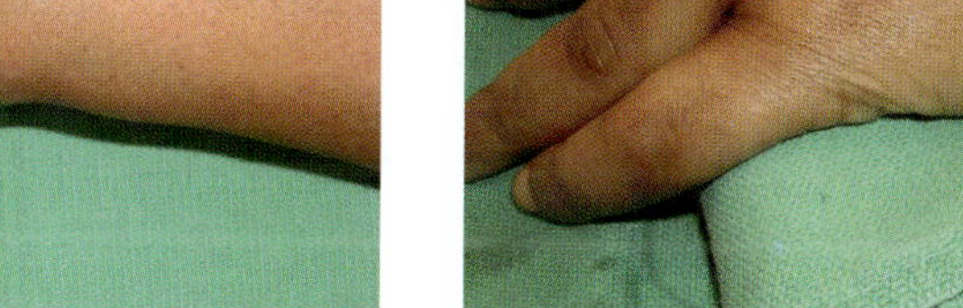

FIGURE 31-8

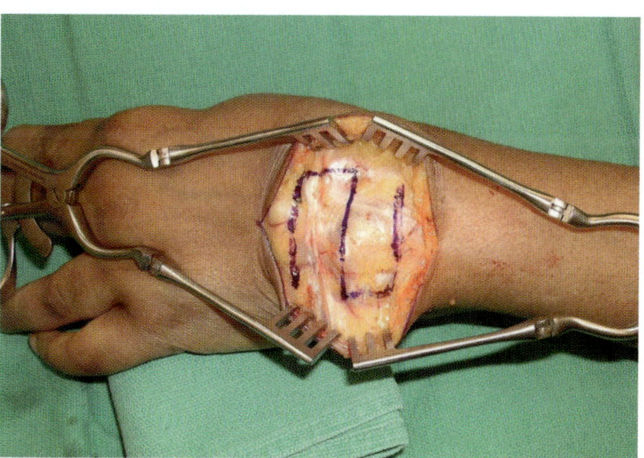

FIGURE 31-9

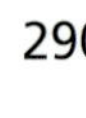

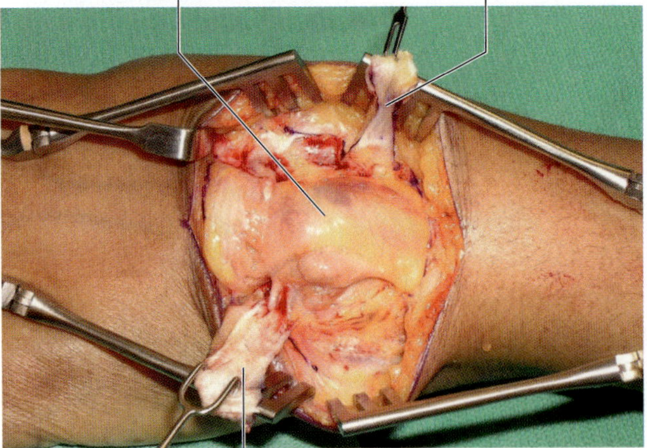

FIGURE 31-10

> **PITFALLS**
>
> *The skin must be handled with great care because vascularity and quality of skin are often impaired by rheumatoid disease and/or rheumatoid medications.*

> **STEP 1 PEARLS**
>
> *Occasionally, tenosynovitis infiltrates into the tendon substance, resulting in a frayed tendon surface. In such cases, the frayed surface should be trimmed.*
>
> *A tendon defect resulting from the excision of a nodule can be closed with a horizontal mattress suture.*

radiocarpal bone erosion, half of the retinaculum can be placed under the extensor tendons to shield the wrist from the extensor tendons, and the other half is used to close over the tendons. The septae are divided between the second and third; third and fourth; fourth and fifth; and fifth and sixth extensor compartments. This converts the multiple extensor compartments into a single compartment and reveals the exuberant amount of synovial tissue encasing the extensor tendons (Fig. 31-10).

Procedure

Step 1: Synovectomy

- Fresh, sharp no. 15 blades are used to excise the synovial tissue from the extensor tendons. Tendons with invading synovial tissue within the extensor tendons must be excised completely (Fig. 31-11).
- After removing the synovial tissue, one can appreciate multiple ruptured extensor tendons that will require reconstruction (Fig. 31-12).

Step 2: Tendon Transfer for the Ruptured Tendons

- The reconstructive plan depends on the number of ruptured extensor tendons (see Table 31-1).
- All the tendon junctures are secured using braided sutures.
- Figure 31-13 shows a separate incision made at the level of the metacarpal to identify the distal EPL tendon. The EIP tendon was transferred to weave into the EPL tendon to restore EPL tendon function.

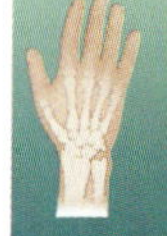

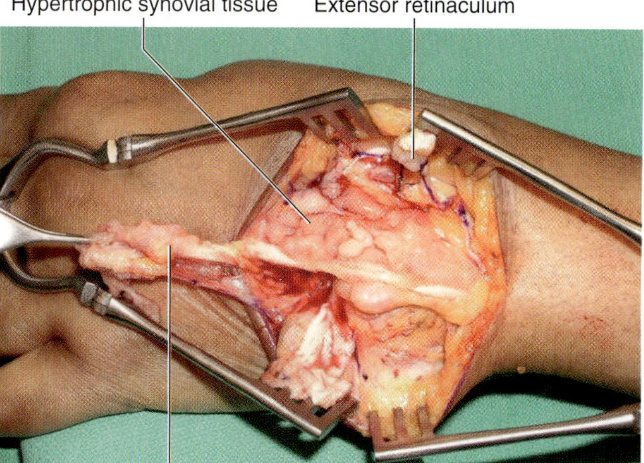

FIGURE 31-11

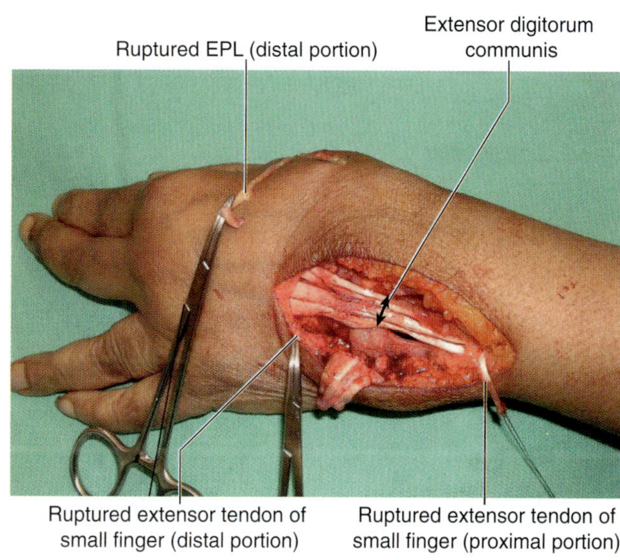

FIGURE 31-12

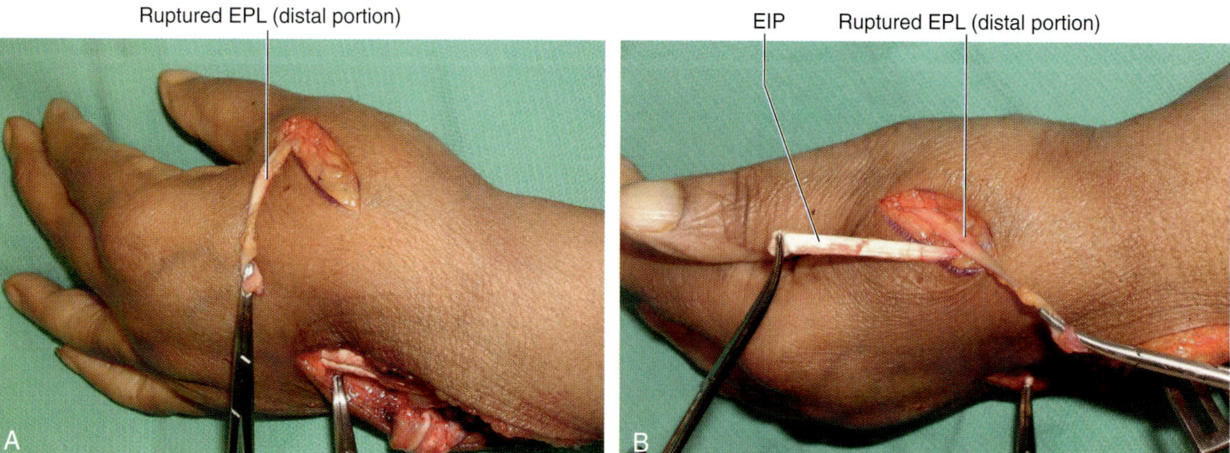

FIGURE 31-13

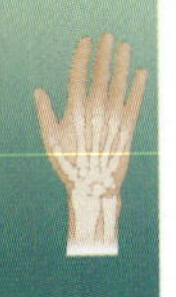

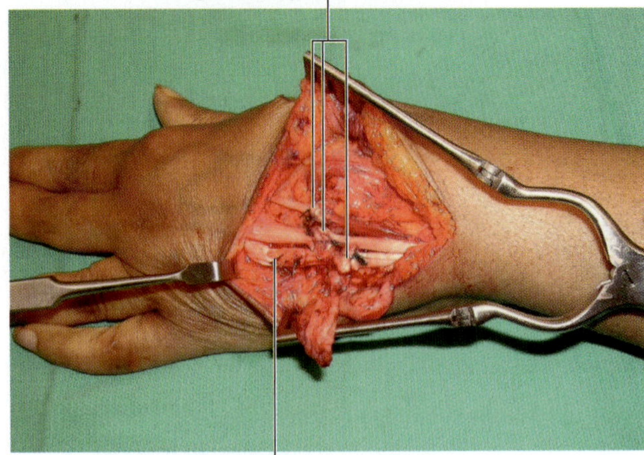

FIGURE 31-14

STEP 2 PEARLS

In patients with both ring and small finger extensor tendon ruptures, an EIP transfer is preferred to an end-to-side repair of the ring and small finger extensor tendons to the long finger extensor tendon because the oblique path of the transferred tendons could result in abduction of the small finger, causing functional problems.

When an FDS tendon is used as a motor, a subcutaneous transfer is preferred to one through the interosseous membrane to reduce the likelihood of adhesions.

It is preferable to transfer the FDS tendons on the radial side of the forearm because the direction of pull will help with correction of the ulnar deviation deformity.

If fusion of the thumb interphalangeal (IP) joint is being considered, it is important to check the strength of the intrinsic muscles and the condition of the MCP joint. A thumb IP joint fusion will be able to give satisfactory pinch strength only if the MCP joint is stable and functional.

- Figure 31-14 shows the repair of the distal end of the small finger extensor tendon to the intact ring finger extensor tendon in an end-to-side fashion.
- When more than three extensor tendons are ruptured, the FDS tendons are used for transfer. The FDS of the ring finger is identified and divided through a transverse incision in the distal palm. This tendon is then retrieved in the distal forearm by a separate longitudinal incision and passed in a subcutaneous tunnel on the radial aspect of the forearm to reach the extensor tendons on the dorsum of the wrist. A single FDS tendon can be used to motorize up to three extensor tendons. If more than three extensors are ruptured, one should consider transfer of both the ring and long finger FDS tendons.

STEP 3 PEARLS

Resection of the head of the ulna (Darrach procedure) is sometimes required at the same time.

Step 3: Imbricate the Lax Dorsal Wrist Capsule

- The dorsal wrist capsule is sometimes quite lax, and it will be imbricated using the braided sutures. The forearm is placed in supination, and the capsule over the distal ulna is closed tightly using horizontal mattress 3-0 braided sutures.

STEP 4 PITFALLS

Tension is set with all the fingers in fully extended posture because some stretching of the tendon repairs will occur during therapy.

Step 4: Tighten the Lax Extensor Tendons

- After synovectomy of the dorsal wrist, we can see the lax extensor tendon because of expansion by the hypertrophic synovitis. In this situation, tightening the lax extensor tendons with the braided sutures should give the patients more power to extend their fingers (see Fig. 31-14).

Step 5: Recreate the Pulley for Extensor Tendons

- The distal end of the extensor retinaculum is placed under the extensor tendons to augment the wrist capsular repair (Fig. 31-15A).
- The proximal extensor retinaculum is sutured over the extensor tendons to recreate the pulley (Fig. 31-15B).

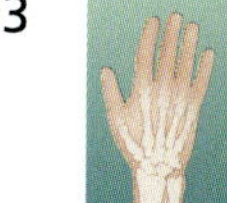

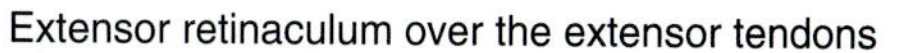

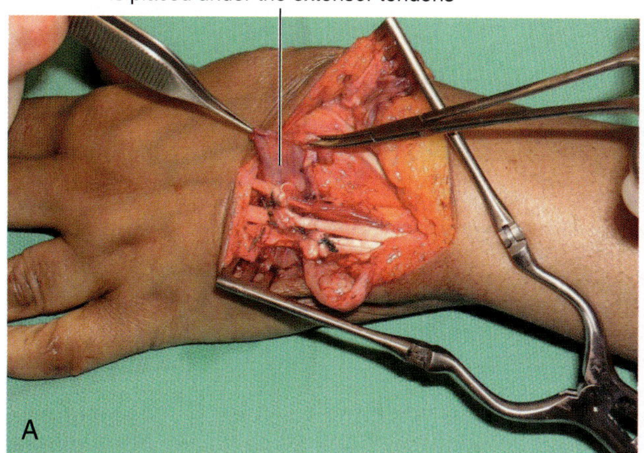

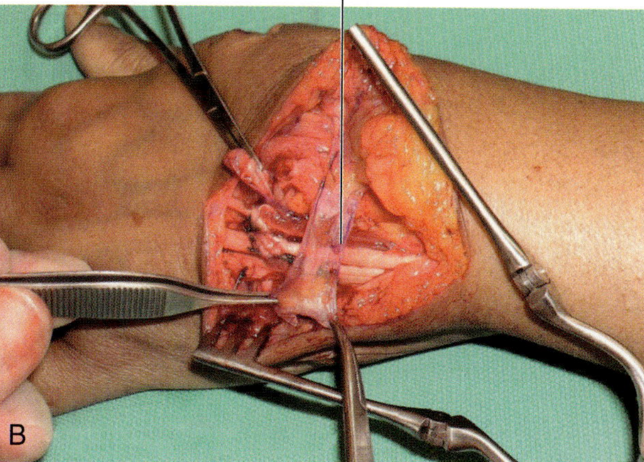

FIGURE 31-15

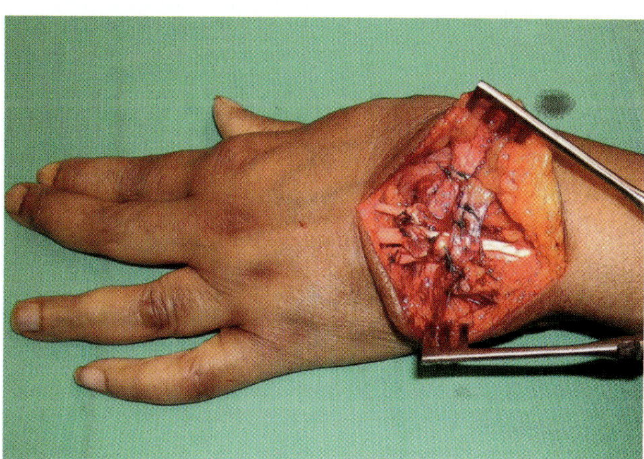

FIGURE 31-16

Step 6: Skin Closure

- The tourniquet is released, and hemostasis is obtained (Fig. 31-16).
- The skin is closed using 4-0 nylon.

Postoperative Care and Expected Outcomes

- If the distal ulna is excised, the patient should be placed in a supination splint for 4 weeks to allow healing of the dorsal capsular repair.
- Fingers are kept in fully extended position for 4 weeks before initiating active range-of-motion exercises.
- With extensor tendon ruptures, the outcome of tendon transfer is good, although an increase in extension lags is observed when more tendons are involved.
- With flexor tendon ruptures, patients with isolated ruptures in the palm or at the wrist had the best functional results. Patients with multiple ruptures within the carpal canal had a worse prognosis.

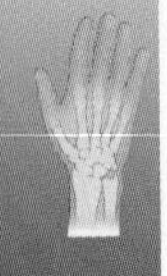

Evidence

Chung US, Kim JH, Seo WS, Lee KH. Tendon transfer or tendon graft for ruptured finger extensor tendons in rheumatoid hands. *J Hand Surg [Am]*. 2010;35: 279-282.

The authors evaluated the clinical outcome of tendon reconstruction using tendon graft or tendon transfer and the parameters related to clinical outcome in 51 wrists of 46 patients with rheumatoid arthritis with finger extensor tendon ruptures. At a mean follow-up of 5.6 years, the mean MCP joint extension lag was 8 degrees (range, 0 to 45), and the mean visual analogue satisfaction scale was 74 (range, 10 to 100). Clinical outcomes did not differ significantly between tendon grafting and tendon transfer. The MCP joint extension lag correlated with the patient's satisfaction score, but the pulp-to-palm distance did not correlate with patient satisfaction. The authors concluded that both tendon grafting and tendon transfer are reliable reconstruction methods for ruptured finger extensor tendons in rheumatoid hands. (Level IV evidence)

Ertel AN, Millender LH, Nalebuff E, et al. Flexor tendon ruptures in patients with rheumatoid arthritis. *J Hand Surg [Am]*. 1988;13:860-866.

The authors presented 115 flexor tendon ruptures in 43 hands with rheumatoid arthritis, one hand with psoriatic arthritis, and one hand with lupus erythematosus. Ninety-one tendons were ruptured at the wrist, 4 ruptures occurred at the palm, and 20 ruptures occurred within the digits. At the wrist level, 61 ruptures were caused by attrition on a bone spur, and 30 were caused by direct invasion of the tendon by tenosynovium. All ruptures distal to the wrist were caused by invasion of the tendon by tenosynovium. Patients whose ruptures were caused by attrition regained better motion than those whose ruptures were caused by invasion by tenosynovitis; however, motion overall was poor. Patients with isolated ruptures in the palm or at the wrist had the best functional results. Patients with multiple ruptures within the carpal canal had a worse prognosis. The severity of the patient's disease and the degree of articular involvement had a great effect on the outcome of surgery. Prevention of tendon ruptures by early tenosynovectomy and removal of bone spurs should be the cornerstone of treatment. (Level IV evidence)

Ishikawa H, Hanyu T, Tajima T. Rheumatoid wrists treated with synovectomy of the extensor tendons and the wrist joint combined with a Darrach procedure. *J Hand Surg [Am]*. 1992;17:1109-1117.

The authors presented a long-term follow-up study to evaluate outcomes of extensor tendon and wrist synovectomy combined with a Darrach procedure. Patients were followed for an average of 11 years. The authors concluded that pain and forearm rotation had improved compared with the opposite untreated side. However, carpal collapse and palmar carpal subluxation continued to progress equal to the opposite untreated side. The authors suggested that in addition to the previously mentioned treatments, stabilization of the wrist using radiolunate arthrodesis in addition to wrist tendon transfer procedures to balance the wrist should be considered early. (Level IV evidence)

Moore JR, Weiland AJ, Valdata L. Tendon ruptures in the rheumatoid hand: analysis of treatment and functional results in 60 patients. *J Hand Surg [Am]*. 1987;12:9-14.

The authors presented 60 cases of tendon ruptures related to rheumatoid disease and discussed the strategies for reconstruction of flexor and extensor tendon ruptures. The authors advocated early treatment of extensor synovitis and distal radioulnar joint disease to prevent extensor tendon ruptures. (Level IV evidence)

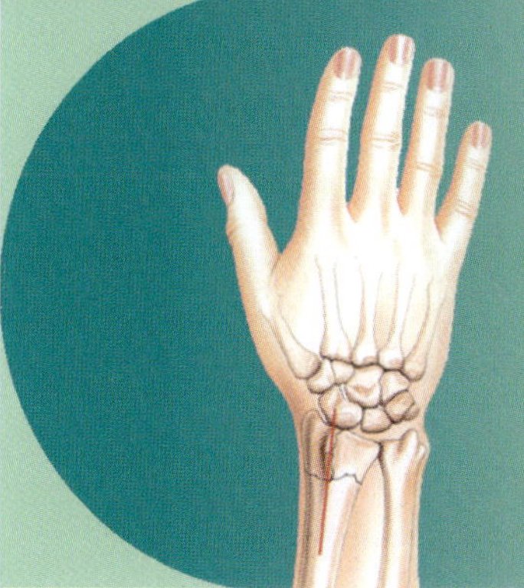

Crossed Intrinsic Tendon Transfer

Shimpei Ono, Sandeep J. Sebastin, and Kevin C. Chung

See Video 24: Crossed Intrinsic Tendon Transfer for Correction of Ulnar Deviation Deformity

Indications

- Performed in rheumatoid arthritis patients who have passively correctable ulnar deviation deformity (Fig. 32-1) with associated ulnar subluxation of the extensor tendon at the metacarpophalangeal (MCP) joint (Fig. 32-2) without arthritis or subluxation
- Ulnar subluxation of extensor tendon in chronic posttraumatic radial sagittal band injury

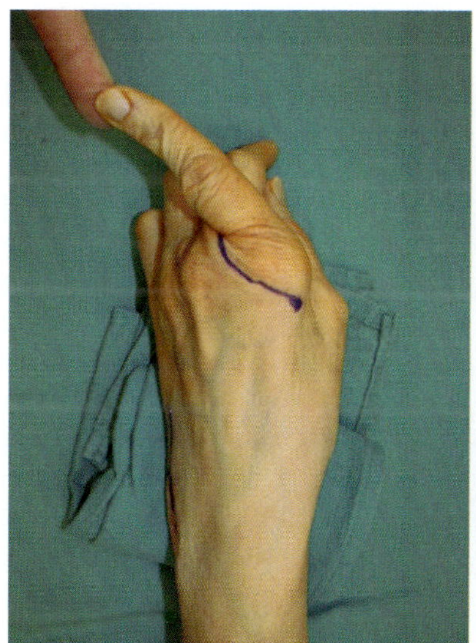

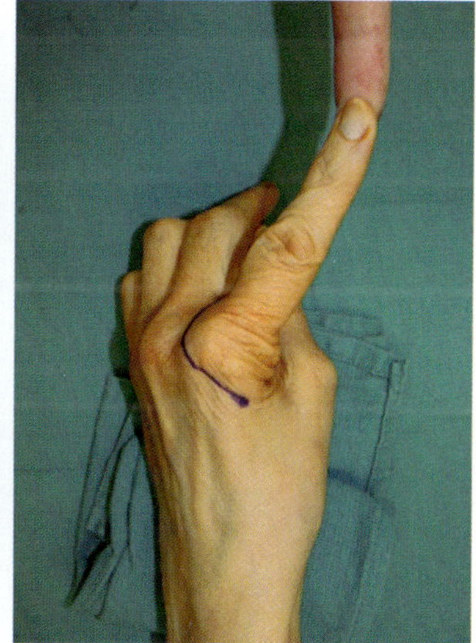

FIGURE 32-1

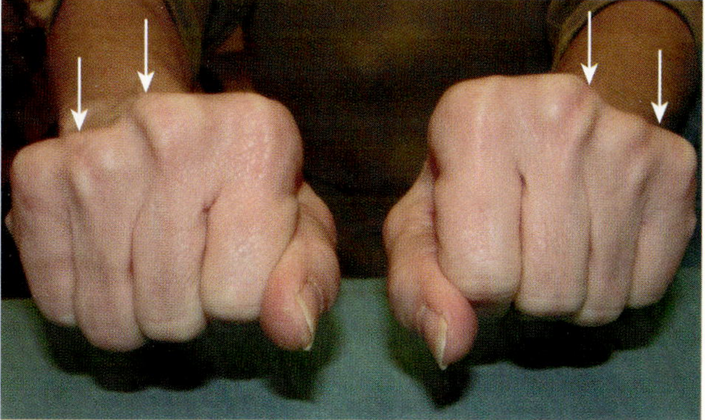

FIGURE 32-2

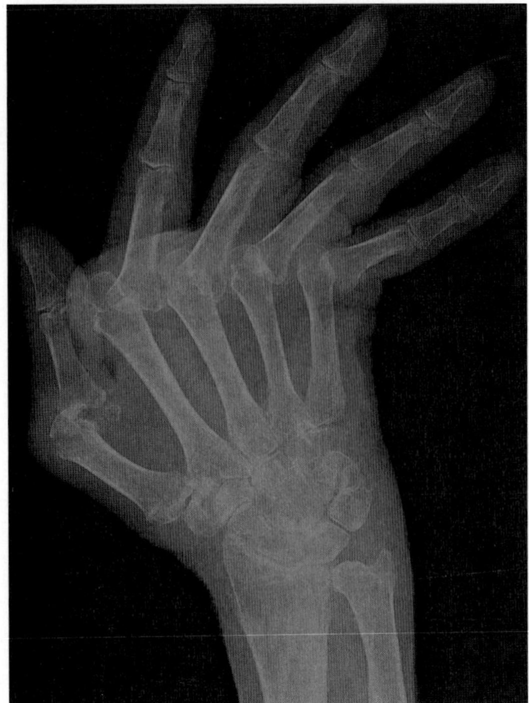

FIGURE 32-3

Examination/Imaging

Clinical Examination

- Clinical examination is to determine the condition of the MCP joint and the intrinsic tendons.
- A crossed intrinsic tendon transfer cannot be done in a patient who has a subluxed or arthritic MCP joint (Fig. 32-3). These patients need implant arthroplasty because a soft tissue procedure will not be able to hold a subluxed MCP joint in position. In addition, the patient is examined for the presence of MCP joint synovitis that can be addressed at the same operation.
- The intrinsic tendons should be examined for the presence of intrinsic muscle contracture (intrinsic tightness). This is done by the Finochietto-Bunnell test, which is performed by passively holding the patient's MCP joint in full extension and attempting proximal interphalangeal (PIP) joint flexion. PIP joint flexion will be restricted in patients with intrinsic tightness (Fig. 32-4A and B).

Imaging

- A radiograph of the hand is useful to determine the condition of the MCP joint.

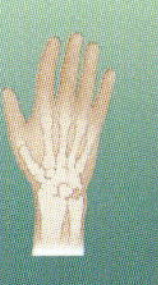

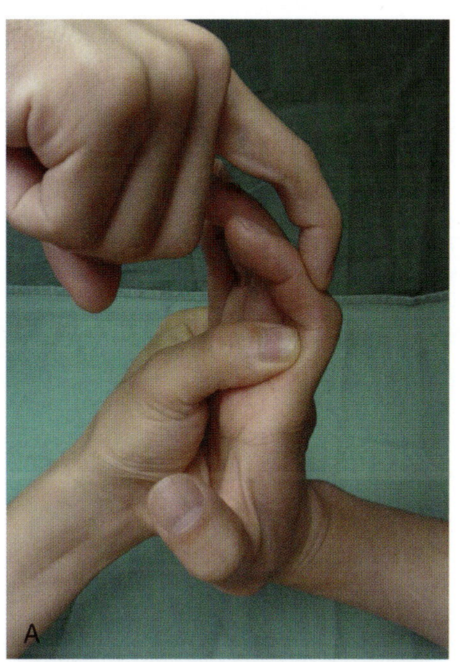

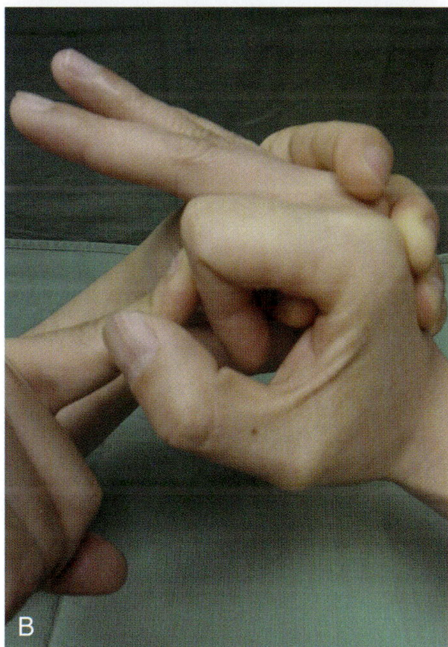

FIGURE 32-4

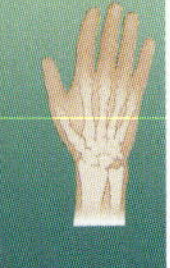

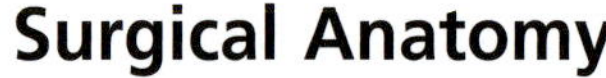

Surgical Anatomy

- The common intrinsic tendon is formed by the tendons of the palmar and dorsal interosseous muscles on the ulnar side of the digit and by the interossei (palmar and dorsal) and the lumbrical tendon on the radial side. These tendons pass palmar to the axis of the MCP joint to form the common intrinsic tendon. This tendon then divides into a medial band that inserts along with the central slip into the dorsal base of the middle phalanx and a lateral band that continues to the dorsal base of the distal phalanx (Fig. 32-5A). Contraction of the intrinsic muscles causes MCP joint flexion and interphalangeal (IP) joint extension. The radial and ulnar sagittal bands stabilize the extensor tendon, keeping it over the dorsal midline of the MCP joint (Fig. 32-5B).

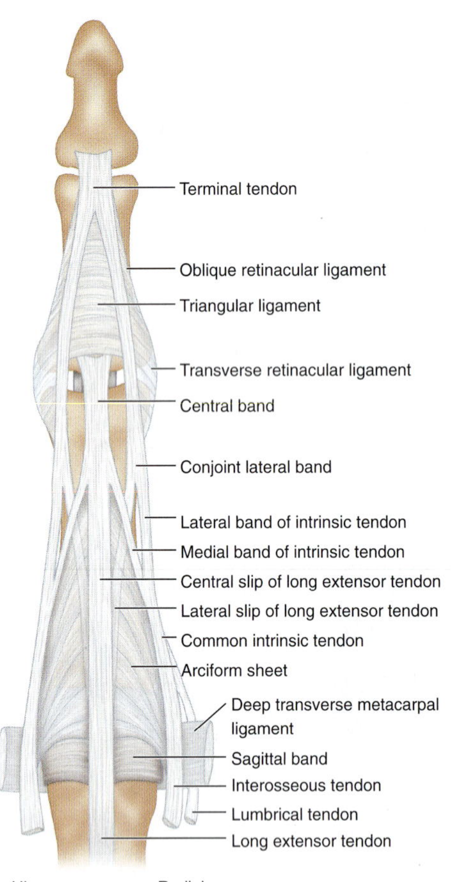

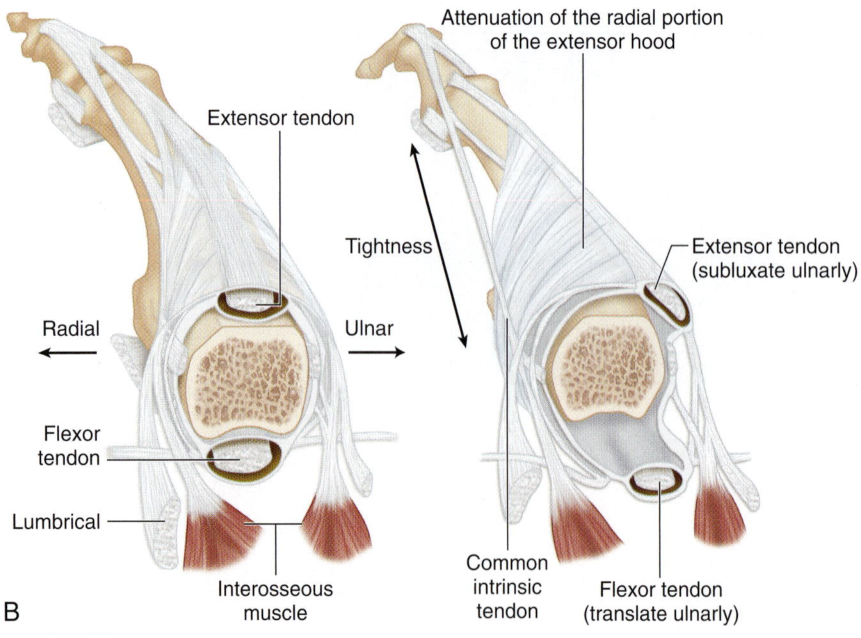

FIGURE 32-5

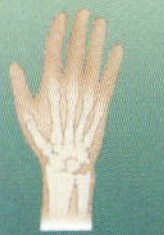

Positioning

- The patient is placed in the supine position, and a pneumatic tourniquet is used.

Exposures

- A dorsal "lazy S"–shaped skin incision over the MCP joint is used if only one finger needs to be addressed (Fig. 32-6).
- For correction of multiple fingers, a dorsal transverse incision is made over the MCP joint of the involved fingers (Fig. 32-7).
- The extensor apparatus over the MCP joint is exposed (Fig. 32-8).

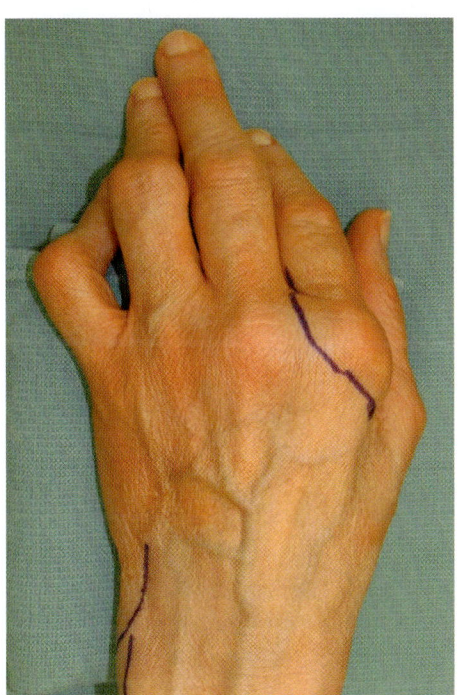

FIGURE 32-6

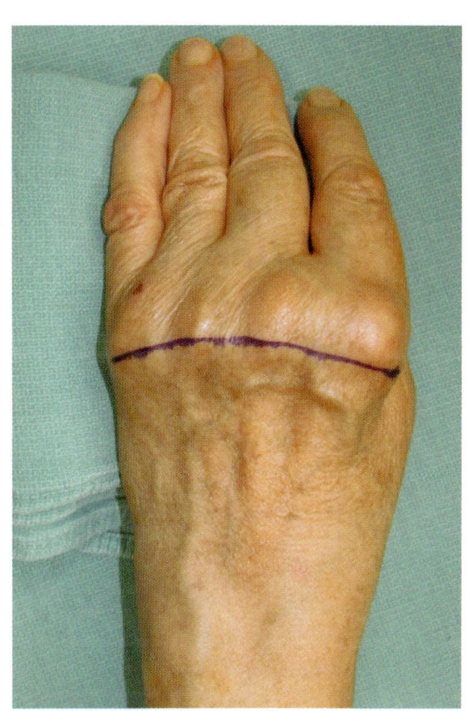

FIGURE 32-7

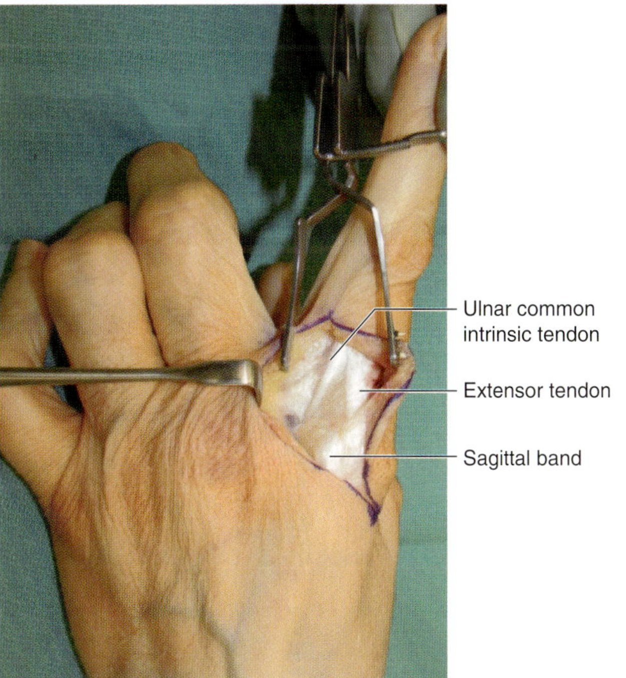

FIGURE 32-8

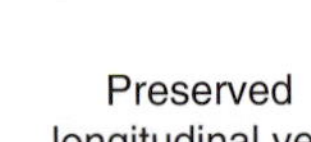

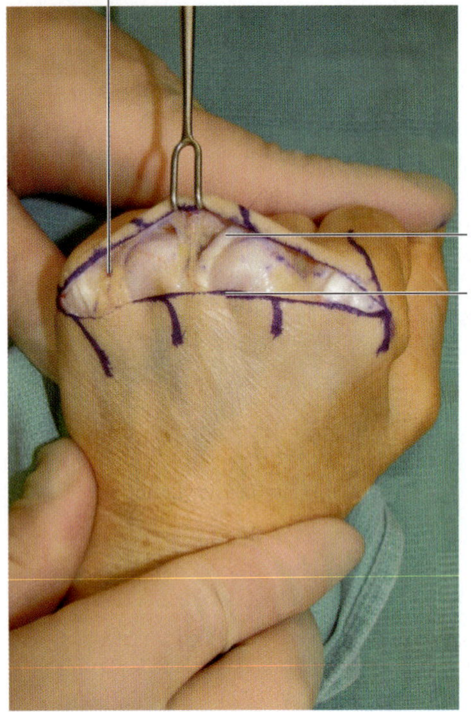

FIGURE 32-9

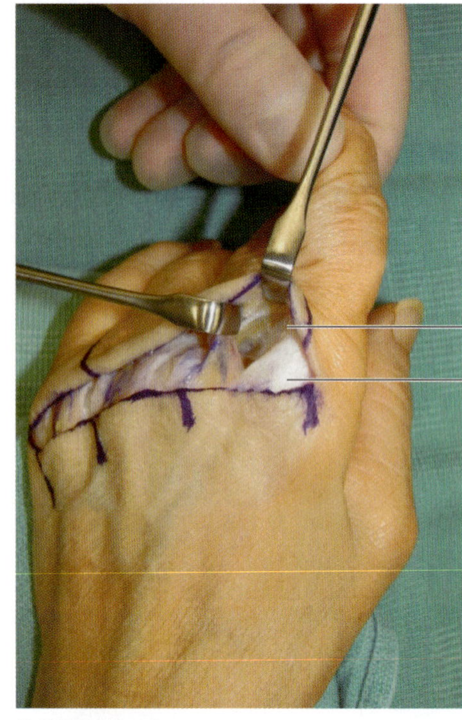

FIGURE 32-10

PEARLS

Care is taken to preserve the longitudinal dorsal veins to limit postoperative swelling (Fig. 32-9).

PITFALLS

The skin must be handled with great care because vascularity and quality of skin are often impaired by rheumatoid disease and/or rheumatoid medications.

STEP 1 PEARLS

A 2- to 3-mm wide portion of the radial sagittal band should be left along with the extensor tendon. This will allow a double-breasted repair of the sagittal band and will help reinforce the transferred intrinsic tendon.

STEP 2 PEARLS

Passing a right-angled retractor around the tendon will help isolate the tendon and will protect the neurovascular bundle volar to it.

Procedure

Step 1: Examination of the Extensor Apparatus and MCP Joint Synovectomy

- The position and condition of the extensor apparatus are noted. Any synovial proliferations are excised.
- A longitudinal incision that parallels the extensor tendon is made through the attenuated radial sagittal band.
- The MCP joint is opened, and a synovectomy is carried out.

Step 2: Elevation of Ulnar Common Intrinsic Tendon

- Dissection is carried out on the ulnar aspect of the proximal phalangeal base in a plane superficial to the extensor apparatus. The interosseous tendons are identified at the base of the MCP joint, and they are followed distally until the formation of the common intrinsic tendon (Fig. 32-10).

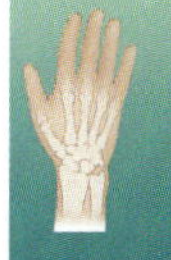

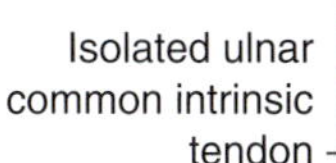

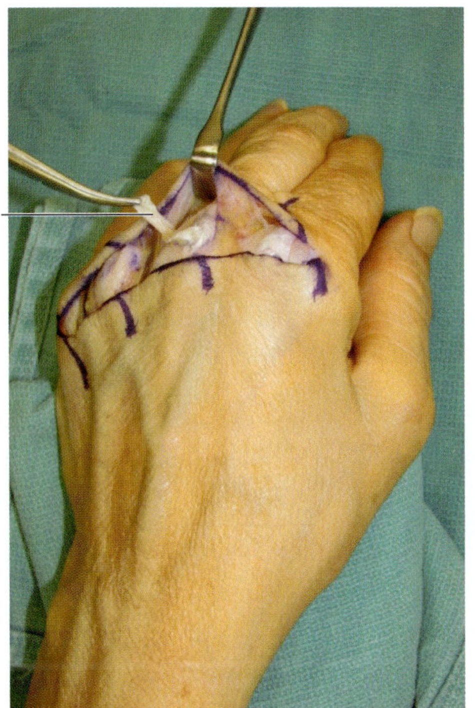

FIGURE 32-11

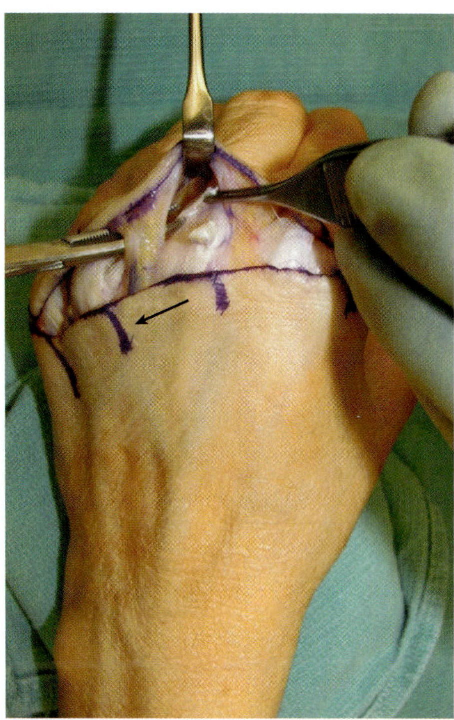

FIGURE 32-12

- The common intrinsic tendon is divided transversely at the midproximal phalanx before it divides into medial and lateral bands. It is then divided longitudinally to separate it from the extensor expansion.
- The common intrinsic tendon is mobilized proximally to the MCP joint (Fig. 32-11).

STEP 2 PITFALLS

If the common intrinsic tendon is divided too proximally, it may not reach the extensor tendon.

Step 3: Transfer of the Ulnar Common Intrinsic Tendon

- The mobilized ulnar common intrinsic tendon is passed under the soft tissue between adjacent MCP joints (it contains longitudinal veins and dorsal sensory nerves) to reach the extensor tendon of the digit ulnar to it (Fig. 32-12).
- The index finger ulnar common intrinsic tendon is used to correct the long finger; the long finger tendon is used for the ring finger; and the ring finger tendon is used for the small finger. Ulnar deviation of the index finger is corrected by double-breasted repair of the radial sagittal band.

STEP 3 PEARLS

The transfer of the intrinsic tendon has two benefits. It reduces the ulnar deviation force acting on the finger and increases the radial deviation force on the adjacent ulnar digit.

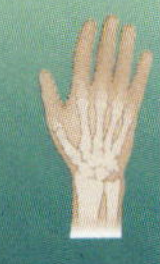

STEP 4 PEARLS

A division of the abductor digiti minimi may be required for the small finger. This is a strong ulnar deforming muscle and is approached from the dorsum around the ulnar side of the MCP joint. One must take care not to divide the ulnar neurovascular bundle or the tendon of the flexor digiti minimi.

Step 4: Centralization of Extensor Tendon

- A 3- to 4-mm longitudinal slit is made in the midportion of the extensor tendon overlying the MCP joint. The ulnar common intrinsic tendon is passed through this slit and sutured to itself using one or two horizontal mattress 3-0 Ethibond sutures. Tension is adjusted by keeping the MCP joint in extension and correcting the ulnar deviation deformity. This centralizes the extensor tendon (Figs. 32-13 and 32-14).
- A double-breasted repair of the radial sagittal band is done using one or two 3-0 Ethibond mattress sutures (Fig. 32-15).

Step 5: Skin Closure

- The tourniquet is released, and hemostasis is obtained.
- The skin is closed using 4-0 nylon (Fig. 32-16).

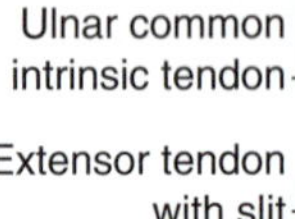

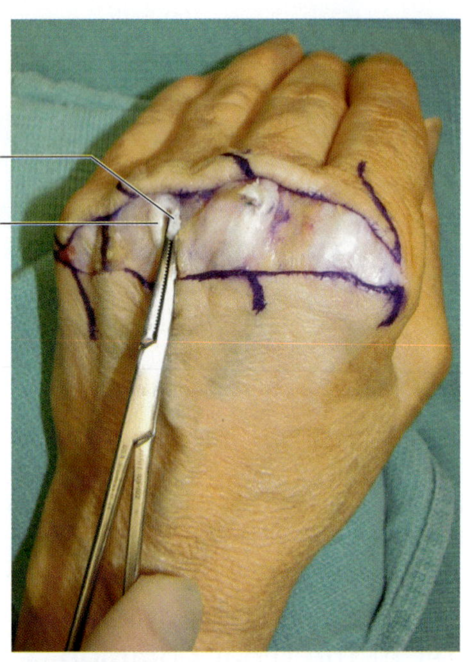

FIGURE 32-13

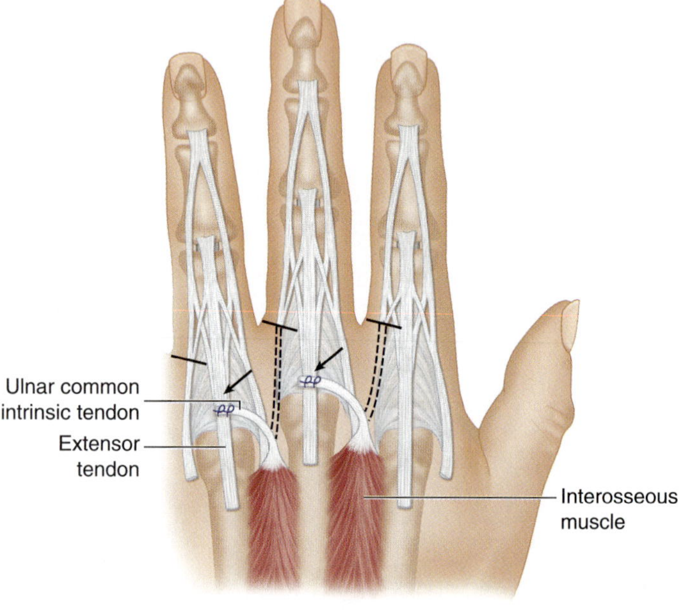

FIGURE 32-14

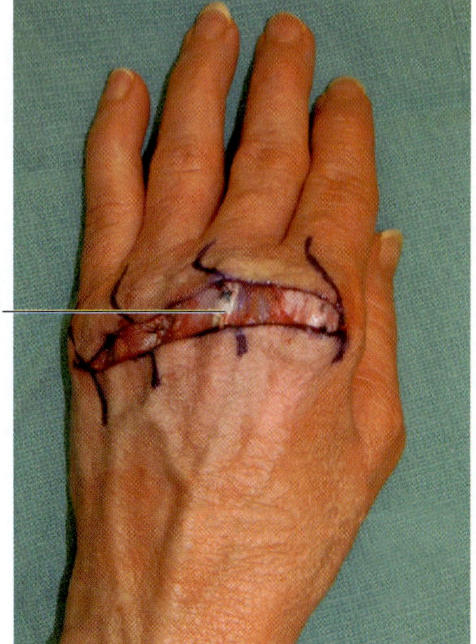

FIGURE 32-15

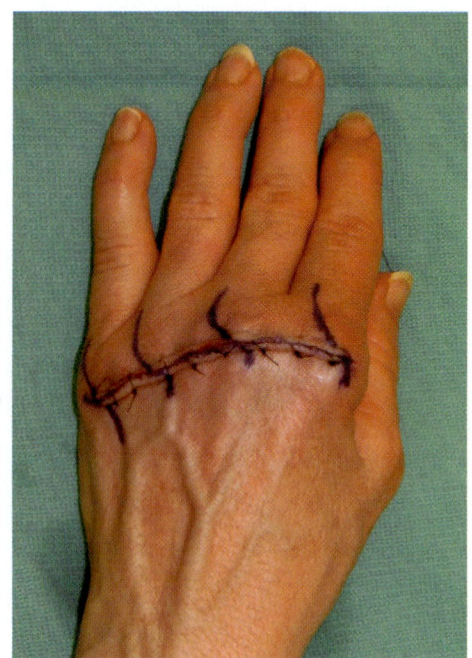

FIGURE 32-16

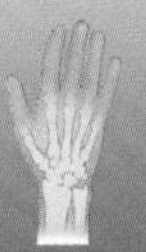

Postoperative Care and Expected Outcomes

- The hand is immobilized with a volar hand splint that keeps the MCP joint extended and corrects the ulnar deviation deformity. The wound is inspected 10 days later, and the sutures are removed. The patient is then given a thermoplastic splint to maintain the MCP joint in extension for another 4 weeks. This is followed by a gradual mobilization protocol and protective splinting for another 4 weeks.
- A crossed intrinsic transfer provides reliable long-term correction of the ulnar drift deformity in patients without MCP joint subluxation. However, it may be associated with a decrease in active range of motion at the MCP joint.

Evidence

Clark DI, Delaney R, Stilwell JH, et al. The value of crossed intrinsic transfer after metacarpophalangeal silastic arthroplasty: a comparative study. *J Hand Surg [Br]*. 2001;26:565-567.

The authors retrospectively studied 73 rheumatoid hands undergoing primary MCP joint replacement. In 28 hands, a crossed intrinsic transfer was performed, and in 45 hands, it was not. A similar splintage and rehabilitation program was followed in each group. The two treatment groups had similar preoperative ulnar drift (crossed intrinsic transfer group mean, 27 degrees; comparative group mean, 29 degrees). After a follow-up of 50 months, the crossed intrinsic transfer group had statistically less ulnar drift (crossed intrinsic transfer group mean, 6 degrees; comparative group mean, 14 degrees; P = .01). There were no other significant differences at follow-up. (Level IV evidence)

Oster LH, Blair WF, Steyers CM, Flatt AE. Crossed intrinsic transfer. *J Hand Surg [Am]*. 1989;14:963-971.

The authors presented a retrospective analysis of the long-term results of the crossed intrinsic transfer. Thirty rheumatoid hands and one hand with systemic lupus erythematosus were examined. The average follow-up was 12.7 years. The average postoperative ulnar drift for all fingers was 5 degrees, and the magnitude of it did not increase over time. The average active range of motion for the MCP joint was 47 degrees, and for the PIP joints, 58 degrees. The outcomes for crossed intrinsic transfer attached to the lateral band were similar to outcomes for transfers attached to the collateral ligament of the MCP joint. The crossed intrinsic transfer procedure effectively provides long-term correction of ulnar drift in the rheumatoid hand. (Level V evidence)

Pereira JA, Belcher HJ. A comparison of metacarpophalangeal joint Silastic arthroplasty with or without crossed intrinsic transfer. *J Hand Surg [Br]*. 2001;26:229-234.

The authors presented 43 hands undergoing Silastic interposition arthroplasty of the index, middle, ring, and little finger MCP joint for rheumatoid arthritis that were randomly allocated to undergo replacement with or without crossed intrinsic transfer. The patients were reviewed at a median of 17 months after surgery. The demographic characteristics and preoperative clinical measurements of the two groups were indistinguishable. Both groups showed improvement in ulnar drift and an altered arc but no change in total range of motion at the MCP joint. Grip strength and pulp-to-pulp pinch were significantly and comparably improved in both groups. There was no difference in pain scores or perceived function between the treatment groups. The authors concluded by saying that crossed intrinsic transfer does not significantly affect the outcome of silicone interposition arthroplasty of the MCP joint in rheumatoid patients. (Level IV evidence)

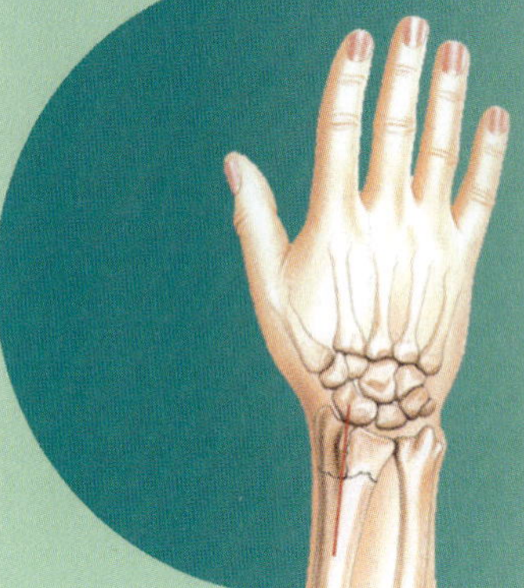

Correction of Swan-Neck Deformity in the Rheumatoid Hand

Yoshitaka Minamikawa and Akio Minami

See Video 25: Lateral Band Release for Rheumatoid Swan-Neck Deformity

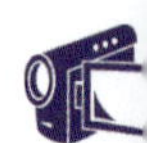

Indications

- Treatment of swan-neck deformity is based on the flexibility of the proximal interphalangeal (PIP) joint and condition of the joint cartilage.
- The Nalebuff classification is the most widely accepted and useful method for surgical decision-making.
  - Type 1: PIP joint is flexible in all positions of the metacarpophalangeal (MCP) joint.
  - Type 2: PIP joint flexion is limited in certain positions of the MCP joint.
  - Type 3: PIP joint flexion is limited irrespective of position of the MCP joint.
  - Type 4: PIP joints are stiff and have a poor radiographic appearance.
- Type I deformities need a procedure to limit PIP hyperextension (e.g., splint, dermodesis, flexor digitorum superficialis [FDS] tenodesis) and restore distal interphalangeal (DIP) extension (e.g., tenodermodesis, fusion).
- Type II deformities require an intrinsic release and/or MCP joint arthroplasty in addition to the procedure for type I.
- Type III deformities require restoration of flexion of the PIP joint by manipulation, lateral band mobilization, and lengthening of the central slip depending on the severity of soft tissue contracture.
- Arthrodesis of the PIP joint is often recommended for type IV deformities with joint destruction; however, implant arthroplasty is always an option.

Examination/Imaging

Clinical Examination

- Active and passive range of motion of the PIP joint is tested with the MCP joint in extension and flexion. This is to evaluate whether the intrinsic muscles are contributing to the restricted PIP joint motion. Restriction in radial and ulnar deviation is also tested with the MCP joint in extension to evaluate which of the intrinsic muscles is responsible for the PIP joint tightness.
- When active motion of the PIP is not nearly equal to passive motion, adhesions of the flexor tendons must be suspected.
- When the PIP joint is flexible regardless of the metacarpophalangeal (MCP) joint position (type I), a PIP extension block splint may correct the deformity while restoring full flexion (Fig. 33-1A).
- When flexion of the PIP joint is restricted with the MCP joint in extension and radial deviation, ulnar intrinsic muscle tightness exists.

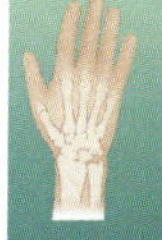

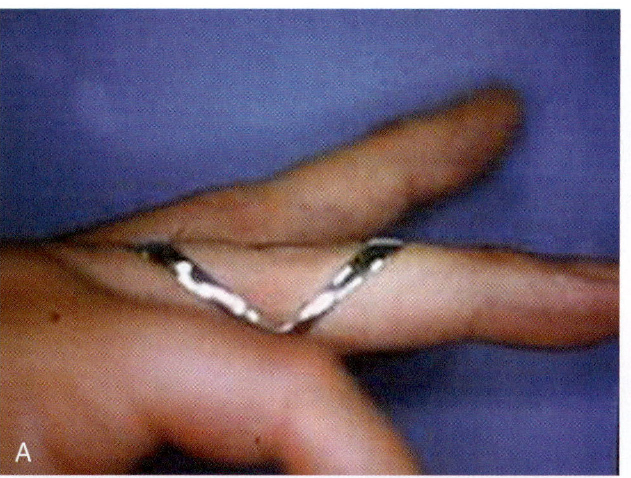

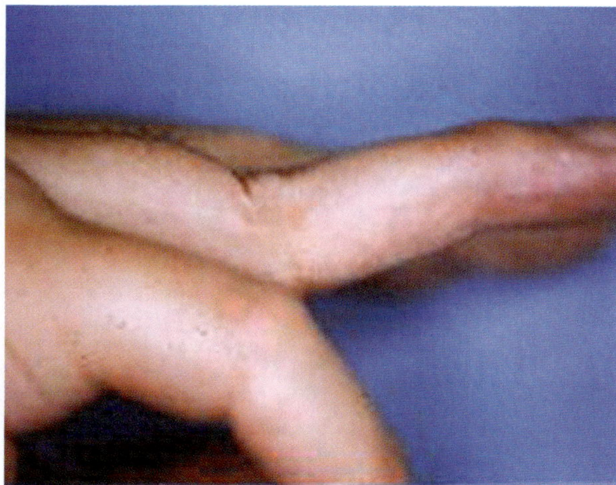

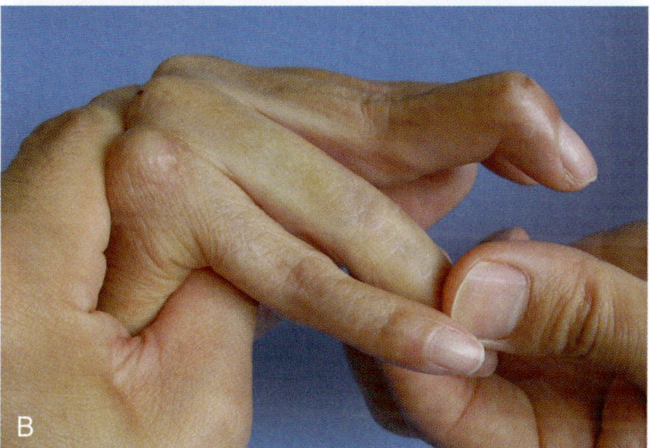

FIGURE 33-1

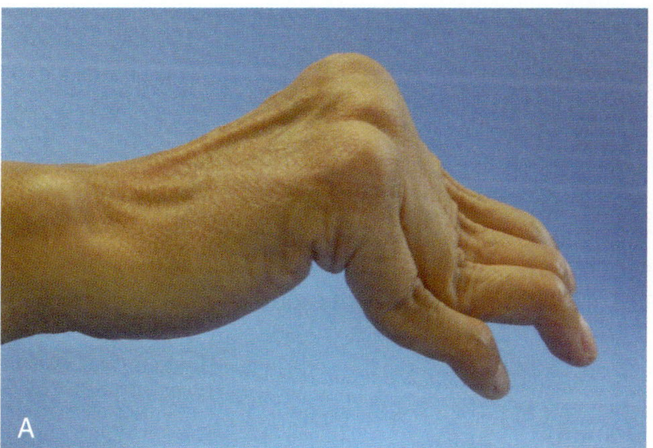

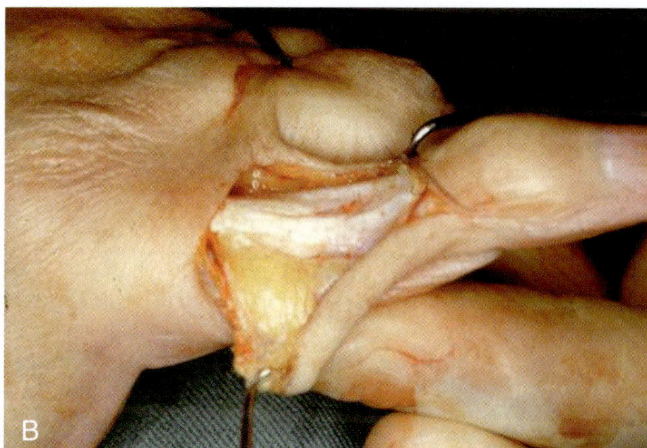

FIGURE 33-2

- When passive flexion of the PIP is limited with the MCP joint in flexion, the pathology is the stiff PIP joint (type III) (Fig. 33-1B).
- The typical swan-neck deformity is associated with flexion contracture of the MCP joint, hyperextension of the PIP joints, and dorsally displaced lateral bands (Fig. 33-2).

Imaging

- A radiograph of the hand is useful to assess the condition of the PIP joint and the MCP joint.

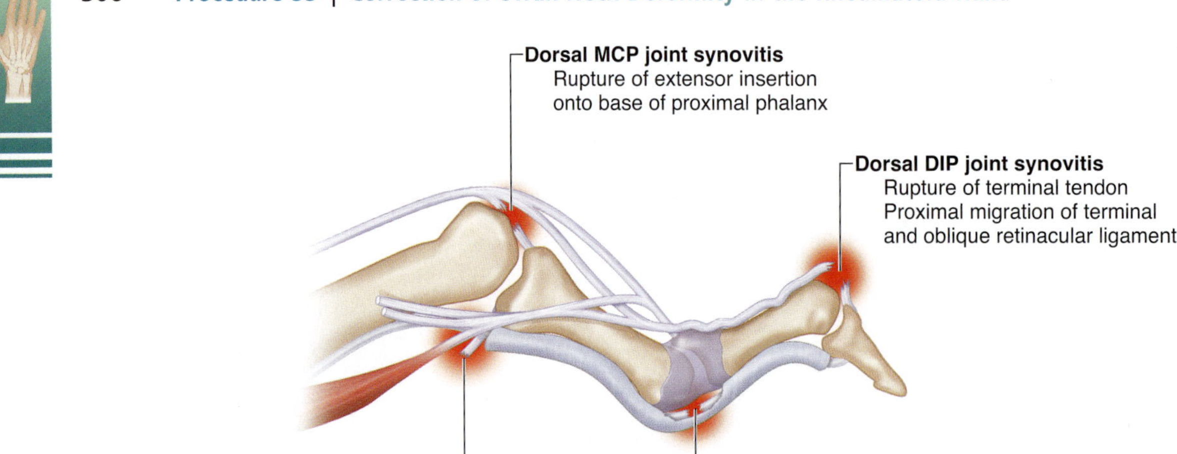

FIGURE 33-3

Surgical Anatomy

- A swan-neck deformity can occur as a result of abnormalities at the wrist, MCP joint, PIP joint, or DIP joint (Fig. 33-3).
- Synovitis within the PIP joint leads to stretching, weakening, and eventually destruction of the volar plate and collateral ligaments and the insertion of the FDS, resulting in the loss of palmar restraint at the PIP joint. This loss allows the normal extensor forces to cause abnormal hyperextension of the PIP joint.
- Synovitis of the MCP joint causes attenuation of the volar plate, resulting in volar subluxation of the MCP joint. Over time, volar subluxation results in shortening of the intrinsic muscles, leading to PIP joint hyperextension and ultimately swan-neck deformity.
- DIP joint synovitis can cause weakening and rupture of the terminal extensor tendon insertion, leading to the development of a mallet deformity. The proximal migration of the terminal extensor insertion causes the lateral bands to become lax. All the power of the common extrinsic extensor is now directed toward the central slip that inserts into the middle phalanx. Over time, the volar supporting structures of the PIP joint are weakened, and the PIP joint is forced into hyperextension, resulting in a swan-neck deformity.
- Synovitis at the wrist joint can lead to carpal collapse, carpal supination, and ulnar translation. Carpal collapse leads to a relative lengthening (relaxation) of the long flexor and extensor tendons. The interosseous muscle can then overpower the action of the extrinsic muscles and lead to MCP joint flexion and PIP joint extension, which over a prolonged period causes a physiologic shortening of the intrinsic muscles.

Procedures to Prevent Hyperextension of the PIP Joint (for Types 1 to 3)

Bone Anchor Repair of the Volar Plate

Step 1

- A zigzag incision is made over the long finger crease (Fig. 33-4A).

STEP 1 PITFALLS

Care must be taken not to injure the digital nerve at the tip of the flap. The nerve is just beneath the skin (Fig. 33-4B). The other digital nerve is identified at the base of the flap and protected (Fig. 33-4C).

Step 2

- The accessory collateral ligament is identified and incised (Fig. 33-5A and B). The volar plate with the entire flexor sheath is retracted laterally to expose the head of the proximal phalanx (Fig. 33-5C).

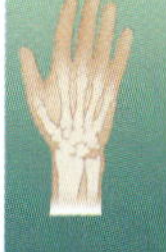

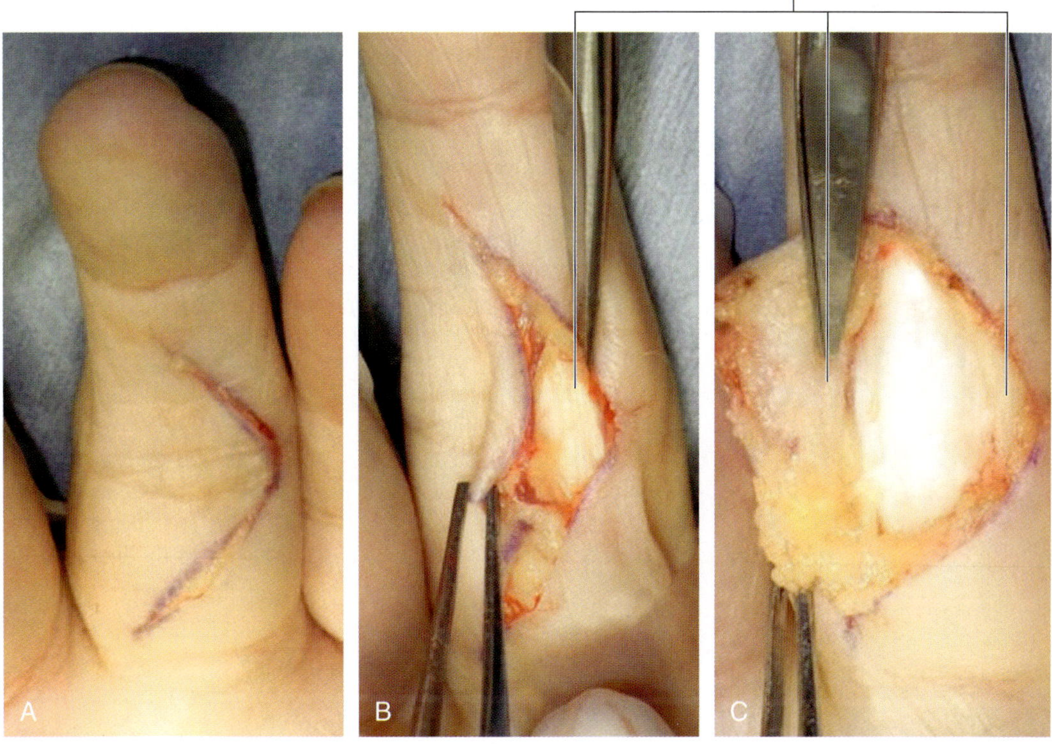

FIGURE 33-4

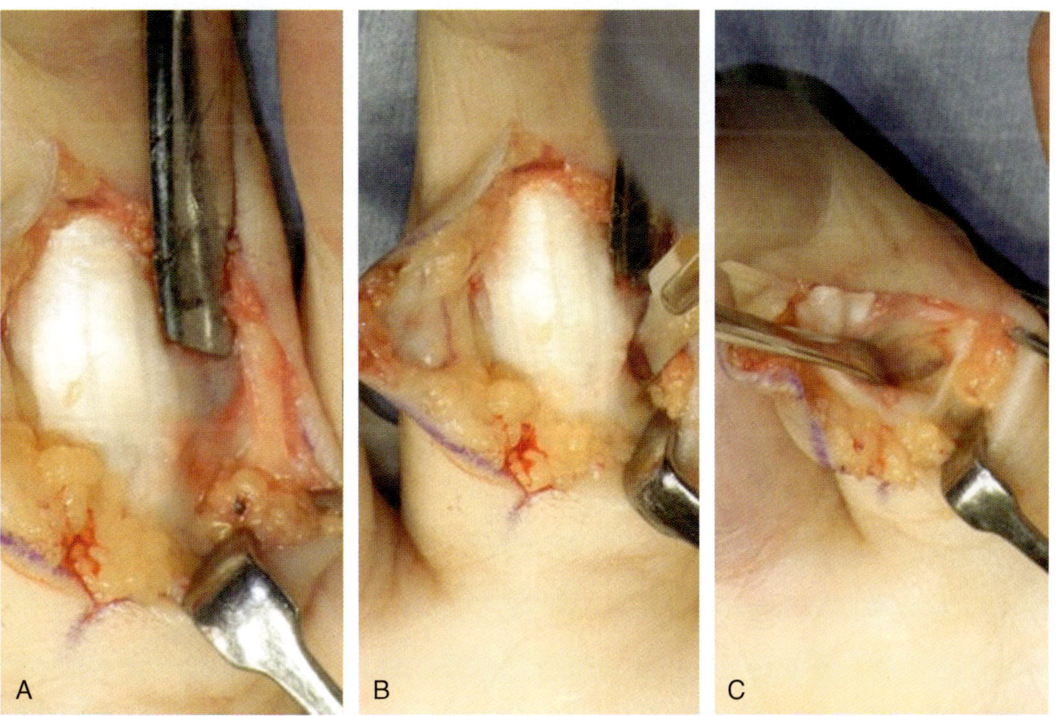

FIGURE 33-5

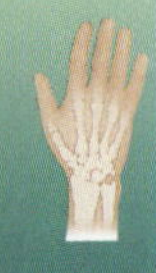

STEP 3 PITFALLS

It is important to visually confirm that the anchor has gone all the way into the drill hole before removing the instrument (Fig. 33-6C).

Step 3

- A drill hole is made in the center of the palmar surface of the proximal phalanx about 5 to 7 mm proximal to the joint line (Fig. 33-6A).
- A bone anchor (Mitek Mini, Mitek Surgical Products Inc., Norwood, Mass) is placed in the hole (Fig. 33-6B).

Step 4

- The bone anchor typically has two needles with sutures. One needle is passed from the dorsolateral aspect of the volar plate (Fig. 33-7A) to emerge at the central portion of the volar plate (Fig. 33-7B). It is then passed through the edge of the previously divided accessory collateral ligament (Fig. 33-7C).

Step 5

- The sutures are tied to each other, aiming to maintain the PIP joint in about 10 degrees of flexion (Fig. 33-8A).
- The other needle is passed in a similar fashion on the other side. After the second suture is tied, the PIP joint should be positioned in about 15 to 20 degrees of flexion. The first suture loop needs to shift medially to develop sufficient tension in the second suture loop (Fig. 33-8B and C).

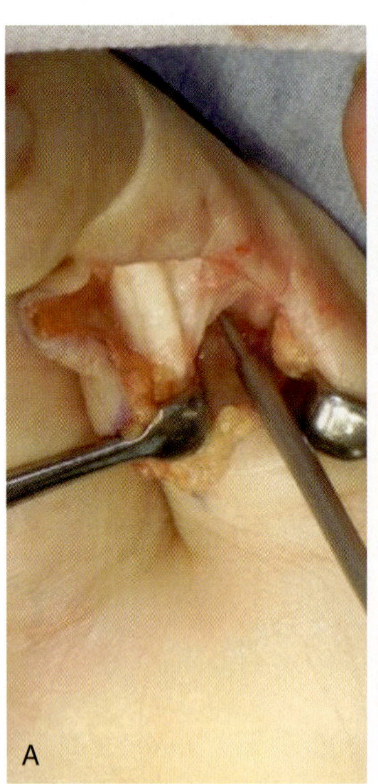

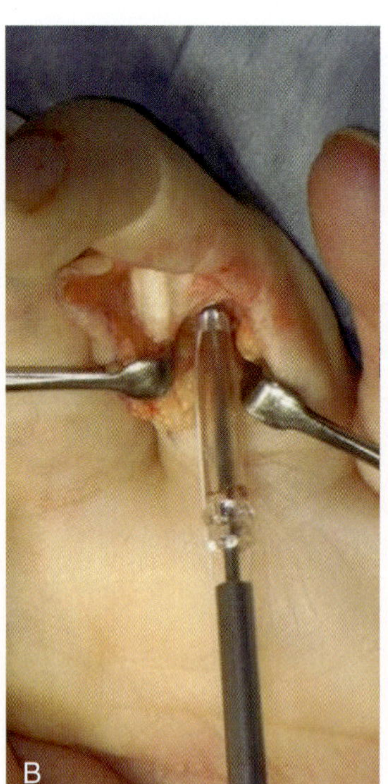

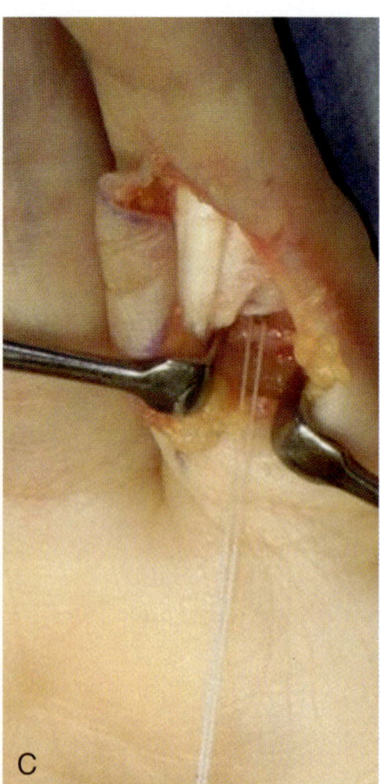

FIGURE 33-6

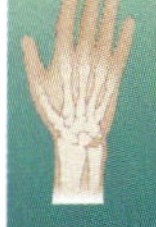

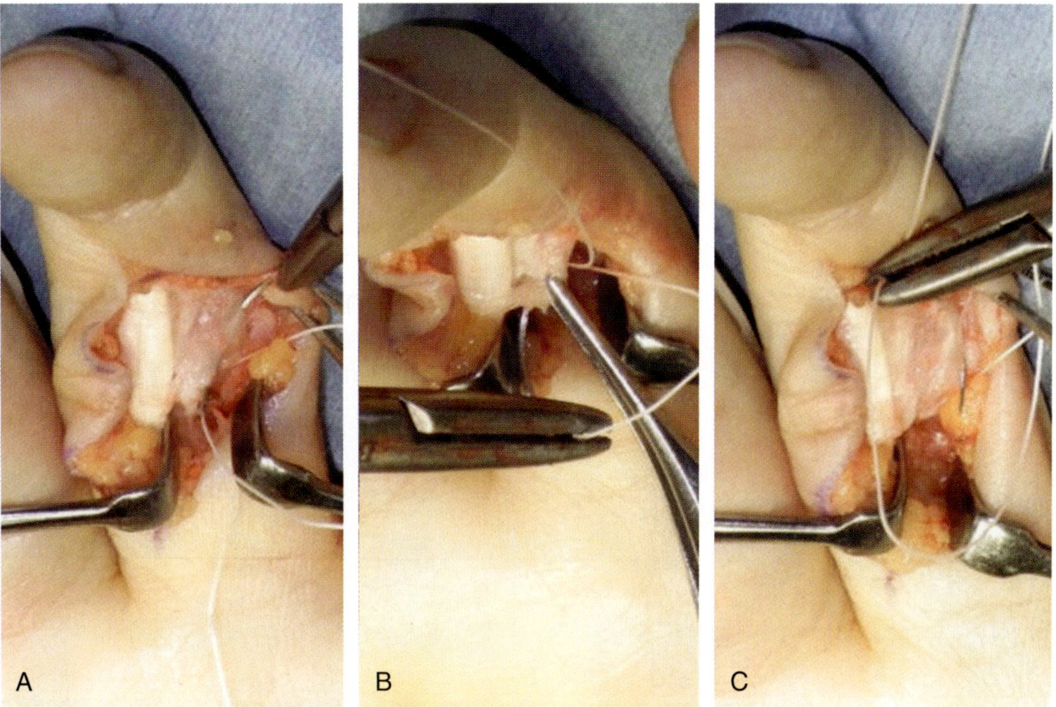

FIGURE 33-7

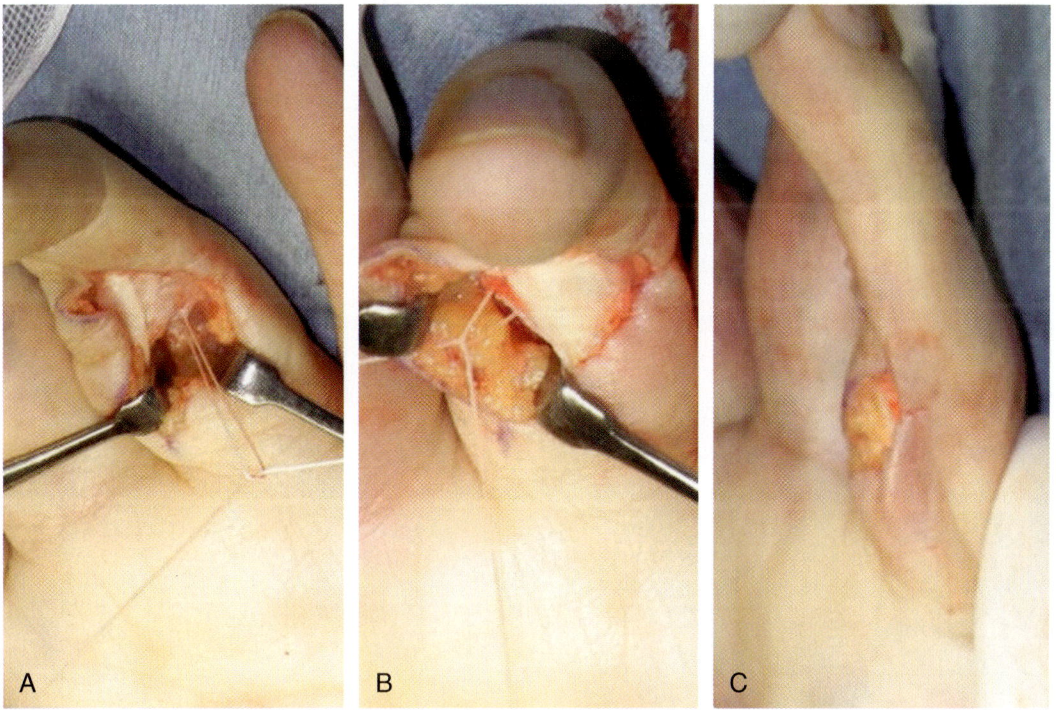

FIGURE 33-8

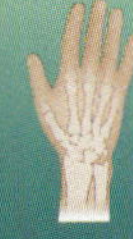

FDS Tenodesis

Step 1

- One of the slips of the FDS is divided proximal to A2 pulley (Fig. 33-9A and B).

Step 2

- A hole is made in the distal third of the proximal phalanx from the volar to lateral surface. The FDS slip is passed through this hole from volar to lateral and is sutured with the PIP joint in slight flexion (Fig. 33-9C).

STEP 2 PEARLS

A single slip of FDS is usually too large to pass through the hole. It is better to use half of the slip instead. Another option would be to pass the entire slip through the A2 pulley.

Retinacular Ligament Reconstruction

Step 1

- The ulnar lateral band is divided at the midproximal phalanx (Fig. 33-10A).

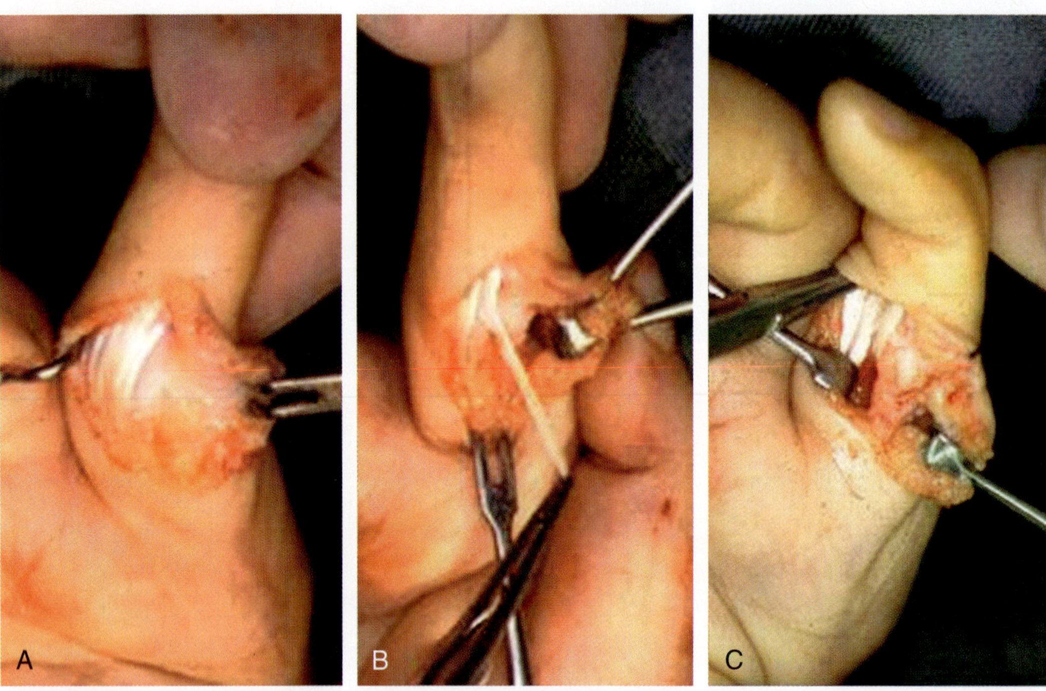

FIGURE 33-9

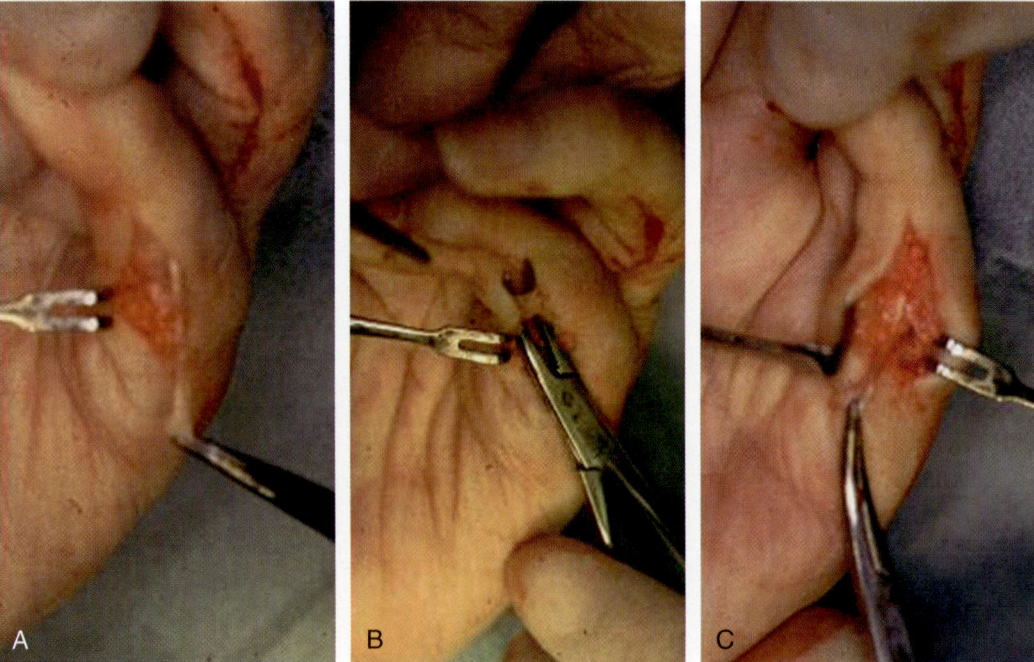

FIGURE 33-10

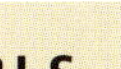

STEP 2 PEARLS

An extension block pin must be used to protect the reconstructed retinacular ligament.

Step 2

- The divided lateral band is dissected distally and passed below the Cleland ligament so that the ulnar lateral band is now volar to the axis to the PIP joint to maintain the PIP joint in flexion. The lateral band is sutured to the A2 pulley or into the bone of the proximal phalanx to maintain the PIP joint in 15 to 20 degrees of flexion (Fig. 33-10B and C).

Procedures to Correct DIP Joint Deformity (for Types 1 to 4)

Dorsal Tenodermodesis of the DIP Joint

Step 1

- An ellipse of skin is excised from the dorsum of the DIP joint (Fig. 33-11A).

Step 2

- A 3-0 nylon horizontal mattress suture is passed such that it holds a good bite of both the skin and the underlying extensor tendon (Fig. 33-11B).

Step 3

- The DIP joint is held in extension, and the 3-0 nylon suture is tied (Fig. 33-11C).

Step 4

- An oblique K-wire is inserted to maintain the DIP joint in extension and is cut off beneath the skin (Fig. 33-11D).

STEP 4 PEARLS

Although soft tissue reconstruction for DIP joint extension is often discouraged and arthrodesis is recommended, tenodermodesis combined with pinning the DIP joint (>2 months) creates a stiff DIP joint that will also allow slight motion.

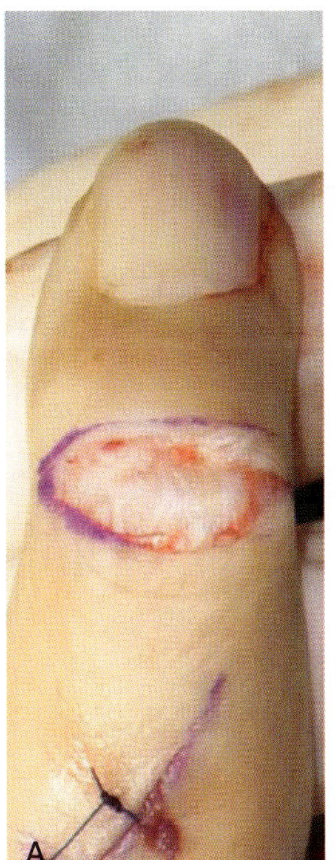

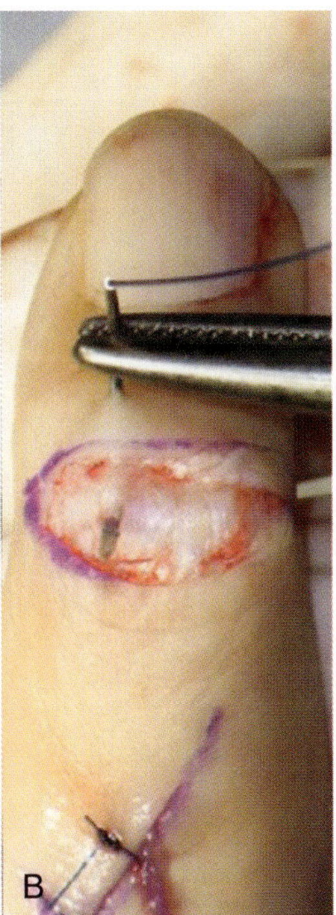

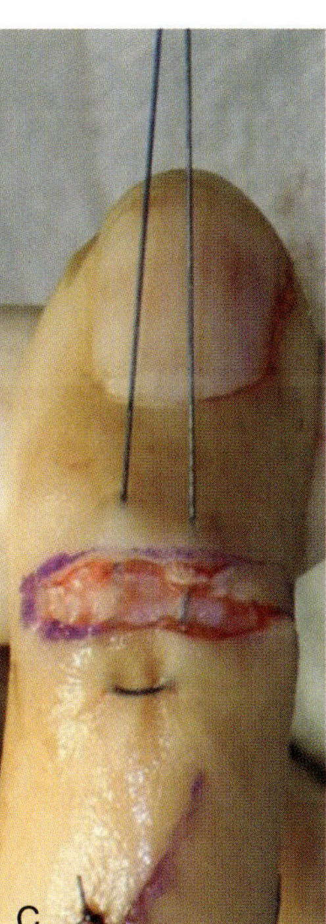

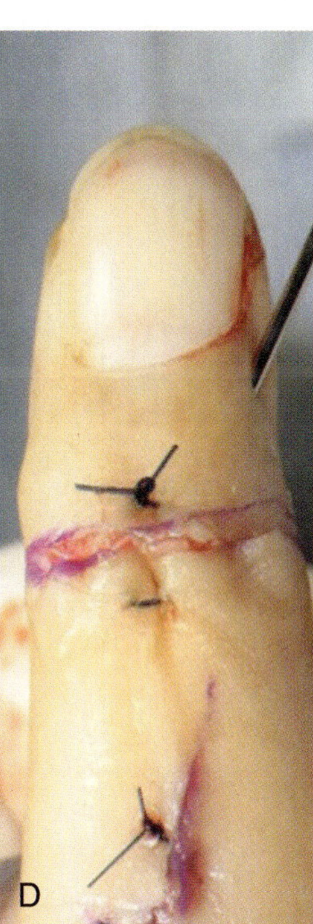

FIGURE 33-11

STEP 2 PEARLS

Try to preserve a wide central slip. Occasionally, the demarcation between the central slip and the lateral bands is unclear. A wider central slip can better resist accidental rupture during joint manipulation and is easier to lengthen.

STEP 3 PEARLS

The dorsal capsule and the dorsal portions of the collateral ligaments may need to be released to obtain good flexion at the PIP joint.

STEP 3 PITFALLS

Tension of the central slip should be monitored carefully during manipulation to prevent rupture.

Procedures to Correct a Stiff Swan-Neck Deformity (Type 3)

Lateral Band Mobilization

Step 1

- The extensor apparatus is exposed by a dorsal curved incision. The lateral bands are dorsally displaced and adherent to the central slip. They do not move laterally or palmar, which causes the extension contracture (Fig. 33-12A).

Step 2

- The lateral bands are separated from the central slip from distal to proximal by sharp dissection (Fig. 33-12B).

Step 3

- The PIP joint is gently flexed to enable the lateral band to move laterally and palmar (Fig. 33-12C).

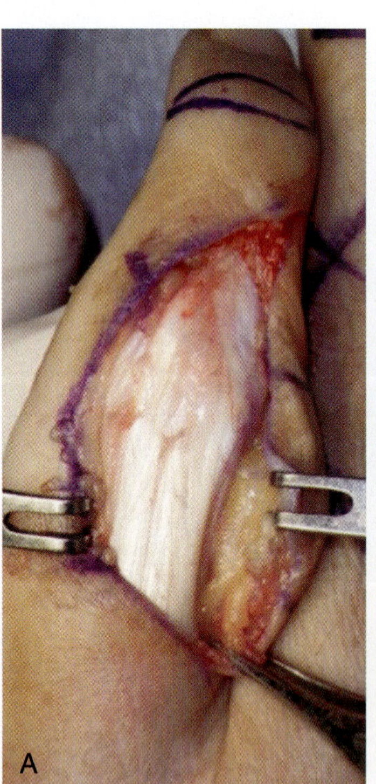

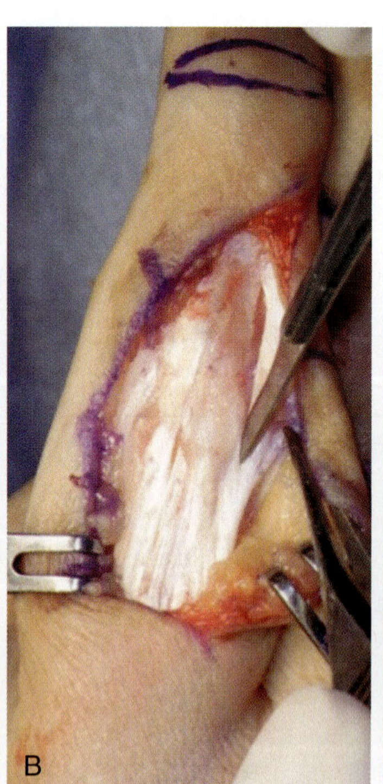

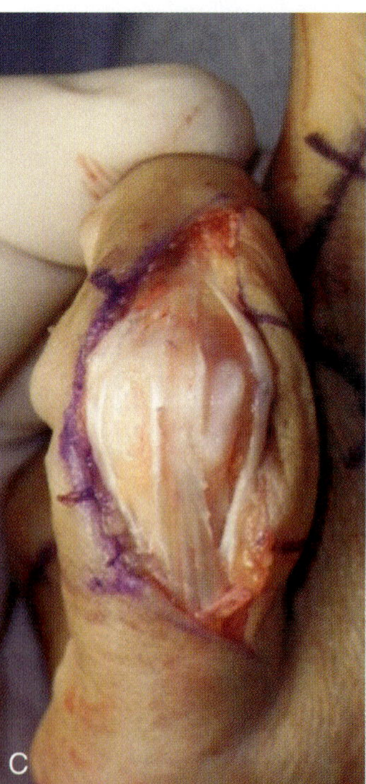

FIGURE 33-12

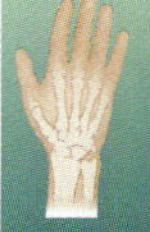

Step-Cut (Z) Lengthening of the Central Slip

Step 1

- A step-cut lengthening of the central slip should be considered if shortening of the central slip restricts PIP joint flexion after manipulation of the PIP joint and mobilization of the lateral bands has been attempted.
- A Z-incision of the central slip is made beginning 3 to 4 mm proximal to the insertion at the middle phalanx (marked as black dot on figures) and extended 1 to 1.5 cm proximally (depending on the severity of the deformity) (Fig. 33-13A).

Step 2

- A dorsal joint release including the capsule and dorsal part of the collateral ligaments is carried out (Fig. 33-13B).

Step 3

- The PIP joint is positioned in slight flexion, and the lengthened central slip is repaired using multiple horizontal mattress sutures (Fig. 33-13C).

STEP 3 PITFALLS

An extension deficit of the PIP joint often develops after step-cut lengthening of the central slip. To prevent rupture of the repair and facilitate early mobilization, the length of the step cut should allow at least three or four sutures.

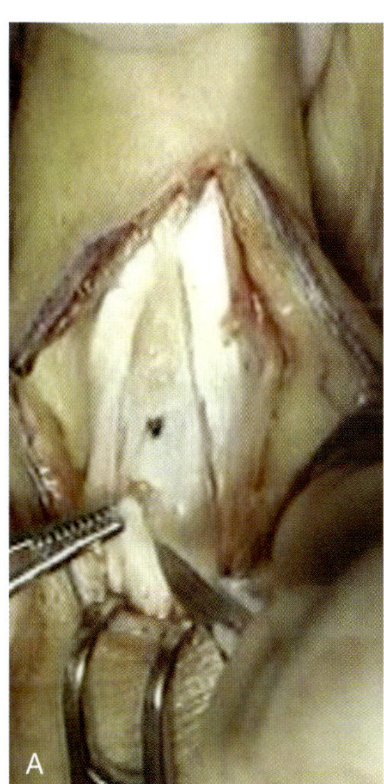

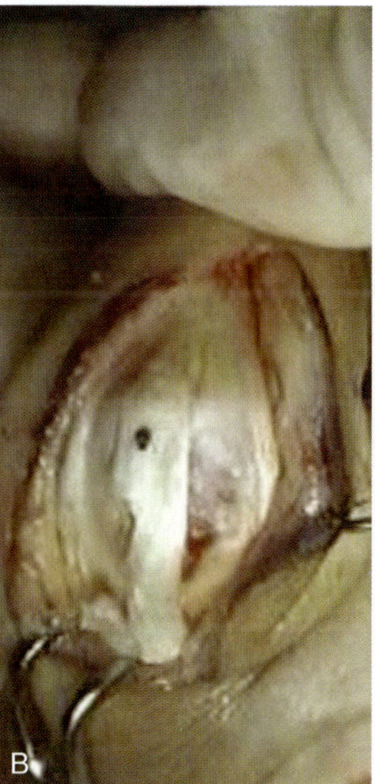

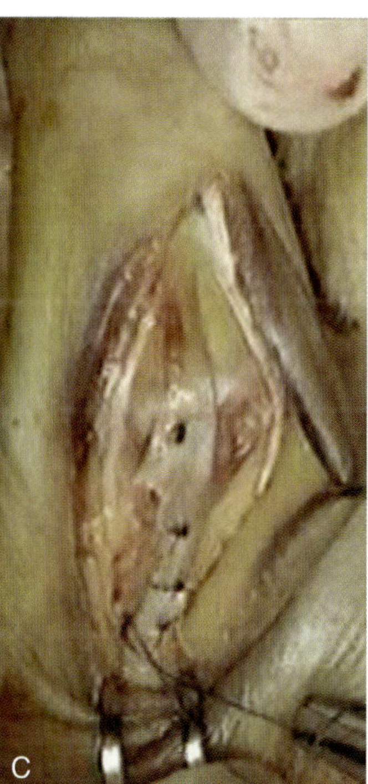

FIGURE 33-13

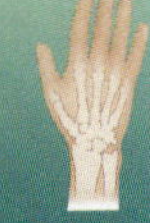

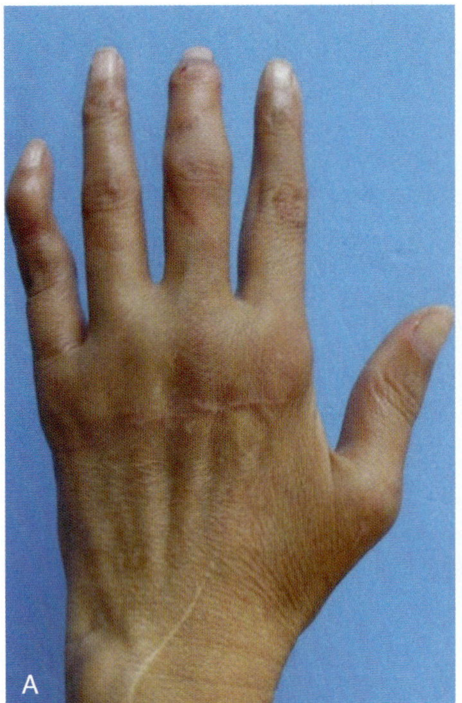

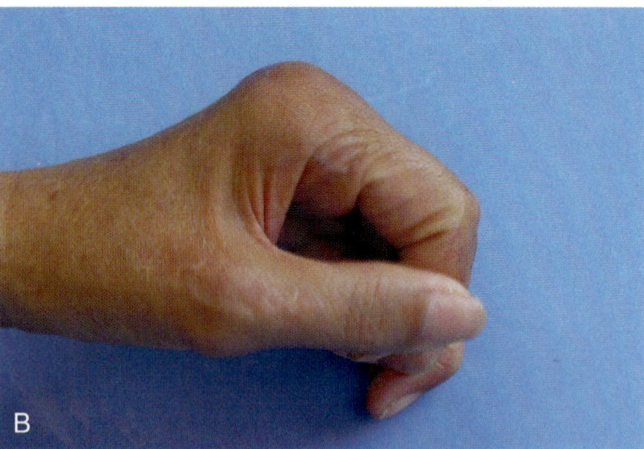

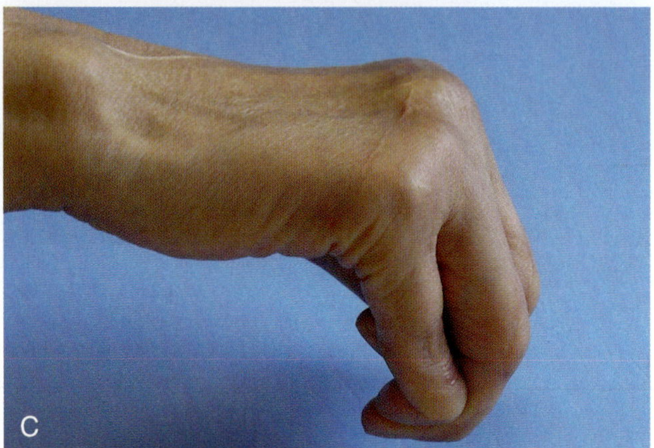

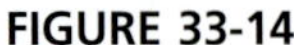
FIGURE 33-14

Postoperative Care and Expected Outcomes

- Active motion should be encouraged as early as the second postoperative day.
- A dorsal extension block splint is used for 2 weeks until the surgical wounds have healed. This is followed by a thermoplastic figure-of-eight splint for an additional 8 weeks.
- After manipulation of the PIP joint or mobilization of lateral bands for a type III deformity, the PIP joint should be kept in flexion with a splint for 1 or 2 weeks to stretch the dorsal soft tissue. Patients should continue active flexion except in cases that also required central slip lengthening. These patients should be immobilized for 3 to 4 weeks.
- The results of surgery are unpredictable for advanced swan-neck deformity, and the percentage of good results is small. However, even if motion is lost, the flexed position of the PIP joint is functionally much better than the hyperextended position. Therefore, one must not hesitate to perform surgery for advanced swan-neck deformity as long as PIP joint hyperextension can be prevented.
- Figure 33-14 shows the appearance of the patient in Figure 33-2 one year after surgery. The patient underwent release of the ulnar intrinsic muscle, manipulation of the PIP joints, tenodermodesis of the DIP joint of the index and small fingers, and lateral band mobilization and volar plate reconstruction using bone anchors for the long and ring fingers. The swan-neck deformity was corrected, and all fingers had reasonable flexion except the small finger where the deformity recurred.

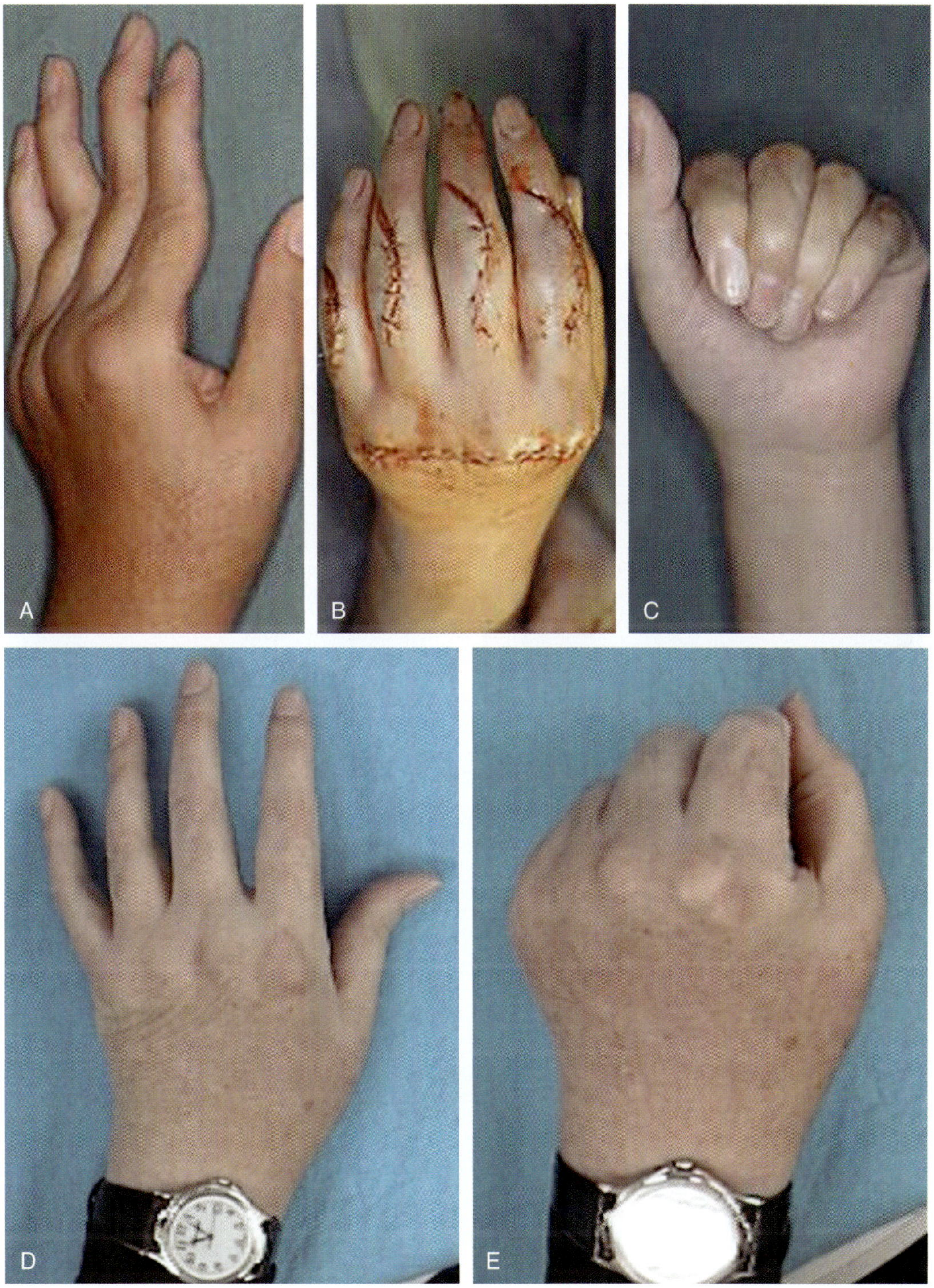

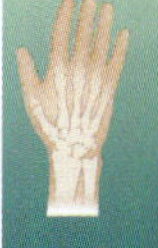

FIGURE 33-15

- Figure 33-15 shows a stiff swan-neck deformity with MP flexion-contractures of all fingers in a 49-year-old woman. She underwent intrinsic muscle release and lateral band mobilization of all fingers. In addition, lengthening of the central slip was done for the long and ring fingers. An extension block pin was inserted into the head of the proximal phalanx to protect the central slip repair, and the distal wounds were left open. Excellent flexion of the PIP joint in 6 months (Fig. 33-15C) and at the10-year follow-up showed that the correction of the deformity was maintained (Fig. 33-15D and 33-15E).

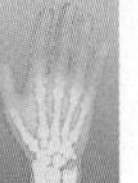

Acknowledgment

We would like to thank Shimpei Ono, MD, for use of Figure 33-3.

Evidence

de Bruin M, van Vliet DC, Smeulders MJ, Kreulen M. Long-term results of lateral band translocation for the correction of swan neck deformity in cerebral palsy. *J Pediatr Orthop*. 2010;30:67-70.
The authors treated 62 fingers with lateral band translocation and reported a 84% success rate at 1 year, which declined to 60% at 5 years. The authors concluded that lateral band translocation should not be considered a long-lasting procedure in the treatment of cerebral palsy. (Level IV evidence)

Kiefhaber TR, Stricland JW. Soft tissue reconstruction for rheumatoid swan-neck and boutonniere deformities: long term results. *J Hand Surg [Am]*. 1993;18:984-989.
Ninety-two swan-neck deformities in rheumatoid patients were treated with dorsal capsulotomy and lateral band mobilization. The authors concluded that the results were unpredictable, and PIP motion deteriorated over time. (Level IV evidence)

Ozturk S, Zor F, Sengezar M, Isik S. Correction of bilateral congenital swan-neck deformity by use of Mitek mini anchor: a new technique. *Br J Plast Surg*. 2005;56:822-825.
Four congenital swan-neck deformities were successfully treated with reinforcement of the volar plate using the Mitek Mini anchor system. Two sutures of the anchor system crossed the PIP joint in a V fashion; the anchor was inserted into the volar surface of the proximal phalanx, and two sutures were passed through two holes created at the palmar proximal aspect of the middle phalanx. The sutures were tied to each other with the PIP joint in 20 degrees flexion. (Level IV evidence)

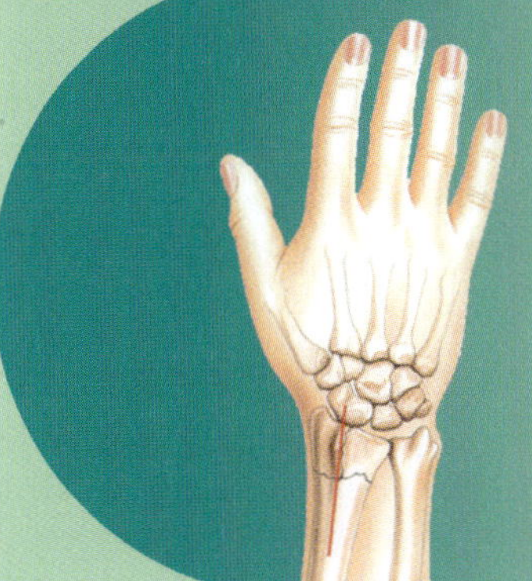

PROCEDURE 34

Reconstruction of the Central Slip with the Transverse Retinacular Ligament for Boutonnière Deformity

Makoto Motomiya and Akio Minami

See Video 26: Correction of Boutonnière Deformity

Indications

- Boutonnière deformity is classified into three stages by Nalebuff, as follows:
  - *Stage 1:* Mild deformity; 10 to 15 degrees of extension lag at the PIP joint, and PIP joint passively correctable
  - *Stage 2:* Moderate deformity; 30 to 40 degrees of extension lag at PIP joint, and PIP joint passively correctable
  - *Stage 3:* Severe deformity that cannot be corrected passively
- *Indication:* Boutonnière deformity of the PIP joint with almost full passive extension (stages 1 and 2) is suitable for this reconstructive surgery.
- *Contraindication:* If articular destruction is evident or if a severe fixed flexion contracture is present (stage 3), arthrodesis or arthroplasty of the PIP joint is recommended.

Examination/Imaging

Clinical Examination

- Boutonnière deformity is seen in a patient with rheumatoid arthritis (Fig. 34-1).
- Passive PIP joint extension should always be evaluated before surgical reconstruction.
- The mobility of the PIP joint is very important for obtaining good results. Therefore, in the case of the boutonnière deformity with severe flexion contracture of the PIP joint, rehabilitation or joint splinting in extension of the PIP joint should be performed before the operation.

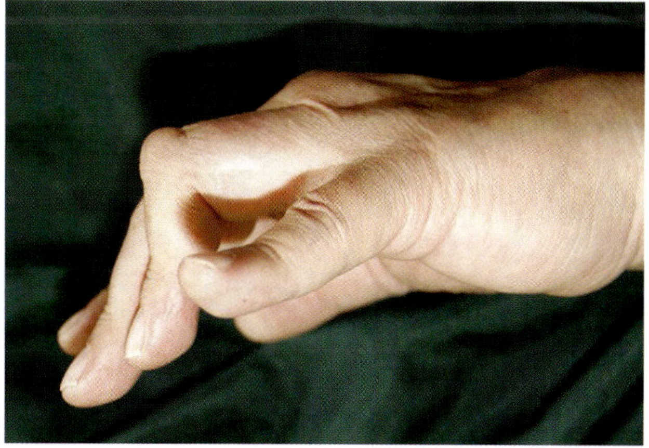

FIGURE 34-1

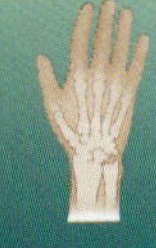

Imaging

- Radiographic examination is required to evaluate the status of the metacarpophalangeal (MCP), proximal interphalangeal (PIP), and distal interphalangeal (DIP) joints.
- If the PIP joint is destroyed, arthrodesis or arthroplasty is recommended.
- Magnetic resonance imaging examination may help to identify synovitis of the PIP joint.

Surgical Anatomy

- Disruption of the central slip of the extensor tendon results in palmar migration of the lateral bands with PIP joint flexion. Proximal displacement of the extensor apparatus results in the DIP joint hyperextension deformity (Fig. 34-2A is normal; B shows boutonnière deformity).
- The transverse retinacular ligament is the key component in this procedure. This ligament holds the lateral bands in the palmar direction during flexion. It inserts into the palmar plate of the PIP joint and flexor tendon sheath (Fig. 34-3).

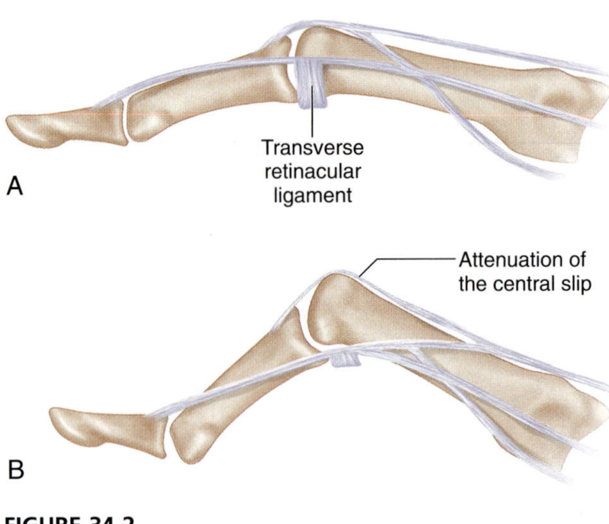

FIGURE 34-2

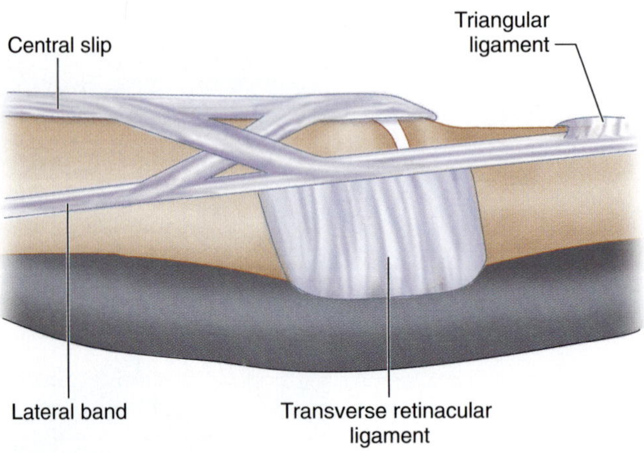

FIGURE 34-3

Exposures

- Extensor apparatus is approached through a dorsal curved incision over the PIP joint. The dissection is carried down to the extensor hood, preserving the dorsal venous system (Fig. 34-4).

Procedure

Step 1

- Both lateral bands and transverse retinacular ligaments are identified first. The central slip is usually attenuated or ruptured, and the capsule of the PIP joint appears directly under the fat tissue. In Figure 34-5, the black arrow shows the transverse retinacular ligament.
- The radial and ulnar transverse retinacular ligaments are cleanly separated from their insertions at the palmar plate.

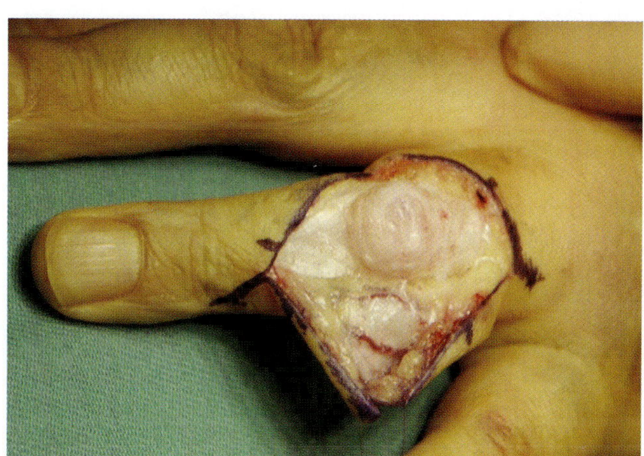

FIGURE 34-4

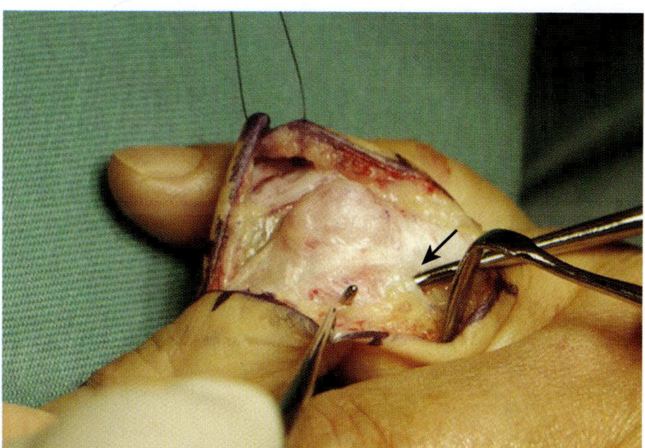

FIGURE 34-5

PEARLS

The surgery is done under wrist block/digital block to confirm the proper tension for the active finger motion during operation.

PITFALLS

The surgeon should be careful to protect any dorsal sensory subcutaneous veins and nerves encountered.

STEP 1 PEARLS

If there is a contracture of the PIP joint, the surgeon should cut the accessory collateral ligament and release the volar plate at the proximal portion to obtain full passive extension of the PIP joints.

Removing adhesion of the lateral band and cutting the oblique retinacular ligament may be necessary to obtain flexion of the DIP joint.

Synovectomy of the PIP joint should be performed for patients with active rheumatoid arthritis.

STEP 1 PITFALLS

Collateral ligaments of the PIP joint should be preserved to prevent instability of the joint.

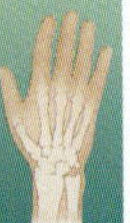

STEP 2 PEARLS

Determining the tension of the suture is very important to obtain good flexion and extension of the PIP and DIP joints.

STEP 2 PITFALLS

If the suture is too tight, it is likely to result in extension contracture of the PIP and DIP joints.

Step 2

- The transverse retinacular ligaments are turned over onto the dorsal aspect on the PIP joint to lift the lateral band dorsally and are then sutured to one another (Fig. 34-6).
- Tension of the suture is determined by noting the nearly full active extension of the PIP joint (Fig. 34-7).
- The schema of this operation is shown in Figure 34-8.

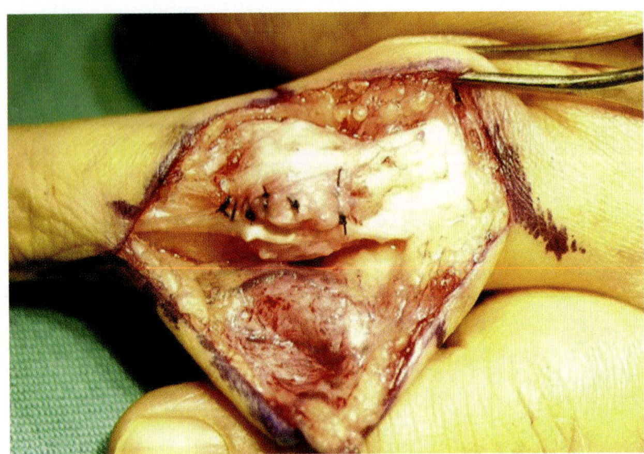

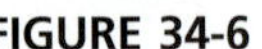

FIGURE 34-6

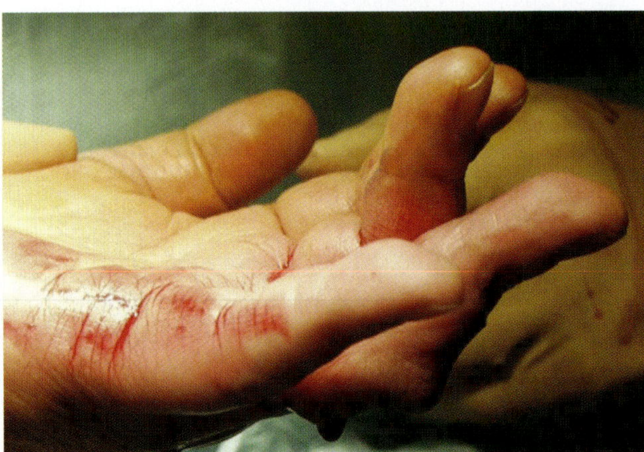

FIGURE 34-7

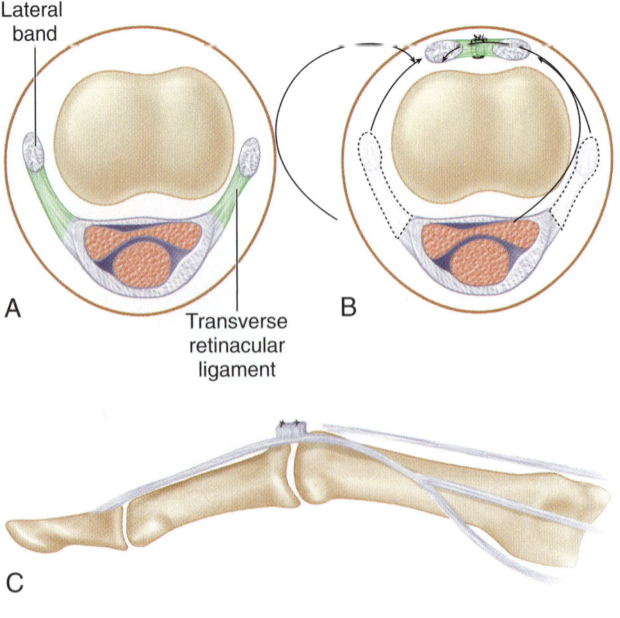

FIGURE 34-8

STEP 3 PEARLS

The release of the lateral band should be done at the level of the distal half of the middle phalanx.

STEP 3 PITFALLS

Releasing the lateral bands too far is likely to result in the extension lag of the DIP joint.

Step 3

- Check active flexion of the DIP joint because the tension of the lateral band is tighter after suturing of the transverse retinacular ligaments (Fig. 34-9).
- If DIP joint flexion is limited, releasing the lateral band between the PIP and DIP joints is recommended.
- Make small transverse cuts in the lateral band until the DIP joint can be actively flexed at 30 degrees (Fig. 34-10).
- After the operation, the PIP joint is immobilized in full extension with a Kirschner wire or volar splint for about 14 days.

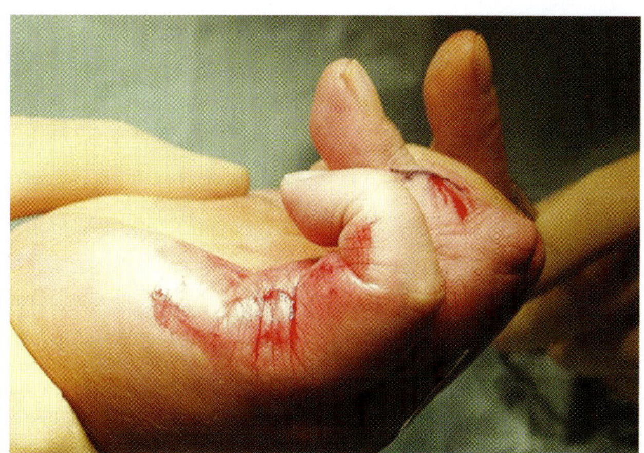

FIGURE 34-9

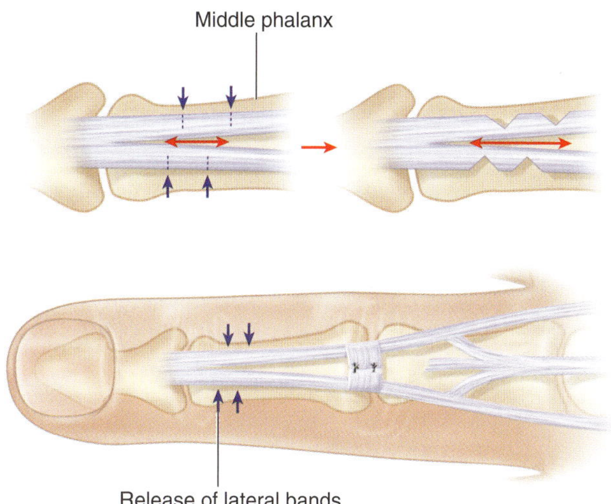

FIGURE 34-10

PITFALLS

Rehabilitation should be performed under the supervision of a hand therapist.

Postoperative Care and Expected Outcomes

- Active flexion exercises of the DIP joint are started within 3 days while the PIP joint remains immobilized.
- About 14 days after surgery, active flexion exercises of the PIP joint are gently started, but active extension exercises of the PIP joint should be avoided at the early stages.
- The PIP joint is held in full extension in the daytime by a dynamic splint and at night by a static splint for several weeks.
- After removing the splint, active finger exercises are started gradually.

Evidence

Kato H, Uchiyama S, Yamazaki H, et al. Treatment for boutonnière deformity in rheumatoid arthritis [Japanese]. *Kansetsugeka*. 2008;27:58-63.
A clinical experience report of a modified Ohshio method of repair of boutonnière deformity using the transverse retinacular ligament. This modification involves releasing the lateral bands between PIP and DIP joints to obtain active flexion of the DIP joint. There was a significant improvement in all seven fingers of six patients, and the DIP joint could be actively flexed by releasing the tight lateral bands. (Level IV evidence)

Nalebuff EA, Millender LH. Surgical treatment of the boutonnière deformity in rheumatoid arthritis. *Orthop Clinic North Am*. 1975;6:753-763.
In this paper, boutonnière deformity in patients with rheumatoid arthritis can be classified into three stages, which serve as a guide to the appropriate management. (Level V evidence)

Ohshio I, Ogino T, Minami A, et al. Reconstruction of the central slip by the transverse retinacular ligament for boutonnière deformity. *J Hand Surg [Br]*. 1990;15:407-409.
A clinical experience report of a new method of repairing boutonnière deformity using the transverse retinacular ligament. There was a significant improvement in all six fingers of five patients, but moderate limitation of flexion of the DIP joint remained in cases with severe contracture of the lateral bands. (Level IV evidence)

Salvi V. Technique for the buttonhole deformity. *Hand*. 1969;1:96-97.
A surgical technique for boutonnière deformity is described using the dorsally based flaps of the PIP joint capsule to reposition the lateral band dorsally. The Ohshio method was modified from this Salvi procedure. (Level V evidence)

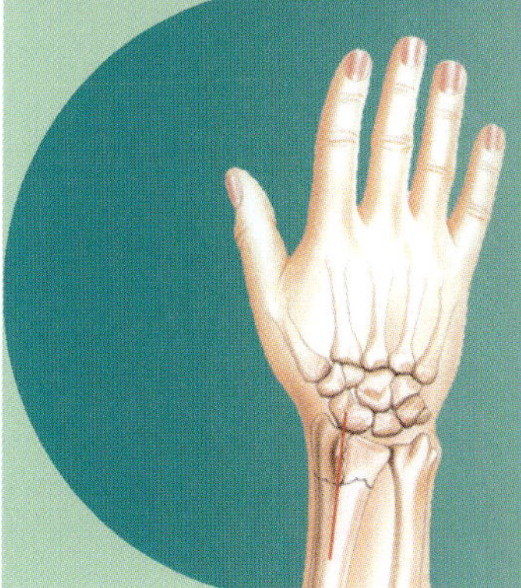

PROCEDURE 35

Silicone Metacarpophalangeal Joint Arthroplasty

Nathan S. Taylor and Kevin C. Chung

See Video 27: Silicone Metacarpophalangeal Joint Replacement Arthoplasty for Rheumatoid Arthritis

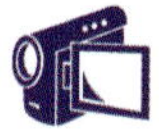

Indications

- Finger metacarpophalangeal (MCP) joint contracture or subluxation in rheumatoid arthritis (RA) patients
- MCP joint contracture or dislocation in patients with other rheumatic conditions, such as scleroderma or systemic lupus erythematosus

Examination/Imaging

Clinical Examination

- The patient's MCP joints should be evaluated for range of motion and stability. If the MCP joints are not dislocated but the fingers are drifted ulnarly, intrinsic transfer may be performed to correct the finger misalignment for the small, ring, and long fingers; the radial sagittal band of the index finger is tightened to centralize its extensor tendon because no ulnar intrinsic tendon is available for transfer.
- With chronic subluxation of the MCP joints, ligamentous contracture around the joints cannot be corrected by soft tissue reconstruction alone. MCP joint arthroplasty is the preferred option in most of these cases.
- The thumb MCP joint laxity should be assessed, which is best treated with MCP joint fusion at the time of silicone MCP arthroplasty (SMPA).
- For patients who have collapse of the wrists and radial deviation of the metacarpals, the wrist problem should be addressed first either by fusion or by arthroplasty. Otherwise, the radial deviation of the metacarpals will cause early postoperative ulnar subluxation of the fingers after SMPA. Realigning the metacarpals by means of the wrist procedures will enhance the outcome of SMPA.

Imaging

- Posteroanterior, lateral, and oblique radiographs of the hand and wrist are essential to identify joint alignment, joint congruity, and bony erosions.

Surgical Anatomy

- The MCP joint is a condylar joint that allows flexion and extension but also radial and ulnar deviation.
- The radial and ulnar sagittal bands stabilize the extensor tendon, keeping it over the dorsal midline of the MCP joint. The sagittal bands are attached to the volar plate.

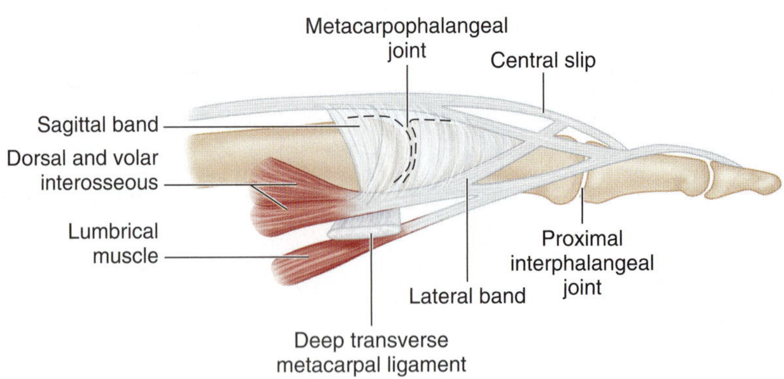

FIGURE 35-1

- The lateral bands pass volar to the MCP joint and dorsal to the proximal interphalangeal (PIP) joint. Contraction of the intrinsic muscles through the lateral bands causes MCP joint flexion and PIP joint extension (Fig. 35-1).
- The cause of tendon subluxation at the MCP joint in RA is joint synovitis altering the ligamentous support in the joint. The hypertrophic synovial tissue distends the ligamentous support of the joint, resulting in stretching of the radial and ulnar sagittal bands. Forceful gripping in daily activity tasks stresses the radial sagittal band, resulting in weakening of the radial support.
- Progressive ulnar subluxation of the extensor tendons causes the ulnar drift seen in RA hands.
- Chronic ulnar subluxation of the extensor mechanism results in ulnar lateral band contracture, which eventually causes fixed contracture of the ulnar lateral bands.

Positioning

- The procedure is performed under tourniquet control with the patient in the supine position and the extremity abducted with the hand on a hand table.

Exposures

- A transverse incision is made over the head of the metacarpals for wide exposure of all affected joints while preserving the dorsal veins and sensory nerves (Fig. 35-2A and B).

Procedure

Step 1

- The radial sagittal bands are incised to expose the MCP joints, and synovial tissues are sharply excised from the joints (see Fig. 35-3, sagittal band incision marked by dotted line).
- The collateral ligaments are divided at the metacarpal neck, and heads of the metacarpals are resected at the proximal origin of the collateral ligament using an oscillating saw (Fig. 35-4). After metacarpal head resections, the fingers can be brought into alignment. Resection of the heads should decrease the tightness of the ulnar intrinsic tendons that contribute to ulnar deviation of the fingers. Therefore, ulnar lateral band release is usually not necessary, if sufficient resection of the head of the metacarpal is performed.

PEARLS

The thin skin over the hand in RA patients must be kept in mind. Gentle traction must be performed with skin hooks and sutures to avoid pinching the skin edges, which may cause postoperative wound complications (Fig. 35-3).

STEP 1 PEARLS

Preserve the radial collateral ligament insertion on the proximal phalanges for later reconstruction.

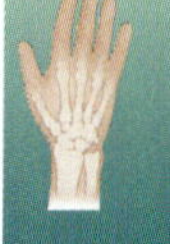

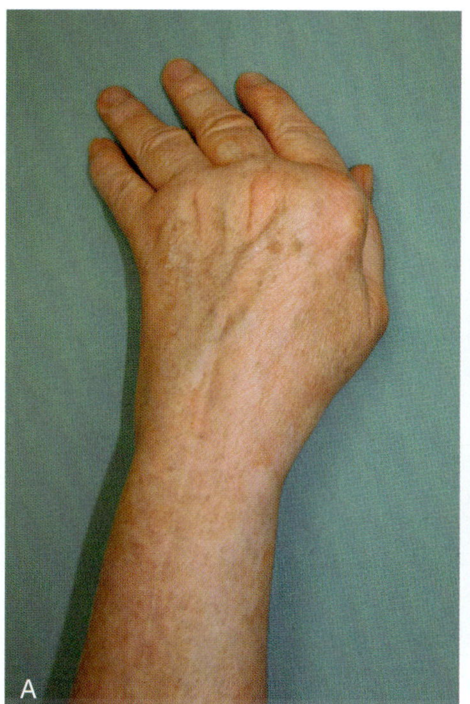

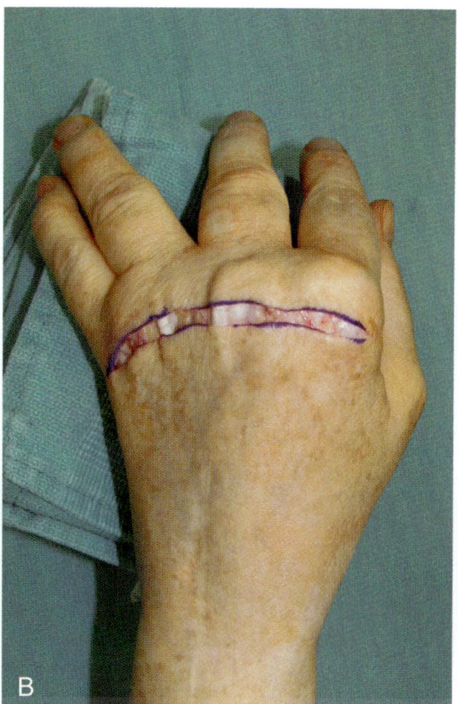

FIGURE 35-2

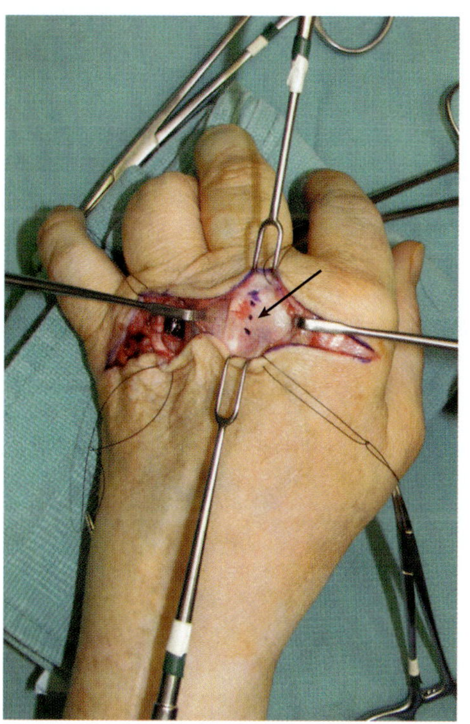

FIGURE 35-3

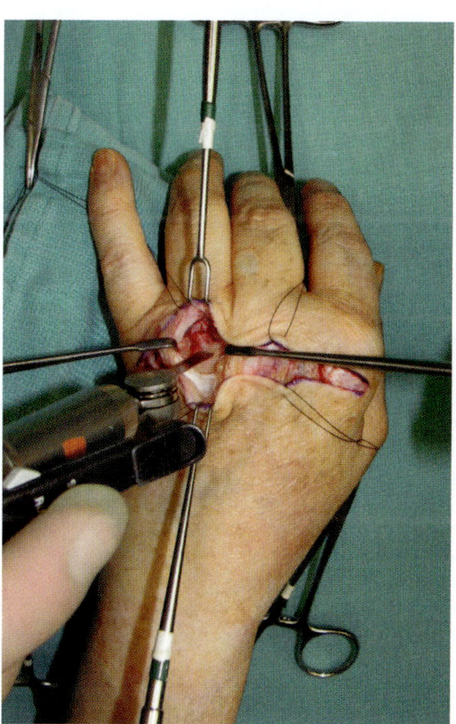

FIGURE 35-4

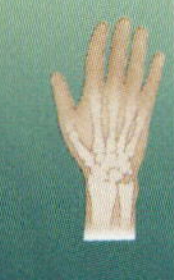

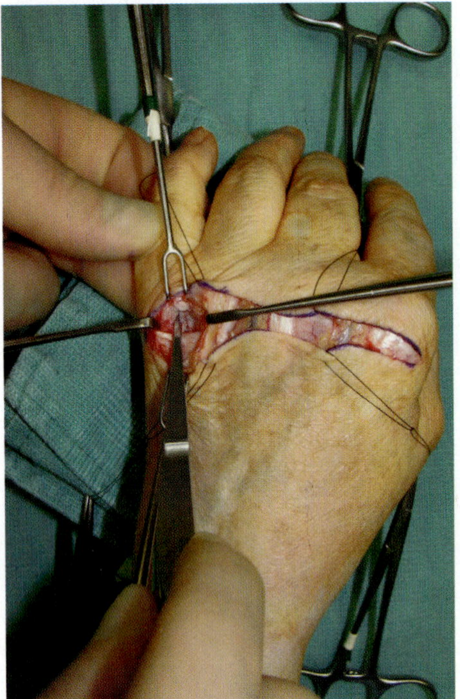

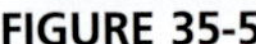

FIGURE 35-5

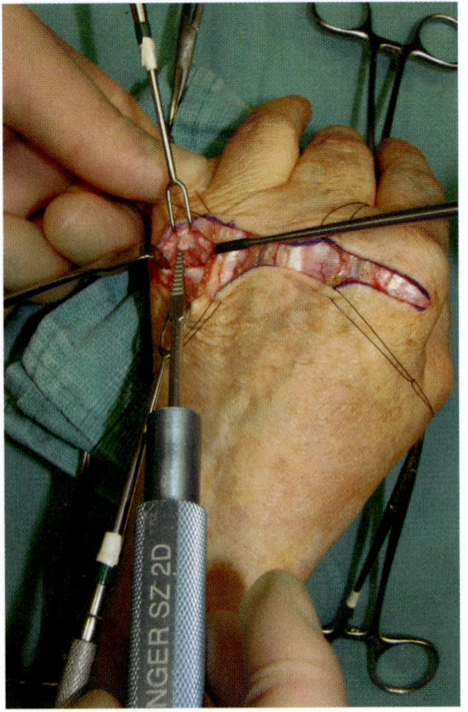

FIGURE 35-6

> **STEP 2 PITFALLS**
>
> *The bases of the proximal phalanges may be quite deformed, and identifying the medullary cavity can be difficult. One must be careful when broaching the proximal phalanges to avoid perforating the cortex.*

> **STEP 3 PEARLS**
>
> *The medullary canals of the proximal phalanges should be prepared first because these usually determine the implant size to be used. The exception to this is the ring metacarpal, which typically has a narrower canal than the ring finger proximal phalanx and should therefore be prepared first to avoid over-reaming the proximal phalanx.*

Step 2

- An awl is used to perforate the medullary cavities of the metacarpals and proximal phalanges (Fig. 35-5). Typically, the medullary cavities of the metacarpals are devoid of bone and are easily broached.

Step 3

- Sequential-sized broaches are used to enlarge the medullary cavity. The largest implants that will fit into the medullary cavity are inserted. Unlike the awl, which should be inserted in a twisting motion to enlarge the medullary cavity, the broach is rectangular in shape and should be inserted straight, without twisting, to make a square trough to accommodate the shape of the silicone implant ends (Fig. 35-6).

Step 4

- Two drill holes are made with a 0.035-inch Kirschner wire (K-wire) on the radial metacarpal, and 3-0 braided permanent sutures are placed through these drill holes for imbricating the radial collateral ligaments. These sutures are placed before insertion of the implants (Fig. 35-7A and B).

Step 5

- The implants are inserted (Fig. 35-8), and the radially placed 3-0 braided sutures are used to reattach the radial collateral ligament and bring the fingers into slight radial deviation (Fig. 35-9A to E). The ulnar lateral bands can be released, if they are still tight and cause the fingers to deviate ulnarly. However, as stated previously, ulnar band release is usually not necessary.

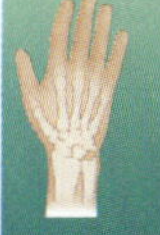

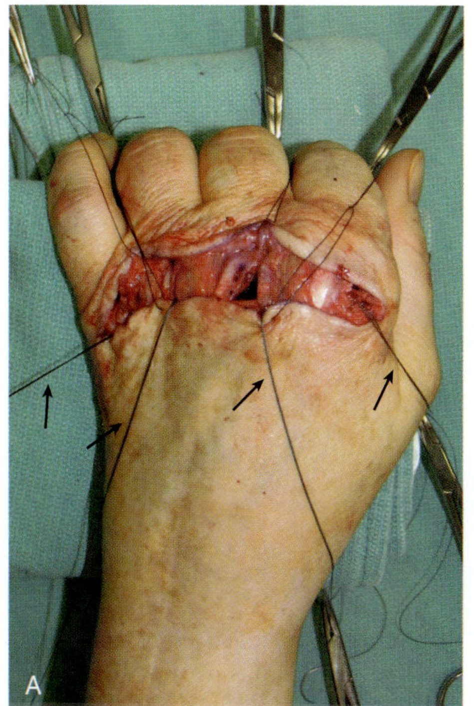

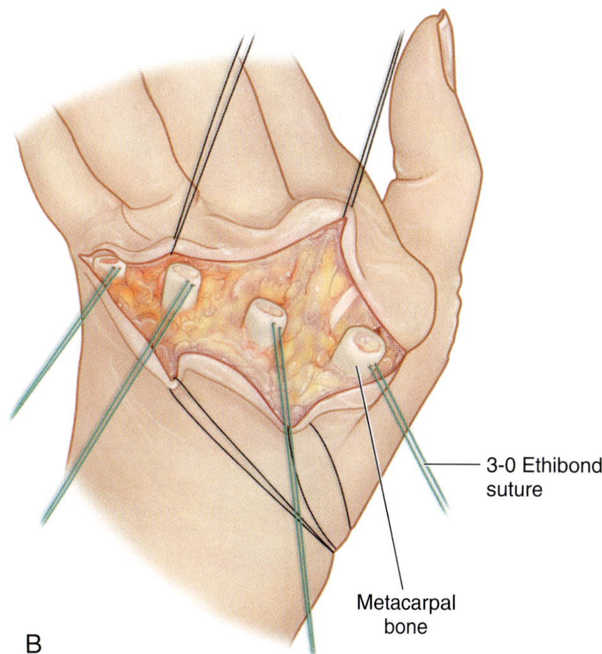

FIGURE 35-7

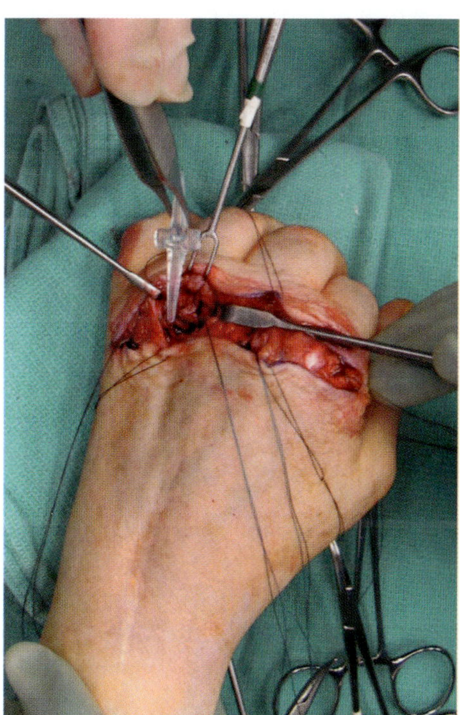

FIGURE 35-8

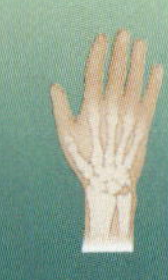

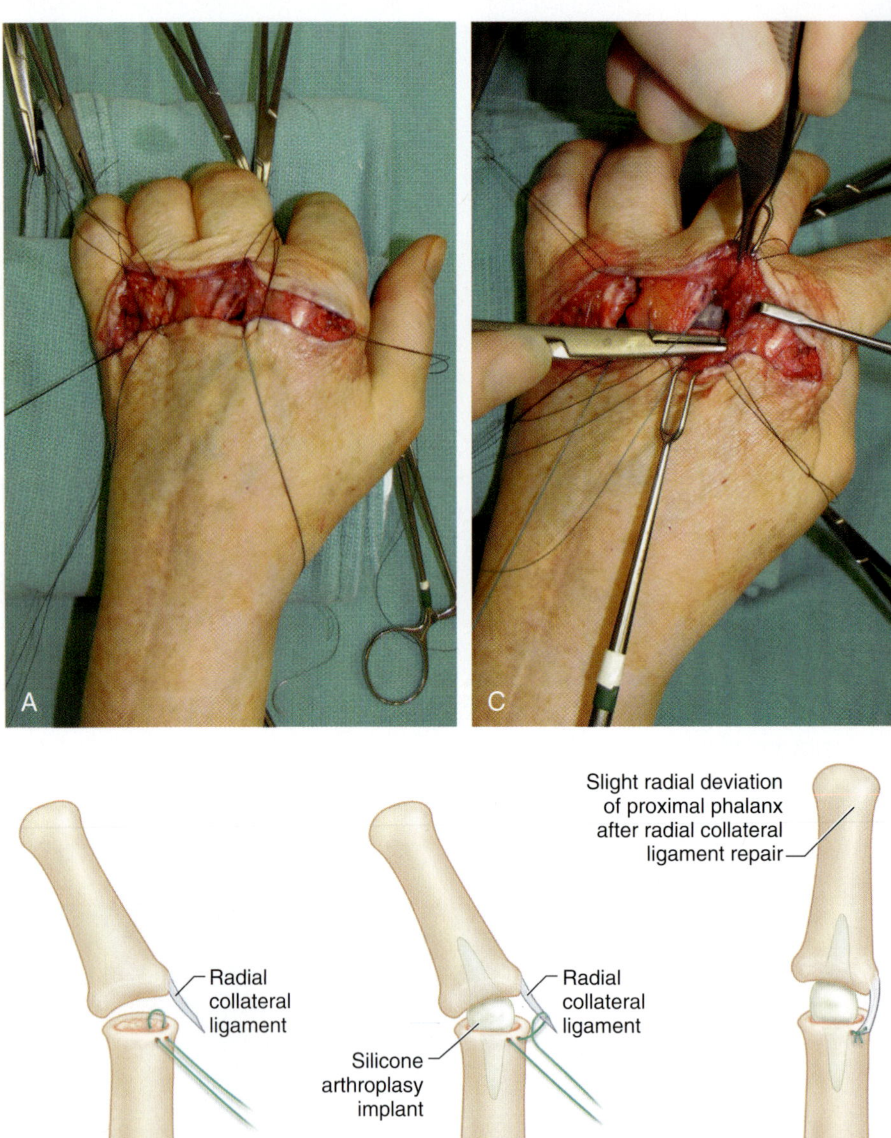

FIGURE 35-9

Step 6

- If the extensor tendons cannot be centralized easily because of tightness of the ulnar sagittal bands, these must be released as well. The extensor tendons are then centralized by imbricating the radial sagittal bands with 3-0 braided horizontal mattress sutures (Fig. 35-10A to D).

Step 7

- The tourniquet is released, and all bleeding points are cauterized. A drain is typically not necessary. The wound is then closed with interrupted absorbable dermal sutures, and the skin is closed with 4-0 horizontal mattress nylon sutures (Fig. 35-11). The hand is immobilized in a volar resting short-arm splint.

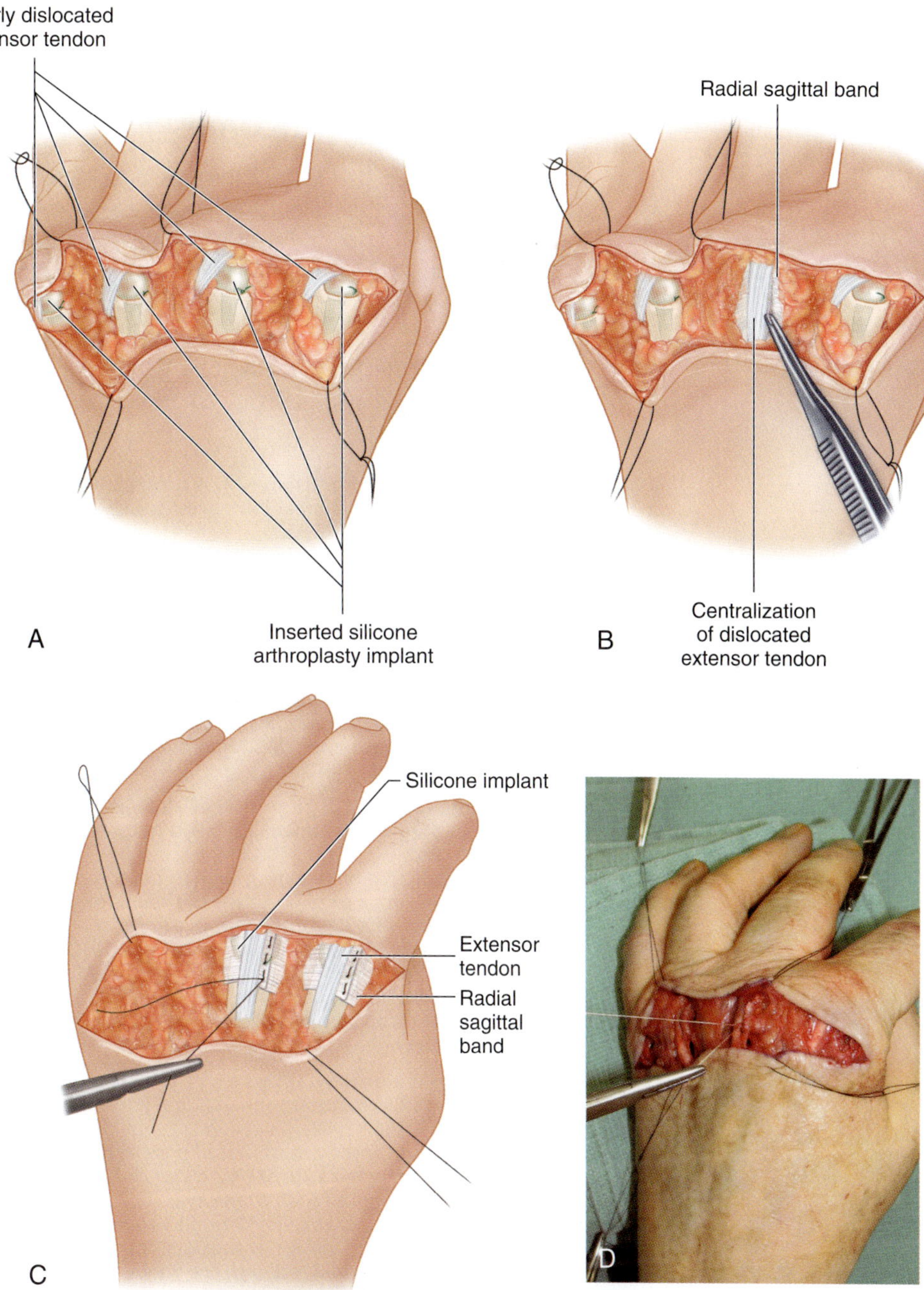

Ulnarly dislocated extensor tendon

Radial sagittal band

A

Inserted silicone arthroplasty implant

B

Centralization of dislocated extensor tendon

Silicone implant

Extensor tendon

Radial sagittal band

C

D

FIGURE 35-10

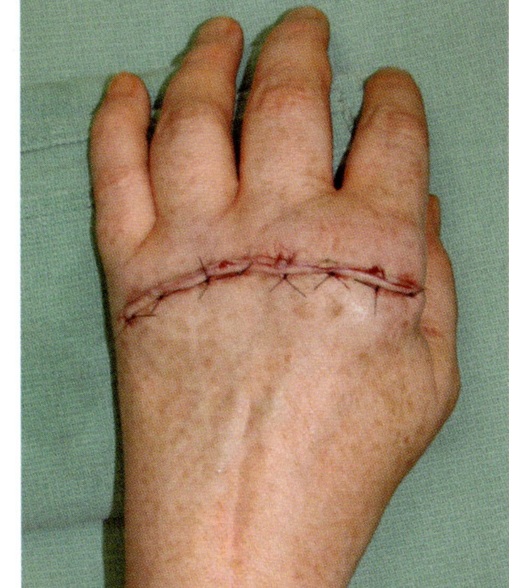

FIGURE 35-11

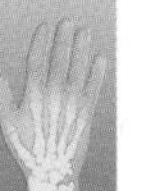

Postoperative Care and Expected Outcomes

- One week after surgery, the patient is placed in a dynamic extension splint. The patient will initiate active flexion exercises while in this dynamic splint for 6 weeks. A hand therapist will evaluate the patient's progress weekly, and the splint is adjusted as necessary to align the fingers.
- Studies have shown that static extension splints may work just as well as dynamic extension splints. However, we have no experience with the static protocol. Patients will typically gain about 30 to 40 degrees of active motion at the MCP joint, favoring an extended arc of motion.

Evidence

Chung KC, Kotsis SV, Kim HM. A prospective outcomes study of Swanson metacarpophalangeal joint arthroplasty for the rheumatoid hand. *J Hand Surg [Am]*. 2004;29:646-653.
This study presented 6-month and 1-year prospective outcomes data from patients who had undergone MCP joint reconstruction. Functional assessment by grip strength, pinch strength, and Jebsen-Taylor test did not improve significantly compared with preoperative values. Subjective assessment by the Michigan Hand Outcomes Questionnaire (MHQ), however, did improve significantly. Ulnar drift significantly decreased 1 year after surgery by an average of 24 degrees, and MCP joint range of motion increased, but this change was not significant. Continued follow-up evaluation of this cohort will determine whether these improvements are maintained in the long term. (Level III evidence)

Chung KC, Kotsis SV, Kim HM, et al. Reasons why rheumatoid arthritis patients seek surgical treatment for hand deformities. *J Hand Surg [Am]*. 2006;31: 289-294.
The purpose of this study was to determine how function, pain, and aesthetics rank in order of importance to rheumatoid arthritis patients who are considering MCP joint arthroplasty for rheumatoid hand deformities. Function, pain, and aesthetic domains from the MHQ were used in a logistic regression model to determine the factors associated with choosing hand reconstruction. Patients with less function and greater pain were more likely to choose MCP joint arthroplasty. Aesthetics was not a statistically significant predictor. (Level III evidence)

Chung KC, Kotsis SV, Wilgis EF, et al. Outcomes of silicone arthroplasty for rheumatoid metacarpophalangeal joints stratified by fingers. *J Hand Surg [Am]*. 2009;34:1647-1652.
This multicenter, international prospective cohort study evaluated 68 patients with RA treated with SMPA. Ulnar drift, extension lag, and arc of motion for the MCP joint of each finger were measured at baseline preoperatively and 1 year postoperatively. All fingers showed an improvement in ulnar drift, extension lag, and arc of motion. The largest improvements were seen in the ulnar digits compared with the radial digits. The authors concluded that despite experiential increased difficulty in maintaining posture of the ulnar digits after SMPA owing to deforming forces, sufficient correction of the deformities in the ulnar fingers is possible if adequate bone resection and realigning of the extensor mechanism are carefully performed during the procedure. (Level I evidence)

Chung KC, Kowalski CP, Kim HM, Kazmers IS. Patient outcomes following Swanson Silastic metacarpophalangeal arthroplasty in the rheumatoid hand: systematic overview. *J Rheumatol*. 2000;27:1395-1402.
This National Institutes of Health R01 study was initiated to determine the outcomes of MCP joint arthroplasty. Although MCP joint arthroplasty had been performed for more than 30 years, the research studies on this procedure varied greatly in length of follow-up, outcome assessments, and study design. (Level III evidence)

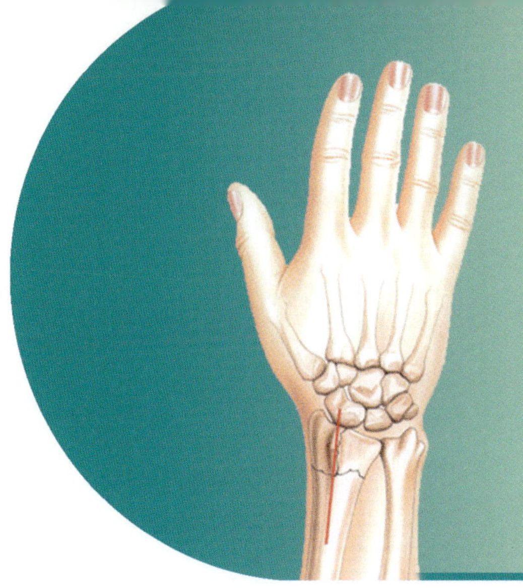

Section VI

CONGENITAL CONDITIONS

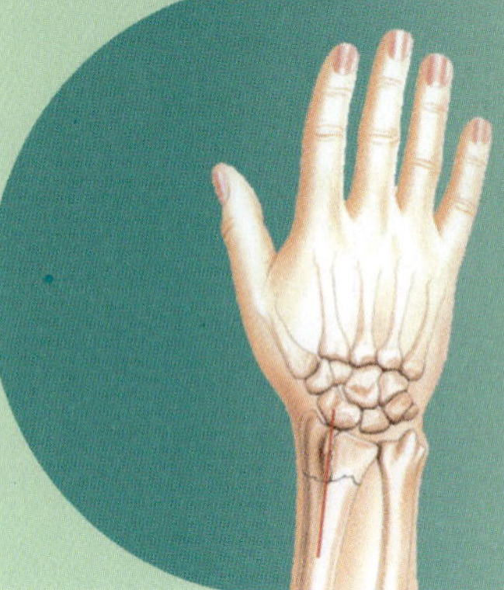

Syndactyly Release

Jennifer Waljee, Sandeep J. Sebastin, and Kevin C. Chung

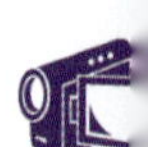

See Video 29: Syndactyly Release and Skin Grafting

See Video 30: Syndactyly Release with Pentagonal Flap

Indications

- Syndactyly release is indicated to improve aesthetic appearance, alleviate functional limitations, and prevent deformity due to growth restriction.
- Syndactyly release is usually performed between 12 and 18 months of age when the anatomic structures are larger and anesthesia is safer compared with younger ages. Long-term results are not compromised by waiting longer, although it is preferable to complete surgery before the child enters nursery school. An earlier release at about 6 months of age should be considered in children with syndactyly of the fourth web because the difference in length of the ring finger and small finger can lead to angulatory and rotatory deformities. Similarly, in children with complicated syndactyly, the first web space should be released at an earlier age.
- If the syndactyly involves more than one web space, it is safer to release contiguous web spaces at separate stages to avoid disrupting the blood supply to the finger between the web spaces.

Examination/Imaging

Clinical Examination

- Syndactyly is classified by the extent of fusion and the elements that are fused. Complete syndactyly involves the entire length of the fingers from the web to the tip (Fig. 36-1), whereas incomplete does not involve the entire length (Fig. 36-2). Simple syndactyly involves fusion of the skin only. Complex syndactyly describes fusion of the phalanges, usually the distal phalanx. Complicated syndactyly refers to fusion of multiple digits and is typically associated with other congenital anomalies such as Apert or Poland syndrome (Fig. 36-3).

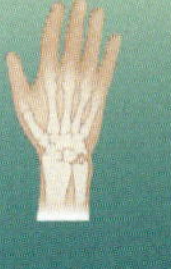

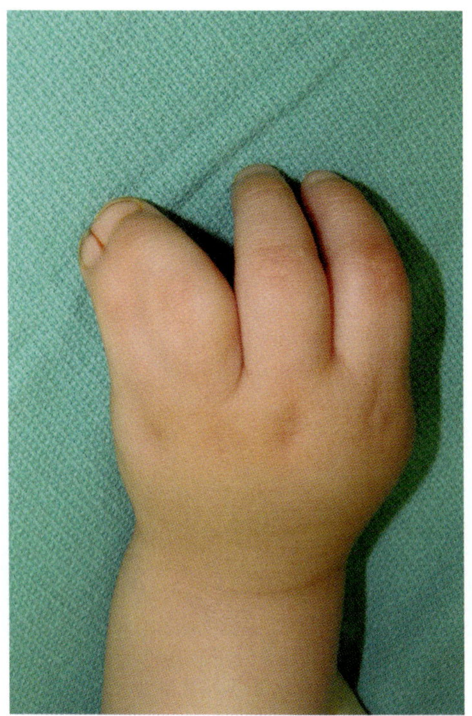

FIGURE 36-1

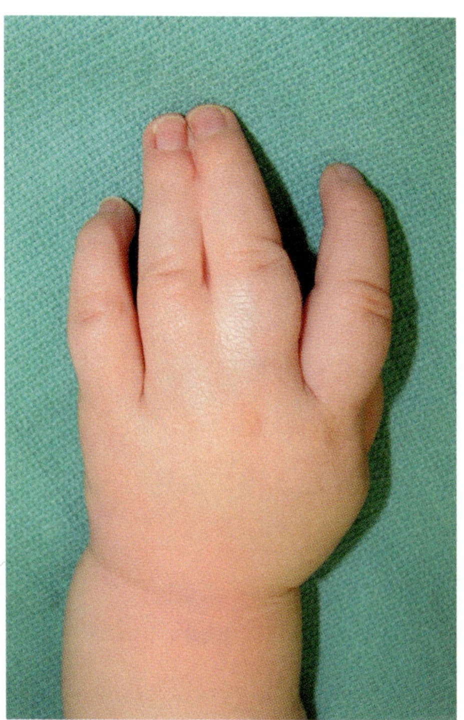

FIGURE 36-2

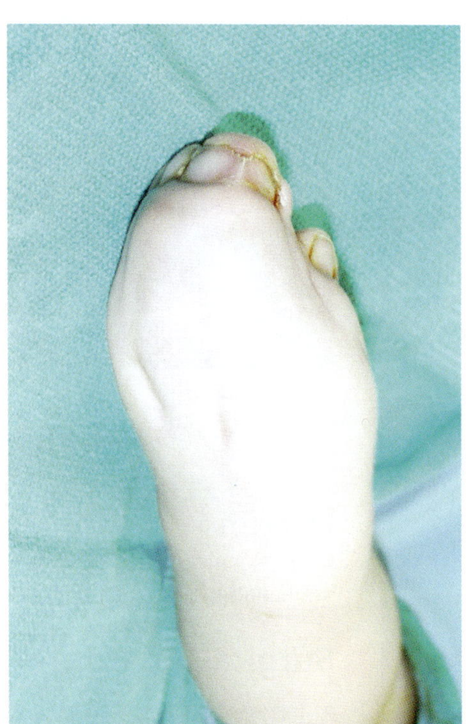

FIGURE 36-3

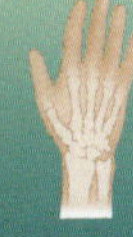

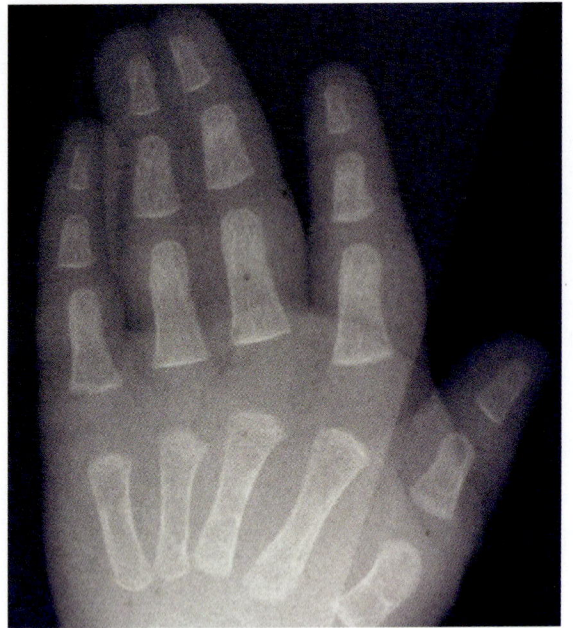

FIGURE 36-4

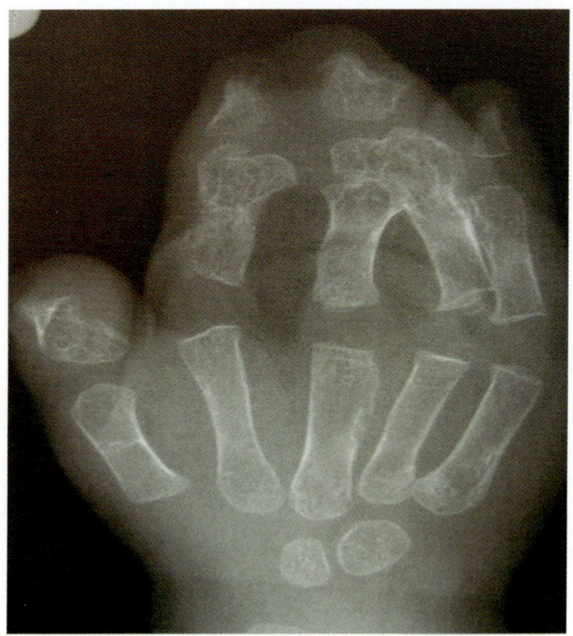

FIGURE 36-5

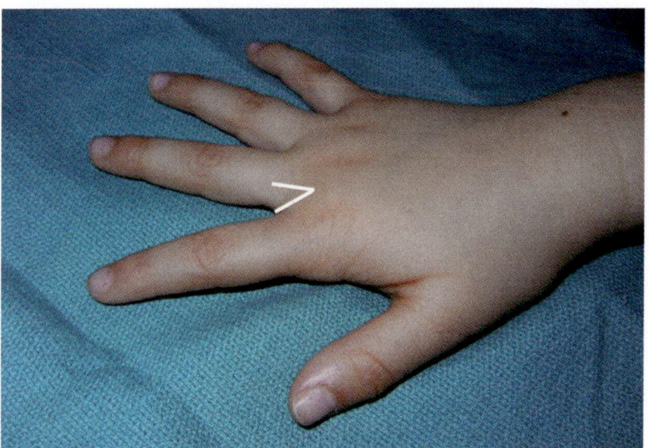

FIGURE 36-6

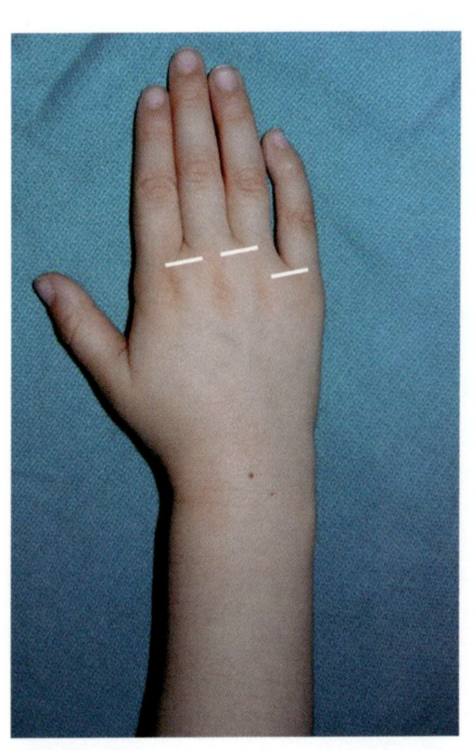

FIGURE 36-7

Imaging

- Preoperative radiographs can distinguish simple and complex syndactyly and the presence of additional skeletal elements (Figs. 36-4 and 36-5).

Surgical Anatomy

- The web space is U shaped, with a 45-degree slope from the metacarpal head to the midproximal phalanx (Fig. 36-6). The web space of the index and long finger is at the same level, whereas the web space of the fourth web is more proximal (Fig. 36-7).

Positioning

- The patient is placed supine on the operating room table with the entire upper extremity prepared into the field. The groin is also prepared into the field in the event that a full-thickness skin graft is needed.

Positioning Equipment

- A tourniquet is applied to the upper extremity.

General Principles

- The new web space should be created more proximal than normal to account for web creep with growth of the child.
- A flap should be used to resurface the web space. The use of skin grafts should be avoided in the web spaces.
- An interdigitating flap design should be used for coverage of digits. However, if primary flap closure is tight, there should be no hesitation in using a full-thickness skin graft.

Procedure

Release of Simple Complete Syndactyly

Exposures

- A proximally based dorsal rectangular flap for web reconstruction, along with interdigitating flaps, is used.
- The proximally based dorsal rectangular flap is designed by marking the metacarpal heads and a point on each digit at the midpoint of the proximal phalanx. The points are connected to form a proximally based flap with its base at the level of the metacarpal heads (Fig. 36-8).

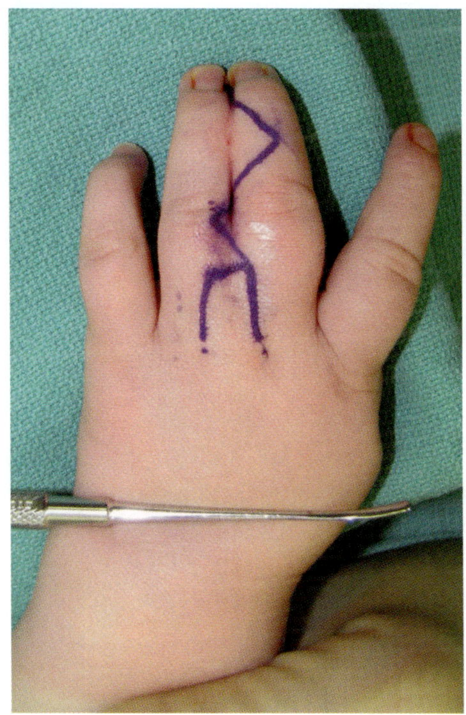

FIGURE 36-8

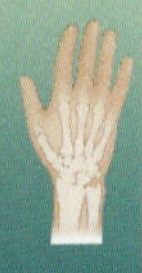

PEARLS

For separation of long and ring finger syndactyly, a rectangular flap is designed over the volar skin to cover the radial side of the ring finger. Having supple skin over the ring finger will make it more comfortable to fit a ring over the finger (Fig. 36-11).

- The interdigitating flaps are designed as two Zs, one on the dorsum and the other on the palmar surface, such that they form mirror images. The dorsal Z is designed first and connects the following four points sequentially (Fig. 36-9):
  - *Point A:* Distal corner of previously designed rectangular flap
  - *Point B:* Midpoint of the proximal interphalangeal (PIP) joint dorsal crease of the adjacent digit
  - *Point C:* Midpoint of mid-middle phalanx of the adjacent digit
  - *Point D:* Midpoint of the distal interphalangeal (DIP) joint dorsal crease of adjacent digit
- For the flaps to interdigitate, the tips of the palmar and dorsal Zs must oppose each other. A 25-gauge needle is inserted through the skin from the dorsum to the palmar surface at the same level as the tip of the proximal dorsal flap (point B), and a palmar flap is designed such that the tip is on the other finger (Fig. 36-10A). The remainder of the mirror palmar incision is then designed (Fig. 36-10B).

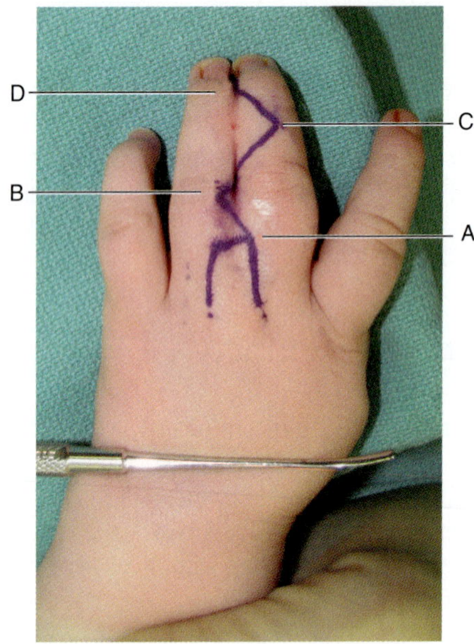

FIGURE 36-9

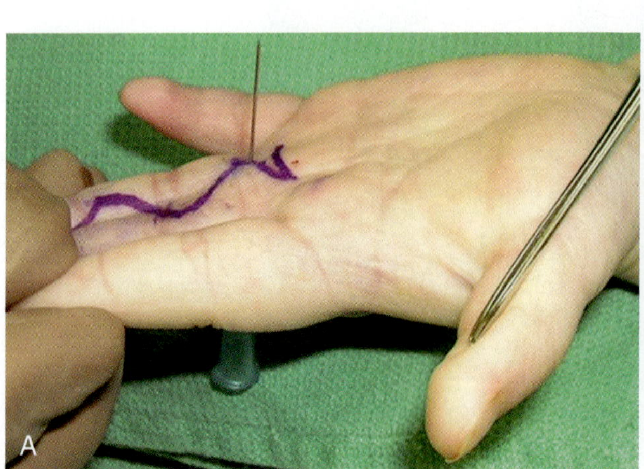

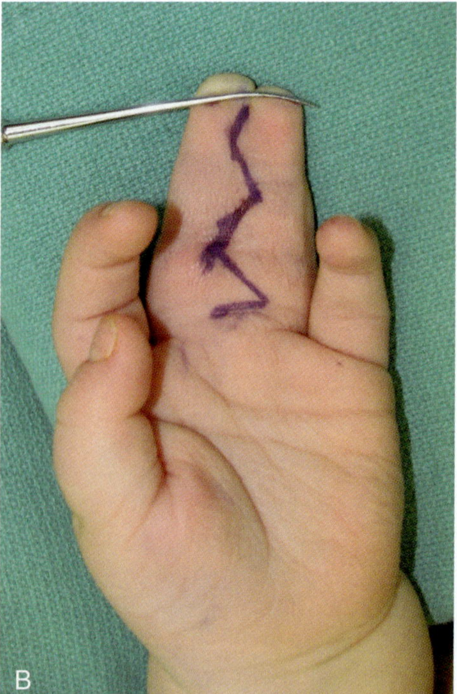

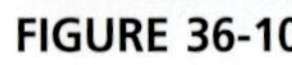

FIGURE 36-10

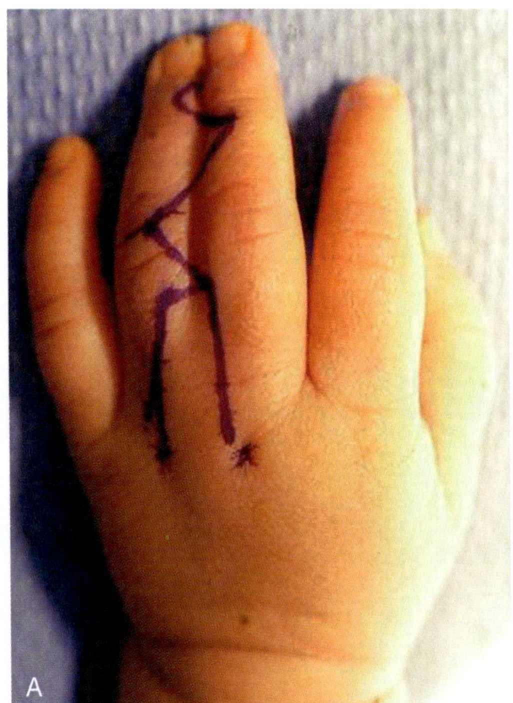

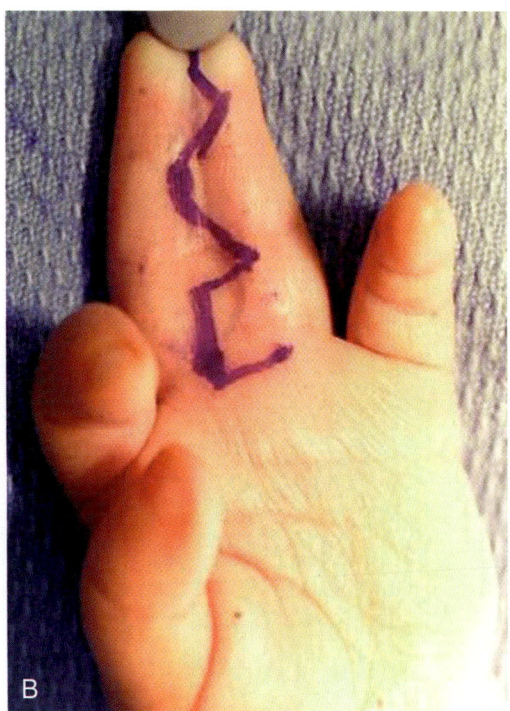

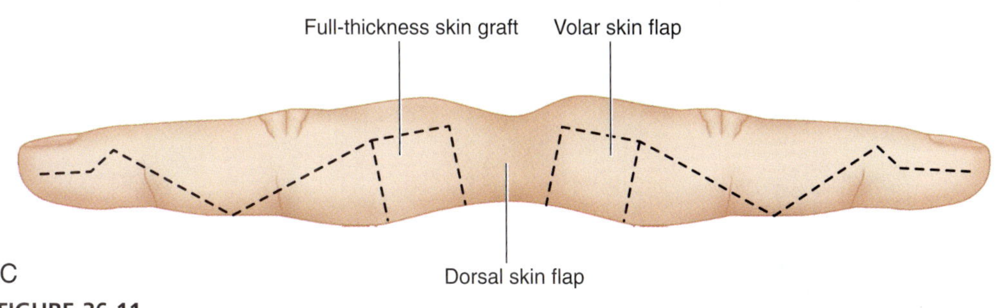

FIGURE 36-11

STEP 1 PEARLS

The dorsal and palmar skin flaps are elevated only to the edge of the finger. Further dissection does not improve movement of the flap significantly and unnecessarily exposes the tendons.

Opposing flaps are designed at the distal fingertip to be inset along the paronychial fold (Fig. 36-12A and B).

STEP 1 PITFALLS

Care is taken not to devascularize the skin flaps by creating flaps that are excessively thin.

Step 1: Flap Elevation

- The incisions are made, and the designed skin flaps are elevated.

Step 2: Separation of Digits

- The distal fingertip with nail plate is divided sharply with tenotomy scissors (Fig. 36-13).
- The longitudinal neurovascular structures are identified and protected (Fig. 36-14).
- Tenotomy scissors are used to spread between the digits in a transverse direction as the fused digits are retracted laterally. The transverse fascial bands are identified and divided sharply. This dissection is begun distally and continued proximally until the digits are completely released at the level of the transverse intermetacarpal ligament, which is spared (Fig. 36-15).

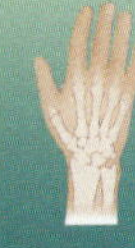

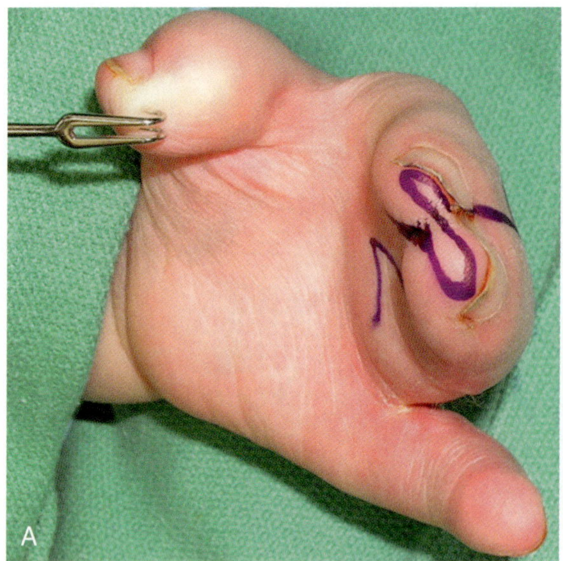

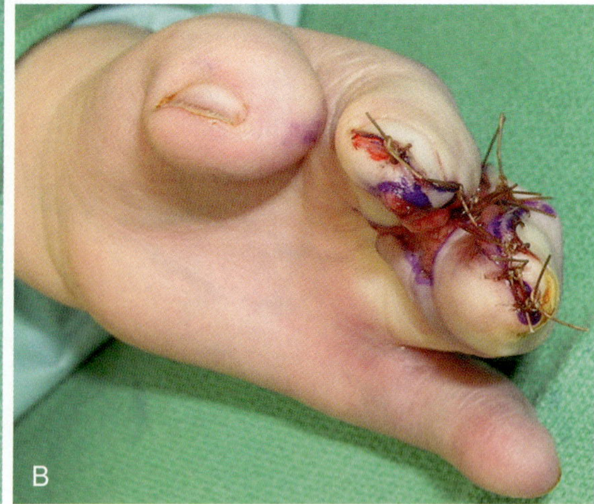

FIGURE 36-12

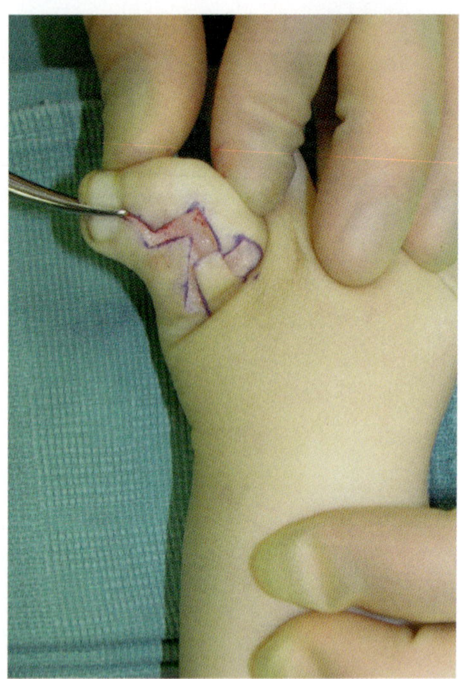

FIGURE 36-13

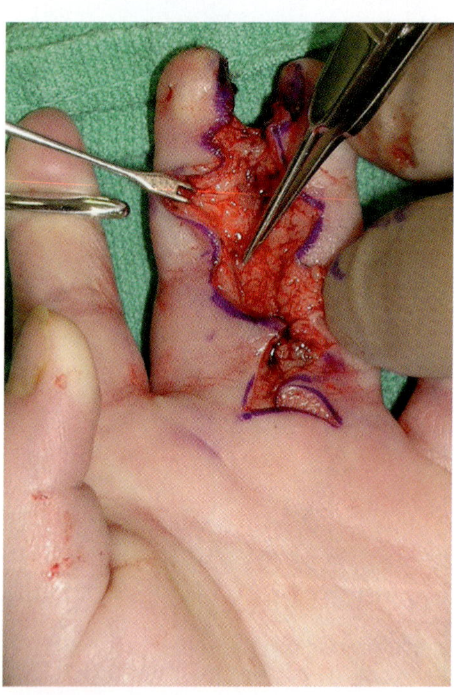

FIGURE 36-14

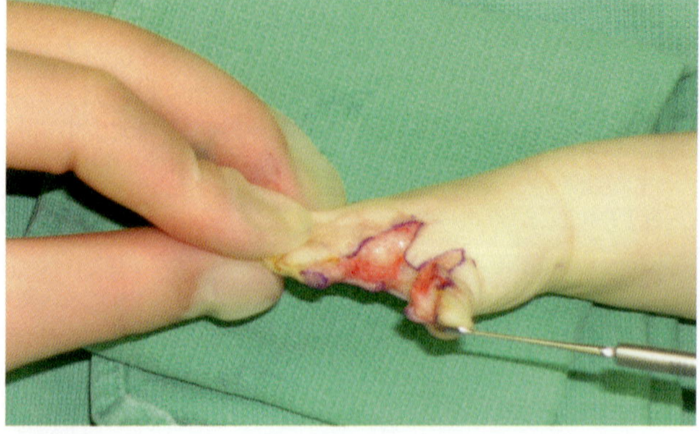

FIGURE 36-15

STEP 3 PEARLS

It is important not to suture the interdigitating flaps under tension. It is preferable to leave small raw areas. These will seal and close over time. Larger raw areas will need a full-thickness skin graft.

Step 3: Inset of Skin Flaps

- The dorsal skin flap is advanced into the new web space and secured with 4-0 absorbable (chromic) suture. The skin flap should easily advance into the new web space without tension (Fig. 36-16).
- The interdigitating flaps are inset across the digits (Figs. 36-17 and 36-18).

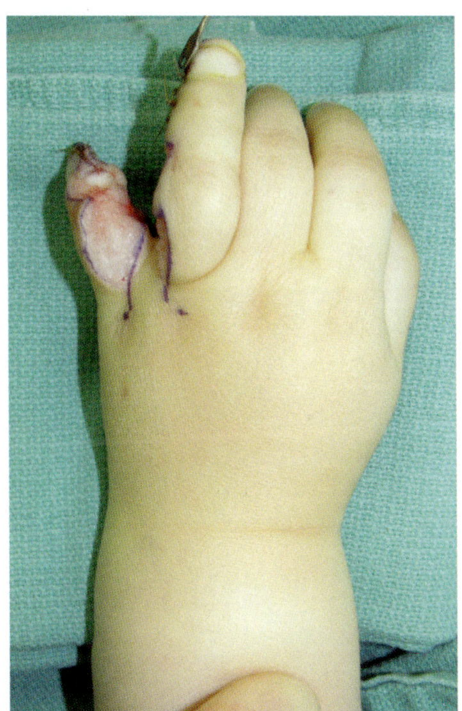

FIGURE 36-16

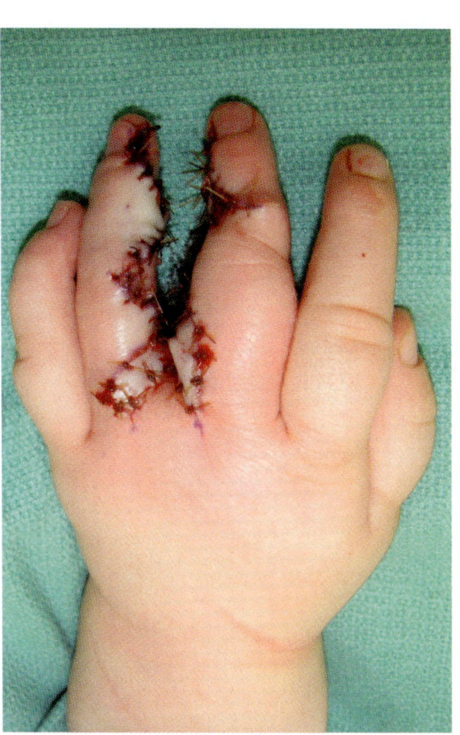

FIGURE 36-17

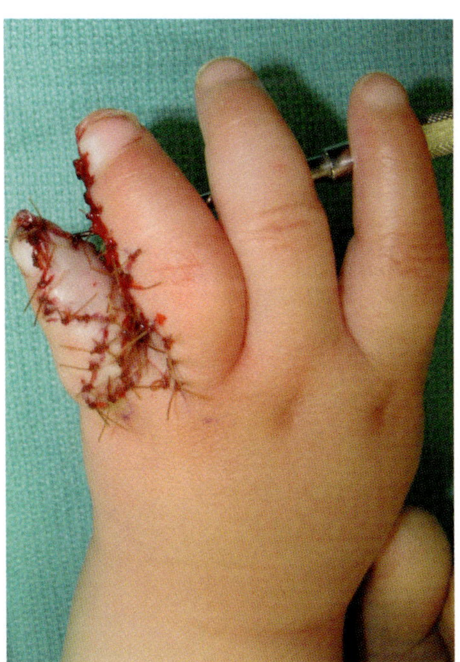

FIGURE 36-18

Step 4: Harvest of Full-Thickness Skin Graft from the Groin

- Areas that are not covered with these skin flaps are grafted with a full-thickness skin graft harvested from the groin (Fig. 36-19). An elliptical incision is made along the groin crease, and the skin and dermis are incised with a no. 15 scalpel.
- The skin and dermis are elevated sharply using a scalpel or tenotomy scissors. Any additional subcutaneous fat that is taken with the graft is removed sharply with tenotomy scissors.
- The skin graft is then cut to fill any additional defects not covered by the interdigitating flaps. It is preferable to leave fewer, larger gaps to be filled by a skin graft, rather than multiple small areas, because these will make it technically easier to contour the skin graft to the defect.
- The skin graft donor site is closed using a few dermal sutures with absorbable suture, and the skin is approximated with chromic suture.

STEP 4 PEARLS

Scars in the groin invariably spread over time, regardless of the manner in which they are closed. Therefore, we prefer to close these wounds with a few dermal sutures and a simple running closure using a chromic suture. These scars can be revised at a later date if the patient desires (Fig. 36-20).

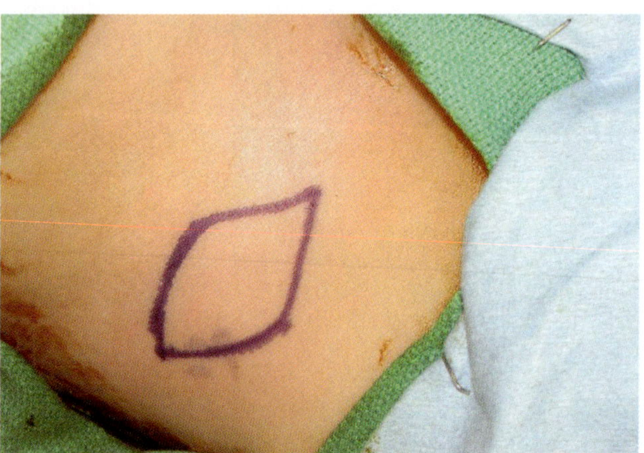

FIGURE 36-19

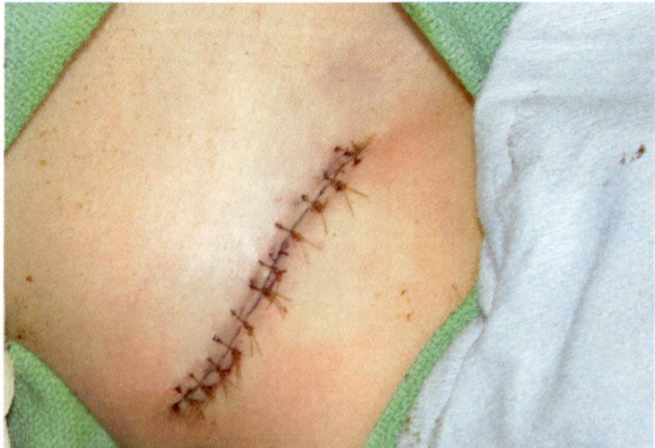

FIGURE 36-20

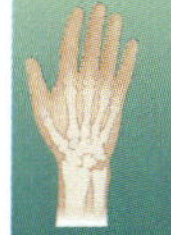

Procedure

Release of Simple Complete Syndactyly and Use of Dorsal Pentagonal Flap

Exposures

- The dorsal pentagonal island flap is based on a constant cutaneous perforator of the dorsal metacarpal artery that arises in the intermetacarpal space at the level of the neck of the metacarpal (Fig. 36-21). This flap design is useful in patients who have a relatively lax simple syndactyly or an incomplete simple syndactyly, where it is felt that a skin graft may not be required for coverage of the digital raw areas. In such cases, the dorsal pentagonal flap is better than the standard proximally based dorsal rectangular flap because (1) a larger flap can be designed on the dorsum of the hand to resurface the web space and sides of the finger simultaneously, (2) the island design allows the flap to advance further than the standard proximally based flap, and (3) the lax dorsal skin permits primary closure of the flap donor site. However, the senior author does not use this flap design if a skin graft is required for coverage of the digit (e.g., tight syndactyly, complex syndactyly) because the time saved by doing this flap is negated by use of skin grafts. Additionally, a prominent dorsal scar is created.

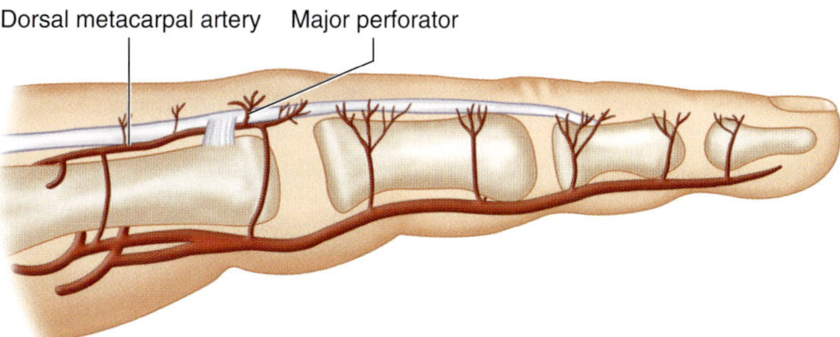

FIGURE 36-21

- The flap is designed by marking the metacarpal heads and outlining a pentagonal flap to incorporate the perforating vessel that arises at the level of the metacarpal neck. This perforating vessel is not visualized in the flap elevation. The V-shaped portion of the flap is designed proximally for primary closure, and a curved incision is made 2 mm distal to the head of the metacarpals to match the curved incision over the volar web space (Fig. 36-22).
- This flap is combined with interdigitating flaps as described previously (Fig. 36-23).

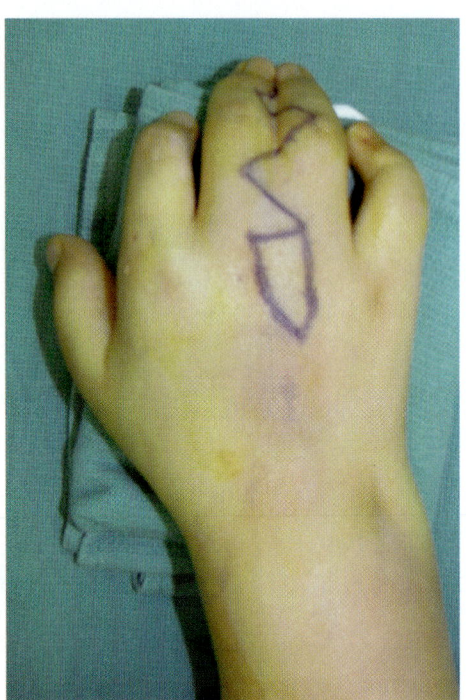

FIGURE 36-22

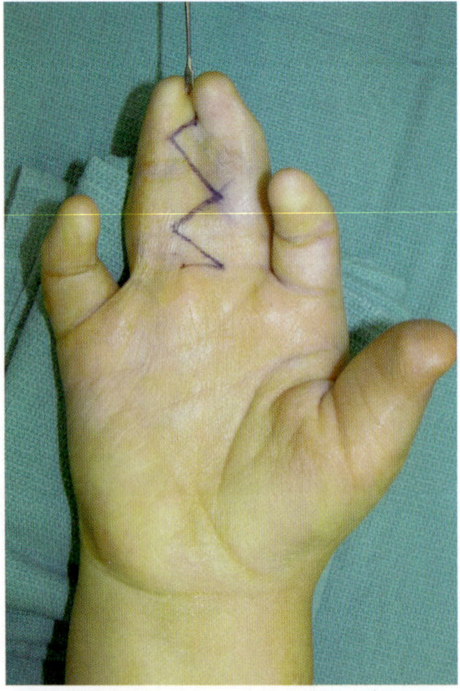

FIGURE 36-23

STEP 1 PEARLS

The fine crossing veins should be preserved (see Fig. 36-24).

Identifying the perforating vessel between the heads of the metacarpals is not necessary.

Step 1: Flap Elevation

- The pentagonal flap is incised, and scissors are used to separate the flap from the adhering septa so that the flap can be more mobile (Fig. 36-24).
- The flap is mobilized in a plane superficial to the paratenon.

Step 2: Separation of Digits

- The digits are separated as described previously (Fig. 36-25).

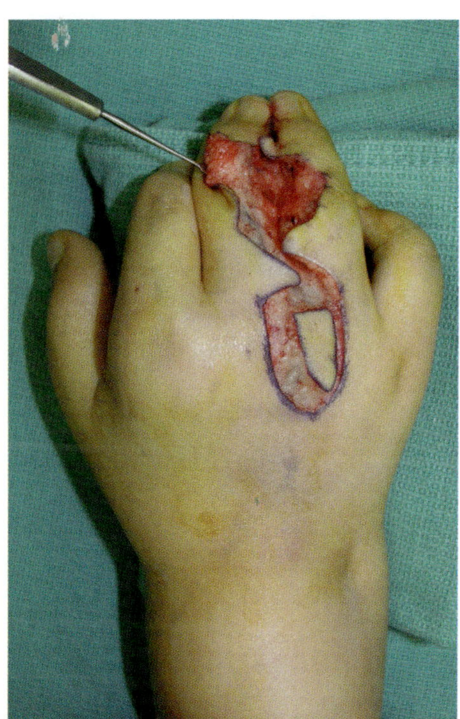

FIGURE 36-24

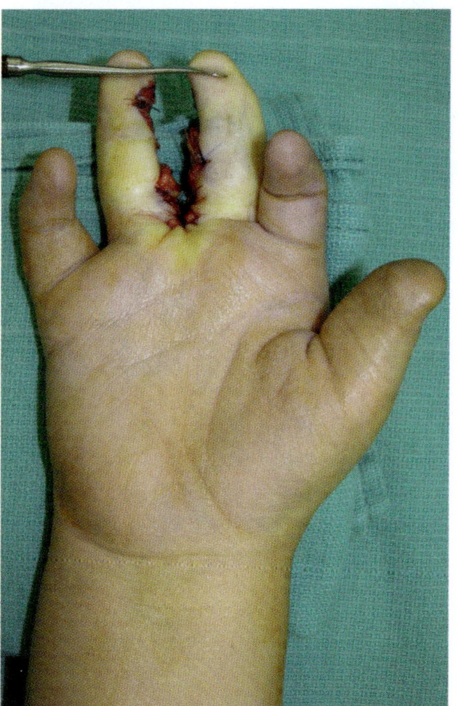

FIGURE 36-25

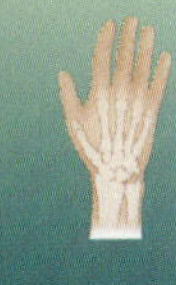

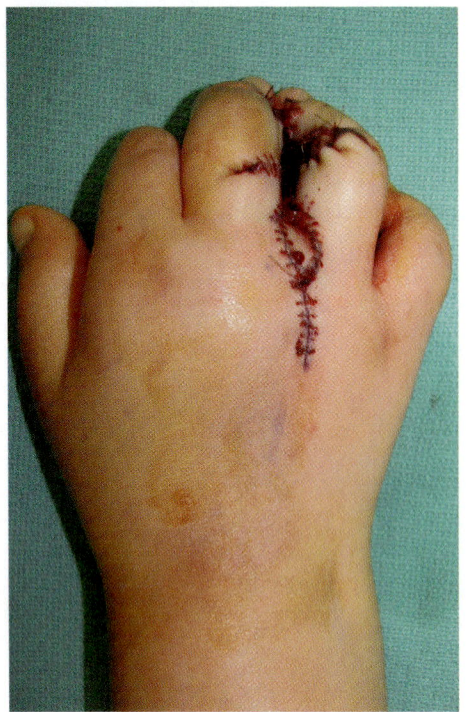

FIGURE 36-26

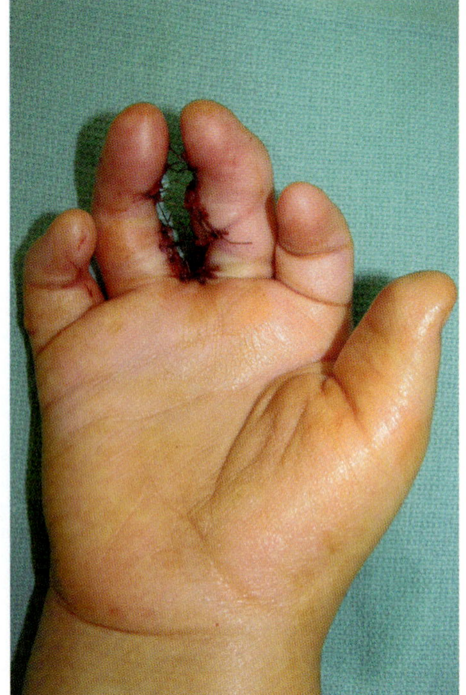

FIGURE 36-27

Step 3: Inset of Skin Flaps

- The flap is advanced and sutured to the volar web skin (Fig. 36-26).
- The interdigitating flaps are inset across the digits (Fig. 36-27).

STEP 3 PEARLS

The flap will be tight during the advancement, and small defects will seal and close over time.

Postoperative Care and Expected Outcomes

- Dressings are applied to provide compression along the skin graft sites.
- The hand is immobilized for 2 weeks to prevent shear injury to the grafts. Hand use may resume in 2 weeks when dressings are removed. No therapy is necessary in children, but scar massage exercises should be taught to the parents when the wound is healed to decrease scar thickness. If the web space is still not fully healed, parents must be taught to put Xeroform gauze between the fingers to prevent the open wounds from healing to each other.

PEARLS

Web creeping can occur with normal hand growth and can be prevented by releasing the border digits early in life and by overcompensating the web space deepening at the time of the procedure.

Arthrodesis can be performed in cases of complex syndactyly with joint instability or skeletal deformity, if the patient has reached skeletal maturity.

PITFALLS

Short-term complications following syndactyly release include skin necrosis, skin graft failure, digital nerve injury, and digital vessel injury resulting in digit ischemia.

In the long term, web creeping and scar contracture may occur, requiring revision surgery, including scar release and skin graft placement.

Keloid scarring has been reported in 1% to 2% of patients.

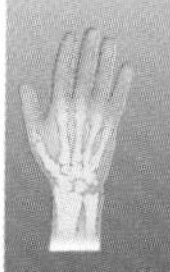

Evidence

Chang J, Danton TK, Ladd AL, Hentz VR. Reconstruction of the hand in Apert syndrome: a simplified approach. *Plast Reconstr Surg*. 2002;109:465-470.
This case series of 10 patients with Apert syndrome and hand deformities provides a concise and thorough summary of the principles of reconstruction and digit release in the patients with complex syndactyly. (Level V evidence)

Lumenta, DB, Kitzinger HB, Beck H, Frey M. Long-term outcomes of web-creep, scar quality, and function after simple syndactyly surgical release. *J Hand Surg [Am]*. 2010;35:1323-1329.
This review of 19 patients with syndactyly describes the incidence of scar contracture and web creep following digit release. The authors used a palmar and dorsal triangular skin flap with interdigitating zigzag incisions for separation of the digits. Full-thickness skin grafting was used in all cases. Over a long postoperative follow-up period (mean, 11.5 years), the incidence of scar contracture and web creep remained low with the use of full-thickness skin grafting. (Level V evidence)

Sherif MM. V-Y dorsal metacarpal flap: a new technique for correction of syndactyly without skin graft. *Plast Reconstr Surg*. 1998;101:1861-1866.
This report details the use of a V-Y island flap for web space reconstruction in 12 patients with syndactyly. The advantages of this approach include reduced operating time and the avoidance of skin grafting. (Level V evidence)

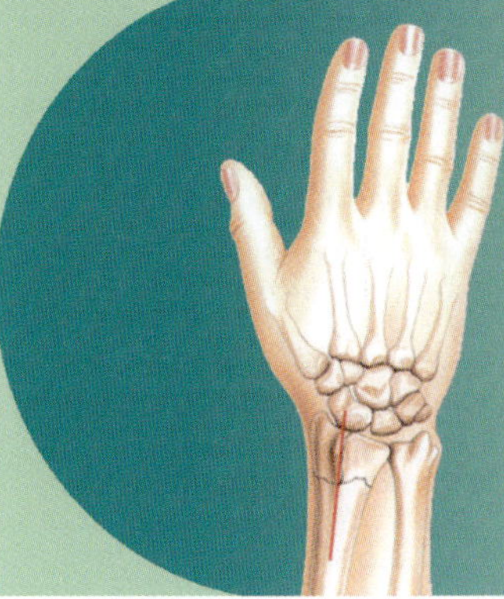

Duplicated Thumb Reconstruction

Jennifer Waljee, Sandeep J. Sebastin, and Kevin C. Chung

See Video 31: Duplicated Thumb Reconstruction

Indications

- The goal of thumb reconstruction is to restore an acceptable appearance without compromising existing function. Although a child with thumb duplication can function perfectly without reconstruction, the stigma associated with an uncorrected deformity may be unacceptable for the child or the parents, or both.
- Reconstruction should be considered at about 12 months of age, before the development of significant deviation deformity and because of the ease of general anesthesia. Furthermore, dissection of anatomic structures is easier compared with younger ages, and the development of pinch grasp occurs at about 12 months.

Examination/Imaging

Clinical Examination

- The classification of duplicated thumb is based on the level of duplication, which ranges from type I, which is partial split of the distal phalanx, to type VII, which is complete split of the metacarpal (Table 37-1). The type corresponds to the number of abnormal skeletal elements present. For example, type III has three abnormal bones (two distal phalanges and a partially split proximal phalanx). Wassel type IV is the most common type (Fig. 37-1).
- Genetic counseling is usually not necessary except for type VII, which is associated with other congenital anomalies and is inherited in an autosomal dominant pattern.
- The duplicated elements are abnormal in size and shape, and the radial duplicate is typically smaller in size. The surgeon should examine the thumb for the level of duplication, the degree of hypoplasia of each component, stability of the involved joints, and position of the thumb with respect to the bony axis and first web space.

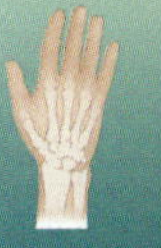

Table 37-1 Classification of Thumb Duplication

Wassel Type	Anatomic Description	%
I	Bifid distal phalanx	4
II	Duplicated distal phalanx sharing common distal interphalangeal joint articulation	16
III	Bifid proximal phalanx	11
IV	Duplicated proximal phalanx sharing common metacarpal articulation	40
V	Bifid metacarpal	10
VI	Duplicated metacarpal sharing common carpal articulation	4
VII	Triphalangeal thumb	20

From Watt AJ, Chung KC. Duplication. *Hand Clin.* 2009;25:215-227.

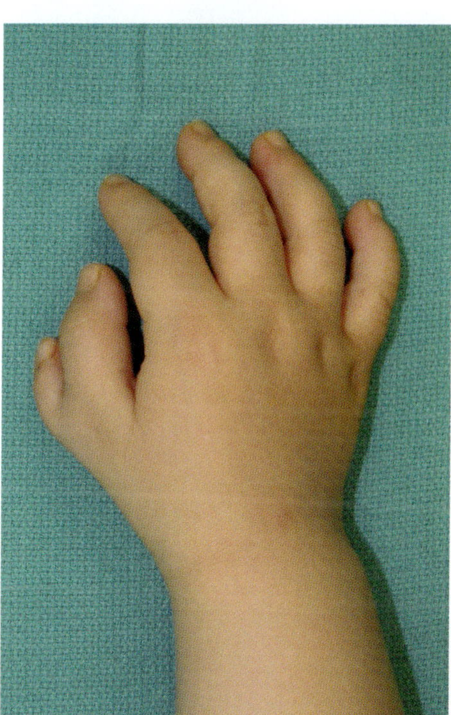

FIGURE 37-1

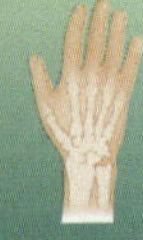

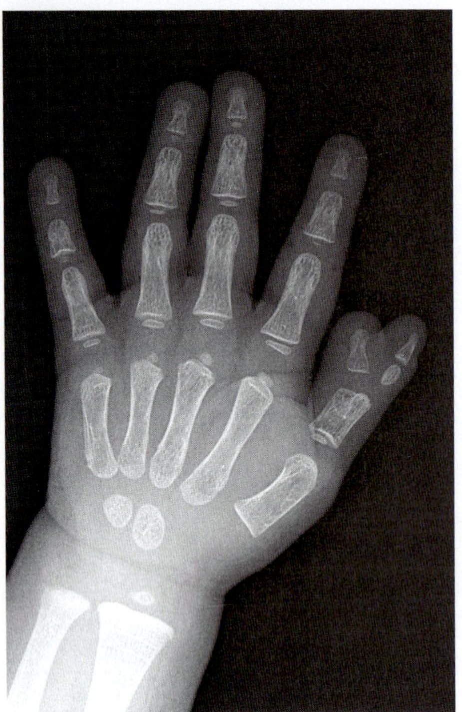

FIGURE 37-2

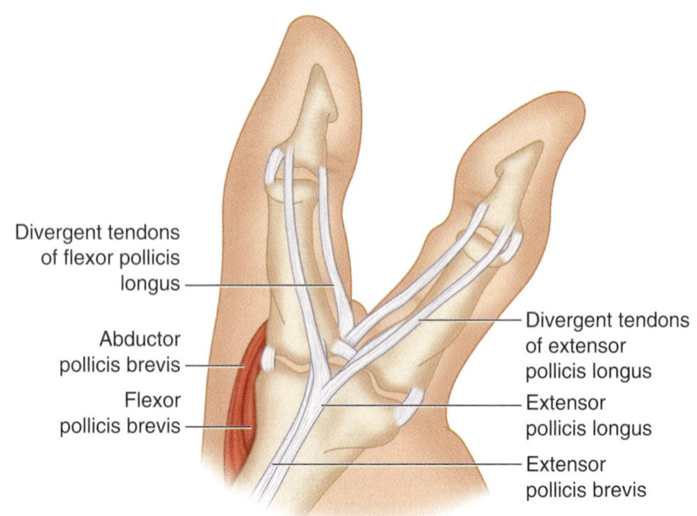

FIGURE 37-3

Imaging

- Preoperative radiographs are indicated to identify the size and number of duplicated skeletal elements and to determine whether the elements are attached (bifid) or separated (duplicate) (Fig. 37-2).
- The osseous anatomy is abnormal, with varying degrees of bony hypoplasia as well as widening and angulation of the articular surfaces.

Surgical Anatomy

- The flexor and extensor tendons are split and insert eccentrically. An abnormal connection between the flexor and extensor tendons on the radial aspect of the thumb often exists as well. The origins and insertions of the thenar musculature, particularly the opponens pollicis (OP), are aberrant in cases of proximal duplication. The abductor pollicis brevis (APB) and flexor pollicis brevis (FPB) insert into the proximal phalanx of the radial duplicate, whereas the OP inserts into the radial metacarpal. The net effect of the long flexor tendons is to pull the distal phalanges into convergence while the thenar insertions create divergence at the proximal phalangeal level, creating a zigzag deformity (Fig. 37-3).
- The arterial supply of the duplicated thumb most commonly consists of a single digital artery located on the ulnar side of the ulnar and radial duplicates, in 74% of cases. Twelve percent of patients exhibit three digital arteries, located on the radial and ulnar sides of the ulnar duplicate and the ulnar side of the radial duplicate. Ten percent of patients exhibit four digital arteries, and 5% maintain a single digital artery associated with the ulnar duplicate.
- Stability of the thumb is maintained by the ulnar collateral ligament, and typically the ulnar thumb is retained to preserve this structure.

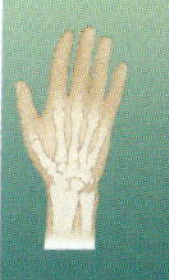

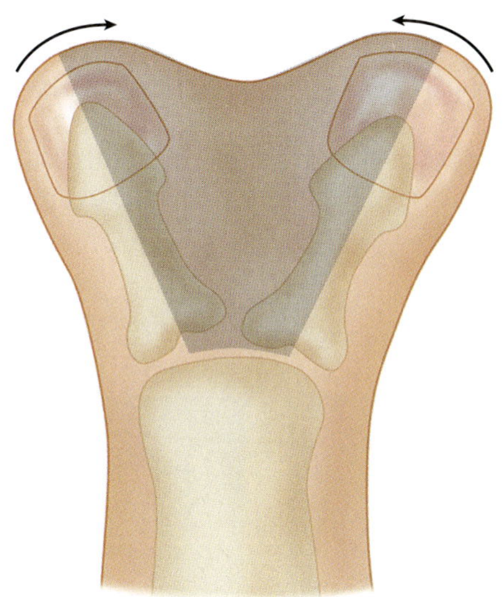

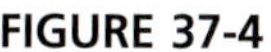

FIGURE 37-4

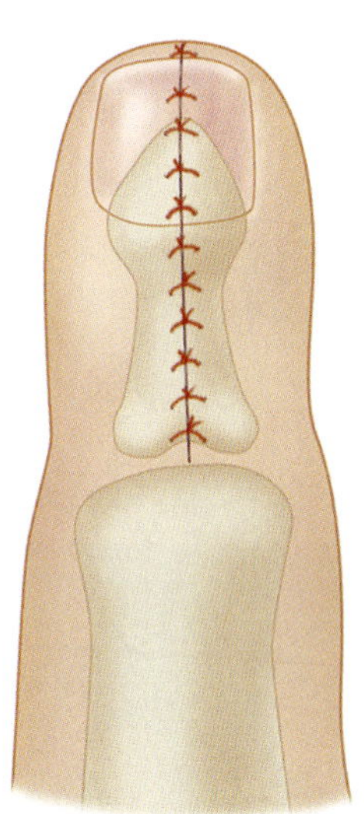

FIGURE 37-5

PEARLS

The Bilhaut-Cloquet procedure attempts to combine both thumbs into a single unit by removing the central portion of both thumbs to create a single thumb (Figs. 37-4 and 37-5). While conceptually appealing, it is exceedingly difficult to create an aesthetically pleasing thumb. A mismatch of the nail fold is common, and the cleft in the central combined thumb can be noticeable. It is preferable to accept a smaller thumb and use the soft tissue from the resected thumb to augment the size of the retained one.

Positioning

- The procedure is conducted under general anesthesia with the patient placed supine on the operating room table. The entire upper extremity is prepared and draped after a tourniquet is applied.
- Intraoperative fluoroscopy is often required, and the operative table is positioned to allow easy access for the C-arm.

Exposures

- When removing the radial thumb, one must retain a periosteal flap from the radial collateral ligament of the resected thumb to reconstruct the radial collateral ligament of the retained thumb. The extensor tendon from the resected thumb can be transferred to the ulnar side of the retained thumb for tendon.
- We describe the reconstruction of a type III and type IV thumb duplication.

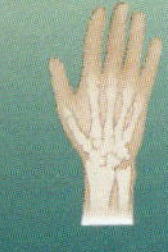

Procedure

Reconstruction of a Type III Thumb Duplication

Step 1

- The radial digit is selected for removal. A curvilinear, Y-shaped incision is made over the radial digit (Figs. 37-6 to 37-8).
- The soft tissues are dissected to the level of the radial aspect of the interphalangeal joint.
- The distal insertions of the flexor tendon, extensor tendon, and radial collateral ligament are carefully elevated off from the base of the distal phalanx of the radial duplicate.

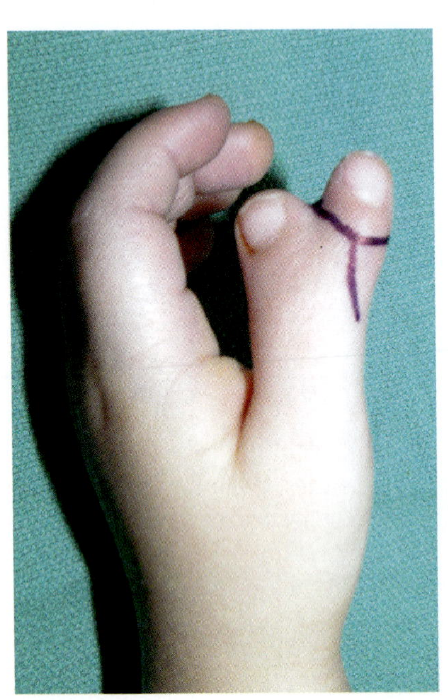

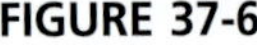

FIGURE 37-6

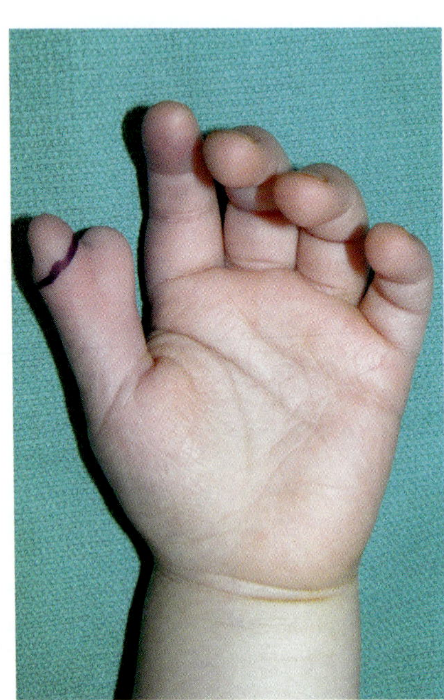

FIGURE 37-7

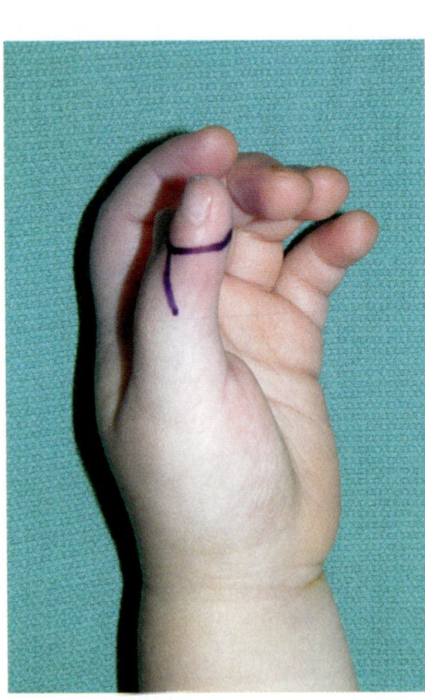

FIGURE 37-8

Step 2

- The radial duplicate thumb is excised at the level of the interphalangeal joint.

Step 3

- The redundant radial head of the proximal phalanx is removed, taking care to preserve the proximal attachment of the radial collateral ligament (Figs. 37-9 and 37-10).

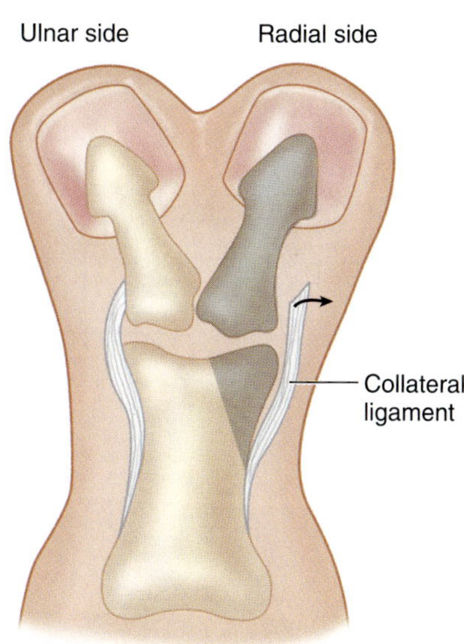

FIGURE 37-9

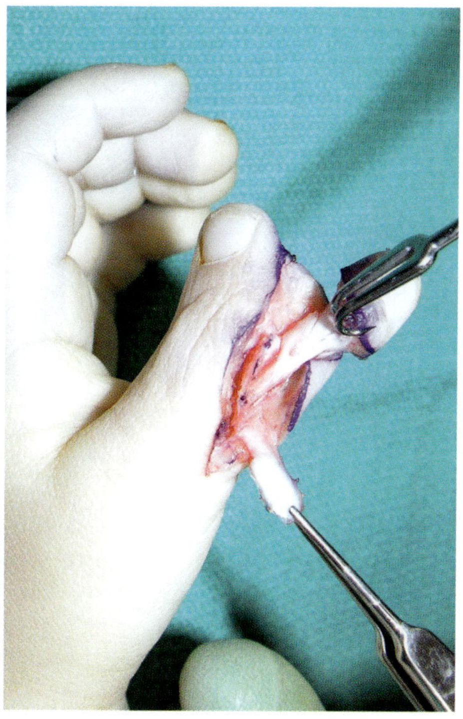

FIGURE 37-10

Step 4

- The retained distal phalanx is centralized over the proximal phalanx. A single longitudinal 0.045-inch Kirschner wire (K-wire) is passed through the distal and proximal phalanx in a retrograde fashion to act as an internal splint.

Step 5

- The radial collateral ligament is reattached to the retained thumb using 3-0 braided nonabsorbable suture (Fig. 37-11).

Step 6

- Deviation of the digit can be corrected by reattaching the previously elevated extensor and flexor insertions to the base of the distal phalanx of the retained thumb (Fig. 37-12).

Step 7

- The tourniquet is released and hemostasis secured. The skin is closed using chromic catgut. A Z-plasty can be designed to rearrange any redundant skin (Figs. 37-13 and 37-14).
- A thumb spica splint is applied to the arm.

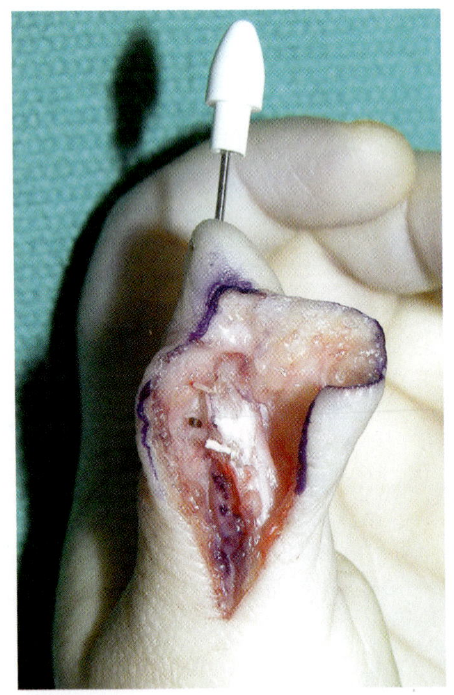

FIGURE 37-11

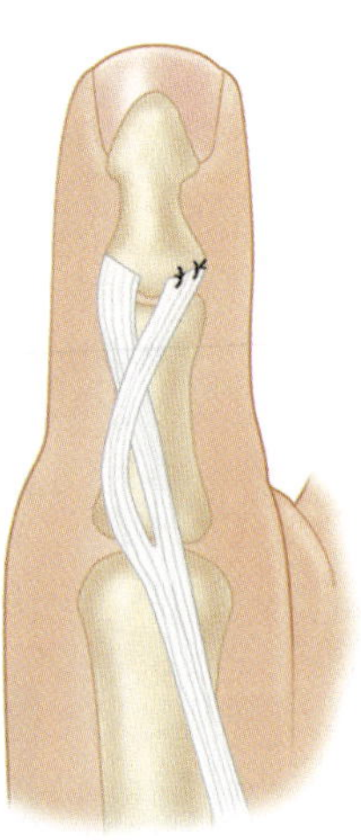

FIGURE 37-12

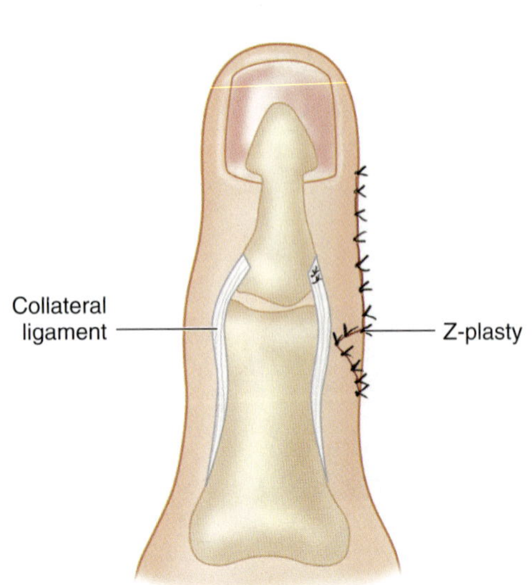

FIGURE 37-13

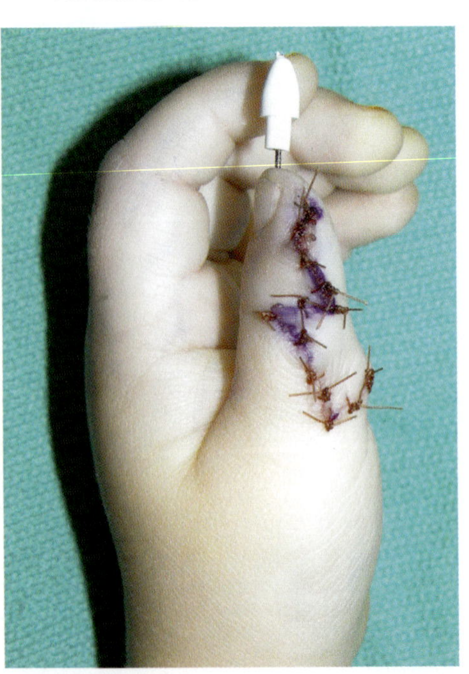

FIGURE 37-14

Procedure

Reconstruction of Type IV Thumb Duplication

Step 1

- The radial digit is selected for removal, and the skin incisions are designed as described previously (Figs. 37-15 and 37-16). The skin flaps are elevated sharply to expose the radial aspect of the metacarpophalangeal joint.
- The insertion of the APB is detached, and the radial collateral ligament is elevated off the base of the radial duplicate on a longitudinal periosteal flap (Fig. 37-17).
- The extensor and flexor tendons going to the duplicate thumb are divided distally at the level of the interphalangeal joint.

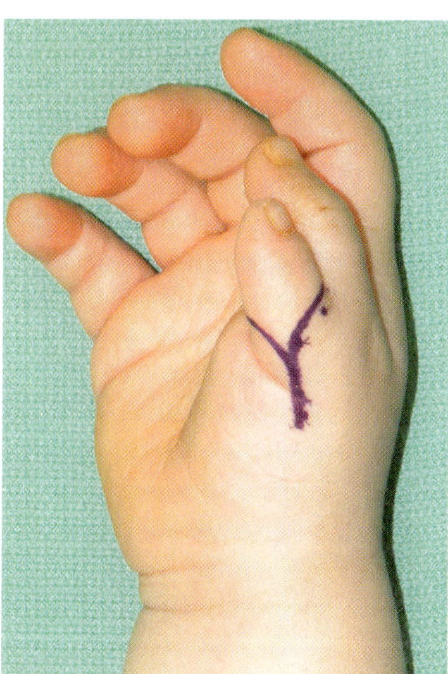

FIGURE 37-15

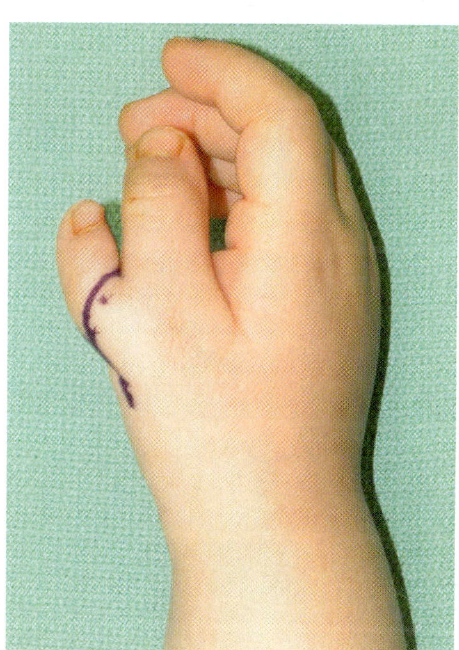

FIGURE 37-16

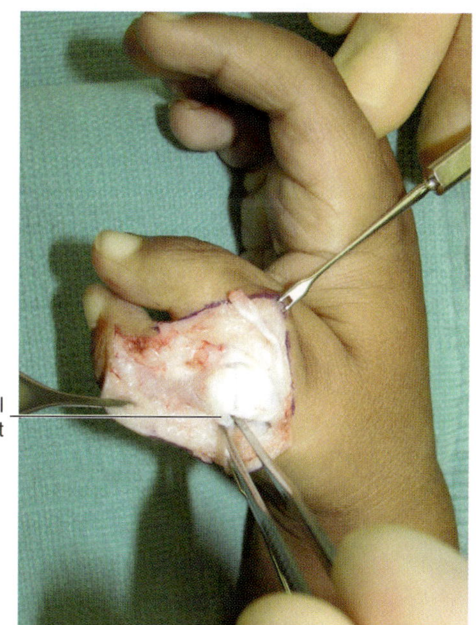

FIGURE 37-17

Step 2

- The dissection continues sharply to divide the attachments between the remaining thumb and the duplicated proximal phalanx, and the radial duplicated digit is removed (Fig. 37-18).

Step 3

- A partial osteotomy of the radial portion of the head of the metacarpal is done to reduce its prominence. This osteotomy is easily performed using the knife blade with a back-and-forth motion over the unossified metacarpal (Figs. 37-19 and 37-20). Care should be taken to preserve the origin of the radial collateral ligament during this osteotomy.

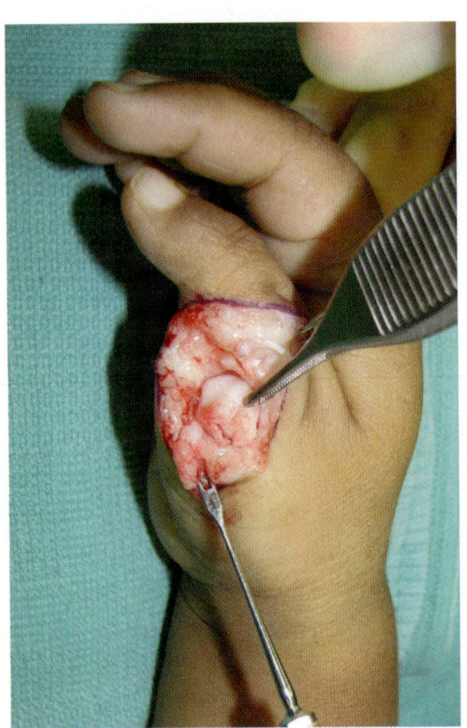

FIGURE 37-18

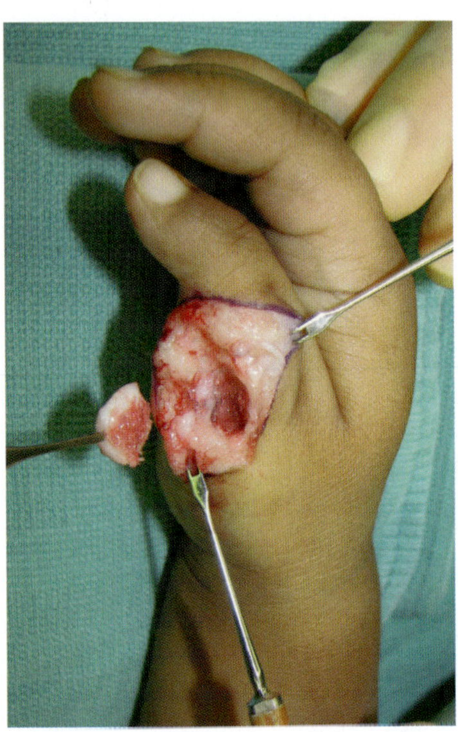

FIGURE 37-19

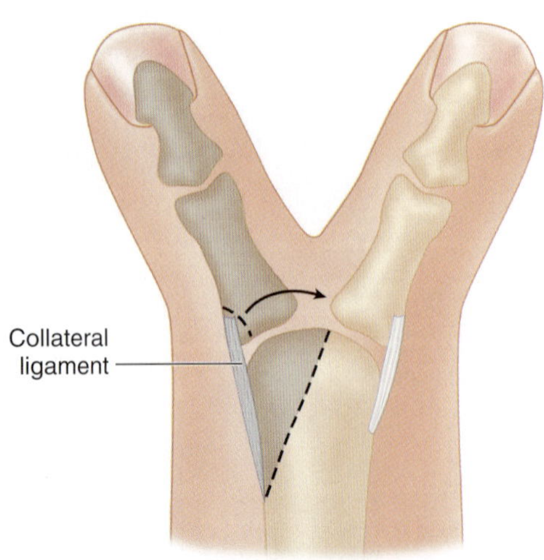

FIGURE 37-20

Step 4

- The thumb phalanges and metacarpal are aligned and pinned with an oblique 0.045-inch K-wire (Fig. 37-21).

Step 5

- The periosteal flap carrying the radial collateral ligament and the APB insertion is sutured to the radial base of the proximal phalanx using nonabsorbable braided suture. Additional sutures may be needed to reinfoirce the origin of the radial collateral liagment at the head of the metacarpal (Fig. 37-22).

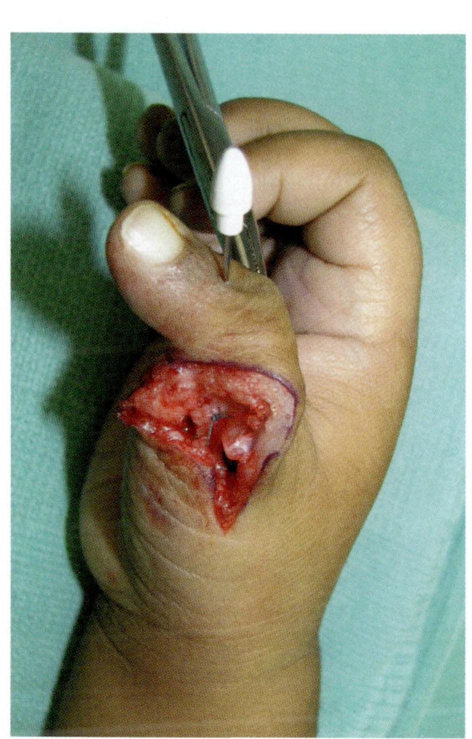

FIGURE 37-21

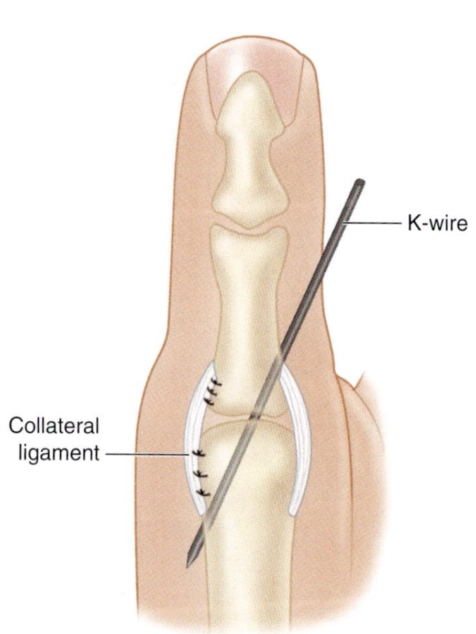

FIGURE 37-22

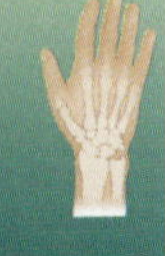

Step 6

- The extensor tendon from the resected thumb is passed subcutaneously from the ulnar incision and sutured to the ulnar distal phalanx of the retained thumb to balance the thumb and counteract the radial deforming force (Figs. 37-23 and 37-24).

Step 7

- The tourniquet is released and hemostasis secured. The skin is closed using chromic catgut. A Z-plasty can be designed to rearrange any redundant skin (Fig. 37-25).
- A thumb spica splint is applied to the arm.

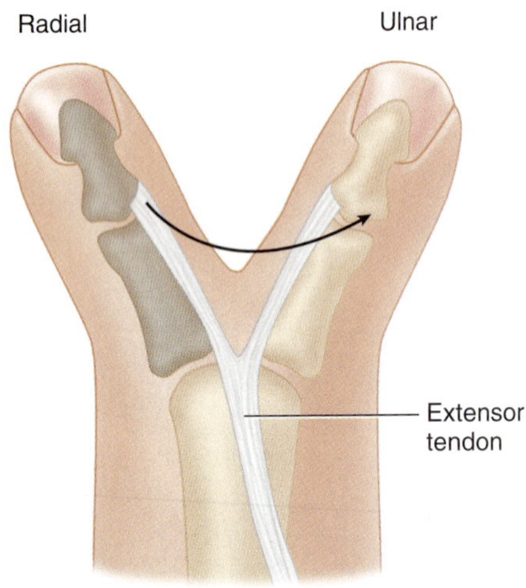

FIGURE 37-23

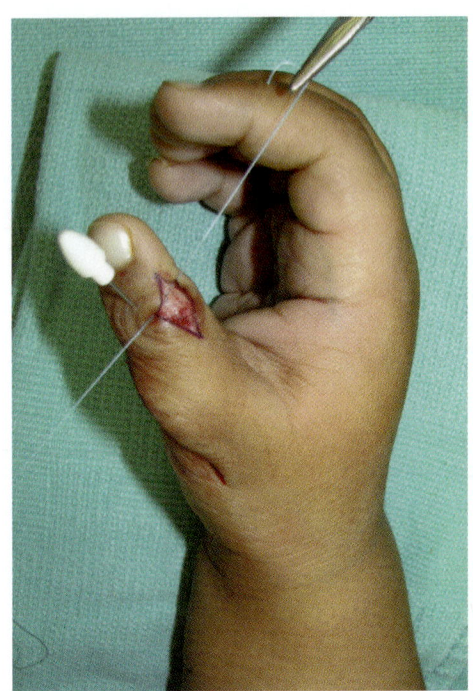

FIGURE 37-24

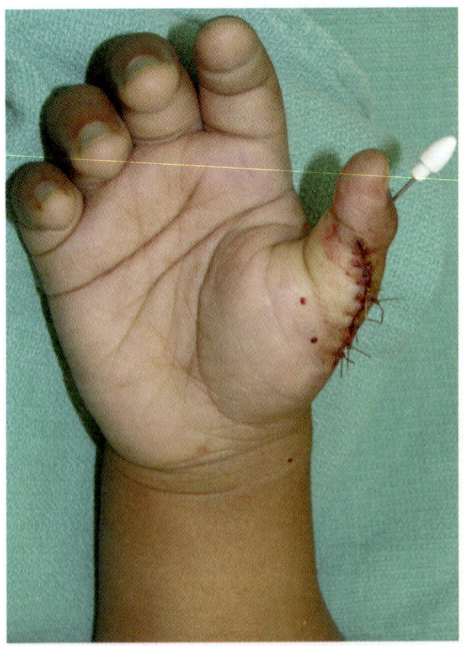

FIGURE 37-25

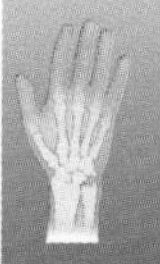

Postoperative Care and Expected Outcomes

- The K-wire is removed at 6 weeks after surgery.
- Development of a zigzag deformity is not uncommon during growth. These children should be followed yearly and corrective osteotomy performed to realign the thumb if progressive deviation is seen.

Evidence

Baek GH, Gong HS, Chung MS, et al. Modified Bilhaut-Cloquet procedure for Wassel type-II and III polydactyly of the thumb: surgical technique. *J Bone Joint Surg [Am]*. 2008;90:74-86.
The authors describe the Bilhaut-Cloquet technique for Wassel types II and III thumb duplication in 7 patients with 52-month follow-up. The authors describe the functional and aesthetic outcomes and their technique performing the procedure. Patients and parents reported satisfaction with the postoperative appearance. Range of motion at the interphalangeal joint was superior for type II duplications compared with type III duplications, and the authors report no episodes of nail deformity or growth arrest. (Level IV evidence)

Goldfarb CA, Patterson JM, Maender A, Manske PR. Thumb size and appearance following reconstruction of radial polydactyly. *J Hand Surg [Am]*. 2008;33: 1348-1353.
This article reviews the outcomes of 26 patients who underwent thumb reconstruction (31 thumbs) for duplication with a 3-year follow-up. Aesthetic appearance was measured by objective measurements and using a visual analogue scale. The authors report nearly symmetrical appearance of the contralateral thumb but decreased nail width. Angulation of the thumb was the most common cause of poor aesthetic outcome. (Level IV evidence)

Horii E, Hattori T, Koh S, Majima M. Reconstruction for Wassel type III radial polydactyly with two digits equal in size. *J Hand Surg [Am]*. 2009;34:1802-1807.
The authors describe their technique for ablation of the accessory radial thumb and collateral ligament reconstruction for thumb duplication in 13 patients with 2-year follow-up. The distal articular surface of the proximal phalanx was maintained, and the authors used the radial EPL to augment the strength of the ulnar EPL. The authors report excellent stability and alignment with this technique, but restricted range of motion at the interphalangeal joint. (Level V evidence)

Ogino T, Ishii S, Takahata S, Kato H. Long-term results of surgical treatment of thumb polydactyly. *J Hand Surg [Am]*. 1996;21:478-486.
The authors report one of the largest series of thumb reconstructions, with long-term follow-up of nearly 4 years. Wassel types III, V, VI, and VII and resection of ulnar-sided thumb yielded more unsatisfactory results. Results improved over the study period. The authors conclude that outcomes improve with surgeon experience. (Level IV evidence)

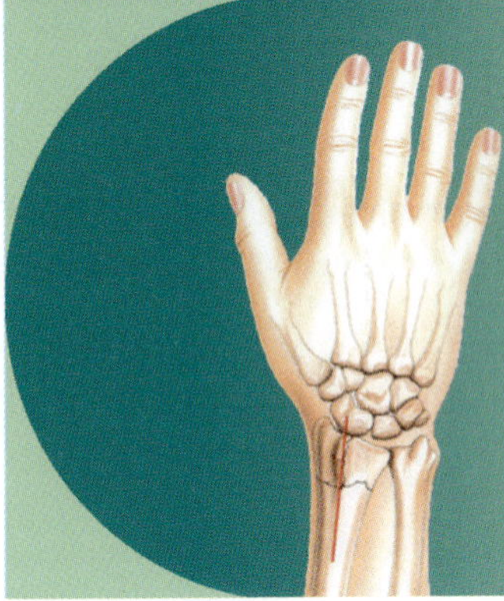

Reconstruction for Congenital Thumb Hypoplasia

Jennifer Waljee, Sandeep J. Sebastin, and Kevin C. Chung

Congenital thumb hypoplasia can vary from mild size discrepancy to complete absence. The Blauth classification is useful for categorizing the degree of development (Table 38-1). It is critical to assess the stability of the thumb carpometacarpal (CMC) joint to determine the appropriate surgical treatment for thumb hypoplasia. The goal of surgical intervention for children with a stable CMC joint (Blauth types I, II, and IIIA) is preservation of the existing thumb and augmentation of the deficient soft tissue elements. Conversely, if the CMC joint is unstable or absent (Blauth types IIIB, IV, and V), any remnants of the existing thumb should be ablated, and reconstruction should proceed by pollicizing the index finger. This chapter focuses on the reconstruction of Blauth types I, II, and IIIA hypoplasia.

Indications

- Congenital thumb hypoplasia is seen with a stable CMC joint with varying degrees of soft tissue deficiency (Blauth types I, II, and IIIA). The important soft tissue deficiencies are the following:
  - Narrow first web space (<50 degrees of radial thumb abduction)
  - Atrophic or absent thenar muscles leading to the inability to oppose the thumb to small finger
  - Attenuated or absent ulnar collateral ligament (UCL) of the metacarpophalangeal (MCP) joint with an unstable MCP joint (>20-degree difference in UCL laxity compared with the normal side)

Table 38-1 Blauth Classification of Thumb Hypoplasia and Treatment Options

Type	Features	Treatment Options
I	Mild hypoplasia with all elements present	No treatment
II	Narrow first web, ulnar collateral ligament insufficiency, and absence of thenar intrinsic muscles	No treatment Z-plasty of first web, UCL strengthening/reconstruction, and opponensplasty
III	Type II plus extrinsic tendon deficiencies and/or skeletal deficiency	
IIIA	Stable CMC joint	Same as type II
IIIB	Unstable CMC joint	Pollicization
IV	Absent metacarpal and rudimentary phalanges "Pouce flottant"	Pollicization
V	Total absence	Pollicization

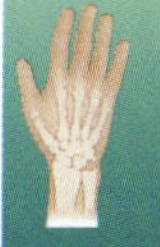

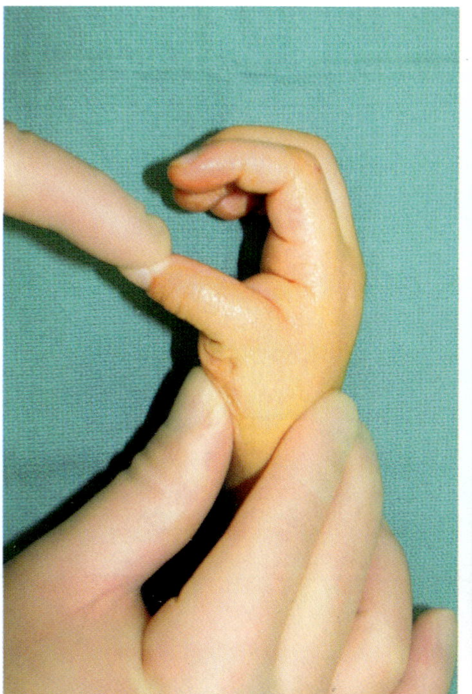

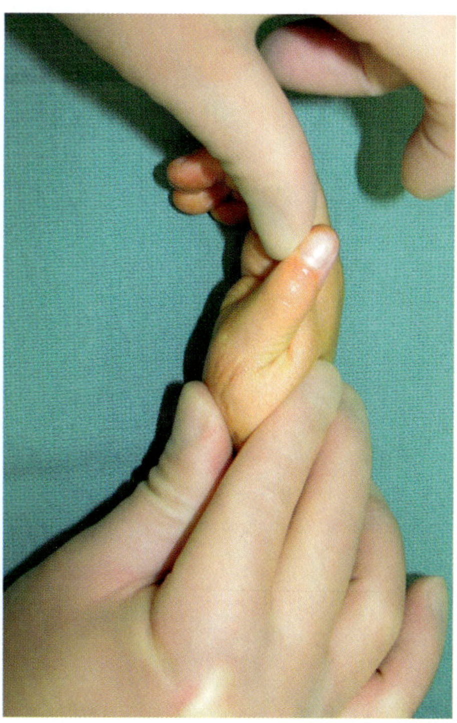

FIGURE 38-1

- Reconstructive procedures for thumb hypoplasia (Blauth types I, II, and IIIA) can be performed at a later age (2 to 4 years) because the child can use the thumb for activities without developing maladaptive compensation patterns. However, it is preferable to correct these deformities before the child enters school to avoid any stigma from an uncorrected deformity.

Examination/Imaging

Clinical Examination

- The child should be examined to assess the degree of first web narrowing, opposition function of the thumb, and stability of the thumb MCP joint (Fig. 38-1). Serial examination of a child is required to differentiate between Blauth types IIIA and IIIB. A newborn child uses digital grasp and begins to use the thumb in grasp at about 1 year of age. If the child uses the thumb in manipulating objects, this suggests that a type IIIA deficiency is present. If the child prefers to grasp objects between the index and long finger web space, this web space appears wider because the index finger is pronated toward the thumb. This suggests type IIIB hypoplasia because the child is incapable of using the unstable thumb for effective pinch.
- The entire upper extremity should be examined for other elements of radial deficiency, and patients should be examined for systemic manifestations of associated hematologic and cardiac syndromes such as Holt-Oram, thrombocytopenia-absent-radius (TAR) syndrome, VACTERL (i.e., *v*ertebral abnormalities, *a*nal atresia, *c*ardiac abnormalities, *t*racheoesophageal fistula and/or *e*sophageal atresia, *r*enal agenesis and dysplasia, and *l*imb defects), and Fanconi anemia.

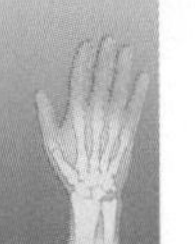

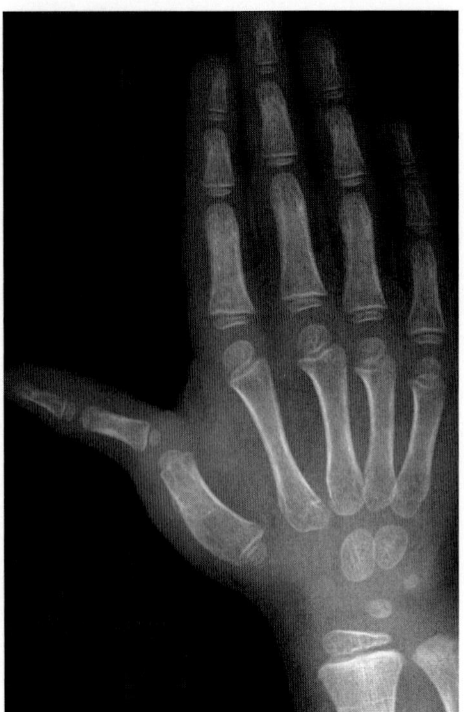

FIGURE 38-2

Imaging

- Radiographs of the hands, wrists, and forearms are useful in determining the degree of metacarpal and phalangeal hypoplasia of the thumb and index finger and can identify the presence of other associated upper extremity anomalies (Fig. 38-2).

Surgical Anatomy

- The anatomic deficiencies associated with thumb hypoplasia are detailed in Figure 38-3. The ulnar collateral ligament spans the MCP joint of the thumb and is lax in type II and type III thumbs.
- The intrinsic muscles of the thumb (abductor pollicis brevis [APB], opponens pollicis [OP], flexor pollicis brevis [FPB], and adductor pollicis [AP]) are deficient in types II and III and absent in types IV and V.
- The flexor pollicis longus (FPL) and extensor pollicis longus (EPL) are hypoplastic in type III thumbs. Often, there may be an anomalous connection between the FPL and the EPL at the level of the MCP joint, known as pollex abductus. This connection can attenuate the UCL over time and prevent active interphalangeal joint motion.

Positioning

- The procedure is conducted under general anesthesia with the patient placed supine on the operating room table. The entire upper extremity is prepared and draped after a tourniquet is applied.

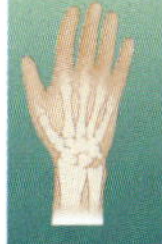

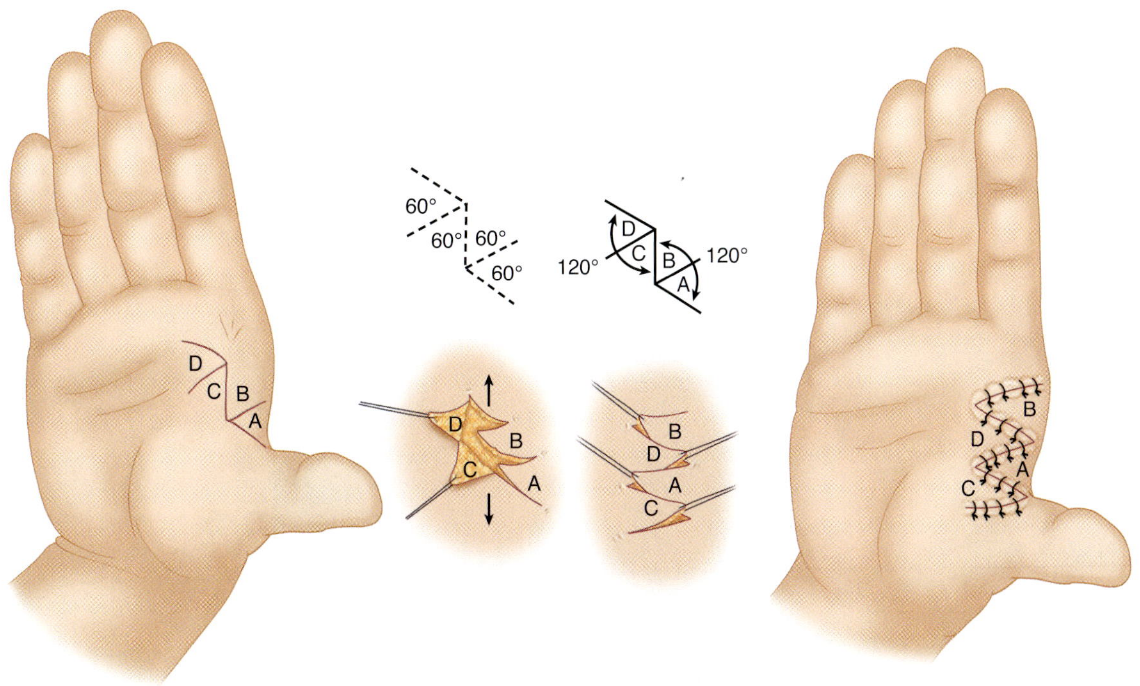

FIGURE 38-5

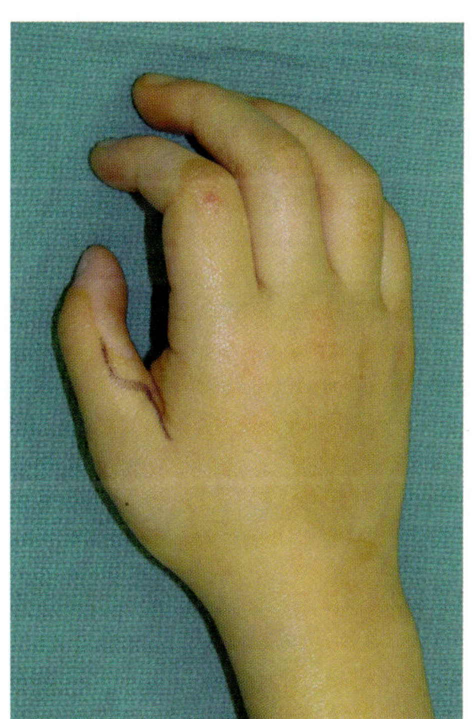

FIGURE 38-6

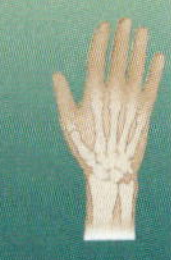

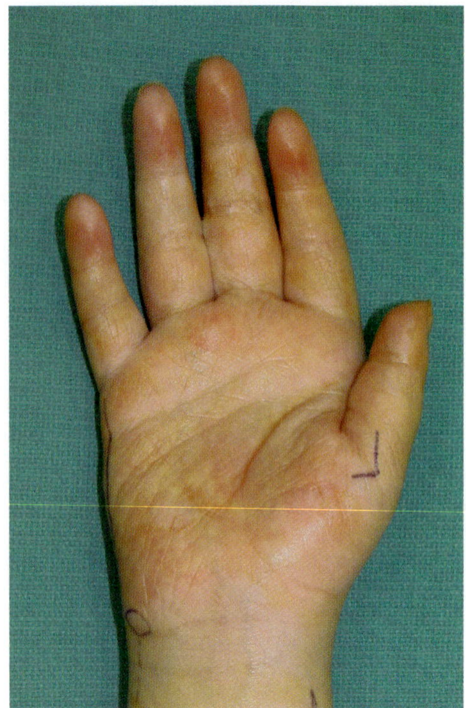

FIGURE 38-7

- A 2-cm chevron incision is marked over the radial aspect of the thumb MCP joint to expose the APB tendon (Fig. 38-7).
- A curvilinear incision is marked from 1 cm proximal and ulnar to the pisiform, along the radial aspect of the hypothenar eminence, to the ulnar aspect of the base of the small finger to expose the hypothenar muscles for thumb abductorplasty (see Fig. 38-7).

Procedure

Step 1: Elevation of Four-Flap Z-Plasty Flaps

- The skin is incised as previously marked, and thick skin flaps are elevated in the loose areolar plane superficial to the muscles.
- Any tight fascial bands overlying the first dorsal interosseous are divided.

Step 2: Exposure of the Ulnar Collateral Ligament

- The ulnar limb of the four-flap Z-plasty is mobilized to expose the tendon of the adductor pollicis and the extensor expansion.
- The adductor pollicis tendon is divided at its insertion into the extensor expansion and reflected ulnarly to expose the thumb UCL.

PEARLS

The radial limb of the four-flap Z-plasty should be designed dorsally, and the ulnar limb should be designed in a palmar direction. This will allow exposure of the thumb MCP joint and UCL through the radial limb incision.

The incision for exposure of the abductor digiti minimi (ADM) should not be along the ulnar border of the hand but slightly palmar, so that the scar is not compressed when the hand is resting.

STEP 1 PITFALLS

Care must be taken to prevent injury to the radial digital nerve to the index finger during elevation of the radial limb and the dorsal sensory branches of the radial nerve during elevation of the ulnar limb of the four-flap Z-plasty.

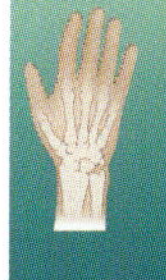

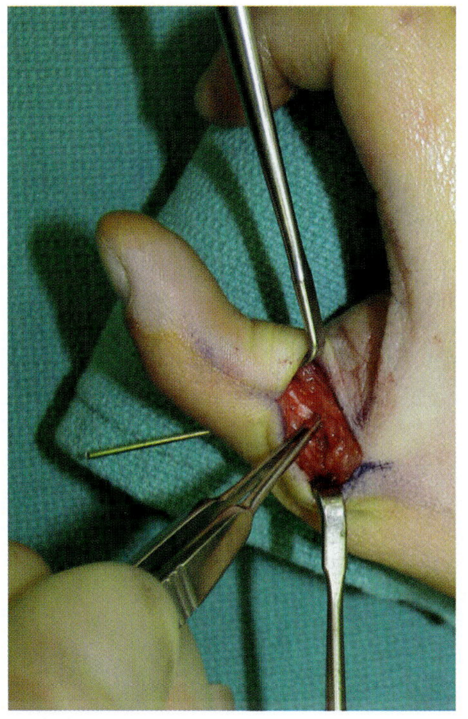

FIGURE 38-8

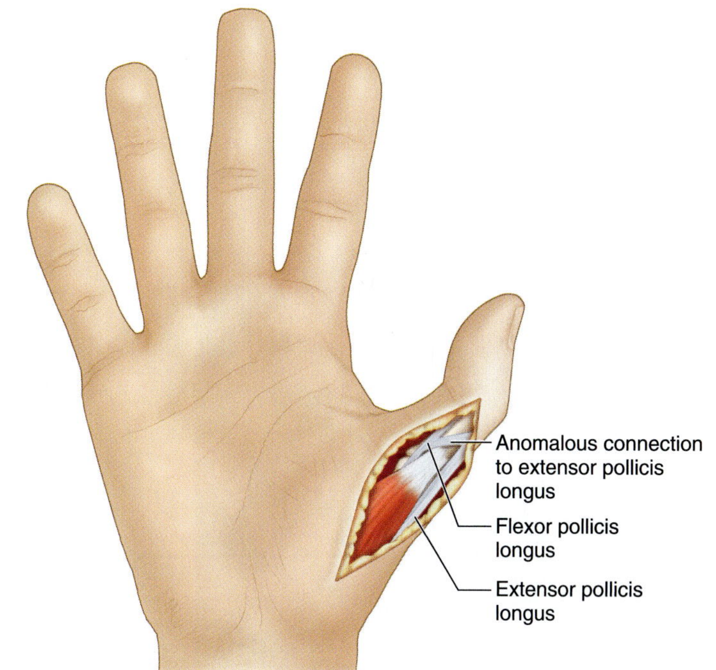

FIGURE 38-9

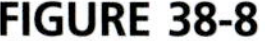

STEP 3 PITFALLS

The K-wire should not exit through the radial aspect of the metacarpal head, where it may impinge on the insertion of the ADM tendon following opponensplasty.

A tip protector should be placed over the end of the K-wire to prevent inadvertent injury during the subsequent portion of the surgery.

STEP 6 PEARLS

Anomalous bands may exist from the FPL on the palmar aspect of the hand to the EPL on the dorsal aspect of the hand (pollex abductus), which should be identified and divided (Fig. 38-9).

Step 3: Pinning of Thumb MCP Joint

- A single 0.045-inch K-wire is passed obliquely from radial to ulnar through the MCP joint to maintain the MCP joint in neutral position (Fig. 38-8).

Step 4: Strengthening of the UCL

- Multiple 4-0 Ethibond sutures are placed in a horizontal mattress configuration to reef the lax UCL.
- The tendon of the adductor pollicis is mobilized, advanced, and sutured to the reefed UCL and extensor expansion to further strengthen the UCL.

Step 5: Transposition of Four-Flap Z-Plasty Flaps

- The Z-plasty flaps are transposed and sutured using 4-0 chromic catgut.
- Figure 38-5 shows the arrangement of the flaps before and after transposition.

Step 6: Exposure of the APB Tendon on the Radial Aspect of the Thumb MCP Joint

- The chevron-shaped incision is used to expose the APB tendon.

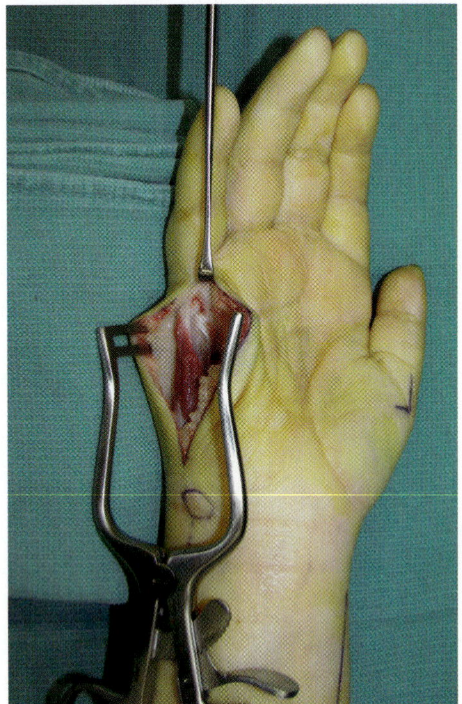

FIGURE 38-10

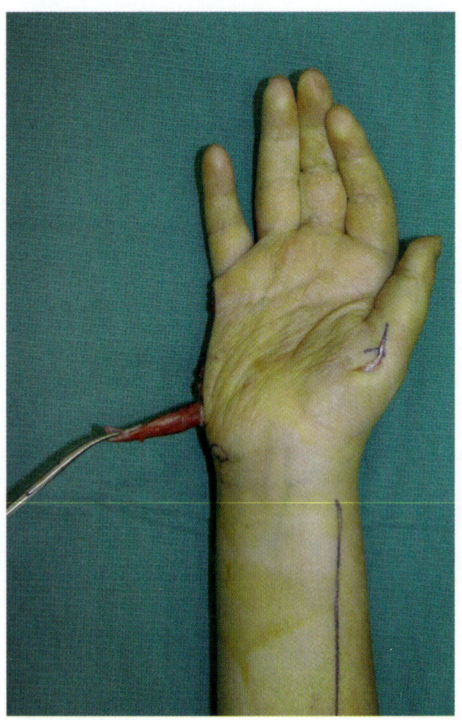

FIGURE 38-11

Step 7: Exposure of the ADM

- The skin is incised in line with the previously marked incision. The ADM is identified in the midportion of the hypothenar eminence and is the most ulnar and superficial of the hypothenar muscles in this location. More proximally, the palmaris brevis overlies the ADM, but it can be differentiated by the transverse orientation of its fibers.
- The ADM is separated from the other hypothenar muscles, including the opponens digiti minimi and the flexor digiti minimi, which are deeper and more radial (Fig. 38-10).

STEP 7 PITFALLS

Care must be taken to identify and protect the digital nerve to the ulnar side of the small finger. This nerve will pass obliquely superficial to the ADM in the distal half of the incision.

The palmaris brevis should be divided to mobilize the proximal portion of the ADM. Care must be taken to protect motor branches of the ulnar nerve during proximal mobilization of the ADM.

Step 8: Division of the Insertion of the ADM

- The ADM has two insertions, one to the ulnar aspect of the base of the proximal phalanx and the other to the extensor expansion. Both of these must be divided to allow the muscle to be elevated (Fig. 38-11).

STEP 8 PEARLS

The ADM barely reaches the APB insertion. Harvesting a slightly longer tendon will make insertion of the transfer easier (Fig. 38-12).

Step 9: Elevation of the ADM

- The ADM is elevated to its origin from the pisiform. The neurovascular bundle to the ADM enters the muscle on the dorsoradial aspect, and care must be taken during proximal elevation of the muscle to prevent injury to the pedicle (Fig. 38-13). The pedicle does not need to be visualized during the harvest. The muscle is dissected to its insertion at the pisiform.

STEP 9 PEARLS

Although the ADM can be elevated off the pisiform to improve the length of the transfer, this maneuver can weaken this delicate muscle. Alternatively, placing the wrist in flexion or using a tendon graft (rarely necessary) can improve the length of the transfer.

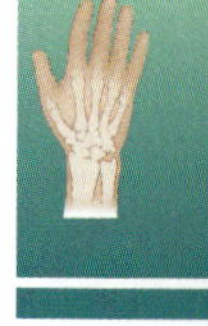

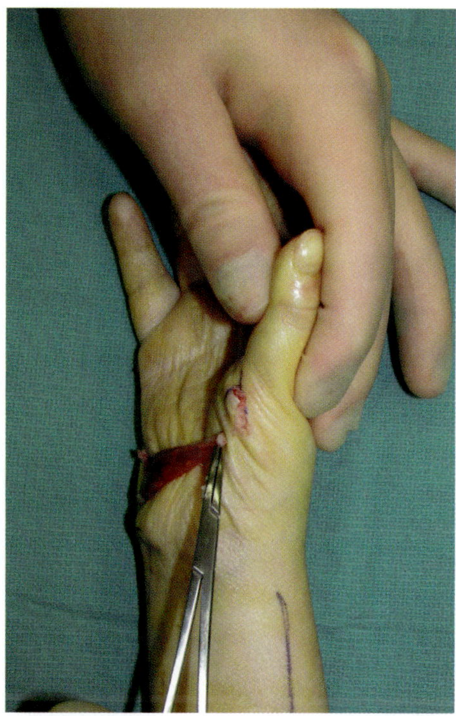

FIGURE 38-12

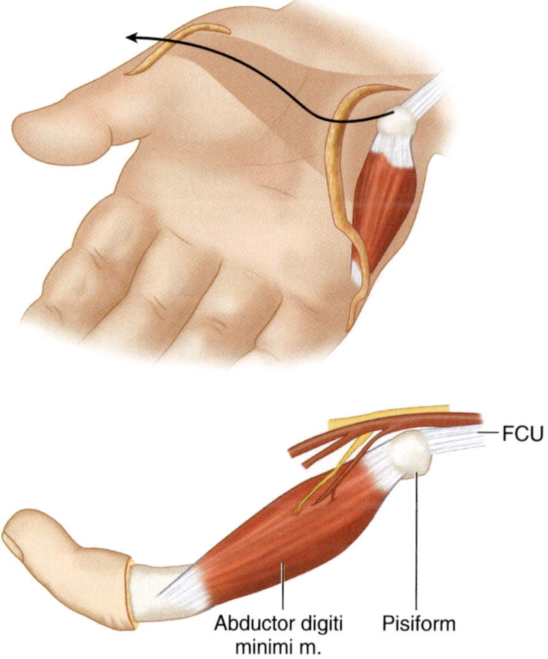

FIGURE 38-13

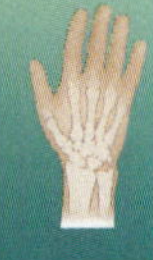

STEP 10 PEARLS

The tunnel must be wide enough to accommodate the ADM without compromising the viability of the muscle or increasing the risk for adhesions. An additional incision can be made at the base of the thenar eminence to ensure a wide tunnel.

Step 10: Creation of a Subcutaneous Tunnel

- A wide subcutaneous tunnel is made from the pisiform to the radial aspect of the thumb MCP joint using a large curved hemostat.

Step 11: Transfer of the ADM

- The elevated ADM is turned 180 degrees like the page of a book, rather than rotating it 90 degrees, to prevent twisting of the pedicle (Fig. 38-14).
- A hemostat passed from the incision at the radial aspect of the thumb through the subcutaneous tunnel is used to bring the ADM to the radial aspect of the thumb MCP joint.
- The ADM tendon reaches the APB insertion with sufficient tension, and overcorrection is unnecessary.
- The ADM tendon is passed under the APB insertion and anchored with 4-0 Ethibond mattress sutures (Fig. 38-15).

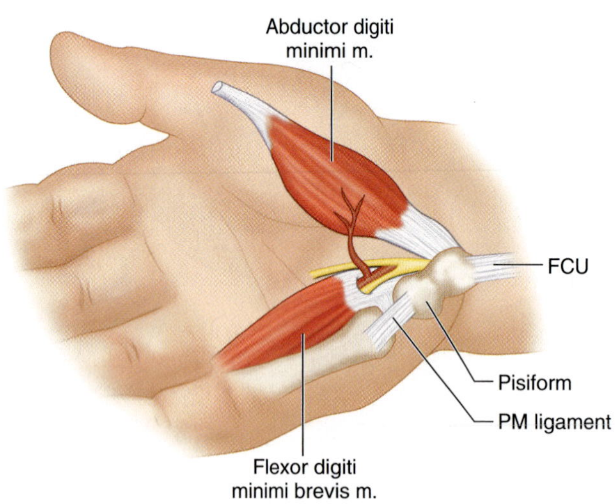

FIGURE 38-14

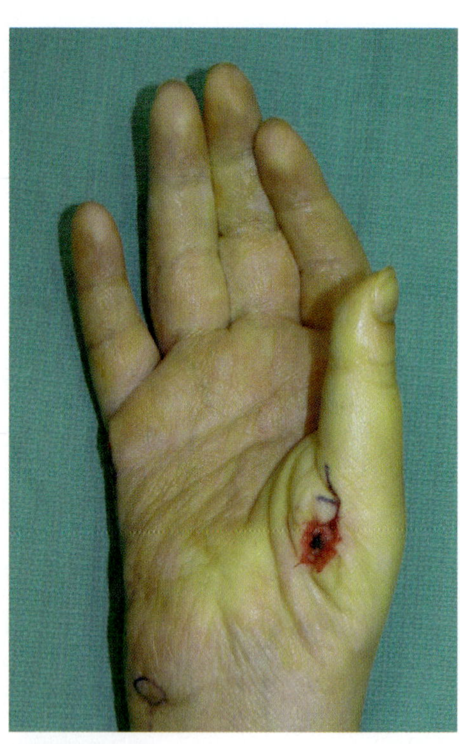

FIGURE 38-15

Step 12: Wound Closure

- The tourniquet is released, and meticulous hemostasis is secured.
- All skin incisions are closed with 4-0 chromic catgut (Fig. 38-16).
- A thumb spica splint to maintain the wrist in slight flexion and to keep the thumb in maximal palmar abduction is provided.

Postoperative Care and Expected Outcomes

- The child is maintained in a thumb spica splint for 4 weeks. The K-wire is removed at 4 weeks and a thermoplastic splint fashioned to maintain the position of the thumb.
- At 4 weeks, children are started on range-of-motion and strengthening exercises and are weaned off the splint gradually over a period of 2 to 4 weeks.
- The results of surgery for thumb hypoplasia are good, and almost all patients have improvements in thumb function.

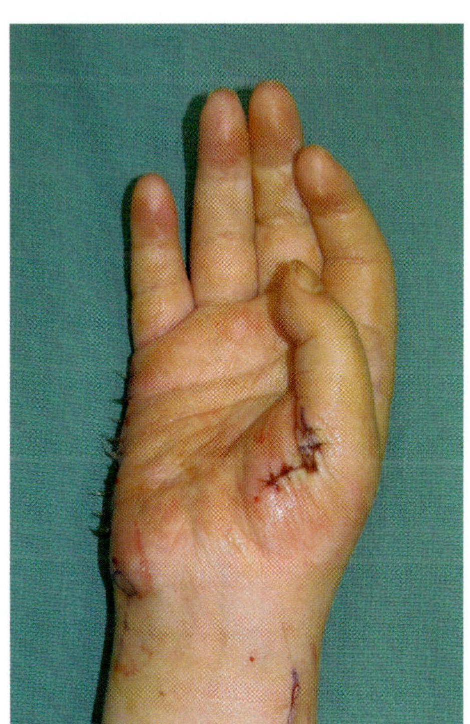

FIGURE 38-16

Evidence

Abdel-Ghani H, Amro S. Characteristics of patients with hypoplastic thumb: a prospective study of 51 patients with the results of surgical treatment, *J Pediatr Orthop*. 2004;13:127-138.
The authors describe the outcomes of 51 patients and 82 hypoplastic thumbs, of whom 18 patients underwent surgical reconstruction with 3-year follow-up. In this series, type V thumb hypoplasia was most common, and the majority (86%) suffered from associated anomalies. Among patients who underwent opponensplasty and UCL reconstruction, the majority achieved stability (70%) at the MCP joint as well as the ability to oppose the finger to the small finger (89%). (Level IV evidence)

Fraulin FO, Thomson HG. First webspace deepening: comparing the four-flap and five-flap Z-plasty. Which gives the most gain? *Plast Reconstr Surg*. 1999;104: 120-128.
The authors use simulated models to determine the anticipated gain between four- and five-flap Z-plasty for web space deepening. The authors conclude that the percentage of deepening achieved by a five-flap Z-plasty is similar to that of a single 60-degree Z-plasty, approximately 75%, and a four-flap Z-plasty using 90-degree angles yields greater deepening (114%). (Level III evidence)

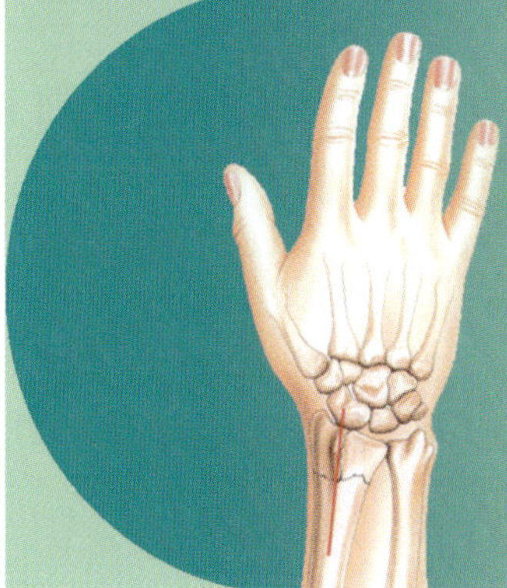

PROCEDURE 39

Pollicization for Congenital Thumb Hypoplasia

Jennifer Waljee, Sandeep J. Sebastin, and Kevin C. Chung

See Video 32: Pollicization

Indications

- Hypoplastic thumb exists with inadequate carpometacarpal joint (Blauth types IIB, IV, and V).
- Pollicization should be considered at about 12 to 18 months of age because at this age general anesthesia is safer and surgical dissection of critical structures is technically easier. In addition, this allows for preliminary correction of any associated radial deficiencies.

Examination/Imaging

Clinical Examination

- The Blauth classification of thumb hypoplasia is useful in determining treatment options. Types IV (floating thumb) (Fig. 39-1) and V (absent thumb) (Fig. 39-2) are straightforward to identify clinically. However, it can be challenging to differentiate type IIIA (stable carpometacarpal [CMC] joint) from type IIIB (unstable CMC joint), and the trapezium and trapezoid are ossified only at 5 to 6 years of age, making radiographs less useful in decision making.

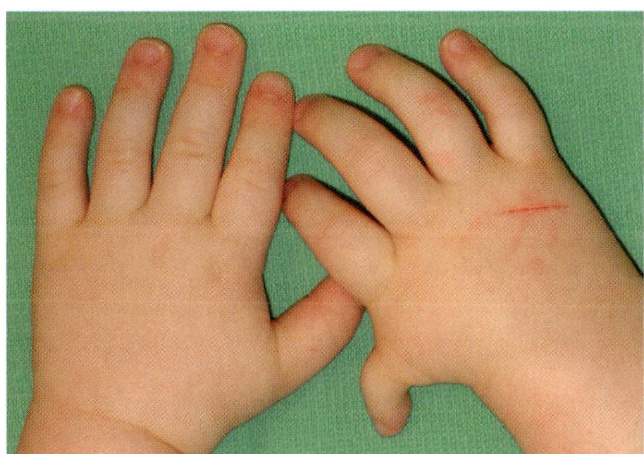

FIGURE 39-1

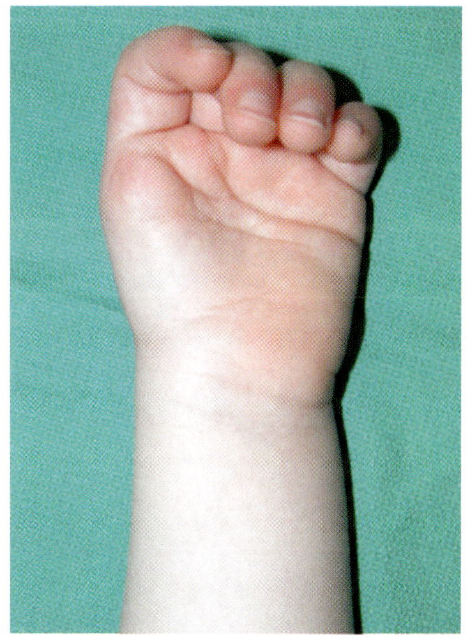

FIGURE 39-2

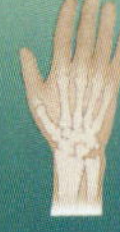

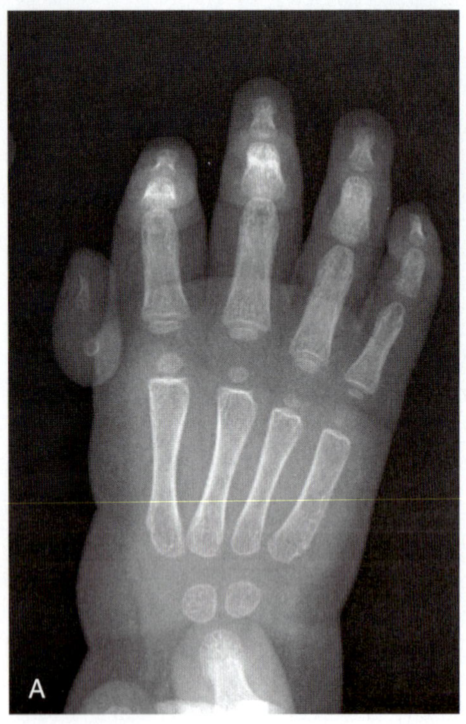

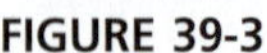

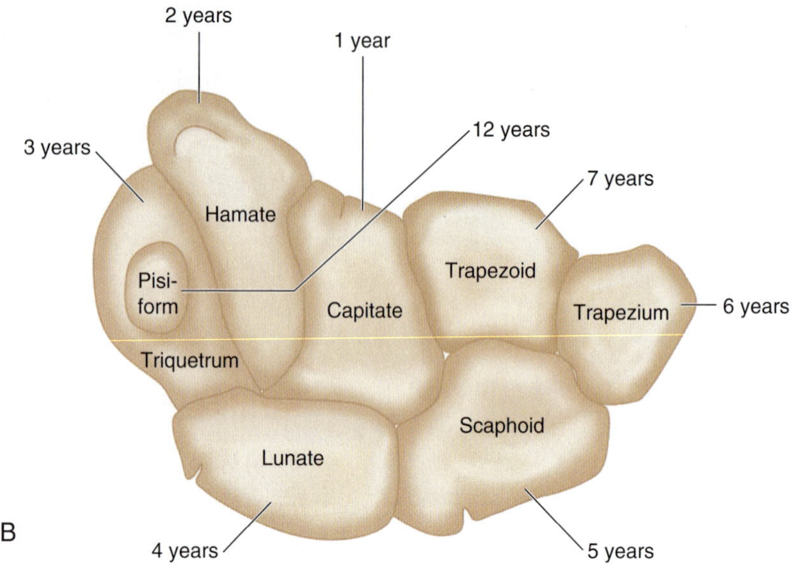

FIGURE 39-3

- Serial examination of a child is required to differentiate between types IIIA and IIIB. A newborn uses digital grasp, and the infant begins to use the thumb in grasp at about 1 year of age. If the child uses the thumb in manipulating objects, this suggests that a type IIIA deficiency is present. If the child prefers to grasp objects between the index and long finger web space, this web appears wider, and the index finger is pronated toward the thumb. This suggests type IIIB hypoplasia.
- The index finger may be stiff and hypoplastic to varying degrees in children with type IV and type V hypoplasia, which will affect the result of pollicization.
- The child should be examined for signs of other systematic abnormalities, such as VACTERL (i.e., *v*ertebral abnormalities, *a*nal atresia, *c*ardiac abnormalities, *t*racheoesophageal fistula and/or *e*sophageal atresia, *r*enal agenesis and dysplasia, and *l*imb defects), Fanconi anemia, and Holt-Oltram syndrome, before considering surgical reconstruction.

Imaging

- Radiographs of the hands, wrists, and forearms are useful in determining the degree of metacarpal and phalangeal hypoplasia of the thumb and index finger. They can also identify other associated upper extremity anomalies, such as radial deficiency.
- The number of carpal bones seen on the radiograph gives a rough estimate of the age of the child (Fig. 39-3A). The order of ossification of carpal bones is detailed in Figure 39-3B. About one center appears per year from the age of 1 year to 7 years.

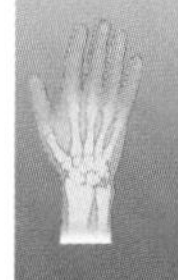

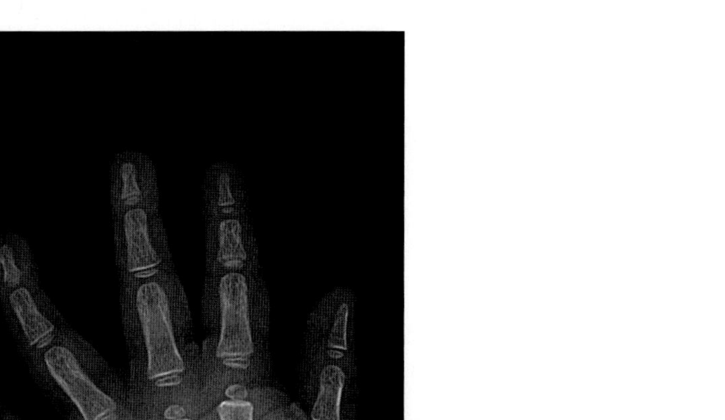

FIGURE 39-4

- The presence of a tapered metacarpal without a base confirms type IIIB hypoplasia. Type IIIA hypoplasia is associated with full length of the metacarpal (Fig. 39-4).

Surgical Anatomy

- After pollicization, the common digital artery to the index and long fingers is the primary blood supply to the transposed digit. The radial digital artery to the index finger may be absent, but the ability to perform index pollicization is not contingent on the presence of the radial digital artery when the main blood supply comes from the ulnar digital artery.

Positioning

- The procedure is conducted under general anesthesia with the patient placed supine on the operating room table. The entire upper extremity is prepared and draped after a tourniquet is applied.
- The limb is exsanguinated fully to permit a completely bloodless field. A well-fitted, small tourniquet is essential because blood in the operative field will jeopardize the operation by obscuring the small structures in the pediatric hand.

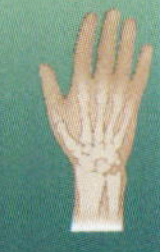

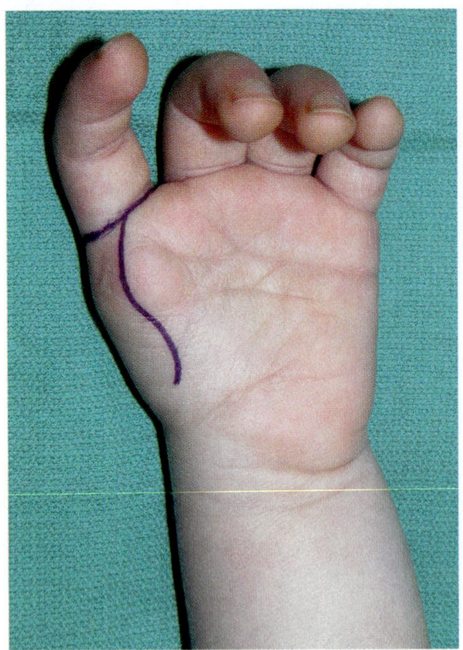

FIGURE 39-5

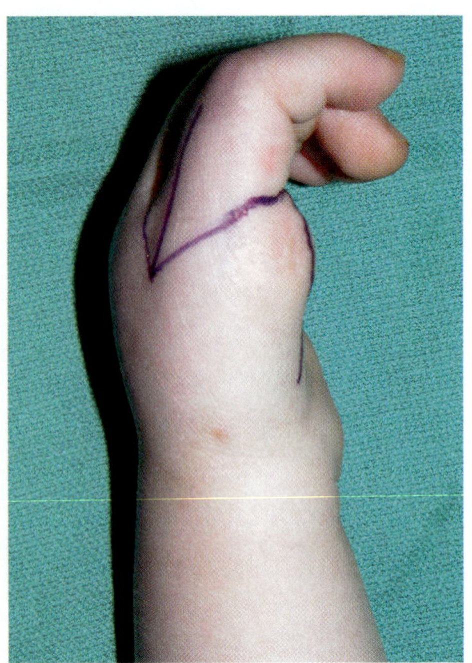

FIGURE 39-6

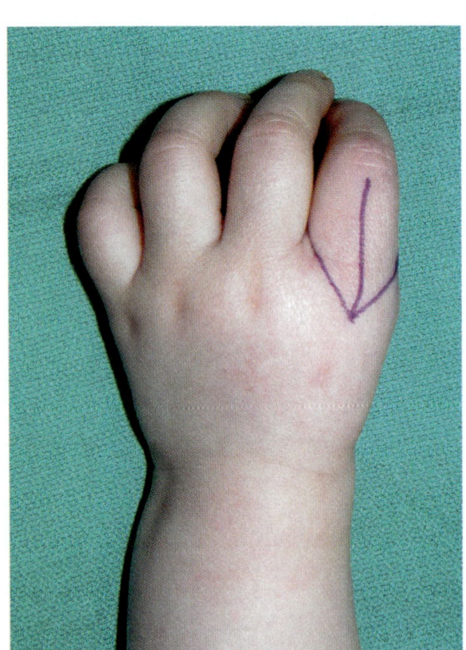

FIGURE 39-7

Exposures

- A longitudinal curvilinear incision is marked over the palmar aspect of the index finger metacarpal (Fig. 39-5). A V-shaped incision is marked over the dorsum of the index finger metacarpal such that the apex is at the level of the neck of the metacarpal (Figs. 39-6 and 39-7). The dorsal and palmar incisions are connected at the base of the finger. A longitudinal incision is marked over the dorsum of the proximal phalanx, extending from the proximal interphalangeal (PIP) joint to the apex of the V.

PEARLS

If the thumb is present, the hypoplastic digit may be filleted and the skin incorporated into the design of the skin flaps or into the first web space for additional soft tissue coverage (Figs. 39-8 and 39-9).

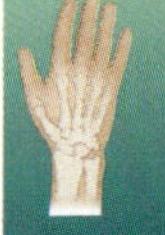

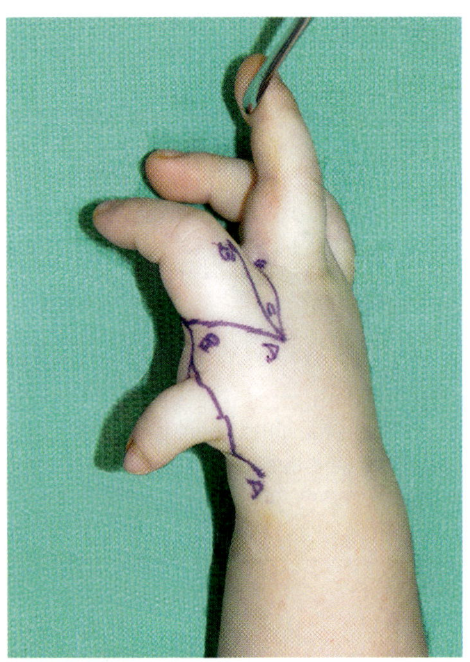

FIGURE 39-8

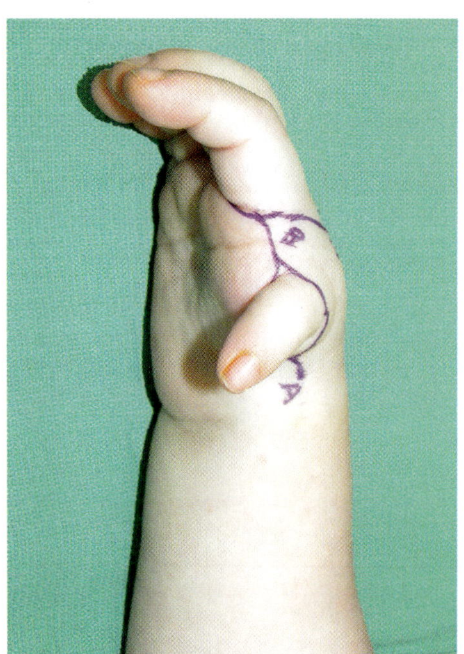

FIGURE 39-9

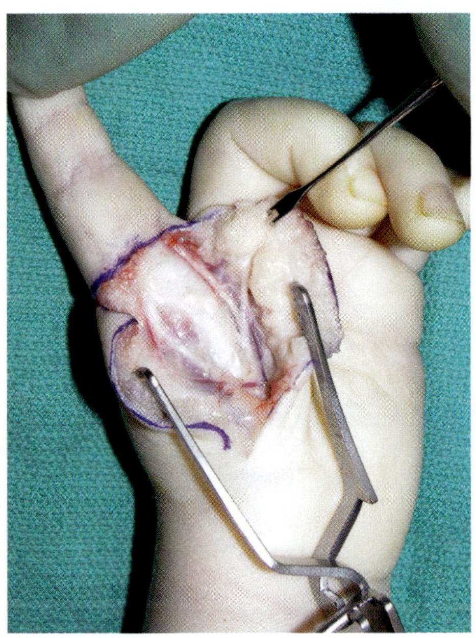

FIGURE 39-10

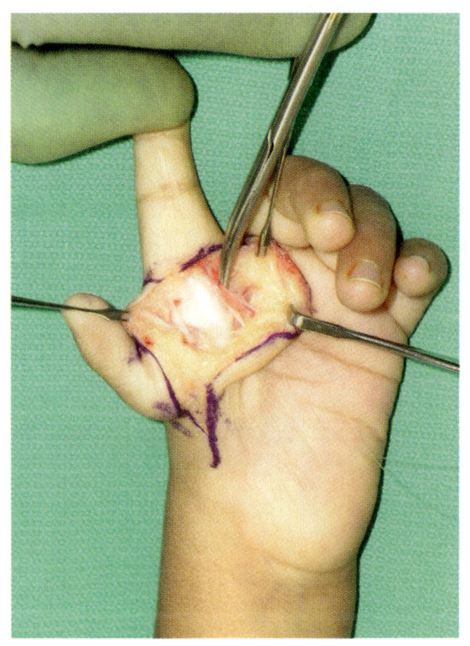

FIGURE 39-11

PITFALLS

Poorly planned skin incisions can lead to inadequate soft tissue coverage of the first web space with difficulty with thumb abduction and need for skin grafting for coverage. The first web space should have supple soft tissue coverage without scars to optimize thumb opposition.

Procedure

Step 1

- The palmar skin incisions are made first, and thick skin flaps are raised.
- The radial neurovascular bundle along the index finger is identified and isolated (Fig. 39-10). The common digital artery to the second web space is then identified. The dissection continues distally to isolate the ulnar digital artery to the index finger and the radial digital artery to the middle finger (Fig. 39-11).

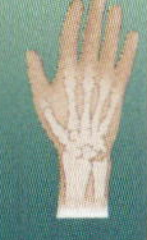

STEP 1 PITFALLS

The radial neurovascular bundle to the index finger may be hypoplastic or absent.

The common digital arteries may arise from the deep arch and may require more extensive dissection.

- The radial digital artery to the long finger is ligated using 6-0 Prolene suture distal to the bifurcation. Dissection of these fine structures will require use of a microscope or loupes with 3.5× or greater magnification. This will allow mobilization of the index finger based on the radial digital artery and the common digital artery. The vessels are mobilized proximally to the level of the superficial arch.
- Intraneural dissection of the common digital nerve is done to separate the fibers of the ulnar digital nerve to the index finger from the fibers of the radial digital nerve to the middle finger. This dissection is carried proximally to the superficial arch as well.

Step 2

- The A1 pulley of the index finger is divided (Fig. 39-12).
- The ulnar neurovascular bundle of the index finger is retracted radially, and the deep transverse metacarpal ligament between the index and long finger metacarpal is divided at the neck of the metacarpal (Fig. 39-13).

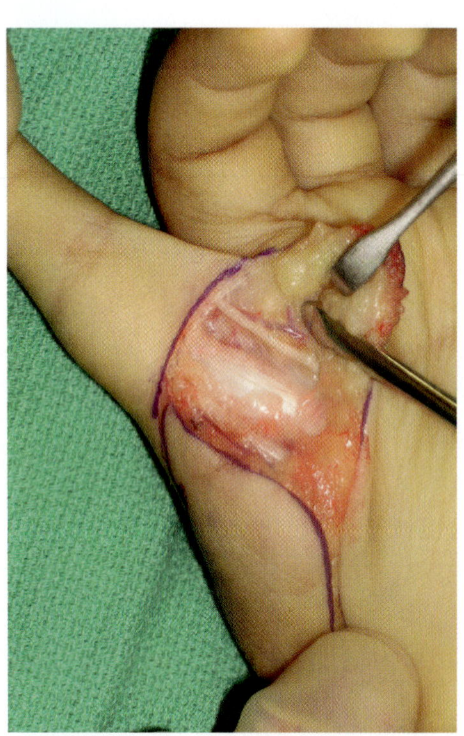

FIGURE 39-12

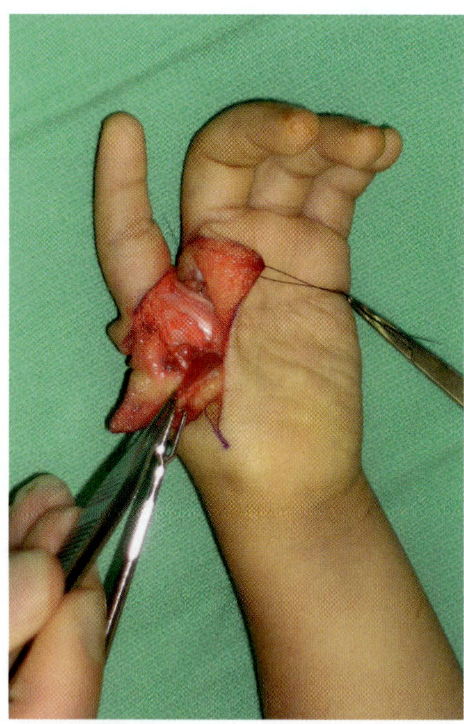

FIGURE 39-13

STEP 3 PITFALLS

The radial and ulnar neurovascular bundles and dorsal veins must be protected during elevation of the origins of the interosseous muscles.

Step 3

- The dorsal skin incisions are made, and flaps are raised. It is important to raise thin flaps, identify the dorsal veins, and protect them (Fig. 39-14).
- The juncturae tendineae between the index and long finger extensor tendons are divided.
- The first dorsal and palmar interossei are elevated off the radial and ulnar aspects of the metacarpal shaft, respectively. Only the proximal portion of these muscles originating from the base of the metacarpal is left intact. The tendons of these two muscles are carefully separated from the metacarpophalangeal (MCP) joint capsule and divided distally along with a small portion of the extensor hood (Fig. 39-15).

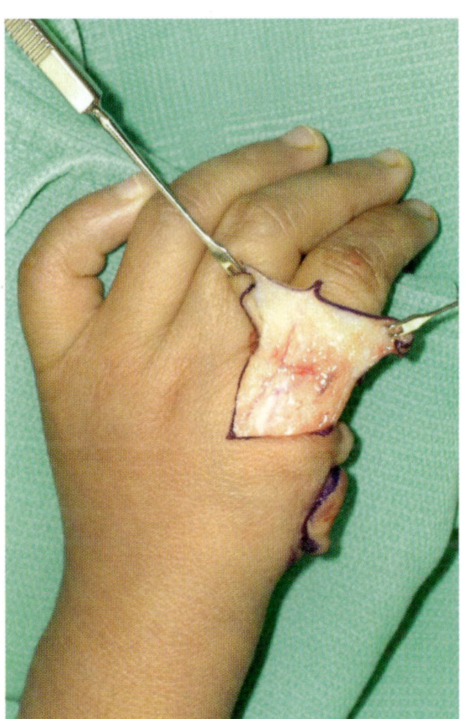

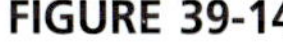

FIGURE 39-14

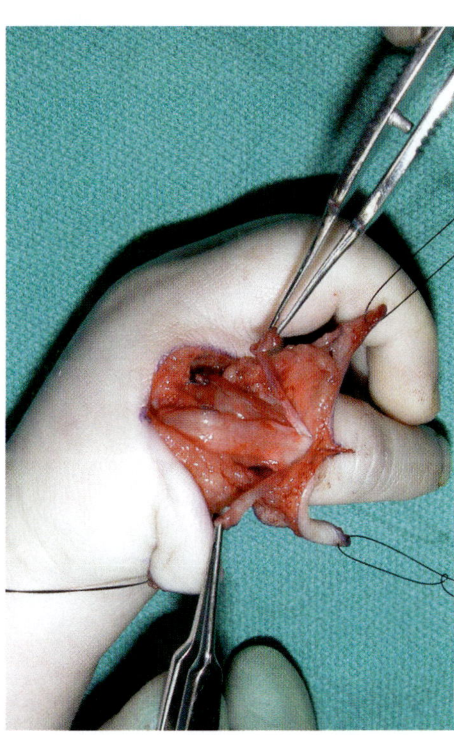

FIGURE 39-15

Step 4

- The skin flaps over the proximal phalanx are raised, and the extensor hood is identified (Fig. 39-16). The radial and ulnar lateral bands are identified on either side of midproximal phalanx.

Step 5

- The index finger metacarpal shaft is shortened by performing two osteotomies.
- The distal osteotomy is done beyond the neck of the metacarpal through the physis (Fig. 39-17 and 39-18). The physis is soft, and a blade can be used for this osteotomy.

STEP 5 PEARLS

The tip of the pollicized index finger should reach the PIP joint of the middle finger to achieve optimal length. However, it is more common for a pollicized finger to be too long rather than too short. Although the metacarpal shaft is removed, the insertion of the flexor carpi radialis and extensor carpi radialis longus proximally and the origin of the collateral ligaments distally must be spared.

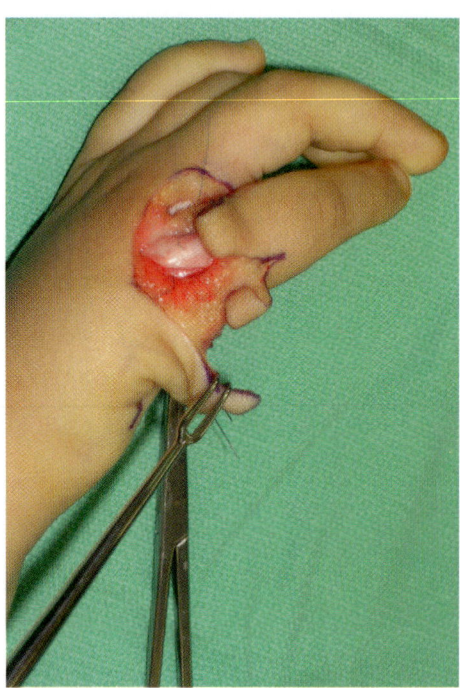

FIGURE 39-16

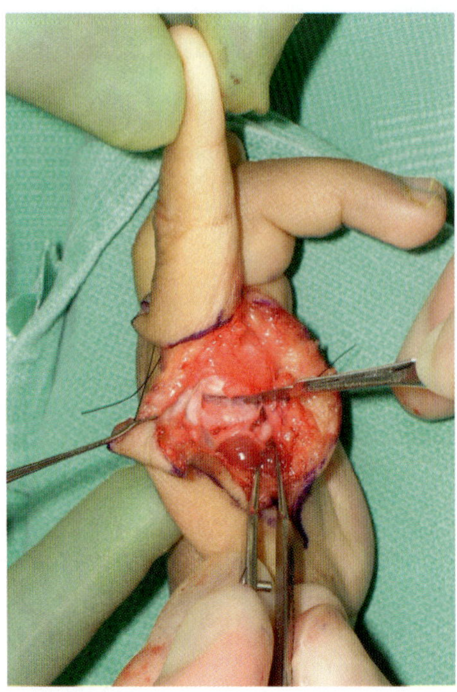

FIGURE 39-17

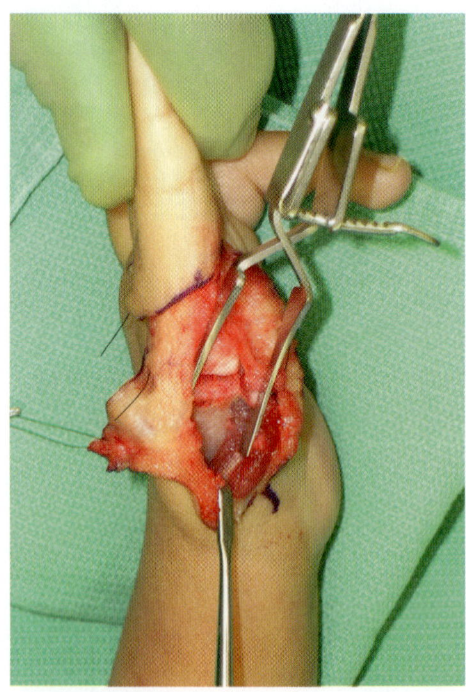

FIGURE 39-18

- The proximal osteotomy is done at the base of the metacarpal using a bone cutter (Fig. 39-19).
- The index finger is now freely mobile and attached only by the dorsal veins, radial and ulnar neurovascular bundles, and flexor and extensor tendons (Fig. 39-20).

Step 6

- At this point, the index finger is positioned over the base of the index metacarpal. The index MCP joint will now function as the new thumb CMC joint. It is positioned in about 45 degrees of abduction and 100 to 120 degrees of pronation to recreate the position of the thumb. The position should be such that the pulp of the index finger is in contact with the radial aspect of the PIP joint and the proximal phalanx of the middle finger (Fig. 39-21).

STEP 6 PEARLS

The normal index finger MCP joint can hyperextend to 20 to 30 degrees beyond neutral. However, this hyperextension is not desirable at the new thumb CMC joint. To prevent further hyperextension, the MCP joint is held in maximal hyperextension, and the dorsal capsule is sutured to the physis with 4-0 nonabsorbable suture to maintain this position.

The index finger metacarpal should be positioned at 45 degrees of abduction relative to the base. An oblique osteotomy of the metacarpal base can be created to improve the position of the thumb.

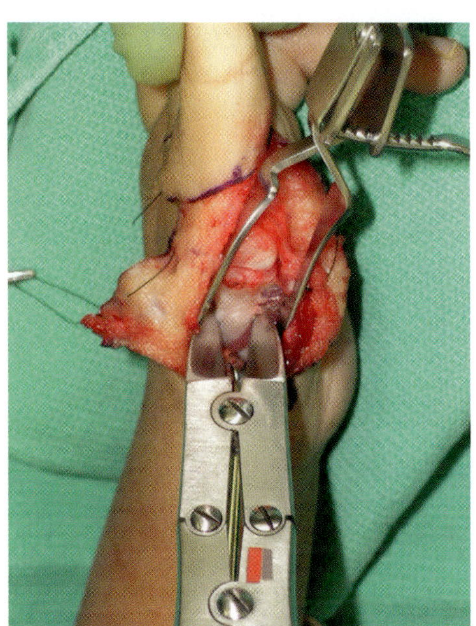

FIGURE 39-19

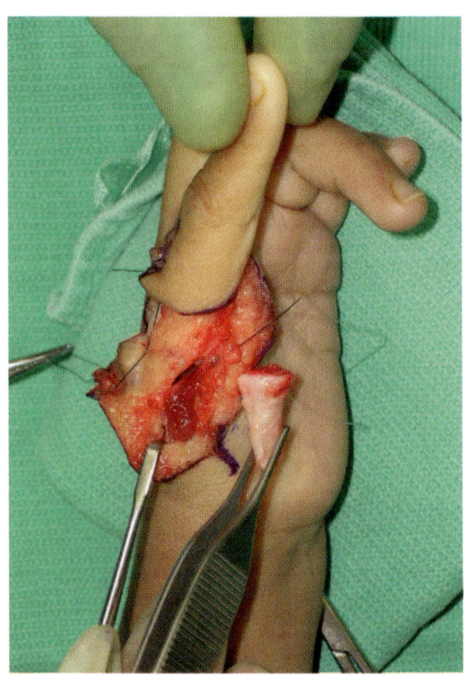

FIGURE 39-20

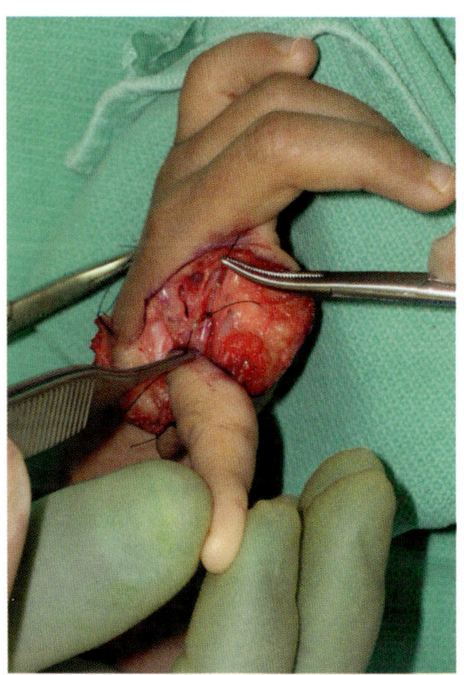

FIGURE 39-21

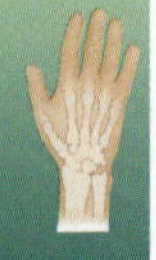

STEP 7 PITFALLS

One must ensure that the palmar incision allows good exposure of the base of the metacarpal. An excessively long pollicized thumb is most often the result of not seating the index finger well proximally.

STEP 8 PEARLS

Some surgeons opt to shorten the extensor and flexor tendons to balance the length owing to the shortened metacarpal. The senior author does not find this necessary and feels that children adapt remarkably well over time.

Step 7

- Additional 4-0 nonabsorbable sutures are placed between the epiphysis and the metacarpal base to stabilize the fixation.

Step 8

- The first dorsal interosseus tendon is attached to the radial lateral band at the level of midproximal phalanx to provide abduction of the pollicized index finger. The first palmar interosseus tendon is attached to the ulnar lateral band and functions as the thumb adductor.
- The extensor and flexor tendons are left attached and will shorten over time. The new anatomic functions of the index finger joints and muscle units are detailed in Table 39-1. The extensor digitorum communis will function as the abductor pollicis longus. The extensor indicis proprius will act as the extensor pollicis longus. The first palmar interosseus will function as the adductor pollicis, and the first dorsal interosseus will function as the abductor pollicis. The index finger distal interphalangeal joint will become the interphalangeal joint; the PIP joint will become the metaphalangeal (MP) joint, and the index finger MP joint will become the pollicized digit CMC joint.

Step 9

- The skin flaps are transposed into position and held with a few tagging 4-0 chromic catgut sutures (Figs. 39-22 and 39-23).
- Figure 39-24 illustrates the movement of the different flaps.

Table 39-1 Functional Units of the Pollicized Thumb

Unit	*New Function*
Skeletal Units	
Distal interphalangeal joint	Interphalangeal joint
Proximal interphalangeal joint	Metacarpophalangeal joint
Metacarpophalangeal joint	Carpometacarpal joint
Musculotendinous Units	
Extensor indicis proprius	Extensor pollicis longus
Extensor digitorum communis (index)	Abductor pollicis longus
First palmar interosseous	Adductor pollicis
First dorsal interosseus	Abductor pollicis brevis

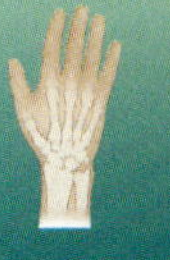

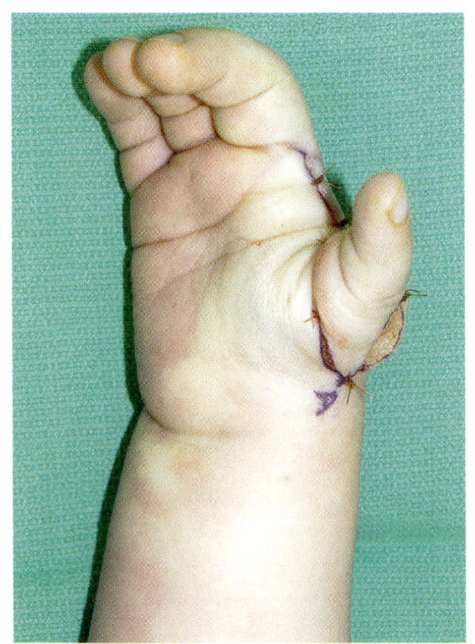

FIGURE 39-22

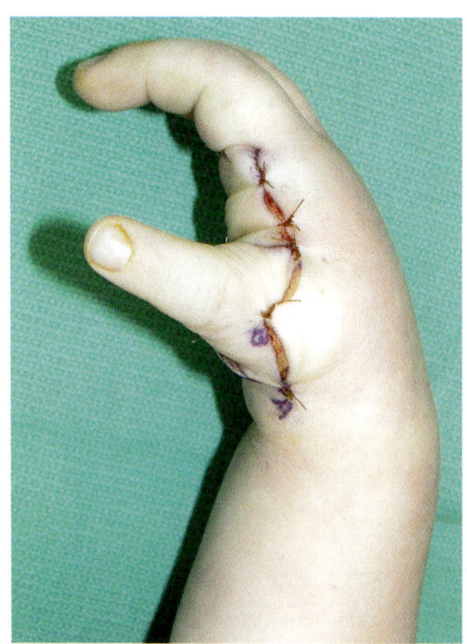

FIGURE 39-23

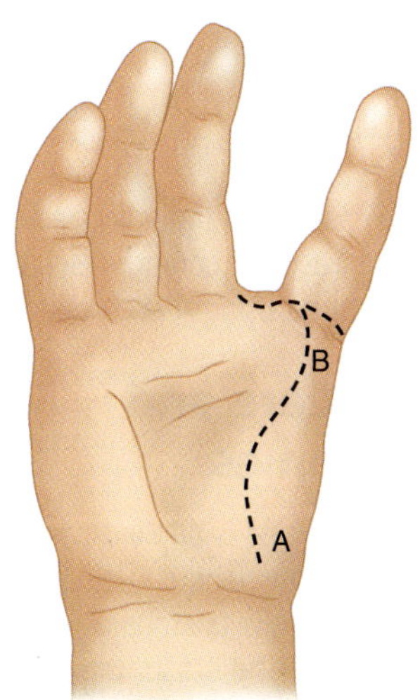

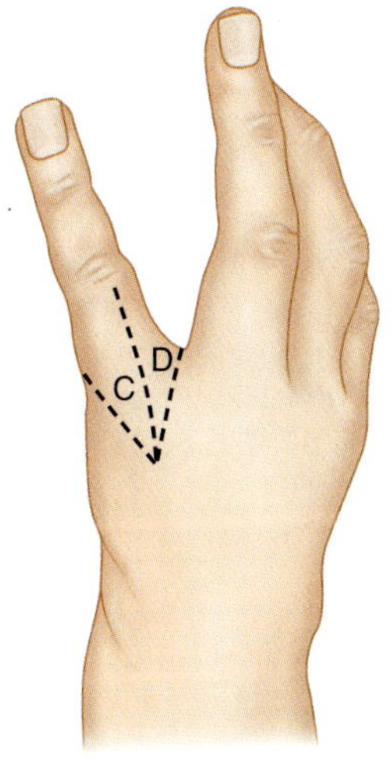

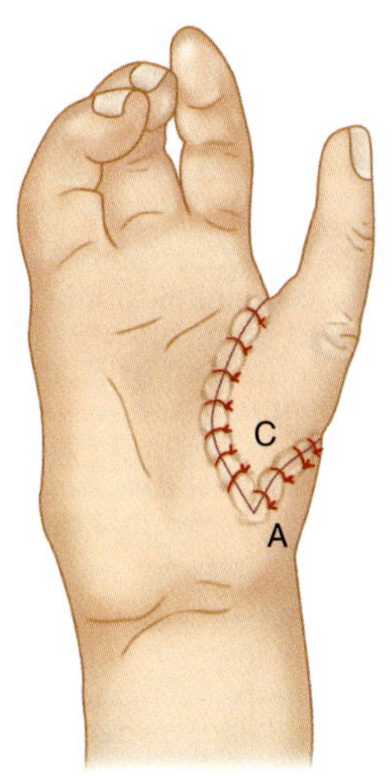

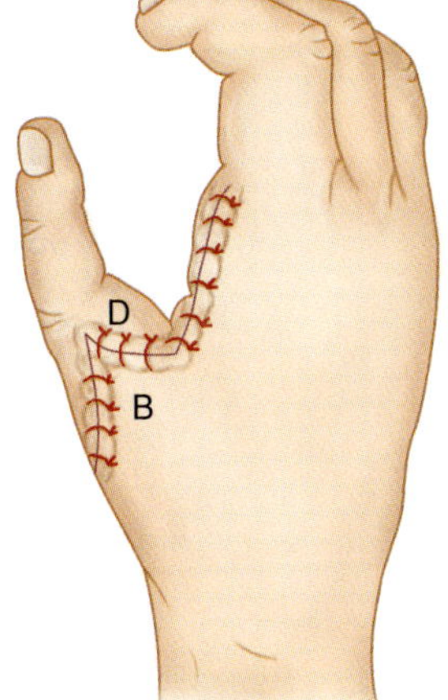

FIGURE 39-24

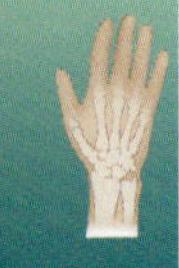

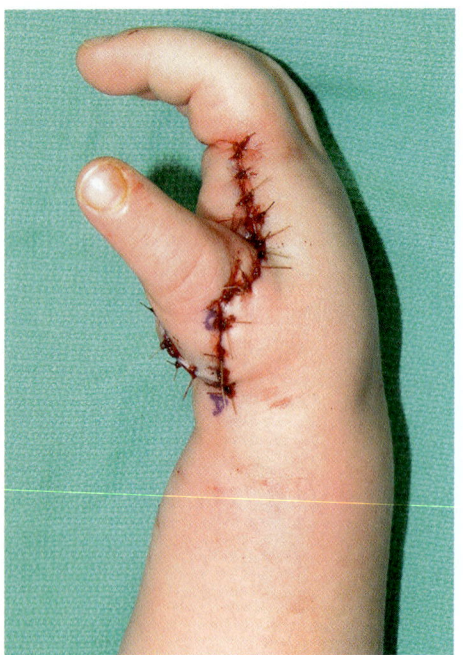

FIGURE 39-25

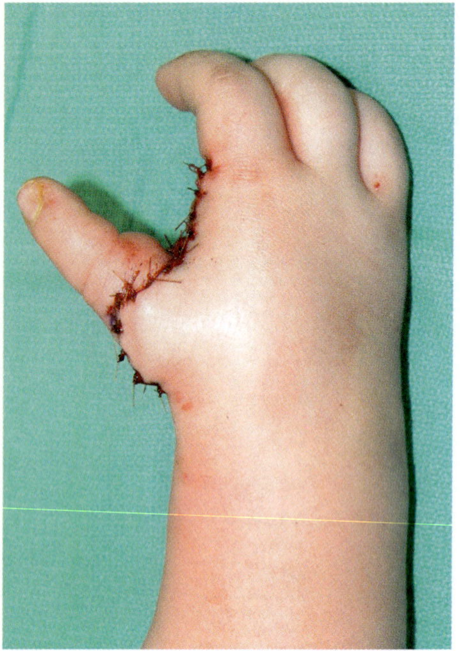

FIGURE 39-26

STEP 10 PITFALLS

The pollicized finger may appear pale after closure, which is usually due to vasospasm and is alleviated with warm soaks. If the perfusion does not improve within 15 to 20 minutes, any constricting closing sutures can be removed and the residual raw area skin grafted. However, persistent failure of perfusion demands exploration of the digital vessels.

Step 10

- The tourniquet is released, and the pollicized digit is inspected for capillary refill and any evidence of vascular compromise. Meticulous hemostasis is secured. The skin flaps are sutured using 4-0 chromic catgut (Figs. 39-25 and 39-26).

Postoperative Care and Expected Outcomes

- A long-arm thumb spica cast is applied with the elbow in flexion, and the arm is kept elevated to promote venous drainage.
- The cast is removed 4 weeks postoperatively, and therapy is initiated to focus on thumb mobility, pinch, and grasp. The patient is transitioned to a short-arm thumb spica splint for protection and stability during this period.
- In general, outcomes following pollicization are directly related to the mobility of the index finger, and pollicization achieves about 30% of grip and pinch strength compared with the contralateral thumb. Figures 39-27 through 39-29 show the postoperative result at 1 year follow-up for the child shown in Figures 39-8 and 39-9.

Evidence

Aliu O, Netscher DT, Staines KG, et al. A 5-year interval evaluation of function after pollicization for congenital thumb aplasia using multiple outcome measures. *Plast Reconstr Surg*. 2008;122:198-205.

This report details the outcomes of 5 patients and 7 hands. The authors examined the rate of improvement following pollicization and assessed patient performance with standardized tasks as well as measures of satisfaction. The results revealed an increase in grip strength and in lateral and tripod pinch strength that compared with normal development. (Level IV evidence)

Buck-Gramcko D. Pollicization of the index finger: methods and results in aplasia and hypoplasia of the thumb. *J Bone Joint Surg [Am]*. 1971;53:1605-1617.

This classic article details the techniques and outcomes for index finger pollicization in 114 patients (100 congenital), with long-term follow-up up to 12 years. The author details his technique and subsequent modifications. (Level V evidence)

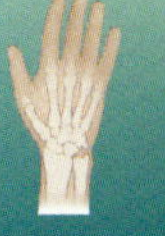

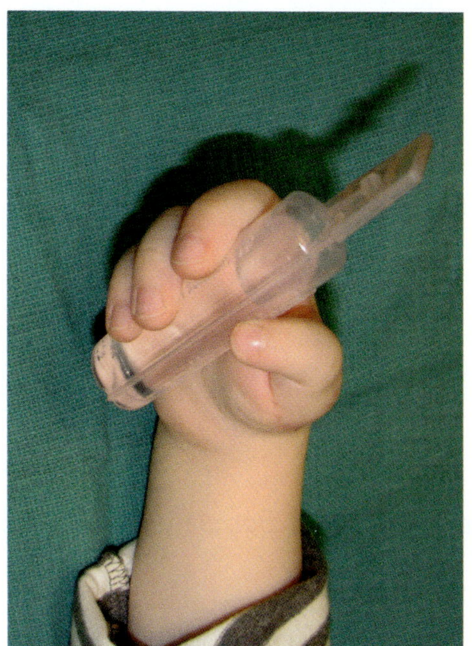

FIGURE 39-27

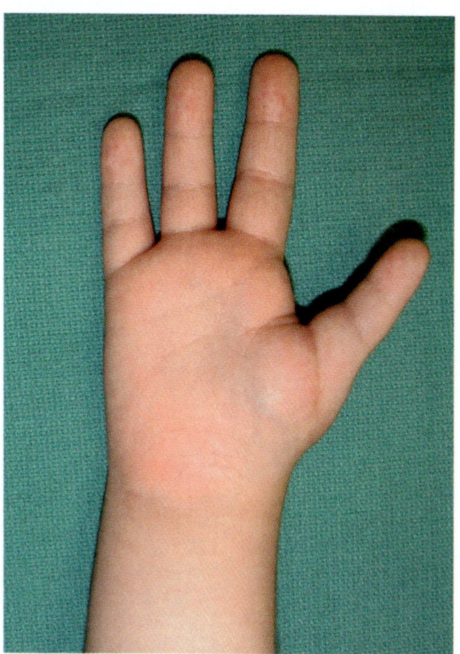

FIGURE 39-28

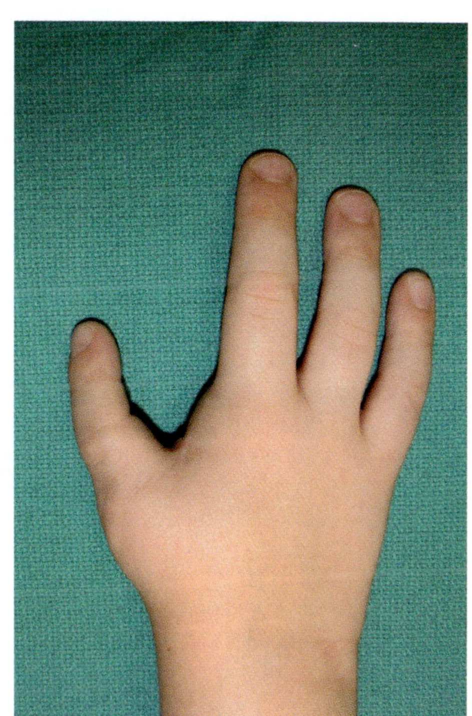

FIGURE 39-29

Manske PR, McCarroll HR. Index finger pollicization for a congenitally absent or nonfunctioning thumb. *J Hand Surg [Am]*. 1985;10:606-613.
The authors presented the functional outcomes in 28 patients who have undergone pollicization for congenitally absent thumbs. In this series, many patients required additional procedures—including opposition transfer, extensor tendon shortening, and arthrodesis—to improve function and cosmesis, particularly among patients with radial club hands or prior centralization. (Level IV evidence)

PROCEDURE 40

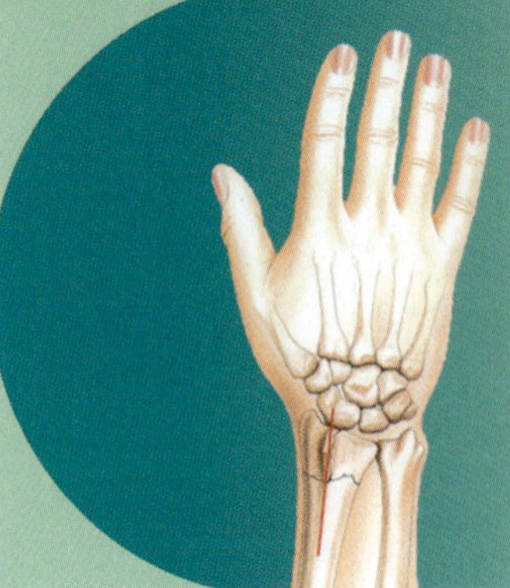

Correction of Constriction Ring

Pao-Yuan Lin, Sandeep J. Sebastin, and Kevin C. Chung

See Video 33: Surgery for Constriction Band Syndrome

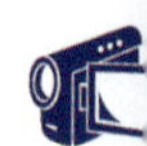

Indications

- Constriction rings may be mild, moderate, or severe.
  - *Mild:* Only skin and a portion of subcutaneous fat are involved, and there is no lymphedema.
  - *Moderate:* The lymphatic channels are interrupted, but the vascular system is intact. Lymphedema can be seen in the portion distal to the constriction ring.
  - *Severe:* The constriction ring interrupts the vascular system so that the distal blood supply is jeopardized and the part distal to the constriction ring is at risk for gangrene.
- Severe constriction rings will need release soon after birth on an emergent basis. Moderate rings can be corrected at a later age (6 to 9 months), when anesthesia is easier and safer and the structures are larger. The correction of mild rings is performed for aesthetic considerations and should be done before the child goes to school (3 to 4 years of age).

Examination/Imaging

Clinical Examination

- The presence of distal lymphedema indicates a lack of sufficient subcutaneous layer to promote the lymphatic flow. Most of the lymphedema will subside within a few months after correction of the constriction ring.
- In children with bilateral constriction ring syndrome, the severity of the deformity of one limb is independent of the other.

Imaging

- Plain radiographs of the affected limb can help identify any associated bony anomalies, especially when the constriction ring is associated with acrosyndactyly.

Surgical Anatomy

- The constriction ring can extend from the skin to as deep as the bone. Affected structures may involve lymphatics, nerves, and the vascular system, and the constriction ring can result in lymphedema, neurologic symptoms, and amputation.

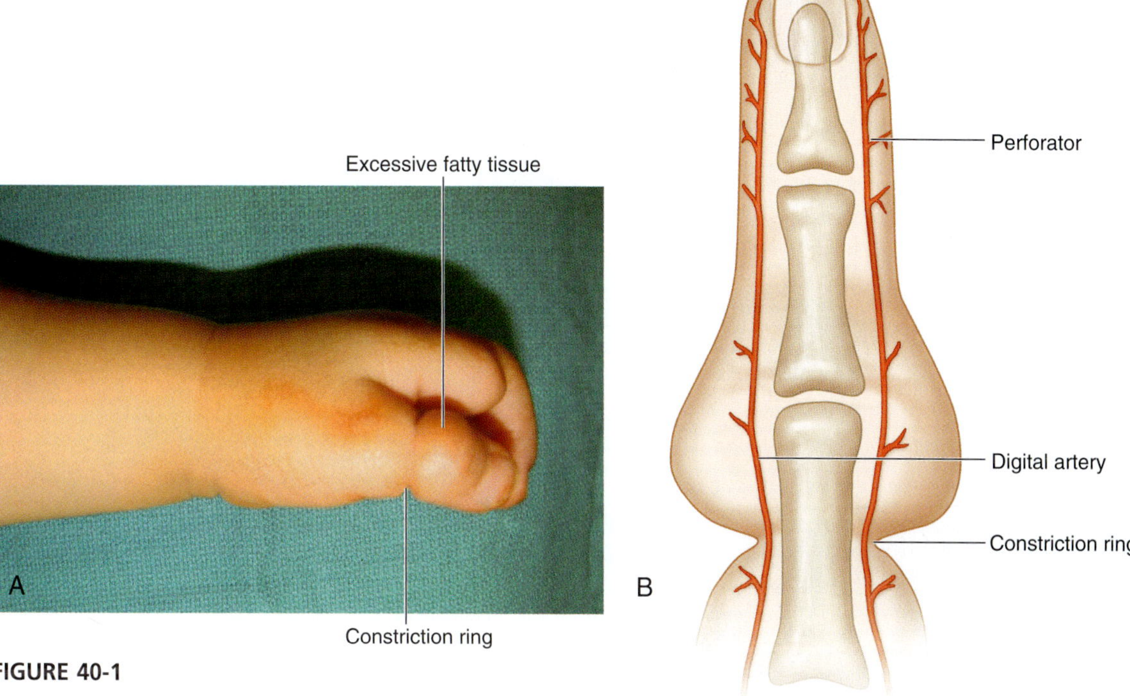

FIGURE 40-1

- The soft tissue and skeletal structures are always normal proximal to the constriction ring, but the soft tissue distal to the ring can present with varying degrees of edema (Fig. 40-1A). The growth centers distal to and just proximal to the constriction can often be injured, resulting in hypoplasia. Nerve palsies have been associated with the bands and are present at birth.
- Excess subcutaneous fat both proximal and distal to the constriction ring should be excised.
- The arterial blood supply of the part distal to the constriction ring arises from perforators that originate from the main artery located in the deep layer. This blood supply can be maintained because of the intact main artery and its venae comitantes (Fig. 40-1B).

PEARLS

For constriction rings of the digits, staged correction is safer. One-stage correction in digits has a greater chance of injuring the vessels and jeopardizing the distal circulation. One-stage correction with circumferential excision of a constriction ring can be performed in the proximal limbs, where injury of deep arterial and venous vessels is less likely.

Positioning

- The procedure is performed under general anesthesia and tourniquet control. The patient is positioned supine with the affected upper extremity on a hand table.

Exposures

- The key principles in surgical correction of constriction rings are the following:
  - The constriction ring is excised, and a Z-plasty is used to transpose skin flaps to prevent a circular scar contracture.
  - Excessive subcutaneous fat is excised and/or transposed to correct the contour deformities.

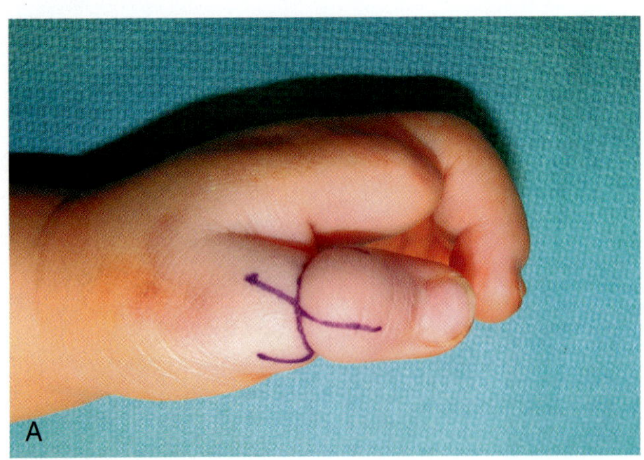
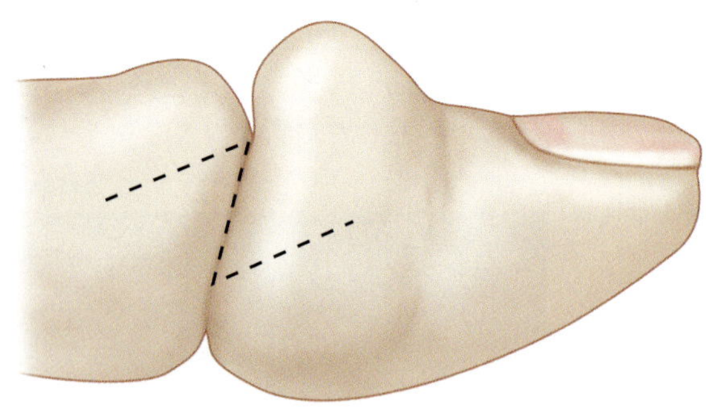

FIGURE 40-2

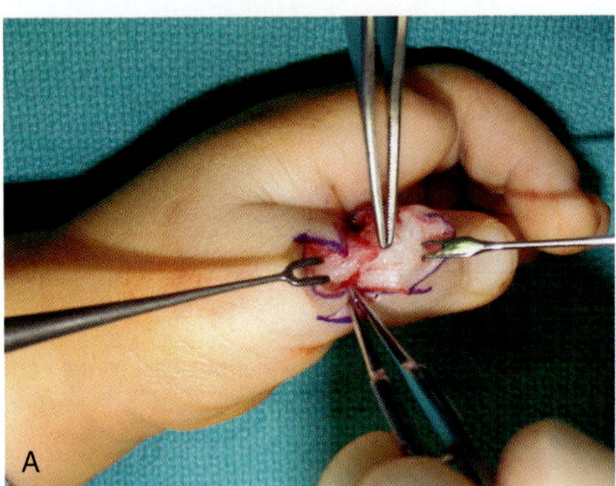
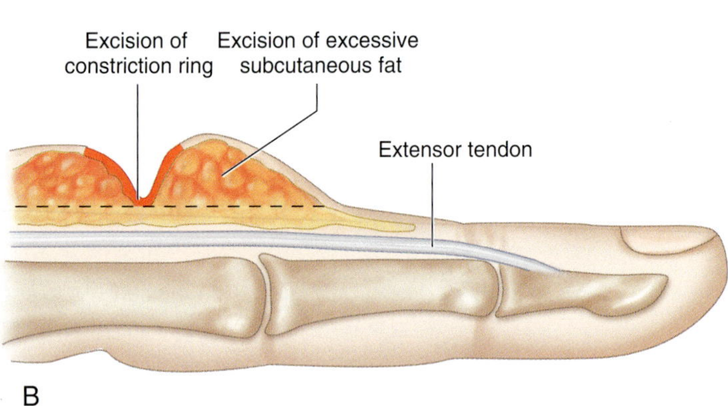

FIGURE 40-3

STEP 1 PEARLS

In finger circumferential rings, it is better to address the dorsal portion first because this improves the aesthetic appearance, and the patient may not need a second stage.

STEP 2 PITFALLS

It is unnecessary to excise the constriction ring; instead, use the skin for closure to avoid skin deficiency during dorsal skin closure.

If the constricted ring involves the palmar side, meticulous dissection should be done to avoid injuring the neurovascular bundles.

Procedure

Correction of Finger Constriction Rings

Step 1: Design of Skin Flaps

- A single Z-plasty is sufficient for correction of finger constriction rings because a one-stage correction is not planned. Either this may be designed on the dorsum, or two single Z-plasties can be designed on both midlateral lines of the finger (Fig. 40-2).

Step 2: Excision of Constriction Ring and Elevation of Skin Flaps

- The constriction ring is incised, and skin flaps are elevated along with a thin layer of fat. This preserves the subdermal plexus and maintains viability of the skin flaps (Fig. 40-3).

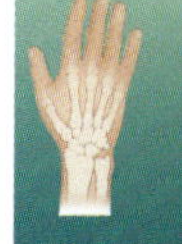

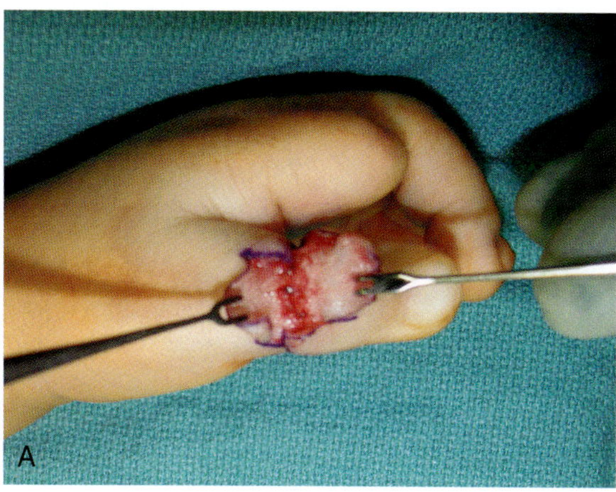

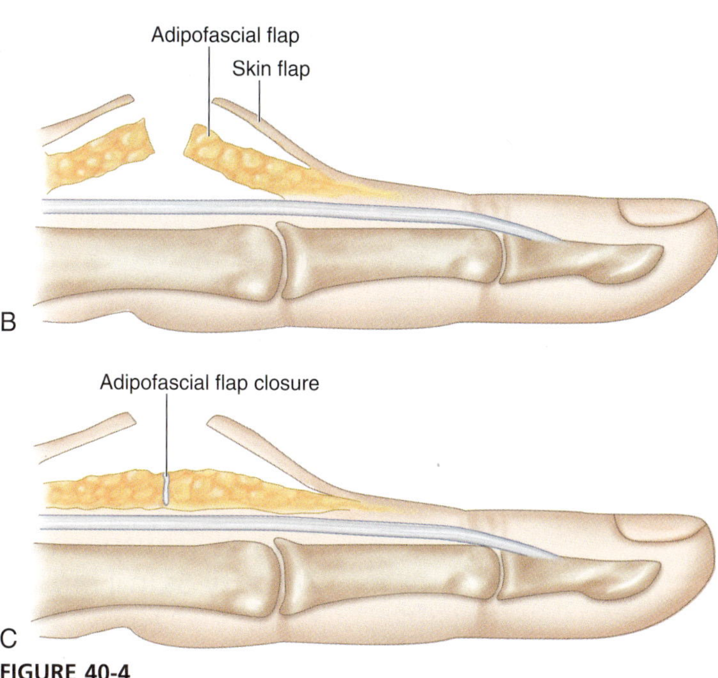

FIGURE 40-4

Step 3: Excision of Excess Subcutaneous Fat

- The subcutaneous fat is elevated proximally and distally superficial to the extensor tendon paratenon or the flexor tendon sheath (Fig. 40-4A and B).
- Excessive dorsal fat, usually on the distal side, should be removed for correction of contour deformity.
- The fat flaps are separated from the skin and sutured to each other using 4-0 Vicryl to correct the contour deformity (Fig. 40-4C).

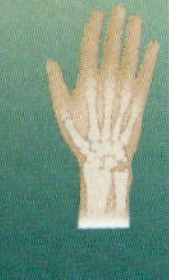

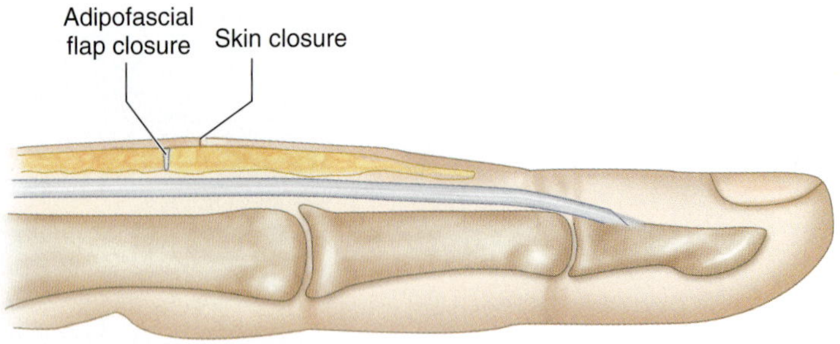

FIGURE 40-5

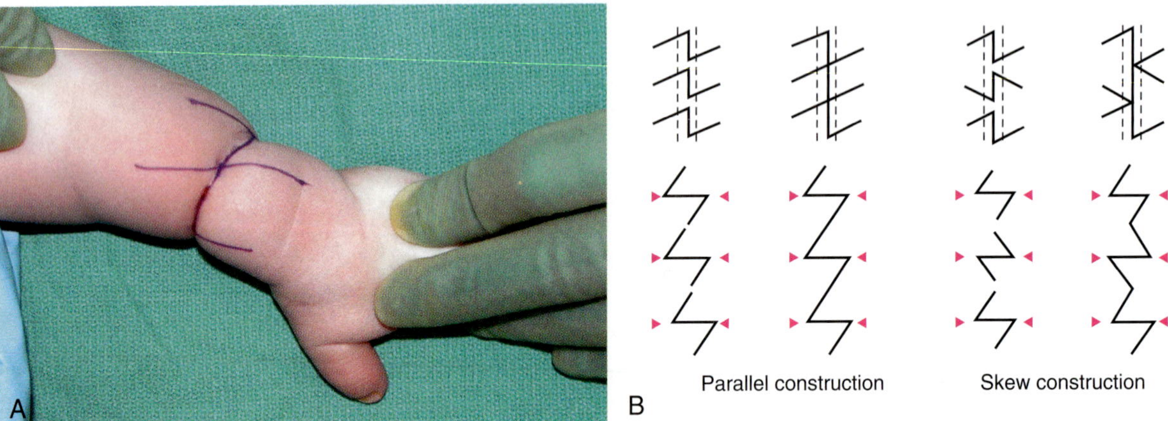

FIGURE 40-6

> **STEP 1 PEARLS**
>
> *Multiple Z-plasties can be constructed in two ways. In a parallel construction, a quadrilateral flap is transposed into a triangular defect, and this results in the formation of dog-ears. A skew construction avoids the formation of dog-ears but results in formation of a broad-tipped flap with a relatively narrow base (Fig. 40-6B).*

Step 4: Transposition and Suture of Z-Plasty Skin Flaps

- Z-plasty skin flaps are transposed and sutured using 4-0/5-0 chromic catgut (Fig. 40-5).

Procedure

Correction of Proximal Limb Constriction Rings

Step 1: Design of Skin Flaps

- Multiple Z-plasty design is used for correction of proximal limb constriction rings because they can be corrected in a single stage (Fig. 40-6A).

Step 2: Excision of Constriction Ring and Elevation of Skin Flaps

- The constriction ring is incised, and skin flaps are elevated.
- Unlike for finger constriction rings, the skin flaps are elevated along with full thickness of the subcutaneous fat in a plane superficial to the deep fascia.

Step 3: Transposition and Suture of Z-Plasty Skin Flaps

- Z-plasty skin flaps are transposed and sutured using 4-0/5-0 chromic catgut (Fig. 40-7).
- Correction of dog-ears may be required if a parallel construction was used for multiple Z-plasties.

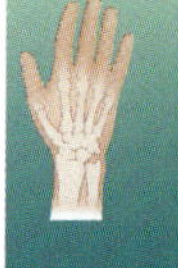

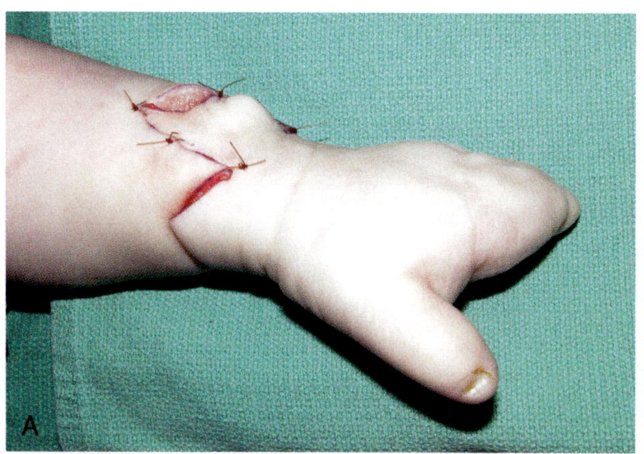

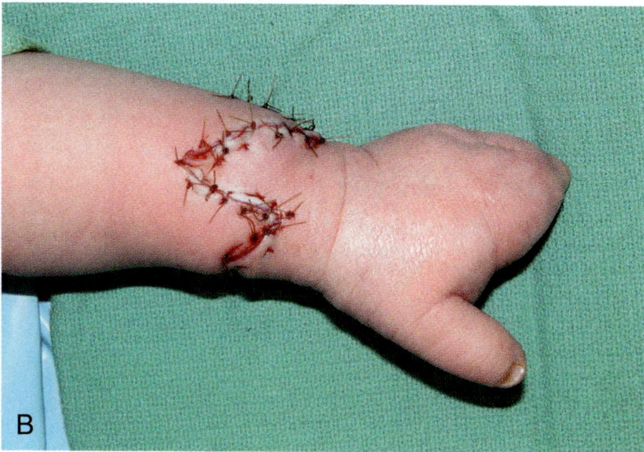

FIGURE 40-7

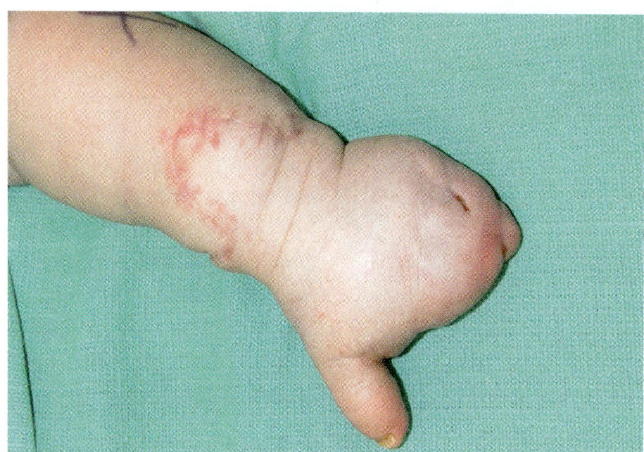

FIGURE 40-8

Postoperative Care and Expected Outcomes

- A soft bulk dressing is applied on the wound. The child's mobility is not restricted postoperatively.
- The lymphedema of the distal part of the affected limb will improve significantly within a few weeks of the surgery, and the contour deformity will improve.
- Figure 40-8 shows the results of the correction of proximal limb constriction rings at 4 months' follow-up.

Evidence

Greene WB. One-stage release of congenital circumferential constriction bands. *J Bone Joint Surg [Am]*. 1993;75:650-655.

In this study, three patients underwent single-stage release of circumferential constriction ring. No wound problems occurred, even when there had been marked swelling of the extremity distal to the band. The single-stage release facilitated postoperative care, and there was no need for additional periods of anesthesia or for additional operations. (Level V evidence)

Upton J, Tan C. Correction of constriction rings. *J Hand Surg [Am]*. 1991;16: 947-953.

A retrospective study of 116 constriction rings in 58 patients who underwent correction of deep and shallow constriction rings. All excellent results occurred in patients with shallow deformities. Improvement of contour was seen; 64% were graded as excellent, 31% as good, and only 5% as poor. (Level IV evidence)

Visuthikosol V, Hompuem T. Constriction band syndrome. *Ann Plast Surg*. 1988;21: 489-495.

A retrospective chart review of 30 cases of constriction band syndrome diagnosed and treated during 1973 to 1986 was conducted. All 30 cases were treated with single-stage Z-plasty surgery. Good results were achieved in 16 of 20 patients with constriction alone. No compromised circulation of the distal limb or total flap loss was encountered in this study. (Level IV evidence)

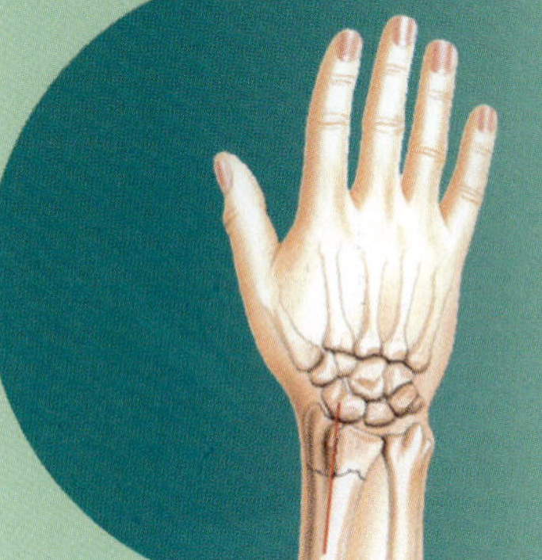

Centralization for Radial Longitudinal Deficiency

Pao-Yuan Lin, Sandeep J. Sebastin, and Kevin C. Chung

See Video 34: Centralization for Radial Deficiency

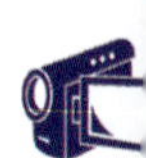

Indications

- Radial longitudinal deficiency (RLD) has been classified into four grades depending on the degree of hypoplasia of the radius (Table 41-1). Centralization is usually performed at 9 to 12 months of age because anesthesia is safer, preliminary soft tissue distraction can be carried out, and subsequent thumb reconstruction can be done before the child develops a maladaptive pattern.
- This procedure may be done first for children with type 0 or 1 deficiencies.
- Children with type 2 or greater deficiencies may need preliminary serial casting or soft tissue distraction using an external fixator.

Examination/Imaging

Clinical Examination

- Sixty percent to 70% of children with RLD have an associated systemic or musculoskeletal abnormality, the most common being scoliosis. Therefore, before surgery, all children with RLD should undergo a thorough musculoskeletal and systemic examination, including spinal radiographs, cardiac echocardiographic evaluation, renal ultrasound, and a complete blood count.
- It is important to assess elbow function. Some children are unable to flex the elbow, and the radial deviation deformity allows them to get the hand to the mouth. Correction of the radial deformity may improve the appearance but will limit function.

Imaging

- Plain radiographs of both hands and forearms (Fig. 41-1) should be obtained.

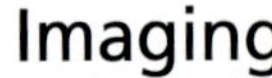

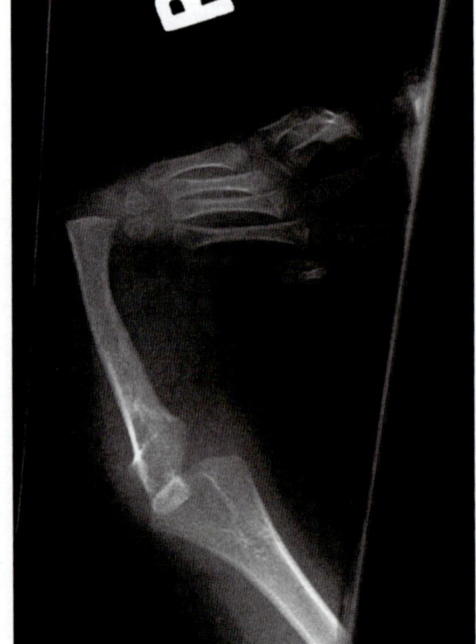

FIGURE 41-1

Table 41-1 Classification of Radial Longitudinal Deficiency

Type	Distal Radius	Proximal Radius
N	Normal	Normal
0	Normal	Normal, radioulnar synostosis, congenital radial head dislocation
1	>2 mm shorter than ulna	Normal, radioulnar synostosis, congenital radial head dislocation
2	Hypoplasia	Hypoplasia
3	Physis absent	Variable hypoplasia
4	Absent	Absent

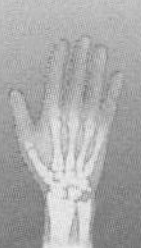

Surgical Anatomy

- Children with RLD have anomalies involving the muscular, vascular, and nervous systems in addition to the obvious skeletal deformity.
- *Skeletal anomalies:* The radius is either absent or partially developed, and the ulna is bowed posteriorly and shortened to two thirds its normal length. The articulation between the carpus and ulna does not form a normal joint. It is usually fibrous but can be lined by hyaline cartilage.
- *Muscle anomalies:* The extensor carpi radialis longus and brevis may be absent or fused to the extensor digitorum communis (EDC). The extensor pollicis longus (EPL), extensor pollicis brevis (EPB), and abductor pollicis longus (APL) are present if the thumb metacarpal is present, or they may be fused to the surrounding tissues. The supinator is generally absent, as is the pronator quadratus. The pronator teres is absent if the radius is absent. The flexor carpi radialis longus and brevis are often absent. The flexor carpi ulnaris is usually present and normal, as is the flexor digitorum superficialis. The palmaris longus is often absent. The flexor pollicis longus is present only if the thumb metacarpal is present. If the thumb is present, the thenar muscles are usually present. The hypothenar, interosseous, and lumbrical muscles are usually normal.
- *Vascular anomalies:* The brachial and ulnar artery are usually present and normal, but the radial artery is absent or attenuated. The interosseous arteries are usually well developed.
- *Nerve anomalies:* The median and ulnar nerves are present, but the median nerve is the most superficial structure on the radial side of the arm and may be confused during surgical dissection with a tendinous structure. The median nerve must be identified first during the exposure. The radial nerve frequently ends at the elbow; thus, the median nerve supplies sensation to the radial side of the arm.

Positioning

- The procedure is performed under general anesthesia and tourniquet control. The patient is positioned supine with the affected extremity on a hand table.

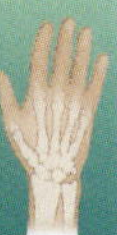

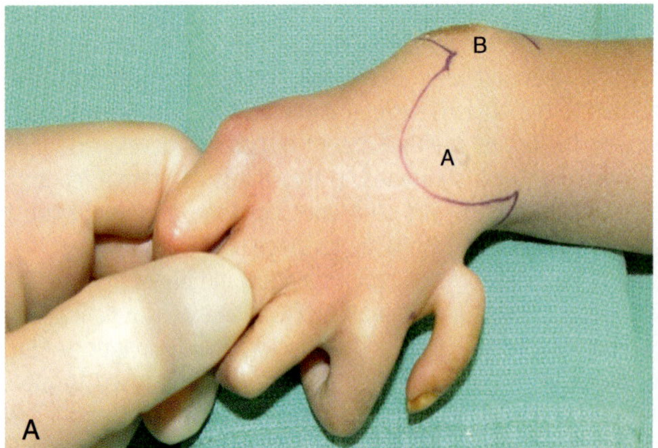

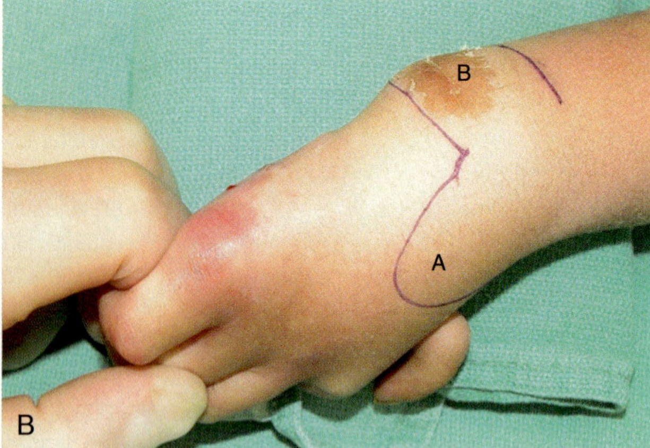

FIGURE 41-2

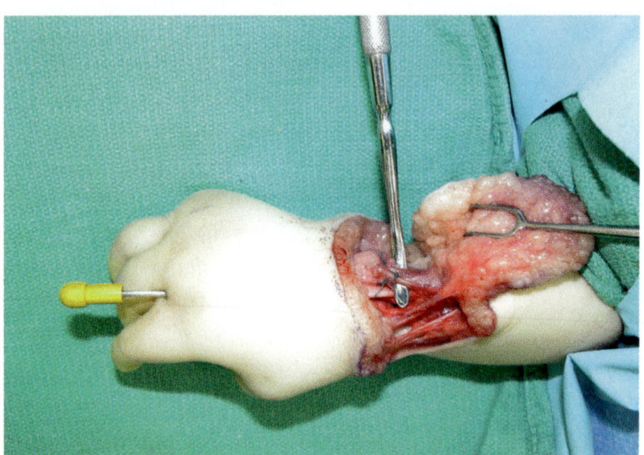

FIGURE 41-3

Exposures

- The four key steps of centralization are the following:
  - Preliminary soft tissue distraction using an external fixator device
  - Design of a bilobed skin flap that transfers the redundant skin on the ulnar side to make up for the skin deficiency on the radial side. The skin incision should start at the point of greatest tension on the radial side of the wrist. The first flap can be marked on the dorsum of the wrist, based proximally (flap A), with another corresponding flap at 90 degrees that lies on the area of greatest skin redundancy on the ulnar side (flap B) (Fig. 41-2).
  - Balancing the tendons to counteract the tendency of radial deviation. This is done by plication of ulnar extensor tendons and transfer of any available radial extensor tendons to the ulnar side (Fig. 41-3).
  - Centralizing the carpus over the ulna.

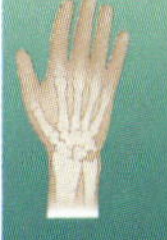

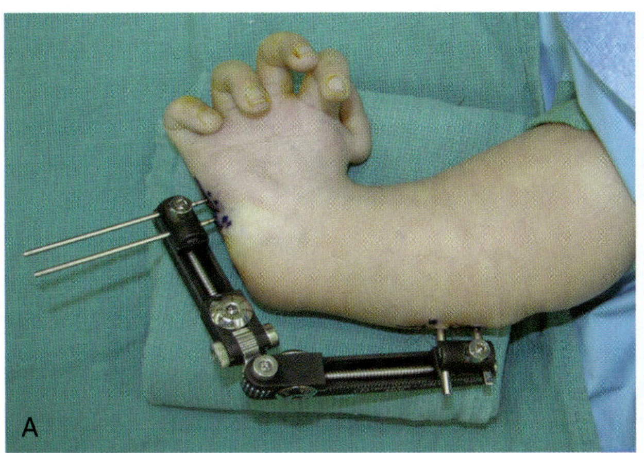

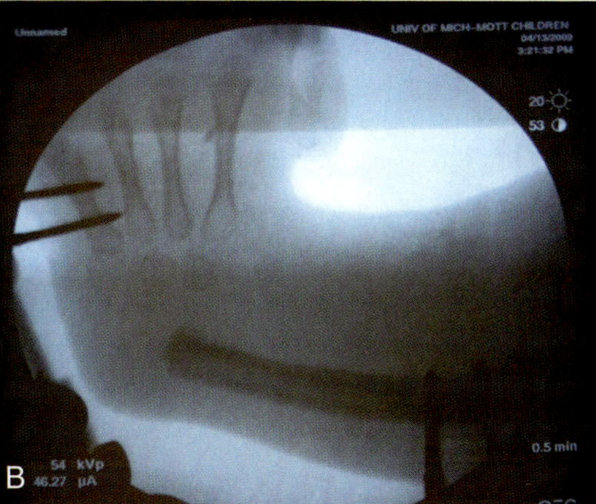

FIGURE 41-4

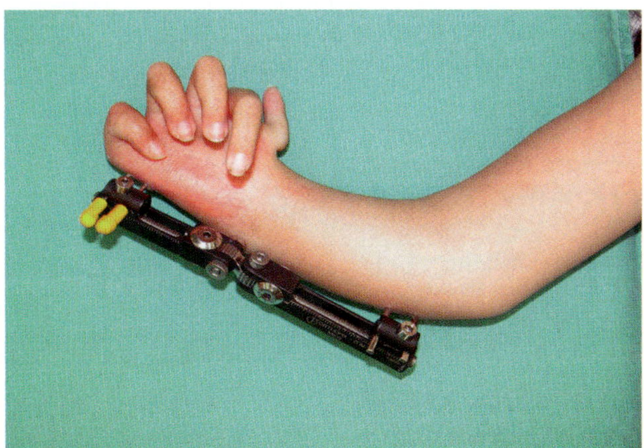

FIGURE 41-5

> **STEP 1 PEARLS**
>
> *Preliminary distraction can lengthen taut radial structures and prevent the need for ulna resection during centralization.*

Procedure

Step 1: Preliminary Soft Tissue Distraction

- A uniplanar external fixator device is applied on the ulnar side of the affected limb (the metacarpal of small finger and ulna of patient shown in Figure 41-4). This is best done at 6 to 9 months of age.
- The parents begin distraction at a rate of 1 mm/day about 4 to 5 days after placement of the device. The patient is observed with a weekly clinic visit and radiograph.
- Distraction is continued until the hand is about in a neutral position. Normally, it takes about 2 months of distraction to achieve this position (Fig. 41-5).
- The external fixator device can be removed at the same time as surgery for centralization.

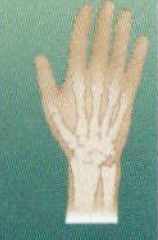

STEP 2 PITFALLS

Care should be taken to preserve the superficial cutaneous nerves and longitudinal veins.

Flaps should be kept as thick as possible to avoid devascularizing the wound edges.

Beware of the large dorsal branch of the median nerve, which replaces the absent superficial radial nerve that supplies sensation to the radial aspect of the hand. This branch is positioned in the subcutaneous fold between the wrist and forearm.

STEP 4 PEARLS

If the carpus cannot be reduced, the radial side of the wrist needs to be reexamined, and any radial fibrous bands should be divided to facilitate reduction of the carpus onto the ulna.

Occasionally, partial carpectomy or limited shaving of the carpus to create a notch in it for seating of the distal end of the ulna may be required to achieve reduction. However, it should be remembered that carpal bones are resected only if reduction is impossible, because excessive resection of the epiphysis will arrest growth. Rather than accepting this risk, preoperative soft tissue stretching using an external distractor is recommended in most cases.

Step 2: Elevation of Bilobed Flap

- The skin is incised along the previously marked bilobed flap.
- The flap is raised in a plane superficial to the extensor retinaculum.

Step 3: Dissection of Nerve and Tendons

- The median nerve must be identified first during the exposure. It is the most superficial structure on the radial side of the distal forearm and can easily be confused with a tendinous structure (Fig. 41-6).
- The extensor carpi ulnaris (ECU) is easier to find distal to the retinaculum. The ECU is shortened by imbrication after centralization, and the ECR is divided at its insertion to facilitate later transfer to the ECU (Fig. 41-7).
- The dorsal ulnar sensory nerve is identified and protected.

Step 4: Ulnocarpal Joint Reduction and Centralization

- The wrist capsule is opened distal to the ulnar physis, and a soft tissue release is carried out until the carpus can be brought over the distal ulna (Fig. 41-8).
- The carpus is mobilized off the palmar capsule until it can be reduced onto the distal ulna for centralization.

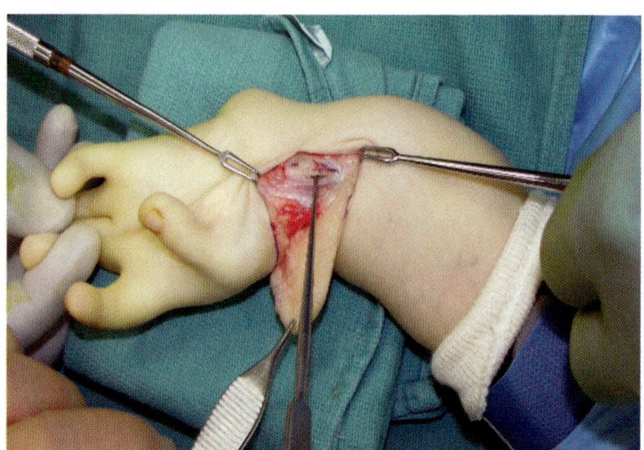

FIGURE 41-6

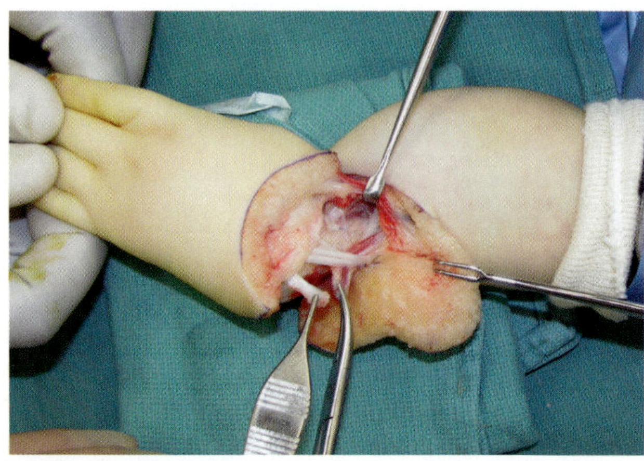

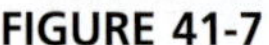

FIGURE 41-7

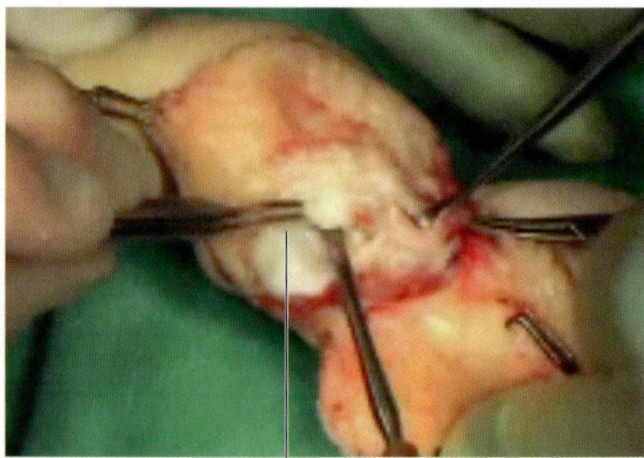

FIGURE 41-8

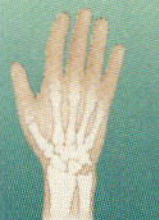

STEP 5 PEARLS

If the ulna has an angular deformity greater than 30 degrees, a diaphyseal closing wedge osteotomy is performed at the apex of the deformity and secured with the same K-wire.

Step 5: Fixation

- The ulnocarpal reduction is maintained by 0.062-inch K-wire placed antegrade through the carpus and then retrograde into the ulnar shaft under fluoroscopic guidance (Fig. 41-9).

Step 6: Wrist Stabilization

- The ECR tendon is transferred to the distal stump of the ECU passing below the EDC (see Fig. 41-3). The proximal end of the ECU is advanced and sutured to the dorsal wrist capsule. Tendon repairs are done using 2-0 Ethibond horizontal mattress sutures.
- The extensor retinaculum is repaired using 4-0 Vicryl, and skin is closed with 4-0 chromic sutures (Fig. 41-10).

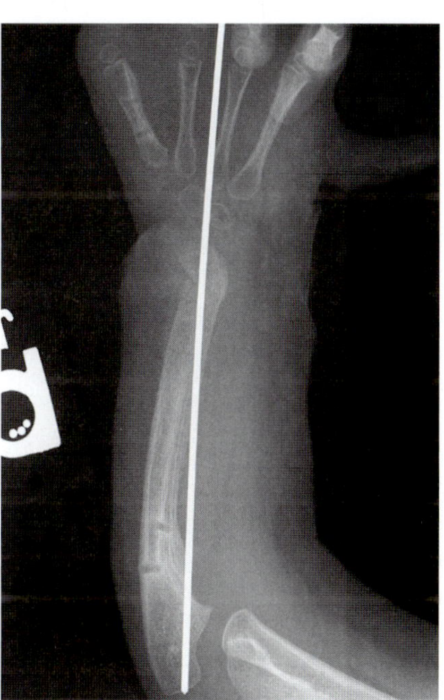

FIGURE 41-9

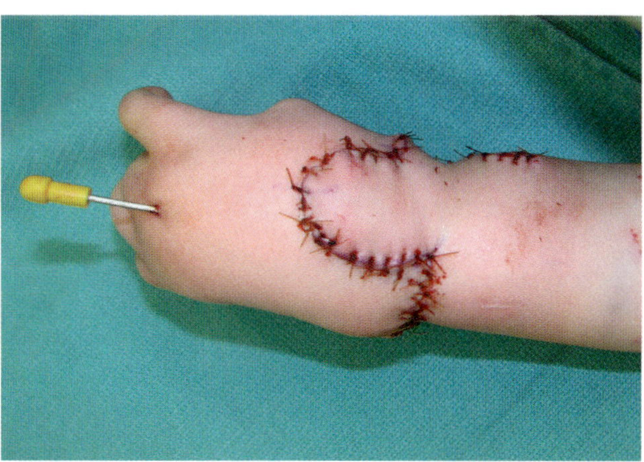

FIGURE 41-10

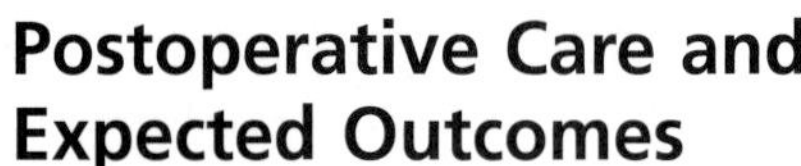

Postoperative Care and Expected Outcomes

- A long-arm cast with the elbow flexed to 90 degrees is provided. The extremity is immobilized for at least 8 weeks, and the pin is kept in place for as long as possible. A long-arm Orthoplast splint to maintain wrist position is worn full-time for 3 months and then at night until skeletal maturity. Prolonged pin fixation followed by long-term splinting is necessary to minimize recurrence.
- Recurrence is the most common source of failure following centralization, and the cause appears to be multifactorial. Operative causes include the inability to obtain complete correction at surgery, inadequate radial soft tissue release, and failure to balance the radial force. Postoperative reasons consist of early pin removal, poor postoperative splint use, and the natural tendency for the shortened forearm and hand to deviate in a radial direction for hand-to-mouth use.
- Even a successful centralization still results in a shortened forearm segment secondary to altered growth of the ulna (60% of normal). The short forearm is both a cosmetic and functional problem for the teenager with radial deficiency. Lengthening of the ulna can be accomplished using uniplanar or multiplanar shaft-distraction devices.

Evidence

Damore E, Kozin SH, Thoder JJ, Porter S. The recurrence of deformity after surgical centralization for radial clubhand. *J Hand Surg [Am]*. 2000;25:745-751.
Preoperative, postoperative, and follow-up radiographs were used to determine the initial deformity, amount of surgical correction, and degree of recurrence in 14 children (19 cases of radial deficiency). The average preoperative angulation measured 83 degrees. Centralization corrected the angulation an average of 58 degrees to an average immediate postoperative total angulation of 25 degrees. At the final follow-up examination, there was a loss of 38 degrees, and the total angulation increased to an average of 63 degrees. (Level IV evidence)

Goldfarb CA, Klepps SJ, Dailey LA, Manske PR. Functional outcome after centralization for radius dysplasia. *J Hand Surg [Am]*. 2002;27:118-124.
Case series of 21 patients (25 wrists) an average of 20 years after surgery who underwent functional outcome assessment. The Jebsen-Taylor scores, a measure of hand function, were significantly altered, with an average total score of 48 seconds compared with an average normal score of 30 seconds (62% increase). The DASH (Disabilities of the Arm, Shoulder, and Hand) questionnaire, a measure of upper-extremity function, showed only a mild disability of 18%. These long-term follow-up data show that hand function remains markedly abnormal, whereas upper extremity disability is mild. Improved wrist alignment and increased ulna length did not correlate with improved upper extremity function. (Level IV evidence)

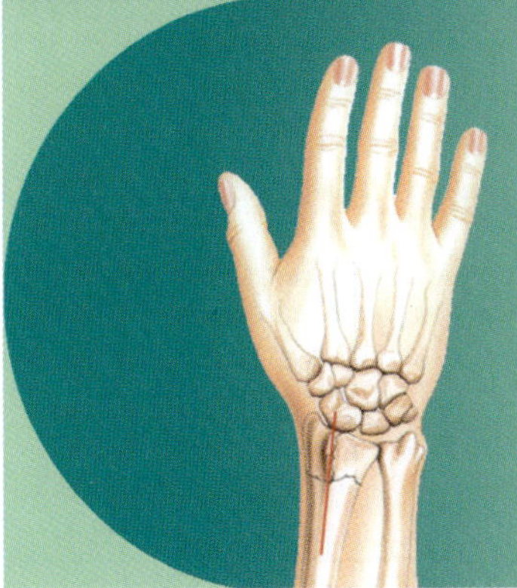

PROCEDURE 42

Cleft Hand Reconstruction

Sandeep J. Sebastin and Kevin C. Chung

A central cleft associated with a tight thumb and index finger web space in a child is probably the strongest indication for cleft hand closure. An isolated central cleft should not create a functional problem, and most pediatric hand surgeons will agree that closure of the cleft is primarily an aesthetic consideration to decrease the stigma associated with a prominent deformity. The indications for the cleft closure procedure must be discussed fully with the parents.

Indications

- Presence of a transverse bone in which growth leads to a progressive deformity
- Syndactyly affecting border rays with progressive deviation of the longer ray
- Constricted first web space
- Closure of the cleft for aesthetic reasons

Examination/Imaging

Clinical Examination

- A cleft hand is considered a longitudinal deficiency affecting the central digits. It is commonly inherited as an autosomal dominant trait with variable penetrance. The condition may be bilateral and may involve the feet. Manske and Halikis have proposed a classification based on the status of the first web space that is useful in planning treatment (Table 42-1).
- Patients with a typical cleft hand present with a V-shaped cleft in the center of the hand. This is occasionally associated with absence, polydactyly, and/or syndactyly of one or more digits. The cleft may be minor or major with absence of one or more digits. The absence progresses from the radial to the ulnar side. Polydactyly/syndactyly involves the digits adjacent to the cleft. Proximal muscle tendon units and nerves may be variably absent.
- There is a strong genetic component associated with hand clefts, and genetic counseling is helpful.

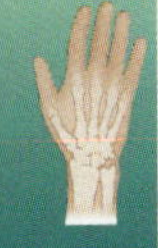

Table 42-1 Classification of Cleft Hand (Manske and Halikis)

Type	Description	Characteristics
I	Normal web	Thumb web space is not narrow
IIA	Mildly narrowed web	Thumb web space is mildly narrow
IIB	Severely narrowed web	Thumb web space is severely narrowed
III	Syndactylized web	Thumb and index rays syndactylized, web space obliterated
IV	Merged web	Index ray suppressed, thumb web space merged with the cleft
V	Absent web	Thumb elements suppressed, ulnar rays remain, thumb web space no longer present

Imaging

- Radiographs of the hand and upper limb are necessary for all congenital hand problems to identify other areas of concern.
- Metacarpal anomalies are frequently noticed. These include absence of metacarpals within the cleft, transverse tubular bones that widen the cleft with growth, bifid metacarpals supporting one finger, and duplication. Phalangeal anomalies include longitudinally bracketed epiphyses or double phalanges.

Positioning

- The procedure is performed under tourniquet control with the patient in the supine position.

Exposures

- In children who have a central cleft with narrow thumb and index finger web, the skin over the dorsum of the cleft is raised as a palmar-based flap. This flap is used to resurface the narrow thumb and index finger web after it is released. Elevating this flap on the dorsum is easier because of a lack of adhering palmar fascia. Additionally, this allows access to the metacarpal heads that can be sutured together to close the cleft.
- A distally based rectangular flap is designed over the midproximal phalanx on one of the fingers adjoining the cleft. This flap will be used to create the web space formed after closure of the central cleft. An important consideration is to create a smooth slope in the web space.
- Figures 42-1 and 42-2 show a 2-year-old boy with a central cleft between the index and long fingers, a tight thumb and index finger web space, and complete complex syndactyly between the long and ring fingers. The syndactyly will need to be released in a second operation.

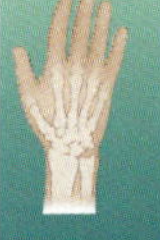

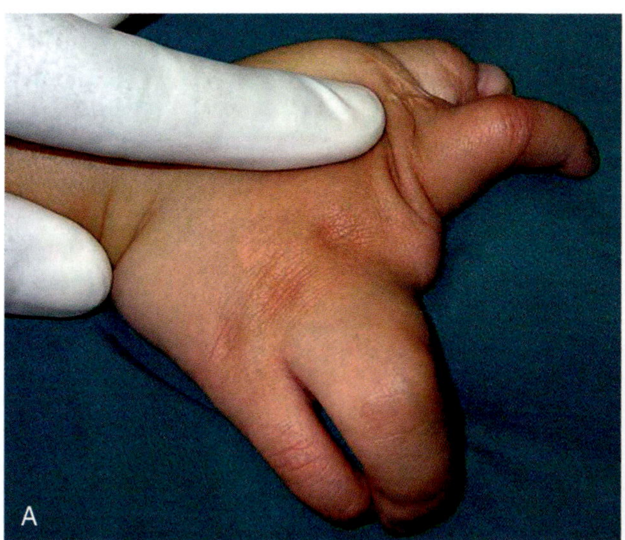

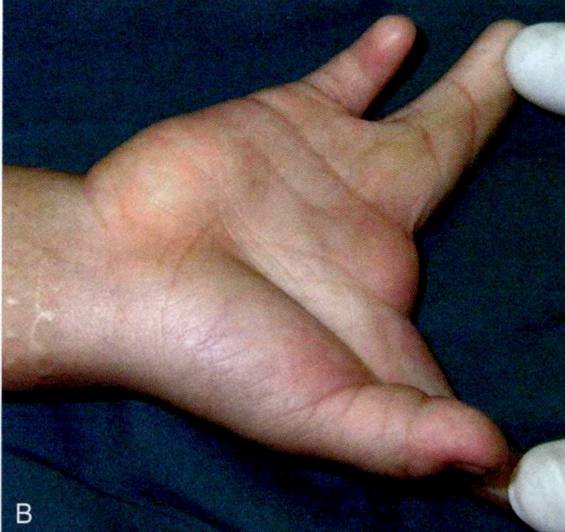

FIGURE 42-1

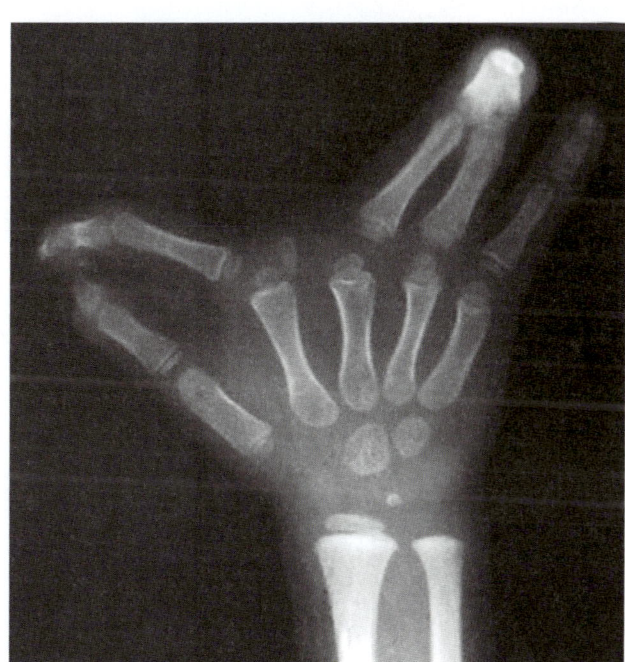

FIGURE 42-2

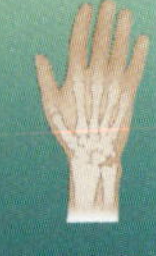

STEP 1 PEARLS

The flap should be mobilized sufficiently to allow easy transposition to the thumb and index finger web space.

The viability of this flap depends on preservation of the intrinsic blood supply, and dissection must maintain the subdermal plexus.

Procedure

Cleft Hand Reconstruction

Step 1: Elevation of Palmar-Based Cleft Flap

- A palmar-based flap is designed, extending to the dorsum of the hand by parallel incisions (Figs. 42-3 and 42-4).
- The parallel incisions are connected on the dorsum, and the dorsal flap is elevated superficial to the extensor tendons (Fig. 42-5).
- The neurovascular bundles are identified on the palmar aspect and protected, and the flap is mobilized by dividing any strands of palmar fascia (Fig. 42-6).

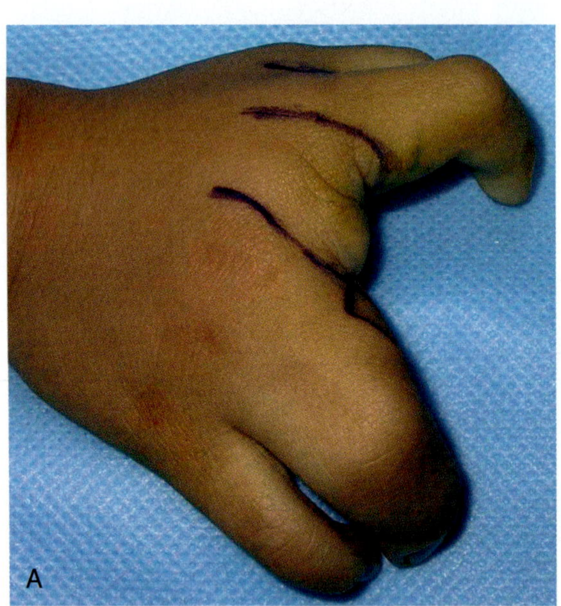

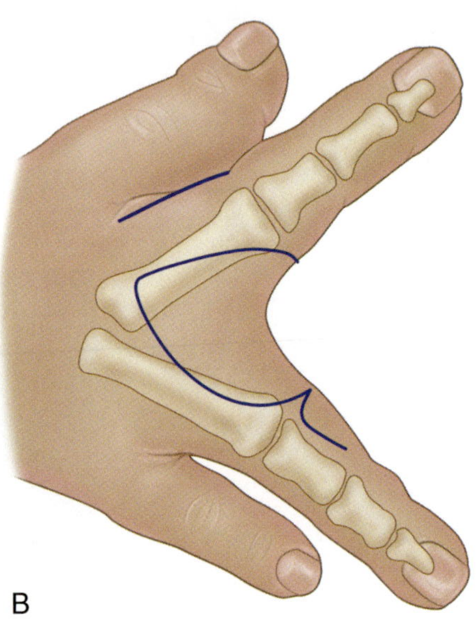

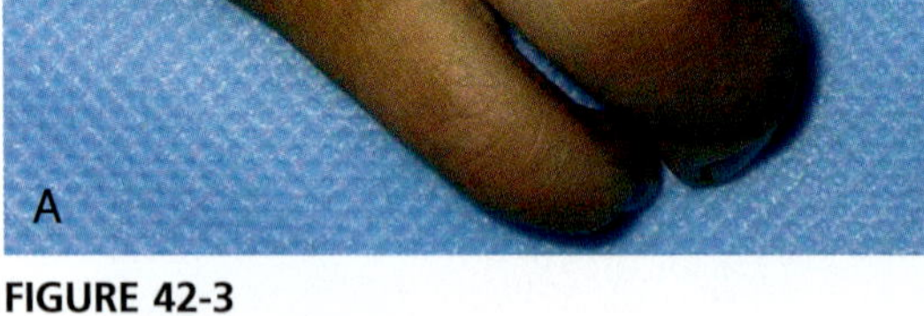

FIGURE 42-3

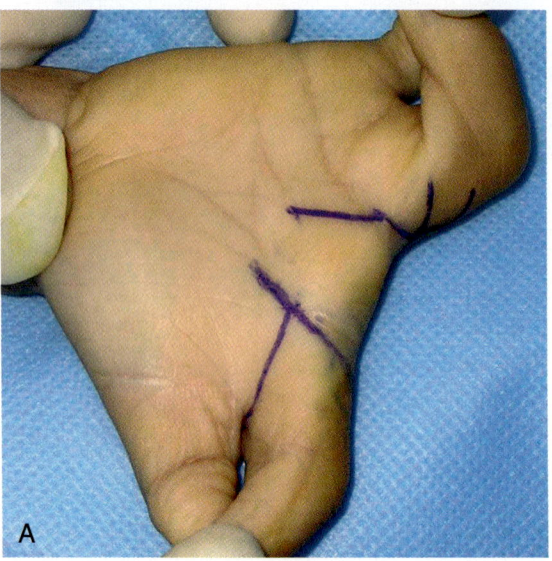

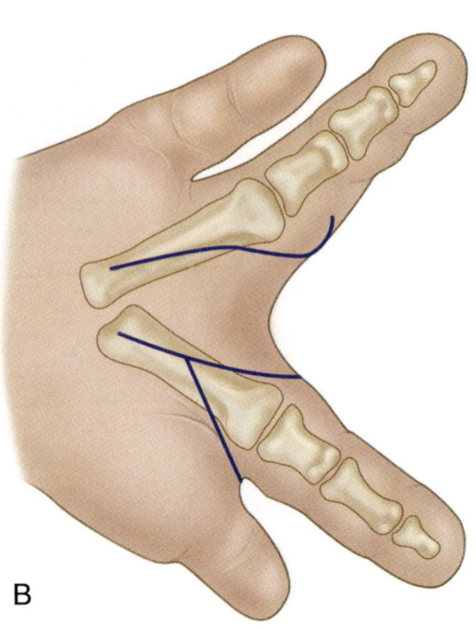

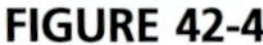

FIGURE 42-4

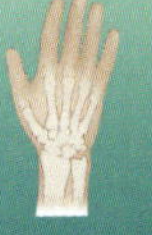

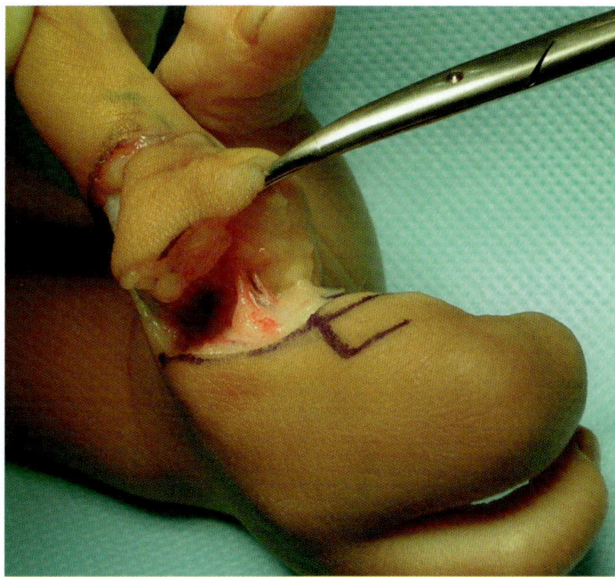

FIGURE 42-5

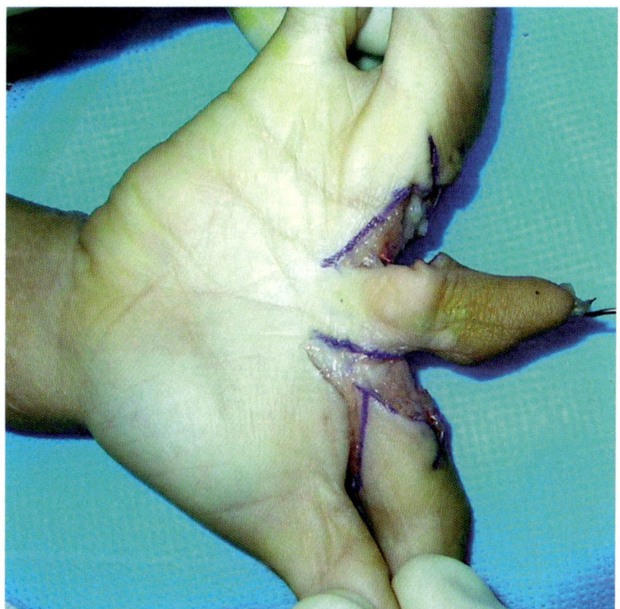

FIGURE 42-6

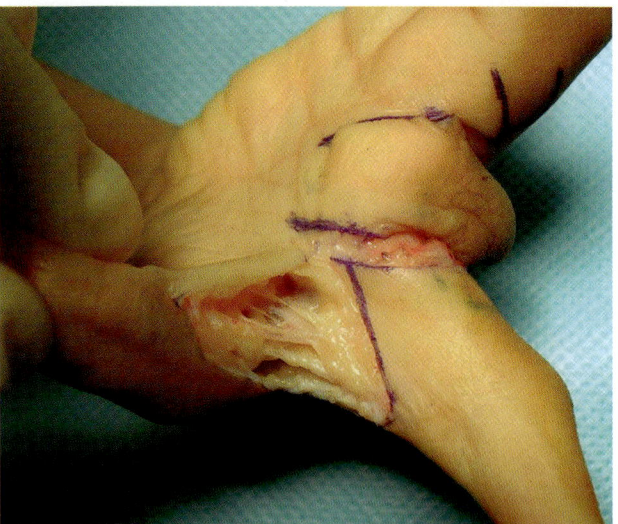

FIGURE 42-7

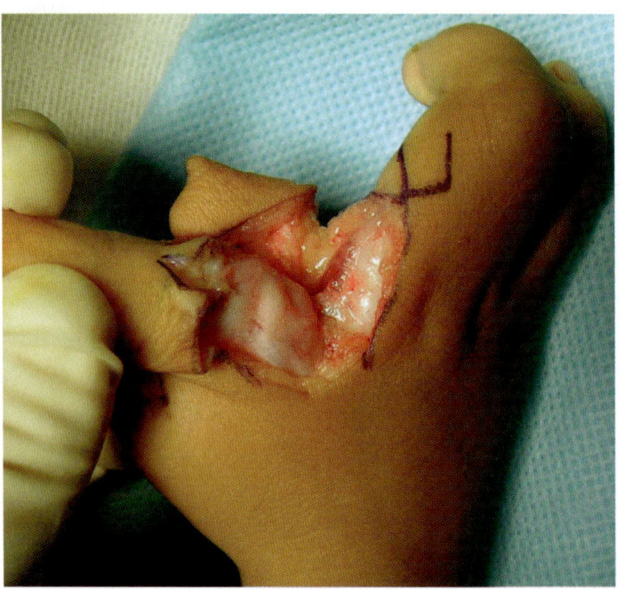

FIGURE 42-8

STEP 2 PEARLS

Depending on the severity of the thumb and index finger web space narrowing, one may need to divide the fascia, the adductor pollicis, and the first dorsal interosseous, and rarely an osteotomy of the thumb metacarpal may be required to realign the thumb.

STEP 3 PEARLS

It is rather easy to place sutures into the bones, which have not fully ossified. Tension is adjusted so that one does not create an overly tight closure, which can cause scissoring of the fingers.

Step 2: Release of Thumb and Index Finger Web Space

- An opening incision is made between the thumb and index finger to release the web space contracture (Fig. 42-7).

Step 3: Closure of Cleft

- The metacarpal heads adjoining the cleft are exposed as a result of elevating the flap (Fig. 42-8).
- Nonabsorbable sutures are placed into the metacarpal heads to bring the metacarpals together (Figs. 42-9 and 42-10).

Step 4: Transfer of Cleft Flap to Resurface Thumb and Index Finger Web

- The previously elevated flap is transposed into the defect created by release of the thumb and index finger web (Fig. 42-11).

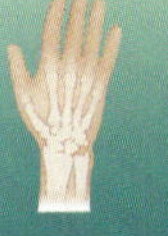

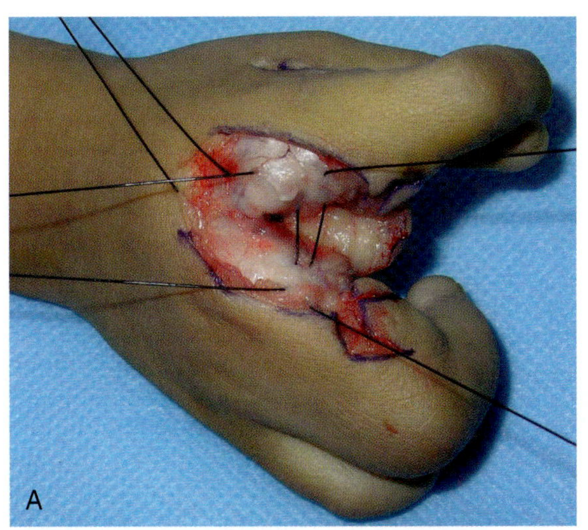

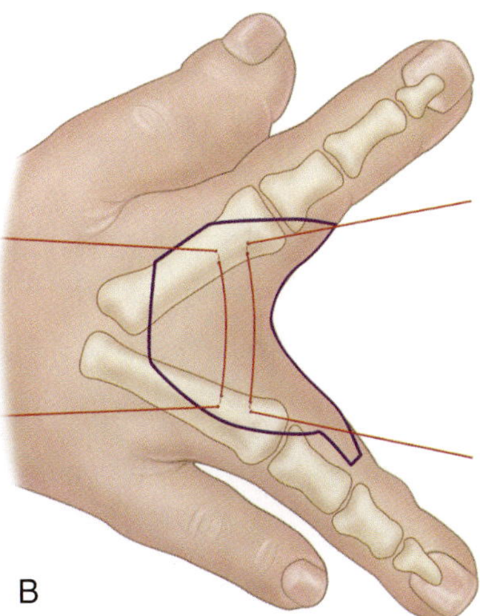

FIGURE 42-9

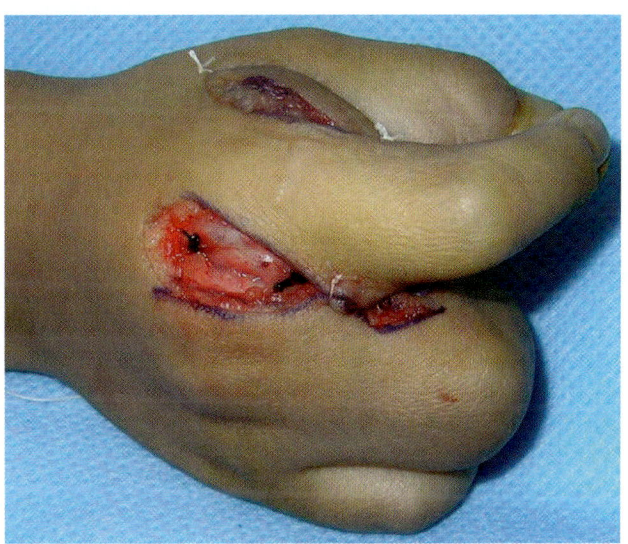

FIGURE 42-10

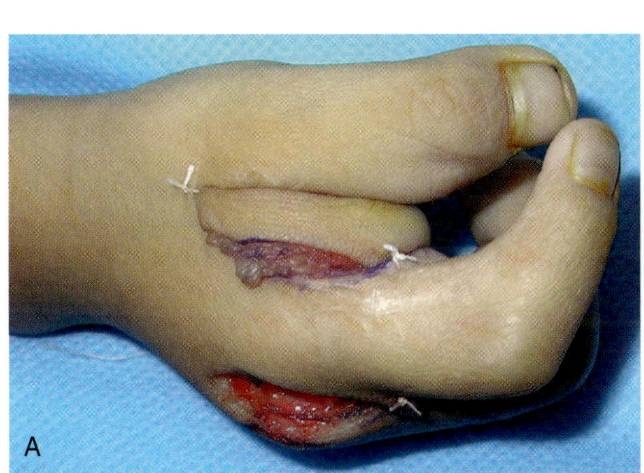

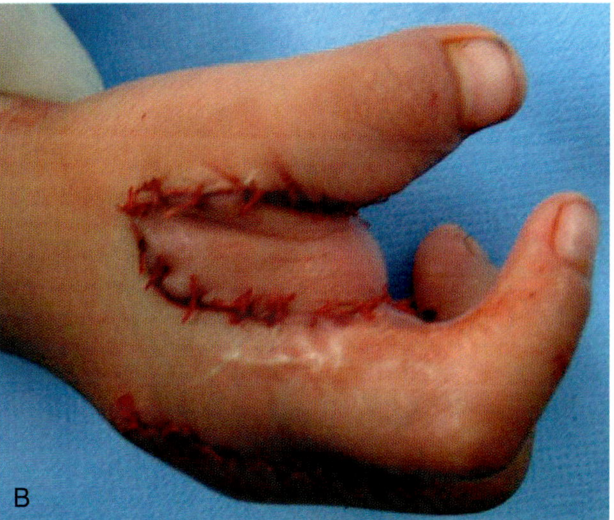

FIGURE 42-11

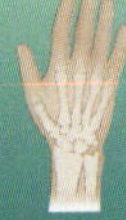

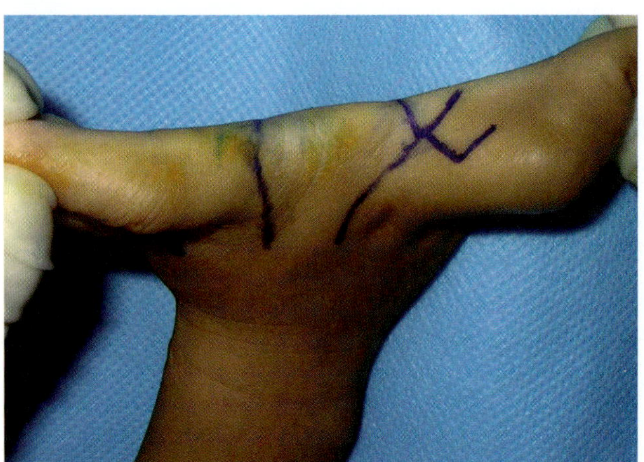

FIGURE 42-12

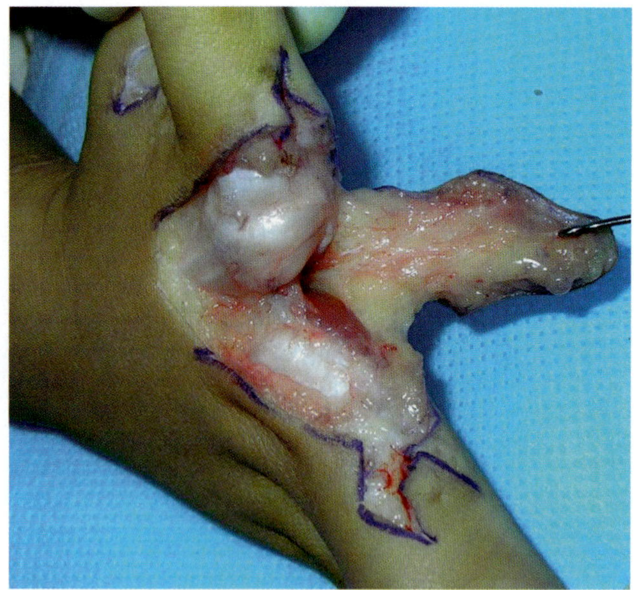

FIGURE 42-13

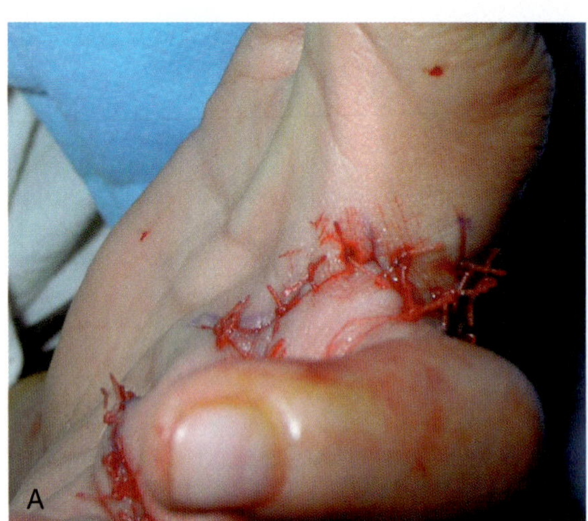

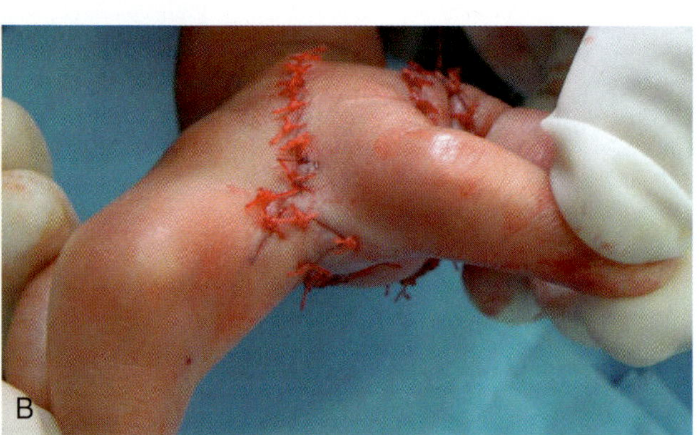

FIGURE 42-14

> **STEP 5 PEARLS**
>
> *It is better to elevate this flap (ring finger) after closing the cleft by suturing the metacarpal heads together. This allows for adjustments to the flap design based on final location of the web space.*

Step 5: Creation of New Web Space in Cleft

- A distally based rectangular flap is designed over the ring finger, which will be sutured to the index finger on cleft closure to re-create the web space (Fig. 42-12).
- The flap is elevated and sutured to the opposite incision to create the gentle slope of the web space (Figs. 42-13 and 42-14).

Step 6

- All skin incisions are closed with absorbable sutures to avoid difficult suture removals in children. Chromic catgut is preferred because it dissolves earlier (Fig. 42-15).

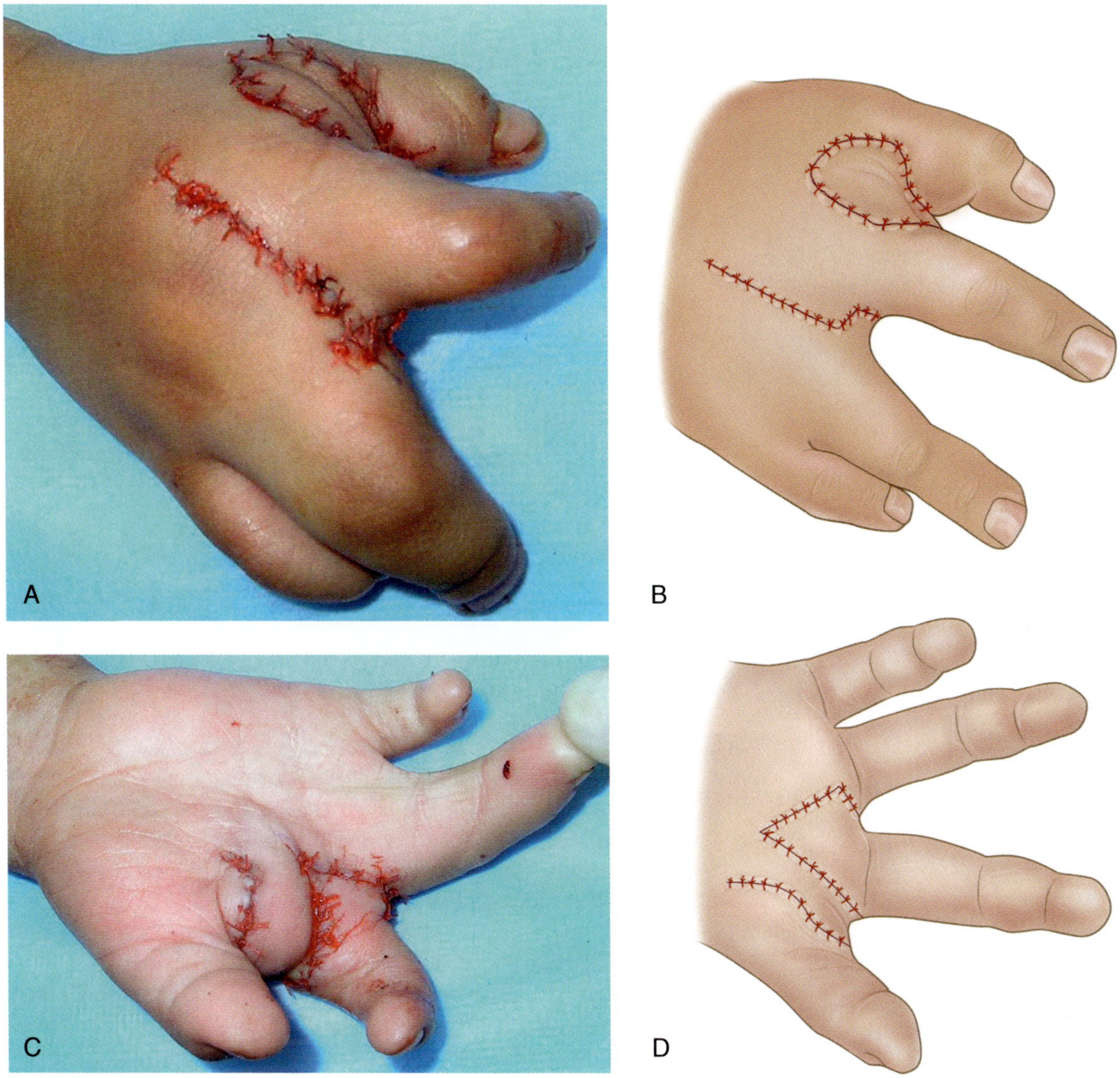

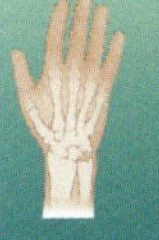

A B C D

FIGURE 42-15

Postoperative Care and Expected Outcomes

- The hand is splinted for 4 weeks to allow healing of the intermetacarpal closure.
- No therapy is necessary after splint removal. The child is followed yearly to evaluate the growth of the hand. Creeping of the web space is not uncommon with cleft surgery. Future web space releases may be needed to enhance the functional and aesthetic results for the hand. The outcome depends on the degree of preoperative deformity, and good function can be achieved in children with a preserved thumb.

Evidence

Rider MA, Grinder SI, Tomkin MA, Wood VE. An experience of the Snow-Littler procedure. *J Hand Surg [Br]*. 2000;25:376-381.

The authors reviewed 12 cases using the Snow-Littler procedure to close hand clefts. The procedure described is similar to the techniques illustrated in this chapter. They concluded that this technique improved the appearance and function for children with hand clefts. (Level IV evidence)

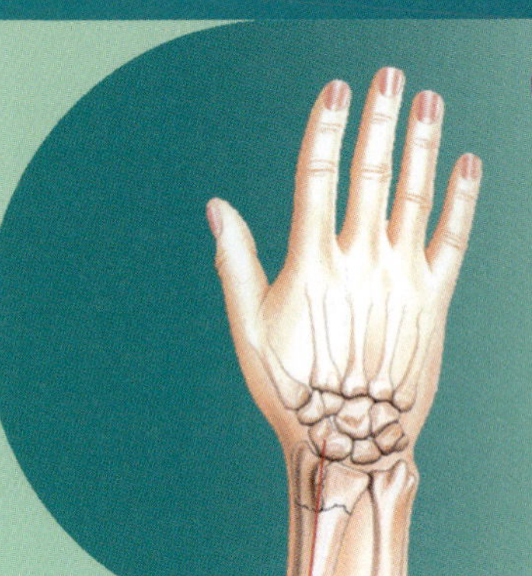

PROCEDURE 43

Carpal Wedge Osteotomy for Congenital Wrist Flexion Contracture (Arthrogryposis)

Sandeep J. Sebastin and Kevin C. Chung

See Video 35: Triceps Lengthening and Elbow Release in Arthrogryposis

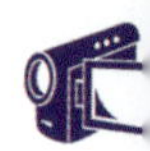

Indications

- Wrist flexion contracture with fixed bony changes (carpal coalition) (Figs. 43-1 and 43-2)

Examination/Imaging

Clinical Examination

- The ability of the child to open and close the fingers should be determined. If the child does not have active finger extension, correction of the wrist flexion contracture will result in loss of ability to passively extend the finger by the tenodesis effect (Fig. 43-3).
- The function of the extensor carpi ulnaris (ECU) should be assessed. A transfer of the ECU to the radial wrist extensors may be required to improve wrist extension and diminish the ulnar deviation deformity.
- It is important to examine the child along with an occupational therapist to evaluate the functional status of the wrist. This will help to determine the optimal wrist position in children who need surgery and to avoid surgery in children who have adapted well to the wrist flexion contracture.
- These children frequently have lower limb anomalies that can be corrected simultaneously to reduce the overall number of procedures.

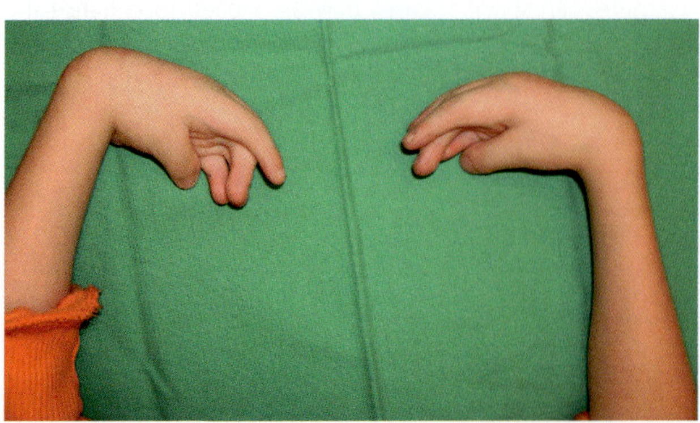

FIGURE 43-1

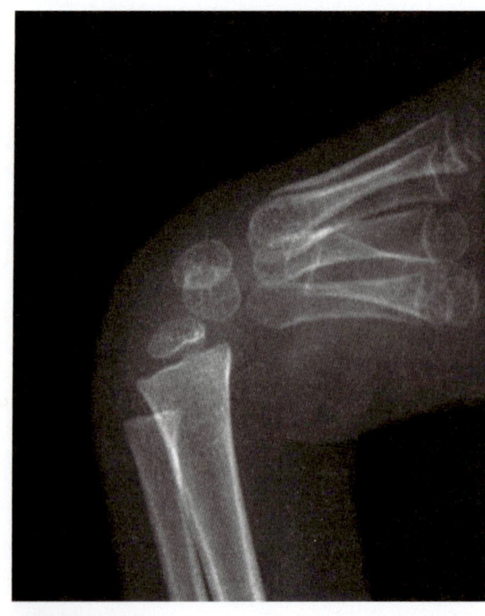

FIGURE 43-2

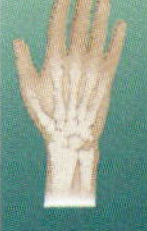

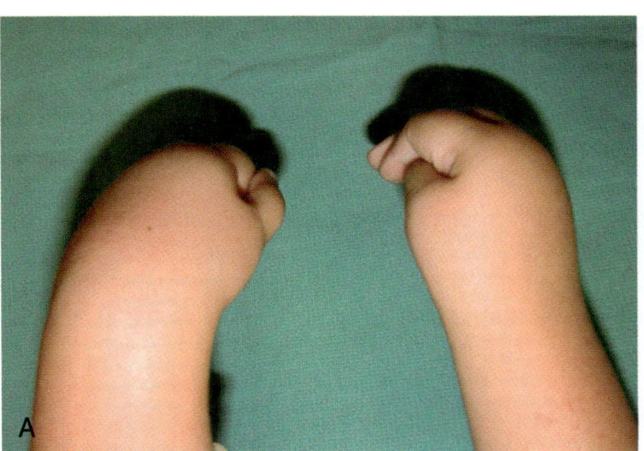

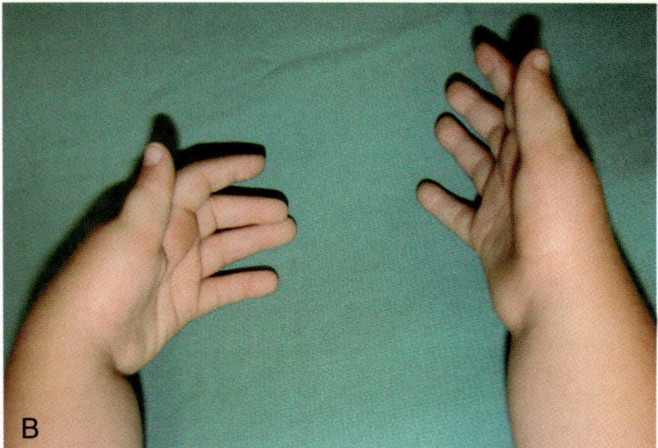

FIGURE 43-3

Imaging

- Radiographs of the wrist can help in planning the location of the wedge resection.

Surgical Anatomy

- The extensor tendons are usually small. The radial wrist extensors (extensor carpi radialis longus and brevis) are usually adherent to the dorsal capsule, and the proximal musculature is absent. The ECU is often the largest extensor tendon.

Positioning

- The procedure is performed under tourniquet control with the patient in the supine position. The degree of elbow contracture may complicate arm position during surgery. The tourniquet should be placed as high as possible to increase the surgical field.
- Intraoperative fluoroscopy will be required to plan the wedge resection and to confirm position of the K-wires that will be used for fixation.

PEARLS

The sensory branches of the radial and ulnar nerve are elevated along with the skin flaps.

The entire midcarpal joint must be visualized and the extensor compartments mobilized sufficiently for full exposure.

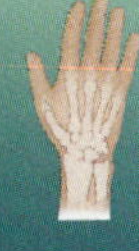

PITFALLS

The EPL is small and must be handled carefully. The radial extensor tendons are atrophic and usually attached to the dorsal capsule.

STEP 1 PEARLS

Intraoperative fluoroscopy can be used to confirm the position of the osteotomy in the older child. In the younger child whose carpus has not yet ossified, the position should be confirmed visually.

A scalpel blade can be used in the younger child because the carpus is relatively soft. An osteotome will be required in the older child. Using a saw is not necessary because there is less control of the cut and the bone is soft.

STEP 1 PITFALLS

Ensure that the wedge resection is over the midcarpal joint and not the radiocarpal joint.

Prevent injury to the volar wrist capsule.

STEP 3 PEARLS

It is easy to pass the K-wires in an antegrade fashion through the osteotomy site to exit at the skin distally between the metacarpals. Then the osteotomy is closed, and the K-wires are passed retrograde across the osteotomy and the radiocarpal joint into the distal radius.

Exposures

- A single 4-cm longitudinal incision centered over the dorsum of the wrist is made. The extensor retinaculum is identified, and skin flaps are raised on both sides superficial to the retinaculum.
- The third compartment is identified by its location ulnar to Lister tubercle and opened. The extensor pollicis longus (EPL) tendon is brought out of the third compartment.
- The wrist capsule is opened in the floor of the third compartment. The second and fourth compartments are elevated extraperiosteally off the distal radius and the carpus to expose the carpus.

Procedure

Step 1

- A wedge of bone is removed from the midcarpal joint using an osteotomy. The amount of bone removed depends on the preoperative flexion and ulnar deviation deformity. The proximal cut is made perpendicular to the long axis of the radius, and the distal cut is made perpendicular to the metacarpals. This results in a wedge because of the flexion deformity. The wedge should be made wider on the radial side if correction of an ulnar deviation deformity is also required (Fig. 43-4).

Step 2

- The aim of the wedge osteotomy is to get the wrist into a posture of slight extension (Fig. 43-5). If the wrist cannot be brought into this position, tendons on the volar side need to be released. A 4-cm volar longitudinal incision is made proximal to the wrist crease and ulnar to the palmaris longus.
- A tight palmaris longus tendon can be divided. Up to 2 cm of lengthening can be obtained by dividing the tendinous portions at the musculotendinous junction.

Step 3

- Two 0.062-inch K-wires are passed to maintain the corrected position of the wrist after wedge excision of the carpus and release of any volar restricting structures (Fig. 43-6).

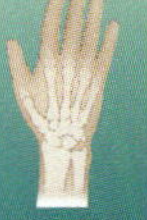

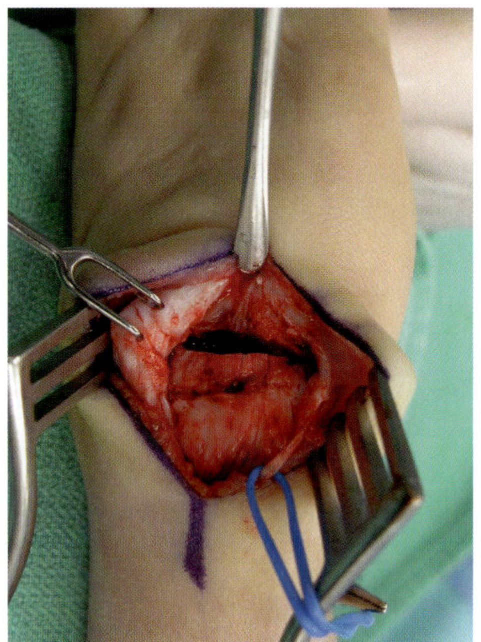

FIGURE 43-4

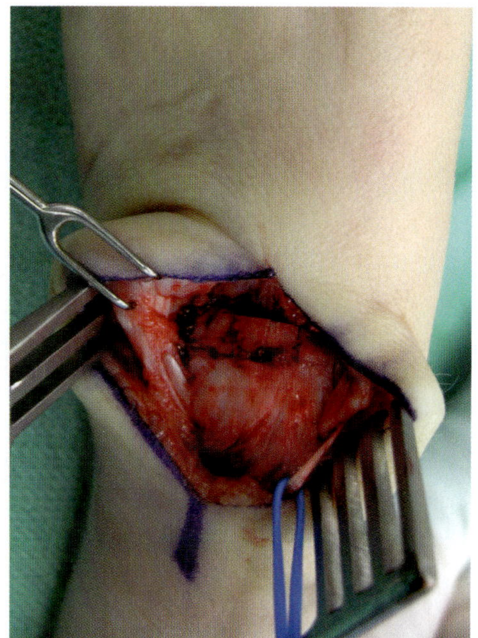

FIGURE 43-5

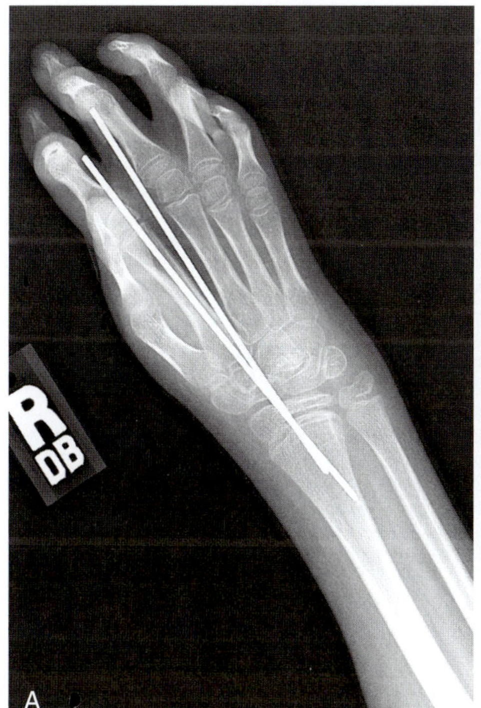

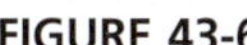

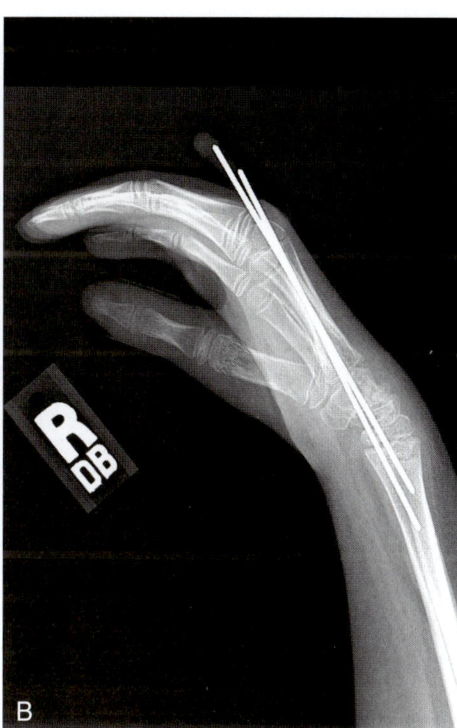

FIGURE 43-6

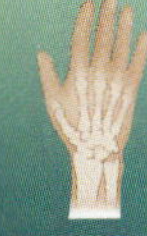

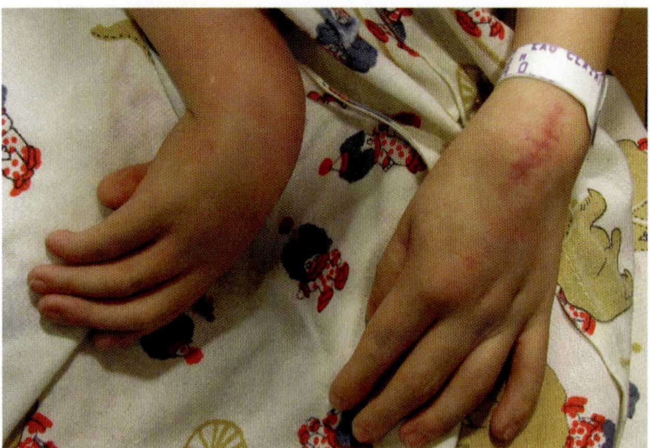

FIGURE 43-7

STEP 3 PITFALLS

The position of the K-wires should be confirmed by intraoperative fluoroscopy. The wires should pass through both midcarpal and radiocarpal joints to ensure a stable fixation.

Step 4

- The dorsal capsule is repaired using 3-0 Vicryl sutures.

Step 5

- If a good-quality ECU tendon is present, it can be divided distally and transferred subcutaneously to reach the radial wrist extensors to provide some radial wrist extension.
- The skin and subcutaneous tissue are closed with absorbable sutures.

Postoperative Care and Expected Outcomes

- The limb is immobilized in an above-elbow fiberglass cast. The cast will be maintained for 6 weeks to allow the osteotomy site to heal. The K-wires are removed at 6 weeks, and the osteotomy site is protected with use of an intermittent splint for 3 months. Finger motion is permitted within the cast.
- Formal therapy is usually not required in younger children who adjust to the repositioned wrist. Surgery reliably repositions the wrist, which improves grasp (Fig. 43-7). Improvements in activities of daily living are dependent on degree of limb involvement and overall status of the child.

Evidence

Bennett JB, Hansen PE, Granberry WM, Cain TE. Surgical management of arthrogryposis of the upper extremity. *J Pediatr Orthop*. 1985;5:281-286.

Case series of 25 patients who underwent 56 operative procedures to correct upper extremity deformities due to arthrogryposis. Functional improvement was observed clinically and reported subjectively by the patients or their parents in 75% of the cases. (Level IV evidence)

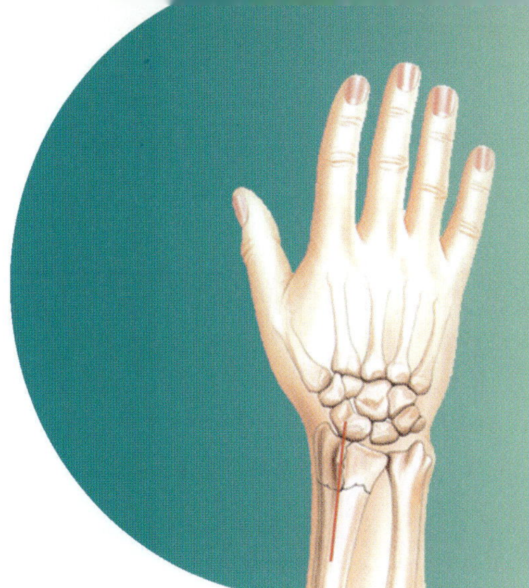

Section VII

SOFT TISSUE COVERAGE

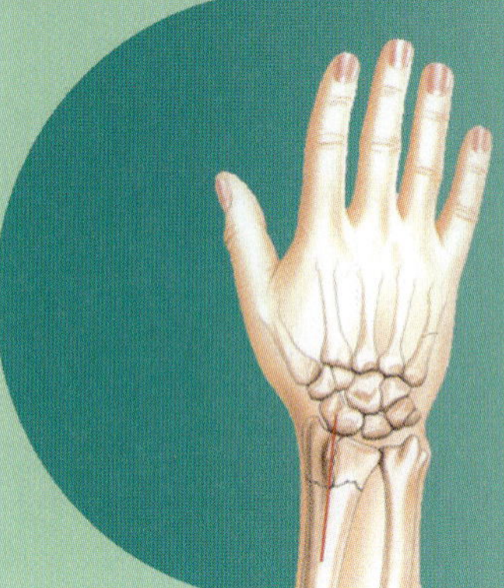

PROCEDURE 44

Dorsal Metacarpal Artery Perforator Flap

Sandeep J. Sebastin and Kevin C. Chung

See Video 36: Dorsal Metacarpal Artery Perforator Flap

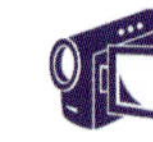

Indications

- Dorsal and lateral finger soft tissue defect proximal to the distal interphalangeal (DIP) joint (Fig. 44-1)
- Palmar finger soft tissue defect proximal to the DIP joint in patients with injuries to multiple fingers that make it difficult to use local flaps from adjacent digits
- Palmar or dorsal soft tissue defects proximal to the DIP joint in more than one finger

Examination/Imaging

Clinical Examination

- *Defect:* The flap should be used for defects that are free of infection. This is determined by looking at the wound bed and the surrounding skin for edema and erythema. This is a low-flow flap that is easily compromised by any residual infection.
- *Perforator:* There should be no injury in the vicinity of the selected perforator. Injuries that may disturb the perforator include metacarpal neck fractures, lacerations extending into the web space, contusion on the dorsum of the hand, and previous injection of local anesthetic agent. The perforator artery may be intact, but the tenuous venae comitantes are easily injured and can result in flap failure owing to venous congestion.
- *Morbidity:* This flap requires division of some dorsal sensory branches during flap elevation. This will result in loss of sensation in the territory of the nerve and, rarely, a painful neuroma. Closure of the flap donor site will result in a visible scar on the dorsum of the hand. Patients should be informed about these problems preoperatively.

Imaging

- A radiograph of the hand is useful in patients with a posttraumatic defect to rule out any associated metacarpal neck fractures.
- A preoperative Doppler assessment of the perforator is not required. It is difficult to separate the Doppler signals of the perforator from the dorsal metacarpal artery (DMA). In our experience, the perforator is always present, and, if the DMA is absent, the perforator should arise directly from one of the branches of the deep palmar arch.

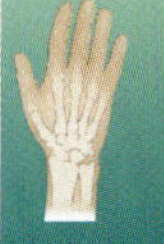

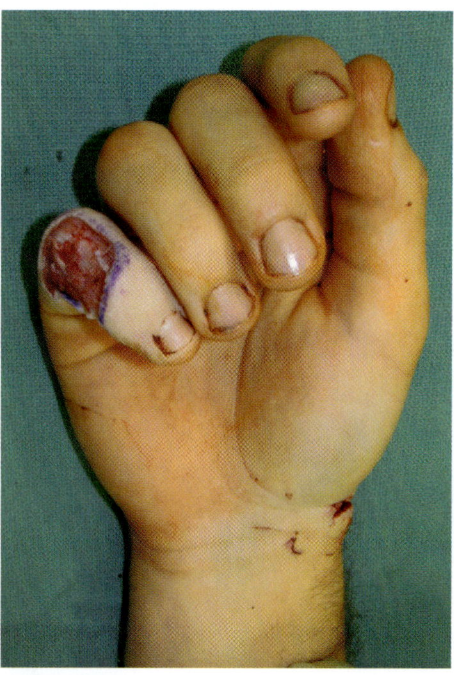

FIGURE 44-1

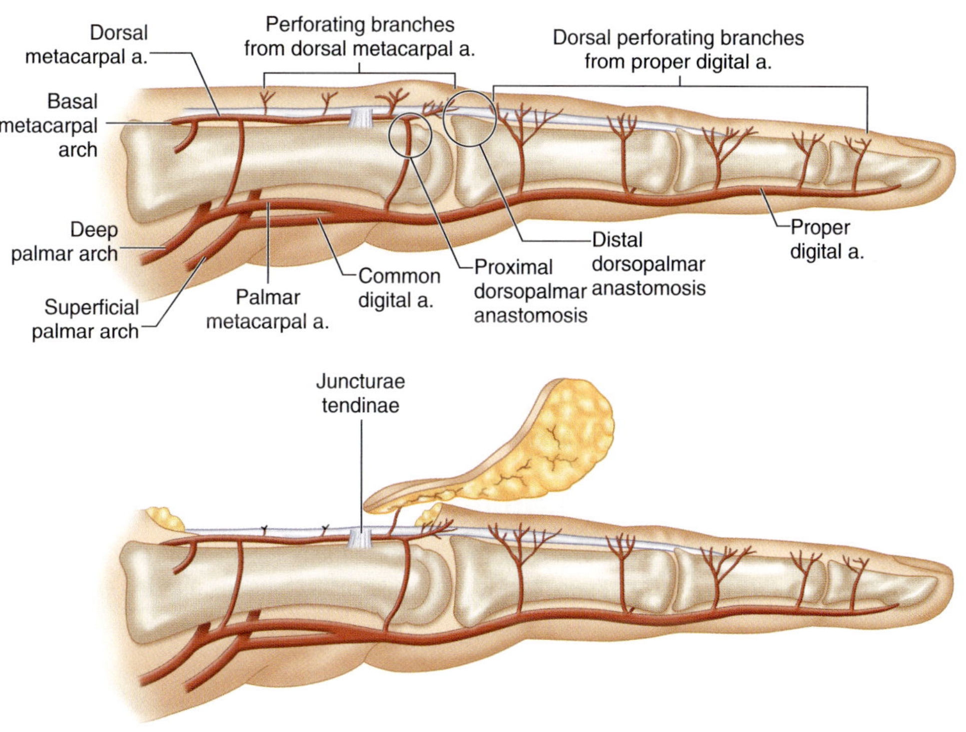

FIGURE 44-2

Surgical Anatomy

- *Vascular basis:* The flap is based on the distal cutaneous perforator of the DMA that arises at the level of the metacarpal neck in the second to fourth intermetacarpal spaces. In addition to the DMA, this flap is also nourished by the palmar arterial system through a dorsopalmar anastomosis. This anastomosis is formed by the dorsal perforating branch of the palmar metacarpal artery (arising from the deep palmar arch) and the DMA at the neck of the metacarpal (Fig. 44-2).

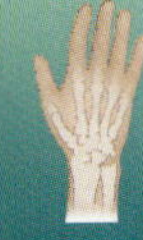

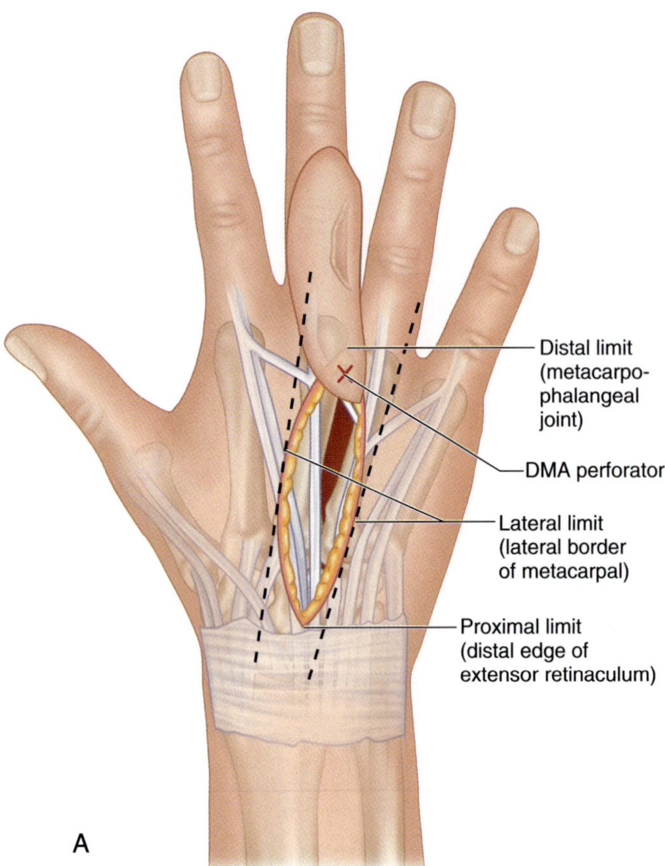

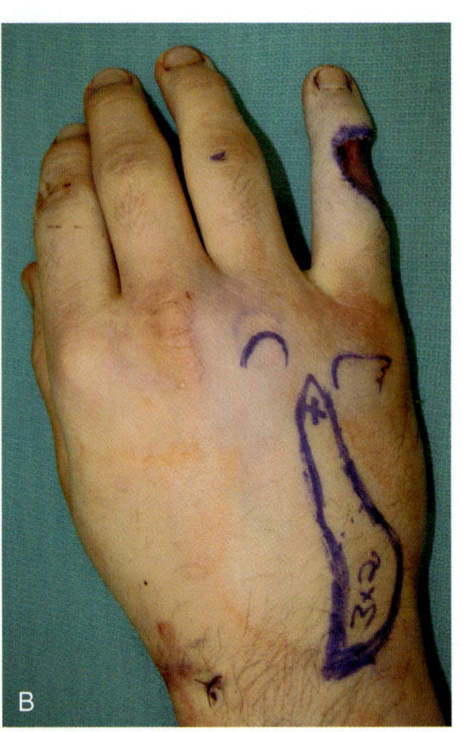

FIGURE 44-3

- *Limits of the flap:* We limit our flaps between the distal edge of the extensor retinaculum, the metacarpophalangeal (MCP) joint, and the outer borders of the adjoining metacarpals (Fig. 44-3A and B).

Positioning

- The procedure is performed under tourniquet control.
- The patient is positioned supine with the affected extremity on a hand table.

Exposures

- *Flap design:* The DMA perforator closest to the defect is marked at the level of the metacarpal neck in the intermetacarpal space. The location of the perforator represents the pivot point of the flap. The distance between the perforator and the proximal edge of the defect represents the bridge segment of the flap. Based on the size of the soft tissue defect, a flap is designed proximal to the perforator at a distance that equals the bridge segment.
- The flap may be designed as wholly cutaneous, cutaneous with a dermoadiposal bridge segment, or wholly adiposal.
- Flaps with a dermoadiposal bridge segment can reach the defect by passing the bridge under a skin tunnel or by laying open the intervening skin segment (Fig. 44-4).

PEARLS

We design the skin island in an oblique fashion when a wider flap is required to accommodate a defect that involves two surfaces (palmar + lateral or dorsal + lateral).

If the flap design extends proximal to the distal edge of the extensor retinaculum, we design the flap as a curved ellipse instead of a straight ellipse. Once the flap is raised, the curved ellipse is straightened out and inset as a straight ellipse. This results in an additional 8 to 10 mm while maintaining the design within the previously mentioned limits (Fig. 44-5).

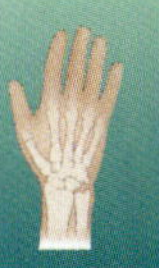

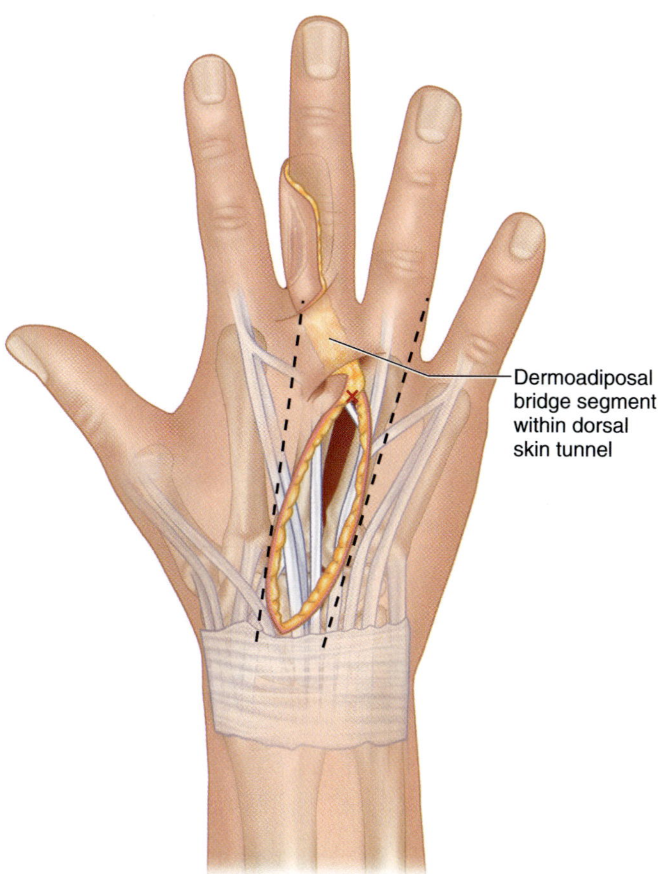

FIGURE 44-4

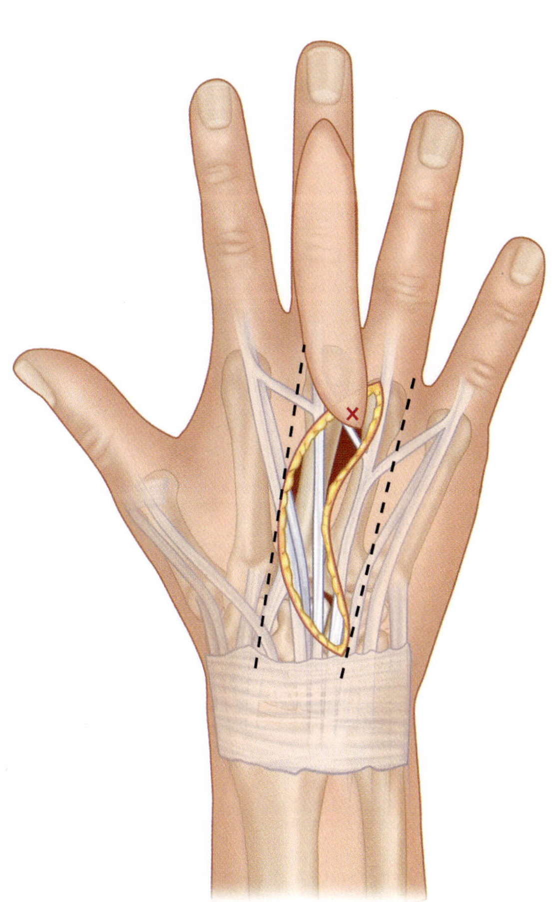

FIGURE 44-5

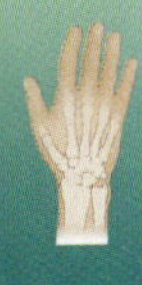

STEP 1 PEARLS

The aim of the lateral incision is to identify the correct plane of flap elevation. The flap is elevated in the loose areolar plane superficial to the extensor tendon paratenon. It is difficult to identify this plane, if we make the proximal incision first.

STEP 1 PITFALLS

Try to preserve the extensor tendon paratenon because this will maintain the gliding of the extensor tendon postoperatively and prevent any adhesions to the overlying tissue.

Procedure

Step 1

- The skin and subcutaneous tissue on one lateral border of the flap are incised until the underlying extensor tendon is seen (Fig. 44-6).

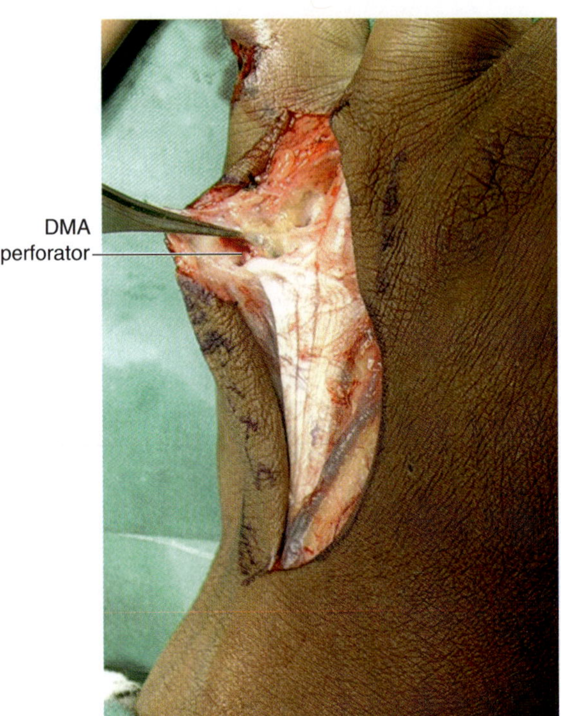

FIGURE 44-6

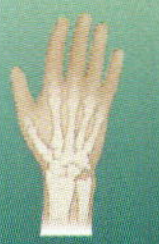

STEP 2 PEARLS

Large veins at the lateral borders of the flap are avoided because these veins only add to stasis within the flap. Veins and dorsal sensory nerve branches that pass though the midsubstance of the flap cannot be avoided, are divided, and are included with the flap.

STEP 3 PEARLS

If the flap is designed with a dermoadiposal bridge segment, it is created by raising thick epidermal skin flaps and keeping the bridge segment as wide as the widest portion of the cutaneous flap.

STEP 3 PITFALLS

The flap can be elevated rapidly in the proximal two thirds; however, once the extensor tendon juncturae are visualized, elevation should proceed slowly as the perforator arises immediately distal to the juncturae tendineae.

Step 2

- The proximal border of the flap is incised using the previously identified plane of elevation.

Step 3

- The remaining lateral border of the flap is incised, and the flap is elevated from proximal to distal (Fig. 44-7).

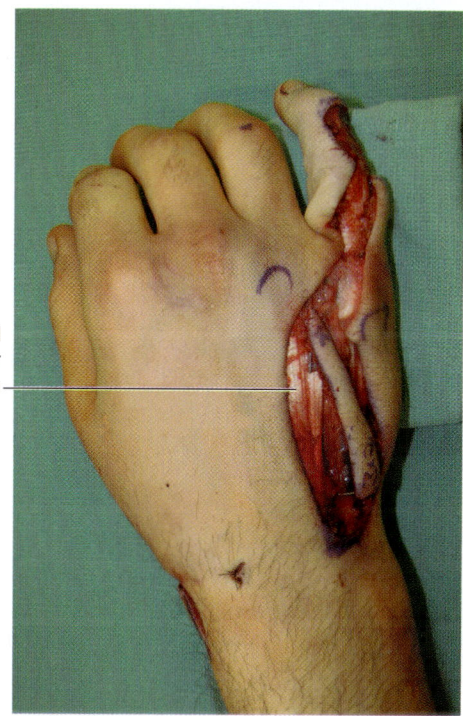

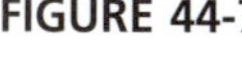

FIGURE 44-7

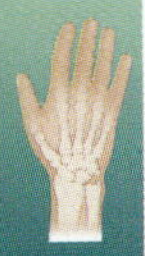

Step 4

- The DMA perforator is identified, and the flap is incised into an island distal to the perforator (Fig. 44-8).

Step 5

- Any intervening normal skin between the flap and defect can be laid open, or a wide tunnel can be made under it to enable the flap to reach the defect (see Fig. 44-7).

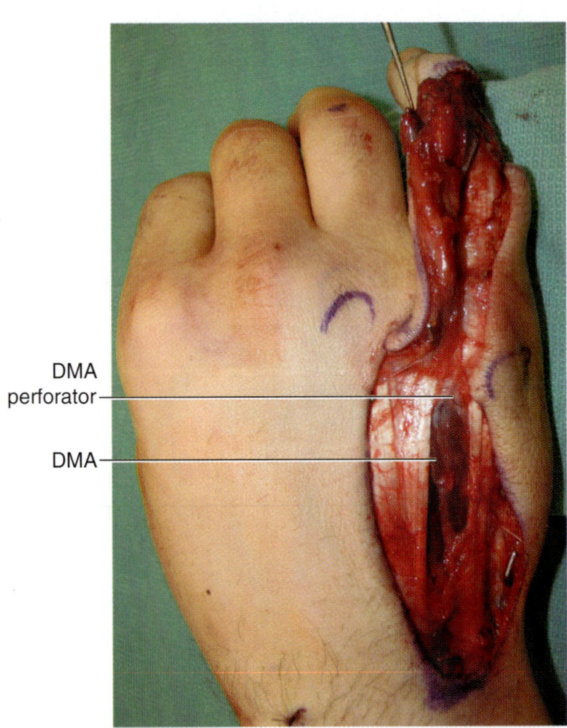

FIGURE 44-8

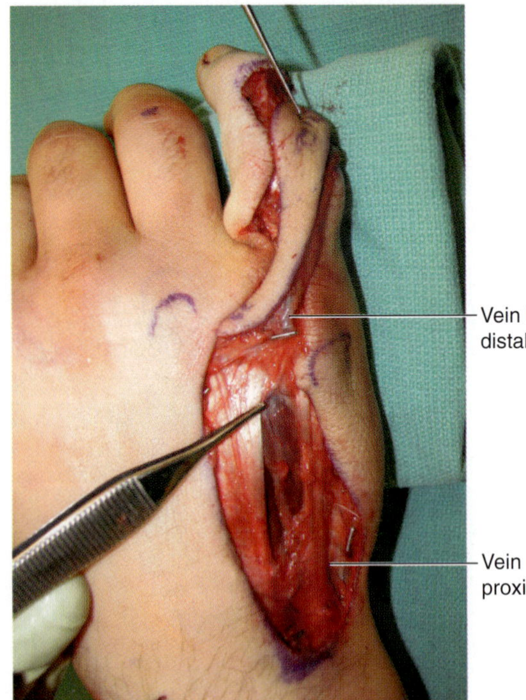

FIGURE 44-9

STEP 4 PEARLS

Large veins that pass through the flap should be carefully divided distal to the flap. This will make pivoting the flap easier and reduce venous congestion in the flap (Fig. 44-9).

STEP 4 PITFALLS

The perforator should not be skeletonized because the connective tissue surrounding the artery contains the draining veins.

STEP 5 PEARLS

We prefer a tunnel for dorsal defects because the lax dorsal skin permits creation of large tunnels. In addition, this preserves the pliable skin over the dorsum of the MCP joint. For palmar defects, we prefer to lay the tunnel open or use a cutaneous bridge segment because making a tunnel in the palmar skin is difficult, and the constrictive fibrous septae can compromise flap vascularity.

STEP 6 PEARLS

This flap is now dependent only on the perforating vessel for blood supply. Allowing it to perfuse for 10 to 15 minutes gives it time to get accustomed to the new vascular flow pattern.

The pedicle of the flap has to be twisted to allow the flap to reach the defect. This should be done after tourniquet release because an empty vessel is more likely to get kinked than a vessel with flow.

STEP 7 PEARLS

Keeping the proximal interphalangeal (PIP) and MCP joints in extension will decrease the stretch on the pedicle.

When the flap is used to cover lateral or palmar defects, a folded gauze placed between the fingers that is incorporated into the final dressing keeps the web open and prevents compression of the bridge segment.

STEP 7 PITFALLS

Flaps wider than 3 cm will require a skin graft for wound closure.

STEP 8 PEARLS

A dermal suture closure will prevent suture hatch marks on the dorsum of the hand and improve the aesthetic appearance.

Primary closure is aided by extension of the wrist.

STEP 8 PITFALLS

Flaps wider than 3 cm will need a skin graft for wound closure.

Step 6

- The tourniquet is released with the flap in its native position, and the flap is allowed to perfuse for 10 to 15 minutes. This time is used to achieve excellent hemostasis.

Step 7

- The flap is then rotated into the defect and loosely anchored to the edges of the defect using 5-0 nylon sutures (Fig. 44-10).

Step 8

- The flap donor site is closed in layers using 4-0 Vicryl and 4-0 nylon.

Postoperative Care and Expected Outcomes

- A volar splint is used for 1 week to keep the fingers and the wrist in extension. Patients are discharged on the first postoperative day and advised to keep the limb elevated. They are started on range-of-motion exercises at 1 week, the sutures are removed at 2 weeks, and patients are then allowed to resume normal activities (Fig. 44-11).
- The DMA perforator flap is easy to raise and has minimal donor site morbidity. It is the ideal flap for resurfacing dorsal soft tissue defects because it provides single-stage "like-for-like" reconstruction (color match, skin thickness, and texture). It provides excellent coverage of defects in the web space and the lateral aspect of the fingers, although the color match is not ideal. It has a valuable role in resurfacing palmar defects, especially in cases when multiple fingers are injured, and it is risky to harvest homodigital/heterodigital vascular island flaps or a cross-finger flap. In addition, more than one flap can be raised at the same time, permitting coverage of multiple fingers simultaneously.

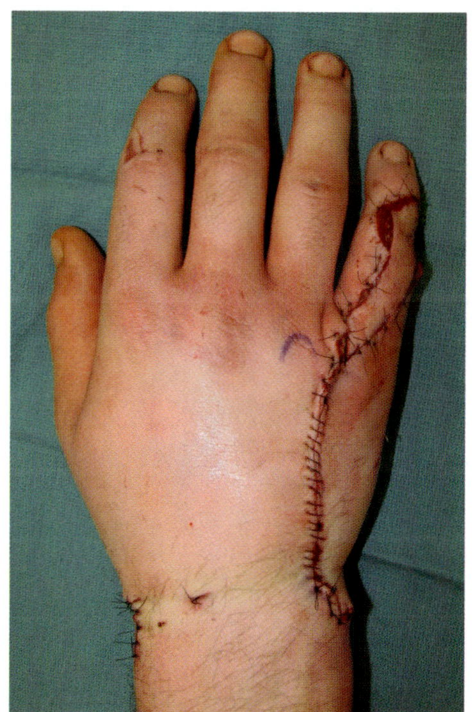

FIGURE 44-10

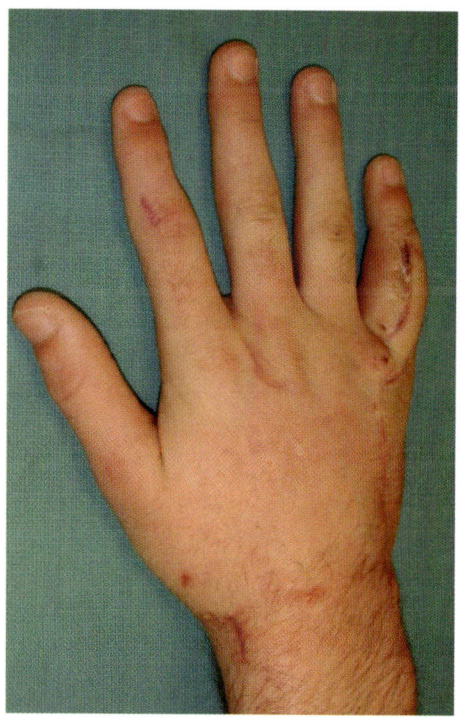

FIGURE 44-11

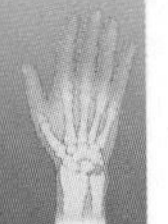

Evidence

Quaba AA, Davison PM. The distally-based dorsal hand flap. *Br J Plast Surg*. 1990;43:28-39.

This is the first description of this flap. The authors carried out dissections in 18 cadavers and noticed the consistent presence of the cutaneous perforator of the dorsal metacarpal artery distal to the juncturae. They used the flap in 21 clinical cases and were able to resurface dorsal defects up to the DIPJ. They reported partial loss of one flap and total loss of one flap. (Level IV evidence)

Sebastin SJ, Mendoza RT, Chong AK, et al. Application of the dorsal metacarpal artery perforator flap for resurfacing soft-tissue defects proximal to the fingertip. *Plast Reconstr Surg*. 2011;128:166-178.

The authors used 56 DMA perforator flaps to resurface 58 finger soft tissue defects in 54 patients. The average flap size was 4.6 × 2.3 cm; 34 flaps were based on the second DMA perforator, 14 were based on the third DMA perforator, and 8 were based on the fourth DMA perforator. Twenty flaps were used to resurface defects distal to the PIP joint, and 36 flaps were used to resurface defects over the PIP joint and proximal to it. Skin graft was needed to close the donor defect in 7 patients. Complications included venous congestion in 6 flaps, arterial insufficiency in 3 flaps with total loss of 2 flaps, and infection in 1 case. The authors felt that this flap could reliably cover soft tissue defects up to the proximal half of the middle phalanx and could be extended to reach the DIP joint by designing it as a curved ellipse or by dividing the DMA proximal to the origin of the perforator. (Level IV evidence)

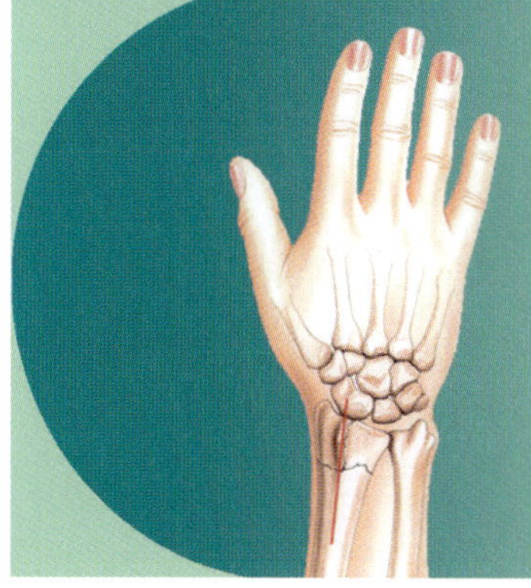

Dorsal Ulnar Artery Perforator Flap

Sandeep J. Sebastin and Kevin C. Chung

Indications

- Palmar soft tissue defects overlying the wrist, carpal tunnel, or hypothenar region (Fig. 45-1)
- Dorsal soft tissue defect overlying the wrist, mid-dorsum of hand, or ulnar border of the hand (Fig. 45-2)

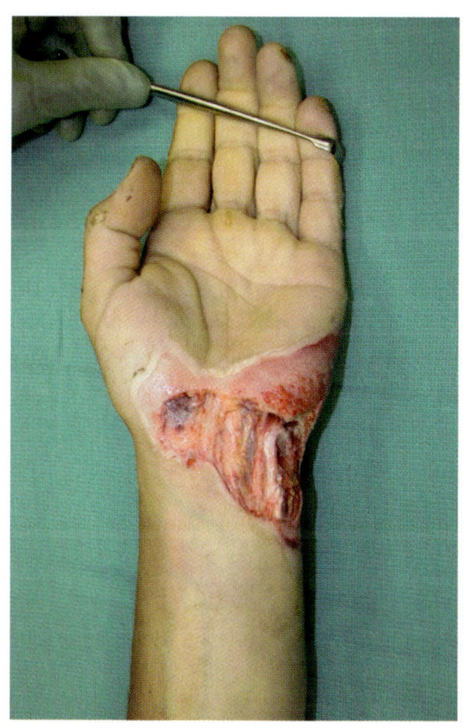

FIGURE 45-1

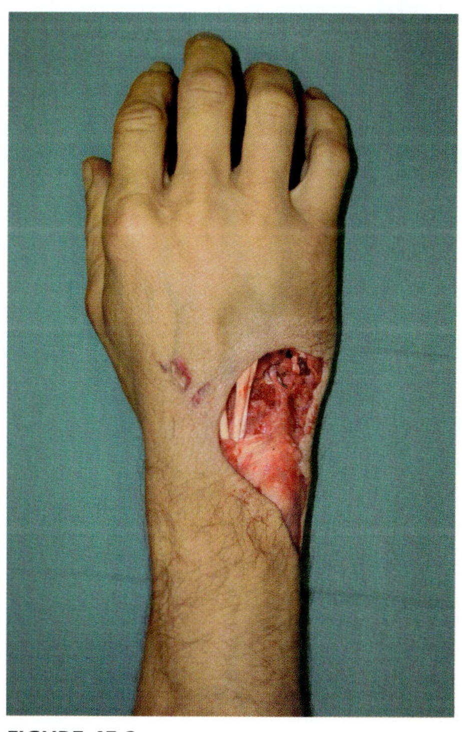

FIGURE 45-2

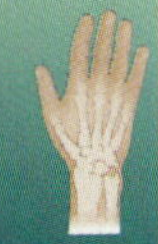

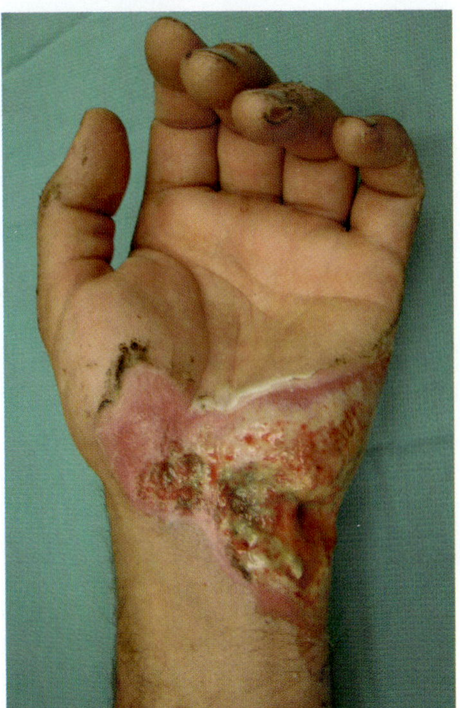

FIGURE 45-3

Examination/Imaging

Clinical Examination

- *Defect:* The flap should be selected for defects that are free of infection. This is determined by looking at the wound bed and the surrounding skin for edema and erythema. This is a low-flow flap that is easily compromised by any residual infection. (Figure 45-3 shows predébridement appearance of the patient in Fig. 45-1.)
- *Perforator:* There should be no injury in the vicinity of the selected perforator. Injuries that may disturb the perforator include ulnar head fractures or lacerations over the distal ulnar forearm with associated tendon, nerve, or vessel injury.
- *Morbidity:* This flap may require division of some branches or the main trunk of the dorsal sensory branch of the ulnar nerve. This will result in loss of sensation in the territory of the nerve and, rarely, a painful neuroma. Patients should be informed about these problems before surgery.

Imaging

- A preoperative Doppler assessment of the perforator is essential to identify the location of the perforator. The Doppler probe is moved from distal to proximal along the ulnar border of the forearm beginning at the pisiform and staying ulnar to the flexor carpi ulnaris (FCU). The perforator is located 2 to 6 cm proximal to the pisiform.

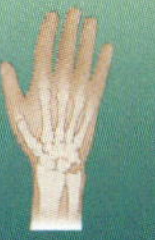

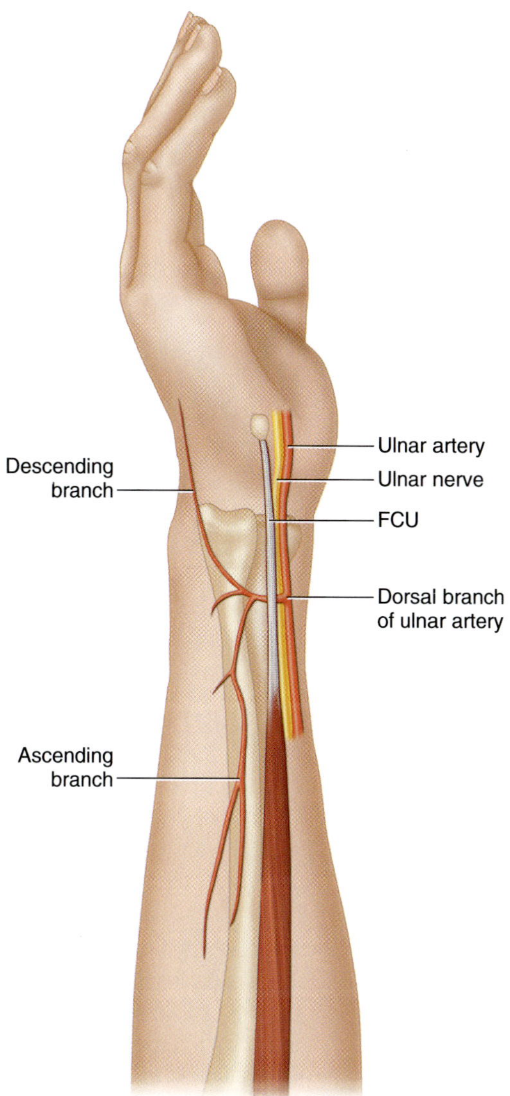

FIGURE 45-4

Surgical Anatomy

- *Vascular basis:* The flap is based on a perforator of the ulnar artery that arises 2 to 6 cm proximal to the pisiform. This vessel passes from palmar to dorsal under the FCU tendon and divides into an ascending branch (directed proximally toward the forearm) and a descending branch (directed distally toward the hand). This flap is based on the ascending branch of the dorsal ulnar artery (DUA) (Fig. 45-4). In addition to the ulnar artery perforator, this flap is also nourished by the dorsal carpal arch through its communications with the descending branch.

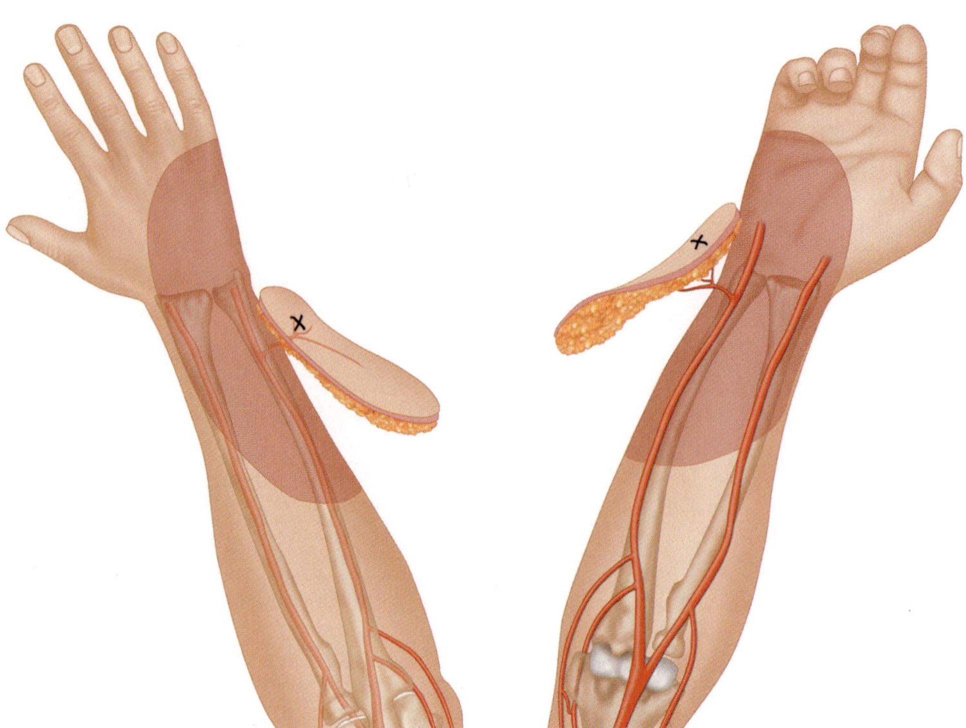

FIGURE 45-5

- *Limits of the flap:* We limit the proximal extent of the flap to the mid-forearm. This results in a 10- to 15-cm long flap, depending on the exact location of the perforator. Selective dye injection studies in cadavers have shown that the staining is limited to the distal third of the forearm skin. The maximum width of the flap is limited to 6 cm because this permits linear closure of the flap donor site. The arc of coverage of the flap is therefore limited to defects within 10 to 15 cm of the perforator (Fig. 45-5).

Positioning

- The procedure is performed under tourniquet control.
- The patient is positioned supine with the affected extremity on a hand table.

Exposures

- *Flap design:* The location of the DUA perforator is determined by Doppler and marked preoperatively. The location of the perforator represents the pivot point of the flap. A line drawn between the pisiform and the medial epicondyle represents the axis of the flap. The distance between the perforator and the proximal edge of the defect represents the bridge segment of the flap. Based on the size of the soft tissue defect, a flap is designed proximal to the perforator at a distance that equals the bridge segment. The flap may be designed as wholly fasciocutaneous, fasciocutaneous with an adipofascial bridge segment, or wholly adipofascial.
- Flaps with an adipofascial bridge segment can reach the defect by passing the bridge segment under a wide skin tunnel or by laying open the intervening skin segment.

PEARLS

An elliptical design makes flap donor site closure easier.

We design the skin island as teardrop shaped, with the widest portion of the flap designed proximally on the forearm (Fig. 45-6).

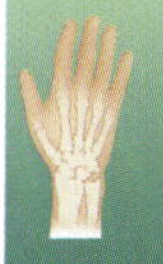

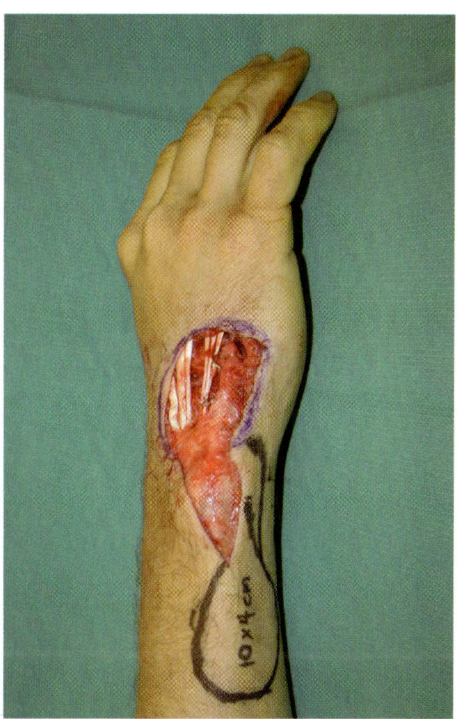

FIGURE 45-6

Procedure

Step 1

- A 4-cm vertical incision centered on a previously marked perforator is made ulnar to the FCU.
- Skin and soft tissue are divided to identify the FCU.
- The FCU is retracted ulnarly to identify the ulnar neurovascular bundle, and the DUA perforator is identified.
- Based on the location of the perforator, the preoperative flap design is confirmed or modified as required.

STEP 1 PEARLS

The aim of the preliminary incision is to identify the DUA perforator.

STEP 1 PITFALLS

Dissection to identify the perforator should stay radial to the FCU (by retracting the FCU ulnarly). The perforator is short (2 to 3 cm) and divides into ascending and descending branches ulnar to the FCU. Dissection ulnar to the FCU can injure the cutaneous branches of the perforator.

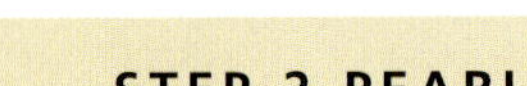

STEP 2 PEARLS

Veins at the lateral borders of the flap are avoided because these veins only add to stasis within the flap. Veins and dorsal sensory nerve branches that pass through the midsubstance of the flap cannot be avoided, are divided, and are included with the flap.

The basilic vein usually travels within the flap. An additional 2 to 3 cm of this vein can be harvested by dissection proximal to the flap margins. This additional length can be used for a venous anastomosis at the recipient site (Fig. 45-8).

STEP 2 PITFALLS

The dorsal branch of the ulnar nerve takes off from the ulnar nerve about 5 to 8 cm proximal to the pisiform. Depending on the course of the nerve, it may occasionally be possible to separate the main nerve trunk or some of the branches from the flap.

A large perforator of the ulnar artery travels along with the dorsal branch of the ulnar nerve, but this will need to be ligated to allow the flap movement (see Fig. 45-8).

Step 2

- The proximal border of the flap is incised, followed by the lateral borders.
- The flap is elevated in the plane superficial to the epimysium of the FCU and extensor carpi ulnaris (ECU) muscle bellies (Fig. 45-7).

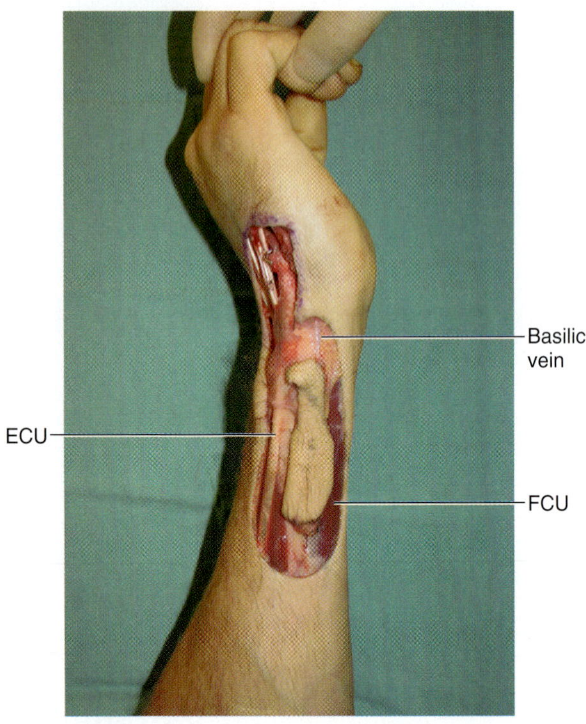

FIGURE 45-7

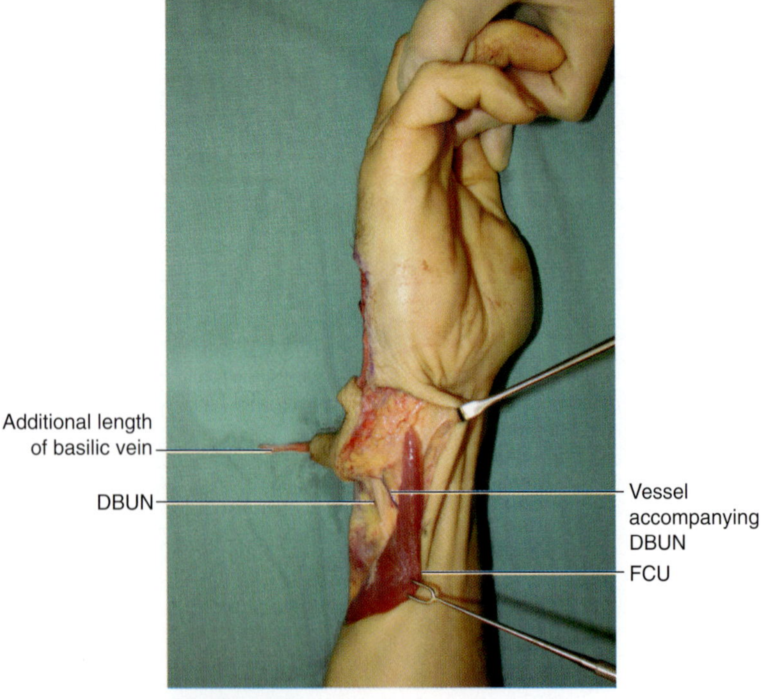

FIGURE 45-8

Step 3

- The flap is made into an island distal to the perforator.

Step 4

- Any intervening normal skin between the flap and defect can be laid open, or a wide tunnel can be made under it to enable the flap to reach the defect.

Step 5

- The tourniquet is released with the flap in its native position, and the flap is allowed to perfuse for 10 to 15 minutes. This time is used to achieve excellent hemostasis (Fig. 45-9).

STEP 3 PEARLS

The flap can be elevated rapidly in the proximal two thirds; however, once the dorsal branch of the ulnar nerve is visualized, elevation should proceed slowly.

A flap designed with a dermoadiposal bridge segment is created by raising thick epidermal skin flaps and keeping the bridge segment as wide as the widest portion of the cutaneous flap.

STEP 3 PITFALLS

Although the cutaneous distal portion of the flap in a teardrop design is narrow, one must elevate a wider adipofascial portion to ensure that the cutaneous branches of the perforator are included.

The perforator should not be skeletonized because the connective tissue surrounding the artery contains the draining veins.

STEP 5 PEARLS

This flap is now dependent only on the perforating vessel for blood supply. Allowing it to perfuse for 10 to 15 minutes gives it time to get accustomed to the new vascular flow pattern.

The pedicle of the flap has to be twisted to allow the flap to reach the defect. This should be done after tourniquet release because an empty vessel is more likely to become kinked than a vessel with flow.

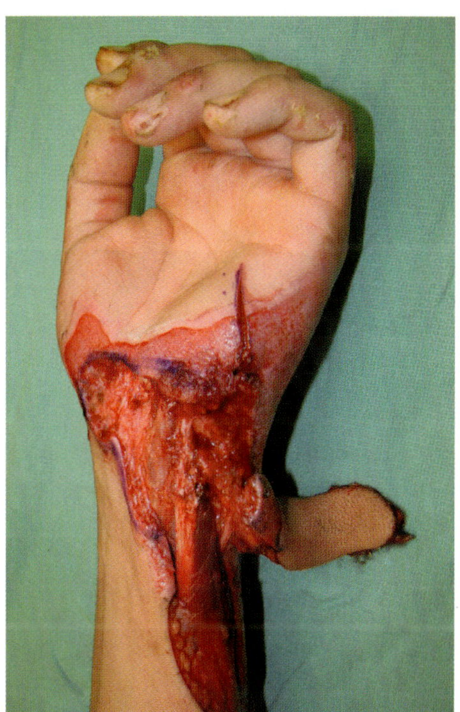

FIGURE 45-9

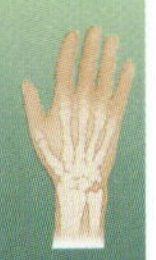

STEP 6 PEARLS

Keeping the wrist in slight flexion will decrease the stretch on the pedicle when the flap is used for palmar defects. The wrist can be maintained in extension, if the flap is being used for dorsal defects.

In larger flaps, it may be better to do a venous anastomosis (Fig. 45-10). If a suitable recipient vein cannot be found for anastomosis, one should consider ligating the large superficial vein within the flap at the level of the wrist (distal to the perforator). This will make rotating the flap easier and decrease the venous congestion caused by these veins (Fig. 45-11).

Step 6

- The flap is then rotated into the defect and loosely anchored to the edges of the defect using 5-0 nylon sutures (Fig. 45-11).

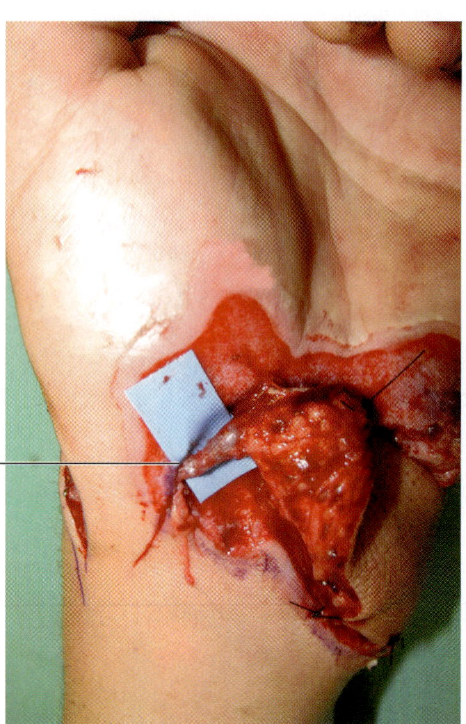

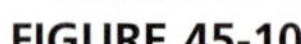

FIGURE 45-10

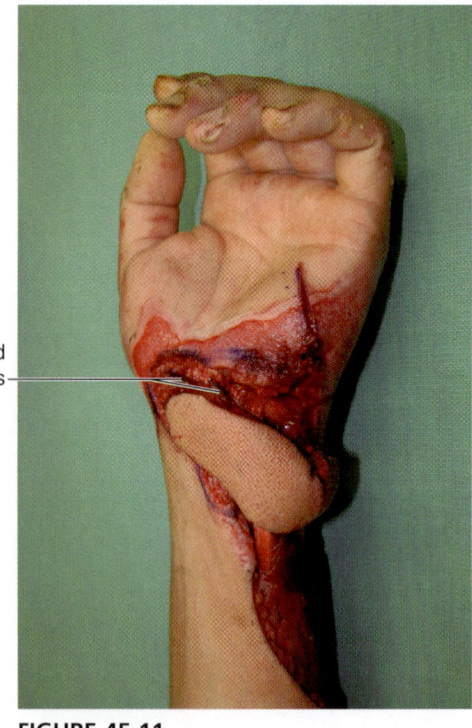

FIGURE 45-11

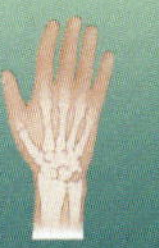

STEP 8 PEARLS

A dermal suture closure will prevent suture hatch marks on the dorsum of the hand and improve the aesthetic appearance.

STEP 8 PITFALLS

Flaps wider than 6 cm will need a skin graft for wound closure.

Step 8

- The flap donor site is closed in layers using 4-0 Vicryl and 4-0 nylon. (Figure 45-12A and B shows the immediate postoperative appearance of patients shown in Figs. 45-1 and 45-2, respectively.)

Postoperative Care and Expected Outcomes

- A volar splint is used for 1 week. Patients are discharged on the first postoperative day and advised to keep the limb elevated. They are started on range-of-motion exercises at 1 week, the sutures are removed at 2 weeks, and patients are then allowed to resume normal activities.

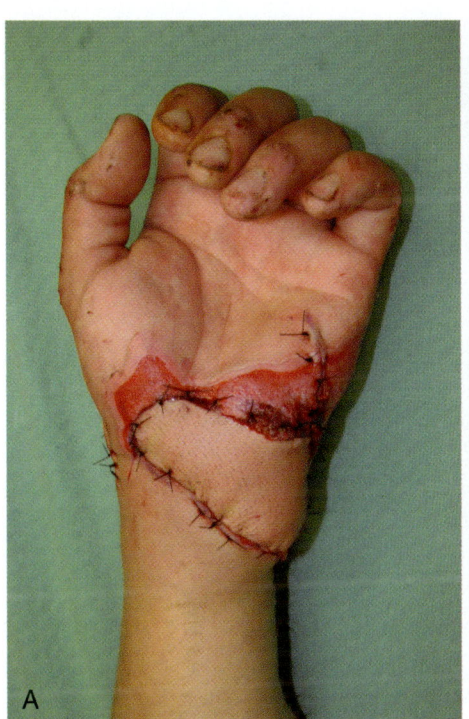

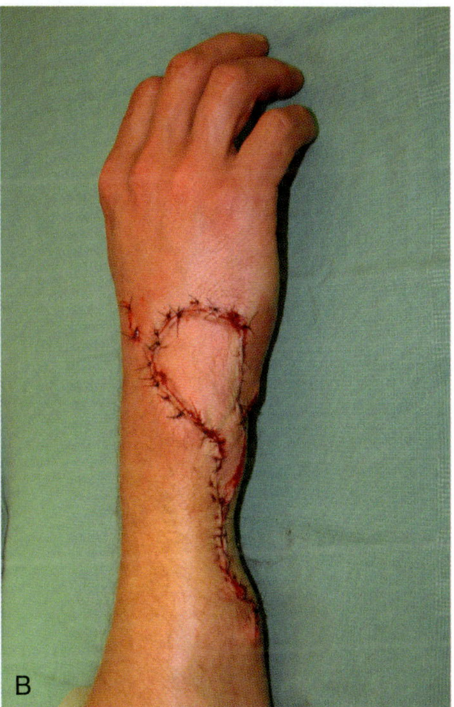

FIGURE 45-12

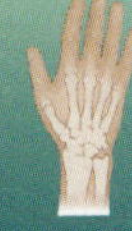

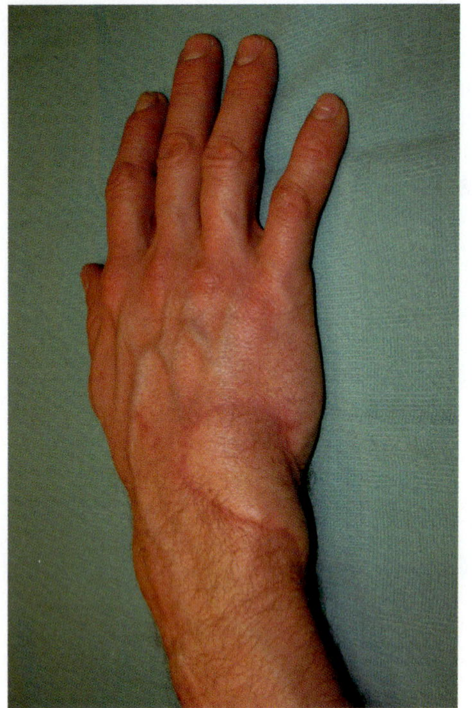

FIGURE 45-13

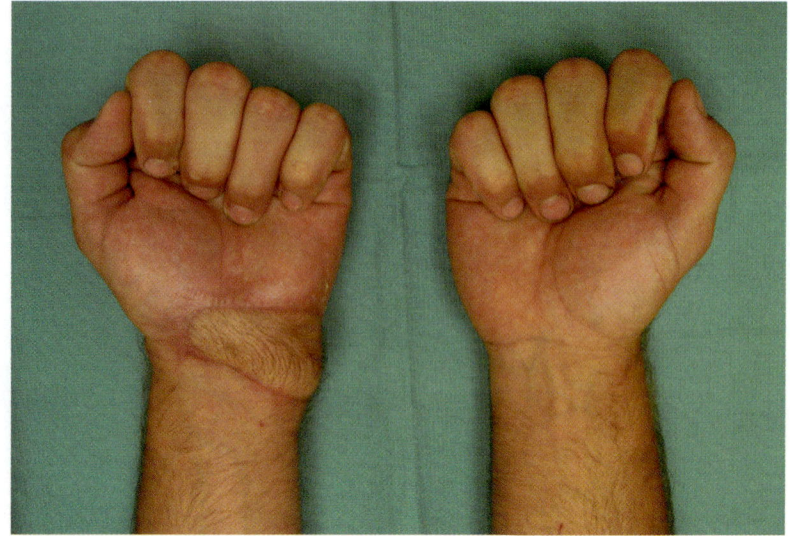

FIGURE 45-14

- The DUA perforator flap is easy to raise and has minimal donor site morbidity. It provides single-stage like-for-like reconstruction (color match, skin thickness, and texture) for dorsal defects. (Figure 45-13 shows the late result of the patient in Figure 45-2.) It has a valuable role in resurfacing palmar defects, especially over the carpal tunnel, although the color match is not very good for palmar coverage. (Figure 45-14 shows the late result of the patient in Figure 45-1.)

Evidence

Antonopoulos D, Kang NV, Debono R. Our experience with the use of the dorsal ulnar artery flap in hand and wrist tissue cover. *J Hand Surg [Br]*. 1997;22: 739-744.

The authors describe a series of six flaps that explored the limits of reliability of the dorsal ulnar artery fasciocutaneous flap. They felt that a larger flap based on the territory of the vessel (10-20 × 5-9 cm) could be harvested. This would allow them to use the flap for defects of the radial side of the wrist and hand. However, they encountered problems with venous drainage and suggested use of larger flaps with caution. (Level IV evidence)

Becker C, Gilbert A. The ulnar flap. *Handchir Mikrochir Plastchir*. 1988;20:180-183.

This is the original description of the ulnar artery perforator flap. The authors carried out 100 anatomic preparations and found the constant branch of the ulnar artery, which named the dorsal branch of the ulnar artery. They reported on eight cases: one was an island flap, four had an intact skin bridge, and there were three fascial flaps. They suggested using the flap for small defects limited to the ulnar side of the hand and to limit flap size to 10 × 5 cm. (Level IV evidence)

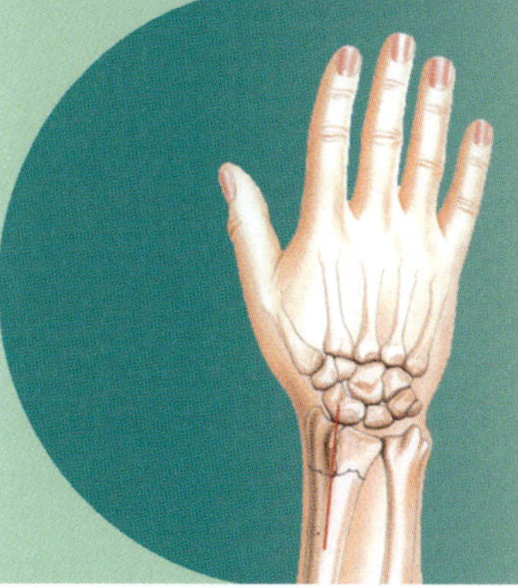

PROCEDURE 46

Pedicled Groin Flap

Sandeep J. Sebastin and Kevin C. Chung

The groin flap used to be the workhorse flap for hand reconstruction, but it has been supplanted by the use of regional flaps (radial forearm and posterior interosseous artery) and free skin flaps (lateral arm and anterolateral thigh). However, it continues to be a safe and reliable alternative for primary coverage of wounds on the hand, particularly when secondary reconstruction is contemplated, such as to add soft tissue for subsequent toe transfer or tendon reconstruction. We use the groin flap as the first choice for dorsal hand coverage, unless there are specific needs to initiate early active motion after fracture fixation and tendon reconstruction. In these select situations, we will cover the wound with a free flap. When the groin flap is used, patients can expect to require several operations after flap division to debulk the flap and to perform tissue rearrangement for contouring the circular flap appearance on the hand.

Indications

- Dorsal or palmar soft tissue defect of the hand (Fig. 46-1)
- In preparation for a toe-to-thumb transfer following traumatic thumb or finger loss

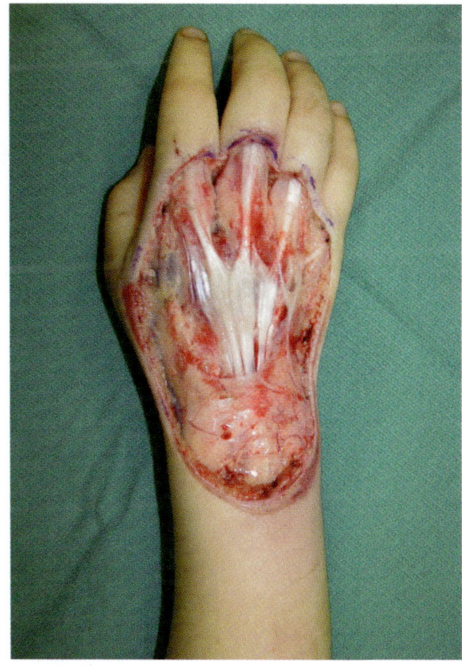

FIGURE 46-1

- Dorsal or palmar soft tissue defects involving multiple fingers
- Circumferential thumb soft tissue defect
- First stage of an osteoplastic thumb reconstruction

Examination/Imaging

Clinical Examination

- Patients should be examined for signs of previous surgery in the groin, including hernia repair, lymph node biopsy, or vein stripping. A higher incidence of thromboembolic and other general complications has been reported in patients older than 50 years with a pedicled groin flap, and an alternative method of coverage may be more suitable in older patients (e.g., a radial forearm flap), provided that the palmar arch is intact and there is no peripheral vascular disease affecting the circulation in the hand.
- The amount of skin required for thumb reconstruction is often underestimated, and the thickness of the flap increases the requirements when circumferential coverage is needed. A rough guideline with regard to the skin requirements in an adult male is as follows:
  - Thumb (circumferential)
    - Distal to the metacarpophalangeal (MCP) joint: 9 × 8 cm
    - Distal to the thenar crease: 13 × 12 cm
  - Palmar hand: 12 × 10 cm
  - Dorsal hand: 12 × 10 cm
  - Finger (circumferential): 7 × 10 cm
- *Morbidity:* This flap requires attachment of the hand to the groin for 3 to 4 weeks, which restricts movements at all joints of the involved upper limb. Patients typically are able to shrug the shoulder, move the elbow minimally, and move the wrist and hand to a greater degree. This period of immobilization will result in stiffness, especially in older patients. In addition, patients will have the use of only one hand and may require help to manage toileting and other activities of daily living. There is a risk for injury to the lateral femoral cutaneous nerve with resultant loss of sensation in the lateral aspect of the thigh and, rarely, a painful neuroma. Patients need a minimum of two surgical procedures (one for inset and another for flap division) and occasionally may need more procedures (for flap delay and flap thinning). Patients must be informed about these issues before surgery.

Surgical Anatomy

- *Vascular basis:* The flap is based on the superficial circumflex iliac artery (SCIA). The SCIA is the smallest branch of the femoral artery and arises about 1 inch below the inguinal ligament. It arises directly from the femoral artery in about 70% of cases; in the remainder, a common trunk is shared with the superficial epigastric artery. The SCIA travels obliquely toward the anterior superior iliac spine (ASIS), becoming progressively superficial as it travels from medial to lateral (Fig. 46-2A and B). At the medial border of the sartorius, the SCIA divides into a deep branch (which remains below the deep fascia and enters the sartorius) and a superficial branch (which pierces the deep fascia, becomes superficial, and supplies the overlying skin on its way to the ASIS). The femoral artery can be palpated immediately below the inguinal ligament at the midinguinal point (midway between pubic symphysis and ASIS). A point is marked 1 inch (2 fingerbreadths) below the inguinal ligament along the femoral artery. This represents the origin of the SCIA. A line drawn from this point to the ASIS represents the course of the SCIA and the vascular axis of the flap. Because of the obliquity of the vascular axis, about two thirds of the flap is designed superior to this axis and one third below this axis.

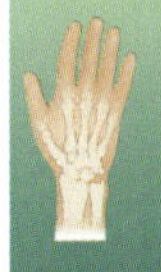

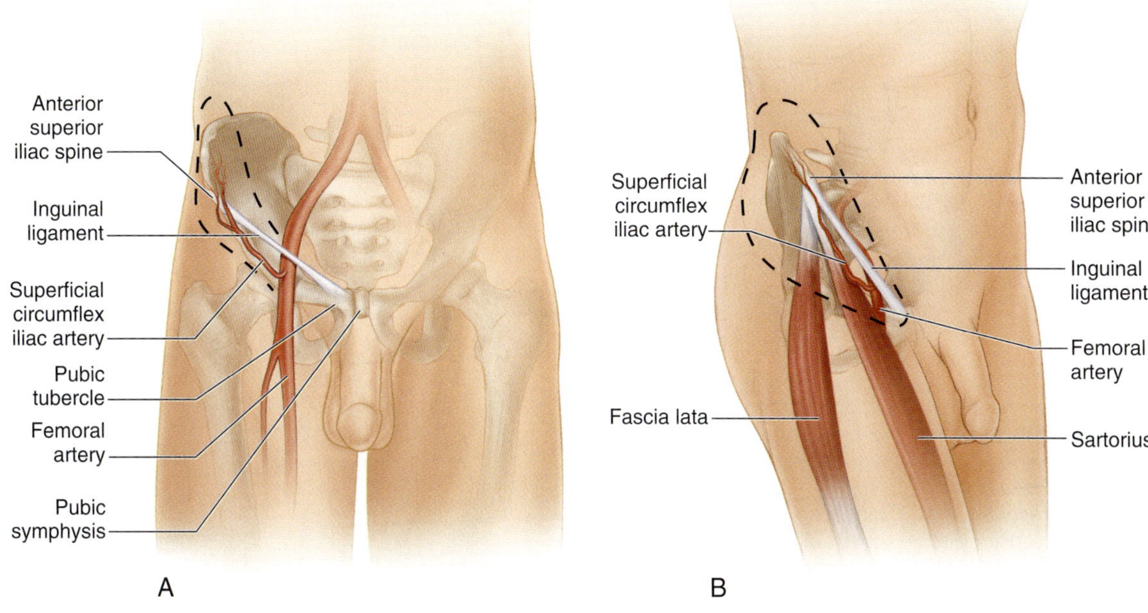

FIGURE 46-2

Beyond the ASIS, the superficial branch divides into three branches that anastomose with the branches of the superior gluteal, deep circumflex iliac, and ascending lateral femoral circumflex arteries. The venous drainage of the flap is by a dual pathway: the superficial circumflex iliac vein (SCIV) representing the superficial venous system, and the venae comitantes of the SCIA representing the deep system. Both of these may drain directly into the femoral vein or indirectly through the saphenous vein.

- *Limits of the flap*
  - *Medial limit:* Although the origin of the SCIA at the femoral artery represents the theoretical medial limit of the flap, it is safer to limit dissection to about 3 to 4 cm lateral to the femoral artery. This is usually 2 to 3 cm medial to the medial border of the sartorius.
  - *Superior and inferior limits:* The maximum width of a groin flap that can be closed primarily is about 10 to 12 cm (about 4 inches). The superior margin is made 4 fingerbreadths above the vascular axis and the inferior margin 2 fingerbreadths below the axis.
  - *Lateral limit:* The portion of the groin flap beyond the ASIS has random pattern vascularization, and it is better to design this portion of the flap with a 1:1 length-to-width ratio. Given that the maximum width of the flap that can be closed primarily is 10 cm, a point 10 cm from the ASIS represents the lateral limit of the flap.
- *Flap size:* The maximum size of a groin flap is about 13 × 10 cm. This is adequate to resurface most soft tissue defects of the hand and thumb. However, this will not allow tubing of the flap in most cases without further medial dissection (Fig. 46-3).

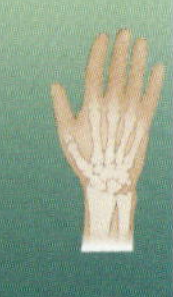

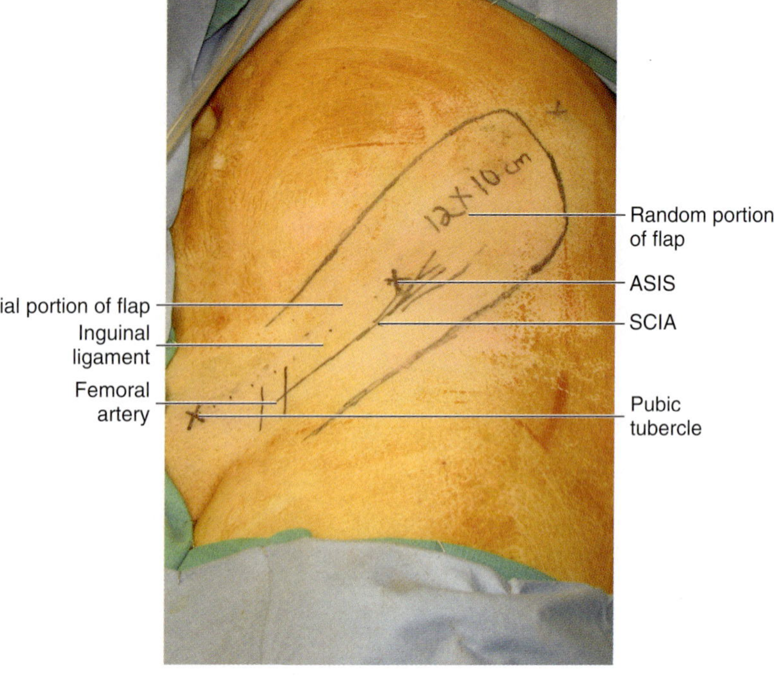

FIGURE 46-3

PEARLS

A bolster placed under the ipsilateral hip allows easier visualization and elevation of the random portion of the flap beyond the ASIS.

PEARLS

Bone and nerve reconstruction can be done at the same time as the groin flap, provided that the wound is ready. It is preferable to delay tendon reconstruction to a later stage because good passive range of joint motion needs to be established before tendon reconstruction.

STEP 1 PEARLS

The flap is raised superficial to the external oblique aponeurosis. It is easy to identify this plane on the superior lateral margin of the flap.

STEP 1 PITFALLS

Full-thickness flaps should be raised, and thinning of the flap is done before inset. This prevents desiccation and injury to the subdermal plexus.

Leaving fat on the abdominal wall will make undermining and subsequent closure difficult.

STEP 2 PEARLS

The inferior portion of the flap is elevated superficial to the fascia lata.

STEP 3 PEARLS

The ASIS should be marked as part of flap design, so that the flap is not elevated in a superficial plane medial to the ASIS.

The junction of the sartorius and the tensor fascia is identified by the slight palpable groove between them.

Positioning

- The patient is positioned supine.

Exposures

- *Flap design:* A template of the defect is made and transferred to the groin within the previously mentioned limits of the flap. The flap design must accurately match the size and shape of the recipient site (Fig. 46-4).

Procedure

Step 1: Elevation of Random Portion of Flap

- The superior lateral margin of the flap is incised first. The incision is deepened until the aponeurosis of external oblique muscle is seen (Fig. 46-5).

Step 2

- The lateral border and the inferior margin of the flap are incised, and the flap is elevated in the previously identified plane from lateral to medial.

Step 3

- The random portion of the flap is elevated rapidly to the ASIS. The lateral border of the sartorius and the fascia lata are identified at the inferior aspect of the ASIS (Fig. 46-6).

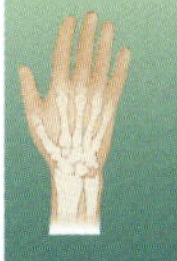

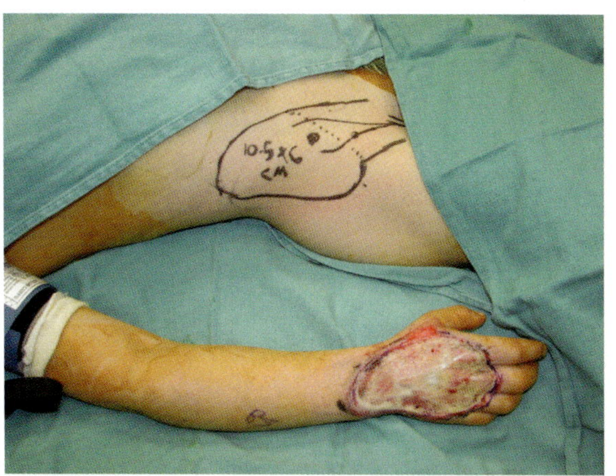

FIGURE 46-4

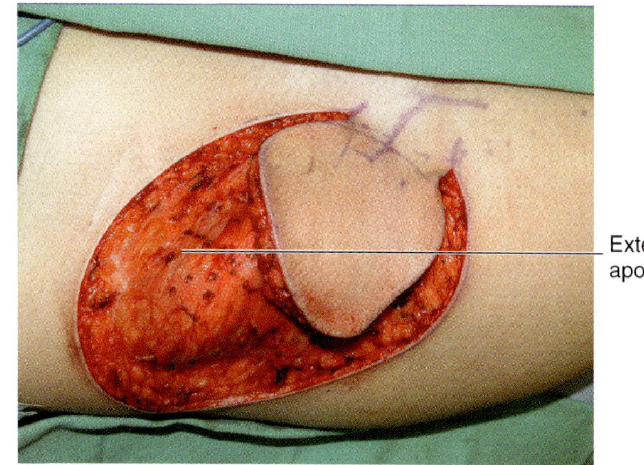

FIGURE 46-5

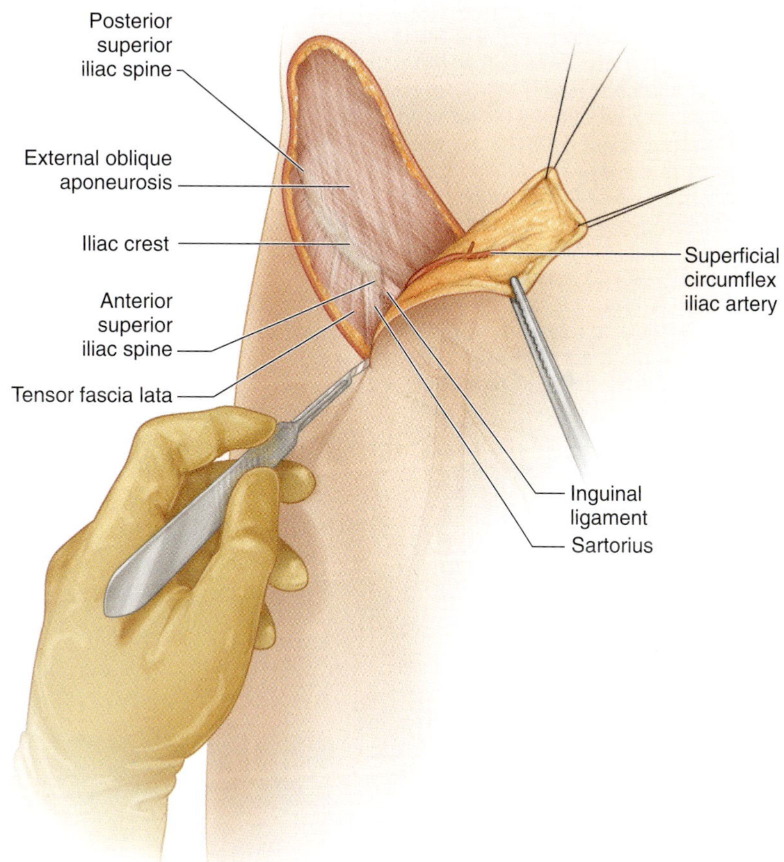

FIGURE 46-6

STEP 5 PEARLS

The SCIA is superficial to the fascia over the sartorius, and the fascia is included to protect the vessel. Transillumination of the flap can help identify the SCIA. The deep branch of the SCIA arises at the medial border of the sartorius and must be identified and ligated carefully without injuring the SCIA before dissection can proceed medially. This branch before it enters the sartorius is very short; it is better to divide it within the substance of the sartorius to prevent injury to the SCIA (Fig. 46-7).

The lateral femoral cutaneous nerve arises beneath the inguinal ligament and passes close to the medial border of the sartorius. It divides into an anterior branch and a posterior branch that pass over the sartorius muscle and pierce the fascia lata at varying distances below the inguinal ligament. Some of these branches may be initially elevated in the flap as a result of including the sartorius fascia and the fascia lata. However, these branches lie deep to the SCIA and can be dissected away from the undersurface of the flap and preserved. Occasionally, it may not be possible to elevate the flap further without dividing it. If further elevation is deemed necessary, the nerve can be divided and repaired (Fig. 46-8).

STEP 6 PEARLS

The connections between the inguinal ligament and fascia lata must be divided to allow the flap to be elevated.

STEP 6 PITFALLS

There is no need to isolate the pedicle, which can be tedious and unnecessarily time consuming.

The pivoting point should be about 2 or 3 cm medial to the sartorius.

Step 4: Elevation of Axial Portion of Flap

- A longitudinal incision is made over the fascia lata and the fascia overlying the sartorius to expose the underlying muscle fibers. The flap is then elevated in a deeper plane, including the fascia over the sartorius, to the medial border of the sartorius.

Step 5

- It is important to identify two structures at this point. The first is the deep (muscle) branch of the SCIA, and the other is the lateral femoral cutaneous nerve.

Step 6

- The flap is dissected medially to 2 to 3 cm from the medial border of the sartorius after separating the lateral femoral cutaneous nerves and dividing the deep branch of the SCIA.

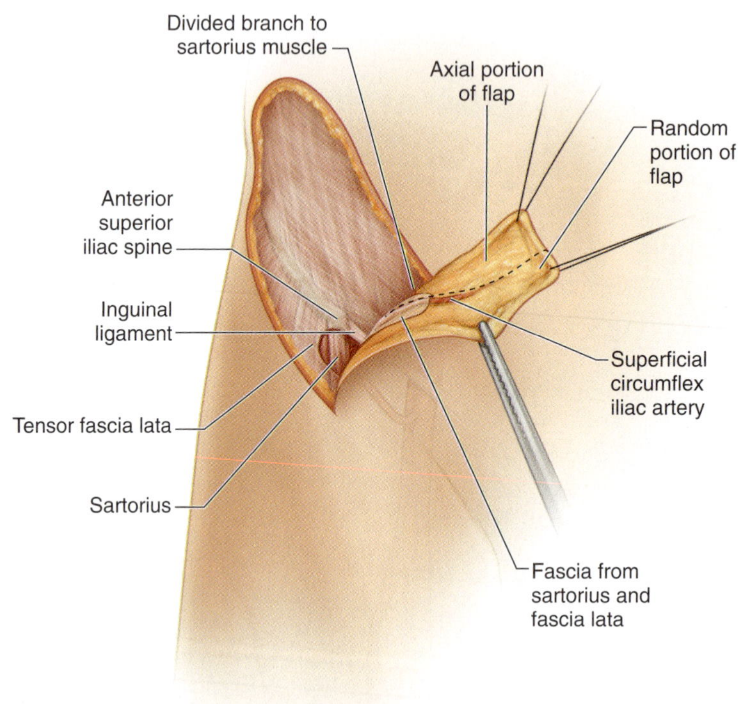

FIGURE 46-7

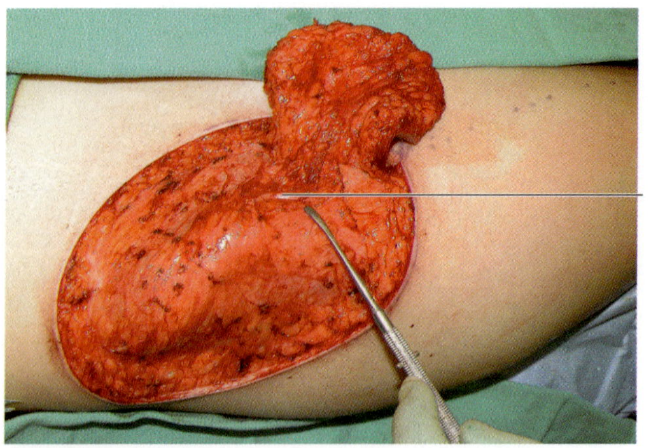

FIGURE 46-8

Step 7: Closure of Flap Donor Site

- The flap donor site is closed from medial to lateral in layers using 2-0 or even 0-0 Vicryl and 2-0 nylon. A drain is usually not required if adequate hemostasis was done because the closure is quite tight and compresses the bed. Even a seemingly large, impossible donor wound can be closed primarily (Fig. 46-9).

Step 8: Thinning of Flap

- The portion of the flap lateral to the ASIS can be thinned safely because the vessel is superficial and the flap relies on the subdermal plexus. Keeping excess fat on the random portion of the flap increases the vascular demands of the flap. The fat is parasitic, brings in no additional circulation, and delays revascularization from the bed.

Step 9: Inset of Flap

- The flap is inset into the recipient defect using simple 3-0 nylon interrupted sutures (Fig. 46-10).

STEP 7 PEARLS

Undermining the skin flaps and hip flexion will facilitate the donor site closure. If a bolster was placed under the hip, it should be removed now.

The scar will always spread, so the large sutures should be left in place until it is time for flap division, about 4 weeks after flap insetting.

STEP 7 PITFALLS

Patients may need to be immobilized with the hip in flexion by keeping a pillow under the knee for a few days, if closure is very tight.

STEP 8 PEARLS

The flap is thinned to match the thickness of the recipient site.

The fat superficial to Scarpa fascia is excised carefully using blunt-point scissors. The aim is to leave a thin layer of fat below the subdermal plexus. The fat lobules in the deeper layers are large, and, as one approaches the subdermal plexus, the lobules of fat become much smaller.

STEP 9 PITFALLS

If areas of the flap appear pale, it has been sutured too tightly, and the offending sutures will need to be removed. Occasionally, the flap may have to be re-inset.

The senior author does not tube the pedicle because the procedure is unnecessarily complicated and the tubing may compress the pedicle. The open area near the pedicle is kept moist with bacitracin ointment and is cleaned twice a day with gauze and then covered with Xeroform gauze.

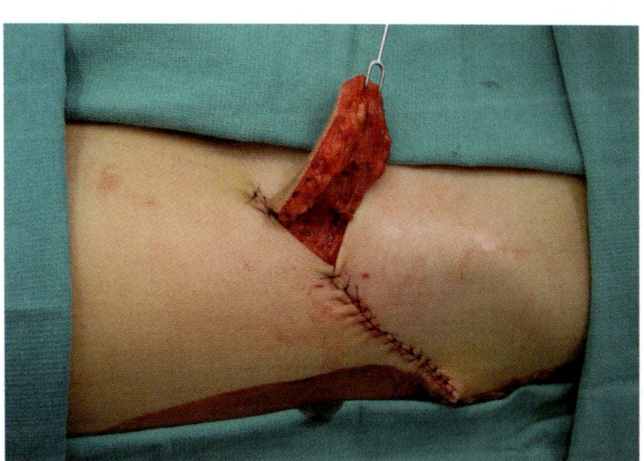

FIGURE 46-9

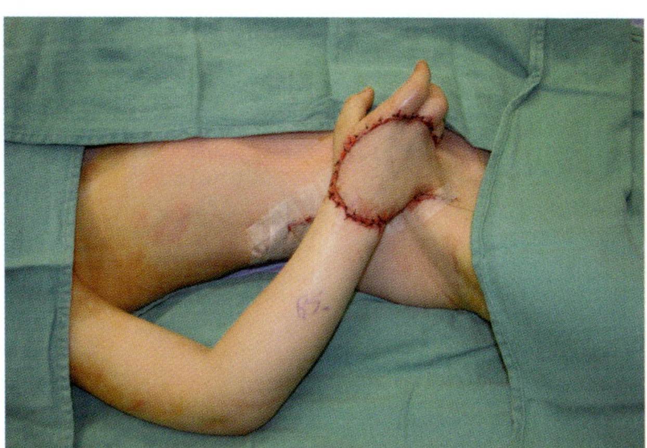

FIGURE 46-10

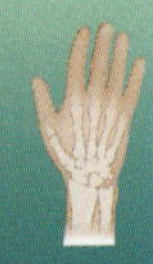

Step 10: Immobilization of the Limb

- The involved upper limb must be immobilized for 2 to 3 days until the patient is comfortable with the flap. This is most critical during the recovery of the patient from anesthesia, when the natural tendency is to take the hand to the mouth to pull the tube out. The surgical team must hold the groin flap arm secure until the patient has emerged from anesthesia.

STEP 10 PEARLS

A pillow placed under the elbow can help place the forearm in the plane of the abdomen and reduce tension on the flap.

STEP 10 PITFALLS

Ensure that neither the flap nor the pedicle is compressed by the dressing.

In the early phase, the flap must be inspected frequently because change in patient position can lead to a kink in the flap or the tubed segment.

If there is full-thickness marginal necrosis of the flap, it is better to wait for 2 to 3 days until the extent of necrosis is demarcated and the initial postoperative swelling comes down. The patient should then be taken to the operating room, the necrosed portion excised, and the flap advanced and re-inset. Waiting longer only delays healing and risks failure on division of the flap.

Step 11: Flap Division

- We divide flaps after 3 weeks (Fig. 46-11).

STEP 11 PEARLS

The joints of the hand, elbow, and shoulder can be mobilized with the patient under anesthesia at the time of flap division. This breaks any flimsy adhesions and makes it easier for the therapist and the patient to recover motion.

Postoperative Care and Expected Outcomes

- Patients should be referred early to the hand therapist to promote passive and active range of motion. For a bulky-appearing groin flap, a compression bandage is provided. Surgery for thinning/defatting the flap should be delayed for at least 3 to 6 months. This can be done by liposuction or as an open technique. We find that the open technique is more effective. Instead of raising half the flap and doing it in stages, we make three incisions around the circumference of the flap at about 120 degrees from each other, while maintaining an intact skin bridge between them. This allows thinning of the entire flap in one stage without risking the vascularity of the flap. (Figure 46-12 shows the late result of the patient shown in Figure 46-1.)
- The groin flap is easy to raise, if dissection is limited lateral to the ASIS. Dissection medial to the ASIS is tricky and needs vigilance. Although the flap brings in a large volume of skin, there are many technical nuances to this flap that need to be addressed for a successful result. Most reports of this flap have mentioned a 15% to 20% incidence of partial flap necrosis.

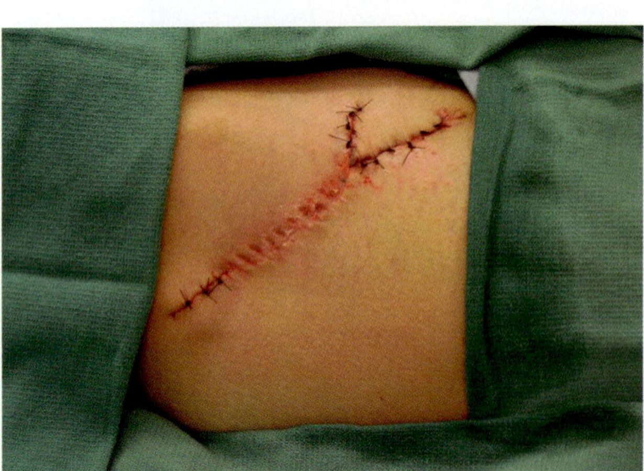

FIGURE 46-11

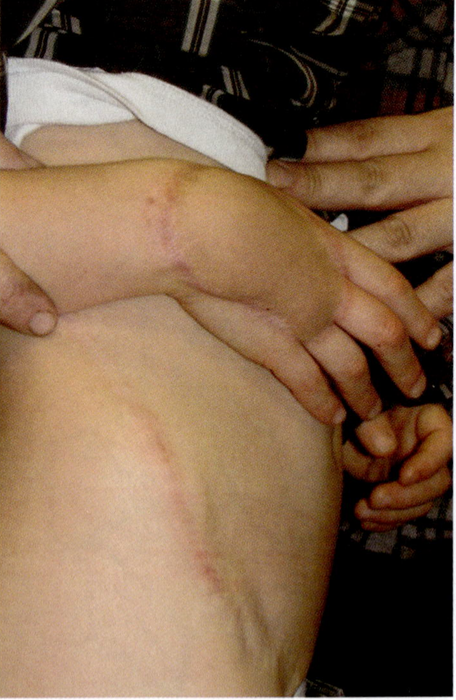

FIGURE 46-12

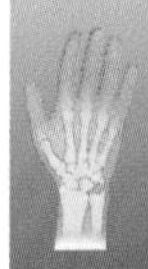

Evidence

Schlenker JD, Averill RM. The iliofemoral (groin flap) for hand and forearm coverage. *Orthop Rev*. 1980;9:57.

The authors retrospectively reviewed 24 groin flaps in 23 patients. The overall complication rate was 38%, and this included 21% infectious complications and a 21% incidence of flap necrosis. (Level IV evidence)

Wray RC, Wise DM, Young VL, Weeks PM. The groin flap in severe hand injuries. *Ann Plast Surg*. 1982;9:459-462.

The authors retrospectively reviewed 27 patients with 28 groin flaps. They reported an 18% incidence of flap necrosis that developed after flap division. The authors could not find a significant difference in necrosis rates between flap division and immediate inset versus flap division and delayed inset. They believed that a preliminary delay procedure before division of the flap would have decreased the incidence of flap necrosis. (Level IV evidence)

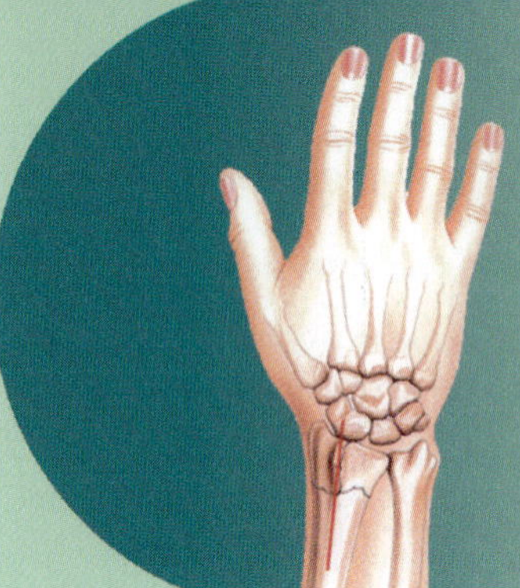

Lateral Arm Flap for Upper Limb Coverage

Lam-Chuan Teoh

Indications

- Procedure is used for soft tissue defects of the hand and wrist. These defects range from a medium size of 3 × 5 cm to a large size of 15 × 20 cm and can include the following:
  - Soft tissue defect from traumatic injuries
  - Soft tissue defect from infections
  - Soft tissue defects from thermal burns
- These skin defects are from loss of the full thickness of the dermis and the entire thickness of the subcutaneous tissues. The deeper tendons and neurovascular bundle could also be lacerated or could have suffered a segmental loss. The underlying bone could also be fractured. These defects include the following:
  - Isolated loss of skin
  - Combined injury with loss of skin, tendon, neurovascular bundle, and bone
- Location of these soft tissue defects could be further classified as follows:
  - Dorsal defect
  - Palmar defect (Fig. 47-1 shows a 10 × 10 cm degloving injury over the palm and thumb in a 35-year-old male fitter.)
  - Radial defect
  - Ulnar defect
  - Distal defect
  - Circumferential
- Free-flap version of the lateral arm flap is always preferred for the resurfacing. The flap is usually harvested from the ipsilateral side. The pedicled version of the flap is harvested from the contralateral side. The pedicled flap is chosen for the following indications:
  - The recipient vessels for anastomosis are not available. (Fig. 47-2 shows a 22 × 4.5 cm circumferential skin defect, following skin necrosis of a trans-metacarpal replant in a 25-year-old carpenter.)
  - The recipient vessels are reserved for subsequent secondary reconstructive procedures, for example, toe-to-thumb/digit transfer.
  - Distal and circumferential defects occur over multiple digits.

Examination/Imaging

Clinical Examination

- Preliminary assessment can be done with inspection of the wound and viewing of the clinical pictures previously taken of the defect. The definitive assessment is performed intraoperatively under anesthesia.
- The recipient defect is assessed to determine the reconstructive requirements.
  - Associated deep tissue injury that requires repair or reconstruction
  - The size, shape, and location of the skin defect (see Figs. 47-1 and 47-2)

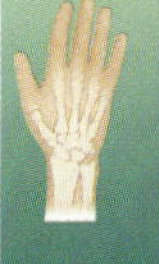

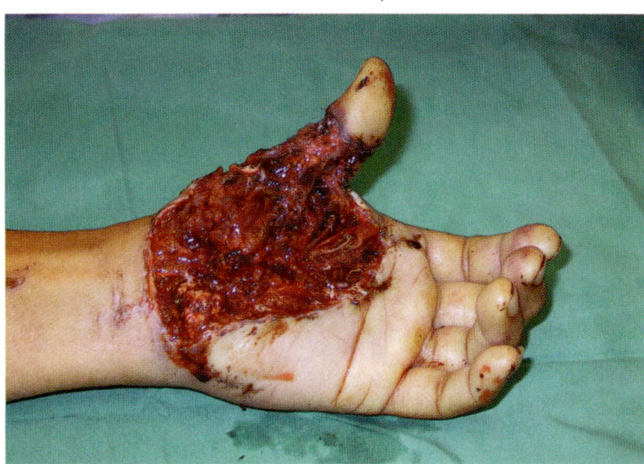

FIGURE 47-1

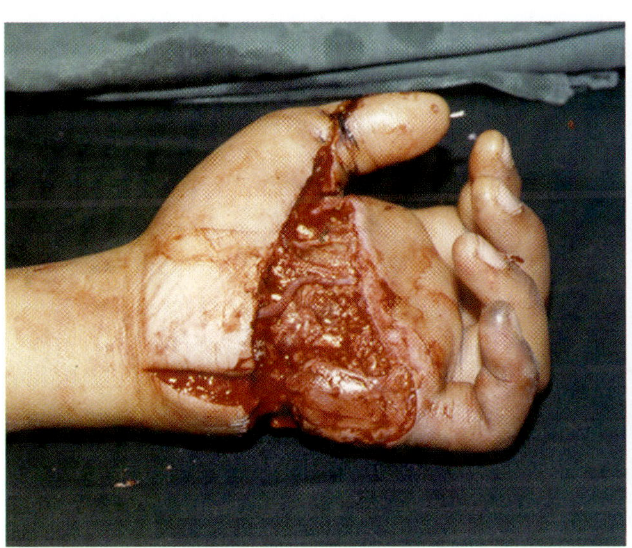

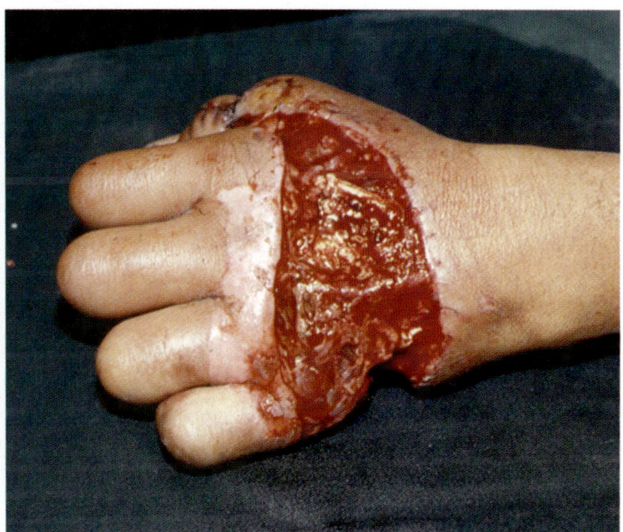

FIGURE 47-2

- Constructing a template of the defect and determining the design of the flap to fit into the defect
- Assessing the availability of the recipient vessels
  - Exclude any previous injury to the intended recipient vessels.
  - Assess the quality of the recipient vessels by direct surgical exposure.
  - Determine the pedicle length from site of the skin defect to the recipient vessels.
- Assessing the donor site
  - Exclude any previous injury to the donor flap territory.
  - Pinch the skin to determine the width of the flap that allows primary closure.
  - Determine obesity and thickness of the flap, which can affect the quality of the flap.

Imaging

- In cases of suspected associated bony injury, radiographs with standard anteroposterior and oblique views of the hand and standard anteroposterior and lateral views of the wrist and forearm are taken.

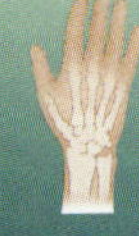

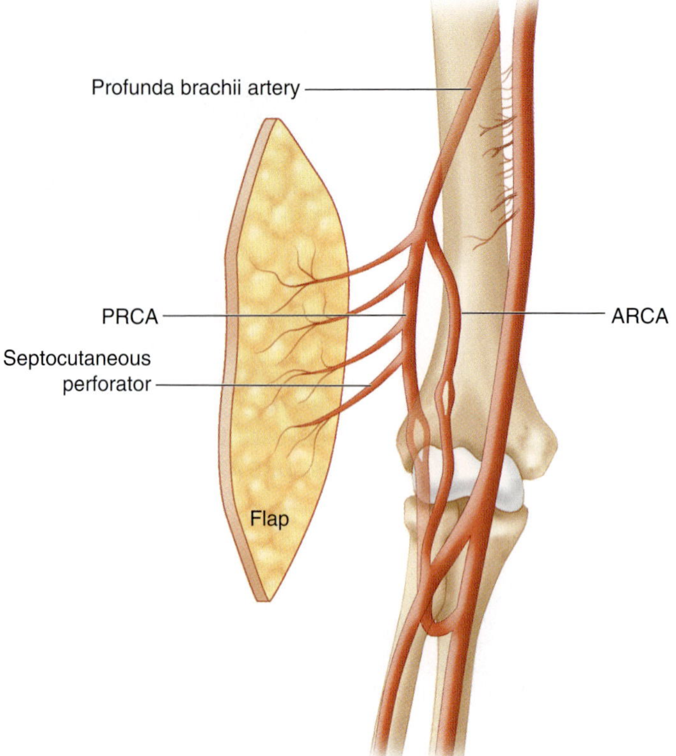

FIGURE 47-3

Surgical Anatomy

- The flap is from the lateral arm region with extension distal to the lateral humeral epicondyle down the lateral side of the forearm. The vascular pedicle is the posterior radial collateral artery (PRCA), a branch of the profunda brachii artery. One to two veins accompany the PRCA artery. The size of the artery is 1.5 to 2 mm in diameter, and the vein 2 to 3 mm in diameter. The vascular pedicle runs in the lateral intermuscular septum accompanied by the posterior antebrachial cutaneous nerve. Three to four septocutaneous perforators supply the lateral arm skin. The most distal branch of the septal vessel is 3 to 5 cm proximal to the lateral epicondyle. There are also three to four small branches of vessels running deep providing periosteal blood supply to the distal lateral humeral bone. The pedicle length of the flap ranges from 5 to 10 cm depending on the design of the flap (Fig. 47-3).
- The flap extends from the deltoid tuberosity to the lateral humeral epicondyle, a length of about 20 cm. The flap can be further extended distally down the lateral aspect of the forearm another 15 cm. The skin over the lateral forearm is thinner than the skin over the lateral arm. The width of the skin flap is limited to 6 cm to allow direct closure of the donor site. Centering the flap over the lateral humeral epicondyle has the advantage of having the thinner distal skin and a longer vascular pedicle.
- In a free-flap version, the ipsilateral flap is preferred. This gives the advantage of confining the wound to the same upper limb. In a pedicled flap version, the flap has to come from the contralateral arm.

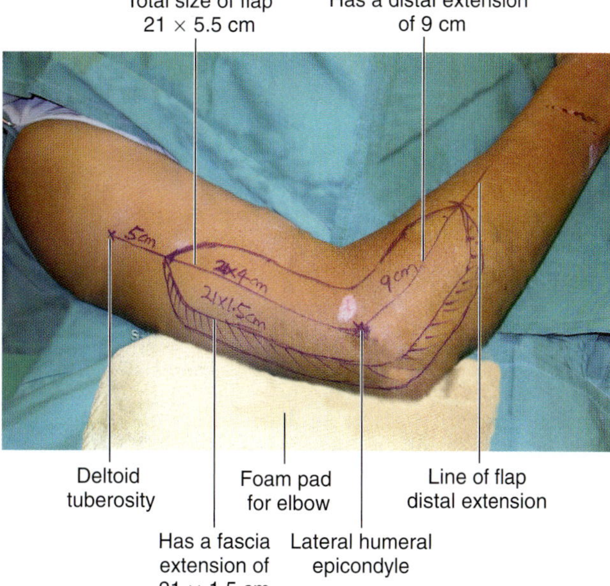

FIGURE 47-4

PEARLS

In patients with a shorter arm, the sterile pressure tourniquet may occupy too much space, making proximal dissection difficult. A narrow manual rubber tourniquet of about 4 cm width can be used in its place effectively. However, the pressure cannot be regulated and is used only for a short duration for the proximal part of the dissection.

Flexion at the elbow and alternatively internal and external rotation at the shoulder facilitate greater reach in dissection of the flap.

PITFALLS

Prolonged pressure on the cubital tunnel during dissection can damage the ulnar nerve. A foam pad is used to cushion the elbow, taking pressure off the cubital tunnel.

PEARLS

The cephalic vein close to the radial artery and the basilic vein close to the ulnar artery are always prepared and made available. Prepare these superficial veins in addition to the venae comitantes. The venae comitantes of the radial and ulnar artery around the wrist are often small and may not be adequate.

The insertion scheme of the flap should be determined before the pedicle length is measured.

Positioning

- The patient is positioned supine with the hand and whole upper limb placed on a hand table.
- The whole upper limb, including the shoulder, is prepared.
- A sterile pressure tourniquet is applied to the arm as proximally as possible.
- A foam pad is used to cushion the elbow, taking pressure off the cubital tunnel and its ulnar nerve. (Fig. 47-4 shows design of 21 × 5.5 cm long and narrow flap design, with fascia extension.)
- For a contralateral pedicled flap, both upper limbs are similarly prepared. The injured hand is brought across the chest to ensure its comfortable reach to the opposite arm.

Preparation of the Recipient Site

- Further débridement may be necessary.
- Skeletal fixation, repair, or grafting of deeper tissues is carried out if necessary.
- Assessment of the skin defect and crafting a template is carried out.
- Exposure, preparation, and assessment of the recipient vessels are undertaken.
- The pedicle length is determined (see Fig. 47-4).

PEARLS

The size of the flap should be about 10% larger than the recipient defect.

Center the flap over the lateral humeral epicondyle, allowing it to include the thinner lateral forearm skin. This also gives the advantage of providing a longer vascular pedicle. However, the flap should extend at least 5 cm proximal to the lateral humeral epicondyle to capture the distalmost septal perforating branch supplying the skin.

Design a long and narrow flap to facilitate direct closure. For a broad and "square-shaped" recipient defect that is much greater than 6 cm, design a flap of half its width and twice its length. The total area of the flap should remain the same. The flap can be inserted to cover the recipient defect by turning it around at about its midpoint; this is the "turn-around technique of flap insertion." (Figure 47-5 shows the appearance of flap after the turn-around technique of flap insertion.)

Fascia extension of up to 4 cm over the anterior and posterior margins of the flap is reliable over the entire length of the flap. The extension provides a substantially broader flap and still allows primary closure of the donor site (see Fig. 47-4).

Design of Free Lateral Arm Flap

- The flap is designed over the lateral arm along an axis extending from the deltoid tuberosity to the lateral humeral epicondyle, extending distally over the lateral forearm to the radial styloid process.
- The flap is centered over the lateral humeral epicondyle, with the long axis lying proximally and distally.
- Connect the most proximal part of the flap to the deltoid tuberosity (see Fig. 47-4).

Harvesting of the Free Lateral Arm Flap

- The flap dissection is performed under exsanguination tourniquet control. Superficial dissection is performed with the skin incision made along the whole perimeter of the flap; proximally, it is extended to the deltoid tuberosity. Sharp dissection is made through the whole thickness of the subcutaneous fat until the deep fascia is reached (Fig. 47-6).
- The deep dissection of the flap harvesting is done in four steps: (1) posterior dissection—elevating the flap from the triceps until reaching the lateral intermuscular septum and exposing the PRCA pedicle; (2) distal dissection—elevating

The turn-around technique of flap insertion

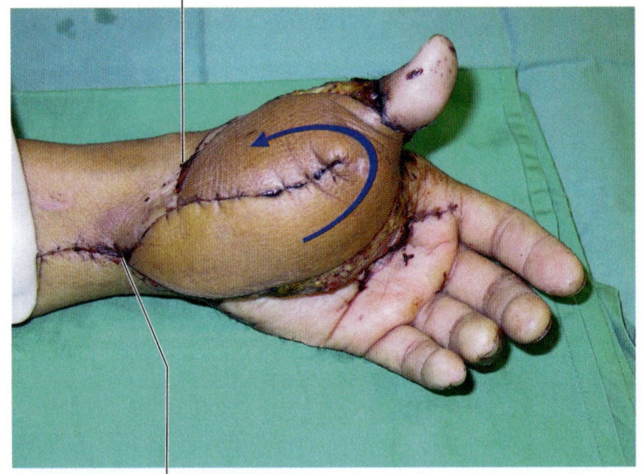

FIGURE 47-5

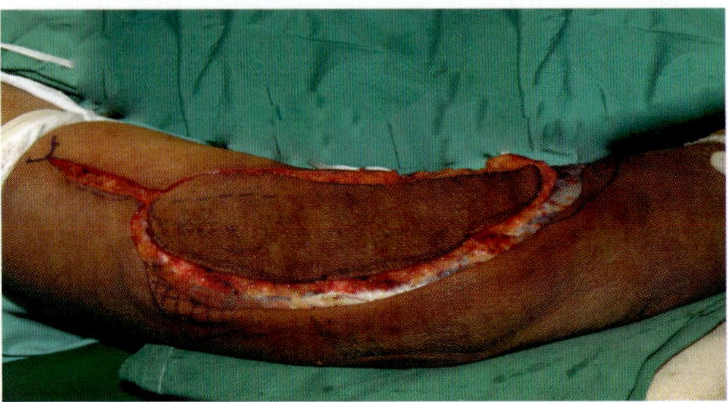

FIGURE 47-6

the flap off the forearm extensor muscles; (3) anterior dissection—elevating the flap from the brachioradialis muscle; and (4) proximal dissection—separating and preparing the proximal PRCA pedicle (Fig. 47-7).

STEP 1 PEARLS

The septocutaneous perforators have multiple small muscular branches to the triceps muscles. These branches should be carefully ligated and divided.

Placing small sharp retractors between the deep fascia and the triceps muscles helps to create space for an easier dissection.

The distal portion of the PRCA pedicle is more visible in the posterior dissection. The proximal portion of the PRCA pedicle is anterior to the intermuscular septum and is less visible.

Procedure

Step 1: Posterior Dissection

- The posterior dissection extends from the lateral humeral epicondyle to the most proximal extent of the flap.
- The deep fascia is incised, exposing the triceps tendon and muscles.
- The fascia is raised from the triceps tendon and muscles from posterior to anterior (Fig. 47-8).
- Three to four septocutaneous perforators supplying the flap visible over the deep fascia are carefully preserved.

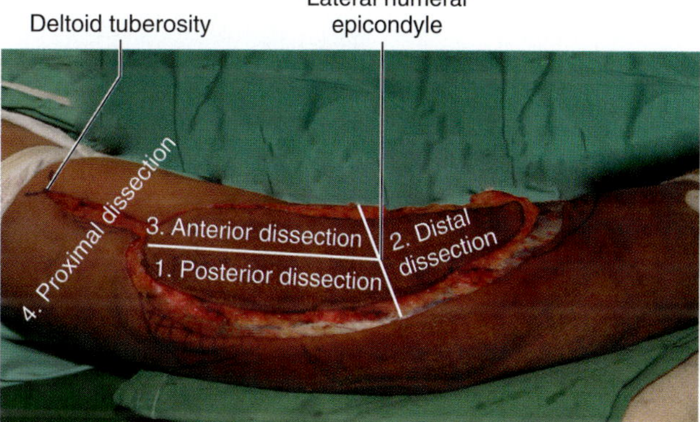

FIGURE 47-7

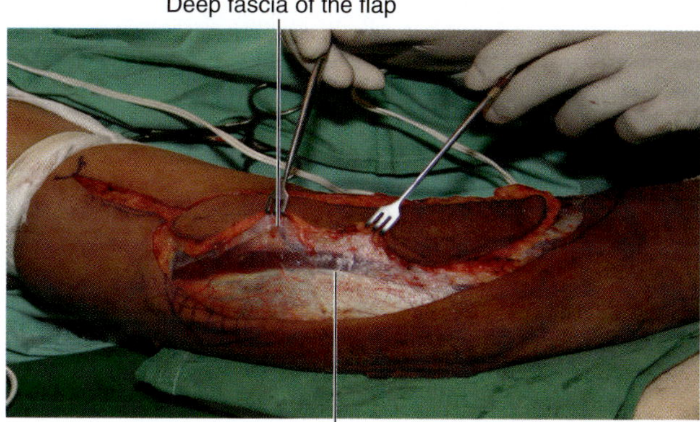

FIGURE 47-8

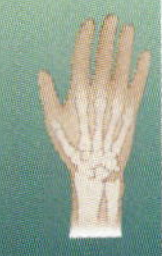

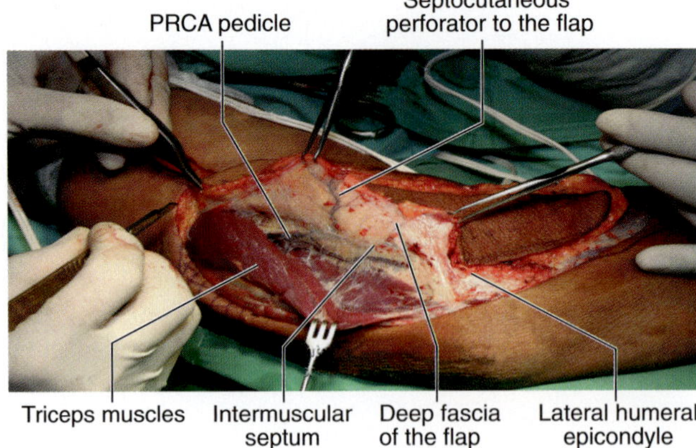

FIGURE 47-9

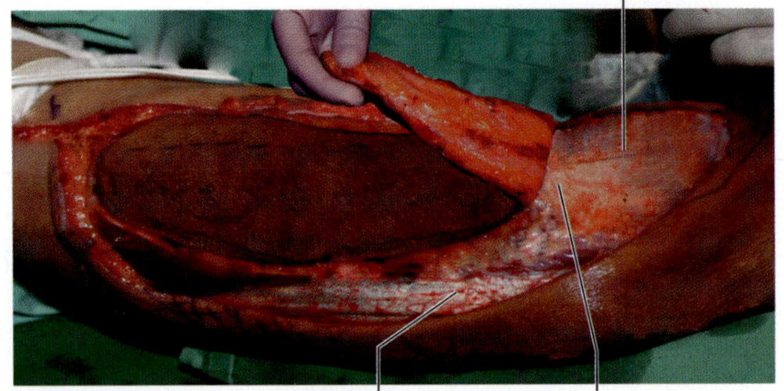

FIGURE 47-10

STEP 2 PEARLS

The distal portion of the flap is thin with less defined deep fascia. Do not include the deeper muscle fascia in the dissection.

STEP 3 PEARLS

The muscles are adherent to the deep fascia in the anterior dissection and require careful dissection.

Multiple muscular branches share the same septocutaneous perforators to the skin; these muscular branches have to be carefully ligated and divided.

In the distal portion, the PRCA pedicle is not well visualized in this anterior location. Its presence has to be continually confirmed by looking at it from the earlier posterior dissection.

In the proximal portion, the PRCA is anterior to the intermuscular septum and is easily identified.

- The fascia is raised until reaching the lateral intermuscular septum, exposing the PRCA pedicle.
- The triceps muscle is separated from the lateral intermuscular septum until the lateral surface of the humeral bone is exposed (Fig. 47-9).

Step 2: Distal Dissection

- The distal dissection is made for the portion of the flap distal to the lateral humeral epicondyle.
- Sharp dissection of the flap is done from distal to proximal, raising the flap from the forearm extensor muscles.
- A few perforating branches from the forearm extensor muscles are cauterized and divided (Fig. 47-10).

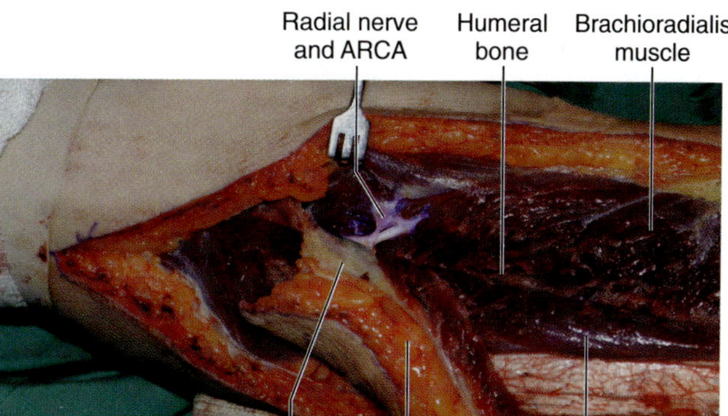

FIGURE 47-11

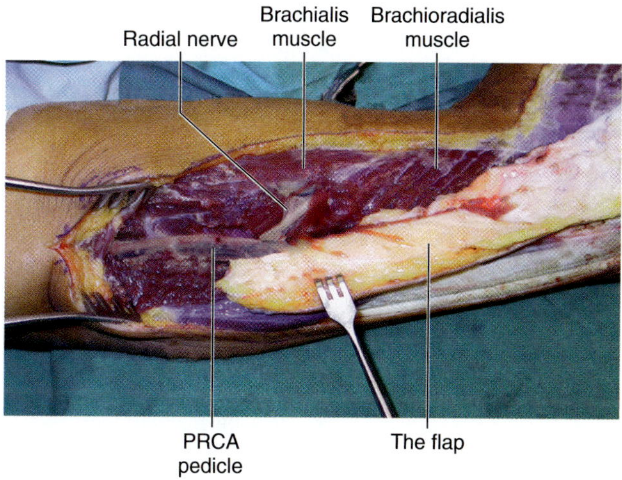

FIGURE 47-12

STEP 4 PEARLS

Placement of a self-retaining retractor on either side of the lateral muscular septum against the triceps muscle posteriorly and the brachialis muscles anteriorly greatly enhances the exposure.

Following the PRCA from its previous distal dissection ensures its easy identification.

The PRCA pedicle in this proximal dissection lies anterior to the lateral intermuscular septum.

The intermuscular septum is divided transversely just proximal to the flap to further free the PRCA pedicle.

The radial nerve comes into view at the midarm level, running distally and anteriorly, and enters between the brachialis and the brachioradialis muscles.

The ARCA accompanying the radial nerve should be ligated and divided to free the PRCA from tethering to the radial nerve.

The posterior cutaneous nerve of the forearm accompanying the PRCA pedicle should be separated and divided.

Step 3: Anterior Dissection

- The anterior dissection extends from the lateral humeral epicondyle to the most proximal extent of the flap.
- Sharp incision is carried through the deep fascia to reach the brachioradialis muscle.
- The deep fascia is dissected away from the muscles from anterior to posterior until the lateral intermuscular septum is reached (Fig. 47-11).

Step 4: Proximal Dissection

- The proximal dissection extends from the proximal tip of the flap to the deltoid tuberosity.
- The triceps muscle is dissected posteriorly and the brachialis muscles anteriorly off the lateral intermuscular septum. Identify the PRCA pedicle, the anterior radial collateral artery (ARCA), and the radial nerve. Continue dissection until the lateral humeral bone is reached.
- The PRCA pedicle is separated and prepared from the proximal end of the flap to its proximal profunda brachii artery origin (Fig. 47-12).

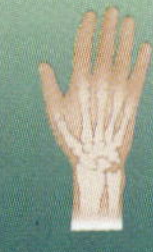

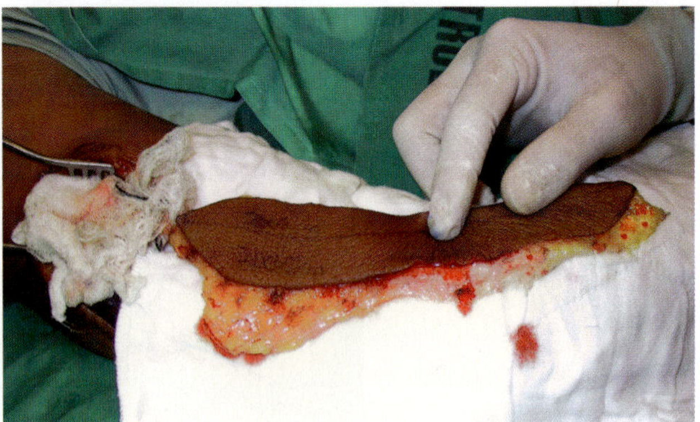

FIGURE 47-13

Step 5: Division of the Vascular Pedicle

- At the conclusion of the dissection, the tourniquet is deflated to check for perfusion to the flap.
- Hemostasis to the bleeding points from the flap should be performed.
- The flap is perfused for the next 10 to 15 minutes before detachment (Fig. 47-13).

Step 6: Closure of the Donor Wound

- The donor site is closed with a closed-suction tube drain.
- The triceps muscle is loosely sutured to the brachialis and brachioradialis muscles.
- Direct closure of the donor wound in two layers is done. Primary split-thickness skin grafting is used for a residual wound that is too tight for a direct closure.

Step 7: Flap Insertion at Recipient Site

- For a defect narrower than 6 cm, the flap is designed to be inserted directly into the defect.
- For a broader defect, the flap can be designed for a turn-around technique of insertion (see Fig. 47-5).

Step 8: Design of the Pedicled Flap

- The design of the flap requires creation of a proximal skin bridge to protect the PRCA vascular pedicle.
- The primary design approach of the pedicle flap is similar the free-flap version.
- However, the flap is extended proximally to the level of the deltoid insertion with two parallel incisions. The width of the skin bridge is the widest width of the flap.
- The proximal end of the flap merges into the proximal skin bridge (Fig. 47-14).

Step 9: Harvesting the Pedicled Flap

- As in the free-flap version, the dissection is performed under exsanguination tourniquet control.
- Superficial dissection is performed with the skin incision along the distal perimeter of the flap. Proximally, the dissection follows the two parallel lines of the skin bridge.

STEP 8 PEARLS

The contralateral injured hand is brought to the flap to assess the comfort of the hand positioning and the adequacy of the flap design.

STEP 9 PEARLS

The step 4 proximal dissection can be less extensive. The dissection is adequate when the PRCA pedicle is sufficiently mobile to allow anterior and posterior movement of the pedicled flap.

The proximal intermuscular septum is not divided, closer dissection of the PRCA pedicle is not necessary, and the posterior cutaneous nerve of the forearm is not divided.

If the proximal skin bridge is not able to be tubed completely, split-thickness skin grafting prevents wound weeping.

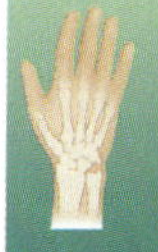

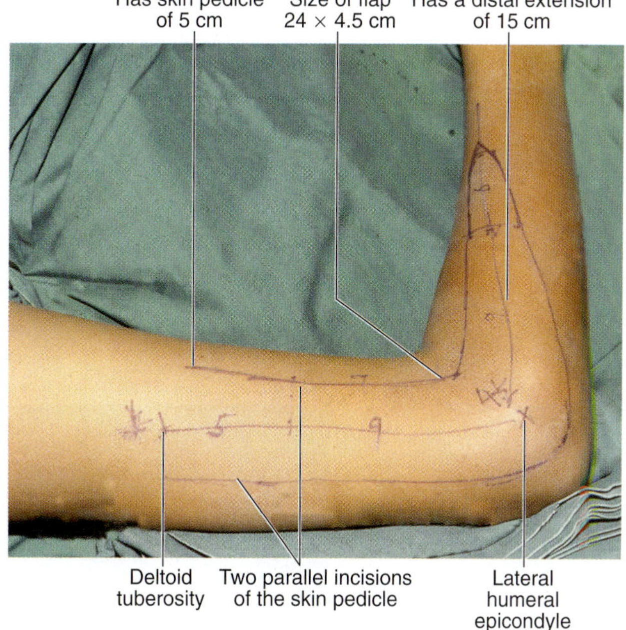

FIGURE 47-14

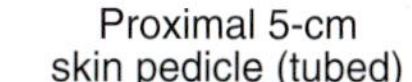

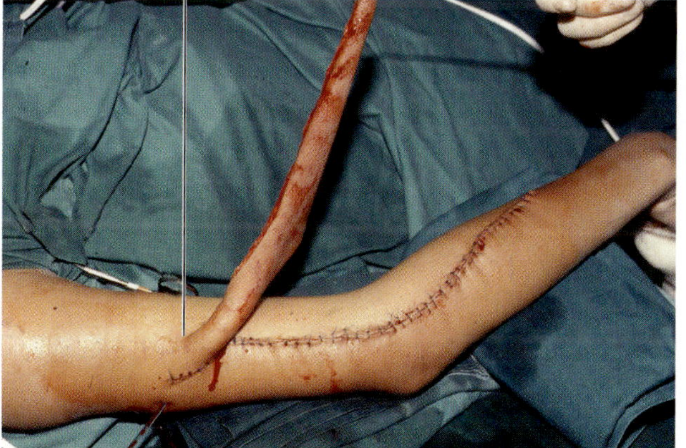

FIGURE 47-15

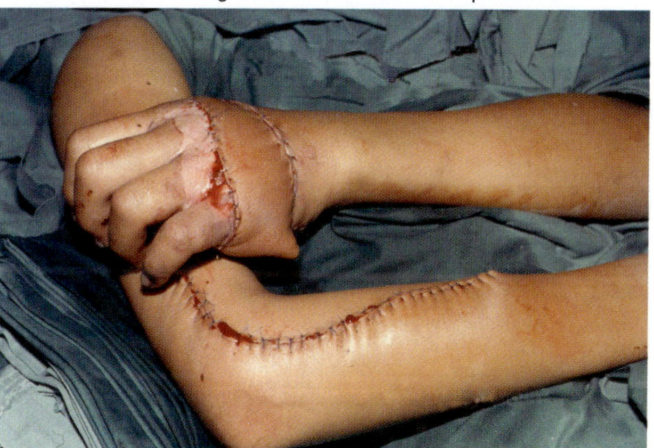

FIGURE 47-16

- Similarly, sharp dissection is made through the whole thickness of the subcutaneous tissues until reaching the deep fascia. The deep dissection of the flap harvesting is done in a fashion similar to the four steps technique. The differences are as follows:
  - The step 1 posterior dissection and step 3 anterior dissection are continued as proximally as possible.
  - The proximal skin bridge is preserved to protect the PRCA pedicle and to attach the contralateral hand to the arm.
  - The proximal skin bridge is tubed to protect the PRCA pedicle (Fig. 47-15).
  - The donor wound is closed primary.
  - The tourniquet is deflated to check for perfusion to the flap.
  - The contralateral hand is brought across the chest for flap insertion (Fig. 47-16).

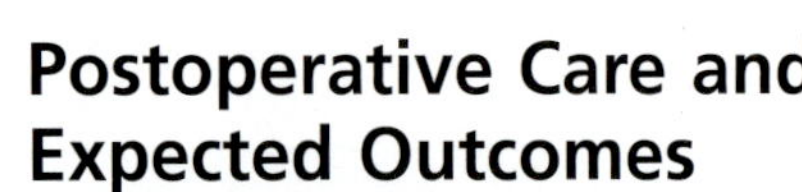

Postoperative Care and Expected Outcomes

- Strapping of both forearms together across the chest is done in the initial 12 hours before surgery while patient is recovering from anesthesia.
- To prevent flap avulsion, the patient is taught to move the upper limbs in unison. Therapy is started the next day to prevent shoulder, elbow, and wrist stiffness.
- All activities of daily living are allowed by the third day (Fig. 47-17).
- Division of flap is performed at 3 weeks (Fig. 47-18).

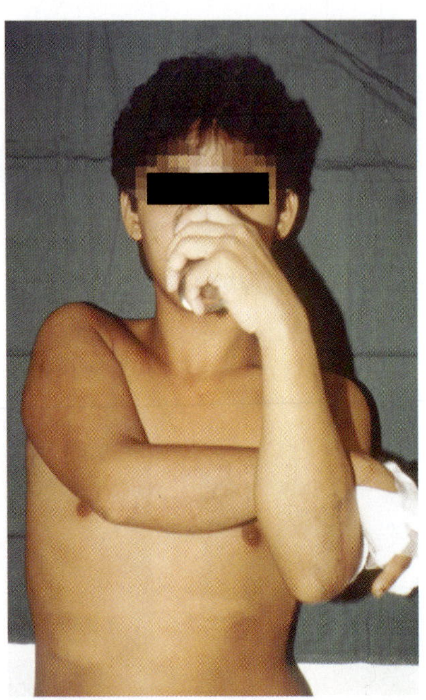

FIGURE 47-17

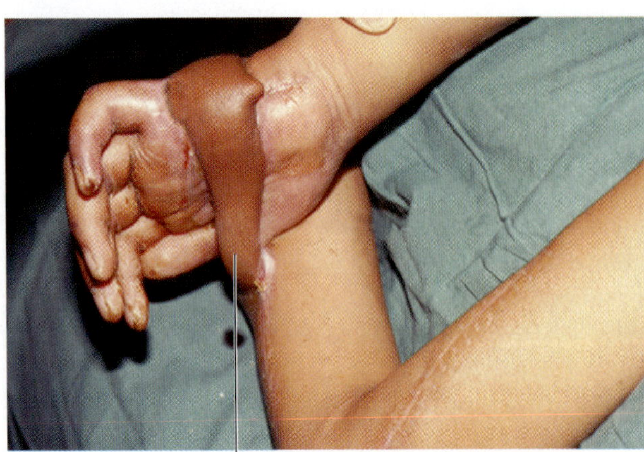

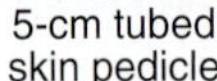

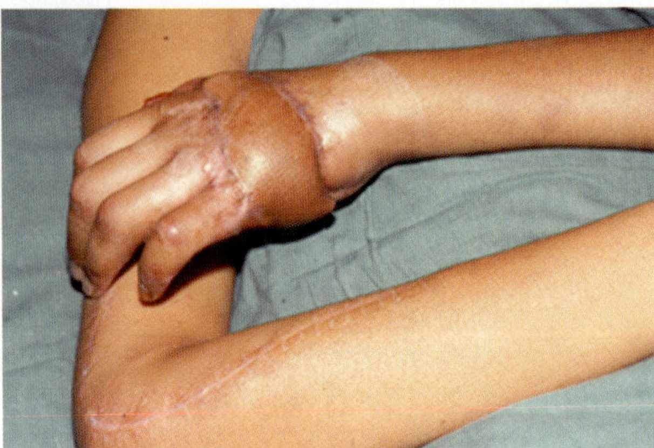

FIGURE 47-18

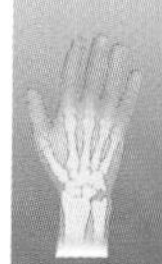

Evidence

Akinci M, Ay S, Kamiloglu S, Ercetin O. Lateral arm free flaps in the defects of the upper limbs—a review of 72 cases. *Hand Surg*. 2005;10:177-185.
Seventy-four free lateral arm flap procedures were performed in 72 patients. Five were performed as emergencies, 12 within 72 hours of injury, and 57 as elective surgery. The size of skin defects ranged from 6 × 4 cm to 20 × 9 cm. There was 7% flap failure rate. One flap dissection was abandoned owing to very thin pedicle and obesity. (Level V evidence)

Katsaros J, Tan E, Zoltie N. The use of lateral arm flap I upper limb surgery. *J Hand Surg [Am]*. 1991;16:598-604.
The lateral-arm free microvascular flap was used for upper limb reconstruction in 20 patients. The size of the flap, modifications to the flap, and complications were documented. There was one flap failure, and nine flaps required surgical thinning at a second procedure. This sole disadvantage was outweighed in clinical use by the advantages and versatility of the lateral arm flap. (Level V evidence)

Ng SW, Teoh LC, Lee YL, Seah WT. Contralateral pedicled lateral arm flap for hand reconstruction. *Ann Plast Surg*. 2010;64:159-163.
Contralateral pedicled lateral arm flaps were used in 22 consecutive patients between 6 and 70 years of age (18 males and 4 females) with hand defects from trauma, infection, burn, and complications of free flap. The flap size ranged from 18 cm^2 to 127.5 cm^2. Eighteen reconstructions were fasciocutaneous, and 4 were osteofasciocutaneous. The flap was divided in 3 weeks. All the flaps survived, with no wound infection. There was no significant shoulder or elbow joint stiffness. (Level V evidence)

Scheker LR, Kleinert HE, Hanel DP. Lateral arm composite tissue transfer to ipsilateral hand defects. *J Hand Surg [Am]*. 1987;12:665-672.
The ipsilateral lateral arm free flap was presented in 29 patients for hand reconstruction. The flap was used in both elective and emergency reconstruction with a success rate of 96.5%. This flap is elevated from the same limb as the injured hand, permitting the entire operative procedure to be performed with the patient under a single regional block anesthesia, both flap and recipient sites being prepared synchronously in a bloodless field. (Level V evidence)

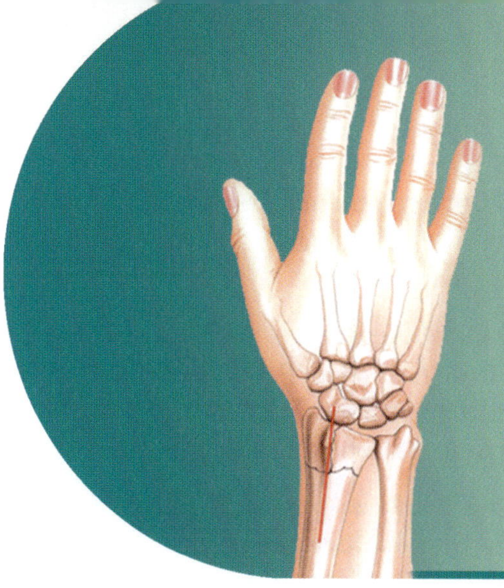

Section VIII

HAND FRACTURES, DISLOCATIONS, AND ARTHRITIS

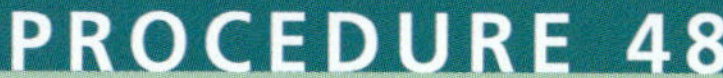

PROCEDURE 48

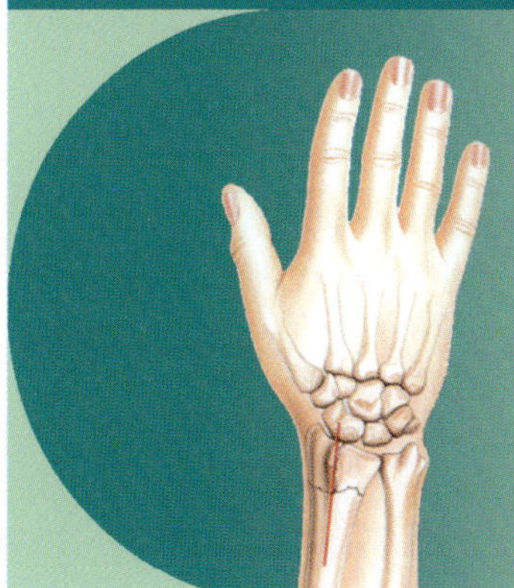

Open Reduction and Internal Fixation of Phalangeal Unicondylar Fractures

Winston Y. C. Chew and Lam-Chuan Teoh

See Video 38: ORIF of Middle Phalanx Volar Avulsion Fracture

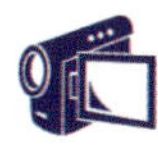

Indications

- Fractures of phalangeal condyles are classified by Weiss and Hastings into various subtypes. The most common is the displaced unicondylar fracture. The obliquity of the fracture line makes it highly unstable and liable to displacement. Nonoperative treatment is often unsuccessful in maintaining the reduction of the fracture. The condylar fragment also bears the origin of the important collateral ligament. The displacement of the fractured condyle therefore results in disruption of articular congruity, joint instability, angular deformity, and loss of joint motion. A displaced condylar fracture is an indication for open reduction and internal fixation.
- Open reduction and internal fixation is aimed at obtaining a perfect reduction of the articular surface. The internal fixation should be as stable as possible to allow early postoperative mobilization, which will encourage cartilage healing.

Examination/Imaging

Clinical Examination

- There is joint swelling from bleeding and soft tissue trauma.
- Angular deformity at the joint results from the fracture displacement.
- Joint motion is painful and restricted.

Imaging

- Standard anteroposterior and oblique views of the hand do not give adequate views of the fracture.
- Standard anteroposterior and lateral views of the affected finger often provide the diagnosis (Fig. 48-1).

Surgical Anatomy

- Midline central tendon splitting approach gives good exposure of the proximal interphalangeal joint. Flexion of the joint and retraction on the tendon allow the extensor tendon to slip around both condyles, giving excellent visualization of nearly the whole dorsal and distal extent of the condyles (Fig. 48-2A).
- To avoid avascular necrosis, blood supply to the fractured condyle should be carefully preserved. The fractured condyle should not be detached from the palmar soft tissue attachment and collateral ligament (Fig. 48-2B).
- These condylar fractures usually have a proximal oblique extension on to the shaft, which is sufficient for placement of the one to two interfragmentary screws for the fixation of the fracture.

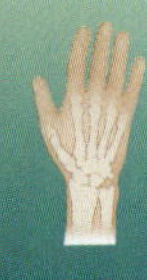

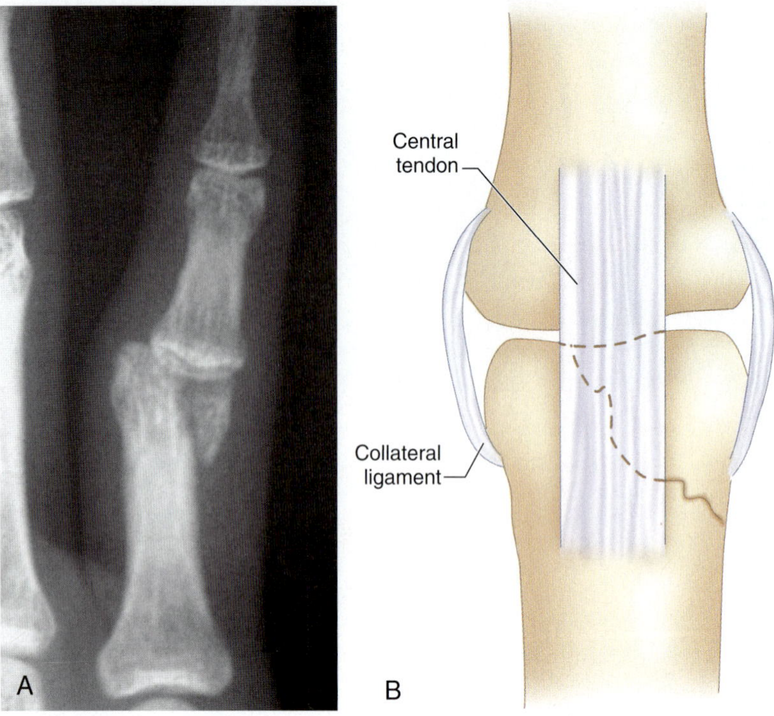

FIGURE 48-1

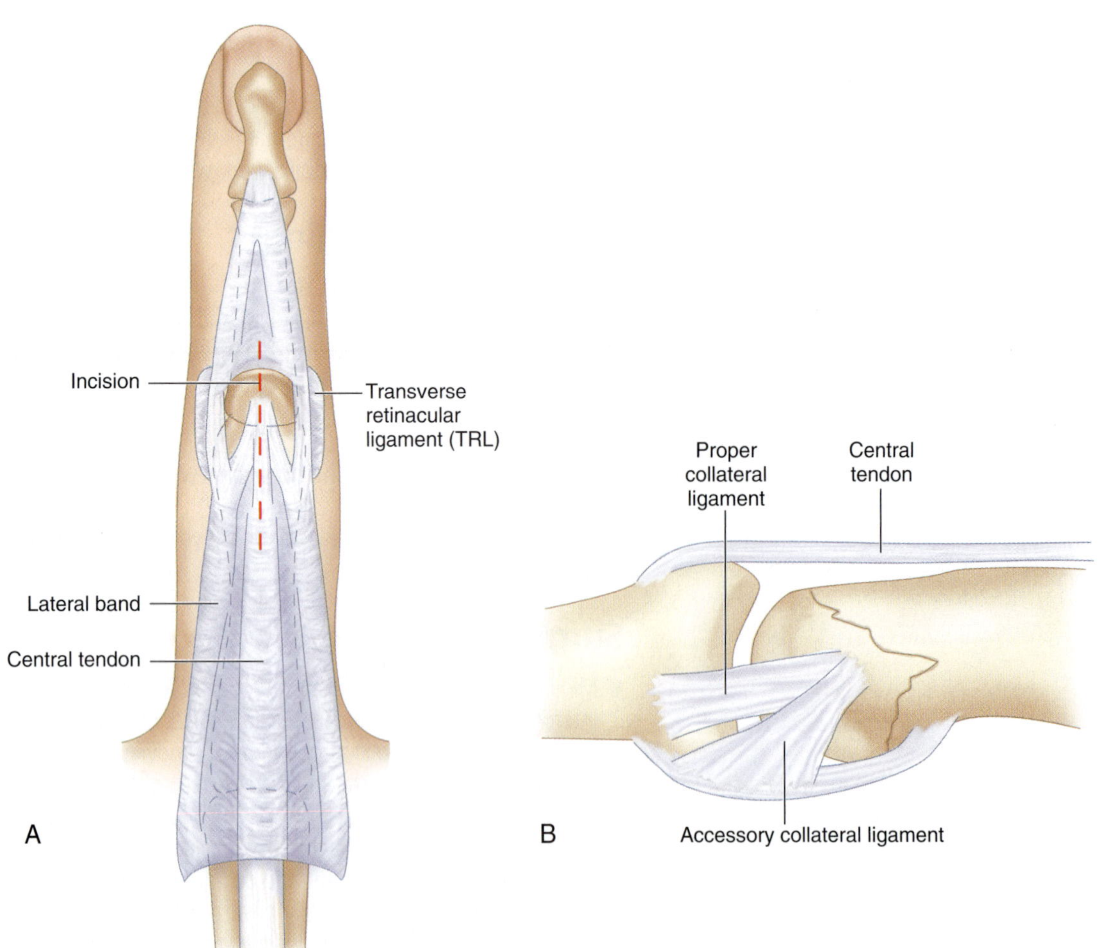

FIGURE 48-2

- Placement of the interfragmentary screws utilizes the nonarticular portion of the bone. When this portion is small, the screw may have to be placed more distally, which may encroach onto the collateral ligament. Care should be taken not to damage the collateral ligament.
- For fractures with little or no metaphyseal extension, intra-articular screw placement with countersunk head may be necessary.

Positioning

- Patient should be positioned supine with a hand extension table.
- The hand should be easily accessible to the mini C-arm for fluoroscopic control during surgery.

Exposures

- A gentle curved incision is made over the proximal interphalangeal (PIP) joint. The proximal limb of the incision extends obliquely over the proximal phalanx. The distal extension over the middle phalanx is much shorter. Figure 48-3 shows marking for the incision, with the proximal extension being longer.
- The extensor tendon is split in the midline and retracted from the midline.
- The loose connective tissue between the extensor tendon and the periosteum allows a plane between them to be developed easily (Fig. 48-4). The periosteum is left undisturbed. Figure 48-4 shows exposure of the joint through a midline incision on the extensor tendon and elevation of the tendon off the periosteum.
- Acutely flexing the joint exposes the articular surface of the proximal phalanx and the fractures widely (Fig. 48-5). Figure 48-5 shows acute flexion of the PIP joint, which allows the split extensor tendon to slip around the condyles, exposing the articular surface and the fracture.
- Joint irrigation with saline in a 20-mL syringe washes away the blood clots and provides a clear visualization of the fracture.
- Any organized clots and debris are gently removed from the fracture site.

PEARLS

Approach to the PIP joint through central splitting of the extensor tendon allows both parts of the tendon to easily slip over the condyles and provide excellent exposure.

Further flexion of the joint gives access to the palmar side of the condyle and provides good visualization of the fracture reduction.

PITFALLS

Do not strip the periosteum from the bone because this will devascularize the bone.

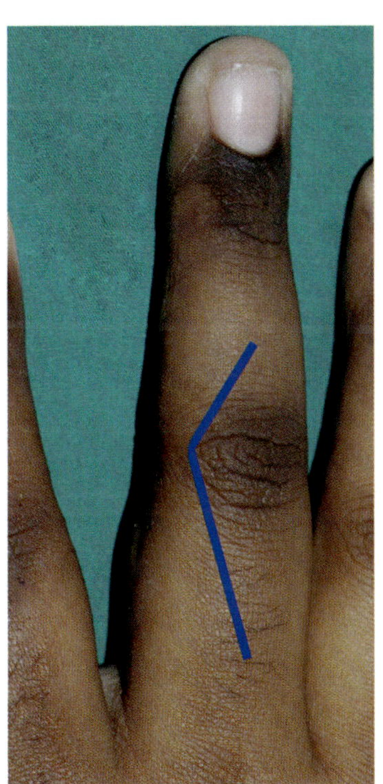

FIGURE 48-3

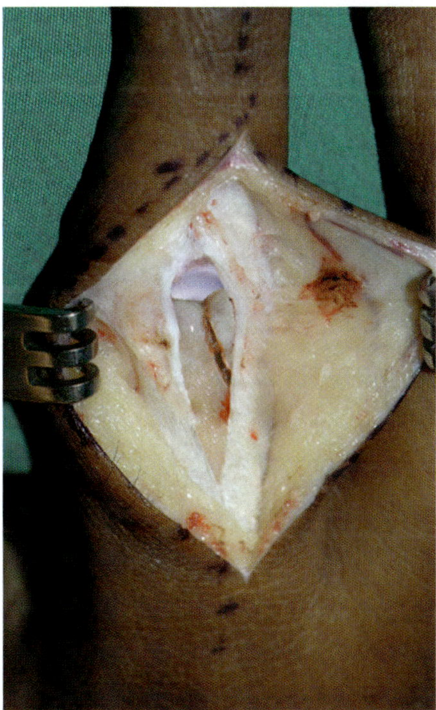

FIGURE 48-4

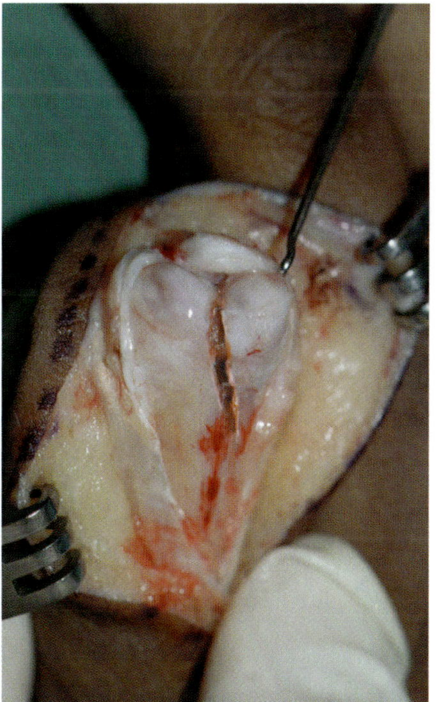

FIGURE 48-5

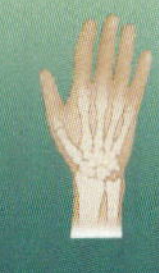

STEP 1 PEARLS

Longitudinal traction on the finger and slight deviation of the finger farther away from the fracture fragment provide a ligamentotaxis-assisted reduction of the fracture.

STEP 1 PITFALLS

Do not detach the fracture fragment from the palmar soft tissues.

Do not denude the fracture bone of periosteum.

Do not apply the reduction clamp too forcefully because this may damage the soft condylar bone.

STEP 2 PEARLS

Plan for insertion of two screws, and place them a good distance apart. For fixation to be effective, the bone surface dimension should be at least three times the diameter of the screw.

Keep the reduction clamp in place until both screws are inserted. If the clamp is in the way of the second screw insertion, reposition the clamp.

The bone on this condylar region is relatively soft, and countersinking of the drill hole is not necessary.

STEP 2 PITFALLS

The screw should not protrude too far out of the opposite cortex because this can irritate the opposite collateral ligament and impede joint motion.

Procedure

Step 1

- Reduction of the fracture is by gentle nudging with a periosteal elevator and bringing the fracture fragment into position with a pair of artery forceps. The reduction should be done in steps, and fine adjustments should be repeated until a perfect congruity of the cartilage surface is achieved.
- A small pointed reduction clamp is then used to hold the reduced fragment in place (Fig. 48-6). For large fragments, two reduction clamps may be used.

Step 2

- The fracture is fixed with interfragmentary (lag screw) fixation technique. The screw is inserted from the fracture fragment to the main bone. The direction of the screw fixation is between perpendicular to the bone surface and perpendicular to the fracture line. The screw size for a proximal phalangeal condyle is usually 1.5 mm in diameter. For smaller bone fragments, 1.3-mm screws are used; for larger fragments, 2.0-mm screws. Ideally, two screws should be used. However, in smaller bone fragments, there may be room for only one screw.
- With the correctly sized drill bit, a drill hole is made in the predetermined entry site and direction. It is a through-and-through drill hole from the fracture fragment to the opposite cortex (Fig. 48-7).
- The near cortex is then overdrilled with a drill bit equal in size to the core diameter of the screw. The correct-length screw is then inserted (Fig. 48-8). With a self-tapping screw, no pretapping is necessary.
- A second screw is then similarly inserted. Figure 48-9 shows insertion of the second interfragmentary screw. Care is taken to avoid the collateral ligament attachment.
- Check with fluoroscopy to ensure correct length of the screws.
- Ranging of the joint is done to check for smooth motion, any soft tissue catching, and stability of the fixation.

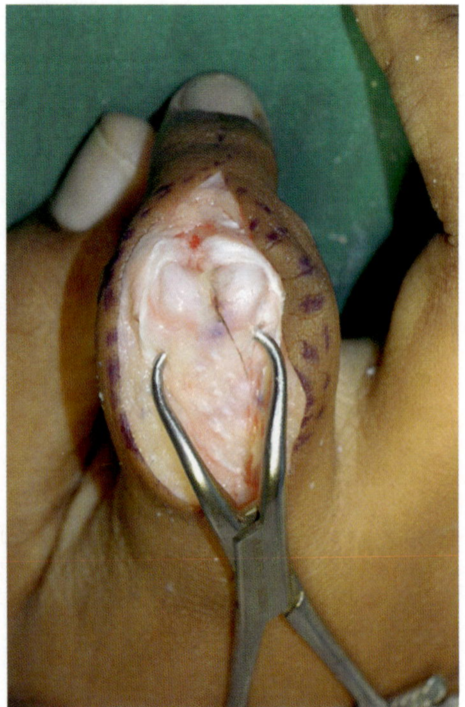

FIGURE 48-6

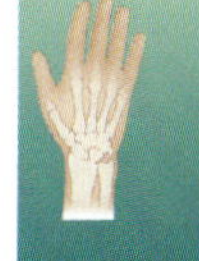

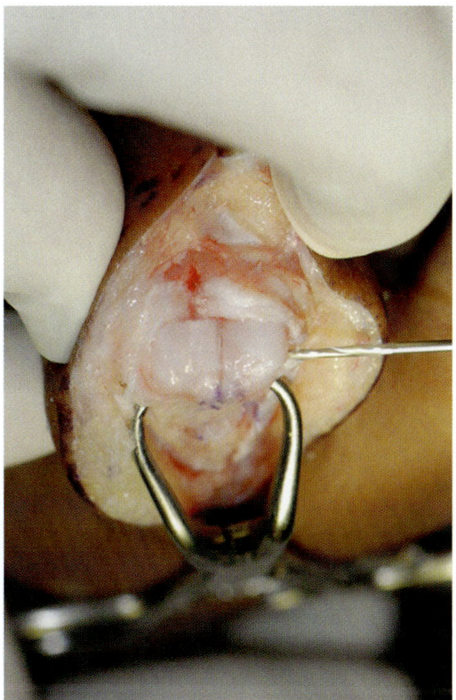

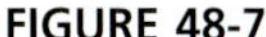

FIGURE 48-7

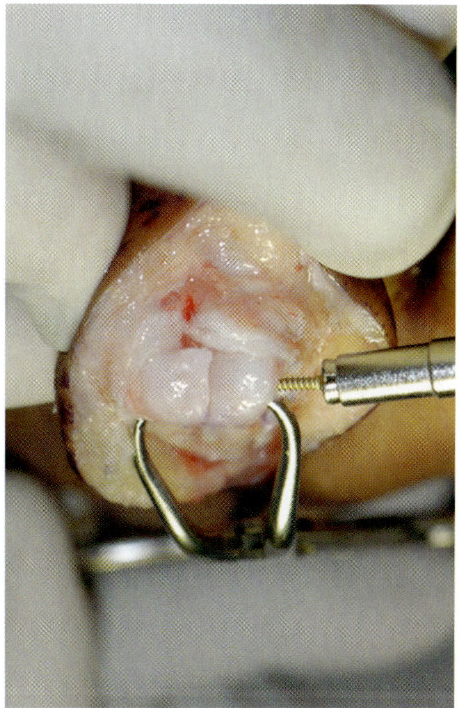

FIGURE 48-8

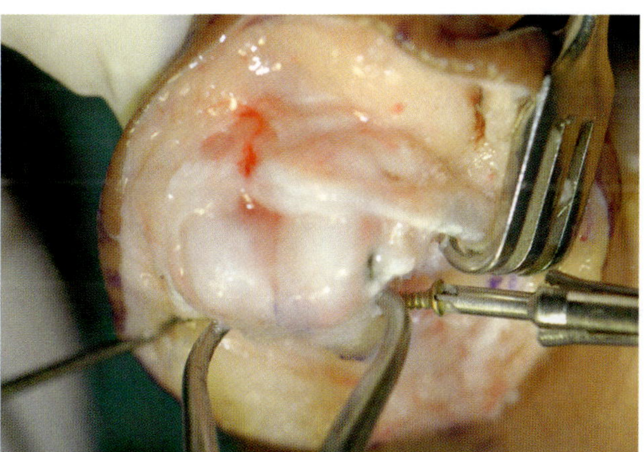

FIGURE 48-9

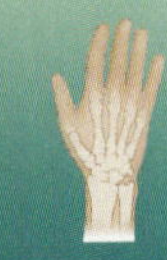

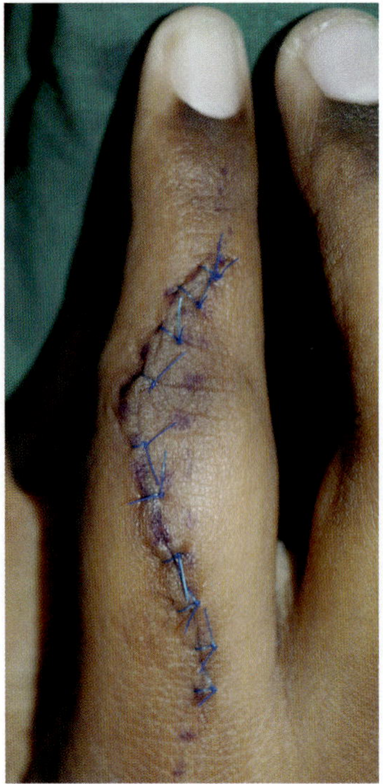

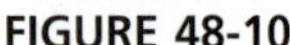

FIGURE 48-10

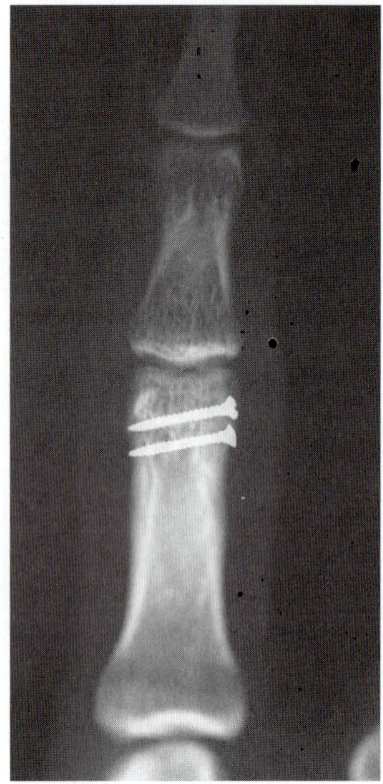

FIGURE 48-11

Step 3

- The extensor tendon is repaired with continuous 4-0 or 5-0 absorbable synthetic sutures. The skin is closed with interrupted nonabsorbable sutures (Fig. 48-10).
- Supplementary regional nerve block of the appropriate nerve territory is done.
- The hand is wrapped in a bulky supportive dressing to include all the fingers for comfort.

PEARLS

Keeping the finger in full extension on a palmar trough splint reduces pain and prevents extension lag from developing. Watch out for flexion contracture of the PIP joint.

Postoperative Care and Expected Outcomes

- Change to a light dressing the next day, and start active range-of-motion exercise four to five times a day. Keep the finger fully extended on a palmar trough splint between exercise sessions for the next 4 weeks.
- The active range of motion is further assisted with passive ranging as tolerated within the limits of pain.
- The fracture unites quickly in 6 weeks, and the joint usually regains near-full range of motion. Figure 48-11 shows uneventful healing of the condylar fracture with good anatomic restoration.

Evidence

Weiss APC, Hastings H. Distal unicondylar fractures of the proximal phalanx. *J Hand Surg [Am]*. 1993;18:594-599.

Thirty-eight patients with unicondylar fractures of the proximal phalanx treated with a variety of fixation techniques (mini screw, screw supplemented with K-wire, single K-wire, multiple K-wires, and loop wire) were reviewed. A commonly used classification of fractures of the distal articular surface of the proximal phalanx is described. The mechanism of injury and results and complications of the treatment were presented. (Level V evidence)

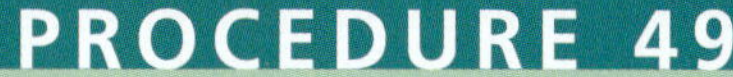

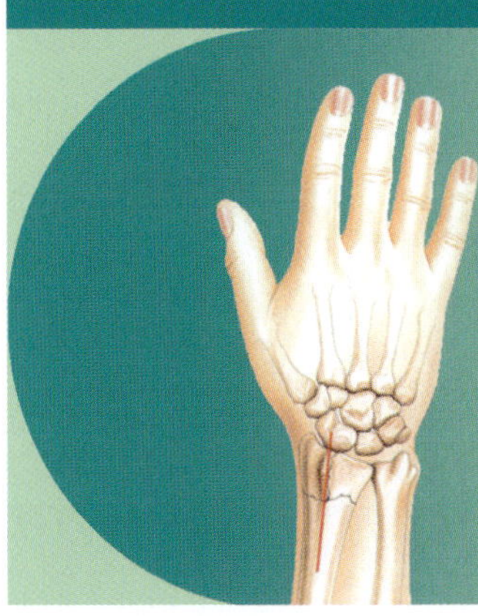

PROCEDURE 49

Open Reduction and Internal Fixation of Phalangeal Shaft Spiral or Long Oblique Fractures

Winston Y. C. Chew

Indications

- Instability as indicated by the following:
  - Rotational deformity causing scissoring
  - Shortening resulting in extensor tendon dysfunction
  - Angulation resulting in pseudoclawing for the proximal phalanx and swan-neck–like deformity for the middle phalanx
  - Significant pain restricting range of motion
  - Displacement during conservative treatment
- Fractures with intra-articular extension resulting in joint incongruity
- Open fractures

Examination/Imaging

Clinical Examination

- Deformity in the form of shortening, rotation, and angulation of the finger (Fig. 49-1)
- Limited range of motion of the affected joint, especially the joint distal to the fracture

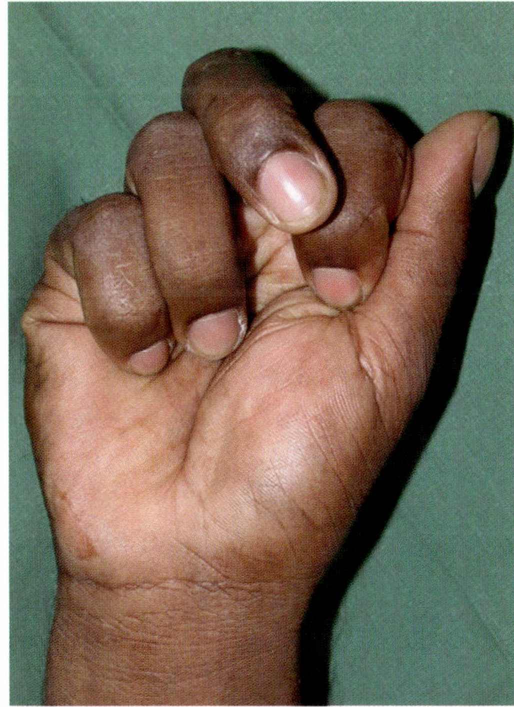

FIGURE 49-1

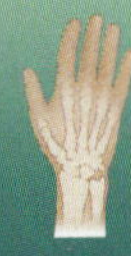

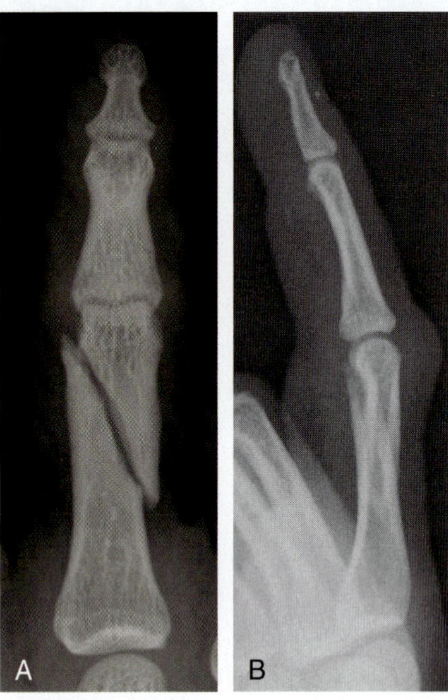

FIGURE 49-2

Imaging

- Standard anteroposterior (Fig. 49-2A) and lateral views (Fig. 49-2B) of the affected finger will often give the diagnosis.
- Oblique views may sometimes be required to give a better understanding of the fracture displacement and degree of comminution, if any.

Surgical Anatomy

- The extensor tendons, consisting of both the extrinsic and intrinsic tendons, form a finely balanced complex over the finger (Fig. 49-3A).
- The central slip inserts to the base of the middle phalanx, and care should be taken not to violate this insertion during exposure.
- The fibrous flexor sheath with its flexor tendons is closely applied to the volar surface of the phalanges (Fig. 49-3B). Hence, all screws must not protrude beyond the cortex, especially on the volar aspect, to avoid attrition of the flexor tendons.

Positioning

- The patient should be positioned supine with a hand extension table.
- The hand should be easily accessible to the mini C-arm for fluoroscopic control during surgery.

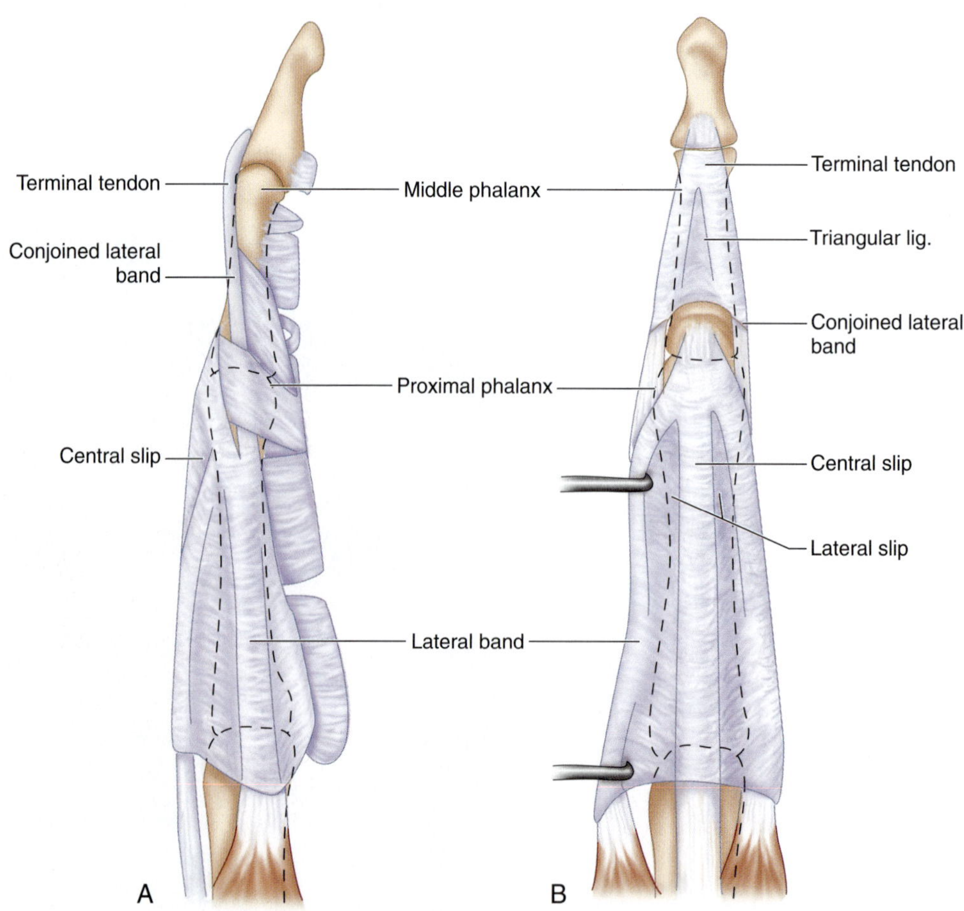

FIGURE 49-3

PEARLS

All clots and debris between the fracture fragments must be débrided to allow anatomic reduction of the fracture fragments.

Exposures

- For the proximal phalanx, the fracture is exposed through a direct dorsal longitudinal incision, splitting the extensor tendon in the midline (Fig. 49-4).
- For the middle phalanx, the fracture is exposed through a direct dorsal longitudinal incision, and the lateral slips of the extensor tendon are mobilized by incising the triangular ligament in the midline and extending distally by splitting the tendon in the midline to its insertion into the distal phalanx.
- The periosteum is incised and elevated. This layer is more prominent if fracture repair is delayed by a few days.

STEP 1 PEARLS

All debris must be cleared because even small amounts can prevent accurate reduction.

STEP 2 PEARLS

Care must be taken to achieve anatomic reduction. Rotational reduction is confirmed by flexing the fingers using the tenodesis effect.

Reduction must be perfect. A very slight malreduction can translate into a rotational deformity.

Procedure

Step 1

- The fracture is exposed, and blood clots and periosteum are débrided from the fracture surface.
- Reduction of the fracture is achieved by longitudinal traction and rotation of the distal fragment toward the proximal fragment to close the fracture.

Step 2

- A small, pointed bone reduction clamp is used to hold the fracture in position (Fig. 49-5). Sometimes, two clamps are required to control rotation.
- Alternatively, artery forceps may be used.

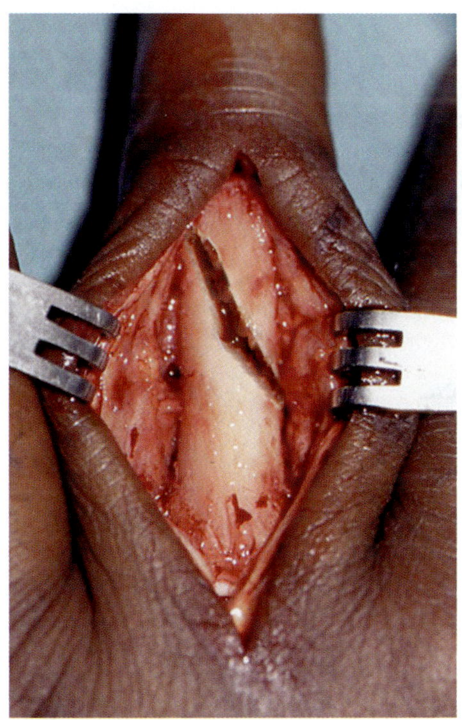

FIGURE 49-4

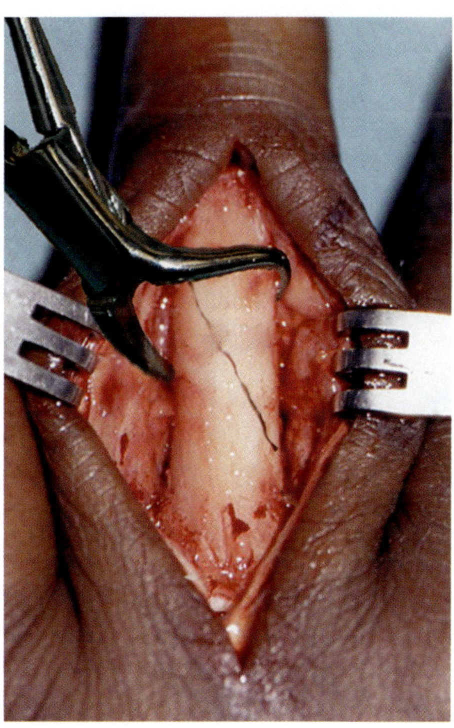

FIGURE 49-5

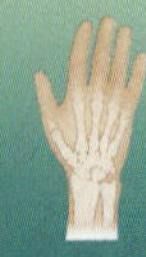

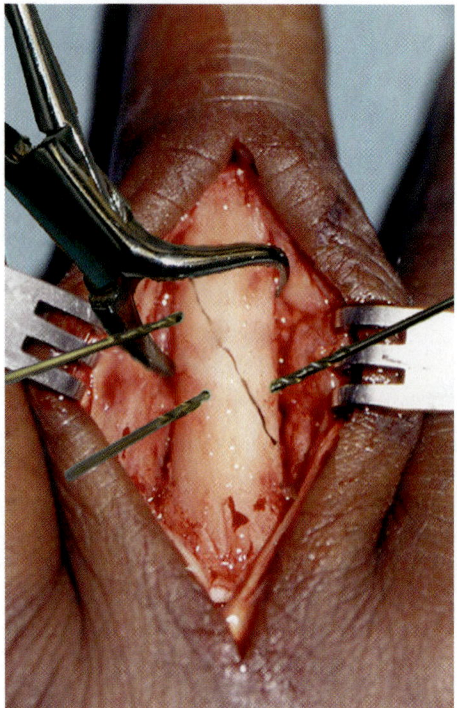

FIGURE 49-6

Step 3

- Precompression of the fracture is achieved by using the pointed bone reduction clamp or artery forceps. This allows a bicortical screw to be inserted instead of a classic lag screw without compromising the compression across the fracture.
- Usually, a 1.5- or 1.3-mm screw is chosen, according to the size of the bone and fragment. Sometimes, for very small fragments, 1-mm screws may be used. Alternatively, for larger bones, 2-mm screws may be used. There should be at least a one-diameter distance from the edge of the fracture to the drill hole.
- The direction of the screw should be perpendicular to the fracture line for maximal compression. Screws should also be placed perpendicular to the rotational plane of the fracture (Fig. 49-6).
- The fracture is held in a precompressed position while the drill hole is made. With precompression, the fracture is not likely to slide and displace during tightening of the screws.

STEP 3 PEARLS

Precompression helps to interdigitate the fracture to lessen the risk for fracture displacement during screw placement.

Smaller screws should be used nearer the apex of the fracture fragments to lessen the risk for fractures.

Ensure that the drill is sharp and that irrigation is done during drilling to reduce the amount of heat produced and the risk for osteonecrosis.

STEP 3 PITFALLS

Care should be taken not to overtighten and fracture the fragments.

Screws that are not perpendicular to the fracture plane may cause the fracture fragments to shear and displace.

Step 4

- The drill hole is countersunk so that the screw head will sit better. This will also lessen soft tissue irritation as well as ensuring that the direction of the screw is maintained, preventing the screw head from being pushed eccentrically when one side of it comes into contact with the phalanx, as is usually the case with a spiral or long oblique fracture.

STEP 4 PEARLS

Countersinking the drill hole will minimize soft tissue irritation and ensure maintenance of the alignment of the screw and, hence, the reduction.

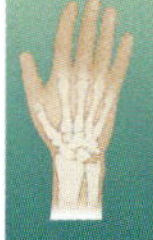

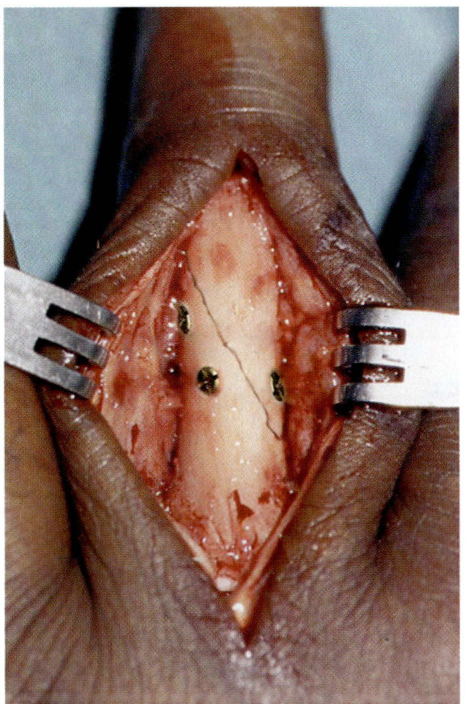

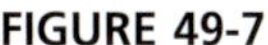

FIGURE 49-7

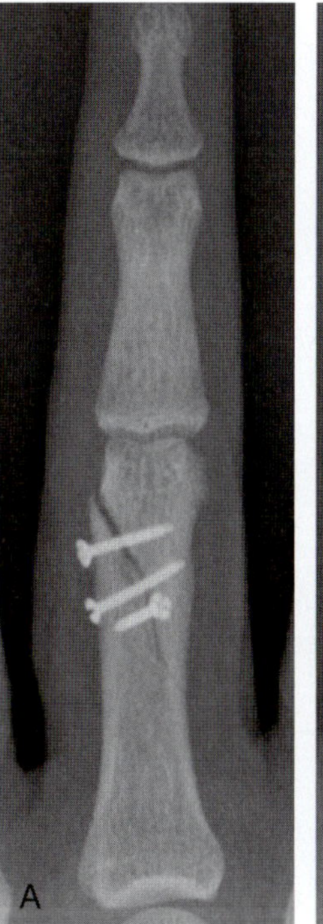

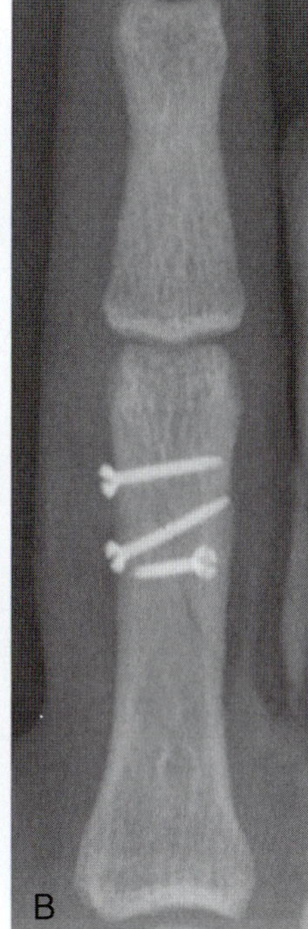

FIGURE 49-8

STEP 5 PEARLS

Rotational alignment of the finger must be regularly checked with each screw inserted.

STEP 5 PITFALLS

The screw length must be perfect. If too long, it may impinge on the flexor tendons. If too short, the fixation will become unstable.

The direction of the screw during insertion must be correctly aligned with the drill hole. Otherwise, the screw will push the distal cortex away and cause a loss of reduction of the fracture (Fig. 49-8A). Figure 49-8B shows screws readjusted with effective interfragmentary compression.

Step 5

- A minimum of two, and, if possible, three, such screws are inserted, each perpendicular to the rotational plane of the fracture (Fig. 49-7).
- The fixation is checked using the mini C-arm to confirm the reduction, positioning, and length of the screws as well as the stability through the full range of motion of the finger.

Step 6

- The periosteum is repaired using absorbable sutures in delayed cases.
- The extensor tendon is repaired using absorbable sutures, usually 4-0 size.
- The skin is repaired using interrupted nonabsorbable sutures, usually 5-0 size.

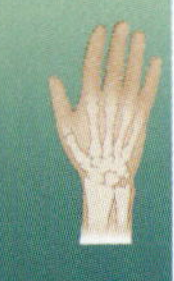

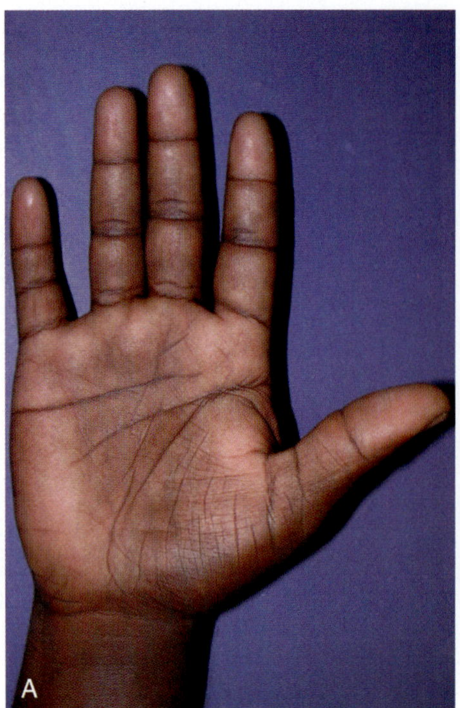

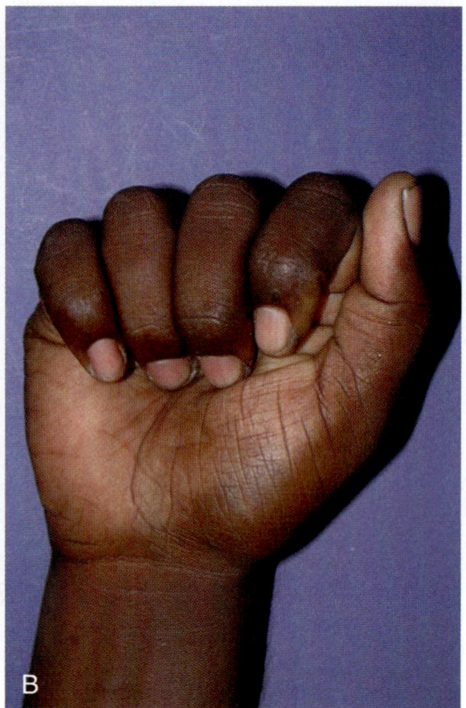

FIGURE 49-9

PEARLS

Early range-of-motion exercise should be started.

Pain control with nerve block may sometimes be required for those who are unable to mobilize the interphalangeal joints because of pain.

Postoperative Care and Expected Outcomes

- Immediate active assisted range-of-motion exercises are started.
- Sutures are removed at 12th to 14th postoperative day.
- Fracture healing is monitored at 2-, 6-, and 12-week intervals with radiographs.
- Progression to passive range-of-motion exercises and strengthening are started as the fracture heals.
- Figure 49-9: Good range of motion of the middle finger is achieved.

Evidence

Black DM, Mann RJ, Constine RM, Daniels AU. The stability of internal fixation in the proximal phalanx. *J Hand Surg [Am]*. 1986;11:672-677.
Five commonly used techniques of internal fixation—dorsal plating, dorsal plating combined with an interfragmentary lag screw, two interfragmentary lag screws, tension-band technique, and crossed Kirschner wires—were tested for rigidity and apex palmar bending. The results showed that both of the techniques that used interfragmentary lag screws across the oblique osteotomies provided significantly more rigidity than did dorsal plating alone or the wired configurations. (Level IV evidence)

Ford DJ, el-Hadidi S, Lunn PG, Burke FD. Fracture of phalanges: results of internal fixation using 1.5 mm and 2 mm A.O. screws. *J Hand Surg [Br]*. 1987;12:28-33.
Thirty-six patients with 38 phalangeal fractures at various levels and with different configurations were treated with open reduction and internal fixation with mini AO screws. Results were satisfactory in 90% of the cases. (Level V evidence)

Kawamura K, Chung KC. Fixation choices for closed simple unstable oblique phalangeal and metacarpal fractures. *Hand Clin*. 2006;22:287-295.
The techniques of percutaneous K-wiring, tension band wiring, lag screw fixation, and plating for fixation of unstable oblique fractures of the proximal phalanx are reviewed. Lag screw fixation is considered the best choice for long oblique phalangeal fractures because this technique provides sufficient rigidity to allow early mobilization. (Level V evidence)

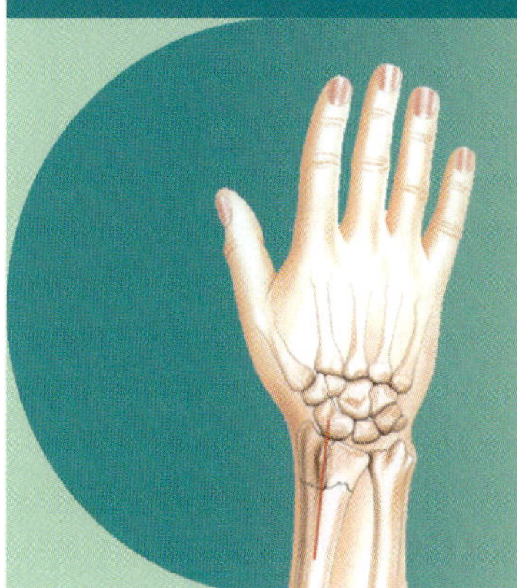

PROCEDURE 50

Open Reduction and Internal Fixation of Phalangeal Shaft Comminuted Fractures

Winston Y. C. Chew and Lam-Chuan Teoh

Indications

- Displaced unstable fracture with angular and/or rotatory deformity is seen, usually with associated shortening.
- Extensive fracture with long segment of shaft involvement occurs, often with intra-articular extension.
- Fracture comminution in the form of multiple butterfly fragments or multiple cortical splits (Fig. 50-1) is suitable for cerclage-wiring–assisted plate fixation technique.
- Comminution with larger butterfly fragments is suitable for interfragmentary screw and plate fixation technique.
- Associated soft tissue injuries need to be addressed at the same time.

Examination/Imaging

Clinical Examination

- Deformity of the finger with angulation, rotation, and shortening
- Grossly unstable and painful with any digital manipulation
- Loss of distal joint active motion
- No neurovascular injuries

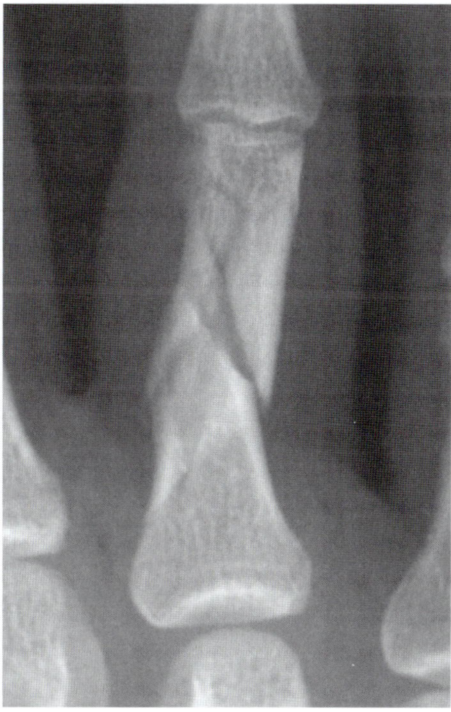

FIGURE 50-1

Imaging

- Obtain standard posteroanterior and lateral radiographs of the finger.
- Intraoperative traction radiographs of the finger will give a better view of the fracture pattern, especially visualization of the overlapping fragments, and help to determine the most suitable method of fixation.

Surgical Anatomy

- The flexor tendons are held by the A2 pulley to the proximal phalanx with very little free space between the tendon and the bone.
- Fracture fragments with extensor tendon or collateral ligament attachments should be reduced and stabilized to preserve optimal joint function.
- Dorsal approach with splitting of the extensor tendon in the midline provides a wide exposure to the dorsal surface of the proximal phalanx, yet leaves sufficient soft tissue attachments on the palmar aspect to maintain blood supply to the bone fragments.

Positioning

- Patient should be positioned supine with a hand extension table.
- The hand should be easily accessible to the mini C-arm for fluoroscopic control during surgery.

PEARLS

The extensor tendon and the periosteum should be incised together down to the bone surface. Do not separate the periosteum from the extensor tendon. The periosteum is thin and friable, and keeping it with the extensor tendon helps to retain its integrity.

The proximal and distal joints usually need to be opened to ensure adequate access to all the fragments and to ensure articular reduction for intra-articular fractures.

Soft tissue attachments to bone fragments should be preserved to ensure the integrity of joint structures and vascularity of the bone fragments.

Soft tissue attachments to the fragments aid in reduction with traction.

Exposures

- For the proximal phalanx, the fracture is exposed through a dorsal longitudinal incision, extending from the metacarpophalangeal (MCP) joint to the proximal interphalangeal (PIP) joint if necessary (Fig. 50-2). The extensor tendon is split in the midline.
- For the middle phalanx, exposure is through a dorsal longitudinal incision extending from the PIP joint to the distal interphalangeal (DIP) joint. The triangular ligament is then divided and the lateral bands of the extensor tendon elevated (Fig. 50-3A and B).
- The periosteum is incised and elevated, sufficient to expose the bone fragments and not to denude the bone fragments totally.
- Collateral ligament, extensor tendon, and tendon sheath attachments should be preserved.

PITFALLS

Forceful elevation of the fragments should be avoided because total detachment may easily occur.

Excessive stripping of the fragments of soft tissue attachments should be avoided to lessen the risk for devascularizing the fragments.

Procedure

- Two techniques are described here. The strategy is to restore the integrity of the cylindrical shape of the shaft to confer stability. The proximal and distal periarticular fragments are then fixed onto this cylindrical construct to obtain overall stability.

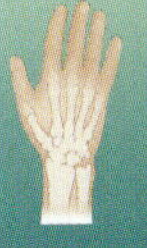

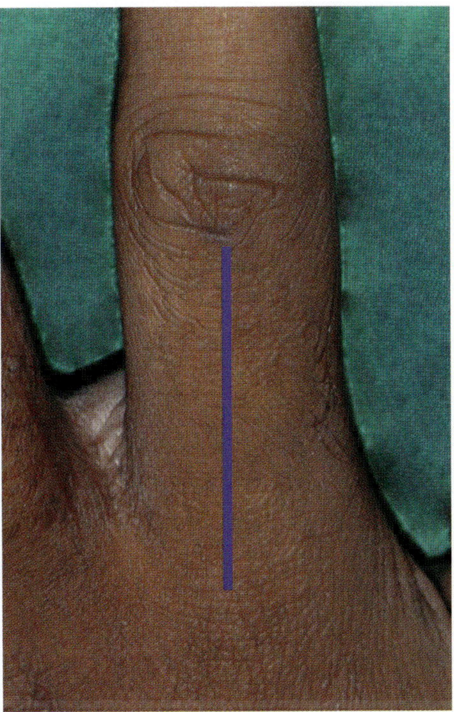

FIGURE 50-2

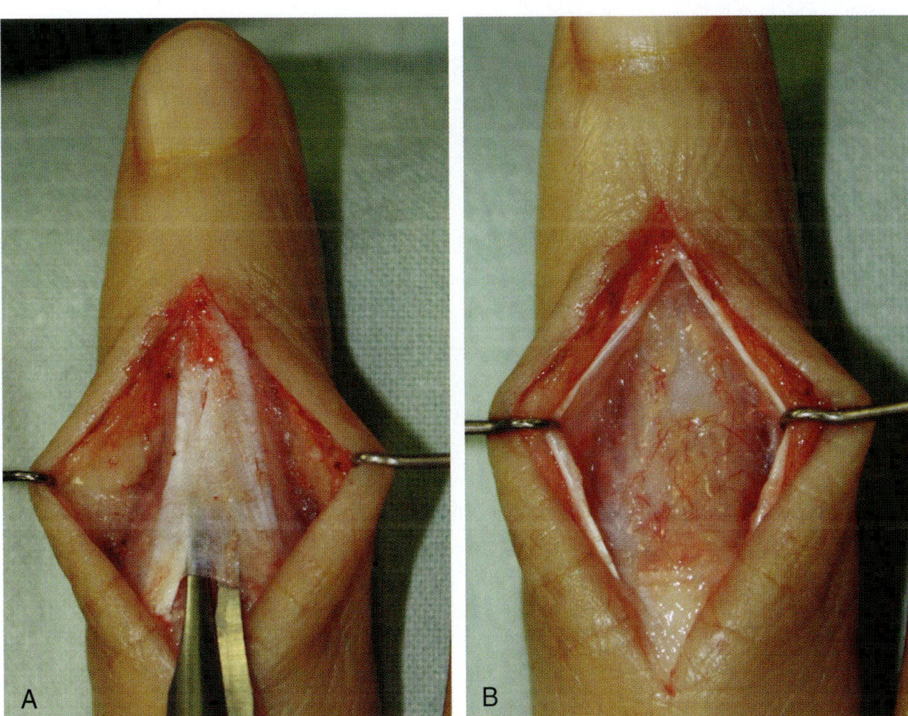

FIGURE 50-3

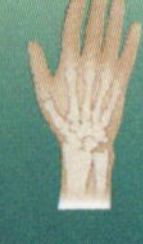

STEP 1 PEARLS

The ideal site of cerclage wire placement is at the midpoint of the fracture fragment. A 1-cm long fragment can accommodate a cerclage wire, and fragments longer than 1 cm may accommodate two.

The C-shaped guide is fashioned using a pair of straight mosquito forceps or small needle holders (with about 4-mm-thick jaws). The 21-gauge needle is gripped firmly, but not so hard as to crush it. Beginning at the tip, the forceps is used to bend the needle by about 30 degrees. The needle is progressively bent from the tip to the hub to create a C-shaped contour. About 5 mm from the hub, the needle is bent 90 degrees in the opposite direction to create a handle that will help in introducing the needle below the phalanx. A 28-gauge wire can easily be inserted into the needle tip for a distance of 1 cm.

STEP 1 PITFALLS

Do not allow the cerclage wire to drop between the fracture fragments because this will fail to secure the fixation.

STEP 2 PEARLS

Rotate the C-shaped guide for the cerclage wire around the palmar surface of the bone. Do not allow any space because this may enter the flexor tendon.

Passively flex the distal joints of the finger and observe the C-shaped guide for the cerclage wire. If the flexor tendon is impaled, the guide will move.

STEP 2 PITFALLS

The flexor tendon can be impaled if the C-shaped guide for the cerclage wire is not kept close to the palmar surface of the bone.

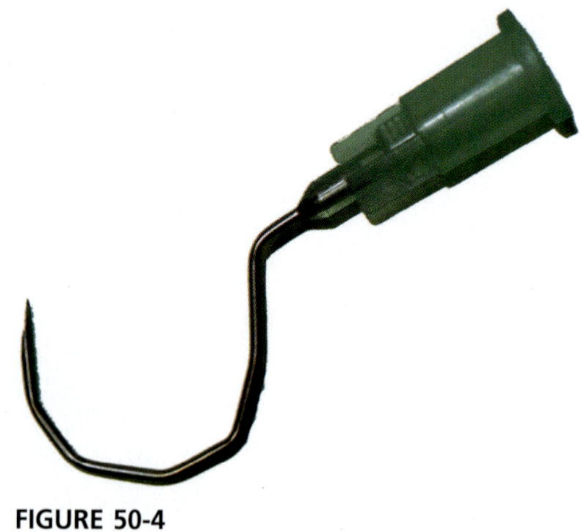

FIGURE 50-4

Cerclage Wiring–Assisted Plate Fixation Technique

Step 1

- The fracture is adequately exposed, and the major fracture fragments are identified.
- The sites for cerclage wire placement are identified.
- A C-shaped guide for the cerclage wire is fashioned from a 21-gauge hypodermic needle (Fig. 50-4).

Step 2

- The C-shaped guide for the cerclage wire is introduced at the predetermined site (Fig. 50-5).
- A 28-gauge stainless-steel wire is threaded through the C-shaped guide. The C-shaped guide is withdrawn, leaving the stainless-steel cerclage wire in position.
- These steps are repeated until all the intended cerclage wires are inserted (Fig. 50-6).

Step 3

- Reduction of the fracture fragments begins by applying longitudinal traction on the finger distally and maintaining the correct rotation position.
- The reduction is further improved by gentle nudging of the fragments with a periosteal elevator. This is further assisted by gentle compression with a hemostat, straight mosquito forceps, and a small pointed reduction clamp.
- The cerclage wires are tightened one at a time from most proximal to distal. The last bit of reduction is achieved by tightening the tension of the cerclage wires. The cerclage wires provide a preliminary stability of the reduction (Fig. 50-7).
- Fluoroscopy images are obtained to ensure the placement of the cerclage wires. These wires should sit close to the palmar surface of the bone. A gap of 5 mm or more indicates that the cerclage wire has passed palmar to the flexor tendon; this should be removed and reinserted correctly.

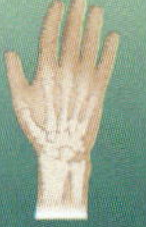

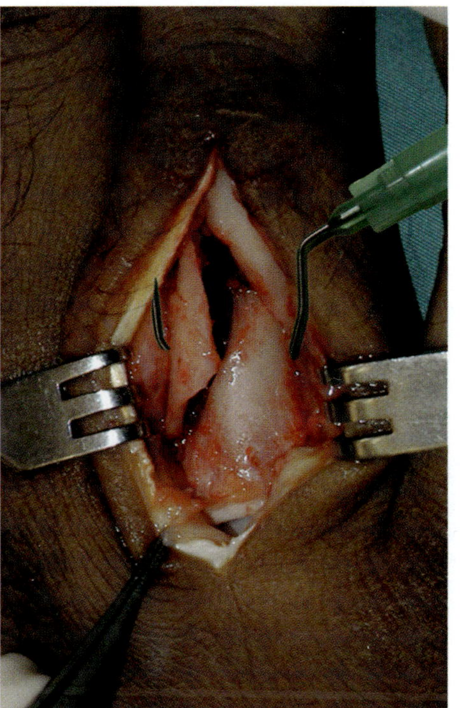

FIGURE 50-5

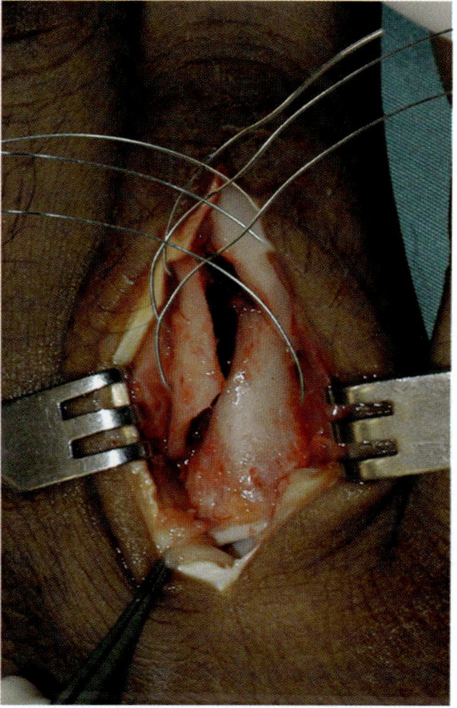

FIGURE 50-6

STEP 3 PEARLS

The tightening tension of the cerclage wires draws the multiple split fragments together and gives a centripetal reduction of the fractures.

STEP 3 PITFALLS

Do not place the knot of the cerclage wire at the midline dorsally. Place the wire knots either medially or laterally for easier placement of the neutralization plate in the next step.

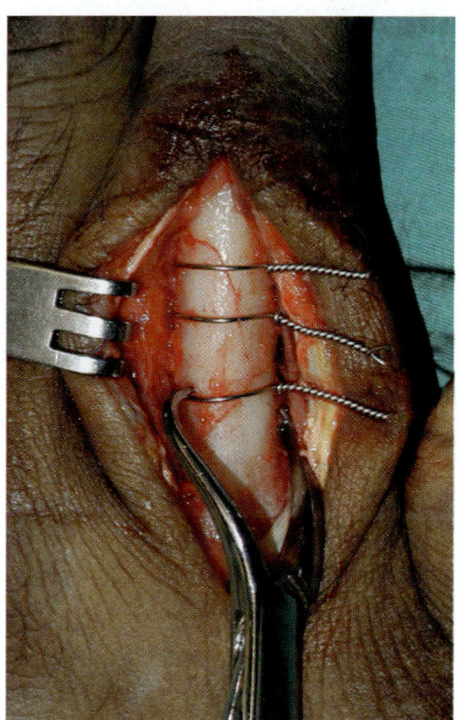

FIGURE 50-7

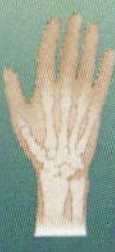

STEP 4 PEARLS

Additional screw fixation in the comminution zone enhances the stability of the fixation construct. The tensioning of the cerclage wires prevents the fragments from separating.

STEP 4 PITFALLS

Measure the screw length accurately. Overpenetration violates the flexor tendon.

Step 4

- Neutralization plating of the fracture with 1.5-mm plate and screws is done (Fig. 50-8).
- The plate should be sufficiently long to bridge the comminution zone and still have two additional holes for fixation at each end of the bone beyond the comminution zone.
- The screw insertion for the plating is on the proximal end first, then the distal end of the bone. Care is taken to ensure that the rotation of the finger is correctly maintained. Additional screw fixation to the comminution zone is possible at the holes where there is no cerclage wire interposing or the presence of fracture line.

Step 5

- After the fixation is completed, fluoroscopy is repeated to confirm the final reduction and to ensure the correct screw placement and length (Fig. 50-9).
- The periosteum is closed with absorbable suture if it is still available. The extensor tendon is also closed with absorbable suture. The skin is closed with interrupted nonabsorbable suture.

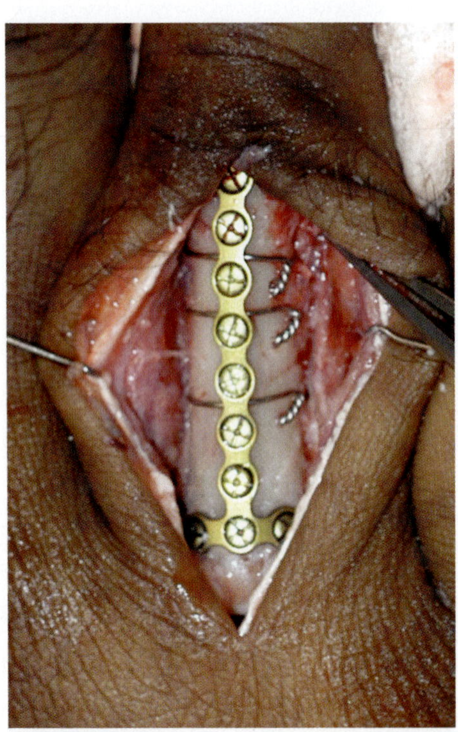

FIGURE 50-8

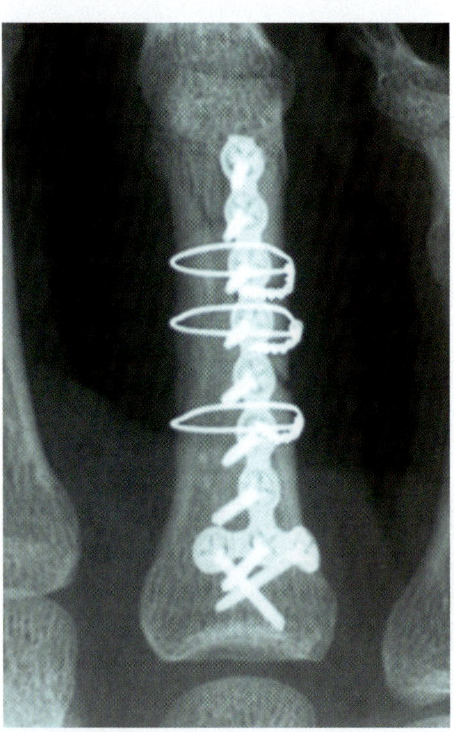

FIGURE 50-9

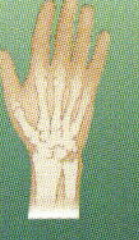

Interfragmentary Screws and Neutralization Plate Fixation Technique

Step 1

- Starting from proximal to distal, the largest fragments are held together with straight mosquito forceps.
- Often, some of these fragments include the proximal or distal articular fragments, and simultaneous articular reduction must be achieved.

Step 2

- The fracture fragments are held in reduction with a compressive force before drilling and screw fixation (precompression) (Fig. 50-10).
- The drill hole is made for the screws, using appropriately sized drill bits without overdrilling the proximal cortex, as is done in conventional interfragmentary screw insertion.
- The drill hole is countersunk.
- Small bicortical screws are inserted using screws ranging from 1 to 1.5 mm, depending on the fragment sizes.

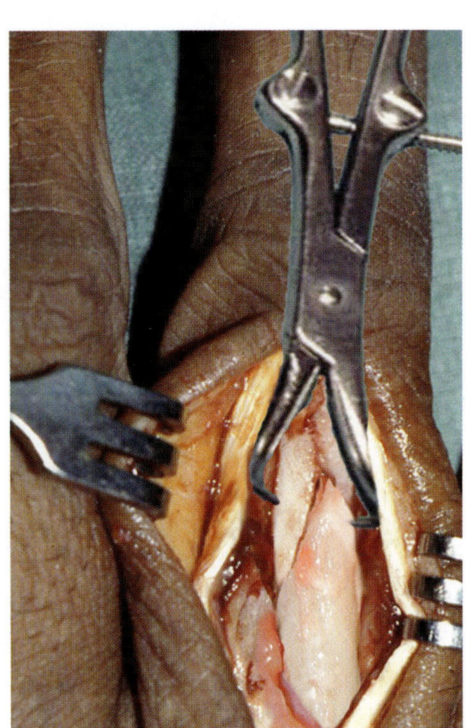

FIGURE 50-10

STEP 1 PEARLS

Traction during surgery aids in reduction of the fragments and uses soft tissue to splint the fragments for fixation.

Straight mosquito forceps with a fine tip are useful for reducing and holding bone fragments while the interfragmentary screws are being inserted, especially for smaller fragments, for which the use of the pointed reduction forceps is not suitable.

Small K-wires may be used to hold some fragments together while other fragments are being reduced.

STEP 1 PITFALLS

Use of the pointed bone reduction forceps is difficult because the fragments are often not in the optimal position or of the appropriate size.

Care must be taken when using the reduction forceps because it may cause further fragmentation of the bone, especially at the apices of the fragments.

STEP 2 PEARLS

Precompression of the fragments with bicortical screw fixation instead of the classic interfragmentary screw fixation technique with overdrilling of the proximal screw hole allows easier screw insertion.

The fragment should be at least the size of three screw diameters.

Countersink the near hole to accommodate the screw head whenever possible.

Ensure that the interfragmentary screws do not catch the collateral ligaments and result in restriction of motion of the involved joint. If passing at the level of the collateral ligaments, longitudinal split of the collateral ligament can be made, and the screw head should be sunk below the ligament to the level of the bone.

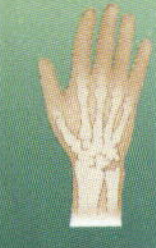

Step 3

- The next closest fragment is then reduced and held in reduction with straight mosquito forceps and fixed with the appropriately sized interfragmentary screw, using the same technique as in step 2.
- Progressively, each subsequent fragment is built onto the first two fragments until the cylindrical shape of the phalangeal shaft is restored and overall alignment is achieved (Fig. 50-11).

Step 4

- The proximal and distal articular fragments are next reduced to the shaft if they have not been previously fixed to the shaft as part of the shaft fragments.
- Intra-articularly placed countersunk screws may be used if necessary for better fixation.

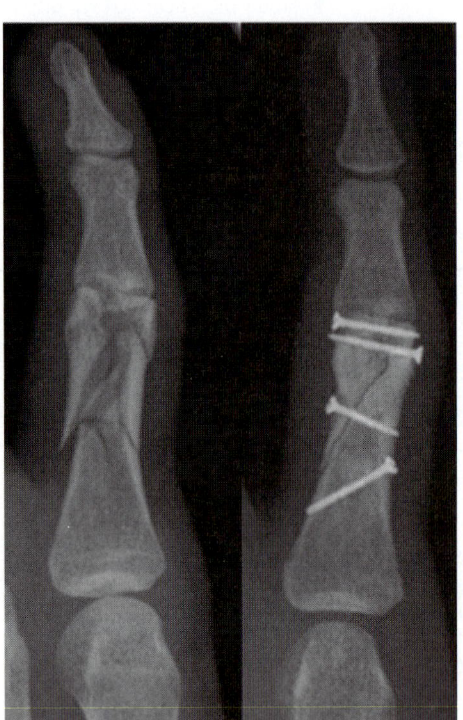

FIGURE 50-11

STEP 2 PITFALLS

Avoid overcompression because this may displace the fracture or even cause fragmentation of the fracture fragments.

The screw length must be exact: if the screw is too short, it does not hold the fragments well; if the screw is too long, there is a risk for impingement of the flexor tendons leading to rupture or stiffness of the finger.

Ensure that the direction of the screw is correct; otherwise, the screw will push away the far cortex instead of holding it in compression, resulting in a loss of reduction.

Avoid overtightening of the screws because this may risk fracture of the fracture fragments.

STEP 3 PEARLS

Constant checking of screw placement and alignment with the mini C-arm should be done to ensure correct position and length.

Some smaller fragments can be left alone so long as the overall integrity of the shaft is restored.

Multiple small screws are preferred over a few large screws.

STEP 4 PEARLS

Intra-articularly placed screws are useful for holding smaller intra-articular fragments without a significant metaphyseal component. Countersunk to just below the level of the subchondral bone, the screw heads do not interfere with joint function.

STEP 5 PEARLS

At least two holes per proximal and distal fragment are necessary for the construct to be stable.

Locking mini-fragment systems with 1.5-mm plates are useful for the phalangeal fractures and, especially in such comminuted cases, increase the stability of the fixation.

STEP 5 PITFALLS

Screws with the wrong lengths may not be accessible once the neutralization plate is fixed and hence should be checked and corrected before the plate is applied.

Some implant systems do not have the appropriate-length plate. This should be verified and the appropriate implants made available before surgery.

STEP 6 PEARLS

For delayed fractures, the periosteum is thickened and can be separated easily from the extensor tendon and repaired as a layer using absorbable sutures.

Step 5

- A neutralization plate is applied dorsally to span the proximal-to-distal condylar region (Fig. 50-12).
- A T- or extended H-plate may be used as deemed suitable (Fig. 50-13).

Step 6

- The extensor tendon is repaired with either absorbable or nonabsorbable sutures.
- The skin is closed with interrupted sutures.

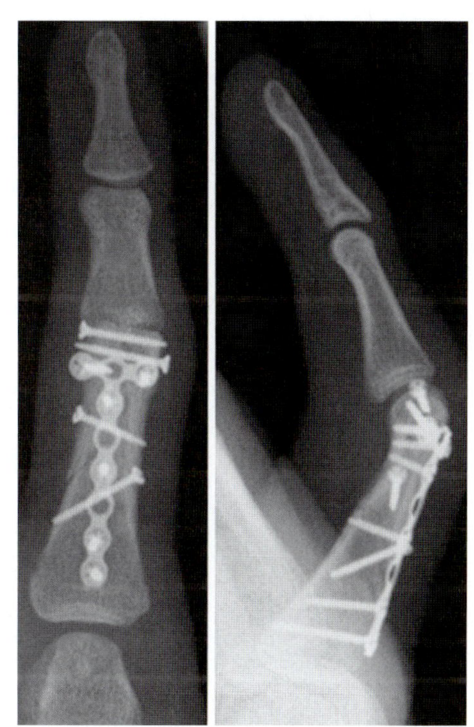

FIGURE 50-12

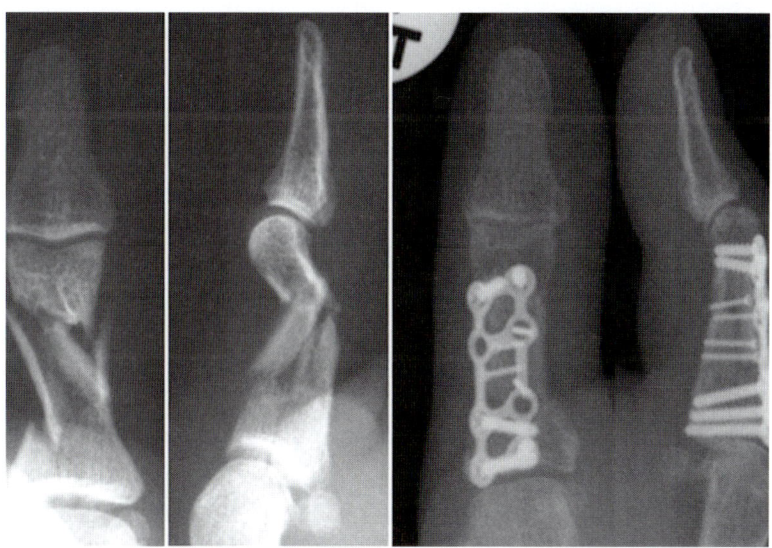

FIGURE 50-13

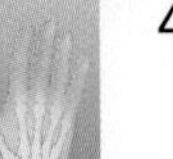

Postoperative Care and Expected Outcomes

- The dressing is lightened the next day, and active range of motion within the limits of pain is initiated.
- The operated finger is splinted in the safe position with the PIP and DIP joints in full extension for 4 to 6 weeks.
- Interval "out-of-splint" active range of motion for 10 to 15 minutes four to five times a day continues. The active range of motion is assisted with passive ranging as tolerated.
- Sutures are removed at 12 to 14 days.
- Strengthening starts after 4 to 6 weeks with radiologic evidence of bone healing.

Evidence

Lu WW, Furumachi K, Ip WY, Chow SP. Fixation for comminuted phalangeal fractures: a biomechanical study of five methods. *J Hand Surg [Br]*. 1996;6;765-767.
The rigidities of five fixation methods in a comminuted phalangeal fracture model were studied: four K-wires, lateral plating with six screws, lateral plating for the triangular butterfly fragment defect with four screws, fixation of butterfly fragment with two screws, and fixation with two crossed intramedullary K-wires. Mechanical testing of compressing, bending, and torsion was performed for each fixation. Lateral plating with six screws provided the most rigid fixation, followed by the four–K-wire technique. (Level IV evidence)

Mitra A, Elahi MM, Spears J, Mitra A. Cerclage clamp: a useful tool in open reduction and internal fixation of complicated metacarpal and phalangeal shaft fractures. *Plast Reconstr Surg*. 2004;114:169-173.
The authors describe the use of a newly designed bone reduction clamp with a channel to facilitate the passing of cerclage wires around the bone for long oblique and spiral fractures of the metacarpal and phalangeal shaft, supplemented with interfragmentary screws. They have used this instrument successfully in 14 cases, although the results were not reported. (Level V evidence)

Teoh LC, Tan PL, Tan SH, Cheong EC. Cerclage-wiring-assisted fixation of difficult hand fractures. *J Hand Surg [Br]*. 2006;31:637-642.
The paper described a technique for difficult hand fractures with multiple butterfly fragments, multiple cortical splits, or intra-articular extension. In 17 difficult hand fractures in 16 patients with an average follow-up of 44.5 months, the average total active range of motion was 247 degrees (range, 220 to 260 degrees). (Level V evidence)

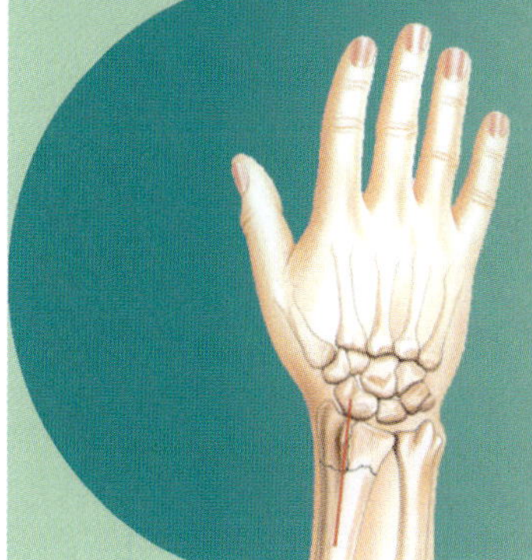

PROCEDURE 51

Volar Plate Arthroplasty for Dorsal Fracture-Dislocations of the Proximal Interphalangeal Joint

Christopher J. Utz and Jeffrey N. Lawton

Indications

- Inability to achieve and maintain a perfect/concentric reduction of an acute/subacute fracture-dislocation of the proximal interphalangeal (PIP) joint is seen.
- Inability to maintain reduction is often due to fracture of a significant volar articular portion of the middle phalanx with comminution that prevents open reduction and internal fixation (ORIF).
- Deitch and colleagues (1999) have shown that dislocations in the absence of fracture, or when less than 30% of the volar articular surface of the middle phalanx is fractured, usually allow a stable concentric reduction of the joint. When 30% to 50% of the volar articular surface of the middle phalanx is involved, a stable concentric reduction is less likely, and when more than 50% of the articular surface is fractured, a stable concentric reduction is unlikely to be achieved with closed means alone.

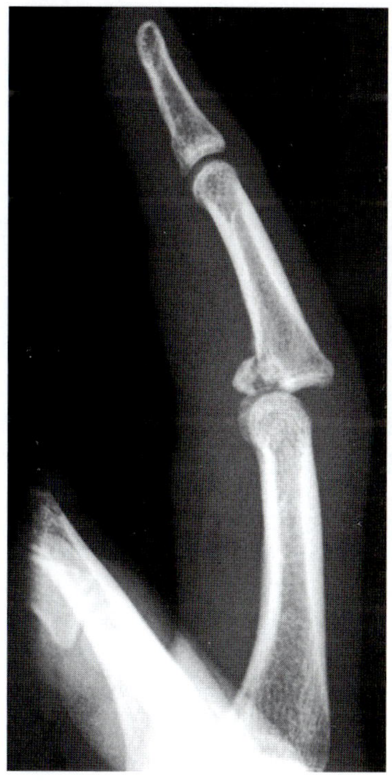

FIGURE 51-1

Examination/Imaging

Clinical Examination

- Acutely, the patient will present with pain to the PIP joint of the affected digit and a clinically obvious deformity and swelling in the digit.
- Alternatively, the patient may present after initial reduction of the dislocation, and the clinical findings may be relatively benign with some mild swelling and pain in the affected PIP joint. If this is the case, it is critical to scrutinize a true lateral radiograph to rule out persistent subluxation because the patient may no longer have clinically evident malalignment. Failure to correct persistent subluxation will result in a poor outcome.

Imaging

- Films of the digit, including a true lateral radiograph of the affected digit centered on the PIP joint, are required. Persistent subluxation can be recognized when the articular surface of the middle phalanx projects dorsal to a line drawn along the dorsal cortex of the proximal phalanx. Additionally, the joint space should be symmetrical both volarly and dorsally (Fig. 51-1).

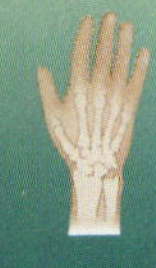

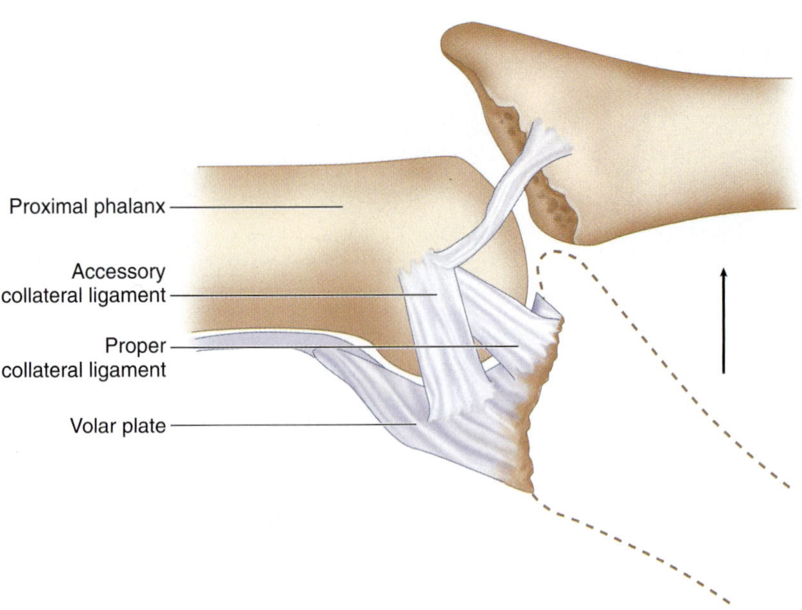

FIGURE 51-2

Surgical Anatomy

- The PIP is a hinge joint with a 100- to 110-degree arc of motion. Its stability is derived from both the bony architecture of the joint and the surrounding ligamentous structures.
- The collateral ligaments are the primary restraints to radial or ulnar joint deviation. They are 2 to 3 mm thick and originate on the lateral aspect of each condyle of the proximal phalanx, passing obliquely and volarly to insert on the volar third of the base of the middle phalanx and the volar plate.
- The volar plate forms the floor of the joint and resists hyperextension of the PIP joint. It originates from the periosteum of the proximal phalanx and the lateral thick, cordlike checkrein ligaments. It inserts across the volar base of the middle phalanx and is confluent with the collateral ligament insertions laterally.
- Because the collateral ligament–volar plate complex inserts on the volar third of the middle phalanx, fractures that involve more than 30% to 40% of the volar articular segment are inherently unstable after reduction. This happens because these ligamentous restraints are attached to the fracture fragment and not to the remaining middle phalanx, which then tends to sublux dorsally. Additionally, a fracture fragment of this size also compromises the inherent bony stability by detaching the volar buttress of the articular surface that cups the proximal phalangeal condyles (Fig. 51-2).

Positioning

- The procedure is performed under tourniquet control on a standard hand table. A lead hand retractor is often useful to maintain retraction of the nonoperative digits.

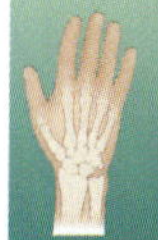

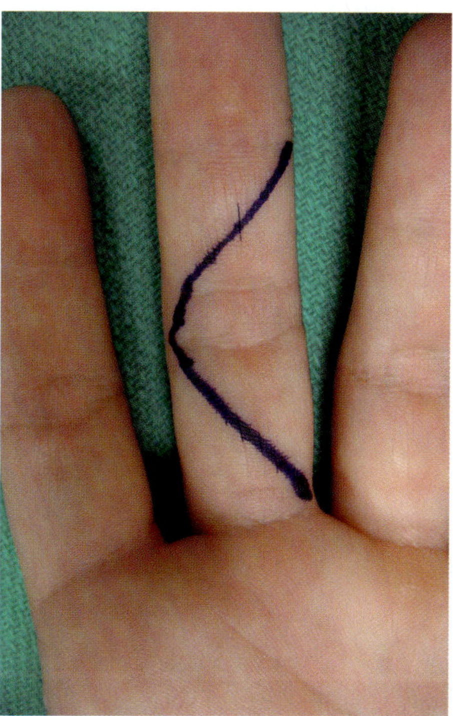

FIGURE 51-3

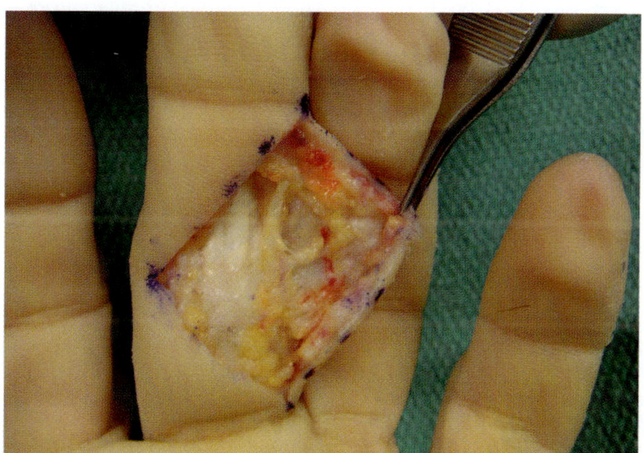

FIGURE 51-4

Exposures

- A standard Bruner incision centered at the PIP flexion crease is used to expose the joint (Fig. 51-3).
- Dissection is carried down bluntly, and the radial and ulnar neurovascular bundles are identified and mobilized (Fig. 51-4).
- The flexor sheath is incised between the A2 and A4 pulleys as a rectangular flap to enable later repair.
- The flexor tendons can then be bluntly retracted radially and ulnarly to expose the volar plate.

PEARLS

Identification and mobilization of the neurovascular bundles is essential to prevent potential traction injuries when hyperextending the PIP joint.

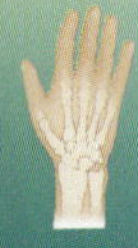

Procedure

Step 1: Incision of the Volar Plate and Joint Exposure

- Incise the volar plate along its lateral margins, freeing it from the accessory collateral ligaments.
- Next, incise and subperiosteally elevate the volar plate at its distalmost aspect on the base of the middle phalanx. This should create a long, broad flap of volar plate (Fig. 51-5).
- The collateral ligaments are then dissected and excised.

STEP 1 PEARLS

Care must be taken in creating the volar plate flap because this determines the stability of the arthroplasty. The flap should be made as broad as possible because a narrow flap will decrease stability.

The flap must also be symmetrical radially and ulnarly because an asymmetrical flap can lead to angular and rotational deformities.

Step 2: Preparation of the Joint and the Volar Plate

- The joint is then hyperextended nearly 180 degrees ("shotgunning") to maximize articular visualization.
- The distal end of the volar plate is sharply detached from any fracture fragments.
- The joint is then inspected with débridement of small fracture fragments and depressed articular cartilage.
- A shallow transverse trough is then created across the base of the middle phalanx at the juncture of the intact articular cartilage and the fracture defect (Fig. 51-6).
- The depth of the trough is such that the thickness of the volar plate may seat within it to allow a smooth transition from the volar aspect of the middle phalangeal articular cartilage onto the repositioned volar plate.
- Sutures are then placed in both the radial and ulnar sides of the volar plate. A 2-0 nonabsorbable suture is used with Bunnell-type pattern.

STEP 2 PEARLS

Similar to creation of the volar plate flap, the trough must be symmetrical in the coronal plane to improve stability and prevent angular deformities.

The depth of the trough at the most dorsal aspect should equal the thickness of the volar plate to provide a smooth transition from articular cartilage to transposed volar plate.

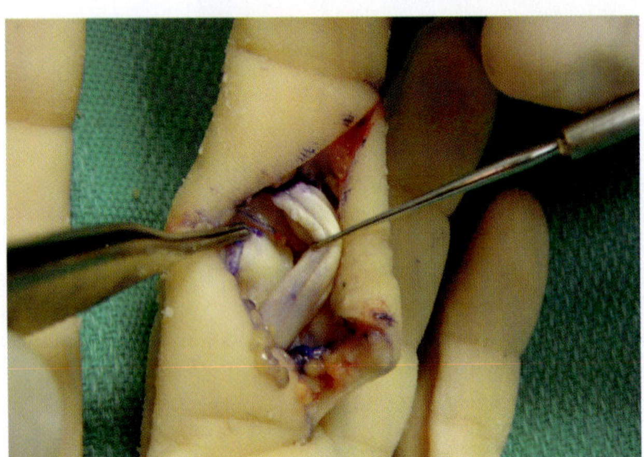

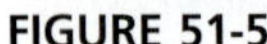

FIGURE 51-5

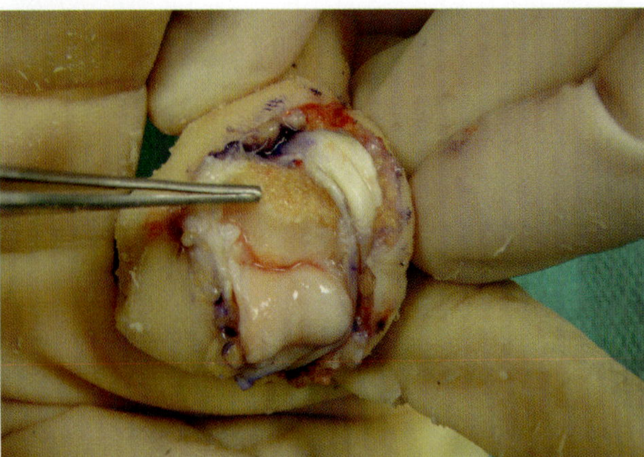

FIGURE 51-6

STEP 3 PEARLS

A concentric reduction of the PIP joint must be achieved and should be critically evaluated both visually and radiographically with a true lateral view on a mini C-arm. If this is achieved, the middle phalanx will glide over the proximal phalanx and not hinge open through the arc or motion.

If additional lateral stability is required, the sides of the volar plate can be sutured to the remnants of the collateral ligaments with a 4-0 braided nonabsorbable suture.

If the PIP joint lacks extension, the volar plate may need to be further mobilized. This can be done by lengthening the checkrein ligaments through step-cutting.

The incidence of postoperative distal interphalangeal (DIP) joint contractures can be decreased by flexing the DIP joint while passing the Keith wires to avoid tethering the lateral bands.

Step 3: Reduction and Fixation

- The free ends of the volar plate sutures are passed through the base of the middle phalanx, using two Keith needles chucked into a wire driver. Volarly, the needles are placed radially and ulnarly in the prepared trough on the middle phalanx, separated by the width of the volar plate. They should also be placed so as to bring the volar plate into the trough—creating a smooth transition from the articular surface to the transposed volar plate. The needles are driven through the middle phalanx to converge centrally on the dorsum of the phalanx distal to the central slip insertion. An incision is made dorsally before pulling the sutures through (Fig. 51-7).
- Tension is then placed on the sutures to bring the volar plate into the prepared trough so as to check joint reduction and range of motion.
- Once a congruous reduction is confirmed with an acceptable range of motion, the sutures are tightened and tied over the periosteum dorsally, ensuring that they do not entrap the lateral bands or central slip insertion.
- Bone graft (harvested from the fracture fragments) can then be placed in the defect of the middle phalanx distal to the insertion of the advanced volar plate to provide support if a large defect exists, thus restoring the bony buttress (Fig. 51-8).

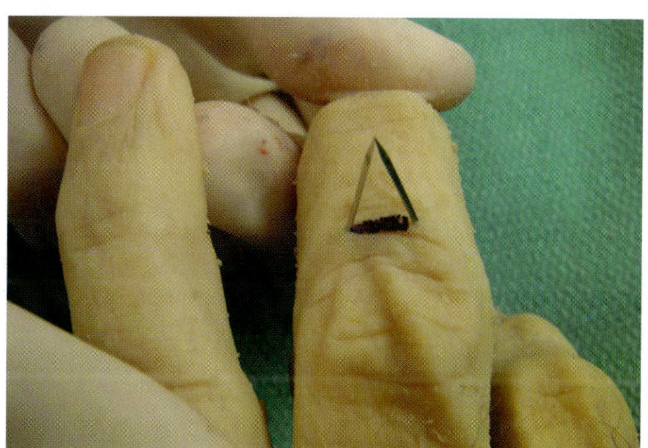

FIGURE 51-7

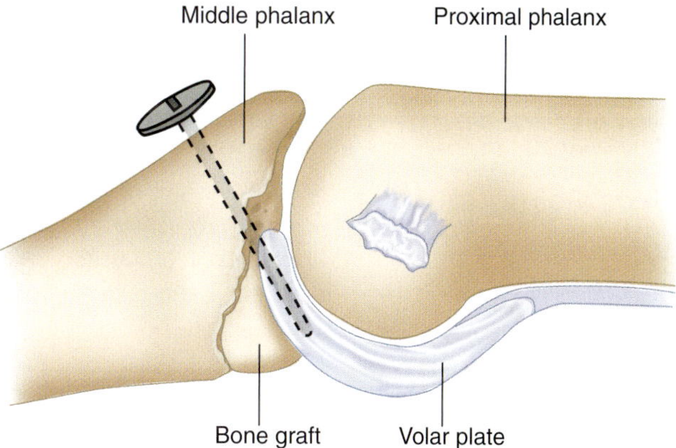

FIGURE 51-8

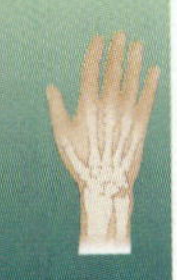

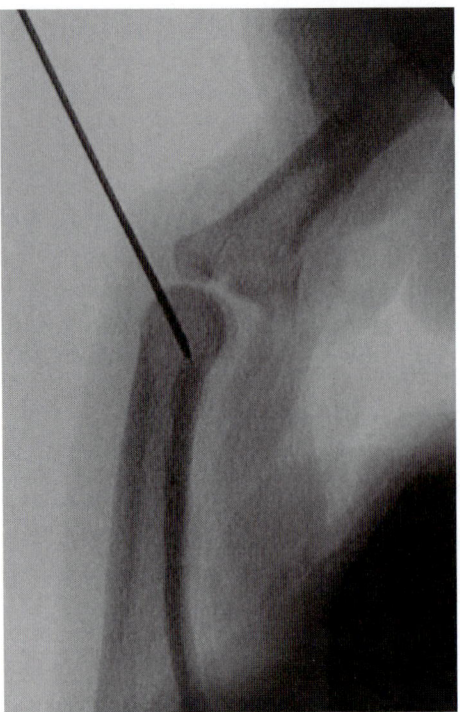

FIGURE 51-9

STEP 4 PEARLS

Use of extension block pinning or an external fixator may be required if the PIP joint lacks stability (most commonly in terminal extension).

Step 4: Extension Block Pinning (Optional)

- The tourniquet is deflated and the incisions closed according to the surgeon's preference after hemostasis has been achieved.
- A 0.035-inch K-wire is then driven into the dorsal aspect of the proximal phalanx in such a way as to prevent hyperextension of the joint (Fig. 51-9). Alternatively, an articulated PIP external fixator may be used, or a K-wire can be placed across the joint in slight flexion to maintain reduction for 3 weeks.
- A soft dressing can be applied to the hand and finger.

PEARLS

Encourage motion of the DIP joint in addition to the PIP because flexion-contractures of this joint have been reported. Patients should also be counseled preoperatively to expect some mild deficits (10 to 20 degrees).

Range of motion can continue to improve up to 1 year postoperatively.

Postoperative Care and Expected Outcomes

- The postoperative dressing is removed within 5 to 7 days, and passive flexion is immediately begun. Active flexion is encouraged over the successive 3 weeks.
- The extension block K-wire is most often removed at 3 weeks. If full extension is not achieved by 6 weeks, a dynamic extension splint may be used.
- Alternatively, if the PIP joint is pinned, the wire is removed at 3 weeks, and active flexion and extension are begun. Often, an extension block splint is used between 3 and 6 weeks to prevent hyperextension.

Evidence

Deitch MA, Keifhaber TR, Comisar BR, Stern PJ. Dorsal fracture dislocations of the proximal interphalangeal joint: Surgical complications and long-term results. *J Hand Surg [Am]*. 1999;24:914-923.
The authors retrospectively analyzed the results of open reduction and internal fixation and volar plate arthroplasty for fracture-dislocations of the proximal interphalangeal joint. They found no differences between the two procedures. Both procedures had good results with no patient-reported pain and minimal functional limitation despite radiographic evidence of degenerative changes. (Level III evidence)

Dionysian E, Eaton RG. The long-term outcome of volar plate arthroplasty of the proximal interphalangeal joint. *J Hand Surg [Am]*. 2000;25:429-437.
The authors examined 17 patients who underwent volar plate arthroplasty for a fracture-dislocation of the proximal interphalangeal joint an average of 11 years postoperatively. All patients reported a pain-free joint with activity and at rest and were able to return to their previous occupation and recreational activities. A statistical difference in total active range of motion was noticed between patients who had surgery within 4 weeks of injury (85 degrees) and those who had it later than 4 weeks after injury (61 degrees). (Level IV evidence)

Durham-Smith G, McCarten GM. Volar plate arthroplasty for closed proximal interphalangeal joint injuries. *J Hand Surg [Br]*. 1992;17:422-428.
The authors review the anatomy and mechanism of proximal interphalangeal joint fracture-dislocations as well as the technique for volar plate arthroplasty. They also reviewed the results of 71 cases of volar plate arthroplasty with follow-up ranging from 6 to 48 months. They report an overall patient satisfaction rate of 94% with an average range of motion of 90 degrees. (Level IV evidence)

Malerich NM, Eaton RG. The volar plate reconstruction for fracture-dislocation of the proximal interphalangeal joint. *Hand Clin*. 1994;10:251-260.
The authors present the original technique for volar plate arthroplasty and review their indications and complications. (Level IV evidence)

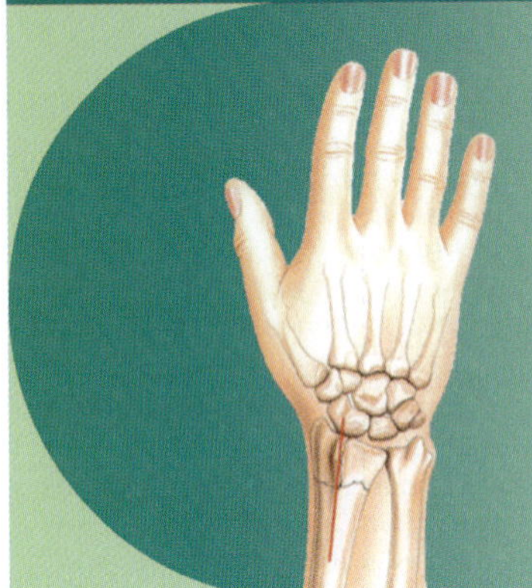

PROCEDURE 52

Hemi-Hamate Arthroplasty

Joyce M. Wilson and Peter J. Stern

Indications

- Unstable PIP joint fracture dislocations in which more than 50% of the palmar base of the middle phalanx is fractured. There must be dorsal cortical continuity.
- Comminuted lateral plateau fractures of the base of the middle phalanx.
- Joint salvage after failed treatment of complex fracture-dislocations of the PIP joint.

Examination/Imaging

Clinical Examination

- Record active range of motion of the affected finger as tolerated.
- Evaluate coronal plane alignment, assessing for lateral deviation that suggests asymmetrical compression of the articular surface.
- Examine the sagittal alignment with the finger extended, looking for colinearity of the proximal phalanx and middle phalanx.

Imaging

- Standard anteroposterior, oblique, and lateral views of the involved digit to assess the amount of articular involvement of the base of the middle phalanx, the integrity of the middle phalangeal dorsal cortex, and other fractures (Fig. 52-1).
- Computed tomography can better delineate the extent of articular cartilage involvement and comminution, but it is rarely necessary.

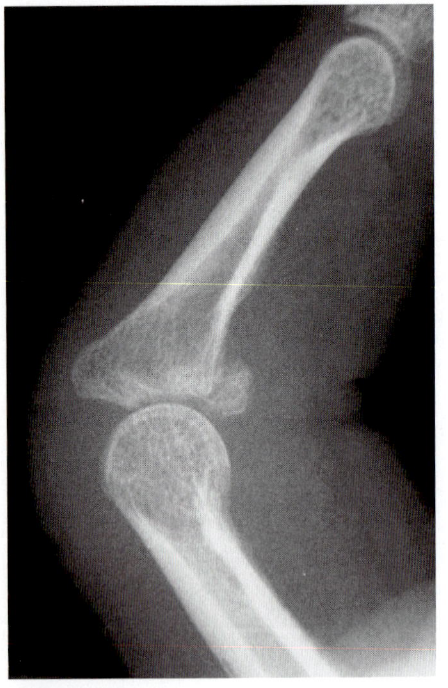

FIGURE 52-1

Surgical Anatomy

- The PIP joint is a complex hinge joint formed by the head of the proximal phalanx and the base of the middle phalanx that moves through a 110-degree arc of motion.
- The volar plate originates from the proximal phalanx periosteum and inserts onto the volar lip of the middle phalanx.
- Lateral joint stability is afforded by the thick collateral ligaments. The proper collateral ligament inserts onto the volar-lateral third of the middle phalanx, and the accessory collateral ligament inserts onto the volar plate.

Figures 52-1, 52-5, 52-7, and 52-8 through 52-11 borrowed with permission from Williams RMM, Kiefhaber TR, Sommerkamp TG, et al. Proximal interphalangeal fracture/dislocations using a hemi-hamate autograft. J Hand Surg [Am]. *2003;28:856-865.*

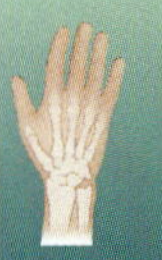

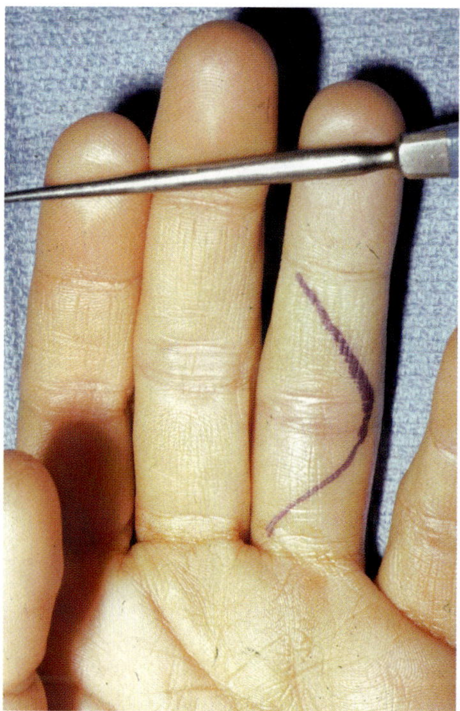

FIGURE 52-2

- Dorsal translation of the middle phalanx is prevented by the volar plate and the cup-shaped articular surface of the middle phalanx, which congruously articulates with the proximal phalanx head.
- Dorsal fracture-dislocations disrupt both of these restraints and result in dorsal subluxation of the middle phalanx.
- The stability of the PIP joint is directly related to the amount of middle phalangeal volar articular surface disrupted. Fractures with as little as 30% of the articular surface involved may be unstable.

Positioning

- The patient is positioned supine on the operating table, with the involved extremity supported by a hand table.
- Intraoperative fluoroscopy is used to confirm a congruous reduction.

Exposures

- Exposure of the PIP joint is gained through a palmar V-shaped incision centered over the PIP joint (Fig. 52-2).
- The skin and subcutaneous tissue are sharply elevated, and both neurovascular bundles are visualized deep to the lateral digital sheet and protected.
- A rectangular flap of the fibro-osseous sheath that includes the entire A3 pulley is developed between the A2 and A4 pulleys.

PEARLS

The V-shaped incision extends from the palmodigital crease to the DIP joint flexion crease, with the apex based either radially or ulnarly centered at the PIP joint.

The neurovascular bundles must be visualized, but it is not necessary to mobilize them; they remain protected deep to the lateral digital sheet.

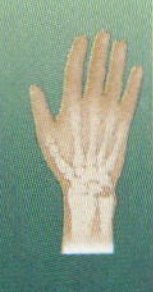

PITFALLS

The collateral ligaments must be released cautiously to avoid injuring the adjacent neurovascular bundles.

- The flexor tendons are retracted to expose the volar plate, which is released from the accessory collateral ligaments at its lateral margins (Fig. 52-3).
- The volar plate is incised transversely from the base of the middle phalanx and reflected proximally (Fig. 52-4).
- Release the collateral ligaments from the head of the proximal phalanx, leaving a small stump attached to the middle phalanx to facilitate volar plate reattachment at the end of the procedure.

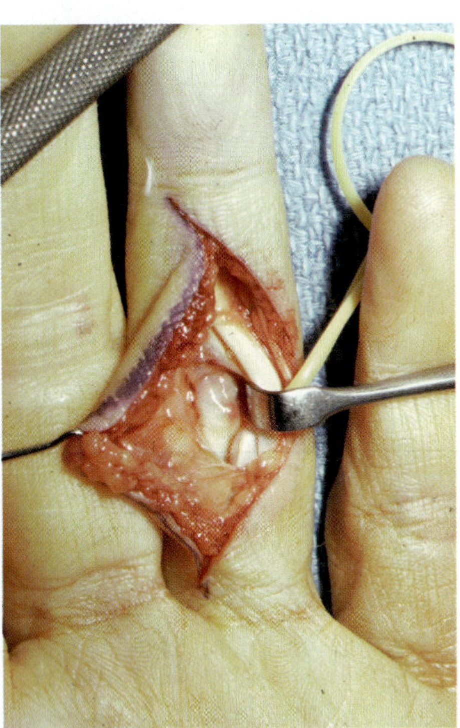

FIGURE 52-3

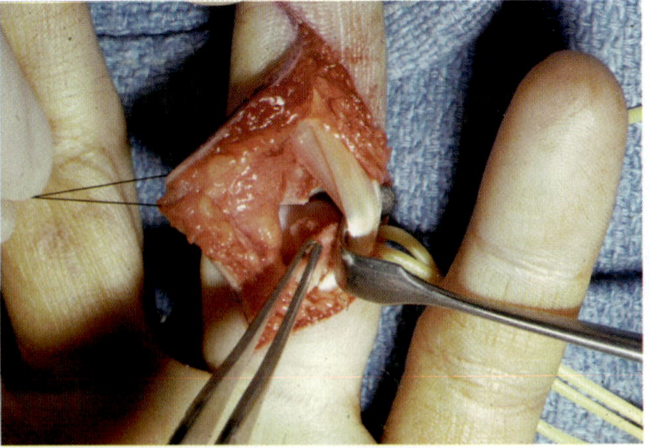

FIGURE 52-4

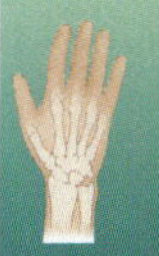

STEP 1 PEARLS

Remove only the minimal amount of the middle phalanx necessary for reconstruction to prevent fracture of the dorsal cortex.

If the height of the defect cannot be measured, it may be estimated by measuring the amount needed to cover the head of the proximal phalanx.

STEP 1 PITFALLS

The dorsal cortex of the middle phalanx can easily be fractured with overly aggressive use of the oscillating saw.

Procedure

Step 1: Preparing the Articular Surface of the Middle Phalanx

- By means of a Penrose drain or moist umbilical tape, the flexor tendons are retracted radially or ulnarly. The PIP joint is hyperextended ("shotgunning") to expose the fracture site. Loose fragments are débrided (Fig. 52-5).
- After the fracture fragments from the articular surface of the middle phalanx are débrided, a 4-mm oscillating saw is used to create a boxlike recipient defect.
- Measure the bony defect, including the width of the articular surface, the dorsal-palmar height, and the proximal-distal length (Fig. 52-6).

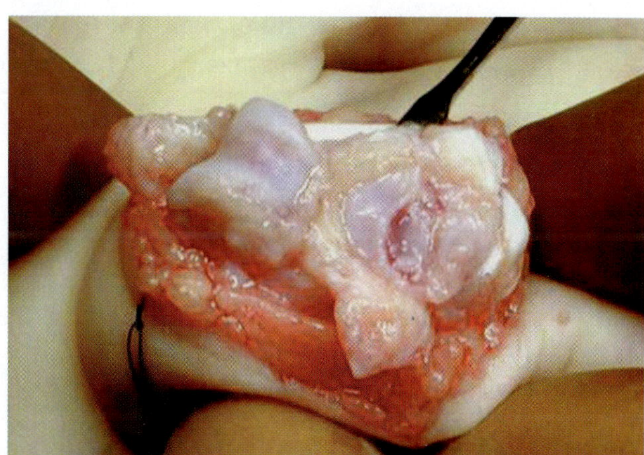

FIGURE 52-5

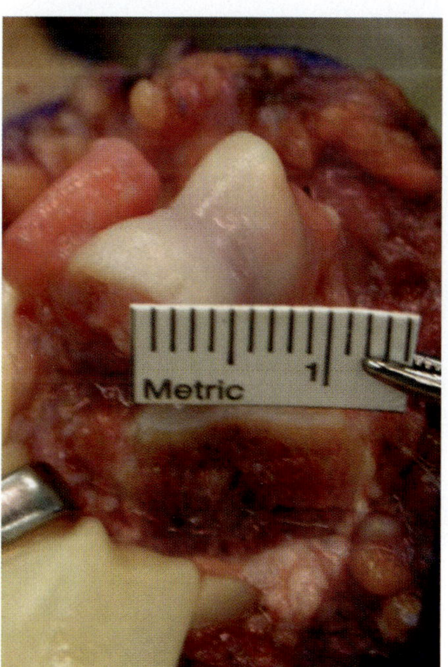

FIGURE 52-6

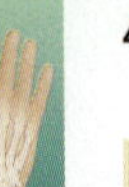

Step 2: Harvesting the Hamate Osteochondral Graft

- Use fluoroscopy to locate the carpometacarpal (CMC) joint at the base of the ring and small finger. Then make a transverse 3-cm incision just proximal to the joint.
- Bluntly mobilize the subcutaneous veins and nerves and retract the extensor tendons.
- Make a longitudinal capsulotomy to expose the ring and small CMC joint (Fig. 52-7).
- Use a fine-tipped marker to outline the donor graft dimension, using the distal articular surface as a reference point.
- Make the axial osteotomy (line A) and the sagittal osteotomies (lines B and C), using an osteotome or an oscillating saw just outside the marked line to ensure that the graft is large enough (Fig. 52-8).
- Make the coronal osteotomy using a curved osteotome, taking care to avoid damage to the articular surface of the ring and small fingers.

STEP 2 PEARLS

Protect the articular surface of the fourth and fifth metacarpals with a Freer elevator when making the osteotomy.

Err on the side of taking an osteochondral graft 1 to 2 mm larger than measured.

The coronal plane osteotomy using the curved osteotome can be facilitated by making an osseous trough in the hamate just proximal to the osteotomy site.

STEP 2 PITFALLS

Failure to leave at least 2 mm of the radial edge of the fourth metacarpal—hamate articulation and 2 mm of the ulnar edge of the fifth metacarpal—hamate joint may lead to CMC joint instability.

Avoid making the coronal osteotomy too obliquely because this might prevent adequate restoration of joint geometry and potentially lead to instability.

The coronal plane osteotomy must be done carefully to avoid fracture of the osteochondral autograft.

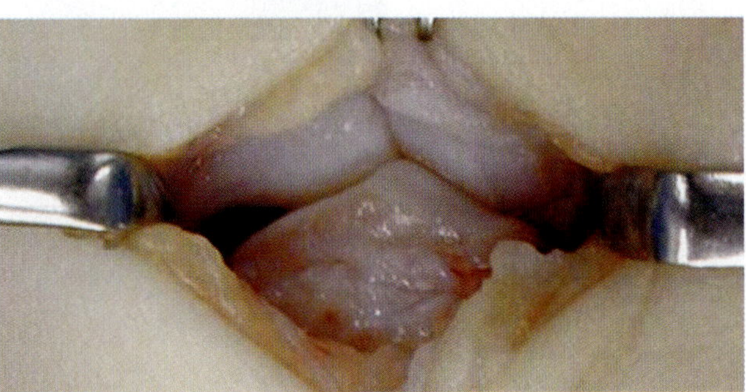

FIGURE 52-7

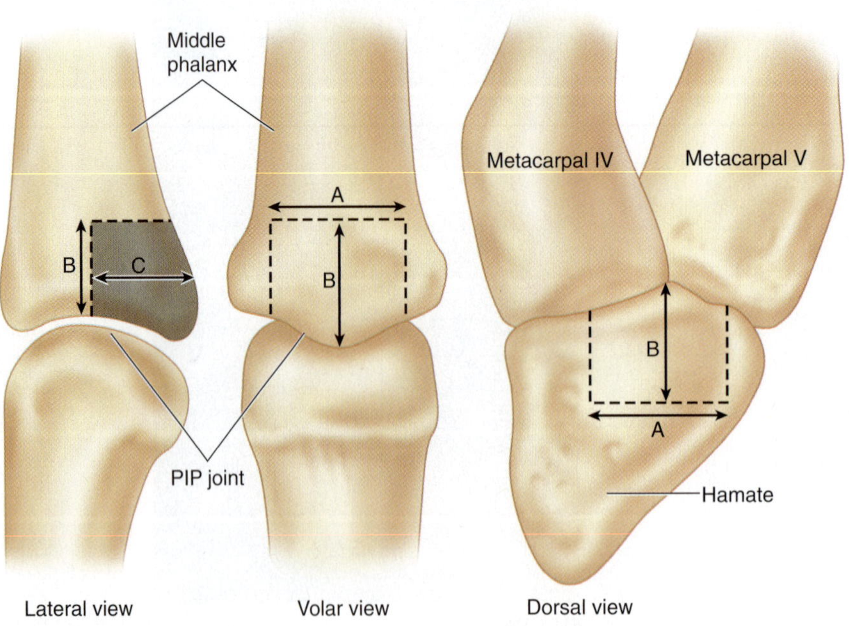

FIGURE 52-8

Step 3: Graft Fixation

- Contour the graft as needed to fill the defect, giving special attention to reconstructing the concave articular surface. Additional bone graft may be used distally if the hamate graft is too vertical (Fig. 52-9).
- Provisionally secure the autograft with a 0.028-inch K-wire.
- Secure the graft with two 1.1- or 1.3-mm screws on either side of the provisional K-wire. A third screw placed into the hole is left once the K-wire is removed if the graft is large enough (Fig. 52-10).
- Reduce the PIP joint and assess rotational alignment and joint stability throughout an arc of motion.
- Assess the screw length under fluoroscopy.
- Trim the distal volar surface of the graft so that there is a smooth transition between the graft and the volar cortex of the middle phalanx.

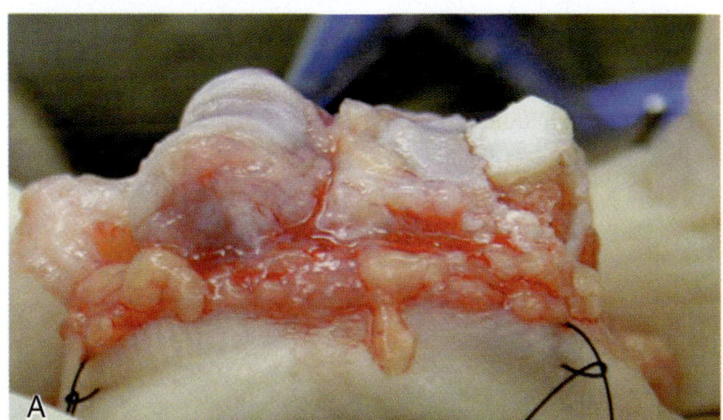

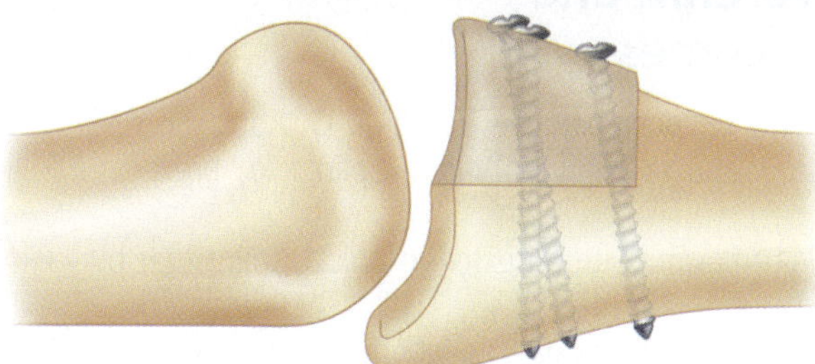

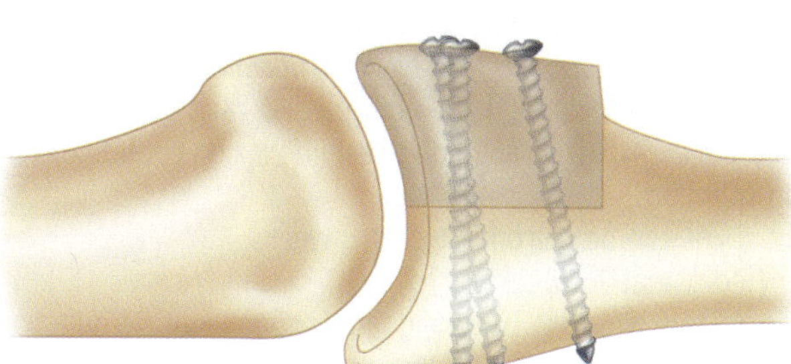

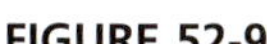

FIGURE 52-9

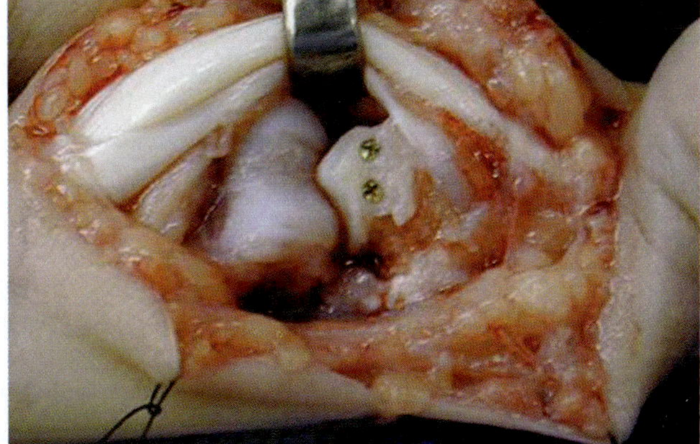

FIGURE 52-10

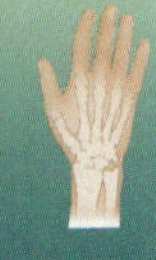

STEP 3 PEARLS

Make every effort to cant the graft into 10 to 15 degrees of extension so as to better restore the cup-shaped contour of the base of the middle phalanx.

The hamate articular cartilage is thicker than the middle phalanx cartilage, which creates an apparent radiographic stepoff (Fig. 52-11). Direct visualization of the joint will confirm the lack of an articular stepoff.

The joint should remain located throughout a full range of motion. Dorsal subluxation suggests that the graft has been set too "flat," failing to restore a concave articular surface.

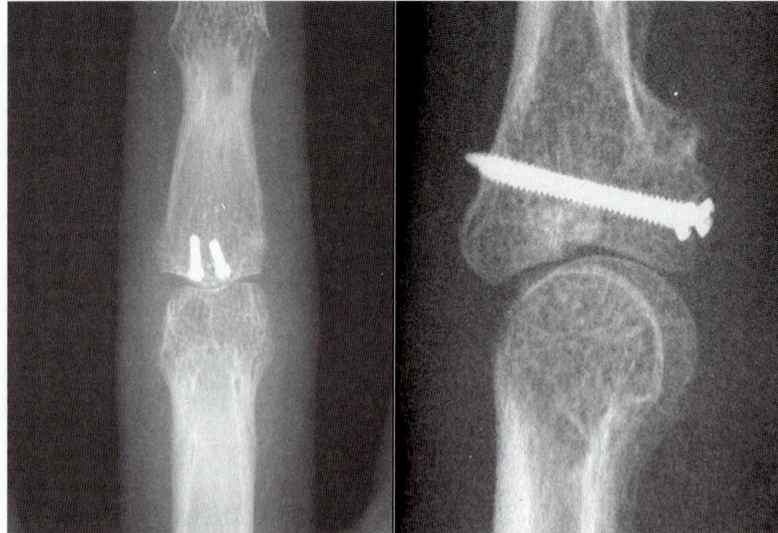

FIGURE 52-11

Step 4: Closure

- Reattach the volar plate to the middle phalanx with a 4-0 nonabsorbable suture. The suture can be secured through small drill holes if necessary.
- Reattach the collateral ligaments to the stumps on the middle phalanx.
- Reapproximate the flexor tendon sheath flap over the PIP joint with a 6-0 absorbable suture.
- Deflate the tourniquet and obtain hemostasis.
- Close the skin and apply a bulky dressing and dorsal splint with the PIP joint in 20 degrees of flexion.

Postoperative Care and Expected Outcomes

- Remove the dressing on postoperative day 3 to 5. Apply an elastic sleeve for edema control and a figure-of-eight splint to prevent PIP joint hyperextension.
- Begin active PIP joint flexion with an extension block splint that prevents full PIP joint extension.
- At the same time, begin active and passive motion of the metacarpophalangeal and distal interphalangeal joints.
- If the radiographs at 3 weeks show concentric joint reduction and solid graft fixation, begin gentle active assisted flexion and extension of the PIP joint.
- Obtain radiographs 6 weeks postoperatively to confirm solid graft fixation and concentric joint reduction (see Fig. 52-11). Begin passive range of motion into flexion and correction of an excessive (>20 degrees) PIP flexion contracture with dynamic extension splinting.
- The figure-of-eight splint can be discontinued at 8 weeks.
- Allow full, unrestricted use at 12 weeks.
- The procedure can restore a stable, well-aligned PIP joint with a functional arc of motion of 90 degrees. A 15- to 20-degree extension contracture is not uncommon.

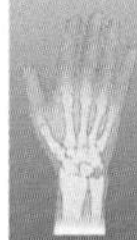

Evidence

Calfee RP, Kiefhaber TR, Sommerkamp TG, et al. Hemi-hamate arthroplasty provides functional reconstruction of acute and chronic proximal interphalangeal fracture-dislocations. *J Hand Surg [Am]*. 2009;34:1232-1241.

The authors retrospectively evaluated 33 patients at an average of 4.5 years after hemi-hamate arthroplasty for both acute and chronic PIP joint fracture dislocations. Patients had an average PIP range of motion of 70 degrees and DIP motion of 54 degrees. The average VAS functional score was 1.4 and DASH score was 5. Ten patients complained of increased pain with cold temperatures. Only one patient required revision surgery. The authors concluded that hemi-hamate arthroplasty restores PIP function after both acute and chronic PIP joint fracture dislocations. (Level V evidence)

Williams RMM, Kiefhaber TR, Sommerkamp TG, et al. Proximal interphalangeal fracture/dislocations using a hemi-hamate autograft. *J Hand Surg [Am]*. 2003;28:856-865.

This retrospective study evaluated 13 consecutive patients with unstable PIP joint fracture-dislocations undergoing a hemi-hamate arthroplasty. Bony union was achieved in all patients. The average arcs of motion at the PIP joint and DIP joint were 85 degrees and 60 degrees, respectively. Average grip strength was 80% of the uninjured side, and the average pain score on the VAS functional score was 1.3. The authors concluded that fracture-dislocations involving greater than 50% of the volar base of the middle phalanx and those that remain unstable even with less articular involvement can be treated effectively with a hemi-hamate arthroplasty. Patients have a stable functional joint with minimal disability. (Level V evidence)

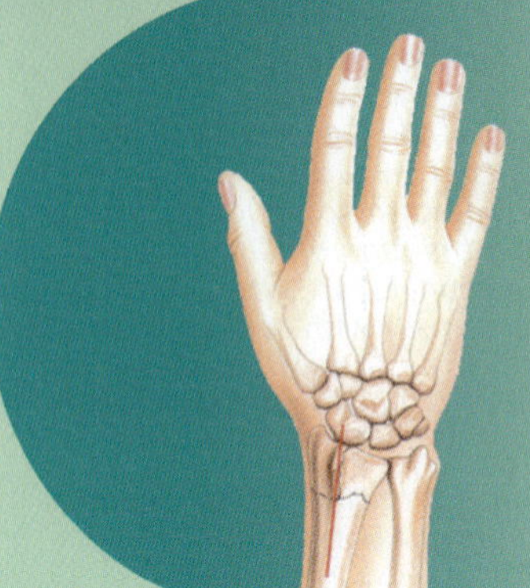

PROCEDURE 53

Metacarpophalangeal and Proximal Interphalangeal Joint Collateral Ligament Avulsion Fractures

Randy R. Bindra and Micah K. Sinclair

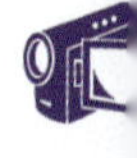

See Video 39: Metacarpal Shaft Fractures

Indications

- Displaced collateral ligament with or without associated joint subluxation or dislocation
- Large avulsion fragment with articular incongruity
- Displaced and interposed fracture fragment within joint
- Border digit injury such as radial border of index finger or ulnar collateral ligament of thumb metaphalangeal (MP) joint
- Injury in athletes

Examination/Imaging

Clinical Examination

- Unilateral swelling and bruising of the injured joint
- Lateral deviation deformity of digit due to loss of collateral ligament integrity (Fig. 53-1)
- Pain with restricted range of motion
- Gentle testing of collateral ligaments to ensure integrity, which may require local anesthetic block. Avoid excessive force to prevent displacement of fragment (Fig. 53-2)
- Patient asked to flex and extend the uninjured joints distal to the injury to evaluate the continuity of the flexor and extensor tendons

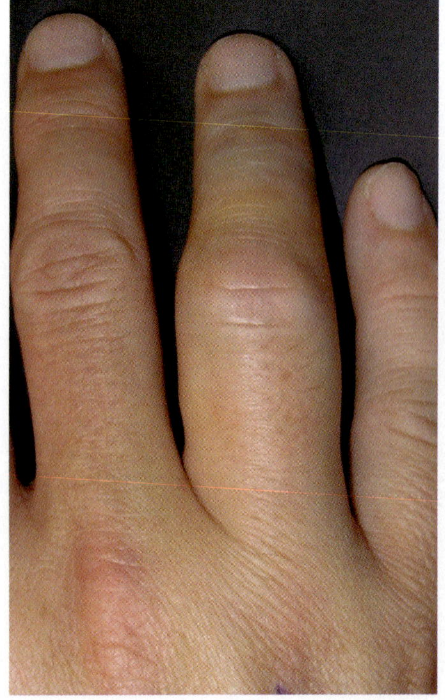

FIGURE 53-1

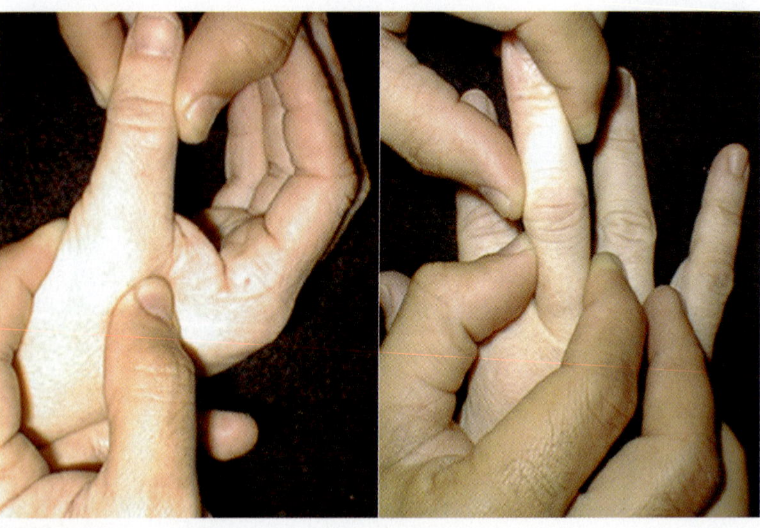

FIGURE 53-2

Imaging

- Posteroanterior, oblique, and true lateral films of the digit for proximal interphalangeal (PIP) joint injuries. At the PIP joint, the most common avulsion fracture is a unicondylar fracture (Fig. 53-3).
- Posteroanterior, oblique, and true lateral films of the hand for metacarpophalangeal (MCP) joint injuries (Fig. 53-4).
- In the immature skeleton, ligament avulsion injuries occur at the growth plate with a fragment of the epiphysis (Fig. 53-5).
- Brewerton view provides a tangential view of the metacarpal head, demonstrating the area of origin of the collateral ligament, which will help to reveal small avulsion fragments from the metacarpal head.
- Computed tomography scanning is useful in cases of suspected involvement of the articular surface for evaluation of joint congruity.

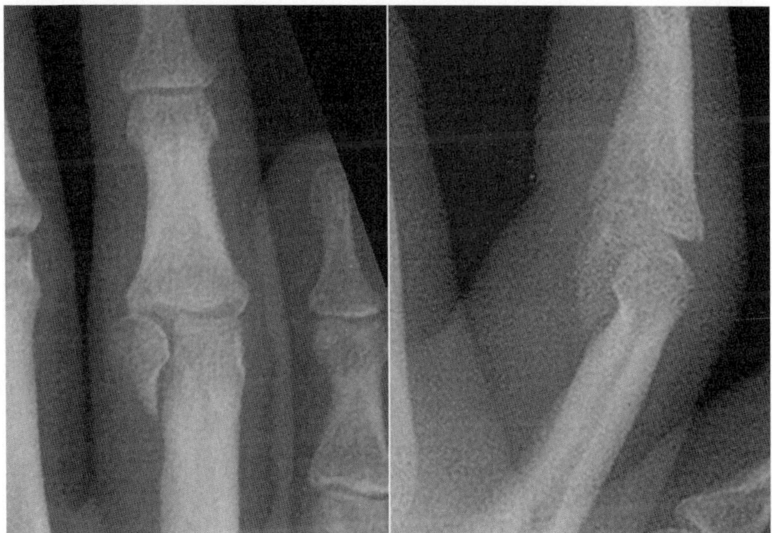

FIGURE 53-3

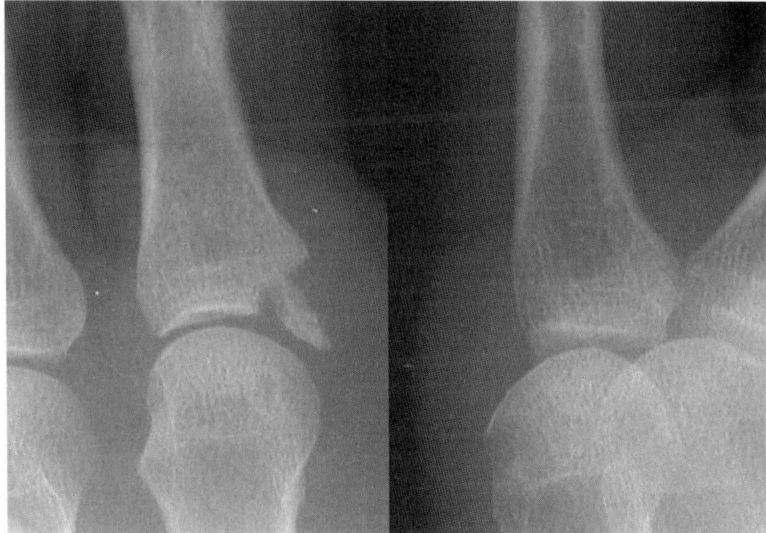

FIGURE 53-4

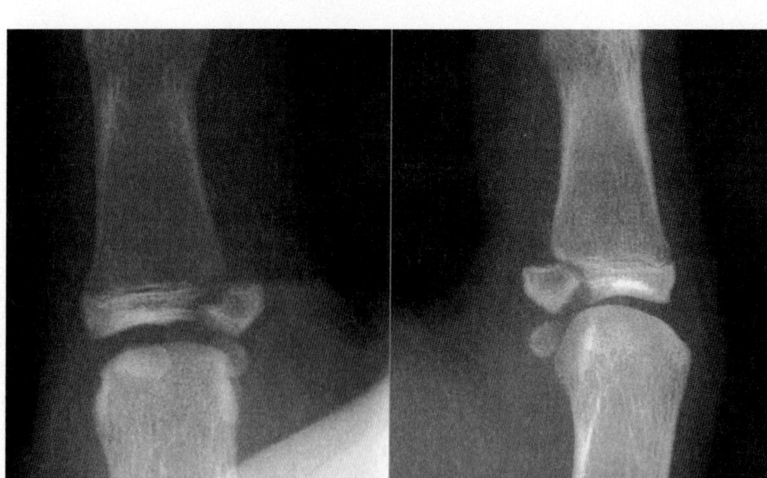

FIGURE 53-5

Surgical Anatomy

- MCP joint collateral ligaments are more commonly avulsed at their distal insertion. An avulsed fragment from the base of the proximal phalanx is lateral and volar to the midaxis.
- Rarely, in more severe injuries, with pure ligamentous avulsions or smaller fragment avulsions, the avulsed ligament lies superficial to the extensor apparatus.
- If avulsed without bone or with a small fragment, the ulnar collateral ligament of the thumb MP joint can come to lie superficial to the adductor aponeurosis (Stener lesion).

Positioning

- The patient is positioned supine with the arm on a hand table.
- The forearm is pronated, and the hand is placed on a towel roll. The surgeon is seated facing the injured side of the digit.
- A tourniquet is used for the procedure.

POSITIONING EQUIPMENT

Intraoperative imaging is critical in this procedure. The mini C-arm is draped sterilely, placed at the axillary side of the table, and brought in when needed during the case.

Exposures

Metacarpophalangeal Joint

- The MCP joint of the thumb and borders of the hand (ulnar side of small and radial side of index finger) can be easily accessed through a lateral approach.
- Cutaneous nerves are located in the subcutaneous plane and must be identified and preserved.
- The oblique fibers of the extensor hood cover the MCP joint and will need to be incised longitudinally for access to the joint; they require meticulous repair on completion.
- Access to the MP collateral avulsion fracture for nonborder digits is achieved by a volar approach that allows reduction and fixation with compression.
- With a volar approach, the digital neurovascular bundle is at risk for injury and must be identified and carefully retracted away from the flexor tendon sheath.
- A Bruner zigzag skin incision is made centered over the proximal digital crease (Fig. 53-6).
- The flexor sheath is kept intact (Fig. 53-7) and retracted subperiosteally off the base of the proximal phalanx and retracted (Fig. 53-8). After fracture fixation, the sheath is allowed to return to its normal position, and no repair is necessary.

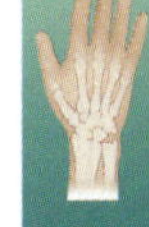

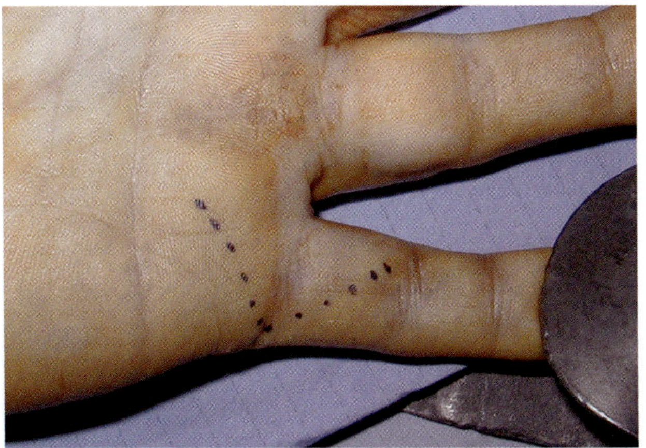

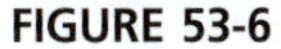

FIGURE 53-6

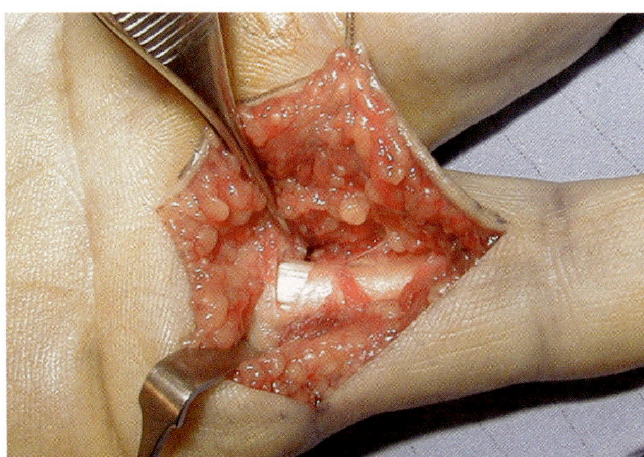

FIGURE 53-7

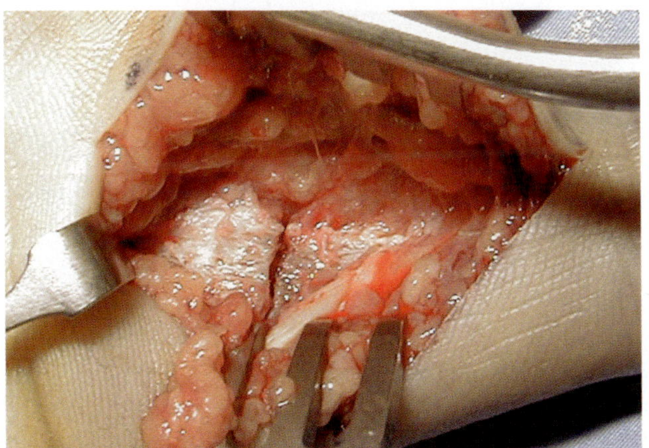

FIGURE 53-8

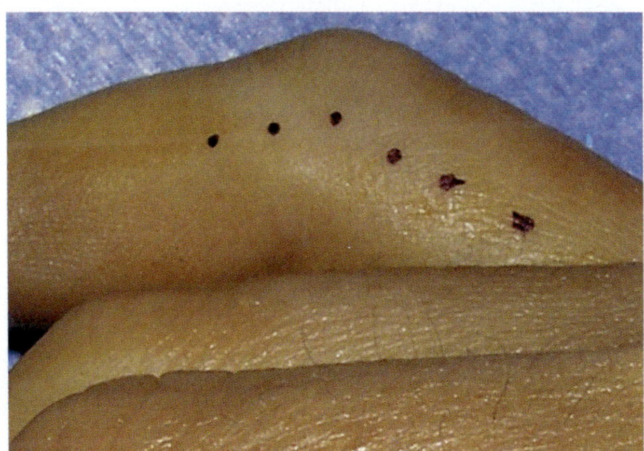

FIGURE 53-9

Proximal Interphalangeal Joint

- At the PIP level, the fracture is approached using a midaxial incision.
- A digital midaxial incision is marked by joining the most dorsal points of the digital creases with the digit in full flexion (Fig. 53-9).
- The transverse fibers of the extensor apparatus at the level of the PIP are released to elevate the lateral band of the extensor mechanism dorsally.

PEARLS

The midaxial skin incision is dorsal to the midlateral line and avoids dissection of the digital neurovascular bundle.

Careful spreading dissection is necessary after skin incision to preserve the subcutaneous nerves.

When exposing the fragments, care must be taken to avoid stripping excessive soft tissue and devascularizing the fragment.

PITFALLS

Injury to cutaneous nerves.

Injury to the collateral ligament insertion on the fragment.

Injury to digital neurovascular bundle or flexor tendon sheath with volar approach to the MP joint.

Procedure

Step 1: Principles and Methods of Fixation

- Type of fixation depends on size of fragment and comminution.
- A single large fragment can be treated with lag screws. If possible, two screws should be employed for rotational stability.

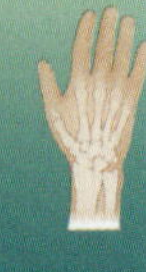

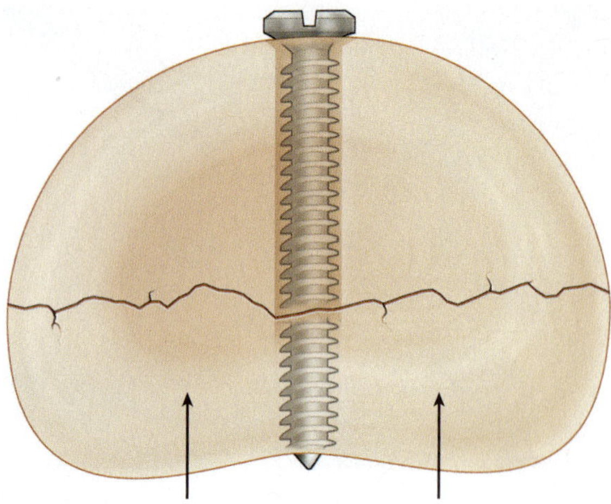

FIGURE 53-10

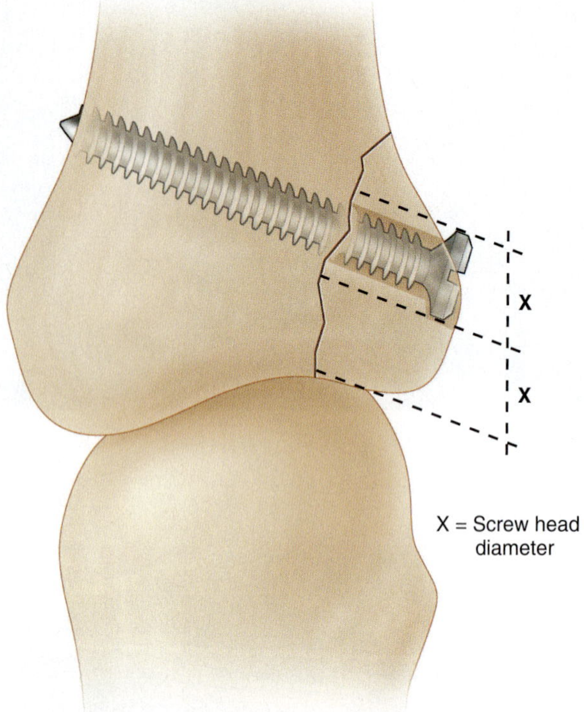

FIGURE 53-11

STEP 1 PEARLS

The screw head must be smaller than one third of the fragment width (Fig. 53-11).

It is preferable to use two small screws for better rotational stability and load distribution rather than a single large screw.

STEP 1 PITFALLS

Using too large a screw can cause comminution of the fragment.

Overtightening the screw can fracture the near cortex.

Countersinking the screw head is not recommended in soft metaphyseal bone because it can result in excessive screw head penetration into the bone to cause loss of compression.

- Lag or compression screw implies a screw that does not have any purchase on the near fragment. This is achieved by drilling a glide hole that exceeds the screw thread diameter in the near cortex. The far cortex is then drilled with the thread hole that matches the screw shaft diameter. As the screw is inserted, it slides through the near cortex and gains purchase in the far cortex. With further tightening, compression between the fragments is generated (Fig. 53-10).
- If screws are not available or lag screw fixation is not possible, tension band fixation of the fragment can be performed. Malleable wire is passed through the collateral ligament close to its bony insertion and passed through a drill hole in the metaphysis in a figure-of-eight loop. The fragment is then reduced, a K-wire is passed through the fragment for longitudinal stability, and the wire loop is tightened to compress the fracture.
- If the fracture fragments are too small for fixation, they may be excised, and direct repair of the ligament to bone is performed using an anchor or pull-through sutures.

Step 2

- The avulsed fragment is carefully handled to maintain the attached collateral ligament.

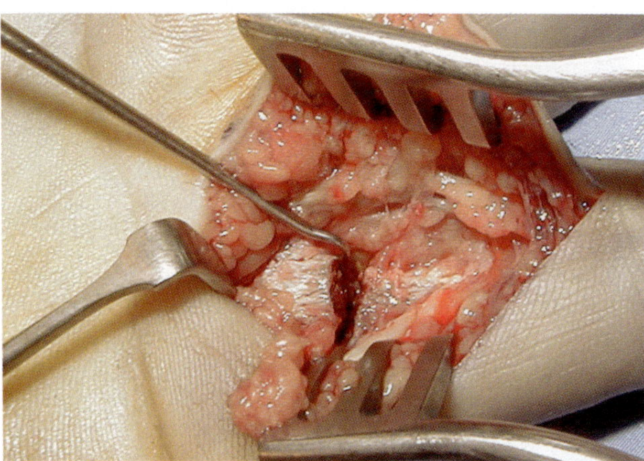

FIGURE 53-12

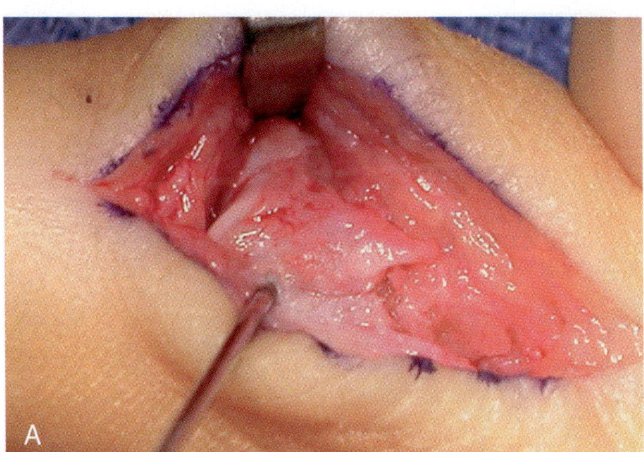

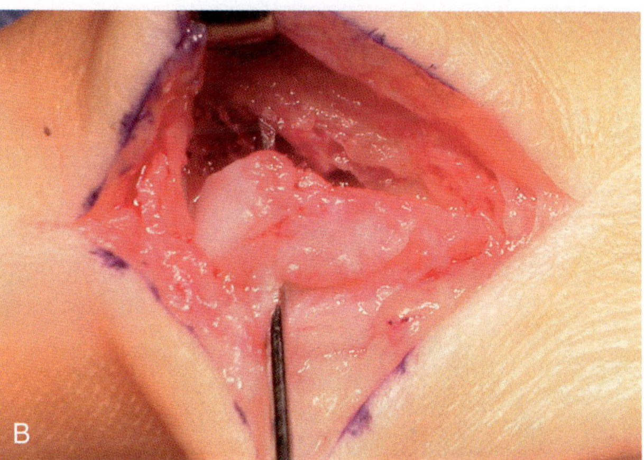

FIGURE 53-13

STEP 2 PEARLS

Ensure that reduction of the joint surface is anatomic before screw insertion.

Use the direction of the K-wire to guide screw placement.

When placing the second screw, apply a reduction forceps to hold reduction to avoid stripping the first screw when tightening the second.

- The fragment must be carefully retracted with a hook, and the joint is subluxated to look for any loose cartilaginous fragments or impaction of the joint surface (Fig. 53-12).
- A 0.035-inch K-wire inserted into the fragment may be used as a joystick to gently manipulate the piece as needed (Fig. 53-13A).
- After reduction, the same wire is advanced distally for temporary fixation (Fig. 53-13B).
- The reduction is then checked by imaging.
- Definitive fixation is then performed. If screw fixation is planned, the appropriate-sized glide hole is drilled through the fragment. The thread hole is then drilled through the far cortex. The screw length is determined, and an appropriate screw is inserted.

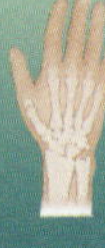

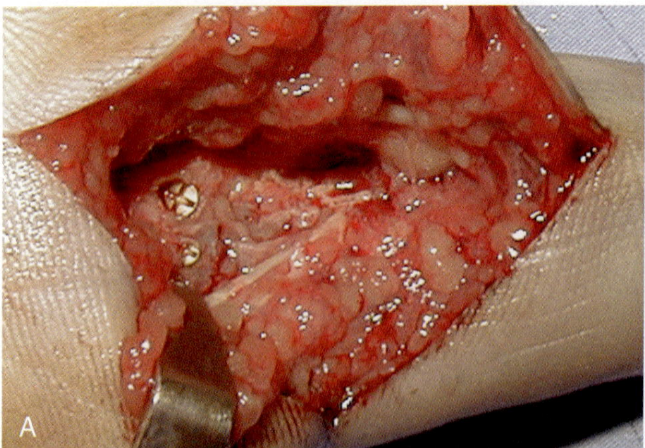

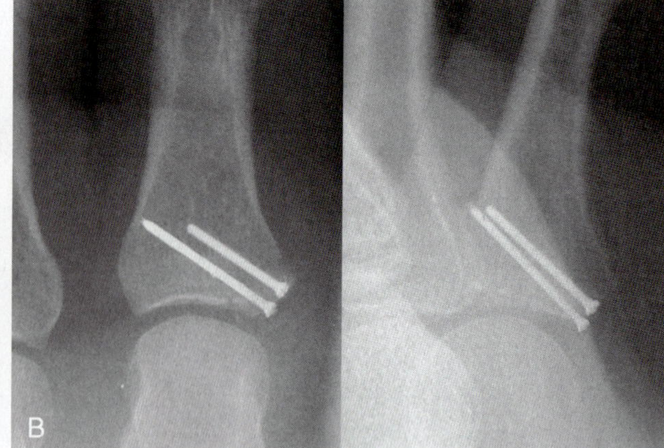

FIGURE 53-14

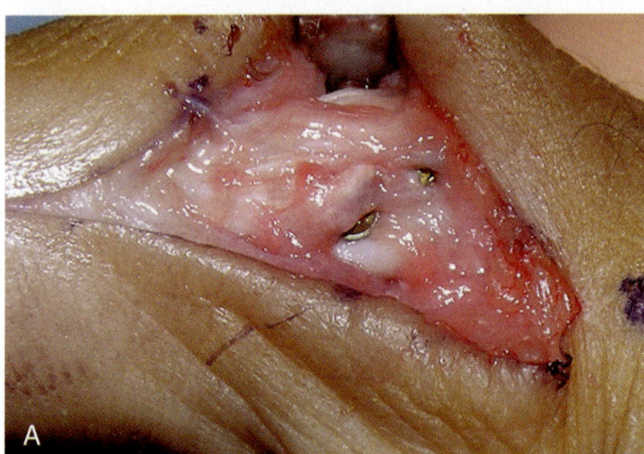

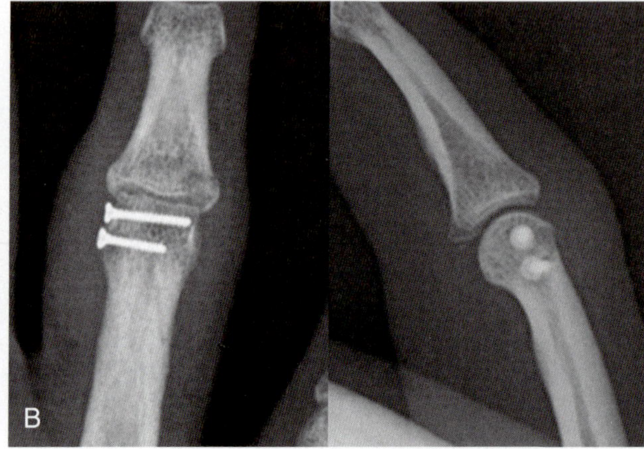

FIGURE 53-15

STEP 2 PITFALLS

The screw may accidentally penetrate the articular surface.

Placement of a long screw may cause irritation of the extensor mechanism at the base of the proximal phalanx.

A long screw at the head of the proximal phalanx may impinge on the collateral ligament at the far end of the joint and lead to joint stiffness.

- The K-wire is then removed, and the second screw is inserted through the K-wire hole, after overdrilling the near cortex (Fig. 53-14).
- At the PIP joint, the screw head may interfere with gliding of the near collateral ligament. This can be avoided by placing one screw at or just proximal to the ligament origin. The second screw is placed between the main and accessory parts of the ligament and tightened until it sinks beneath the ligament complex (Fig. 53-15).

Step 3

- Screw length and position are checked by intraoperative imaging.
- At the MCP joint, the flexor tendons with surrounding sheath are replaced, and no suture is necessary.
- At the PIP joint, the extensor mechanism is then repaired with a continuous nonabsorbable suture.
- The tourniquet is released to secure hemostasis.
- Skin edges are approximated with sutures.

PEARLS

Pain and edema control are essential in the immediate postoperative period.

Resting the hand with the MCP joint in flexion and PIP joint in full extension will prevent extension contracture of the joint.

PITFALLS

Aggressive motion in the face of pain and swelling in the immediate postoperative period will only exacerbate symptoms and cause loss of patient cooperation.

Postoperative Care and Expected Outcomes

- The hand is rested in a plaster splint for the first 5 to 7 days after surgery.
- The hand is placed in a removable splint, and active motion is commenced by the end of the first week after surgery. The ligament repair is protected by buddy taping to the digit adjacent to the injured ligament.
- Splinting is discontinued by 4 to 6 weeks when tenderness and swelling have subsided.
- Strengthening is commenced after full range of motion has returned.
- Most patients with PIP joint injuries can expect residual swelling and flexion contracture that is usually mild.
- MCP joint injuries have a better prognosis, and patients usually can regain full motion. Swelling around the joint is less noticeable than in the finger.

Evidence

Bischoff R, Buechler U, De Roche R, Jupiter J. Clinical results of tension band fixation of avulsion fractures in the hand. *J Hand Surg [Am]*. 1994;19:1019-1026.
This case study included 100 patients from two surgeons at separate institutions with a variety of avulsion fractures in the hand: 51 bony mallet fractures, 38 bony gamekeeper's fractures of the thumb, 8 fractures of the lateral phalange base, and 3 fractures of the dorsal aspect of the middle phalanx. Twenty-one of 51 bony mallet fractures had poor clinical and radiographic outcome. The remainder of the fractures included bony gamekeeper's fractures, fractures of the lateral phalangeal base, and fractures of the dorsal aspect of the middle phalanx. All had excellent radiographic outcome, with only one nonunion, and excellent or satisfactory clinical result. (Level V evidence)

Kozin SH, Bishop AT. Tension wire fixation of avulsion fractures at the thumb metacarpophalangeal joint. *J Hand Surg [Am]*. 1994;19:1027-1031.
In this retrospective case series, nine patients underwent acute open reduction and tension wire fixation of displaced or rotated avulsion fractures. All healed with anatomic alignment without instability or articular incongruity. Mild pain, stiffness, and loss of pinch occurred in three of nine patients. MP motion averaged 77% of the respective opposite hand. IP motion, grip, pinch, and opposition were 96% to 99% that of the contralateral hand. (Level V evidence)

Schubiner JM, Mass DP. Operation for collateral ligament ruptures of the metacarpophalangeal joints of the fingers. *J Bone Joint Surg [Br]*. 1989;71:388-389.
This retrospective case series studied 10 patients who underwent operative fixation of MP collateral ligament rupture of a finger, most commonly the radial collateral ligament of the small finger. Joint instability with lack of end point with applied force was the operative indication. Operative fixation was performed at an average of 6 weeks after injury with pullout suture in 9 patients, and reconstruction with palmaris longus was used in 1 patient. All patients returned to preoperative level of function, free of pain and edema, by 3 months postoperatively. (Level V evidence)

Shewring DJ, Thomas RH. Avulsion fractures from the base of the proximal phalanges of the fingers. *J Hand Surg [Br]*. 2003;28:10-14.
Thirty-three patients had avulsion fractures from the base of the proximal phalanx due to abduction injury. Twelve percent to 28% of the joint surface was involved. Twenty-five patients underwent operative fixation with a single lag screw through the palmar approach. Immediate mobilization with full range of motion by 3 weeks was achieved. Eight patients initially chose nonoperative management and went on to nonunion clinically or radiographically by 2 months. All of these patients subsequently achieved union after operative fixation. (Level IV evidence)

Shewring DJ, Thomas RH. Collateral ligament avulsion fractures from the heads of the metacarpals of the fingers. *J Hand Surg [Br]*. 2006;31:537-541.
Nineteen patients with collateral ligament avulsion fractures from the metacarpal head were reviewed. Eleven patients with displaced fractures were treated with internal fixation through the dorsal approach within 5 days of injury. All went on to union. Seven of these regained full range of motion at 3 months, and 4 had persistent loss of flexion of the MP joint with arc of motion of 34 degrees. Seven patients with nondisplaced fractures were initially treated nonoperatively with buddy strapping. Of these, 4 achieved healing and full range of motion at 6 weeks. Three with nonunion underwent delayed operative fixation in the same fashion. All went on to union and full range of motion. (Level IV evidence)

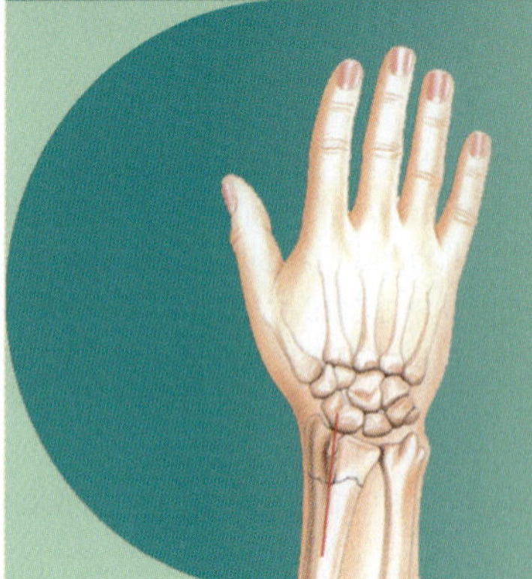

Metacarpal Neck Fractures

Randy R. Bindra and Micah K. Sinclair

Indications

- Angulation greater than 30 degrees
- More angulation acceptable in ulnar rays
- Any rotational deformity
- Displacement
- Multiple fractures
- Polytrauma patient

Examination/Imaging

Clinical Examination

- Note swelling and bruising over the dorsum of the hand.
- Look carefully for any wounds—may indicate an open fracture (Fig. 54-1).
- Look carefully for rotational deformity with fingers flexed and compared with opposite hand (Fig. 54-2).
- Ensure circulation is adequate by checking capillary refill.
- Test and document digital sensation.
- Ask patient to flex and extend interphalangeal joints within limits of pain to confirm continuity of flexor and extensor tendons.

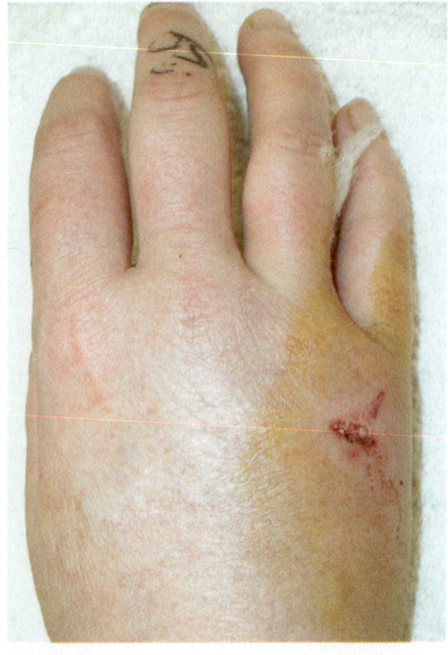

FIGURE 54-1

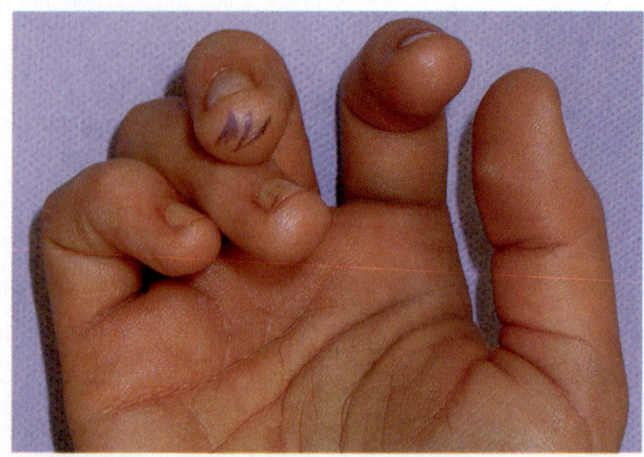

FIGURE 54-2

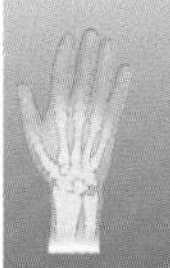

Imaging

- Obtain posteroanterior, oblique, and true lateral films (Fig. 54-3).
- Angulation must be measured against the dorsal cortex on a true lateral view (Fig. 54-4).

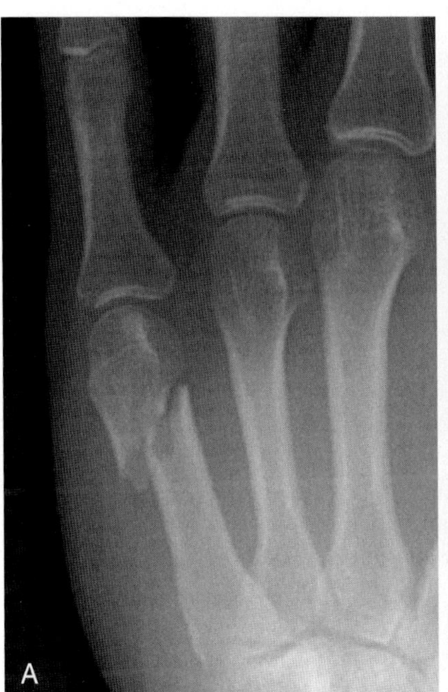

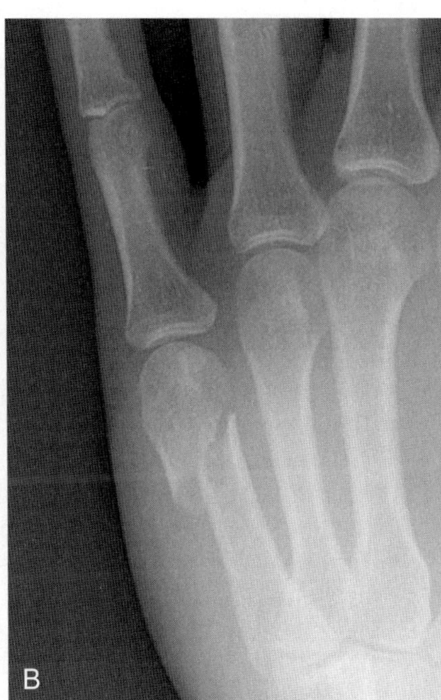

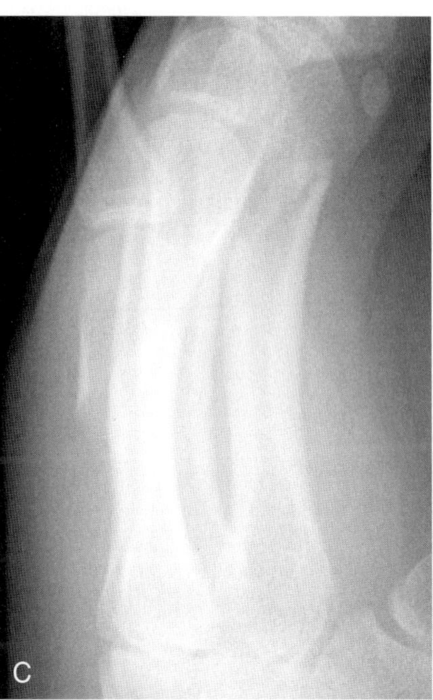

FIGURE 54-3

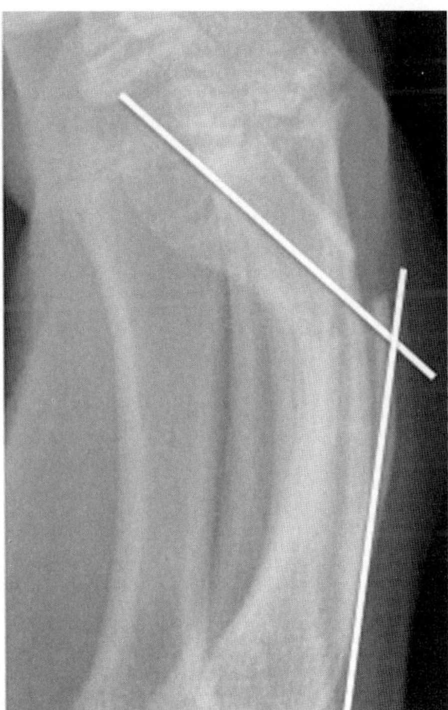

FIGURE 54-4

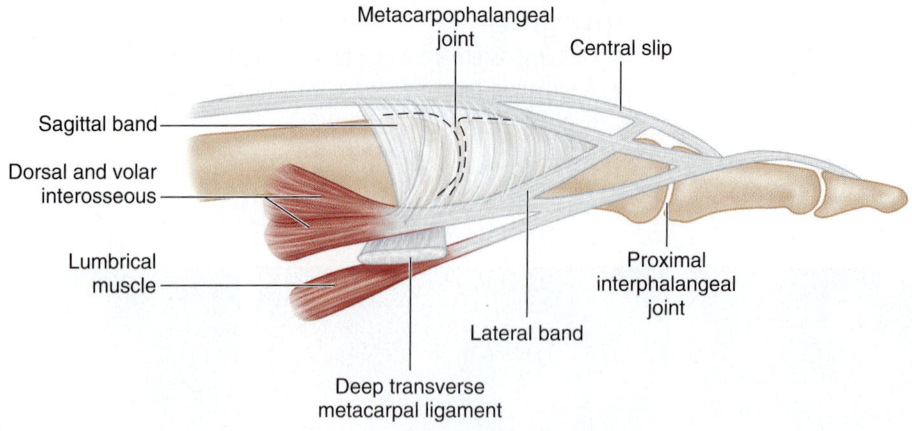

FIGURE 54-5

Surgical Anatomy

- Metacarpals can be easily accessed through the dorsal approach.
- Dorsal cutaneous nerves are located in the subcutaneous plane. The dorsal cutaneous branch of the ulnar nerve winds around the ulnar border of the hand 1 cm distal to the ulnar head and then divides into its branches at the level of the small finger carpometacarpal joint.
- The extensor tendons are surrounded by paratenon and can be easily separated by dividing the juncturae tendinum that interconnect them at the level of the metacarpal necks.
- The extensor hood envelops the distal part of the metacarpal. Plate placement at this level can interfere with gliding of the hood (Fig. 54-5).

POSITIONING EQUIPMENT

- Intraoperative imaging is critical in this procedure. The mini C-arm is draped sterilely and placed at the axillary side of the table and is brought in when needed during the case.

Positioning

- The patient is positioned supine with the arm on a hand table.
- The surgeon is seated on the cephalad side of the table with the forearm pronated to allow access to the dorsum of the hand.
- A tourniquet is used for the procedure.

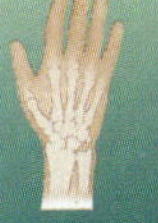

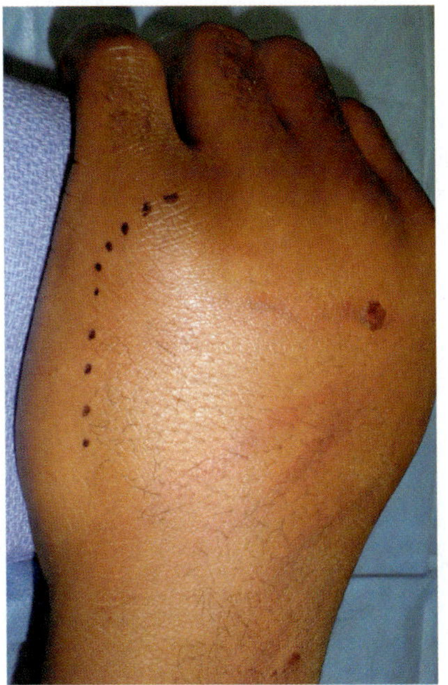

FIGURE 54-6

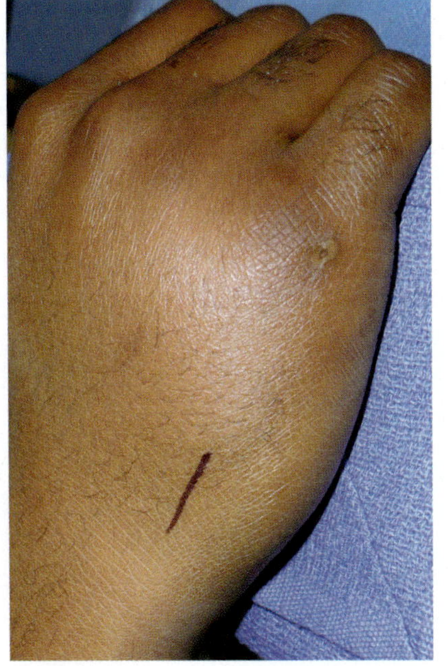

FIGURE 54-7

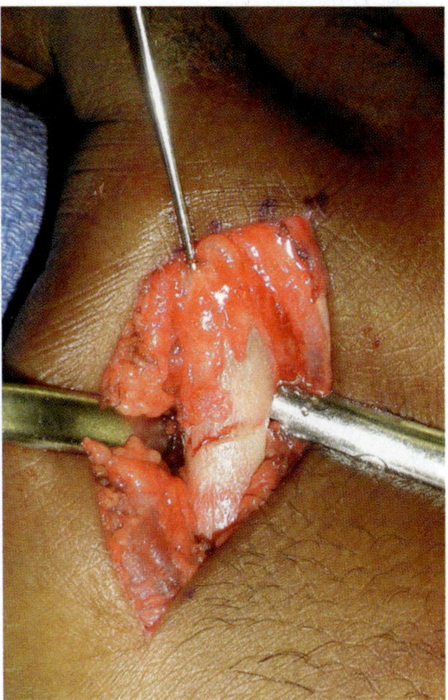

FIGURE 54-8

PEARLS

For plating of adjacent metacarpals, a single skin incision between the metacarpals will allow access to both fractures.

Careful spreading dissection is necessary after skin incision to preserve subcutaneous nerves and veins.

Paratenon around extensor tendons must be preserved to minimize postoperative tendon adhesions.

With exposure for intramedullary pinning of the small finger, particular care must be taken to identify and preserve the dorsal branch of the ulnar nerve.

In case of excessive comminution, the periosteum around the fracture is left intact, and the implant is secured distally and proximally (bridge plating).

PITFALLS

Injury to cutaneous nerves.

Exposures

- For open plating, a longitudinal incision is centered over the metacarpal neck. The incision is on the dorsum for the long and ring fingers. For the border digits—index and small fingers—the incision is on the midlateral line and then curves dorsally at the metacarpophalangeal joint (Fig. 54-6).
- For intramedullary pinning, the incision is placed at the metacarpal base (Fig. 54-7).
- The periosteum at the fracture site is elevated circumferentially to allow accurate reduction without soft tissue interposition.

Procedure

Step 1: Preparation of Plate and Insertion of Blade

- Achieve provisional reduction and stabilize with a K-wire (Fig. 54-8).
- Select the appropriate-sized condylar plate.

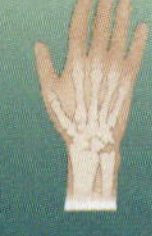

STEP 1 PEARLS

Initial stabilizing K-wire is helpful in fractures for which anatomic reduction is possible.

In the face of comminution, the distal fragment is stabilized with the blade first, and the plate is then reduced to the shaft.

STEP 1 PITFALLS

If the blade hole is drilled at an incorrect angle, the plate stays off the shaft. In this case, it is preferable to bend the blade rather than drill a second hole.

If the blade is left long, it interferes with the collateral ligament on the far side of the joint.

- The plate is held against the fracture, and the required length of plate is determined. The plate is cut to appropriate length (Fig. 54-9).
- The blade hole is drilled first in the metacarpal head. The plate is rotated such that the blade is pointing away from the bone, and the plate hole adjacent to the blade is drilled with the drill directed parallel to the blade (Fig. 54-10).
- The hole is measured, and the blade is cut to the appropriate length.
- The blade is inserted into the hole, and the plate is approximated with the shaft using a bone clamp (Fig. 54-11).

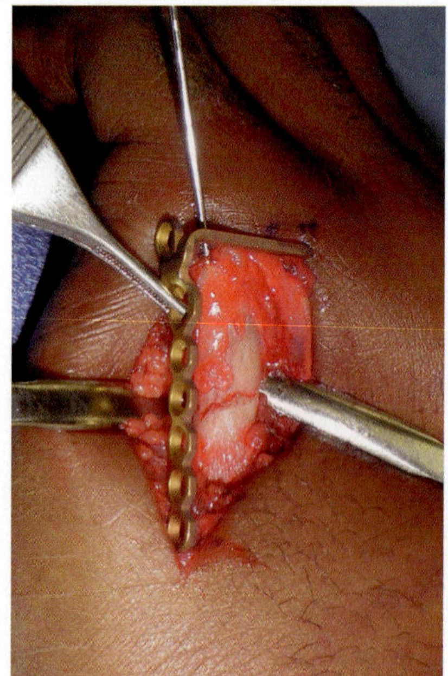

FIGURE 54-9

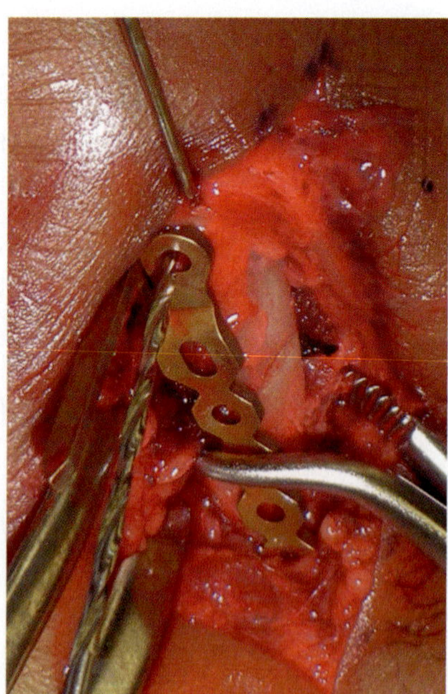

FIGURE 54-10

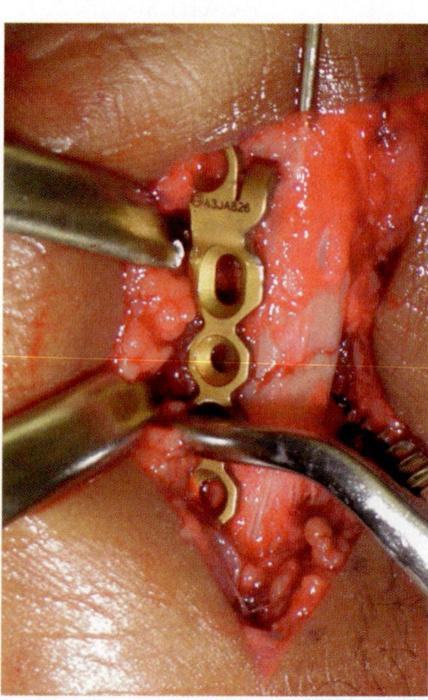

FIGURE 54-11

STEP 2 PEARLS

It is critical to follow the sequence of screw insertion as recommended earlier. Insertion of the most proximal screw first ensures that the plate is aligned with the bone.

STEP 2 PITFALLS

Insertion of distal screws in the shaft or insertion of the screw close to the blade before the shaft screw will not allow correction of the plate position with relation to the shaft.

If the plate is not prebent, the fracture may gap open at the far side of the plate as the plate is secured.

Step 2: Alignment of Plate with Shaft

- The plate is aligned with the shaft, and fracture reduction is confirmed (Fig. 54-12).
- The plate must be contoured well along the shaft.
- The most proximal screw in the shaft is inserted first to secure the plate to the shaft (Fig. 54-13).
- Rotational alignment of the finger is checked clinically, and reduction and plate position are checked radiographically (Figs. 54-14 and 54-15).
- The screw adjacent to the blade is then inserted after drilling.

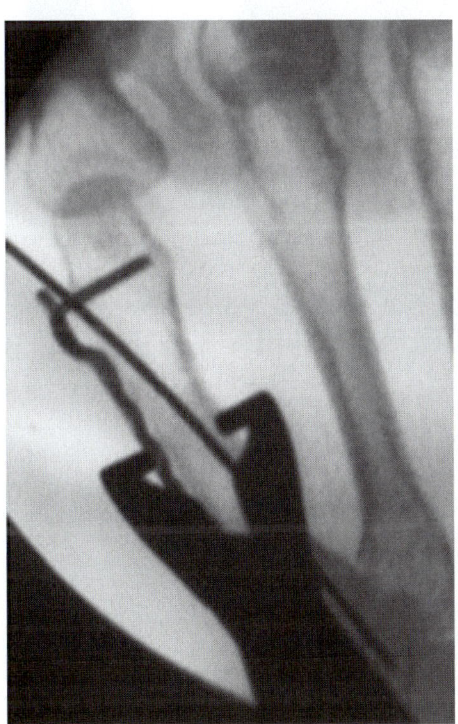

FIGURE 54-12

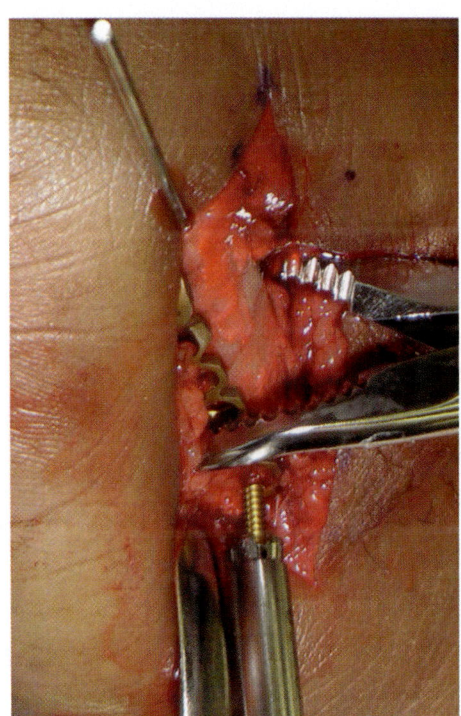

FIGURE 54-13

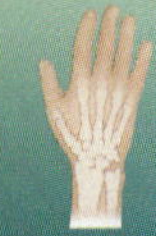

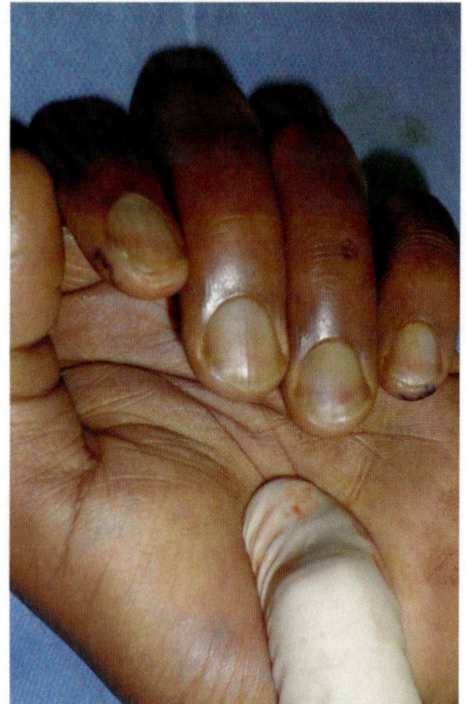

FIGURE 54-14

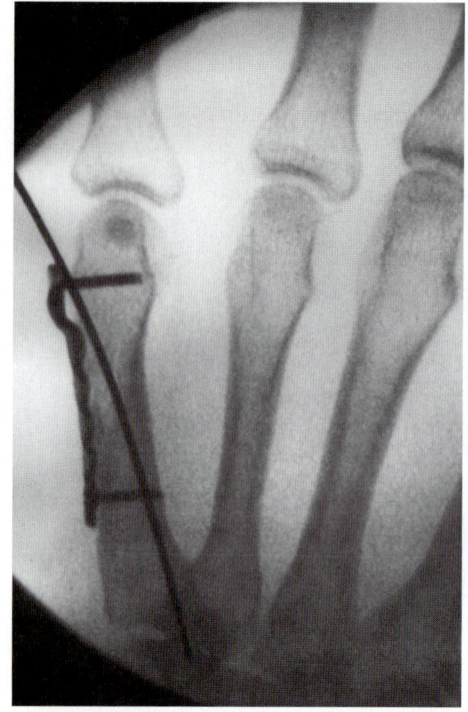

FIGURE 54-15

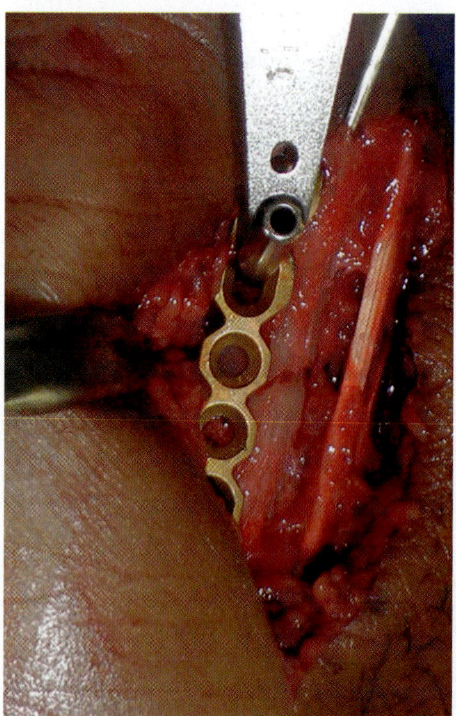

FIGURE 54-16

STEP 3 PEARLS

Try to achieve as much compression as possible with eccentric screw placement and interfragmentary screw whenever possible.

Lag screw and prebending prevent fracture gapping open at the far side of the fracture away from the plate.

Step 3: Compression of the Fracture

- It is helpful to gain compression of a short oblique or transverse fracture to enhance stability.
- Longitudinal compression is achieved by eccentric drilling in the oval hole of the plate. If the screw hole is drilled away from the fracture site, compression is achieved as the screw is inserted and tightened (Fig. 54-16).

STEP 3 PITFALLS

When placing a screw across the fracture for compression, failure to drill near the cortex with a gliding hole may result in distraction rather than compression.

Axial compression with eccentric screw placement is not possible if done later in the fixation as the fragments are fixed rigidly to the plate.

- The screw adjacent to the blade is inserted after drilling (Fig. 54-17).
- In a short oblique fracture, additional compression can be achieved with a lag screw inserted through the plate. To insert a lag screw, the gliding hole is drilled in the near cortex (same diameter as the outer screw diameter—2.0 mm drill for a 2 mm screw). The thread hole (1.5 mm for a 2 mm screw) is drilled in the far cortex (Fig. 54-18).
- Compression is achieved when the screw is fully seated.

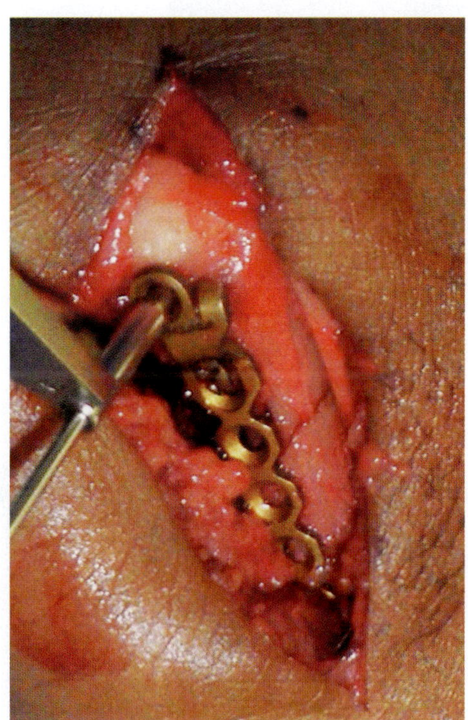

FIGURE 54-17

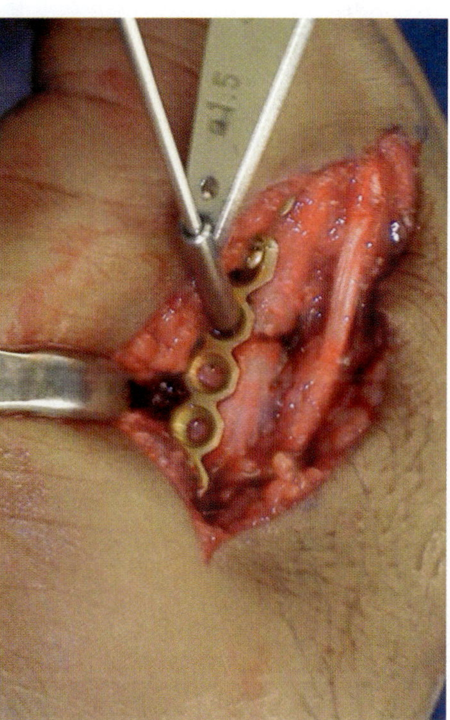

FIGURE 54-18

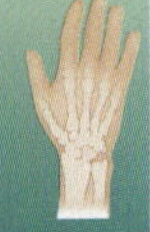

Step 4: Completion of Fixation

- Remaining screws are inserted (Fig. 54-19).
- Radiographs are obtained to confirm that the fracture is reduced and compressed and the screw lengths are correct (Fig. 54-20).
- The fingers are moved passively to ensure that full range and rotational alignment is confirmed.

STEP 4 PEARLS

Once compression is achieved, care must be taken to insert the remaining screws in neutral position (center of hole) to avoid inadvertent distraction.

STEP 4 PITFALLS

The lag screw may get stripped if adjacent screws are not inserted in neutral mode and may distract the fracture.

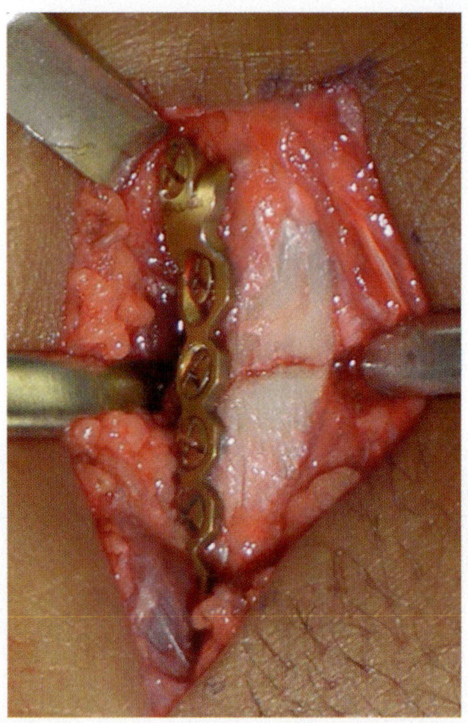

FIGURE 54-19

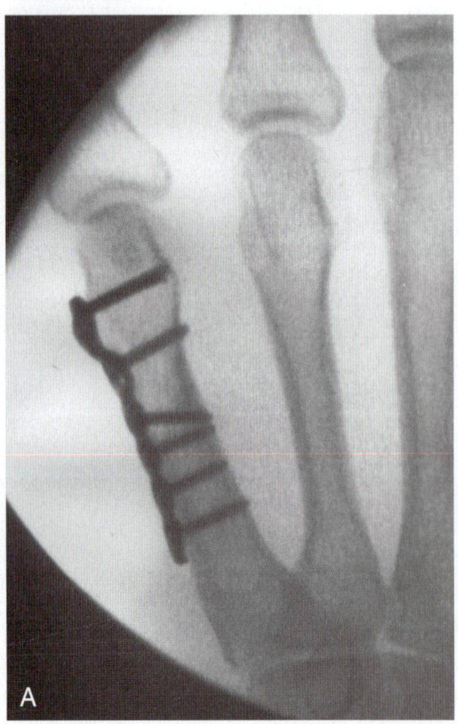

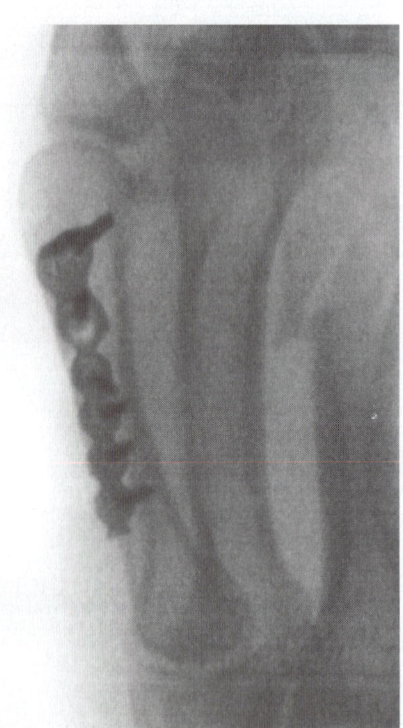

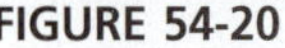

FIGURE 54-20

STEP 5 PEARLS

If preoperative swelling is minimal, subcuticular closure may be performed.

STEP 5 PITFALLS

Failure to release tourniquet and secure hemostasis may result in a hematoma postoperatively.

PEARLS

Initial drilling must be directed obliquely to engage the medullary cavity of the bone.

Attention to the bending of the wires is essential to allow easy passage.

Manual insertion ensures that the wires engage the medullary cavity.

When negotiating the fracture, the wire tends to exit the dorsal side of the fracture. This can be avoided by turning the pin so that the curve points in a palmar direction.

PITFALLS

Insertion of the wires using a power instrument will result in cut-out of the far cortex of the metacarpal head and should be avoided.

Step 5: Wound Closure

- The tourniquet is released, and hemostasis is secured.
- Juncturae tendinum are repaired if required using nonabsorbable sutures.
- Skin edges are approximated with interrupted sutures.

Additional Steps

- Intramedullary pinning of a metacarpal subcapital fracture provides an alternative to open plating with an advantage of percutaneous fixation.
- A 2-cm incision is made just proximal to the base of the metacarpal.
- Cutaneous nerves are identified and protected.
- Using a soft tissue protector, a 2-mm hole is drilled obliquely aiming distally and centrally toward the medullary cavity. A small awl can be used to enlarge the hole (Fig. 54-21).
- A 1.5-mm K-wire is selected and cut to 1 cm longer than the estimated length of the metacarpal. A gentle 30-degree curve is made over a distance of 1 cm at the blunt end of the wire. A 90-degree bend is made over a 1-cm segment in the opposite end of the wire. Both bends are in the same plane (Fig. 54-22).
- The prebent wire is introduced manually into the medullary cavity and passed up to the fracture site under radiographic control (Fig. 54-23). The fracture angulation is then corrected by dorsally directed force on the maximally flexed metacarpophalangeal joint (Fig. 54-24).
- The wire is then advanced across the fracture and right up to the subchondral bone of the metacarpal head while the corrective force is maintained (Fig. 54-25).
- Rotational alignment is clinically examined, and reduction is confirmed radiographically.
- A second wire is then passed in a similar fashion with the curve facing opposite the first wire (Fig. 54-26).
- In a large or osteopenic bone with wide medullary cavity, insertion of three or four pins may be possible.
- The wires are cut close to the bone, and skin is closed with interrupted sutures.

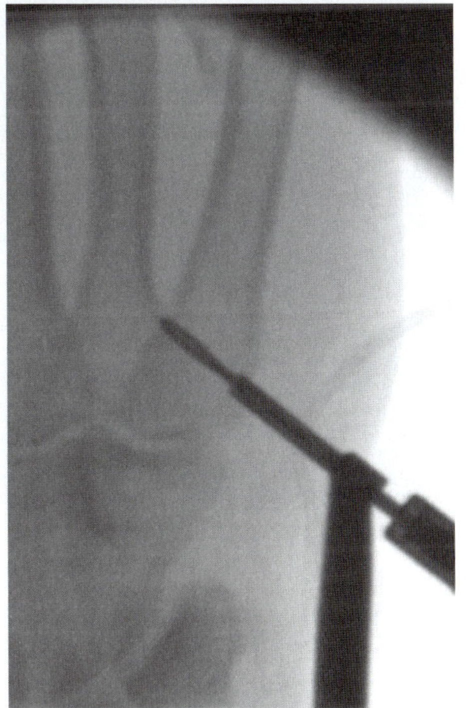

FIGURE 54-21

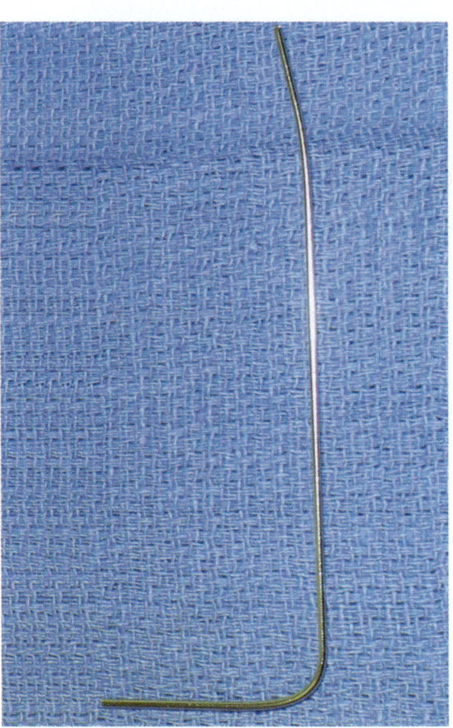

FIGURE 54-22

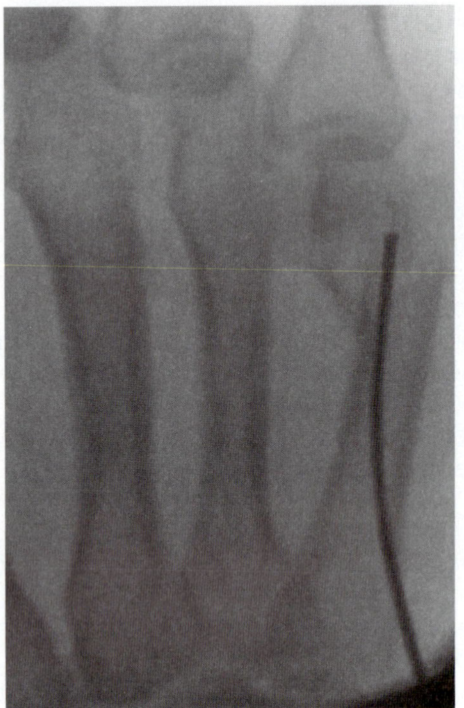

FIGURE 54-23

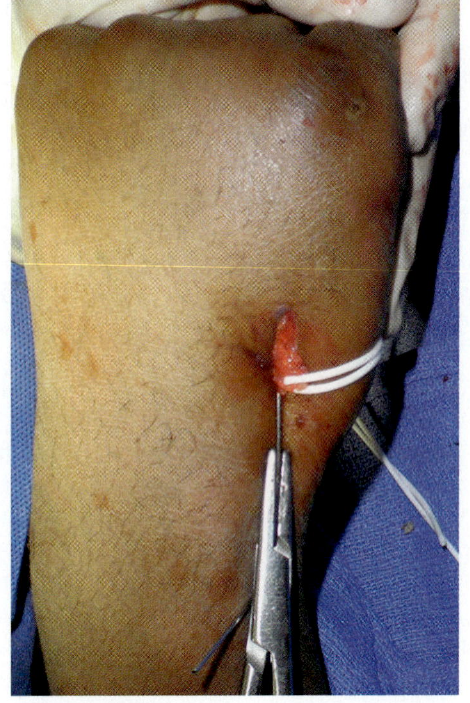

FIGURE 54-24

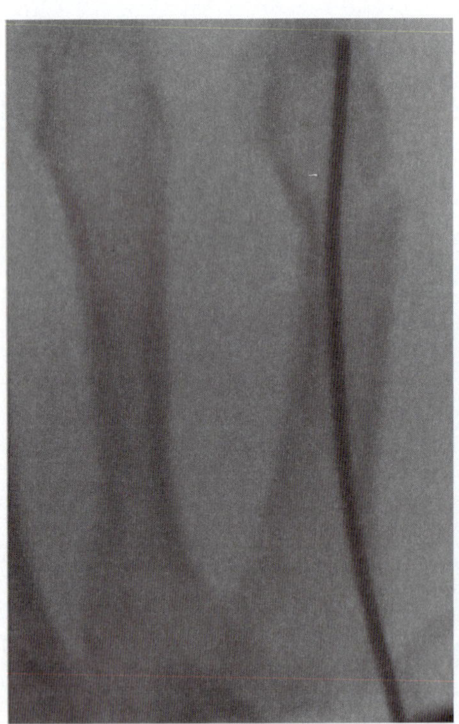

FIGURE 54-25

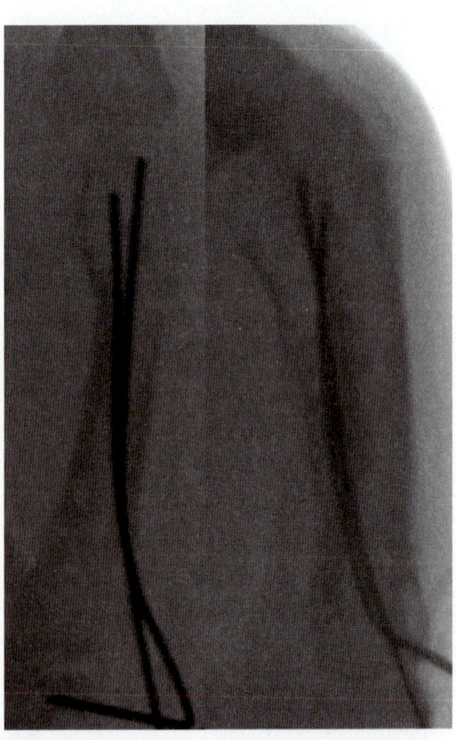

FIGURE 54-26

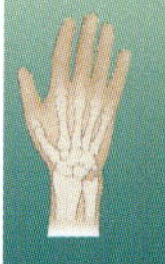

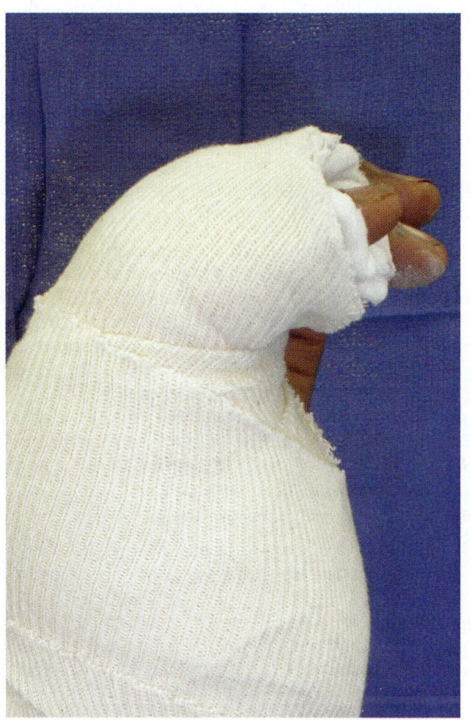

FIGURE 54-27

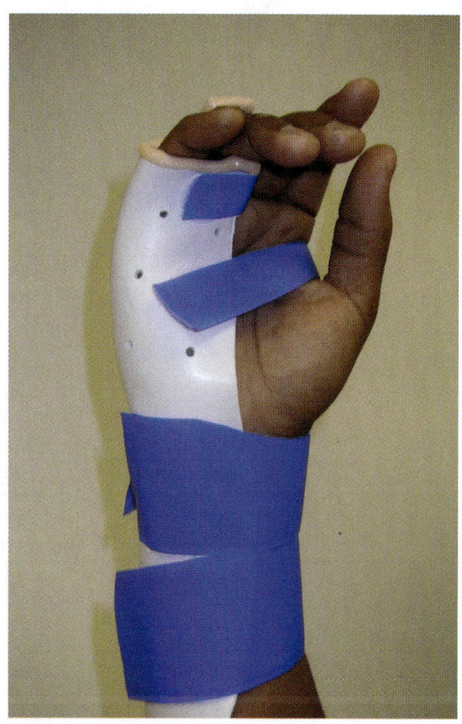

FIGURE 54-28

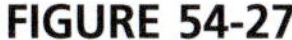

PEARLS

Attention to pain and edema control is essential in the early postoperative period.

Splinting with metacarpophalangeal joints is essential to prevent contracture.

Postoperative Care and Expected Outcomes

- The hand is rested in a splint for the first 5 to 7 days after surgery (Fig. 54-27).
- Following open reduction and plate fixation, active motion is commenced by the end of the first week after surgery. Between exercises, the hand is rested in a thermoplastic splint in a functional intrinsic-plus position (Fig. 54-28).
- If the fracture is treated with closed reduction and percutaneous fixation, the hand is immobilized in a cast for 3 weeks. Motion is started as described previously with a protective splint thereafter.
- Most patients can be expected to regain functional motion after about 6 weeks and nearly full range of motion by 3 months.
- Strengthening exercises are commenced after about 2 to 3 months when the fracture is nontender and the patient has satisfactory motion.

Evidence

Foucher G. "Bouquet" osteosynthesis in metacarpal neck fractures: a series of 66 patients. *J Hand Surg [Am]*. 1995;20:S86-S90.

This is a clinical series of 66 patients with follow-up of 4.5 years. It describes an open-technique anterograde intramedullary fixation of a fifth metacarpal fracture with two to three prebent Kirschner wires inserted into the reduced metacarpal head in divergent directions. All patients returned to full activity, with normal strength in 92% of cases, decreased by 11% in remaining 5 patients. MP extension lag averaged 12 degrees in 12 patients, and only 1 patient had related functional complaints. Disadvantages include removal of wires and possibility of wire protruding through the metacarpophalangeal joint or the dorsal fracture line. (Level V evidence)

Ouellette EA, Freeland AE. Use of the minicondylar plate in metacarpal and phalangeal fractures. *Clin Orthop Relat Res*. 1996;327:38-46.
This is a retrospective review of the treatment of 68 total fractures, 41 of which were metacarpal fractures: 12 proximal fractures, 12 shaft fractures, and 17 distal fractures. Open fractures were included in this study. Follow-up period was an average of 17 months. Range of motion was excellent in 52% and good/fair in 51% of the metacarpal fractures. All fractures went on to union, the infection rate was low (12% of all patients, including phalangeal fractures), and most complications were minor. (Level V evidence)

Schädel-Höpfner M, Wild M, Windolf J, Linhart W. Antegrade intramedullary splinting or percutaneous retrograde crossed pinning for displaced neck fractures of the fifth metacarpal? *Arch Orthop Trauma Surg*. 2007;127:435-440.
*Retrospective cohort clinical series of 30 patients with displaced fifth metacarpal neck fractures. Fifteen patients had antegrade intramedullary splinting, and 15 patients had retrograde percutaneous pinning. Median times for follow-up were 17 and 18 months, respectively. Range of motion of the fifth metacarphophalangeal joint was significantly (*P *= .016) decreased after retrograde pinning (−15 degrees; range, −45 to +5 degrees) compared with antegrade splinting (0 degrees; range, −25 to +10 degrees). VAS was significantly lower in antegrade pinning. Grip strength was equal and equivalent to the contralateral hand. (Level IV evidence)*

Wong TC, Ip FK, Yeung SH. Comparison between percutaneous transverse fixation and intramedullary K-wires in treating closed fractures of the metacarpal neck of the little finger. *J Hand Surg [Br]*. 2006;31:61-65.
Nonrandomized controlled clinical trial of 59 clinical cases to compare percutaneous transverse K-wire fixation and intramedullary K-wires in treating closed fifth metacarpal neck fractures with greater than 30 degrees of angulation. All patients were found to have radiologic union, and there were no statistically significant differences found with relation to range of motion, grip strength, or pain score with greater than 1 year follow-up. (Level IV evidence)

PROCEDURE 55

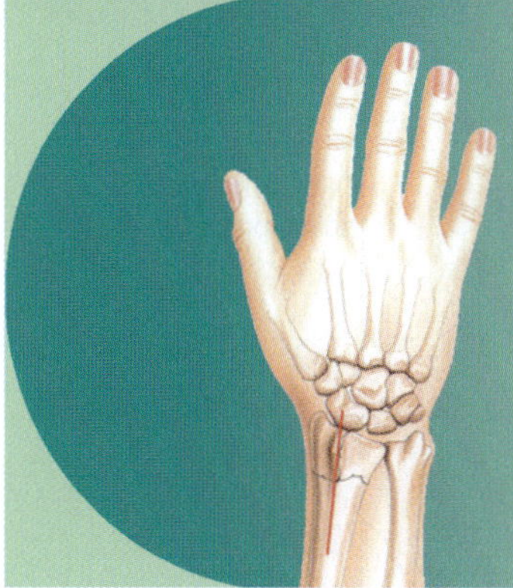

Metacarpal Shaft Fractures

Randy R. Bindra and Micah K. Sinclair

See Video 39: Metacarpal Shaft Fractures

Indications

- Displaced fracture
- Unstable fracture pattern (long spiral oblique)
- Multiple metacarpal fractures
- Angulation greater than 15 degrees
- Rotational deformity
- Shortening with loss of normal cascade
- Open injuries
- Polytrauma patient
- Early rehabilitation in the athlete

Examination/Imaging

Clinical Examination

- Note swelling and bruising over the dorsum of the hand.
- Multiple metacarpal fractures predispose to compartment syndrome of the hand.
- Look carefully for any wounds—may indicate an open fracture.
- Look carefully for rotational deformity with fingers flexed as much as possible and compare with opposite hand.
- Ensure circulation is adequate by checking capillary refill.
- Test and document digital sensation.
- Ask patient to flex and extend the interphalangeal joints within limits of pain to confirm continuity of flexor and extensor tendons.

Imaging

- Obtain posteroanterior, oblique, and true lateral films.
- Angulation must be measured against the dorsal cortex on a true lateral view.
- Shortening is assessed by evaluating alignment of the metacarpal heads—the distal ends of the small, ring, and long fingers form a straight line.

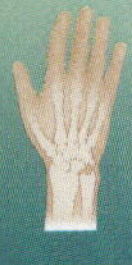

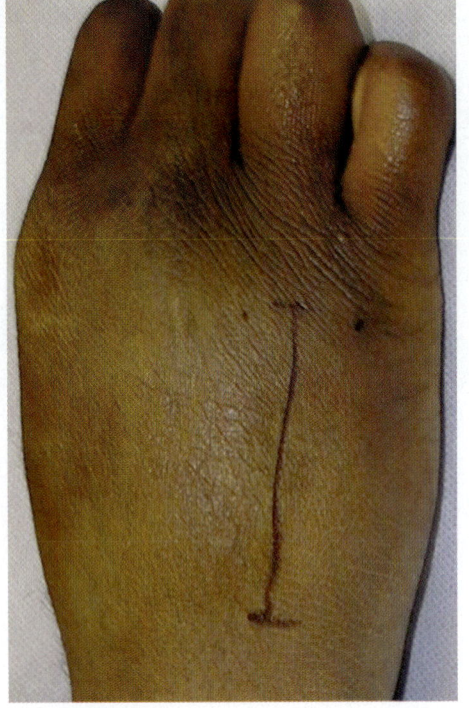

FIGURE 55-1

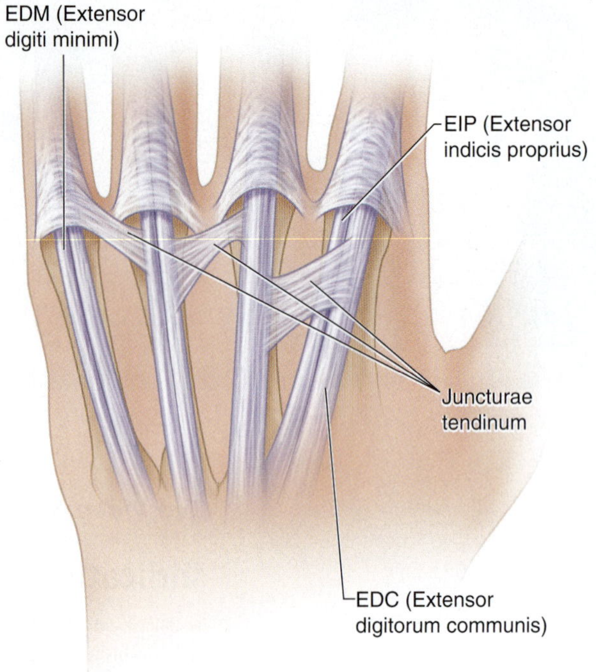

FIGURE 55-2

Surgical Anatomy

- Metacarpals can be easily accessed through the dorsal approach (Fig. 55-1).
- Dorsal cutaneous nerves and veins are located in the subcutaneous plane and must be identified and preserved.
- The extensor tendons are surrounded by paratenon and can be easily separated by dividing the juncturae tendinum that interconnect them at the level of the metacarpal necks (Fig. 55-2).

POSITIONING EQUIPMENT

Intraoperative imaging is critical in this procedure. The mini C-arm is draped sterilely and placed at the axillary side of the table and is brought in when needed during the case.

Positioning

- The patient is positioned supine with the arm on a hand table.
- The surgeon is seated on the cephalad side of the table with the forearm pronated to allow access to the dorsum of the hand.
- A tourniquet is used for the procedure.

Exposures

- A longitudinal incision is marked along the dorsum of the metacarpal. The incision is centered over the fracture and equals the length of the plate.
- In open injuries, the open wound is incorporated in the incision and excised as needed.
- For fixation of multiple fractures, two incisions on the dorsum in the second and fourth web space will provide access to adjacent metacarpals and allow decompression of the interosseous compartments if needed. Alternatively, a transverse incision across the back of the hand may be used as an extension of a preexisting traumatic wound (Fig. 55-3).
- After spreading dissection, the extensors are exposed and retracted (Fig. 55-4).
- The periosteum at the fracture site is elevated circumferentially to allow accurate reduction and remove any interposed soft tissue.

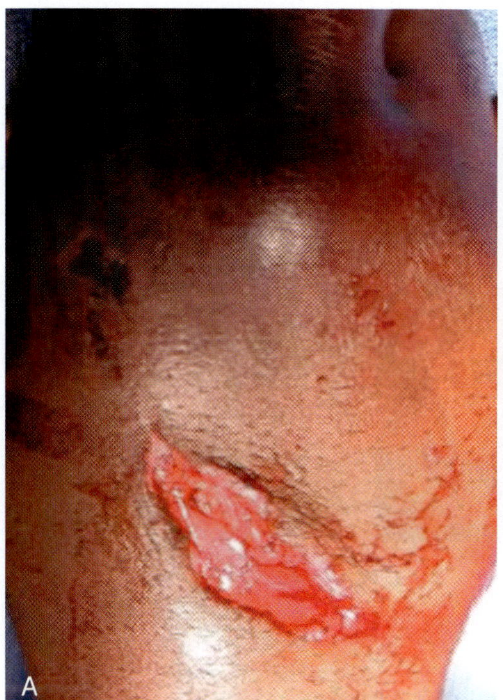

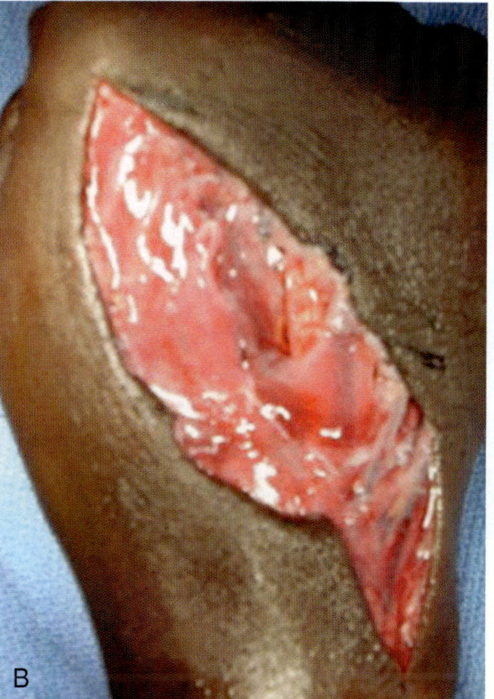

FIGURE 55-3

PEARLS

For plating of adjacent metacarpals, a single skin incision between the metacarpals will allow access to both fractures (Fig. 55-5).

Careful spreading dissection is necessary after skin incision to preserve subcutaneous nerves and veins.

Paratenon around the extensor tendons must be preserved to minimize postoperative tendon adhesions.

Juncturae tendinum between tendons may need to be divided to facilitate retraction of the extensor tendons.

In case of excessive comminution, periosteum around the fracture is left intact, and the implant is secured distally and proximally. Figure 55-6 shows the bridge plating technique used in a comminuted metacarpal fracture due to a gunshot wound.

PITFALLS

Injury to cutaneous nerves.

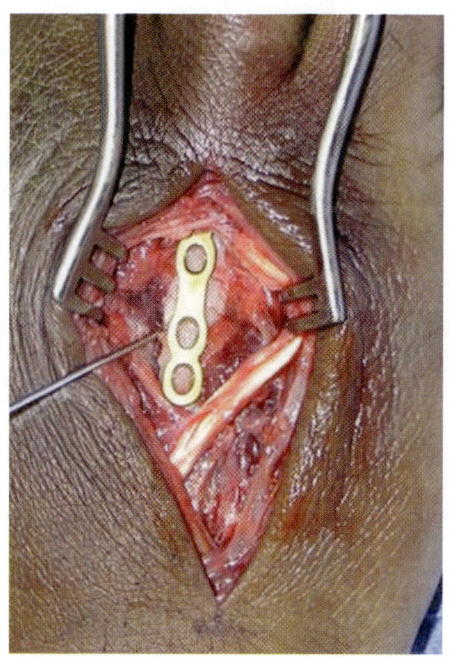

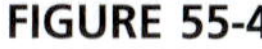

FIGURE 55-4

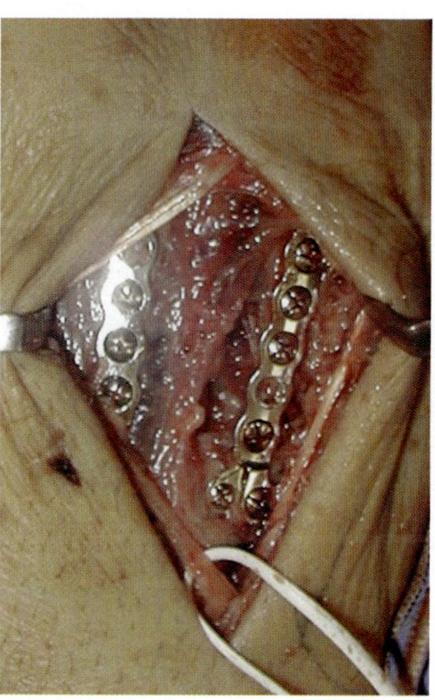

FIGURE 55-5

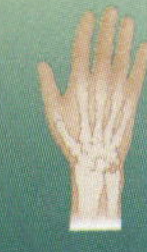

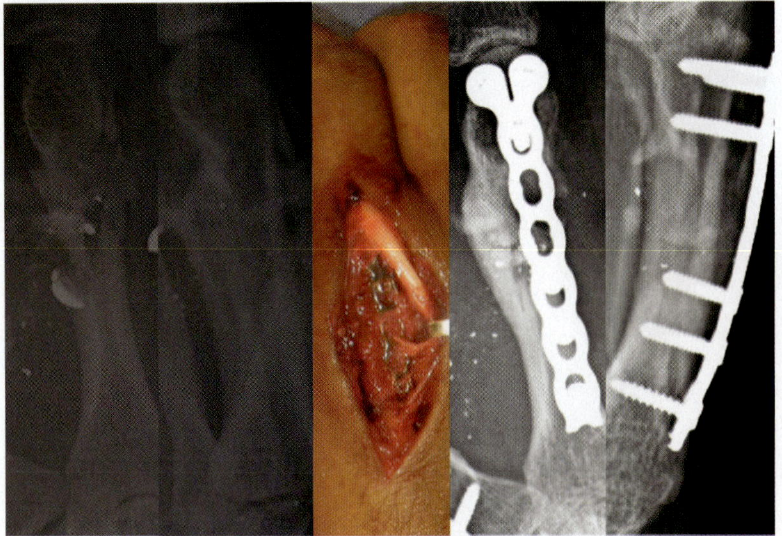

FIGURE 55-6

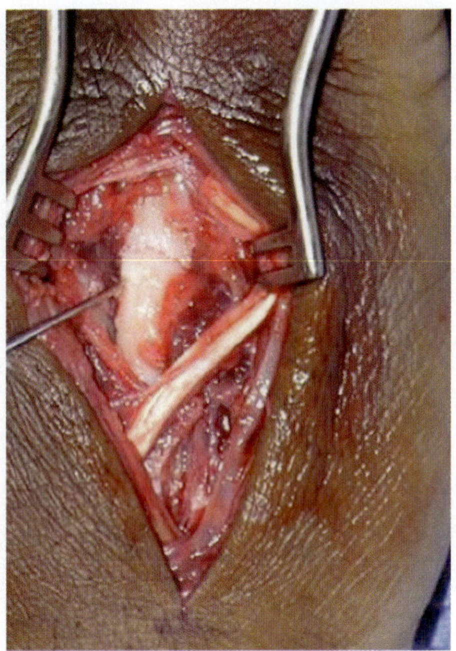

FIGURE 55-7

Procedure

Step 1: Principles and Methods of Fixation

- In oblique and spiral fractures, achieve provisional reduction and stabilize with a K-wire (Fig. 55-7).
- Temporary fixation of transverse fractures is not usually possible. After a trial reduction is performed, proceed with fixation of the plate to one fragment.
- Type of fixation depends on the fracture geometry.
- Transverse fractures are treated with compression plating (Fig. 55-8).
- Short oblique fractures are held with reduction forceps and stabilized with a lag screw. The fixation is then reinforced with a contoured plate without additional compression through the plate (neutralization plate). If the plane of the fracture allows insertion of the lag screw through the plate, this is preferred.
- For insertion of a lag screw, first drill the thread hole through both cortices. Then drill near the cortex with a lag hole and countersink near the cortex. Countersinking minimizes the risk for fracture of the near cortex when the screw is tightened by distributing force more evenly the around screw hole. Screw length is measured and the appropriate screw inserted.
- Long oblique and spiral fractures that are longer than two times the diameter of the bone are stabilized with a series of lag screws. Plating is not necessary (Fig. 55-9).
- When multiple lag screws are to be placed, generally the smaller fragment is lagged to the larger piece.

STEP 1 PEARLS

Initial stabilizing K-wire is helpful in fractures in which anatomic reduction is possible.

In the face of comminution, the proximal shaft fragment is stabilized with the plate first, and then the metacarpal is distracted to its correct length and rotation before fixation to the distal fragment.

STEP 1 PITFALLS

In a short oblique fracture, the lag screw placement interferes with plate placement. If the fracture is in the coronal plane, the plate is fixed to bone first, and then the lag screw is passed through the plate.

Avoid aggressive countersinking of the near cortex using powered instruments to prevent weakening the cortex.

Placing a screw too close to the fracture line may result in additional comminution. Stay at least two screw head diameters away from the fracture line.

Step 2: Dynamic Compression Plate

- A transverse diaphyseal fracture without comminution is best treated with compression plating.
- A dynamic compression plate of adequate length is selected to ensure a minimum fixation of four cortices (two screws) on either side of the fracture.
- The plate is prebent slightly so that it stands off the fracture by 2 mm to ensure that the far cortex does not gap when compression is applied.

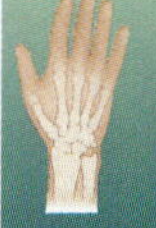

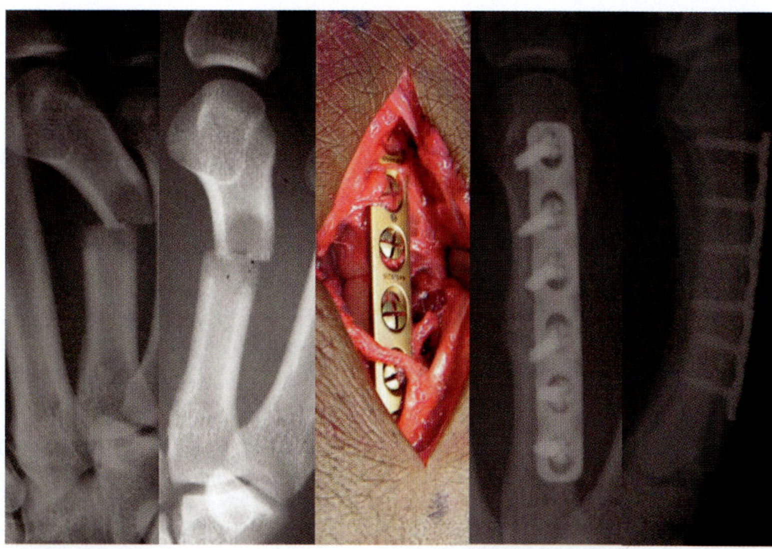

FIGURE 55-8

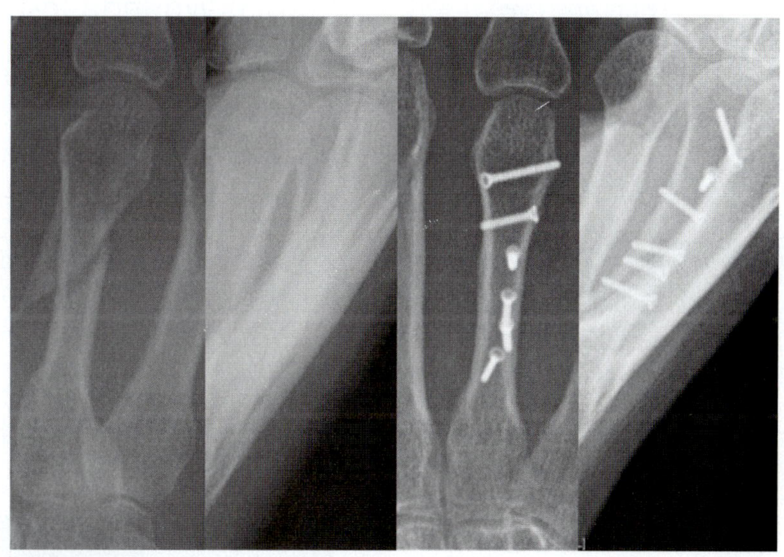

FIGURE 55-9

STEP 2 PEARLS

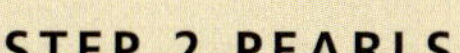

- Ensure that the plate is aligned with the shaft before fixation.
- Use a drill guide to make all drill holes to ensure that the neutral and compression holes are drilled accurately.
- To achieve added compression, compression holes can be drilled on either side of the fracture.

STEP 2 PITFALLS

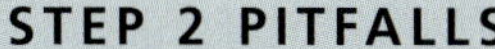

Failure to prebend the plate will result in gapping at the fracture site at the opposite surface. If this situation occurs, it can be addressed with insertion of cancellous bone graft into the gap.

Inaccurate drilling of screw holes can result in distraction at the fracture when the screws are fully seated.

Axial compression with eccentric screw placement is not possible if done later in the fixation because the fragments already are fixed rigidly to the plate.

- The oval holes in the plate enable application of compression as the screws are tightened.
- A trial reduction is first performed, and then the plate is fixed to one fragment with a single screw close to the fracture site. The screw is drilled and inserted in the center of the drill hole.
- The plate is then aligned with the long axis of the bone, and the opposite fragment is fixed. Using an eccentric drill guide, the drill hole for the screw is made at the edge of the oval hole away from the fracture.
- As the screw is inserted and centers within the plate hole, it moves the fragment closer to the fracture, thereby compressing the fracture by about 1 mm.
- The remaining screws are then drilled in the center of each hole (neutral position).

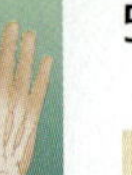

STEP 3 PEARLS

When seating the plate, position plate holes carefully—avoid leaving an empty hole alongside the fracture, which creates a weak spot for potential failure.

If a lag screw through the plate is planned, position the plate to ensure that a hole is situated at the optimal spot for lag screw insertion.

STEP 3 PITFALLS

When placing a lag screw across the fracture for compression, failure to drill near the cortex with a gliding hole may result in distraction rather than compression.

STEP 4 PEARLS

Once compression is achieved, care must be taken to insert the remaining screws in neutral position (center of hole) to avoid inadvertent distraction.

STEP 4 PITFALLS

The lag screw may get stripped if adjacent screws are not inserted in neutral mode and may distract the fracture.

STEP 5 PEARLS

If preoperative swelling is minimal, subcuticular closure may be performed.

STEP 5 PITFALLS

Failure to release the tourniquet and secure hemostasis may result in a hematoma postoperatively.

Step 3: Neutralization Plate

- A neutralization plate is applied after initial fracture compression with a lag screw.
- If the lag screw is to be applied through the dorsal surface of the metacarpal for a coronal fracture, the plate is applied first, and the lag screw is inserted through the plate hole.
- The neutralization plate is contoured to adapt exactly to the dorsal surface of the bone. No prebending is necessary because the lag screw will prevent fracture distraction at the far cortex.
- All screws must be inserted through the center of each hole to avoid inadvertent distraction at the fracture and stripping of the lag screw.
- The screws farthest from the fracture are inserted first to ensure alignment of the plate with the bone.
- If a lag screw is to be inserted through the plate, it is done after initial stabilization of the plate and before completion of fixation.

Step 4: Completion of Fixation

- Remaining screws are inserted.
- Radiographs are obtained to confirm that the fracture is reduced and compressed and the screw lengths are correct.
- The fingers are moved passively to ensure full range and to confirm rotational alignment.

Step 5: Wound Closure

- The tourniquet is released, and hemostasis is secured.
- Juncturae tendinum are repaired if required using nonabsorbable sutures.
- Skin edges are approximated with interrupted sutures.

Additional Steps

- Transverse pinning of a metacarpal shaft fracture is an alternative treatment for fractures that can be reduced by closed manipulation (Fig. 55-10).
- Fractures are usually angulated with the apex dorsal.
- Reduction is achieved by closing the fingers into a fist and stabilizing the hand with all digits in corrected rotation. A dorsally directed force is applied to the flexed proximal interphalangeal joint to push the distal metacarpal fragment dorsally.
- Reduction is achieved by resolution of the palpable bump and confirmed with an image intensifier.

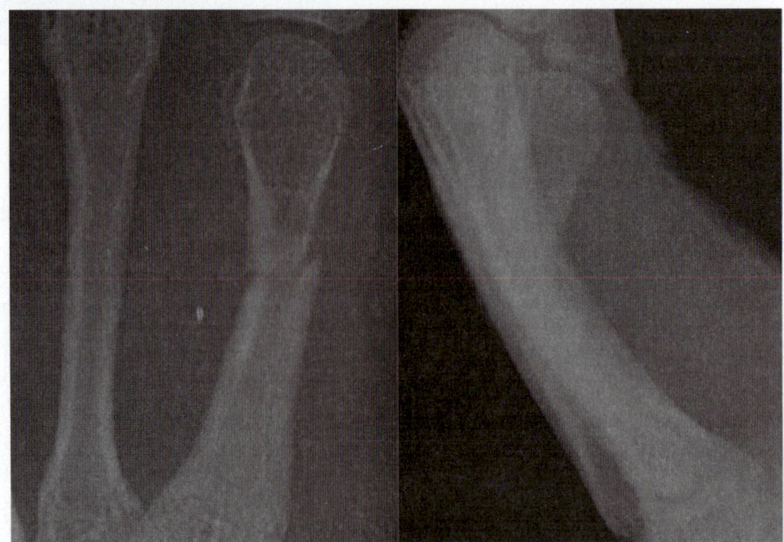

FIGURE 55-10

PEARLS

Attention to pain and edema control is essential in the early postoperative period.

Splinting with metacarpophalangeal joints in flexion is essential to prevent contracture.

When passing K-wire, it is important to count the number of cortices drilled to avoid incorrect trajectory of the K-wire. It should be confirmed that four cortices are passed and the K-wire stops at the outer cortex of the next intact metacarpal (fifth cortex).

PITFALLS

The tip of the K-wire, if it is not abutting the cortex of the adjacent (fifth cortex) metacarpal, may migrate.

PEARLS

Pain and edema control are essential in the immediate postoperative period.

Resting the hand with the metaphalangeal joint in flexion will prevent extension-contracture of the joint.

- With the surgeon holding the patient's fingers in a closed fist with one hand, wires are introduced with the other.
- A stab incision for each K-wire is made over the subcutaneous border of the metacarpal shaft (ulnar for small finger and radial border of hand for index finger), followed by blunt dissection.
- Using a power driver, a K-wire is inserted transversely from the ulnar side of the small finger into the ring finger metacarpal close to the metaphalangeal joint. The wire is stopped at the ulnar cortex of the long finger metacarpal. Reduction and wire position are checked with imaging. Rotational alignment of the digit is checked again.
- Two pins are inserted distal to the fracture site, and a third is inserted proximal to the fracture (Fig. 55-11).
- Each K-wire should capture both cortices of the injured and neighboring uninjured metacarpal and abut against the next metacarpal shaft. The K-wire should go through four cortices and stop at the next intact one (Fig. 55-12). This will prevent late migration of the wire and ensure easy retrieval of the wires after 3 weeks.
- Maintenance of reduction and pin placement are confirmed fluoroscopically.
- K-wires are cut short and bent outside the skin for removal in the clinic.

Postoperative Care and Expected Outcomes

- The hand is rested in a plaster splint for the first 5 to 7 days after surgery.
- Following open reduction and plate fixation, active motion is commenced by the end of the first week after surgery. Between exercises, the injured digit and adjacent finger are immobilized in a thermoplastic splint in a functional intrinsic-plus position.

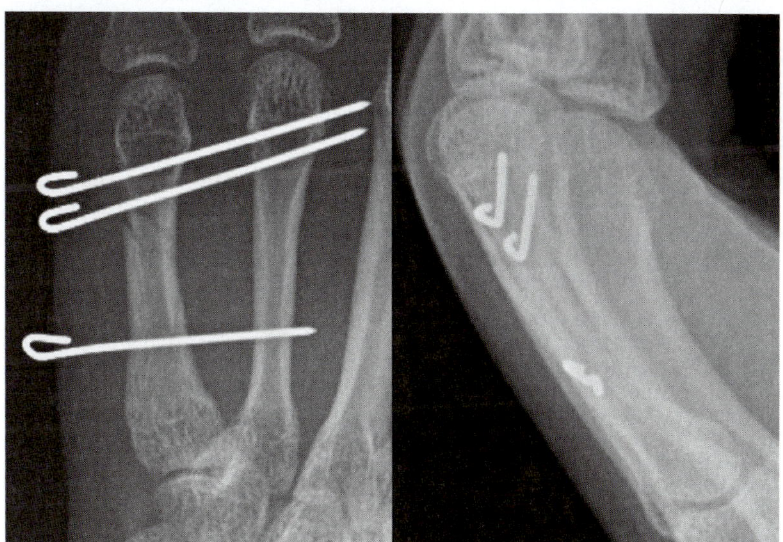

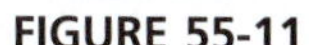
FIGURE 55-11

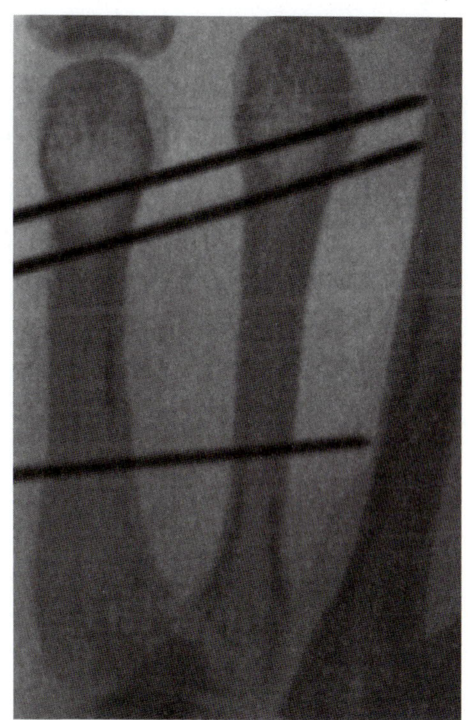

FIGURE 55-12

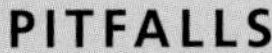

PITFALLS

Aggressive motion in the face of pain and swelling in the immediate postoperative period will only exacerbate symptoms and lose patient cooperation.

- If the fracture is treated with closed reduction and percutaneous fixation, the hand is immobilized in a cast for 3 weeks, with the concern that this mode of fixation is not rigid enough to initiate active motion within 1 week. Motion is started as described previously with a protective splint thereafter. The K-wires are removed in the clinic after 3 weeks.
- Most patients can be expected to regain functional motion after about 6 weeks and nearly full range of motion by 3 months.
- Strengthening exercises are commenced after about 2 to 3 months when the fracture is nontender and the patient has satisfactory motion.

Evidence

Fusetti C, Meyer H, Borisch N, et al. Complications of plate fixation in metacarpal fractures. *J Trauma*. 2002;52:535-539.
Retrospective review of 81 patients with 104 extra-articular finger metacarpal fractures treated with open reduction and plate fixation according to AO technique. Follow-up interval was an average of 13.6 months. Surgical indications included fractures that were unstable, open, multiple, or associated with multiple injuries, or additional fractures on ipsilateral extremity. Plates used included straight plates, T plates, and condylar plates. They found that 32% of fractures treated with open reduction and plating had at least one complication. Nineteen percent of patients had one or more major complications, including nonunion, stiffness, plate loosening, CPRS, and infection. Sixteen percent of patients had one or more minor complications. None could be correlated with the type of plate or fracture morphology. All were correctable. (Level V evidence)

Omokawa S, Fujitani R, Dohi Y, et al. Prospective outcomes of comminuted periarticular metacarpal and phalangeal fractures treated using a titanium plate system. *J Hand Surg [Am]*. 2008;33:857-863.
This is a prospective study with 51 patients with isolated comminuted metaphyseal, metacarpal, or phalangeal fractures and a 1-year follow-up period. Open fractures were included in this study. Twelve patients with metacarpal fractures achieved 91% of total active motion (TAM). Decreased TAM had significant correlation to patient age and intra-articular fracture. Grip strength was 87% of the contralateral uninjured side postoperatively. All fractures went on to union. Plates were removed from 30 patients owing to discomfort, joint stiffness, infection, and hardware breakage. (Level IV evidence)

Ouellette EA, Freeland AE. Use of the minicondylar plate in metacarpal and phalangeal fractures. *Clin Orthop Relat Res*. 1996;327:38-46.
Retrospective review of the treatment of 68 total fractures, 41 of which were metacarpal fractures: 12 proximal fractures, 12 shaft fractures, and 17 distal fractures. Open fractures were included in this study. Follow-up period was an average of 17 months. Range of motion was excellent in 52% and good/fair in 51% of the metacarpal fractures. All fractures went on to union, the infection rate was low (12% of all patients, including phalangeal fractures), and most complications were minor. (Level V evidence)

Page SM, Stern PJ. Complications and range of motion following plate fixation of metacarpal and phalangeal fractures. *J Hand Surg [Am]*. 1998;23:827-832.
Retrospective review of open reduction and internal fixation of metacarpal and/or phalangeal fractures over an 8-year period that included 66 metacarpal fractures. Surgical indications used for plate fixation included multiple fractures, open fractures with soft tissue damage, unstable fractures, bone loss, and malalignment. Thirty-six percent of patients with metacarpal fractures experienced complications, half of which were major, which included four cases of extensor lag/stiffness greater than 35 degrees and five cases of major contracture greater than 35 degrees. Plate fixation yielded a total active motion of greater than 220 degrees in 76% of fractures. Higher complication rates were associated with open fractures, periarticular fractures, and use of minicondylar plates. (Level V evidence)

Soeur JS, Mudgal CS. Plate fixation in closed ipsilateral multiple metacarpal fractures. *J Hand Surg [Br]*. 2008;33:740-744.
Retrospective review of 19 patients with 43 displaced and/or angulated multiple metacarpal fractures treated by early open reduction and internal fixation with 2-mm plates. Eighteen patients recovered full range of motion within 2 months of surgery; 1 patient was lost to follow-up. Implant removal was performed in two metacarpals in 2 patients, owing to extensor tenosynovitis or inhibited adjacent joint range of motion, resulting in complete resolution of symptoms. (Level V evidence)

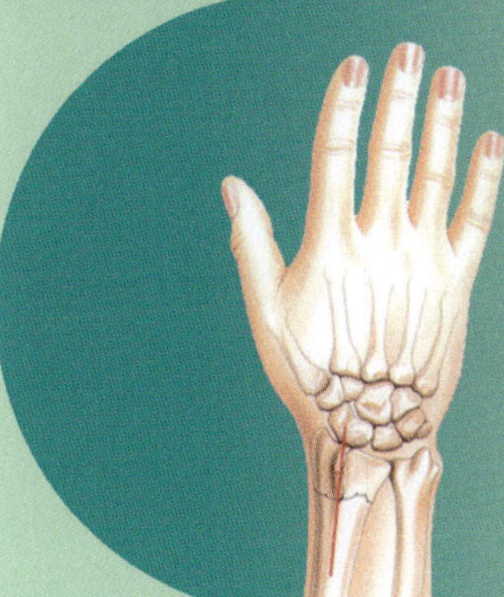

PROCEDURE 56

Percutaneous Pinning of Bennett Fracture and Open Reduction and Internal Fixation of Rolando Fracture

Douglas Sammer

Indications

- If the fracture is nondisplaced at initial presentation (uncommon), it can be treated with splint or cast immobilization for 6 weeks, followed by protected motion.
- Surgery is indicated for failure to maintain acceptable reduction with splint or cast (articular step-off of <1 mm).
- Most Bennett and Rolando fractures are unstable and require surgical intervention.
- In most cases, closed reduction and percutaneous pinning is indicated for Bennett fractures.
- Open reduction is indicated when reduction cannot be achieved by closed means (more common with Rolando fracture).
- If open reduction is required, large fragments can be fixated by a variety of methods (plate, lag screw, percutaneous K-wires), whereas small fragments are best treated with K-wire fixation.

Examination/Imaging

Clinical Examination

- Standard sensory, motor, and vascular examination of the thumb
- Examination for lacerations that may indicate open fracture

Imaging

- Three view radiographs of the thumb: anteroposterior (Robert's view), lateral, and oblique
- Computed tomography rarely indicated

Surgical Anatomy

- A Bennett fracture is a two-fragment intra-articular thumb metacarpal base fracture.
- A Rolando fracture is a three-fragment intra-articular thumb metacarpal base fracture.
- The thumb carpometacarpal (CMC) joint geometry is similar to two interlocking saddles, with their surfaces at 90 degrees to each other.
- The volar beak ligament is deep to the superficial anterior oblique ligament (SAOL) and is an important stabilizer of the thumb CMC joint.

Figures 56-9 through 56-11 provided courtesy of Kevin C. Chung, MD; Figures 56-14 through 56-17 provided courtesy of Sandeep J. Sebastin, MD.

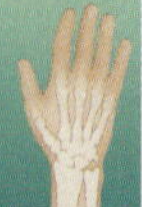

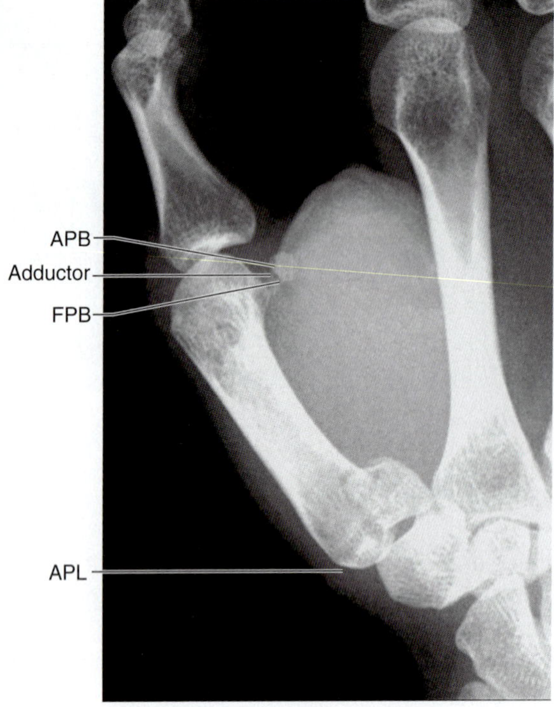

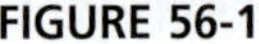

FIGURE 56-1

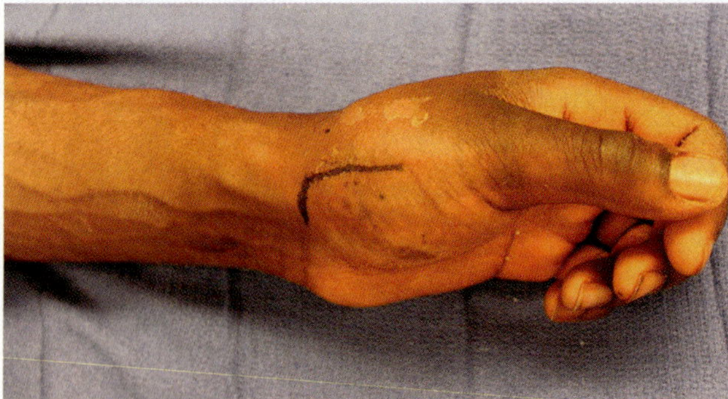

FIGURE 56-2

- In a Bennett fracture, the volar beak ligament stabilizes the Bennett fragment, which is located volarly and ulnarly.
- The larger fragment, consisting of the remainder of the metacarpal, must be reduced to the Bennett fragment.
- The abductor pollicis longus (APL) tendon inserts on the dorsal base of the thumb metacarpal and causes dorsal subluxation and proximal displacement of the metacarpal (Fig. 56-1).
- The adductor pollicis inserts on the metacarpal shaft and causes CMC flexion and adduction (see Fig. 56-1).
- In a Bennett fracture, the metacarpal is supinated, adducted, and flexed, with proximal displacement and dorsal subluxation of the base.

Positioning

- The patient is supine.
- A pneumatic tourniquet is placed on the arm in case closed reduction is not possible and open reduction is required.
- The extremity is placed on a hand table, with the thumb pointing upward.
- The surgeon or assistant placing the K-wires sits at the patient's axilla, facing the palm.
- The surgeon or assistant performing the reduction sits at the patient's shoulder, facing the dorsum of the hand.

Exposures

- If open reduction is required, the exposure is through a modified Wagner incision (Fig. 56-2).
- The longitudinal limb of the incision is along the glabrous/nonglabrous skin border.
- At the thumb base, the incision turns ulnarly and extends to the flexor carpi radialis (FCR) tendon.

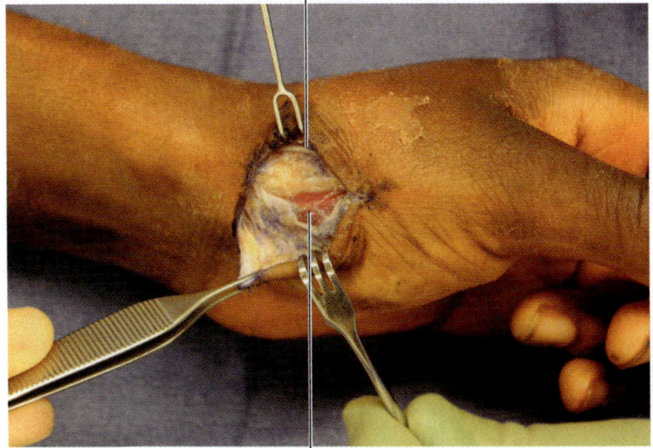

FIGURE 56-3

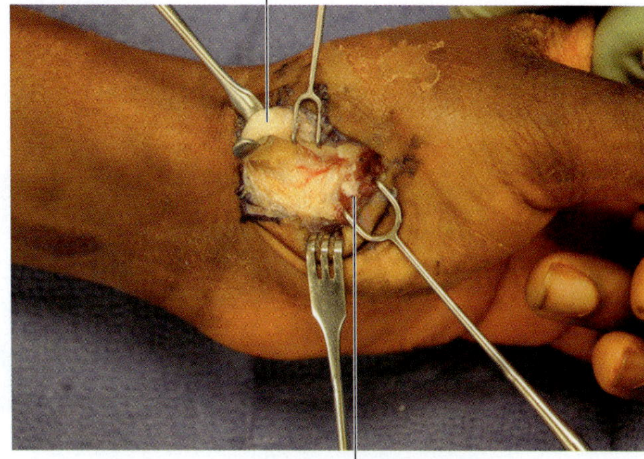

FIGURE 56-4

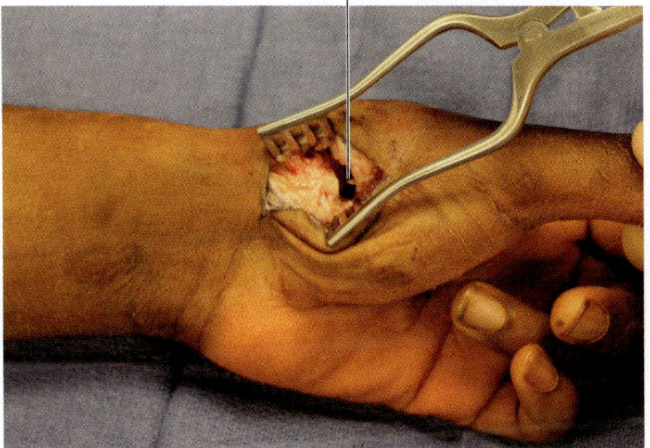

FIGURE 56-5

PEARLS

It is important not to extend the Wagner incision ulnar to the FCR tendon, to avoid injury to the palmar cutaneous branch of the median nerve.

It is important to protect sensory nerves, such as the superficial sensory branches of the radial nerve, and smaller branches of the lateral antebrachial cutaneous nerve (LABC).

Fluoroscopy can be used to confirm joint location before capsulotomy.

PITFALLS

Injury to the palmar cutaneous branch of the median nerve by extending the incision ulnar to the FCR.

Injury to the LABC or superficial sensory branch of the radial nerve.

Excessive soft tissue elevation at the metacarpal base resulting in disinsertion of the APL—care should be taken to preserve the APL insertion.

- Dissection is carried down to the border of the thenar musculature, protecting sensory nerve branches in the subcutaneous tissue (Fig. 56-3).
- A no. 15 blade is used to elevate the thenar muscles off of the metacarpal base and trapezium (Fig. 56-4).
- The APL tendon is reflected ulnarly.
- The joint is then exposed with a transverse capsulotomy, in the interval between the APL and the reflected thenar musculature (Fig. 56-5).

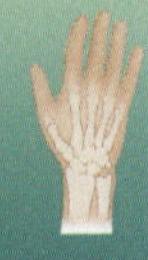

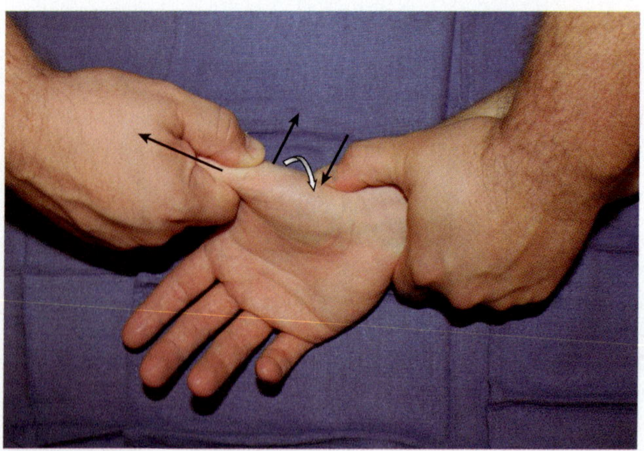

FIGURE 56-6

STEP 1 PEARLS

Fracture reduction should be checked in multiple planes and with live fluoroscopy to ensure correct reduction of articular surface.

STEP 2 PEARLS

- If placing the initial K-wire while maintaining fracture reduction proves difficult, the K-wire can be placed into the metacarpal base, but not across the fracture, with the fracture unreduced.
- Once the K-wire is in position, the fracture is reduced, and the K-wire is advanced across the fracture and into the Bennett fragment.
- K-wires should be advanced using oscillating mode on the K-wire driver, to avoid injury to sensory nerve branches.

Procedures

Closed Reduction Percutaneous Pinning of Bennett Fracture

Step 1

- The Bennett fracture is reduced by radial abduction of the thumb metacarpal, longitudinal traction and pronation of the thumb metacarpal, and direct pressure applied to the dorsal base of the metacarpal (Fig. 56-6).
- Reduction is checked with fluoroscopy.

Step 2

- While reduction is maintained, K-wires are placed.
- Multiple patterns of K-wire fixation are acceptable (Fig. 56-7); the author's preference follows.
  - A 0.045-inch K-wire is advanced across the fracture, entering the radial base of the thumb metacarpal and terminating in the Bennett fragment.
  - A second 0.045-inch K-wire is placed between the thumb and index metacarpals (Fig. 56-8).

Alternative 1

- A 0.045-inch K-wire is inserted into the thumb metacarpal shaft, beginning at the middle or distal third.
- It is advanced proximally down the medullary canal and across the CMC joint into the trapezium.
- The leading tip of the K-wire should enter the subchondral bone of the proximal trapezium, without entering the scaphotrapezial joint (Fig. 56-9).

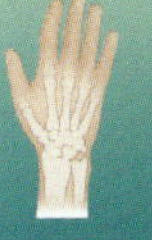

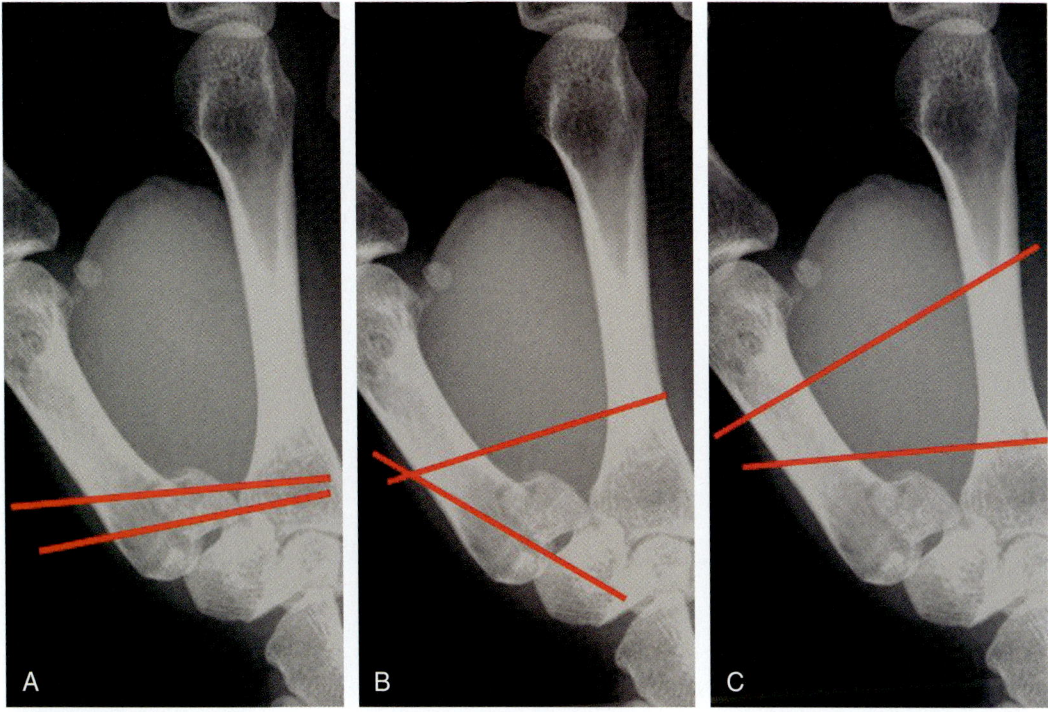

FIGURE 56-7

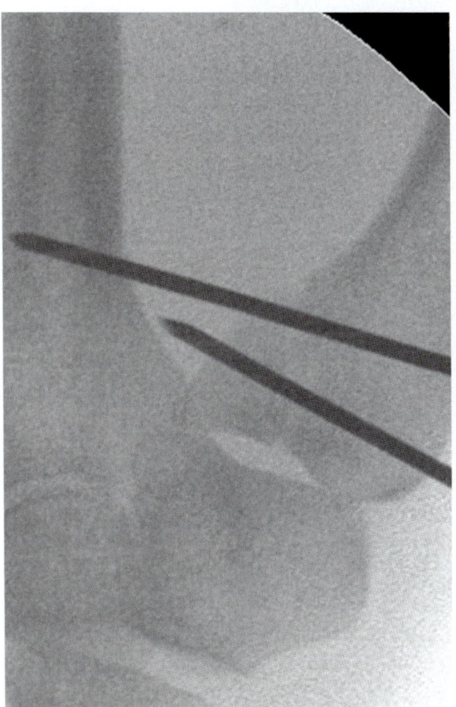

FIGURE 56-8

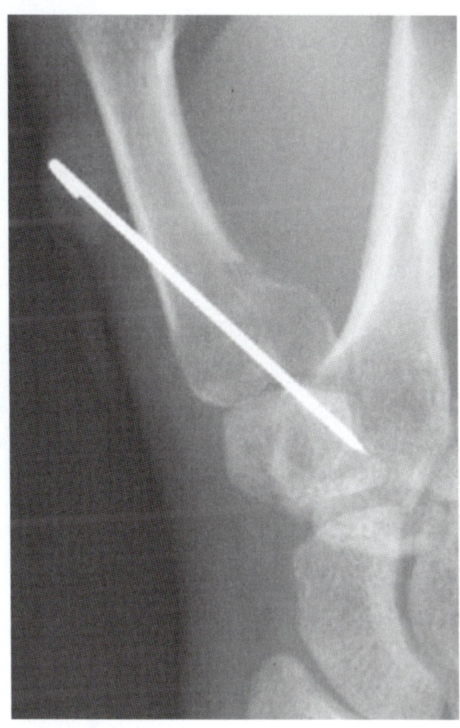

FIGURE 56-9

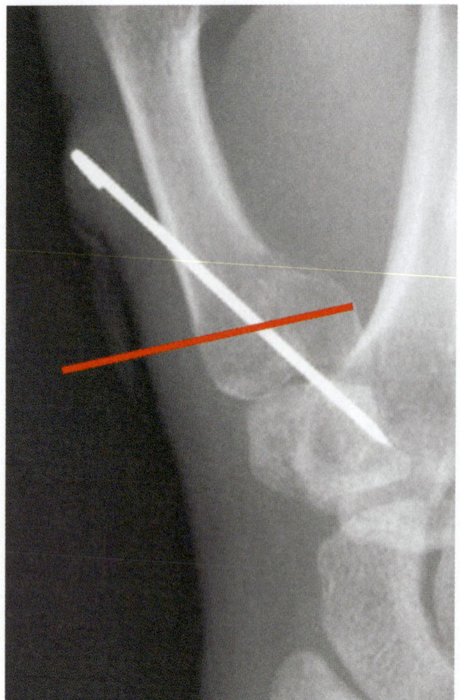

FIGURE 56-10

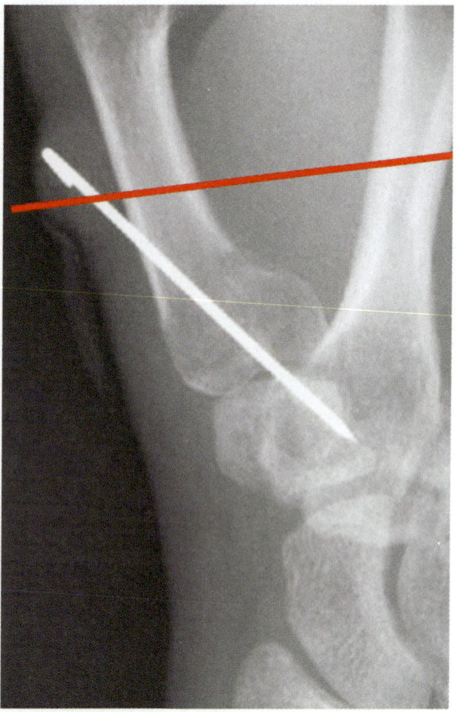

FIGURE 56-11

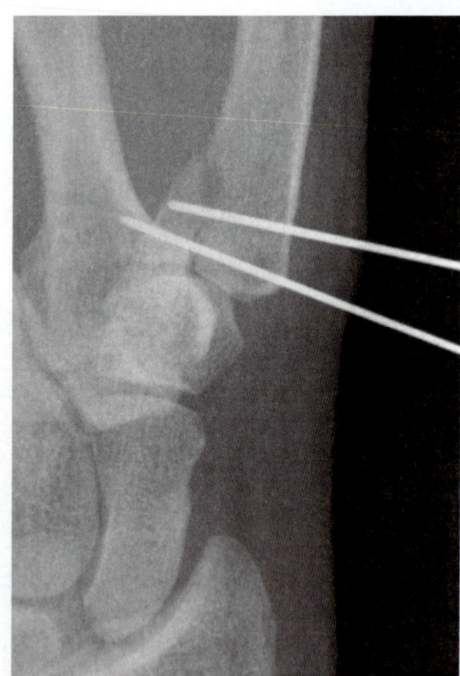

FIGURE 56-12

- The second K-wire is then advanced from the radial metacarpal base, across the fracture, and into the Bennett fragment (Fig. 56-10).
- Alternatively, it can be placed from the thumb metacarpal into the index metacarpal (Fig. 56-11).

Alternative 2

- Two 0.045-inch K-wires are advanced from the radial metacarpal base, across the fracture, and into the Bennett fragment (Fig. 56-12).

Step 3

- Final images are taken to confirm fracture reduction and K-wire position.
- K-wires are cut and capped.
- A forearm-based thumb spica splint is applied, with the interphalangeal joint free.

Postoperative Care and Expected Outcomes

- Pins are removed 6 weeks after surgery.
- Mobilization is begun 6 weeks after surgery under the guidance of a hand therapist.
- Posttraumatic arthritis may develop, particularly if articular reduction is not achieved. This may or may not be clinically significant.
- Radiographic and clinical outcomes are likely superior in patients who heal with less than 1 mm of articular step-off.

Open Reduction and Percutaneous Pinning of Bennett Fracture

Step 1

- The fracture is reduced by the reduction maneuver described previously, combined with direct fragment manipulation.
- Either 0.035- or 0.045-inch K-wires can be used as joysticks if necessary.
- Fracture reduction may be maintained with a bone-reduction clamp.

Step 2

- While visualizing the reduced articular surface, percutaneous K-wires are placed for fracture fixation (Fig. 56-13).

Step 3

- K-wires are cut and capped.
- A volar forearm-based thumb spica splint is placed, with the interphalangeal joint free.

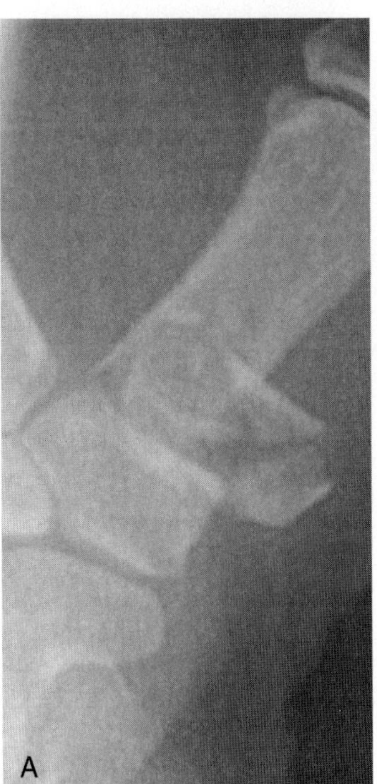

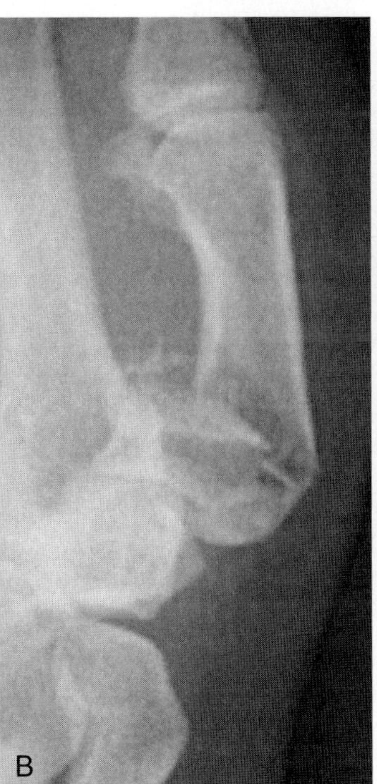

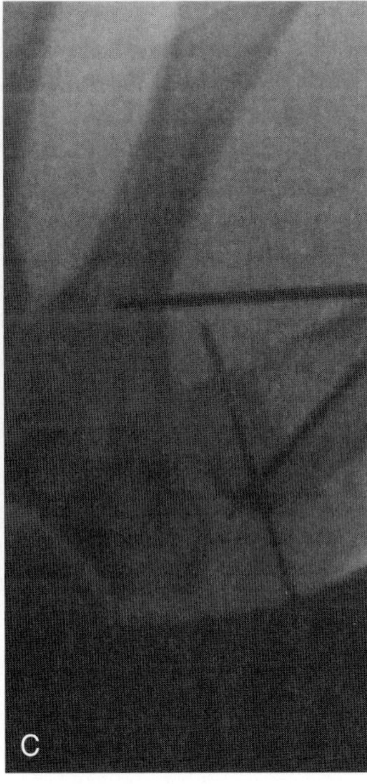

FIGURE 56-13

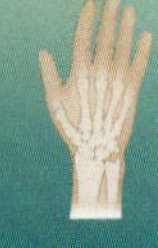

Postoperative Care and Expected Outcomes

- Pins are removed 6 weeks after surgery.
- Mobilization is begun 6 weeks after surgery under the guidance of a hand therapist.
- Posttraumatic arthritis may develop, particularly if articular reduction is not achieved. This may or may not be clinically significant.
- Radiographic and clinical outcomes are superior in patients who heal with less than a 1-mm step-off.

Open Reduction and Internal Fixation of Rolando Fracture

Step 1

- Fracture is exposed as described previously (Fig. 56-14).

Step 2

- Fracture is reduced as described previously, and reduction is maintained with a bone reduction clamp or piercing towel clamp (Fig. 56-15).

Step 3

- A T- or Y-shaped plate is placed across the fracture and secured with bicortical screws (Figs. 56-16 and 56-17).

STEP 3 PEARLS

Locking screws may be used in metaphyseal bone, where the cortex is thin.

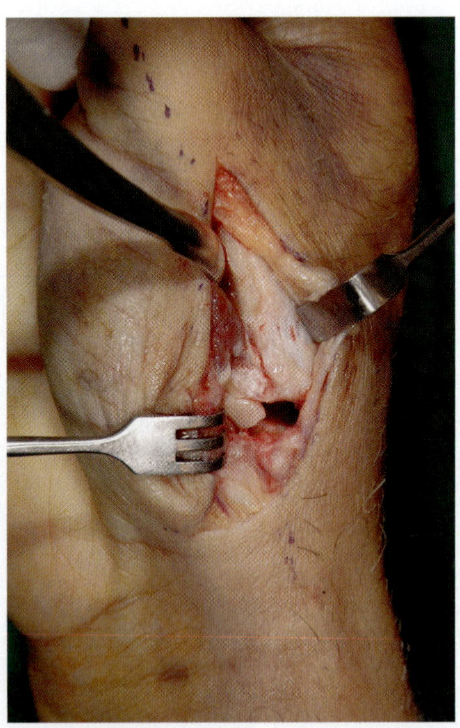

FIGURE 56-14

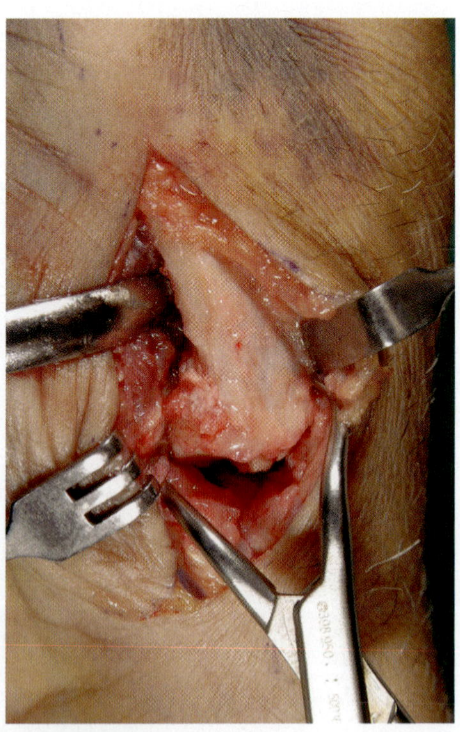

FIGURE 56-15

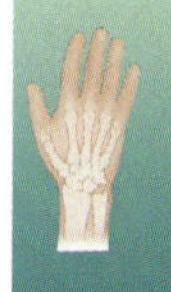

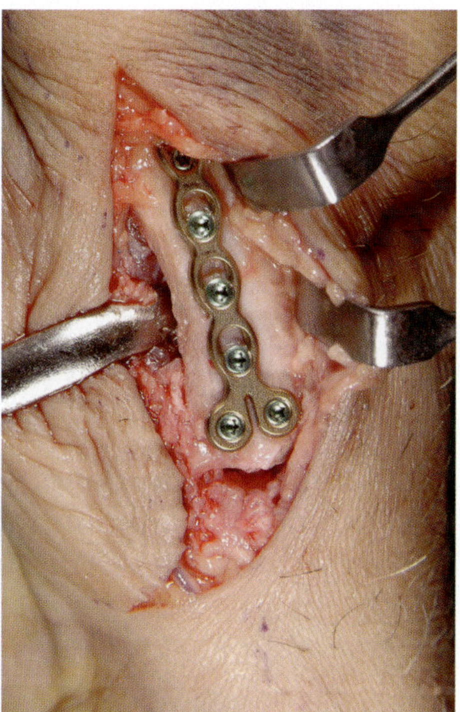

FIGURE 56-16

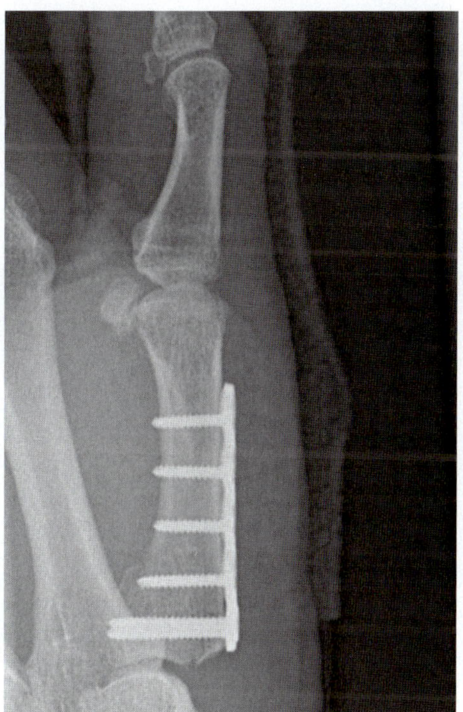

FIGURE 56-17

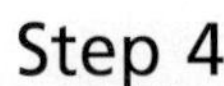

Step 4

- The skin is closed with simple interrupted sutures.
- A sterile dressing is applied, followed by a forearm-based thumb spica splint.
- The interphalangeal joint may be left free.

Postoperative Care and Expected Outcomes

- Sutures are removed in 10 to 14 days, and an Orthoplast splint is made.
- Active range of motion begins at 10 to 14 days, and passive range of motion when tolerated.
- Strengthening begins at 6 weeks.
- Good outcomes are expected if the fracture heals with acceptable articular reduction (step-off of <1 mm).

Open Reduction and Percutaneous Pinning of Comminuted Thumb Metacarpal Base Fracture

Step 1

- Preoperative imaging is obtained, which demonstrates a comminuted intra-articular thumb metacarpal base fracture (Figs. 56-18 and 56-19).

Step 2

- Exposure of the fracture is performed as described previously (see Figs. 56-2 through 56-5).

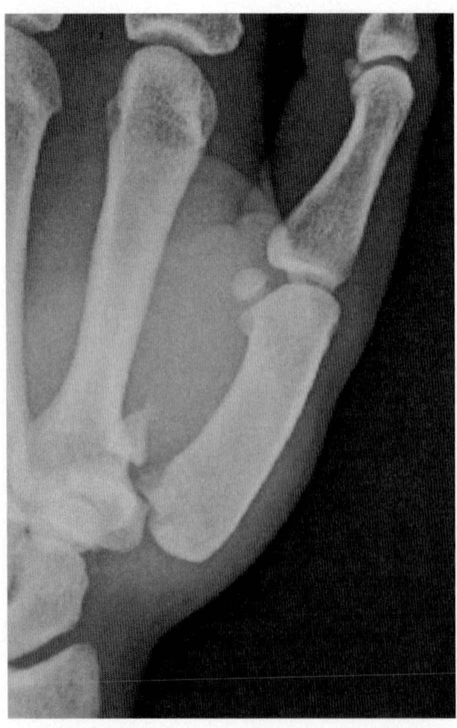

FIGURE 56-18

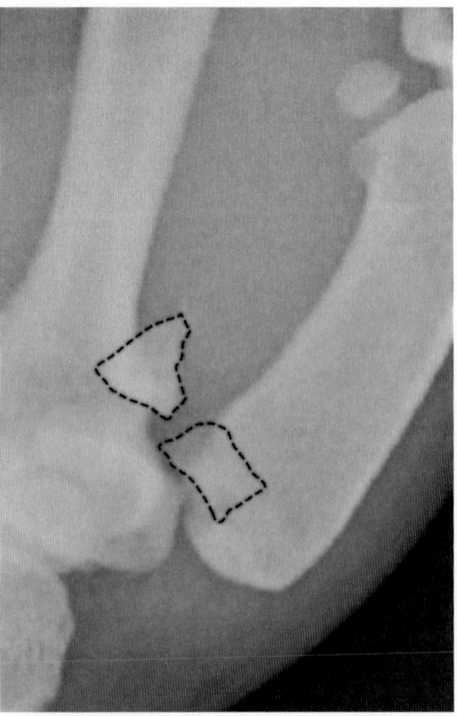

FIGURE 56-19

Step 3

- The fracture is débrided as necessary with a curet, defining the fracture fragments (Figs. 56-20 and 56-21).

Step 4

- The fracture is reduced by direct fragment manipulation, and K-wires are used to stabilize the fracture (Fig. 56-22).

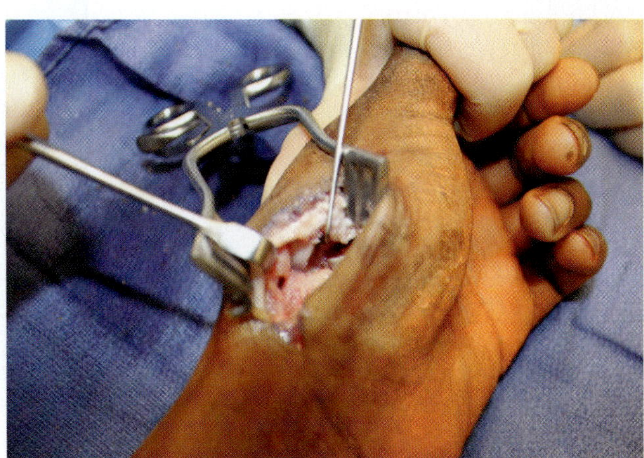

FIGURE 56-20

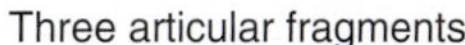

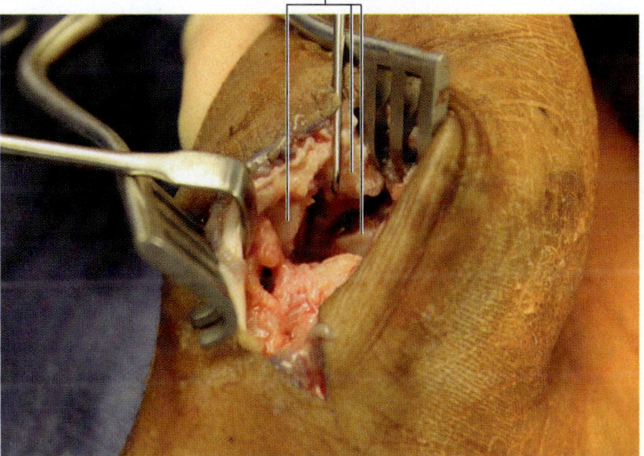

FIGURE 56-21

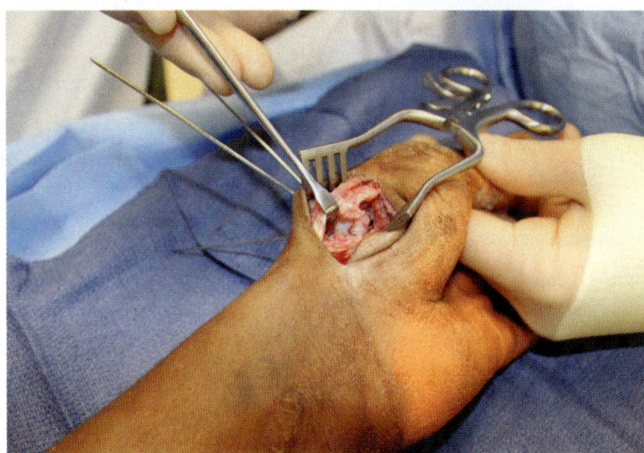

FIGURE 56-22

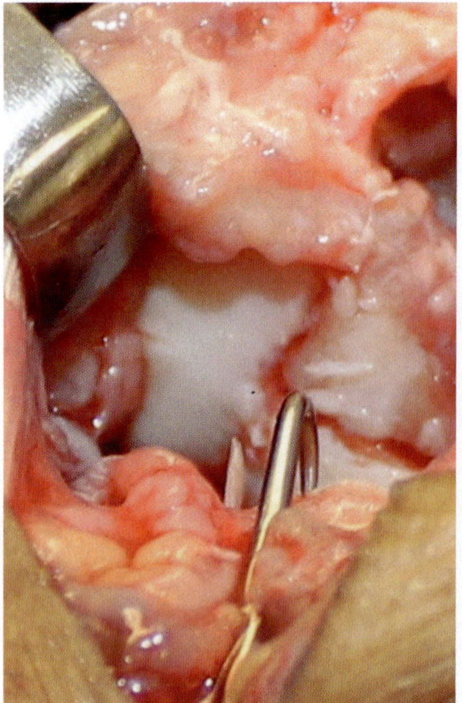

FIGURE 56-23

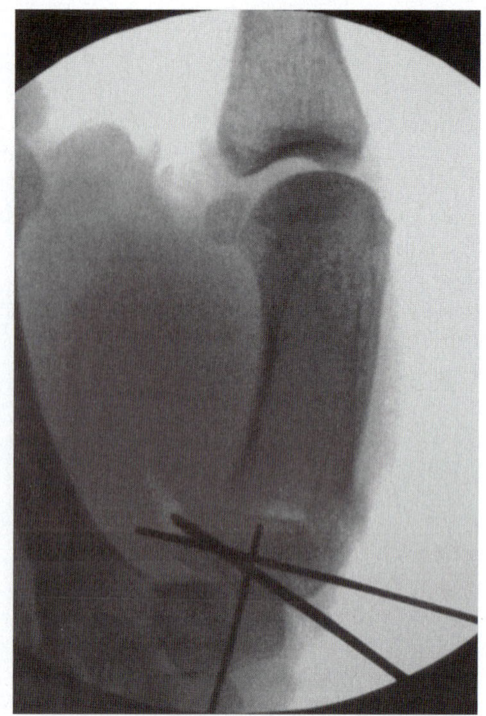

FIGURE 56-24

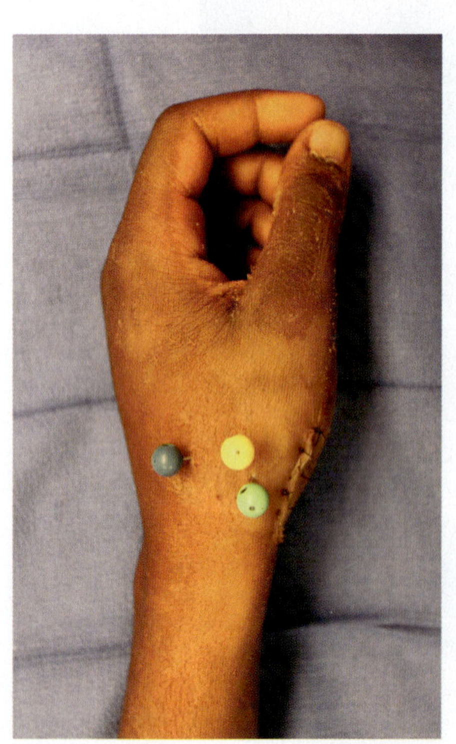

FIGURE 56-25

Step 5

- Direct inspection of the joint is used to confirm articular reduction without step-off (Fig. 56-23).
- Fluoroscopy is used to confirm K-wire placement and fracture reduction (Fig. 56-24).

Step 6

- The wound is irrigated, the capsule is closed with 4-0 absorbable sutures, and the skin is closed.
- Pins are cut and capped, and the patient is placed in a thumb spica splint (Fig. 56-25).

Postoperative Care and Expected Outcomes

- Same as described previously

Evidence

Green DP, O'Brien ET. Fractures of the thumb metacarpal. *South Med J.* 1972;65:807-814.

Classic article describing extra-articular and intra-articular thumb metacarpal base fractures. The authors advocated operative stabilization for intra-articular fractures. (Level IV)

Kjaer-Petersen K, Langhoff O, Andersen K. Bennett's fracture. *J Hand Surg [Br].* 1990;15:58-61.

Long-term follow-up (7.3 years) of 41 patients with a Bennett fracture. A higher percentage of patients with good outcomes (asymptomatic) were found to have an articular step-off of less than 1 mm. (Level IV)

Timmenga EF, Blokhuis TJ, Maas M, et al. Long-term evaluation of Bennett's fracture: a comparison between open and closed reduction. *J Hand Surg [Br].* 1994;19:373-377.

Long-term follow-up (10.7 years) of 18 patients with a Bennett fracture. Posttraumatic arthritis correlated with the quality of the reduction, and was a common occurrence. (Level IV)

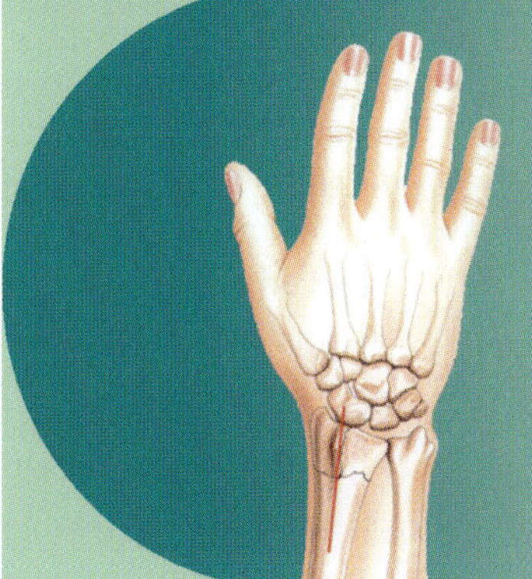

PROCEDURE 57

Open Reduction of Metacarpophalangeal Joint Dislocation

Douglas Sammer

Indications

- Irreducible (complex) metacarpophalangeal (MCP) dislocation

Examination/Imaging

Clinical Examination

- The MCP joint region will be swollen and tender.
- A neurovascular examination of the finger should be performed to document perfusion and sensory changes.
- Simple subluxation should be distinguished from a complete dislocation.
- In simple subluxation, the proximal phalanx is locked in a hyperextended position (Fig. 57-1).
- In a complete dislocation, the proximal phalanx may be less hyperextended and may even be in a bayoneted position (Fig. 57-2).

Imaging

- Obtain three-view radiographs of the hand and involved digit.
- Assess for associated fractures—a dorsal metacarpal shear fracture is not unusual (Fig. 57-3).
- Note the position of the sesamoids, which indicate the location of the volar plate.

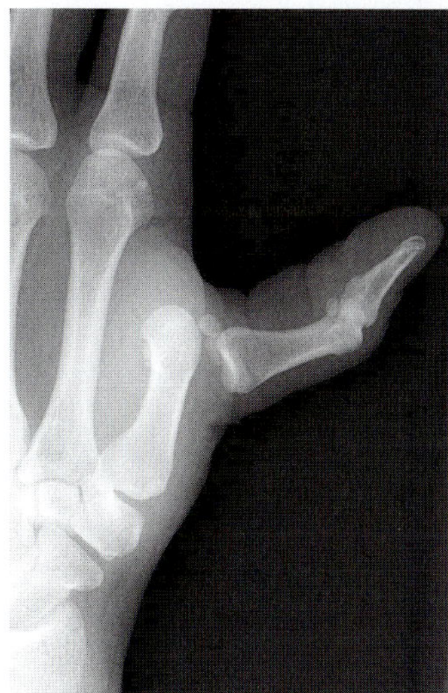

FIGURE 57-1

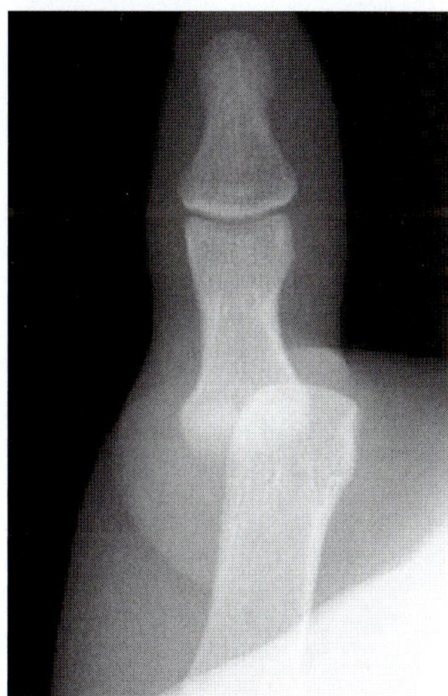

FIGURE 57-2

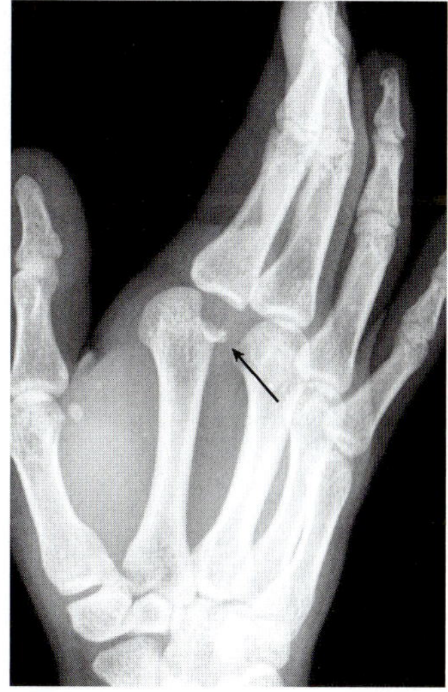

FIGURE 57-3

Figures 57-3 and 57-9 provided courtesy of Sandeep J. Sebastin, MD.

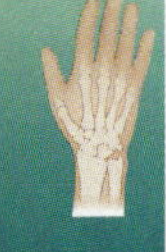

Surgical Anatomy

- The MCP volar plate has a weaker proximal insertion and tends to avulse from the metacarpal, remaining attached to the base of the proximal phalanx.
- In a simple subluxation, the proximal phalanx is hyperextended. In this case, the volar plate remains draped over the articular surface of the metacarpal head and does not lie on the dorsal cortex of the metacarpal head (Fig. 57-4A).
- In a complete or complex dislocation, the proximal phalanx is less hyperextended and may be in a bayonet position. In this case, the volar plate is no longer draped over the metacarpal articular surface but rather lies completely dorsal to the metacarpal head (Fig. 57-4B).
- The dislocation is made complex (irreducible) not only by the volar plate but also by the flexor tendons and lumbrical, which form a noose around the metacarpal neck (Fig. 57-5).

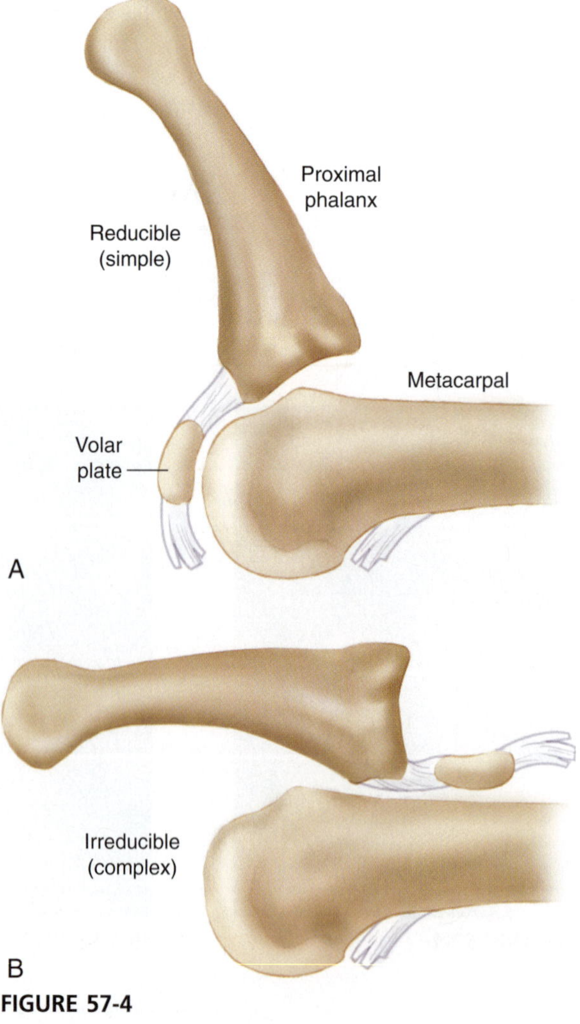

FIGURE 57-4

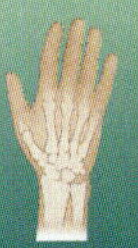

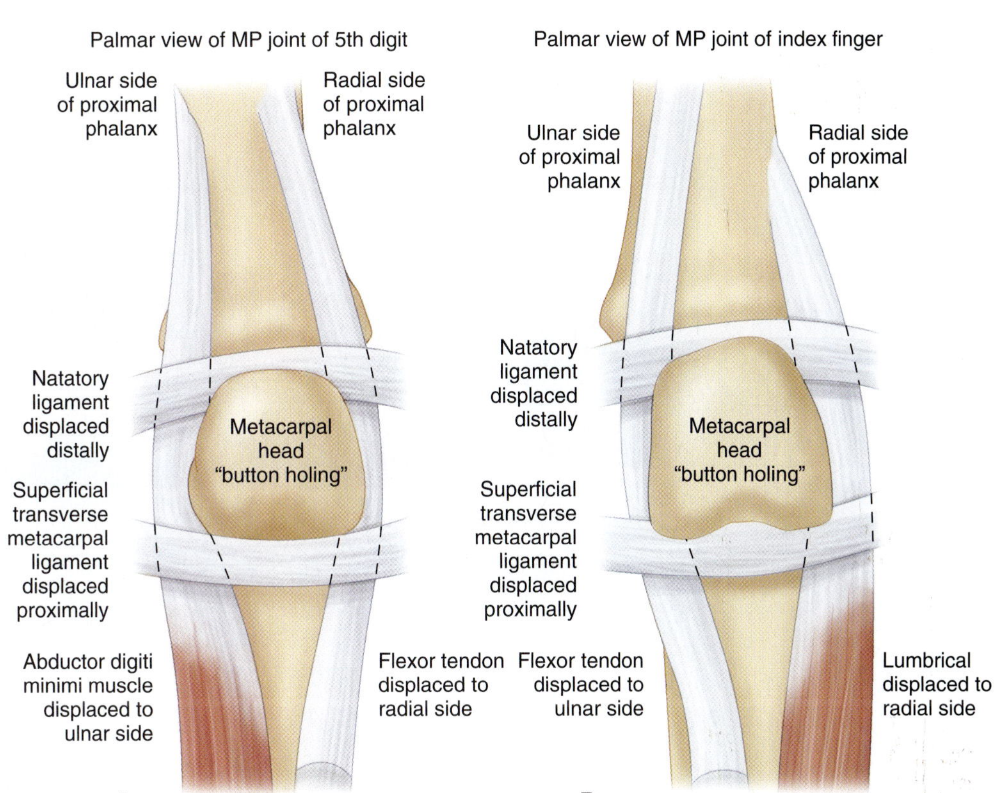

FIGURE 57-5

PEARLS

Dorsal and volar exposures have been described and work equally well.

The dorsal exposure is safer because it avoids potential injury to the neurovascular bundles, which do not lie in their normal anatomic position.

Exposures

- A longitudinal incision is made dorsal to the MCP joint.
- In the thumb, the interval between the extensor pollicis brevis (EPB) and extensor pollicis longus (EPL) is incised.
- In the index and small fingers, the interval between the extensor digitorum communis (EDC) and the more ulnar proprius or minimi tendon is incised.
- In the long and ring fingers, the extensor tendon is split longitudinally in its midline.
- The dorsal capsule is torn, but further capsulotomy and retraction or dorsal capsulectomy may be necessary to visualize the pathology.
- The base of the proximal phalanx with attached volar plate is noted to lie on top of the metacarpal head (Fig. 57-6).
- The flexor tendon can be seen dorsal to the metacarpal head, resulting in a complex (irreducible) dislocation (Fig. 57-7).
- The sesamoids within the volar plate can be seen dorsal to the metacarpal head (see Fig. 57-7).

Procedure

Step 1

- Closed reduction should be attempted one more time after induction of anesthesia, before opening.

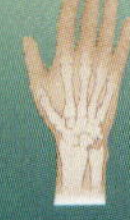

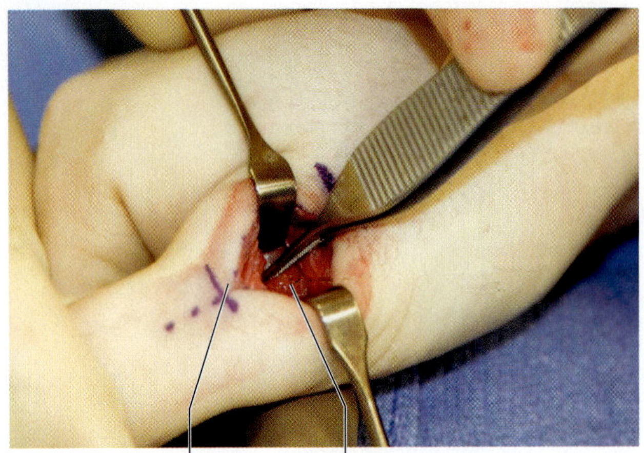

FIGURE 57-6

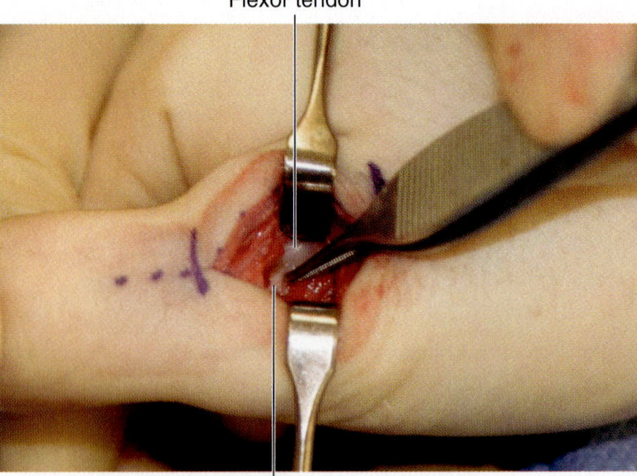

FIGURE 57-7

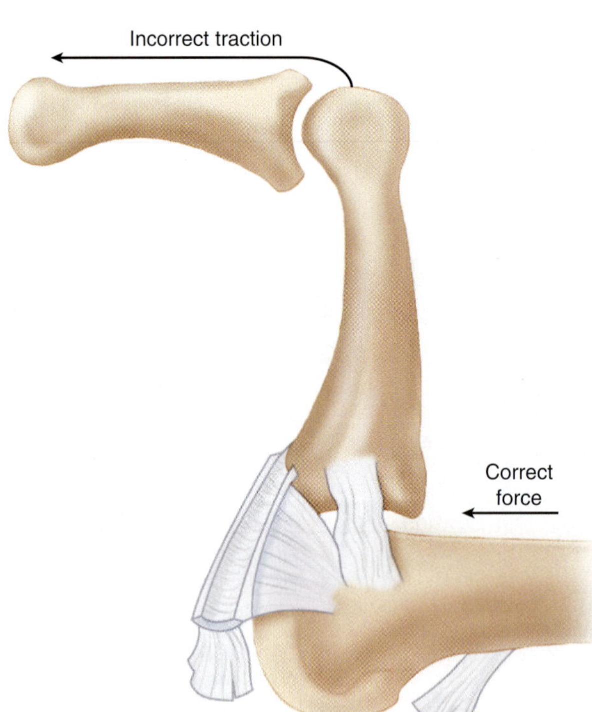

FIGURE 57-8

STEP 1 PITFALLS

Traction should be avoided during reduction maneuvers for both simple subluxation and complex dislocation (see Fig. 57-8).

Traction simply tightens the noose in a complex dislocation.

Traction can convert a simple subluxation to a complex dislocation.

Hyperextension should be avoided during reduction maneuvers for simple subluxation because it can convert this to a complex dislocation.

- The wrist is flexed to take tension off the flexor tendons, which may be preventing reduction.
- Pressure is applied to the base of the proximal phalanx, pushing it distally and volarly, sliding it over the metacarpal head (Fig. 57-8).
- If this is unsuccessful, hyperextension may be required before applying pressure to the base of the proximal phalanx.
- If attempt at reduction under anesthesia is not successful, proceed with open reduction.

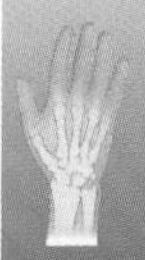

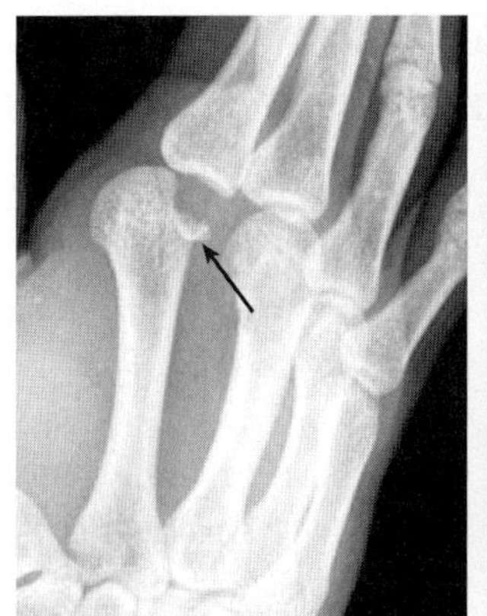
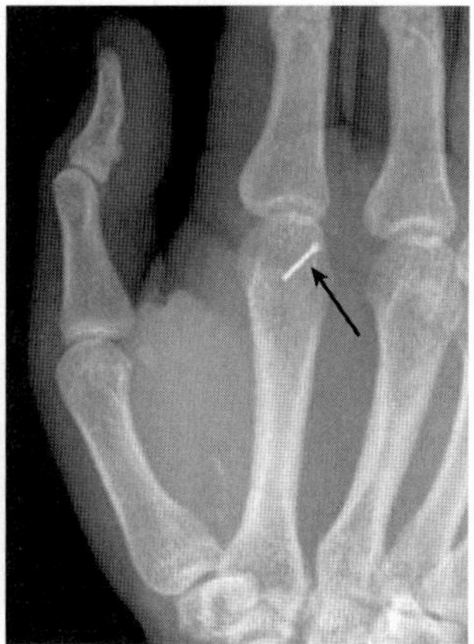

FIGURE 57-9

Step 2

- The dislocation is exposed as described previously (see Fig. 57-6).

Step 3

- The wrist is flexed to relax the noose formed by the flexor tendons and lumbrical.
- A Freer elevator is used to push the volar plate distally and volarly, pushing it back into the joint space.
- Simultaneously, the proximal phalanx is gently pushed distally and volarly, sliding it over the metacarpal head.
- If necessary, the flexor tendon is manipulated gently with a pick-up, pushing it back around the lateral aspect of the metacarpal head and into its normal volar position.

Step 4

- Fluoroscopy is used to confirm concentric reduction of the joint.
- The split extensor tendon is repaired with horizontal mattress 4-0 absorbable sutures.
- The skin is closed with simple interrupted sutures.
- A dorsal block splint is applied, placing the MCP joint in 10 degrees of flexion.

Additional Steps

- Occasionally, reduction cannot be achieved by the previous technique.
- In this situation, the volar plate is divided longitudinally in its midline.
- The split volar plate then spreads out of the way of the metacarpal head as the joint is reduced.
- Alternatively, it can be tucked back into the joint, one side at a time, while radially and ulnarly deviating the proximal phalanx.
- If a dorsal metacarpal head shear fracture is present, it can be fixed with a K-wire or a small screw (Fig. 57-9).
- The MCP joint is usually stable after reduction, and K-wire fixation is not routinely necessary.

Postoperative Care and Expected Outcomes

- Within 3 to 5 days, the patient should begin range of motion.
- An Orthoplast dorsal block splint is fabricated to prevent MCP hyperextension, and active flexion and extension within the splint are encouraged.
- The interphalangeal joints can be left free.
- The splint is weaned and light activity allowed at 4 to 6 weeks.
- No sports or heavy use is allowed for 3 months.
- Patients tend to have very good motion and hand function, although mild residual stiffness is not uncommon.
- Posttraumatic arthritis may occur.

Evidence

Afifi AM, Medoro A, Salas C, et al. A cadaver model that investigates irreducible metacarpophalangeal joint dislocation. *J Hand Surg [Am]*. 2009;34:1506-1511.
The authors developed a cadaveric dorsal MCP dislocation model and then examined the anatomy of irreducible MCP dislocations. The study demonstrates that although there are multiple structures involved in irreducible dislocations, the key structure that inhibits reduction is the volar plate. (Level V evidence)

McLaughlin HL. Complex "locked" dislocation of the metacarpophalangeal joints. *J Trauma*. 1965;5:683-688.
This classic paper is a retrospective review of 160 MCP dislocations, 22 of which required open reduction. Proper closed reduction technique is emphasized. (Level V evidence)

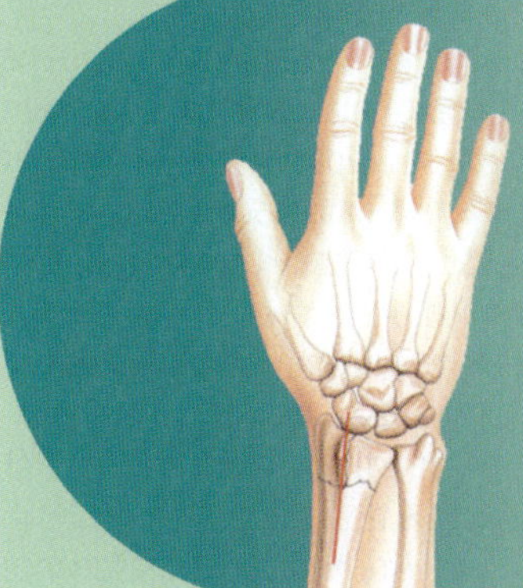

PROCEDURE 58

Skier's Thumb: Repair of Acute Thumb Metacarpophalangeal Joint Ulnar Collateral Ligament Injury

Christopher J. Utz and Jeffrey N. Lawton

See Video 40: Repair of Acute Thumb MCP Joint Ulnar Collateral Ligament Injury

See Video 41: Thumb Radial Collateral Ligament Repair

Indications

- Acute, complete tear of the ulnar collateral ligament (UCL) of the thumb metacarpophalangeal (MCP) joint, particularly if a Stener lesion is present
- Contraindicated in patients with significant arthritic changes in the joint or underlying inflammatory conditions such as rheumatoid arthritis

Examination/Imaging

Clinical Examination

- In the acute presentation, the patient typically has a swollen painful thumb MCP joint. Occasionally, a lump may be palpated on the ulnar side of the thumb MCP joint, representing the avulsed and retracted UCL stump.
- Stress testing of the UCL is performed by applying a valgus force to the extended MCP joint while holding the head of the metacarpal fixed. If the joint deviates more than 30 degrees total or 15 degrees more than the contralateral uninjured thumb, it represents a complete UCL tear. A significant deviation in extension represents a more comprehensive injury that includes the dorsal capsule in addition to the UCL. A similar deviation of 30 degrees of flexion represents an injury to the UCL in isolation. If it deviates less than 25 degrees, it may represent a ligamentous strain that would be amenable to nonoperative treatment. (Fig. 58-1 shows clinical and fluoroscopic examination demonstrating significant ulnar collateral ligament laxity on stress testing.)

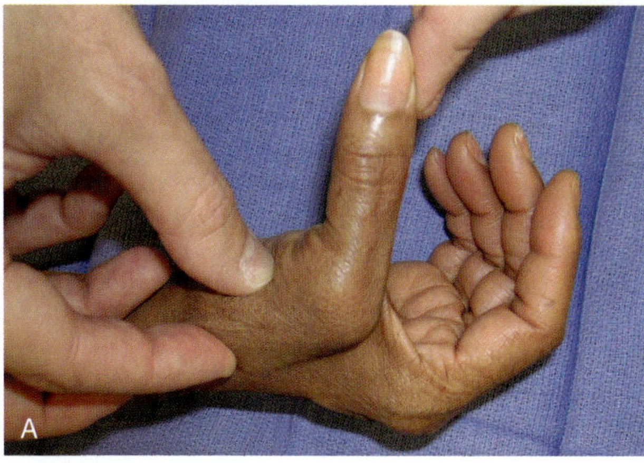

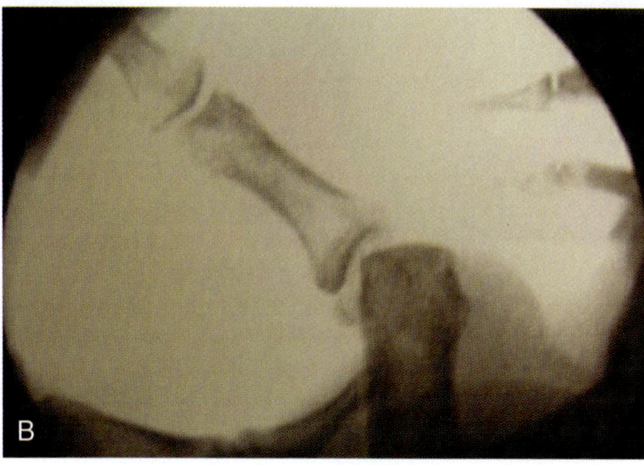

FIGURE 58-1

Imaging

- Standard anteroposterior and lateral radiographs of the thumb should be obtained to check for an avulsion fracture of the proximal phalanx. Volar subluxation of the proximal phalanx suggesting a dorsal capsular tear that might need repair can be seen on the lateral radiograph. Comparison views of the opposite uninjured thumb can be obtained to ensure that subluxation is pathologic and not due to the patient's inherent ligamentous laxity.
- In the absence of a fracture, radiographic stress testing can be performed to evaluate joint laxity; however, this is not necessary because the clinical examination is usually sufficient. This may require a local anesthetic block in order for the patient to cooperate with the examination (see Fig. 58-1).
- In rare instances when the clinical examination is equivocal, magnetic resonance imaging or ultrasound can be used to assess the extent of a UCL tear.

Surgical Anatomy

- The MCP joint has characteristics of both a condyloid and a ginglymus joint, which allow a relatively large range of motion. Consequently, there is little inherent stability in the bony architecture.
- Stability of the joint depends largely on a complex arrangement of ligamentous and musculotendinous structures.
- The ulnar collateral ligament is composed of two units. The proper UCL originates on the ulnar lateral condyle of the metacarpal and traverses obliquely to insert on the volar third of the ulnar proximal phalanx. It is tight in flexion and loose in extension. The accessory UCL originates volar to the proper collateral ligament and inserts on the ulnar sesamoid and volar plate. It is tight in extension and loose in flexion.
- The adductor pollicis inserts on the ulnar sesamoid embedded in the volar plate. It has an aponeurosis that extends obliquely across the MCP joint, inserting into the extensor mechanism distal to the sagittal bands.
- A Stener lesion results from a forceful radial deviation of the proximal phalanx, resulting in a distal avulsion of the UCL from its insertion on the proximal phalanx. Because of the extensive radial deviation of the proximal phalanx, the UCL becomes displaced from its insertion point deep to the adductor aponeurosis and comes to lie superficial and proximal to the adductor aponeurosis, which prevents the ligament from anatomic alignment. The lesion is created with forced radial deviation of the proximal phalanx with displacement of the UCL superficial to the adductor aponeurosis to prevent its anatomic alignment (Fig. 58-2).
- Branches of the superficial radial nerve often cross the operative field and need to be identified and protected.

Positioning

- The procedure is performed under tourniquet control. It can be done under regional or general anesthesia. The patient is usually positioned supine with the affected extremity on a radiolucent hand table.

Exposures

- The lazy S-shaped skin incision is centered over the ulnar side of the MCP joint. It should start distally on the ulnar volar aspect of the proximal phalanx, curve over the joint, and continue proximally just ulnar to the extensor pollicis longus (EPL) tendon (Fig. 58-3).

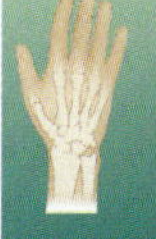

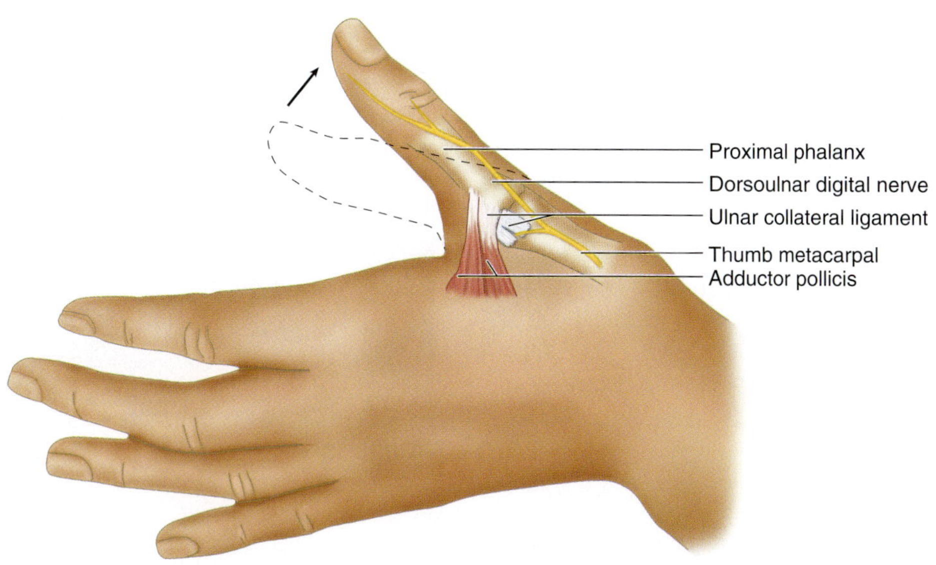

FIGURE 58-2

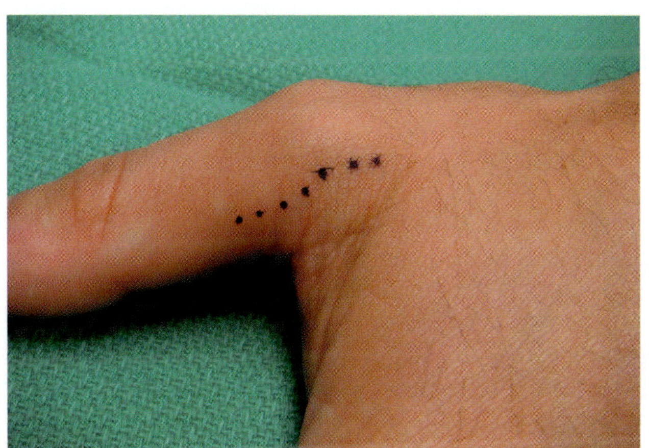

FIGURE 58-3

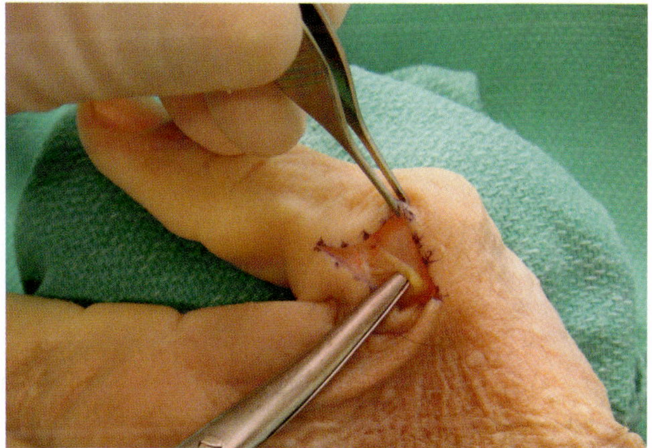

FIGURE 58-4

PEARLS

Care must be taken during exposure to identify and protect branches of the superficial radial nerve that can often be found in this area (see Fig. 58-4).

It is often helpful to use retraction sutures to hold back the skin flaps during the procedure.

If a Stener lesion is not present, an incision in the dorsal MCP capsule is made at the dorsal margin of the UCL. Passing a blunt instrument such as a Freer elevator along the ulnar aspect of the proximal phalangeal base and the metacarpal head will confirm whether the lesion represents a distal avulsion (most commonly), a midsubstance tear, or a proximal avulsion from the metacarpal origin.

- The dissection is carried down through the subcutaneous tissue bluntly to protect branches of the superficial radial nerve, with elevation of full-thickness skin flaps dorsally and volarly. This should expose the EPL tendon, extensor hood, and adductor aponeurosis. Branches of the superficial radial nerve are often found in the operative field and need to be protected (Fig. 58-4).
- At this point, a mass of tissue may be seen at the proximal edge of the adductor aponeurosis. This represents a Stener lesion and consists of the retracted UCL.
- The extensor hood is then incised just ulnar to the EPL tendon, leaving a cuff of tissue on the tendon for later repair. Although there is often scarring that can obliterate the tissue planes, the EPL can then be retracted radially, and the adductor aponeurosis is elevated from the underlying MCP joint capsule and reflected volarly. If a Stener lesion is not present, the torn end of the UCL should be found underneath the adductor aponeurosis.
- If the capsule is not already torn from the injury, an incision should be made in the capsule at the dorsoulnar aspect at the approximate junction of the dorsal capsule and the proper collateral ligament. The MCP joint is then examined for chondral injuries.

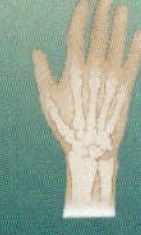

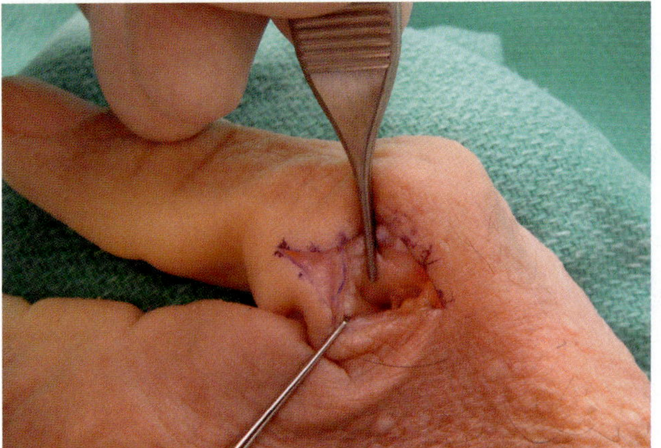

FIGURE 58-5

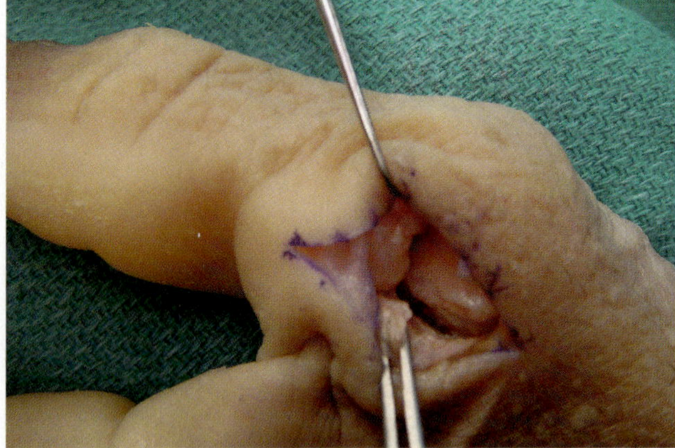

FIGURE 58-6

Procedure

Step 1: Preparation of the UCL and Insertion Site

- The reconstruction technique depends on the pathologic changes observed. Rarely, there is a midsubstance tear of the UCL. If this is found, it can be repaired primarily using a nonabsorbable braided 4-0 suture with interrupted figure-of-eight sutures.
- More commonly, the ligament is avulsed from its distal insertion on the proximal phalanx and requires reattachment using either a pull-out suture (traditional) or bone anchors (the authors' preferred method). In preparation for this, the torn end of the UCL must be mobilized by dissecting it free from adjacent soft tissue, scar, and hematoma (Fig. 58-5).
- The insertion point of the UCL on the volar ulnar aspect of the proximal phalanx is prepared by clearing it of soft tissue with a curette. (In Fig. 58-6, the bone has been cleared of soft tissue and prepared for suture anchor placement. Forceps are holding the mobilized UCL.)
- Microsuture anchors preloaded with a 3-0/4-0 braided permanent suture are used. There are various anchors (both permanent and absorbable) that can be used; each contains a drill to create an appropriate pilot hole for the anchor.
- The pilot hole for the anchor is drilled at the prepared site just distal to the subchondral bone at the articular surface. The authors place two anchors. The first anchor targets the volar one third of the phalangeal base. Anchor placement, which is suitably volar to restore the insertion position of the UCL, is confirmed fluoroscopically. By doing this, if the initial anchor is found not to be sufficiently volar, additional dissection can be performed to place the second anchor appropriately. If the first anchor placement is acceptable, a second anchor is placed more dorsal to the first anchor.
- The bone anchors are placed into the hole with the appropriate introducers, and tension is placed on the sutures to ensure solid fixation in the bone.

STEP 1 PEARLS

To place the first anchor in its appropriate volar location, supination of the thumb to rotate the proximal phalangeal base by an assistant can be most helpful.

STEP 1 PITFALLS

The proper insertion of the UCL, relatively volar on the phalangeal base, is important to restore the appropriate kinematics of the MCP joint.

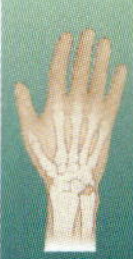

Step 2: Reattachment

- The ends of the suture attached to the anchor are then brought through the distal end of the UCL in horizontal mattress fashion. The MCP joint is held in a neutral or slight ulnarly deviated position in the radioulnar plane, and the sutures are tied.
- This repair is supplemented by suturing the distal volar aspect of the UCL to the volar plate. Additionally, sutures may be placed through the distal UCL and local tissue or periosteum.
- If the dorsal capsule has been torn, it is repaired with 3-0 or 4-0 braided suture to prevent volar subluxation of the joint.
- The MCP joint can be transfixed with a Kirschner wire by correcting palmar subluxation and establishing a slightly overcorrected ulnar-deviated position to prevent tension on the repair. Ideally, the MCP joint is first stabilized and then the sutures placed.

STEP 2 PEARLS

Be sure to identify and attach the UCL to its anatomic insertion point. If the ligament is reattached more distally or dorsally than its normal insertion point, MCP joint range of motion can be decreased.

Be sure to identify and repair dorsal capsule tears to reduce and prevent recurrent volar subluxation of the joint.

STEP 2 PITFALLS

Do not overtighten the dorsal capsule because this can reduce flexion of the MCP joint.

Step 3: Closure

- The adductor aponeurosis is closed using 4-0 absorbable suture with inverted knots to prevent subdermal prominence.
- The skin is closed with a series of horizontal mattress sutures using 4-0 Prolene.
- A dressing is applied and the thumb immobilized in a radial gutter thumb spica splint.

STEP 3 PEARLS

If a proximal disruption is encountered, the UCL origin is similarly created with two suture anchors spaced over the midaxis of the metacarpal head origination point.

Postoperative Care and Expected Outcomes

- Seven to 10 days after surgery, the skin sutures are removed, and the patient is placed in a short-arm thumb spica cast.
- Four weeks after surgery, the cast and K-wire (if used) are removed. After 6 weeks of immobilization, the patient is referred to occupational therapy for a thumb spica splint and initiation of range-of-motion exercises.
- Patients are encouraged to remove the splint and do flexion and extension range-of-motion exercises six to eight times a day. Any radially directed force that would stress the repair is avoided at this time.
- The splint is discontinued except for strenuous activities 2 weeks after the cast is removed.
- After 8 weeks, strengthening exercises focusing on pinch and grip strength in the plane of the flexor pollicis longus (FPL) are initiated.
- Unrestricted activity, including lateral pinch, is allowed after 12 weeks.

PITFALLS

Many patients develop transient neurapraxia of the branches of the superficial radial nerve owing to traction on the nerve during the procedure. This can result in numbness or tingling on the dorsal ulnar aspect of the thumb distal to the incision. This is usually self limiting and resolves over the first several weeks with progressive desensitization exercises.

Patients (and some therapists) must be cautioned against being too aggressive in pinch and grip strengthening early in the postoperative period to prevent attenuation of the repair.

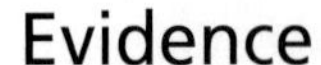

Evidence

Downey DJ, Moneim MS, Omer GE. Acute gamekeeper's thumb: quantitative outcome of surgical repair. *Am J Sports Med*. 1995;23:222-226.
The authors reviewed 11 complete ulnar collateral ligament tears that underwent early surgical repair at an average of 42 months' follow-up. The results showed good stability with slight decrease in motion (50.9 degrees arc of motion at the MCP joint vs. 73.7 degrees in the contralateral uninjured thumb). There were no significant differences in mean grip strength or key pinch between the repaired and uninjured thumbs. (Level IV evidence)

Katolik LI, Friedrich J, Trumble TE. Repair of acute ulnar collateral ligament injuries of the thumb metacarpophalangeal joint: a retrospective comparison of pull-out sutures and bone anchor techniques. *Plast Reconstr Surg*. 2008;122: 1451-1456.
The authors retrospectively compared two cohorts of 30 patients with complete ruptures of the thumb MCP joint ulnar collateral ligament at an average of 29 months' follow-up. One cohort of 30 underwent repair of the ulnar collateral ligament with an intraosseous suture anchor followed by early mobilization, and the other cohort underwent repair with a pullout suture tied over a button with cast immobilization. The authors found that suture anchors with early mobilization resulted in improved range of motion and pinch strength compared with suture buttons. There was no statistical difference in grip strength. (Level III evidence)

Kozin SH. Treatment of thumb ulnar collateral ligament ruptures with the Mitek bone anchor. *Ann Plast Surg*. 1995;35:1-5.
Seven patients who underwent thumb ulnar collateral ligament repair with Mitek bone anchors were reviewed at an average follow-up of 1 year. All patients had a stable MCP joint at follow-up. There was an average of a 7% loss of MCP motion and a 21% loss of IP motion when compared with the contralateral uninjured thumb. Pinch strength and grip strength were 98% and 96% of the contralateral thumb, respectively. (Level IV evidence)

Weiland AJ, Berner SH, Hotchkiss RN, et al. Repair of acute ulnar collateral ligament injuries of the thumb metacarpophalangeal joint with an intraosseous suture anchor. *J Hand Surg [Am]*. 1997;22:585-591.
Thirty patients with complete tears of the thumb MCP ulnar collateral ligament who underwent primary repair with suture anchors were reviewed at an average follow-up of 11 months. All thumbs were stable on stress testing compared with the contralateral thumb. Loss of MCP joint motion averaged 10 degrees compared with the uninjured thumb, and loss of IP joint motion averaged 15 degrees. (Level IV evidence)

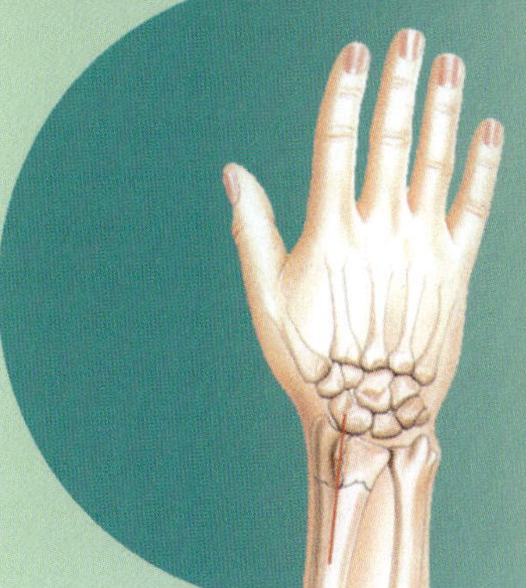

Pyrocarbon Implant Arthroplasty of the Proximal Interphalangeal and Metacarpophalangeal Joints

Nathan S. Taylor and Kevin C. Chung

See Video 42: Pyrocarbon Implant Arthroplasty (Proximal Interphalangeal Joint)

See Video 43: Pyrocarbon Implant Arthroplasty (Metacarpophalangeal Joint)

Indications

- Painful osteoarthritis of the proximal interphalangeal (PIP) and metacarpophalangeal (MCP) joints is found.
- The patient should understand that normal full motion of the joint cannot be restored; therefore, surface replacement arthroplasty should be performed when the arthritic pain has become intolerable.

Examination/Imaging

Clinical Examination

- The patient's joints are assessed for the following:
  - Intact extensor apparatus
  - Intact collateral ligaments
  - Good bone stock of the finger
- If the extensor tendon is not intact, it should be reconstructed at the time of surface replacement arthroplasty.

Imaging

- Three views of the hand are essential to evaluate the structural integrity of the small joints of the hand and adequate bone stock.
- Occasionally, computed tomography scans of the joints may be necessary to assess the articular cartilage.

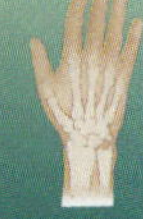

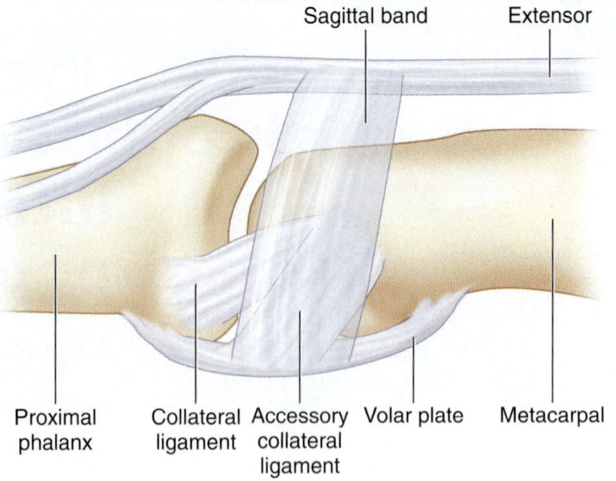

FIGURE 59-1

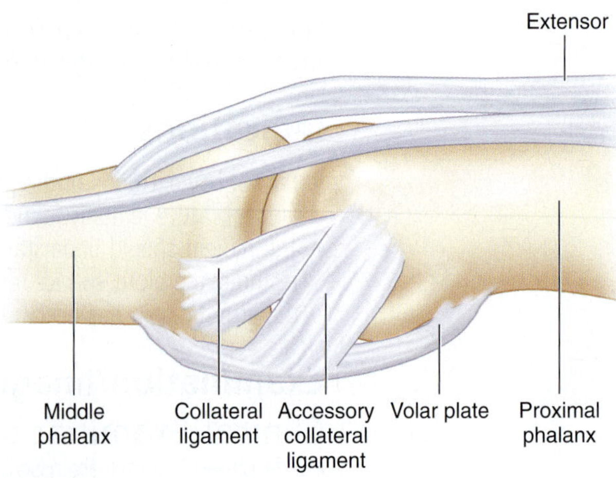

FIGURE 59-2

Surgical Anatomy

- The MCP joints of the fingers are condylar joints (Fig. 59-1), and specific MCP pyrocarbon implants are designed to mirror the anatomic construct. At the MCP joint, excellent soft tissue support and stability provided by the intermetacarpal ligaments give its stable construct. The best indication for pyrocarbon implant arthroplasty is an osteoarthritic MCP joint. Unfortunately, this situation is not often encountered. We generally do not recommend placing pyrocarbon implants in the rheumatoid hand because of the lack of adequate ligamentous support.
- The PIP joints for the fingers are ginglymoid joints that function essentially as hinge joints (Fig. 59-2). Destruction of the PIP joints often weakens the soft tissue support around the joints and may not be sufficiently tight to stabilize the pyrocarbon implants.
- Preserving bone and collateral ligament origins and insertions helps stabilize the arthroplasty.

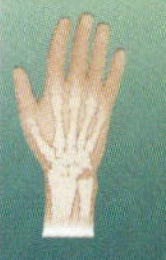

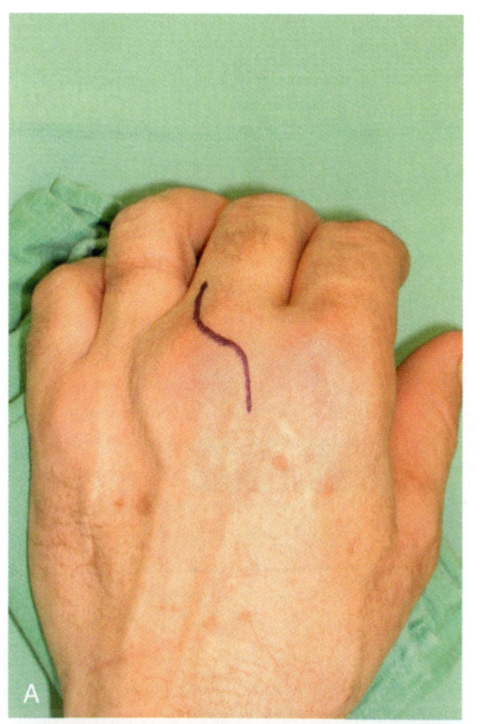

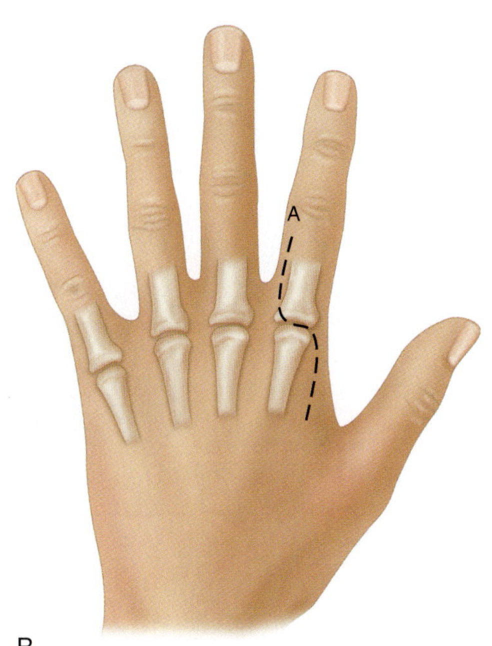

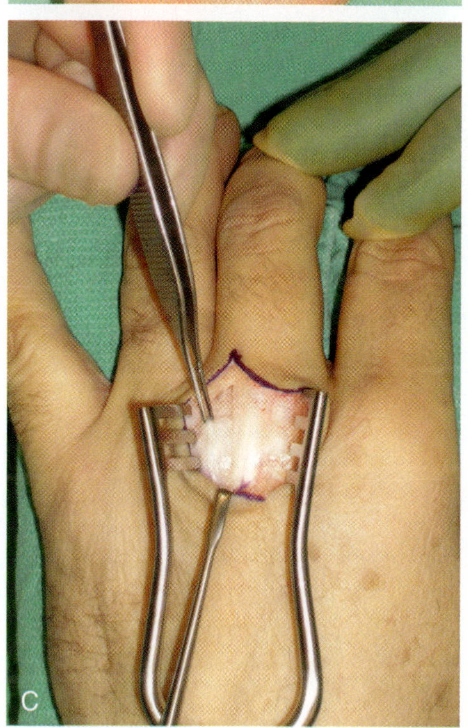

FIGURE 59-3

Positioning

- The procedure is performed under tourniquet control with the patient in the supine position and the extremity abducted with the hand on a hand table.

Exposures

MCP Joint Approach

- A dorsal lazy S-shaped incision is made over the MCP joint for single joint replacement (Fig. 59-3A and B).
- If there is no subluxation of the extensor mechanism, it can be split in the midline to expose the joint capsule. We prefer to incise the radial sagittal band to expose the joint so that the extensor tendon is not disrupted (Fig. 59-3C). The incised sagittal band should be imbricated to centralize the extensor mechanism at the conclusion of the procedure.

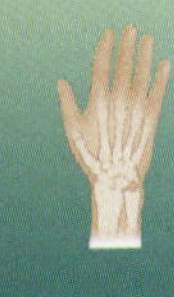

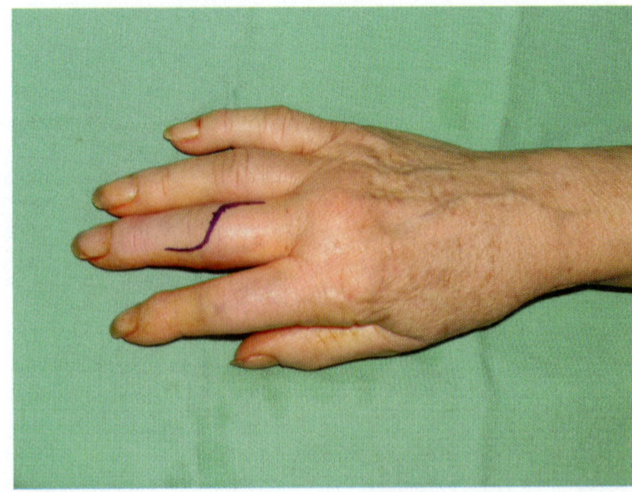

FIGURE 59-4

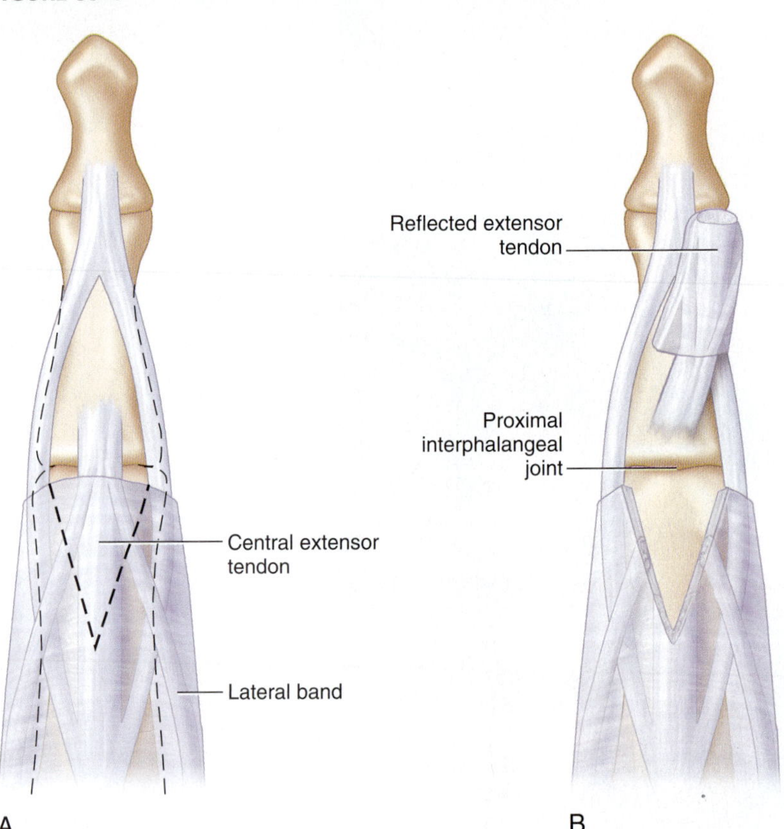

FIGURE 59-5

PEARLS

After the PIP joint arthroplasty, the lazy S-shaped incision can be closed by recruiting lateral skin to decrease tension of the skin flap during flexion of the PIP joint.

PITFALLS

The chevron incision exposure must be performed cautiously because the subsequent tendon repair may stretch out during therapy, resulting in an extension lag.

PIP Joint Approach

- The PIP joint is approached using a lazy S-shaped incision (Fig. 59-4), which provides wide exposure of the joint.
- Two incisions may be used to expose the extensor mechanism.
  - The widest exposure is obtained with a chevron incision that detaches the extensor tendon proximally, with the central tendon remaining inserted distally (Fig. 59-5A). The tendon is reflected distally, and the entire joint is fully exposed (Fig. 59-5B).

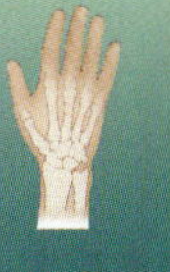

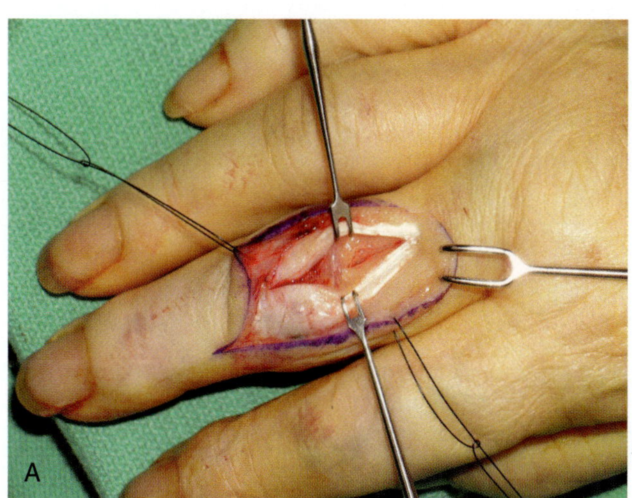

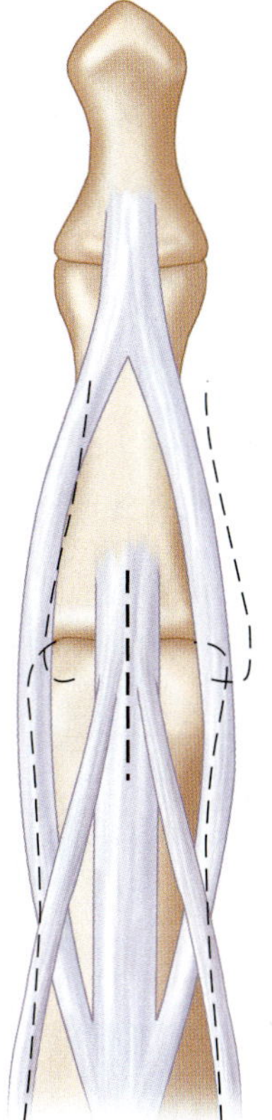

FIGURE 59-6

STEP 1 PEARLS

One must be careful to identify the proximal insertion of the collateral ligaments to avoid damaging these during the vertical proximal osteotomy.

Preservation of as much bone stock as possible will help stabilize the implant.

STEP 1 PITFALLS

Injury to the collateral ligaments will contribute to instability of the construct.

- Our preference is to split the extensor tendon in the midline to maintain tendon integrity and provide adequate exposure (Fig. 59-6A and B). This incision will require traction on the split extensor tendon during the surgical procedure, but the tendon can be closed in a side-to-side fashion that will not stretch out during therapy.

Procedure

PIP Joint Arthroplasty

Step 1

- The manufacturer's manual recommends placing the starter awl first to make the tunnel ready for broaching. However, the osteoarthritic PIP joint is usually very tight, and getting precise placement of the awl is difficult. We have modified this key step by making a freehand cut of the head of the proximal phalanx first, which will fully expose the medullary cavity for precise broaching. Experience is necessary to avoid too much head resection, cutting just at the distal neck of the proximal phalanx (Fig. 59-7A to D).

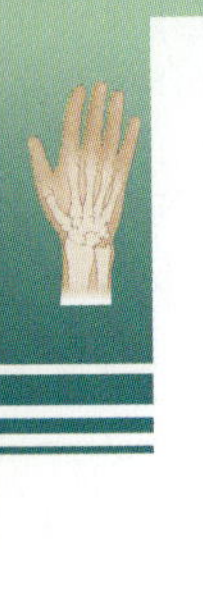

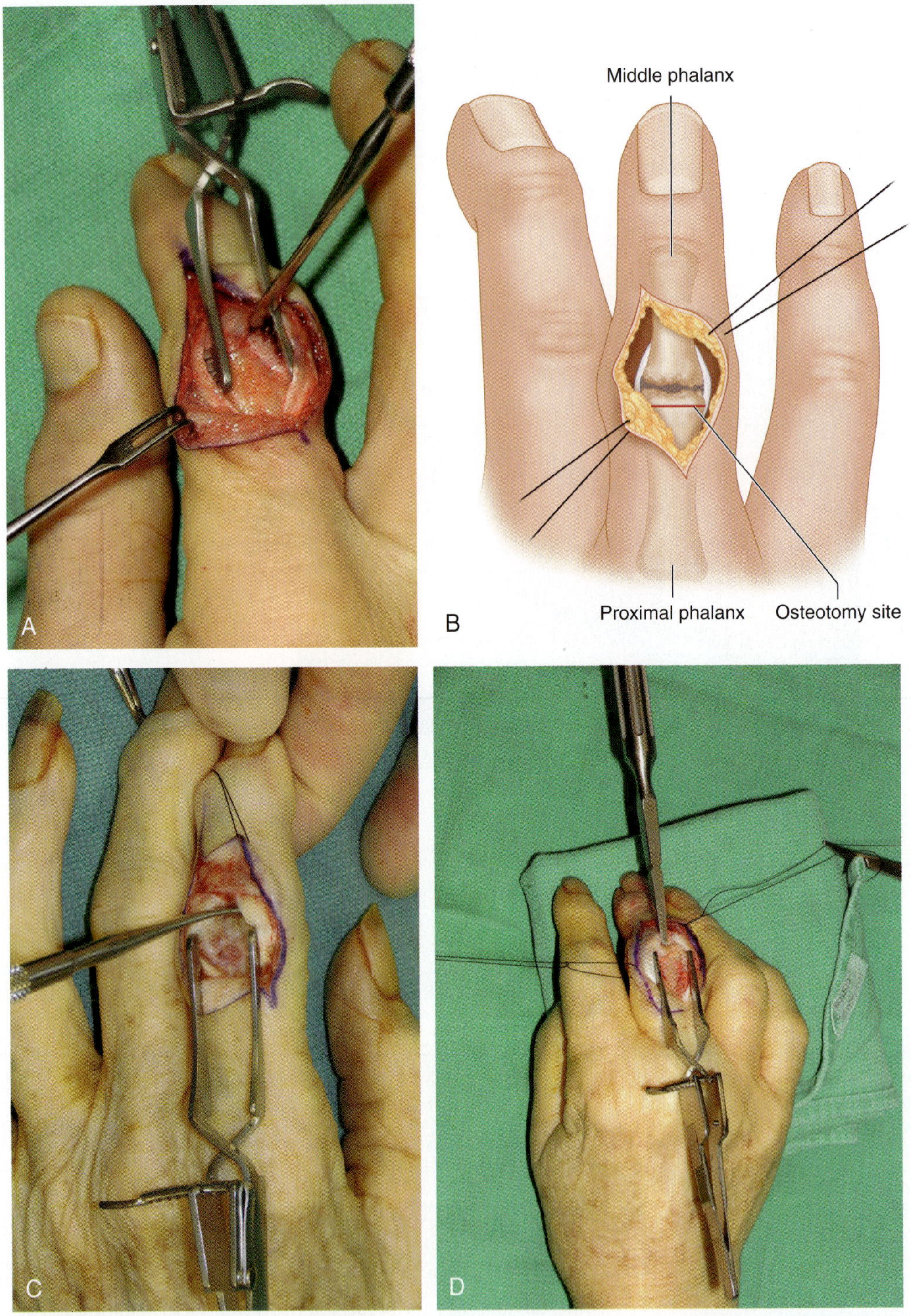

A

Middle phalanx

Proximal phalanx

Osteotomy site

B

C

D

FIGURE 59-7

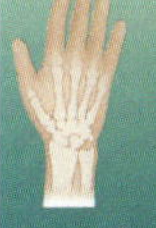

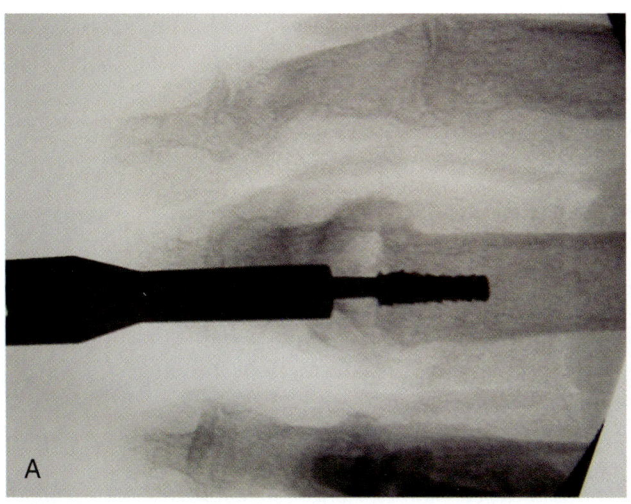

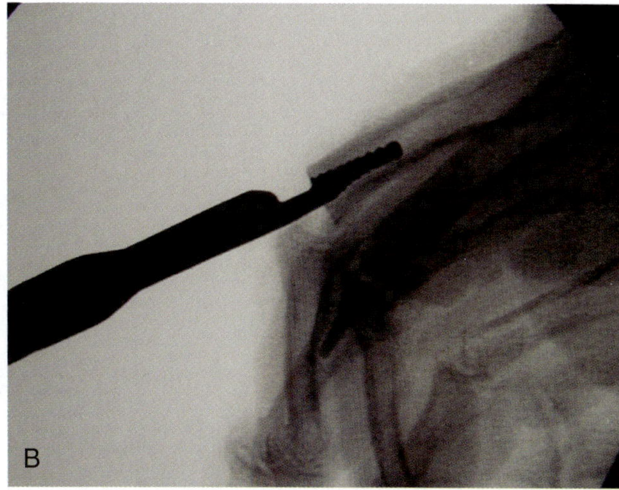

FIGURE 59-8

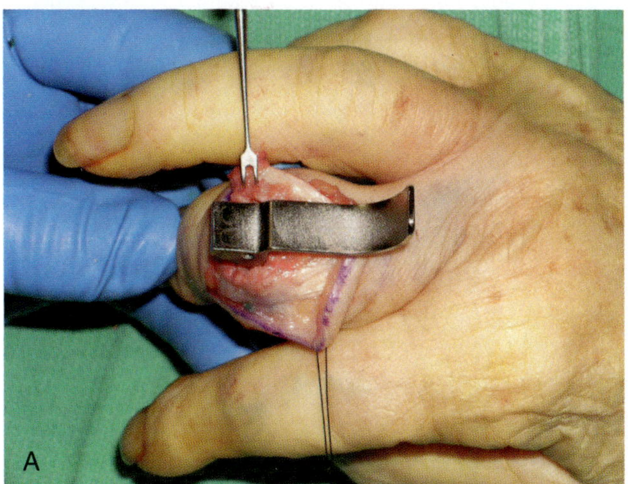

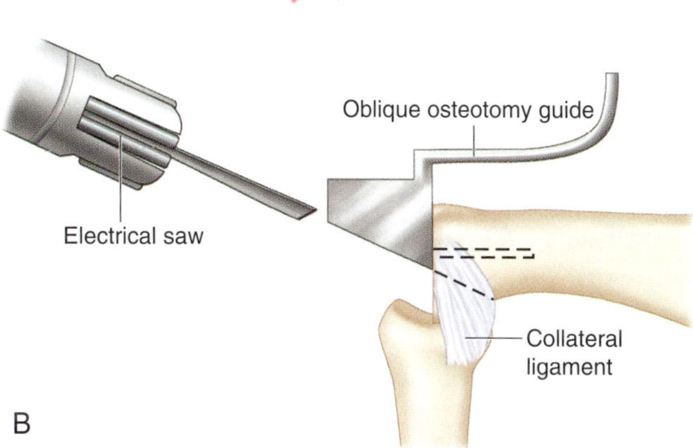

FIGURE 59-9

STEP 2 PEARLS

The hard bone in osteoarthritis makes broaching difficult. Using a mallet to tap the broach into the bone can be helpful to facilitate seating the broach at the required depth, but tapping must be done carefully to avoid fracture.

STEP 3 PEARLS

The PIP pyrocarbon implant components can be mixed one size up or one size down. For example, a no. 30 proximal implant may fit with a no. 20 distal implant, and vice versa.

The middle phalanx can be difficult to broach to a larger size. Therefore, the size of the distal component is often one size down from the proximal component.

Step 2

- A series of broaches are sequentially inserted into the proximal phalanx, starting with a no. 10 broach and increasing to the largest broach that can be accommodated within the medullary canal. The broach must be fully inserted into the medullary canal to fully accommodate the implant, which can be confirmed fluoroscopically (Fig. 59-8A and B).

Step 3

- An oblique cutting guide is then placed into the cut proximal phalanx to complete the volar oblique osteotomy (Fig. 59-9A and B). The proximal phalanx is now ready to accommodate the trial proximal phalanx implant. The pyrocarbon implant is press-fit, and cement is not used.

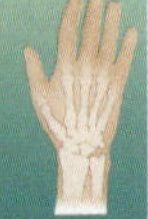

STEP 5 PEARLS

Using a side-cutting bur can enlarge the hole in the middle phalanx sufficiently to make broaching a bit easier. The bone is hard, and the bur can widen the medullary cavity to seat a larger implant.

STEP 6 PEARLS

If the implant is excessively tight, additional bone should be resected from the proximal phalanx, taking care to preserve the collateral ligaments.

Step 4

- A small oval bur is used to remove the articular surface of the middle phalanx and create a gentle trough that can accommodate the middle phalanx implant. Bone is not resected from the middle phalanx.

Step 5

- The medullary canal is broached sequentially to obtain the largest implant that can be accommodated within the medullary cavity.

Step 6

- After adequate placement of the trial implant with the PIP joint moving smoothly, the implant is press-fit into the medullary cavity by tapping it in gently (Fig. 59-10A to C).

Step 7

- The extensor tendon is closed with 3-0 horizontal-mattress braided permanent suture. The tourniquet is released, and all bleeding points are cauterized. The skin is closed with 4-0 horizontal mattress nylon suture, and the finger is splinted in full extension.

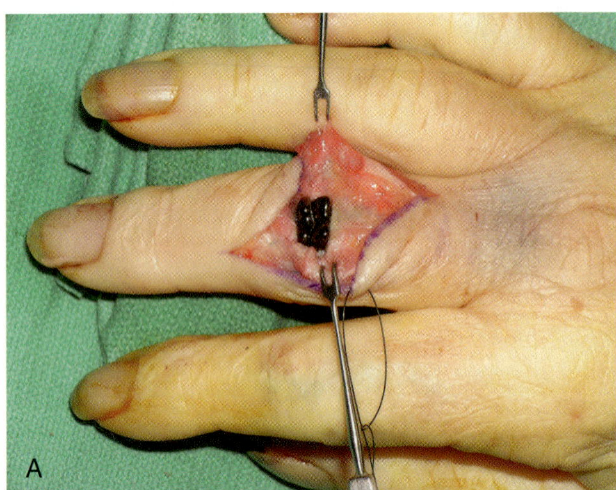

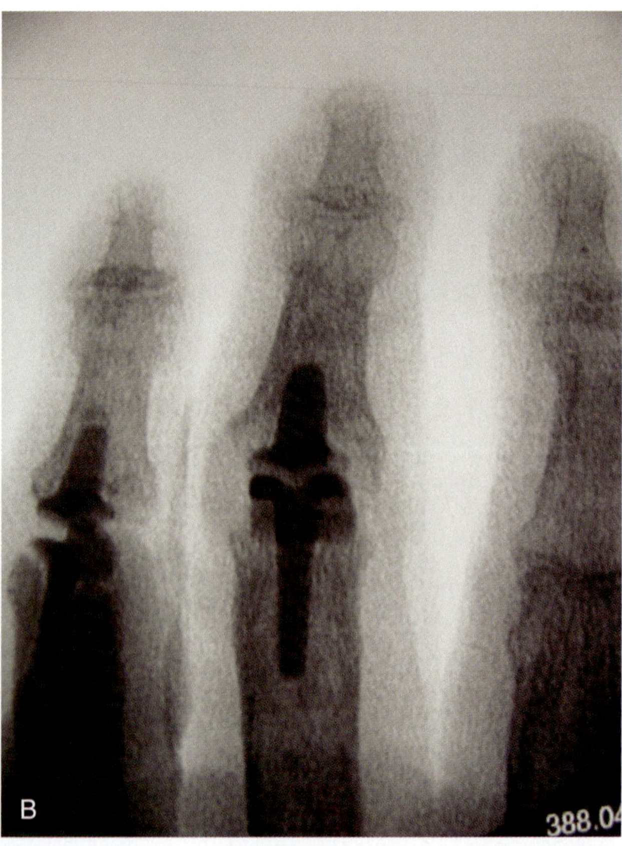

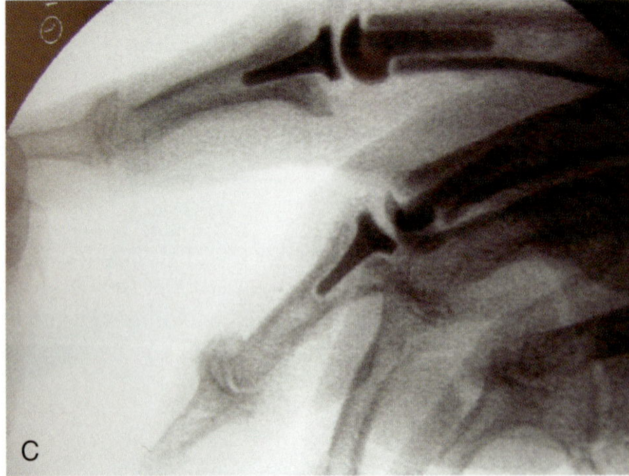

FIGURE 59-10

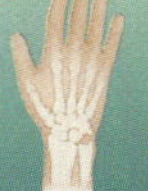

STEP 1 PEARLS

Radial positioning of the metacarpal component should be avoided because this will further increase the radial deviating moment arm and contribute to ulnar drift. Fluoroscopy must be used liberally to ensure that all the instruments are in the precise location to permit perfect seating of the implant.

Procedure

MCP Joint Arthroplasty

Step 1

- The sequence of steps for the MCP joint arthroplasty is similar to that for PIP joint arthroplasty. A starter awl enters the metacarpal head one third of the distance from the dorsal cortex and slightly ulnar to the midline and can be advanced to one half or two thirds of the metacarpal bone length (Fig. 59-11A to D). The implant fits the anatomic shape of the head of the metacarpal, and the cam design of the implant requires the center of axis to enter one third from the dorsal cortex. The proximal implant has a condylar shape, and its stem will reside more dorsally from the midaxis of the joint.

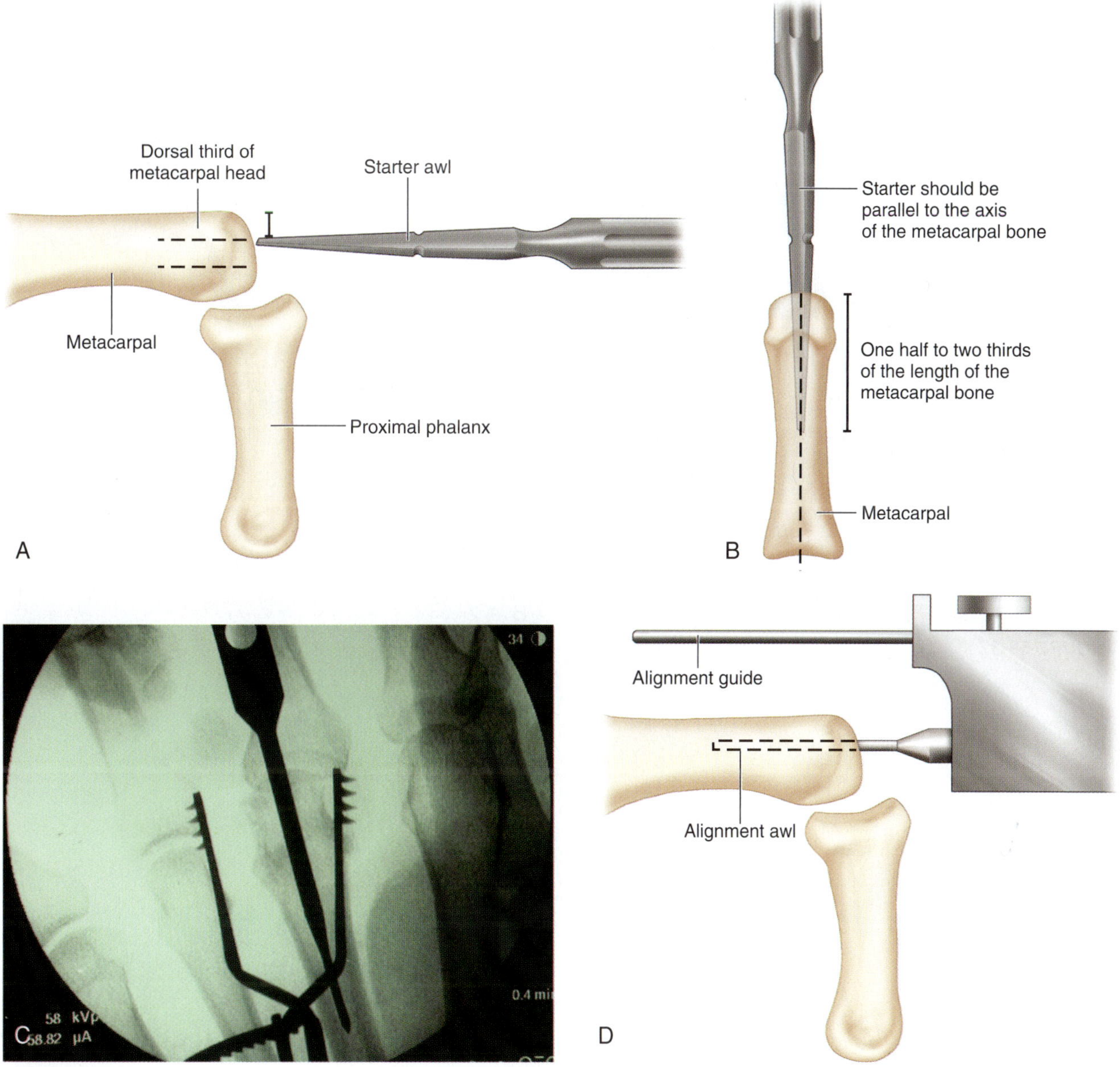

FIGURE 59-11

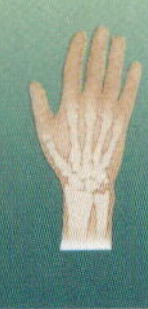

STEP 2 PEARLS

One should identify the proximal insertion of the collateral ligaments and protect these to maintain ligamentous support.

Every effort should be made to preserve as much bone stock as possible.

Step 2

- A proximal osteotomy is made using a proximal osteotomy guide, which has a 27.5-degree distal tilted axial slot for the saw blade (Fig. 59-12A). A conservative osteotomy 1.5 mm distal to the collateral ligament attachment site is recommended to protect the collateral ligaments. The osteotomy is partially made over the dorsal cortex, and complete osteotomy is performed freehand after removal of the alignment guide (Fig. 59-12B).

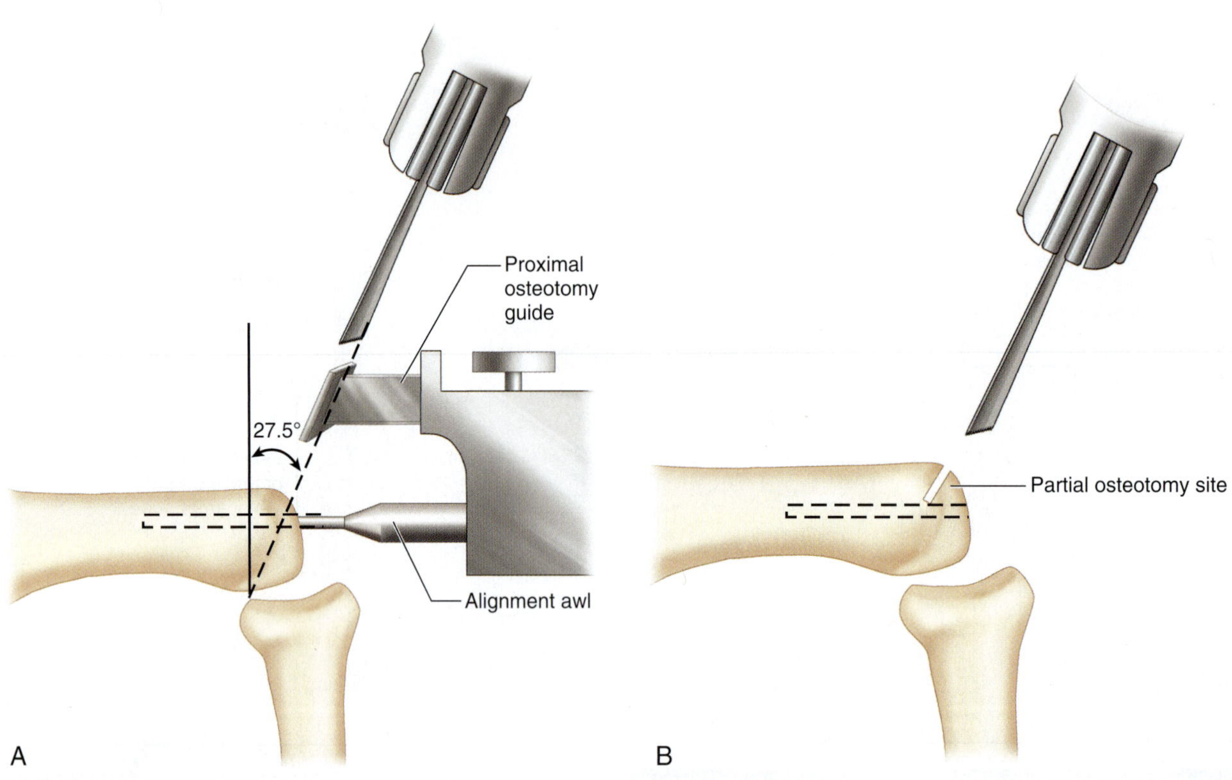

FIGURE 59-12

Step 3

- A medullary canal is created over the base of the proximal phalanx using the starter awl. The starter can be advanced one half to two thirds of the length of proximal phalanx (Fig. 59-13A and B).

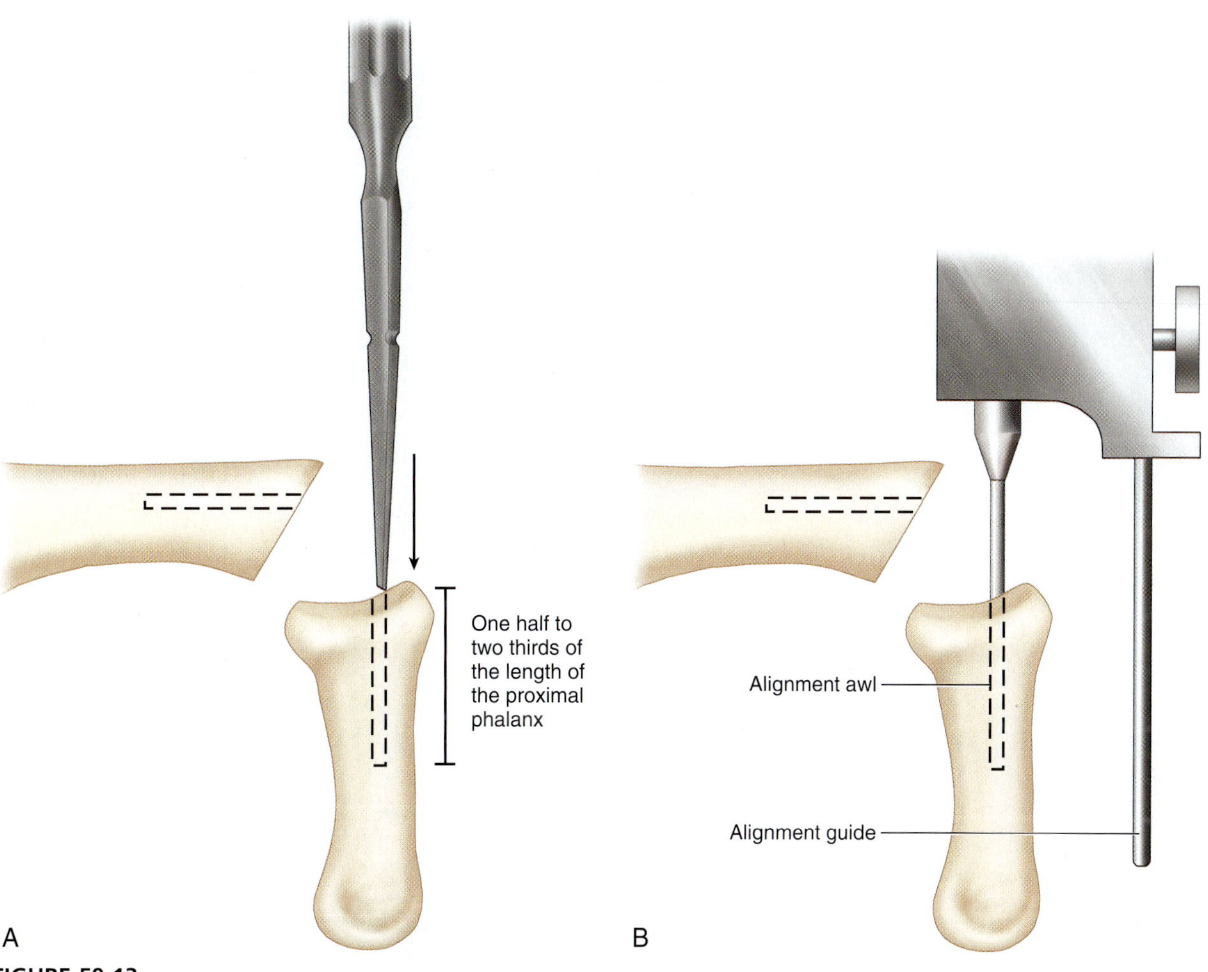

FIGURE 59-13

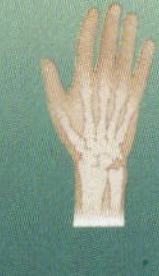

Step 4

- A 5-degree distally tilted osteotomy is made using the osteotomy guide (Fig. 59-14A and B).

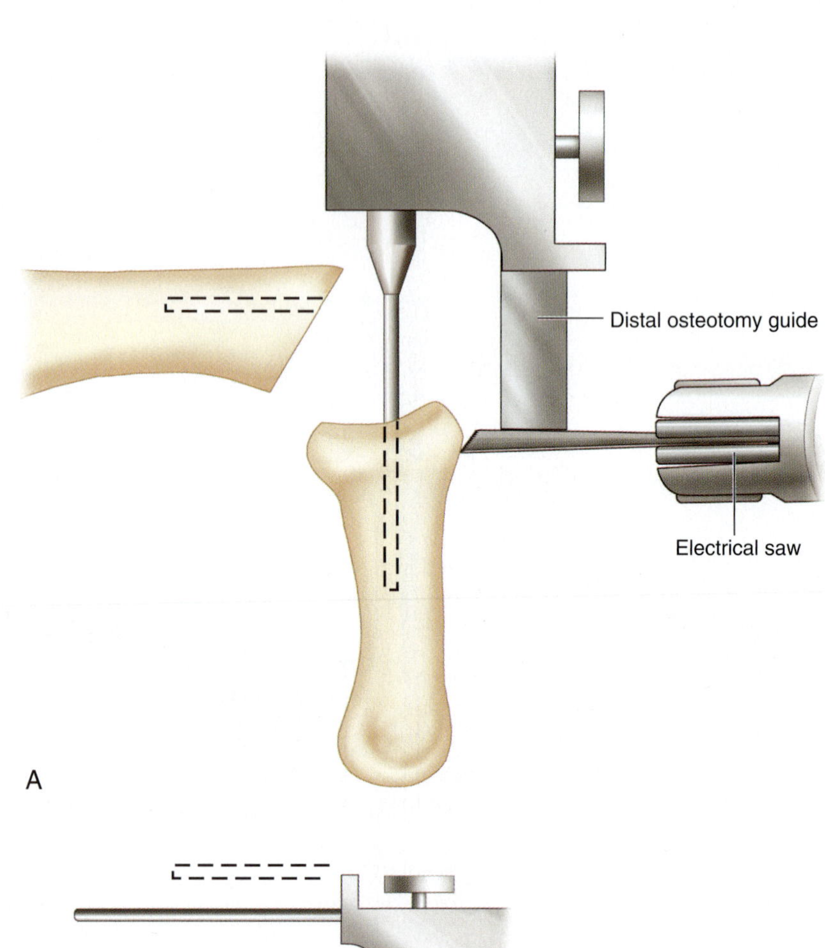

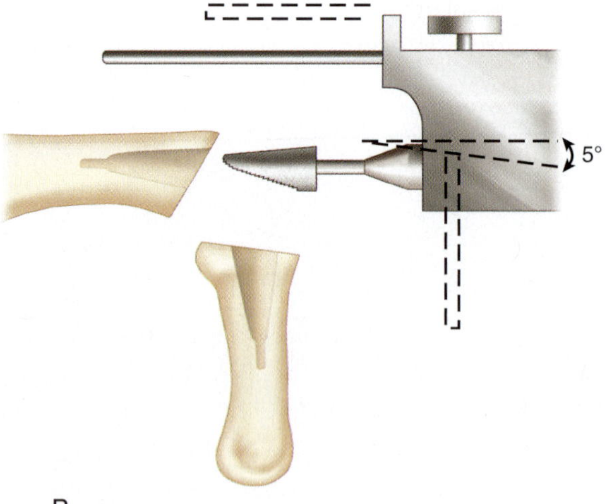

FIGURE 59-14

STEP 5 PEARLS

In cases of significantly sclerotic bone, such as in osteoarthritis, the canal may need to be enlarged with a side-cutting bur.

Broaching is stopped when the reamer is seated just below the bone edge.

Step 5

- A broach is inserted as described previously (Fig. 59-15A and B). Mismatch is not permitted between the proximal and distal components of the implant in MCP joint pyrocarbon arthroplasty.

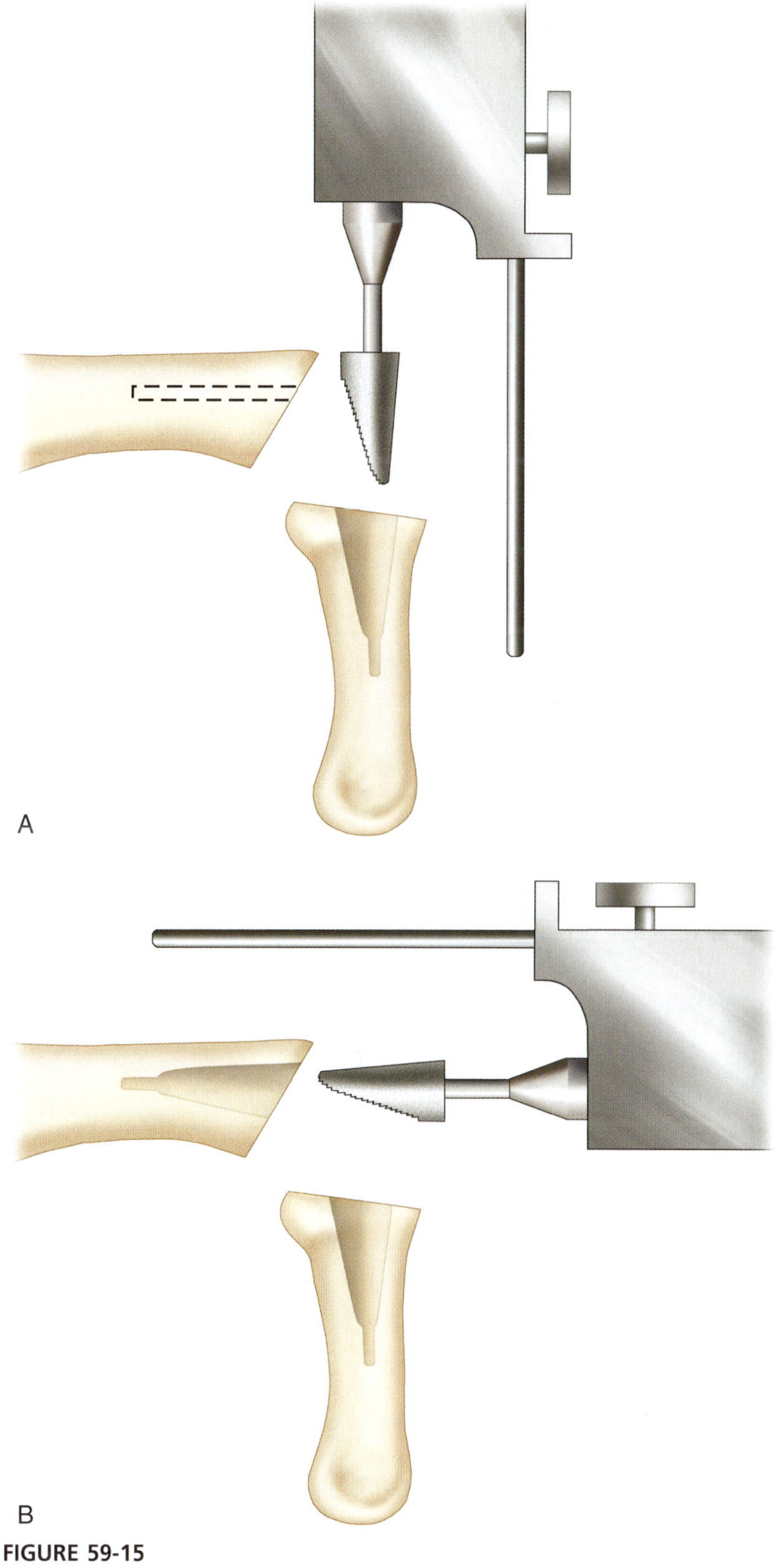

FIGURE 59-15

STEP 6 PEARLS

Final implants tend to be slightly larger than trial components to be press-fit securely.

The MCP joint should move passively through a 0- to 90-degree arc without significant tension.

Step 6

- A trial implant is inserted using a proximal and a distal impactor (Fig. 59-16A and B). The implant is press-fit into the medullary cavity by tapping it in gently (Fig. 59-17A and B).

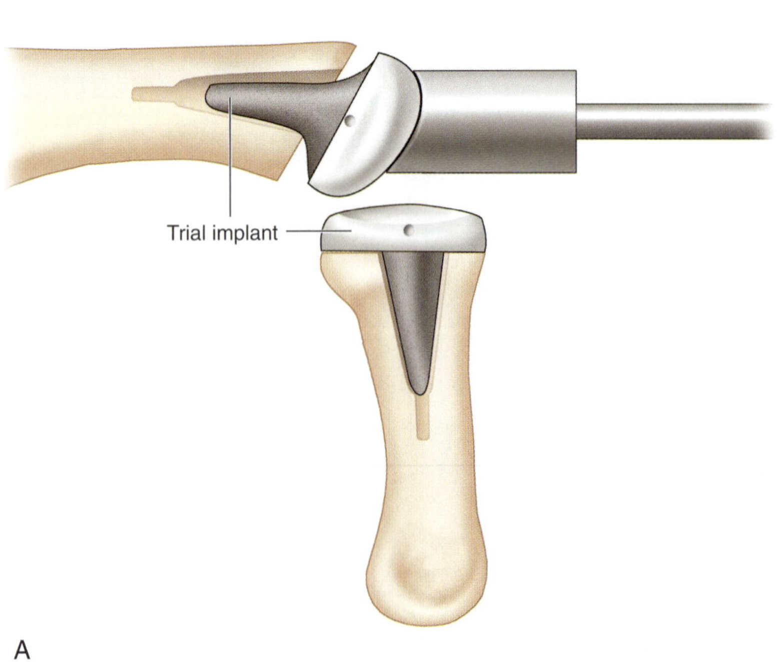

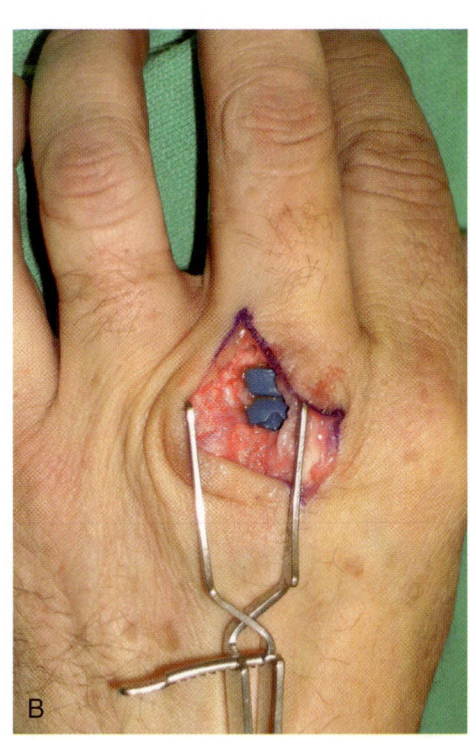

FIGURE 59-16

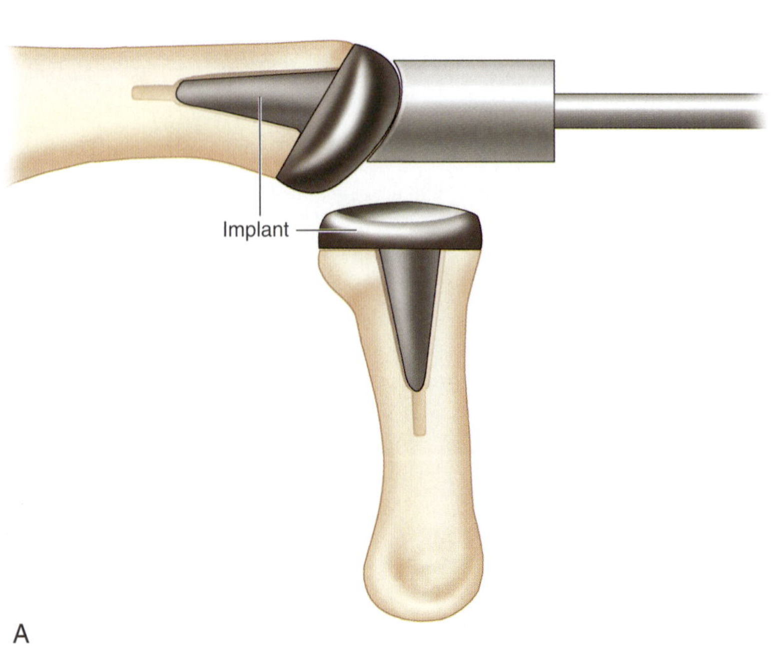

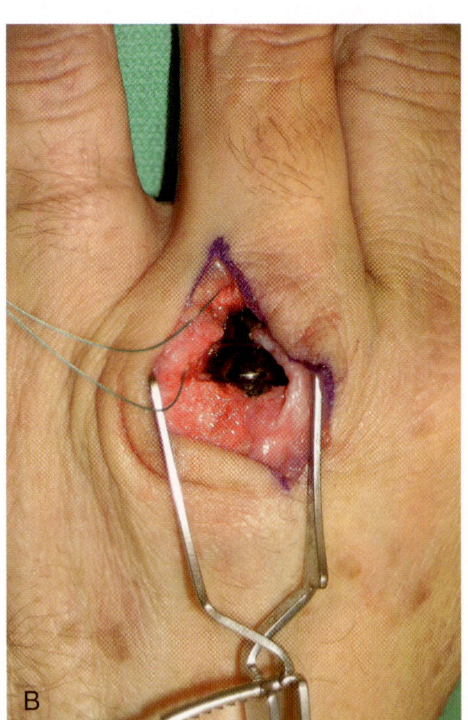

FIGURE 59-17

STEP 7 PEARLS

The dorsal capsule can be trimmed to provide a better-fitting repair over the prosthesis.

A final fluoroscopic examination should be performed to ensure that there has been no subluxation during dressing application.

Step 7

- The incised sagittal band is repaired with 3-0 horizontal-mattress braided permanent suture (Fig. 59-18). The tourniquet is released, and all bleeding points are cauterized. The skin is closed with 4-0 horizontal mattress nylon suture, and the finger is splinted in full extension.

Postoperative Care and Expected Outcomes

- The joint should be kept in extension for 3 weeks after the operation to consolidate the soft tissue support.
- One week after the operation, flexion and extension exercises are started in a dynamic splint. A static resting splint can be worn at night for 2 months after the 3-week exercise program.
- Expected outcomes of this procedure include improvement in pain, improved aesthetic appearance of the hand and fingers, increased ability to perform activities of daily living, improved key pinch strength, minimal change in active arc of motion, and minimal improvement in grip strength.

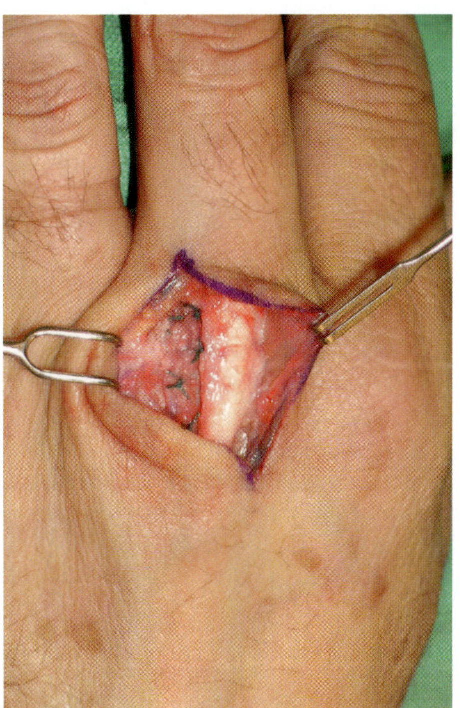

FIGURE 59-18

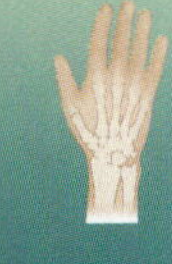

Case Studies

- Figure 59-19 (A to F) shows the long-term result of a PIP joint pyrocarbon implant arthroplasty in a 53-year-old man with severe osteoarthritis and pain over the left index finger PIP joint limiting motion. The patient refused PIP joint fusion; therefore, a pyrocarbon implant arthroplasty was performed.

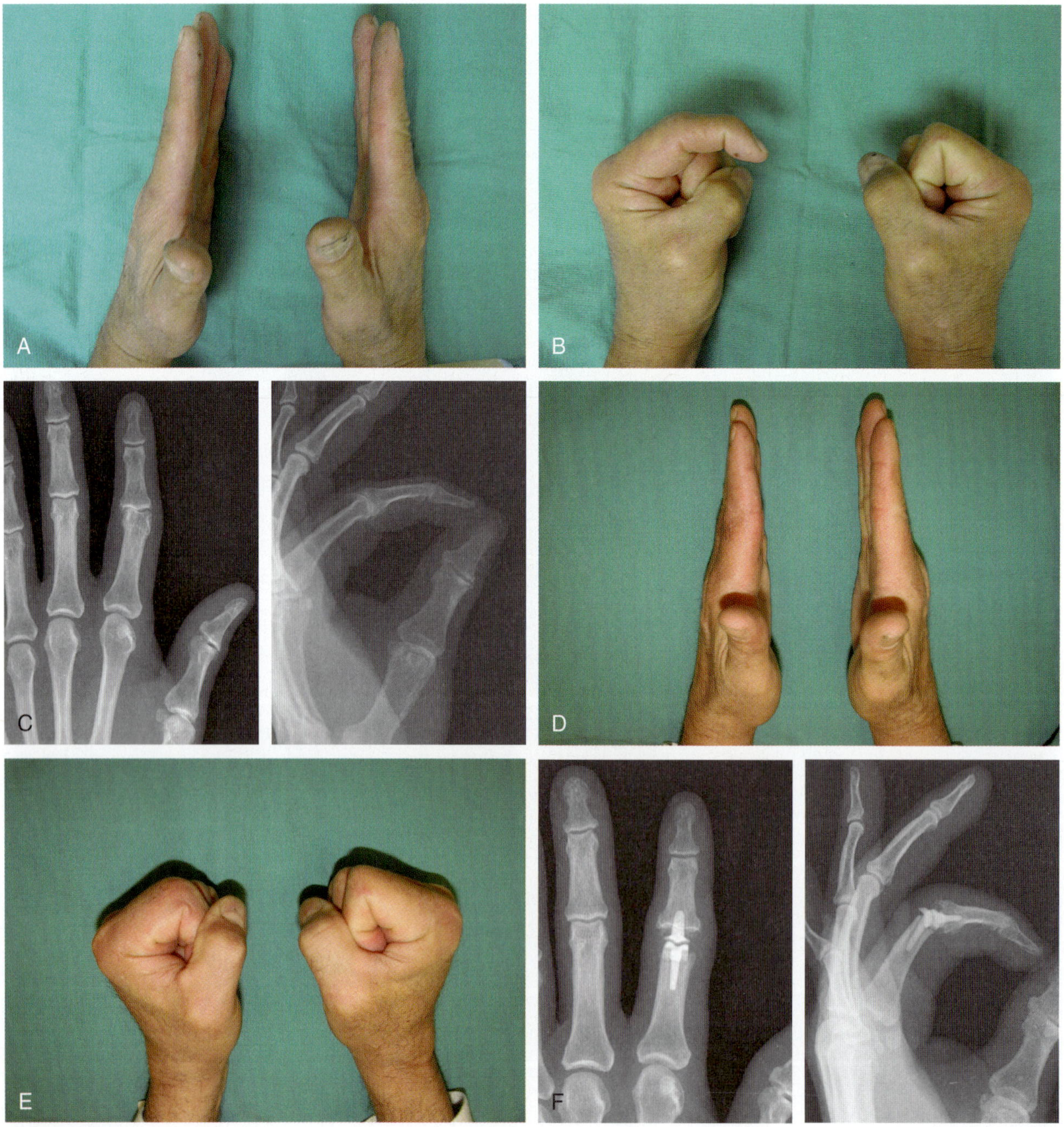

A B C D E F

FIGURE 59-19

- A 70-year-old woman presented with right index finger severe osteoarthritis and pain. She refused PIP joint fusion and opted for a pyrocarbon implant arthroplasty to preserve some motion (Fig. 59-20A). About 18 months after pyrocarbon arthroplasty, she began to experience chronic pain and swelling related to instability and recurrent dislocation of the joint that she was always able to reduce herself (Fig. 59-20B). Because of her persistent symptoms related to the recurrent dislocation, the implant was removed, and a PIP joint fusion was performed. This case illustrates that pyrocarbon arthroplasty can cause long-term problems relating to implant subsidence and dislocation. These complications must be explained carefully to the patient. Because there is no better alternative, and silicone implant for the PIP joint is often associated with joint instability, the pyrocarbon arthroplasty option is still a reasonable solution in lieu of joint fusion.

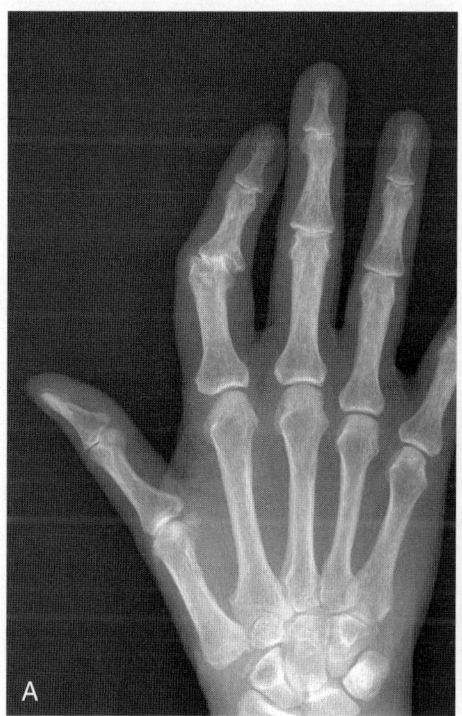

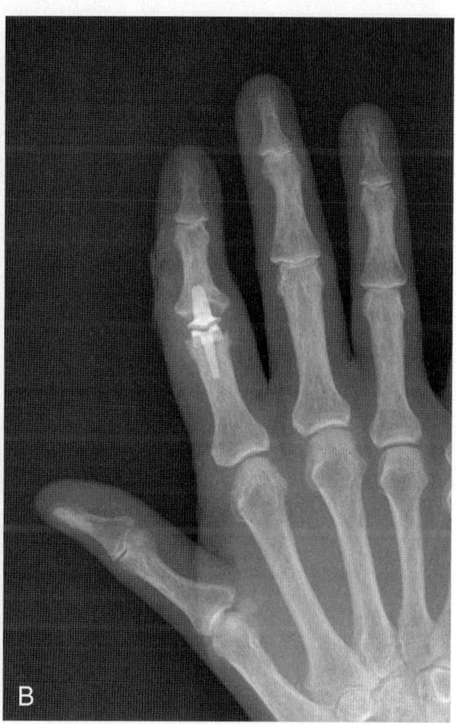

FIGURE 59-20

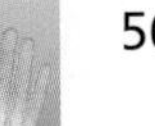

- A 59-year-old woman with a history of severe osteoarthritis of all finger joints presented for pyrocarbon arthroplasty of her right ring finger PIP joint (Fig. 59-21A). Two weeks after the arthroplasty, the joint was dislocated (Fig. 59-21B). The joint was reduced, and an external fixator was used to maintain reduction for 6 weeks (Fig. 59-21C). After removal of the external fixator, the joint was stable and had good motion (Fig. 59-21D). This case illustrates that poor ligamentous support in the PIP joint is unable to maintain joint reduction after implant arthroplasty. The use of an external fixator to reduce the joint permits tightening of the ligament support and can remedy the dislocation complication, if this complication is detected within the first 2 weeks after surgery.

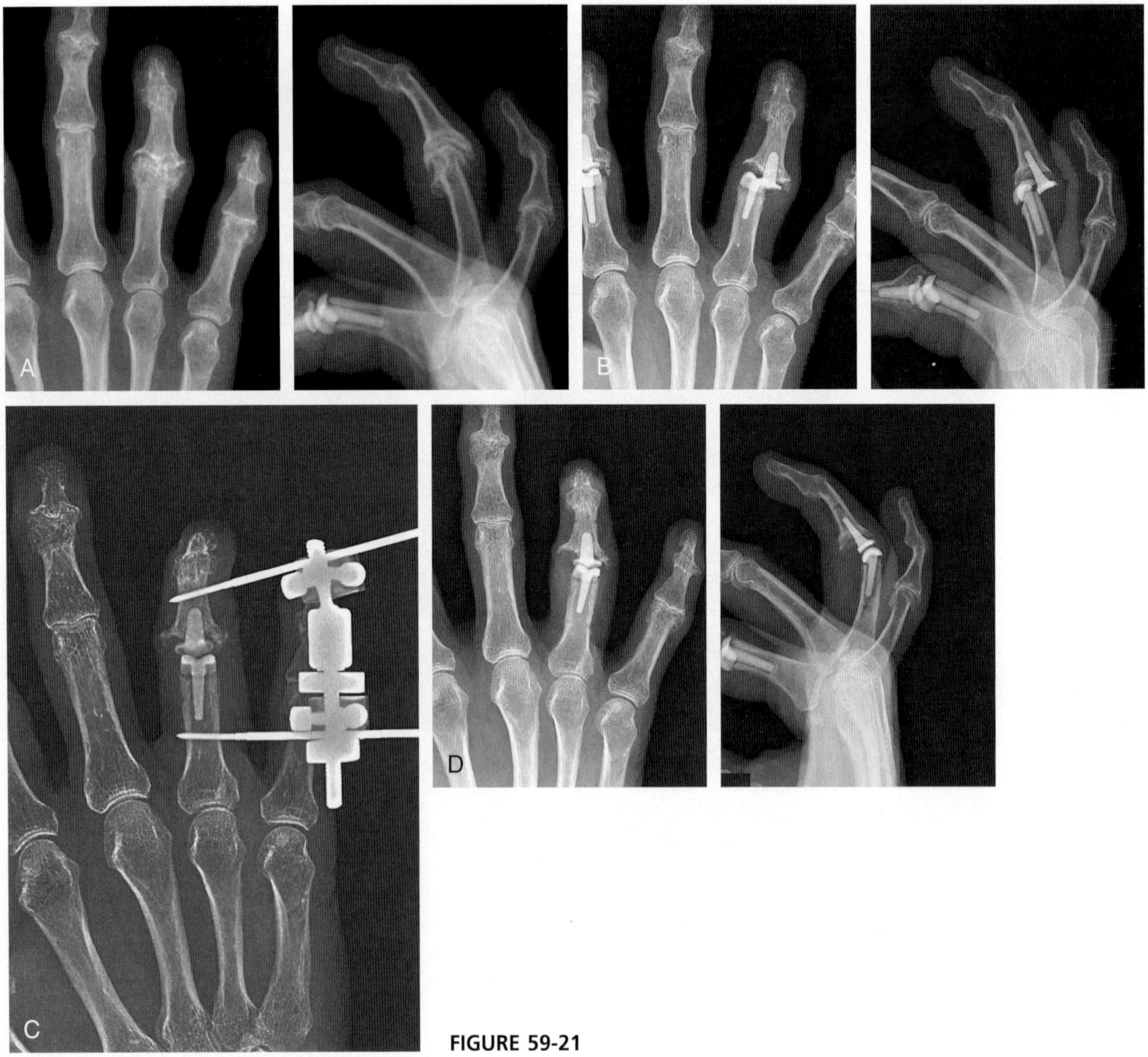

FIGURE 59-21

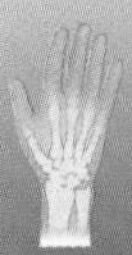

Evidence

Chung KC, Ram AN, Shauver MJ. Outcomes of pyrolytic carbon arthroplasty for the proximal interphalangeal joint. *Plast Reconstr Surg*. 2009;123:1521-1532.
In this case series, 14 patients treated with 21 implants were evaluated prospectively. At 12-month follow-up, mean active arc of motion was 38 degrees, which was slightly decreased from the preoperative value. Mean grip strength improved from 11.3 to 15.1 kg, although the difference was not statistically significant. Mean key pinch values improved significantly from 6.6 kg preoperatively to 9.2 kg at one year (P = .03). Three patients experienced dislocation of the pyrocarbon joint. The authors concluded that PIP pyrocarbon arthroplasty shows encouraging results with regard to patient satisfaction and pain relief but is associated with complications related to implant dislocation that requires prolonged treatment with external fixators. (Level IV evidence)

Cook SD, Beckenbaugh RD, Redondo J, et al. Long-term follow-up of pyrolytic carbon metacarpophalangeal implants. *J Bone Joint Surg [Am]*. 1999;81:635-648.
In this case series, 151 pyrolytic carbon MCP joint implants were inserted in 53 patients: 44 with rheumatoid arthritis, 5 with posttraumatic arthritis, 3 with osteoarthritis, and 1 with systemic lupus erythematosus. Twenty-six patients (71 implants) were followed for an average of 11.7 years after the operation. The arc of motion was improved 13 degrees on average. The authors reported no bony remodeling or resorption, and 94% of the cases showed osseointegration on radiologic examination. The average annual failure rate was 2.1%, and the 5- and 10-year survival rates were 82.3% and 81.4%, respectively. The authors concluded that the pyrolytic carbon MCP joint implant is a durable material for MCP joint arthroplasty. (Level IV evidence)

Parker W, Moran SL, Hormel KB, et al. Nonrheumatoid metacarpophalangeal joint arthritis. Unconstrained pyrolytic carbon implants: indications, technique, and outcomes. *Hand Clin*. 2006:22:183-193.
In this case series, a total of 21 MCP joint arthroplasties were performed in 19 patients. Of these, 10 patients were followed prospectively, and 9 were reviewed retrospectively. Ten index finger MCP and 11 long finger MCP joints were treated. The average duration of follow-up was 14 months. Postoperatively, average MCP joint flexion increased 12.8% (P = .17), MCP extension lag decreased 28.0% (P = .18), oppositional pinch increased 125.9% (P = .02), grip strength increased 38.2% (P = .04), and pain decreased 88.4% (P = .0004), with only 2 patients reporting pain at 1 year. None of the implants demonstrated evidence of loosening or migration. The authors concluded that pyrolytic carbon arthroplasty may be a reasonable option for joint salvage in patients suffering from MCP joint osteoarthritis. (Level IV evidence)

Squitieri L, Chung KC. A systematic review of outcomes and complications of vascularized toe joint transfer, silicone arthroplasty and pyrocarbon arthroplasty for post-traumatic joint reconstruction of the finger. *Plast Reconstr Surg*. 2008;121:1697-1707.
This paper presents a formal systematic review comparing the three currently available techniques—vascularized toe joint (VTJ), silicone, and pyrocarbon implants—to critically evaluate outcomes and complication rates for these three options. Five hundred twenty papers were identified, reviewed, and screened through multiple inclusion and exclusion criteria. The final numbers of papers and joint counts, respectively, are VTJ (13, 85), silicone (14, 181), and pyrocarbon (2, 18). The mean PIP active arc of motion (AAM) for VTJ, silicone, and pyrocarbon were 36.9 (SD 9.2), 45.9 (SD 8.8), and 43.6 (SD 10.9), respectively. The mean MCP AAMs for VTJ and silicone were 34.5 (SD 10.0) and 47 (SD not available and no data available for pyrocarbon). Major complication rates requiring joint revision procedures for VTJ, silicone, and pyrocarbon were 29%, 6%, and 28%, respectively. VTJ transfer has worse AAM and a higher complication rate compared with implant arthroplasty for both PIP and MCP joints. Pyrocarbon has better AAM than VTJ for PIP joints and the best AAM for MCP joints. However, early data suggest a high rate of major complications, and long-term outcomes data are still pending. VTJ transfer is indicated for maintaining the growth plate in a young patient, but its poor outcome does not justify its wide application for reconstructing posttraumatic sequelae of finger joints. Given the lack of improvement in outcomes for posttraumatic finger joint reconstruction in the past 40 years, research efforts should focus on future development of novel arthroplasty devices. (Level III evidence)

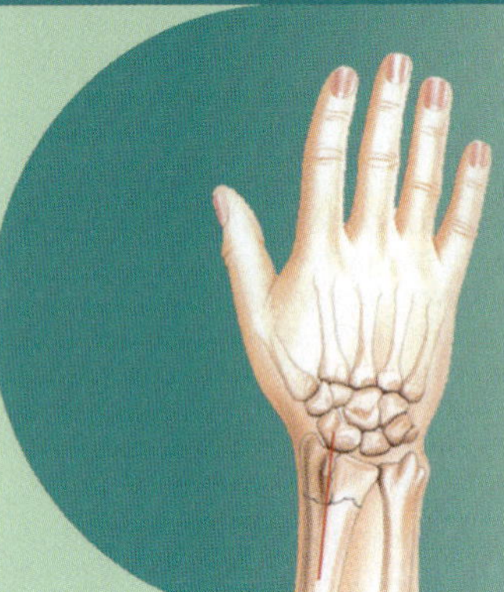

Arthrodesis of Finger and Thumb Interphalangeal and Metacarpophalangeal Joints

Winston Y. C. Chew and Lam-Chuan Teoh

See Video 44: Arthrodesis of Thumb Metacarpophalangeal Joint

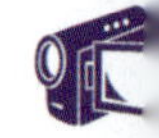

Indications

- Unstable and painful arthritic joints of the fingers and thumb.
- Interphalangeal (IP) joints are suitable for the oblique interfragmentary screw fixation technique, whereas the tension band wiring technique can be used for both IP and metacarpophalangeal (MCP) joints.

Examination/Imaging

Clinical Examination

- Angular deformity of the joints. Assess for possible passive correction as an indication of the degree of soft tissue contracture that may restrict surgical correction.
- Instability with subluxation and dislocation of joints (Fig. 60-1)
- Rheumatoid arthritis of the hands with unstable carpometacarpal and MCP joints of the right thumb with Z-deformity, subluxation of the left index and small finger proximal interphalangeal (PIP) joints, and deformity of the distal interphalangeal (DIP) joints of the right hand (see Fig. 60-1)

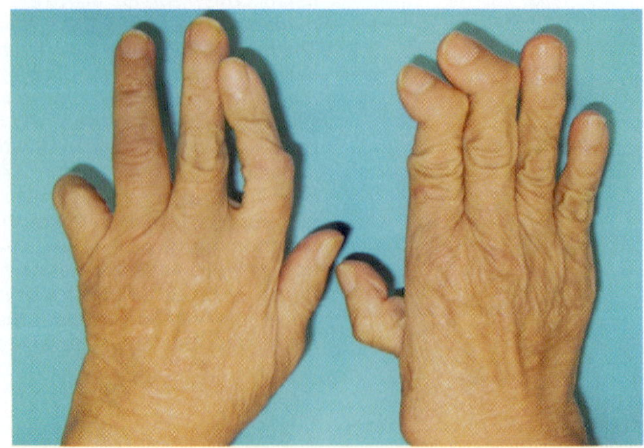

FIGURE 60-1

- Swelling and tenderness of the joints from effusion and osteophytes
- Presence of ganglion cysts
- Restricted active range of motion
- Decreased pinch and grip strength

Imaging

- Obtain standard posteroanterior and lateral radiographs of the involved finger and thumb.
- The alignment and bone stock around the involved joint should be noted (Fig. 60-2).
- Figure 60-2 shows posteroanterior radiographs of the same hands, confirming the clinical findings in Figure 60-1. In addition, there is dislocation of the MCP joint of the left thumb.

Surgical Anatomy

- The cartilage destruction leads to loosening of collateral ligaments and instability of the IP joint. The pinch and grasping stresses lead to angular deformity at the involved joint. Irritation from osteophytes and synovitis leads to pain, joint effusion, and loss of pinch and grasping strength. The extensor tendon, in particular at the DIP joint, may be attenuated, causing mallet deformity, which in chronic cases results in fixed flexion deformity.
- The joint and adjacent bones have to be adequately exposed for débridement and removal of residual cartilage, fashioning of the bone ends, and placement of the implants.
- The fusion angle of the joint is determined preoperatively.

Positioning

- The patient should be positioned supine with a hand extension table.
- The hand should be easily accessible to the mini C-arm for fluoroscopic control during surgery.

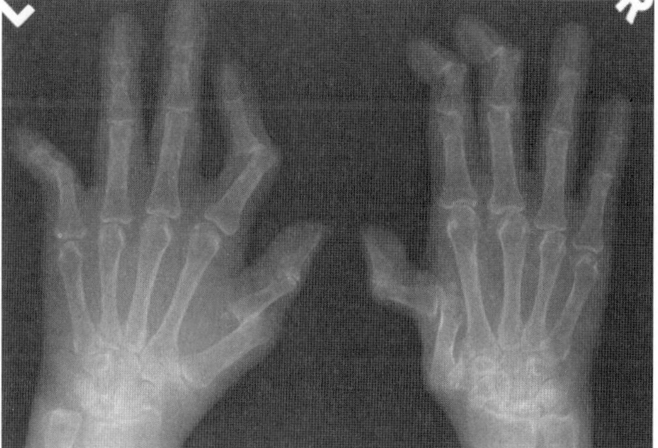

FIGURE 60-2

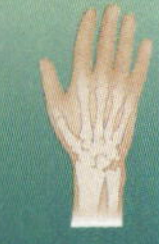

Exposures

Metacarpophalangeal Joint

- Straight dorsal incision from about the midproximal phalanx to the midmetacarpal region. Alternatively, a dorsal curvilinear incision may be used.
- Extensor tendon split in the midline from the proximal phalanx proximally over the MCP joint. For the thumb and index and small fingers with two extensor tendons, the incision on the tendon is carried proximally between the two tendons. For the long and ring fingers, the incision is carried proximally to either the radial or ulnar side of the extensor tendon, taking with it a sliver of the tendon for easy repair during closure.

Proximal Interphalangeal Joint

- The PIP joint is exposed through a gentle curve over the joint and extended over the adjacent bones (Fig. 60-3).
- Figure 60-3 shows the dorsal curvilinear incision over the PIP joint.
- The extensor tendon is split in the midline from proximal to distal, splitting and elevating the central slip attachment and cutting the triangular ligament over the middle phalanx, elevating the lateral bands.
- The collateral ligament on one side is cut to allow the articular surfaces to be exposed adequately in a "shotgun" fashion. If necessary, both collateral ligaments may be cut.

PEARLS

In joints with fixed deformity, release of the soft tissue needs to be performed to reposition and reduce the joint in an optimal position.

The volar plate, especially at the DIP joint, may tent the joint apart, preventing compression of the bones for arthrodesis, and needs to be adequately released.

Distal Interphalangeal Joint

- The DIP joint of the fingers and the IP joint of the thumb are exposed with an H incision, with the transverse part of the H directly over the dorsum of the joint (Fig. 60-4). Alternatively, a Y incision centered over the DIP joint may be used.
- The extensor tendon is divided transversely leaving a 5-mm-long distal stump for subsequent repair. The extensor tendon is repaired at completion of the arthrodesis to maintain the balance of the intricate extensor mechanism.
- The collateral ligaments on both sides are divided, allowing the joint to be hinged open dorsally.

PITFALLS

Care is taken to ensure that the germinal matrix of the nail fold is not violated.

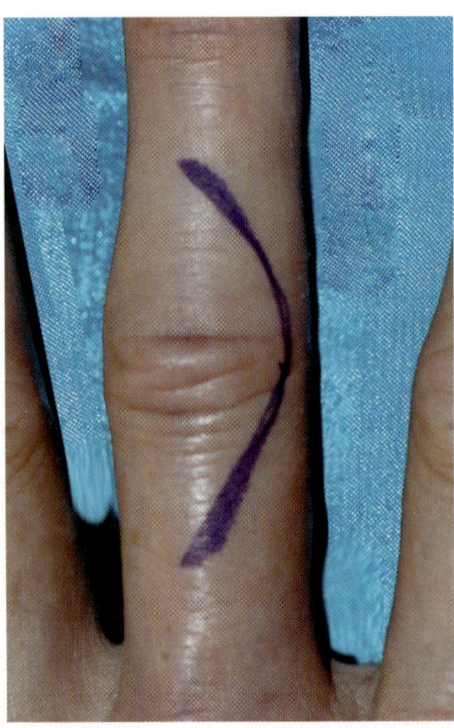

FIGURE 60-3

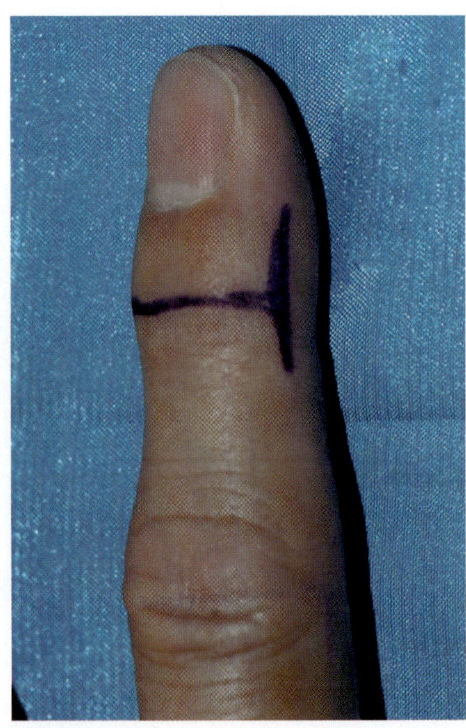

FIGURE 60-4

STEP 1 PEARLS

Scraping the joint surface with a sharp periosteal elevator or small osteotome is effective in removing the residual cartilage.

STEP 1 PITFALLS

In fixed deformity, without soft tissue release, reduction of the joint may not be possible.

STEP 2 PEARLS

Fashioning of the bone ends with the crest-and-trough technique requires minimal removal of bones. It allows preservation of much of the subchondral bone and improves the stability of the fixation. This fashioning technique effectively controls the axial alignment and corrects any preexisting deviational deformity. The large area of bone contact that the technique confers is maintained over a wide range of joint flexion.

Alternatively, the bone ends can be cut using a saw, with the distal bone at 0 degrees and the proximal bone at the desired angle of fusion.

Procedure

Preparation of Joint Surfaces (Crest and Trough Method)

Step 1

- The joint and its adjacent bone ends are adequately exposed.
- Joint débridement using a small bone rongeur is performed. This is aimed to remove the inflamed joint capsule, associated ganglion, osteophytes, and residual cartilage.
- Soft tissue release is done to reduce and realign the joint.

Step 2

- The bone ends are fashioned with the aim of a "crest-and-trough" fitting.
- Figure 60-5 shows the use of the bur to create the crest-and-trough shape of the joint.
- Fashioning the distal bone end is done using a small bur, following the concave shape of the articular surface (see Fig. 60-5). Running the bur transversely over the articular surface creates a gentle trough. The bone surface is burred evenly until the subchondral bone is reached and all the residual cartilage removed.
- Fashioning the proximal condyle is done similarly using a small bur. By following the convex shape of the condylar surface, running the bur transversely creates a crest shape.

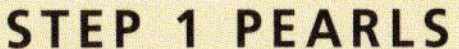

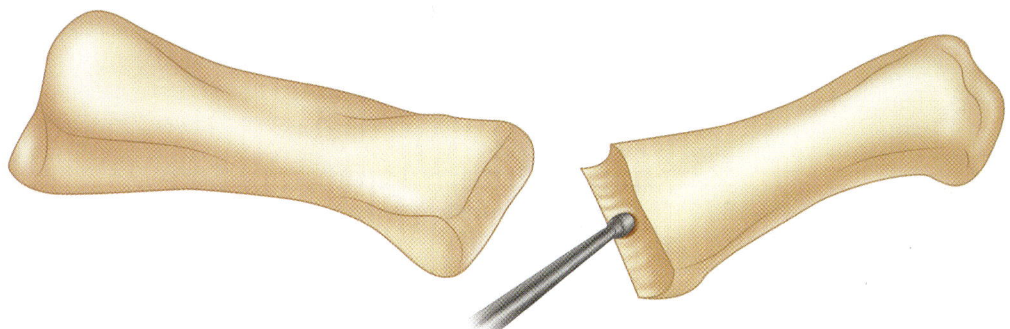

FIGURE 60-5

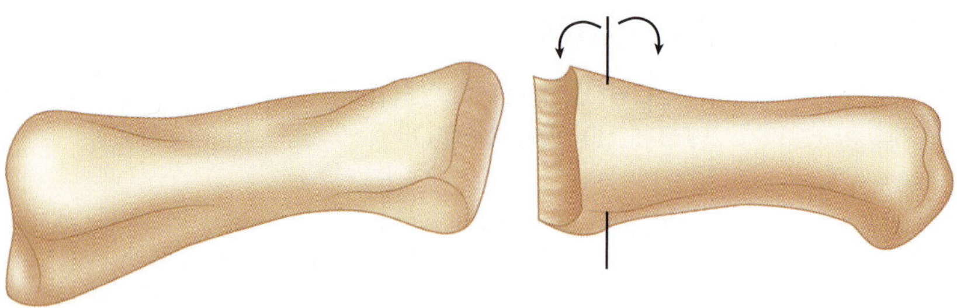

FIGURE 60-6

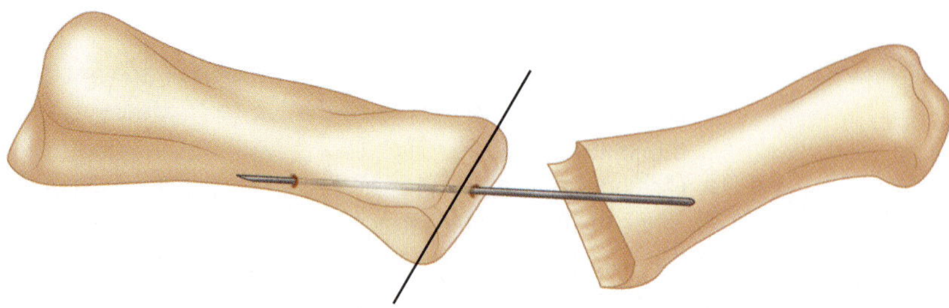

FIGURE 60-7

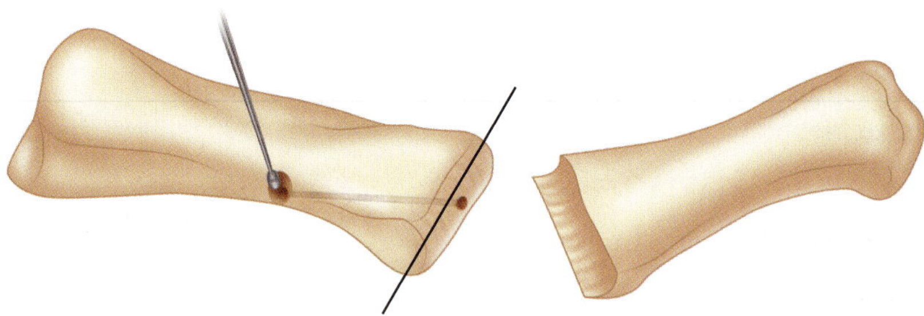

FIGURE 60-8

STEP 2 PITFALLS

Avoid excessive removal of bones by adjusting the shape of the bone surfaces in small steps until the surfaces are fitting. This helps to preserve length and retain good-quality cancellous bone for optimal bony union.

- Trial reduction of the joint is done to ensure a proper surface fitting and axis alignment. Adjust the shape of the bone surfaces in small steps until the surfaces fit well and axis alignment is achieved (Fig. 60-6).
- Figure 60-6 shows that the crest-and-trough configuration of the joint allows fine adjustment of the fusion angle around the axis as shown.

Oblique Interfragmentary Screw Fixation Technique

Step 3

- Fixation of the bone ends is done with an oblique interfragmentary screw, using a 2-mm screw for the PIP joint and the thumb IP joint and a 1.5-mm screw for the DIP joint.
- The proximal drill hole is made over the proximal bone end. The drill hole is set at 45 degrees to the transverse joint surface, using the retrograde drilling technique (Fig. 60-7). The entry point is at "dead center" of the condylar surface for a fusion angle set at 0 degrees. For a joint fusion angle of 10 to 30 degrees of flexion, the entry point is set at 1 to 1.5 mm (the diameter of the drill bit) more palmarly.
- Countersink the exit point of the drill hole over the proximal shaft, and further recess the proximal cortex of the drill hole with a small bur to ensure proper seating of the screw head (Fig. 60-8).

STEP 3 PEARLS

Temporary pinning of the joint with a 0.8-mm K-wire parallel to the drill hole allows compression of the joint before insertion of the screw.

The joint can be readjusted to the correct angle without refashioning the bone ends, yet maintaining similarly good bone contact through a wide range of fusion angles.

Perform the antegrade drilling of the distal bone end after the correct angle of fusion has been confirmed.

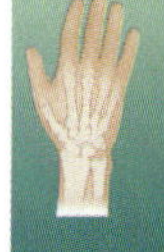

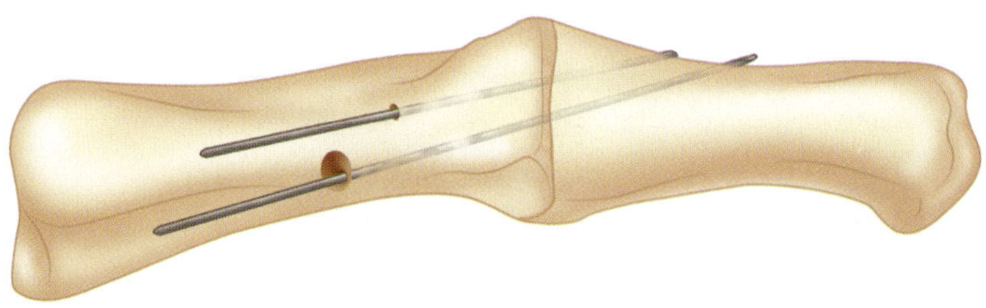

FIGURE 60-9

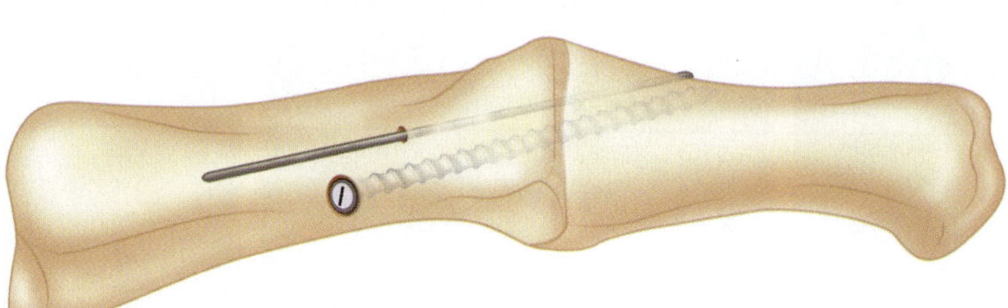

FIGURE 60-10

STEP 3 PITFALLS

The bone can be displaced when introducing the interfragmentary screw. Counterpressure on the distal bone during screw introduction is always necessary. Remove the temporary K-wire after the fixation is completed.

For fusion of the finger DIP joints and thumb IP joint, aim the screw from proximal to distal and slightly palmarly. This will avoid having the screw tip encroach onto the nail matrix.

- Figure 60-8 shows widening of the screw entry point with a bur to accommodate the screw head.
- Reduce the joint, set it to a predetermined angle of fusion, and ensure proper axial alignment and lateral reduction. Temporary pinning of the fusion is done with 0.8-mm K-wire parallel to, but at the same time avoiding encroaching on, the drill hole and intended direction of the screw (Fig. 60-9).
- Figure 60-9 shows a parallel K-wire driven across the joint before drilling.
- Perform a visual assessment of the finger and the whole hand to ensure that the fusion angle and alignment are according to plan. Perform a fluoroscopic check to confirm.
- Antegrade drilling of the distal bone end is then done. Insert the drill through the previous drill hole on the proximal bone, and complete the drilling into the distal bone end.
- Fixation is completed with the required interfragmentary screw (Fig. 60-10). Compression across the joint is achieved by precompressing with a small bone clamp before insertion of the screw.
- The K-wire is then removed (Fig. 60-11).

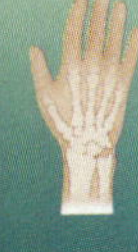

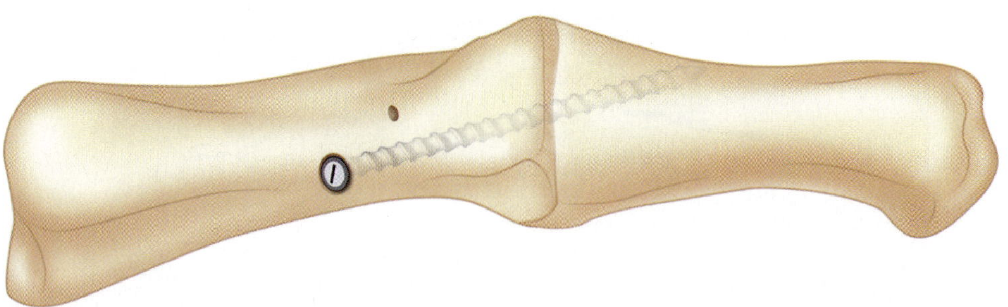

FIGURE 60-11

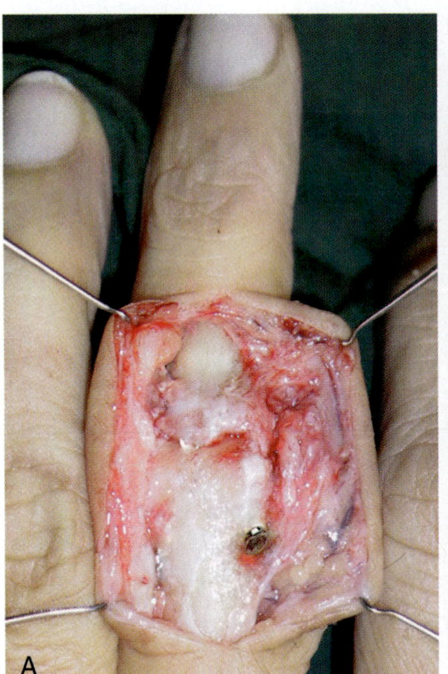

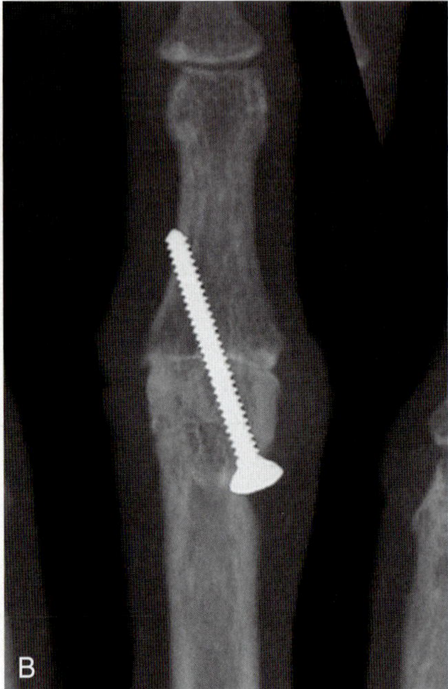

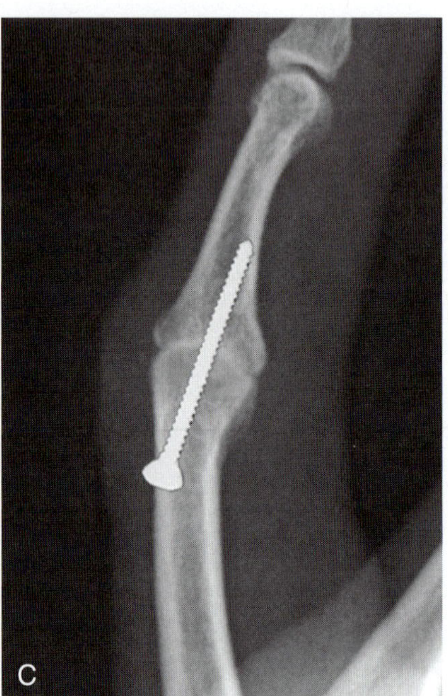

FIGURE 60-12

STEP 4 PEARLS

Repairing the extensor tendon maintains the balance of the intricate extensor mechanism.

The divided collateral ligament, if still available, can be repaired; this will further enhance the stability of the fusion.

Step 4

- After completion of the fixation, fluoroscopy is repeated to confirm the final reduction and the screw position and length (Figs. 60-12 and 60-13).
- Figure 60-12A shows the intraoperative appearance of PIP joint fusion; parts B and C show the radiographic appearance of the joint.
- Figure 60-13A and B shows the radiographic appearance of the DIP joint fusion.
- The extensor tendon is repaired with running 5-0 absorbable suture.
- The skin is closed with interrupted nonabsorbable suture.

Tension Band Wiring Technique (Parallel Wiring)

STEP 1 PEARLS

Appropriately sized K-wires should be used.

Frequent irrigation of the bone should be done during insertion of the K-wires to prevent bone necrosis.

Leaving the K-wires protruding 1 to 2 mm at the fusion surface allows the K-wires to engage into the middle phalanx during positioning before they are driven in.

Step 1

- Two parallel K-wires, sized 1 or 1.25 mm (depending on the size of the bone), are driven retrograde from the joint into the head of the proximal phalanx at an angle equivalent to the desired angle of fusion (Fig. 60-14).
- They are then withdrawn proximally until about 1 to 2 mm of the wire tip is left protruding in the joint.
- Figure 60-15 shows two K-wires driven retrograde from the PIP joint into the proximal phalanx in the long axis of the middle phalanx and parallel to each other.

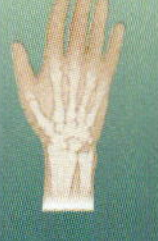

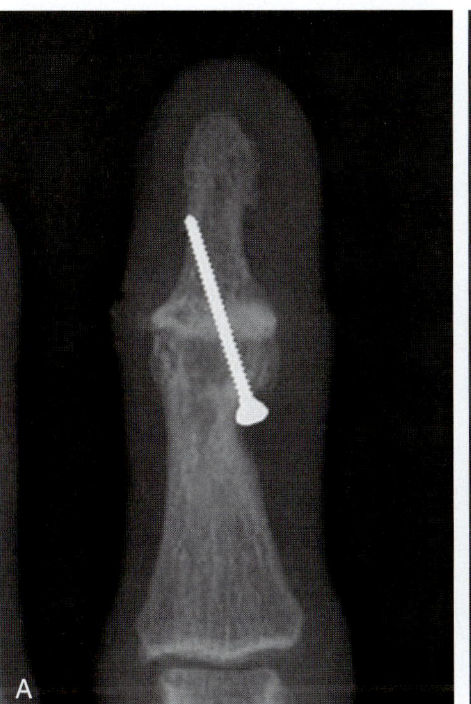

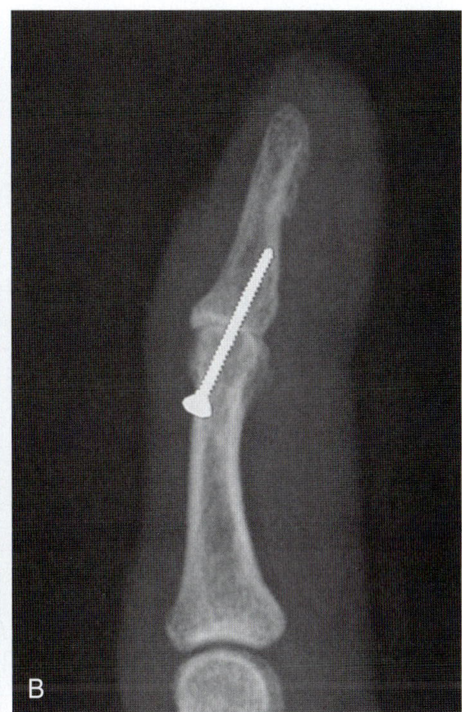

FIGURE 60-13

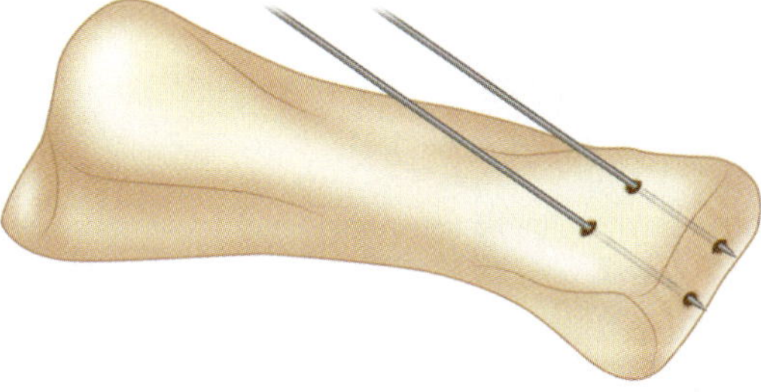

FIGURE 60-14

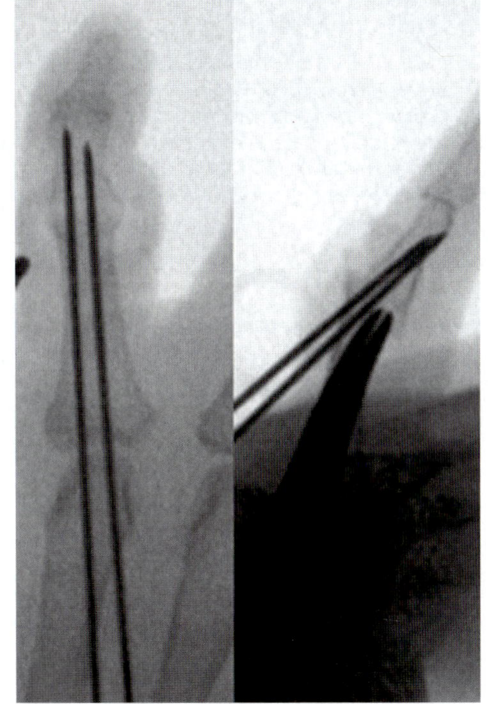

FIGURE 60-15

STEP 1 PITFALLS

The angle at which the K-wires are driven into the proximal phalanx should be the fusion angle. Otherwise, either the fusion angle will be wrong, with the middle phalanx having to accommodate the angle of the K-wires, or the K-wire will not be along the length of the middle phalanx, resulting in a less stable fixation.

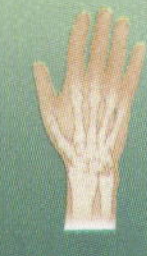

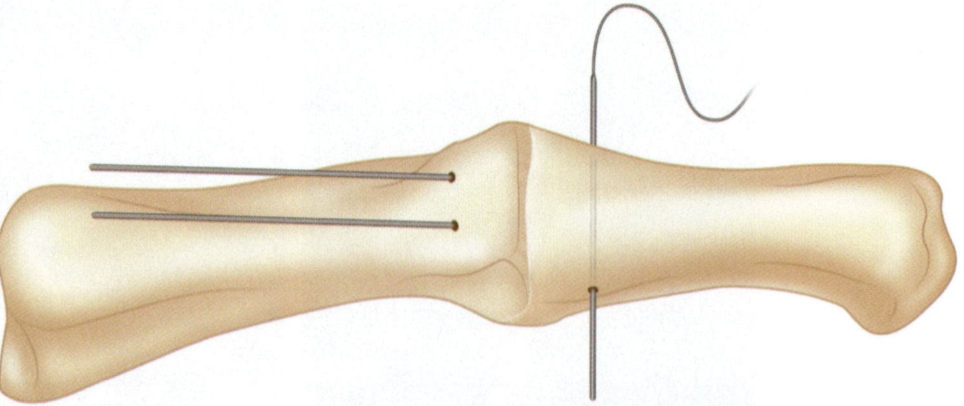

FIGURE 60-16

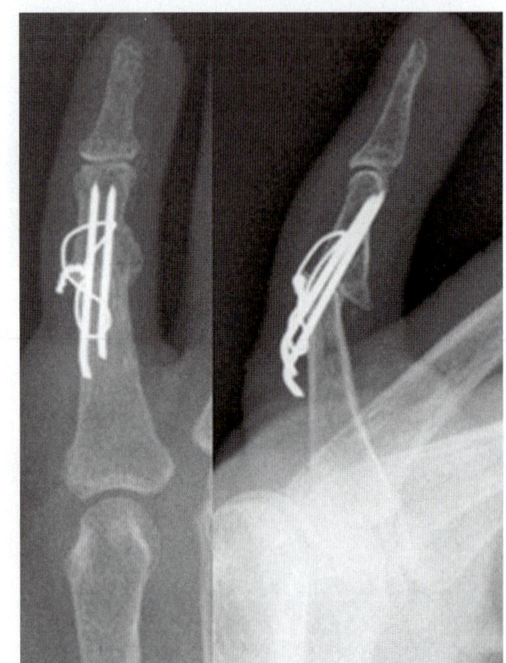

FIGURE 60-17

Step 2

- The middle phalanx is apposed and adjusted to the desired angle of fusion, and the K-wires are driven into the shaft of the middle phalanx.
- The placement of the K-wires is then checked with the mini C-arm to ensure that the tips are not impinging into the distal phalanx or the flexor tendons (see Fig. 60-15).

Step 3

- The hub of an 18- or 19-gauge needle is removed and the needle is used as a cannulated drill to drive a pilot hole transversely across the base of the middle phalanx, about 1 cm from the PIP joint (Fig. 60-16).
- Figure 60-16 shows a 19-gauge needle used to drive a hole in the coronal plane of the middle phalanx about 1 to 1.5 cm from the PIP joint.
- A 24-gauge cerclage wire is passed through this hole and wound dorsally around the two K-wires in a figure-of-eight pattern and tightened, ensuring that the knot of the wire is toward the side of the construct.
- The K-wires are then bent and cut short, and the tips are twisted down against the bone to avoid soft tissue irritation (Fig. 60-17).

Step 4

- The extensor tendon is repaired over the joint, and the skin is closed.

STEP 2 PEARLS

It is desirable but not necessary to engage the volar cortex with the K-wires.

STEP 2 PITFALLS

Care must be taken to ensure that the K-wires are not too long because they may splint the DIP joint or, if driven through the volar cortex, skewer the flexor tendons.

Figure 60-15 shows parallel K-wires driven across the PIP joint from the proximal phalanx into the shaft of the middle phalanx of the small finger under radiographic control.

STEP 3 PEARLS

Ensure that the cerclage wire is tightened evenly on both sides of the PIP joint around the K-wires.

The bent part of the K-wire should be turned toward the bone. This lessens soft tissue irritation as well as helping to hold the wire better.

The knot of the cerclage wire should be put at the side of the PIP joint to lessen soft tissue irritation.

Figure 60-17 shows the cerclage wire tightened around the K-wires, which are then bent to hold the cerclage wire and prevent irritation of soft tissues.

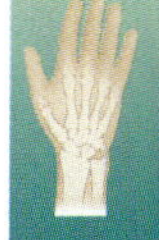

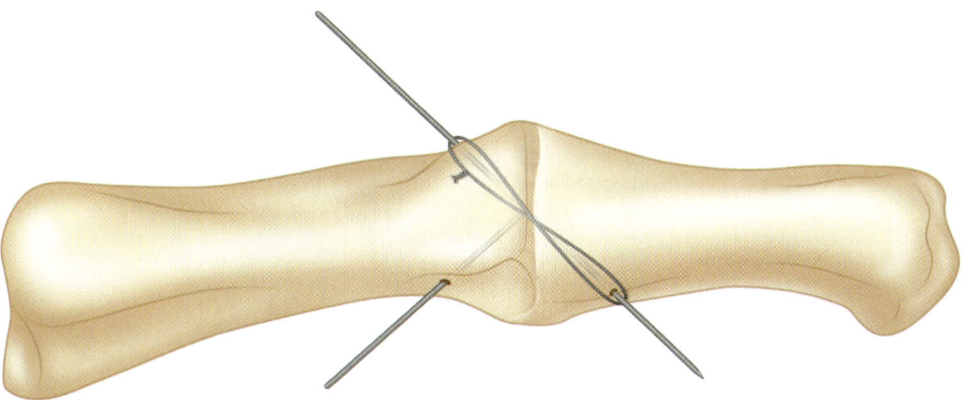

FIGURE 60-18

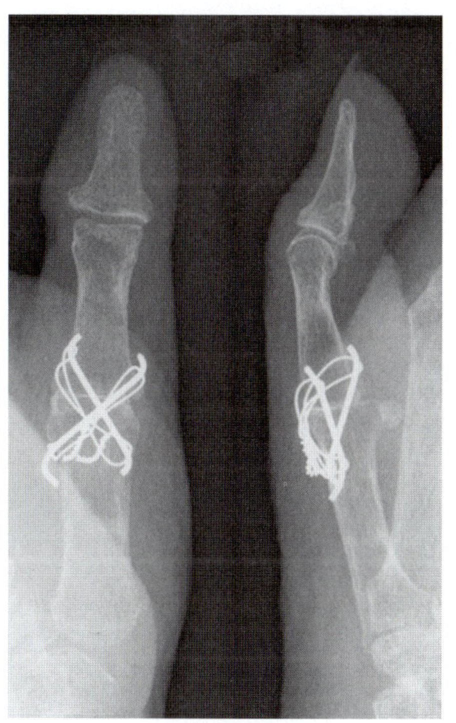

FIGURE 60-19

STEP 1 PEARLS

The rotational alignment of the joint should be checked before driving in the second wire because fine adjustments can still be made.

STEP 1 PITFALLS

Inadequate compression before driving in the second K-wire may result in the joint being splinted apart by the cross K-wires, with risk for delayed union or nonunion.

Tension Band Wiring Technique (Cross Wiring)

Step 1

- The joint is positioned at the angle of fusion, and a 1- or 1.25-mm K-wire (depending on the size of the bone) is inserted obliquely to hold the position of the joint.
- Once the position of the joint (flexion angle and rotational alignment) is confirmed, a 24-gauge cerclage wire is used as a figure-of-eight tension band across the joint around the two ends of the oblique wire. It is tightened to achieve adequate tension and compression across the joint (Fig. 60-18).
- Figure 60-18 shows tension band wiring applied over the first K-wire before driving in the second K-wire.

Step 2

- The alignment of the joint is checked again before another K-wire is inserted obliquely on the opposite side in a crossed fashion.
- Another 24-gauge cerclage wire is then used as a figure-of-eight tension band over the second K-wire.
- The knot of the cerclage wire is then placed at the side of the joint, well bent to avoid irritation of the soft tissue.

Step 3

- The K-wires are cut short and bent toward the bone to hold the cerclage wires in place as well as to avoid soft tissue irritation. They may also be cut just short enough to hold the cerclage wires without being bent (Fig. 60-19).
- Figure 60-19 shows the final radiographic appearance of MCP joint fusion using the cross-tension–band wiring technique.

Step 4

- The capsule and extensor tendon are repaired over the arthrodesed joint, and the skin is closed with interrupted sutures.

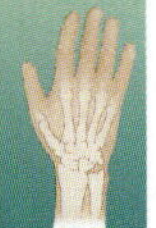

STEP 2 PEARLS

The position of the cross K-wires should be in the midaxial plane. This will ensure that the tension band effect is applied appropriately across the arthrodesis site.

The second K-wire could be driven first into the proximal bone without penetrating across the joint, then driven through only after tension band wire has been tightened over the first wire.

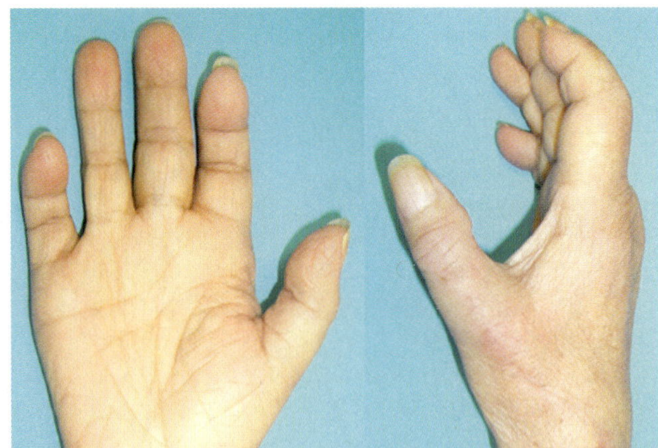

FIGURE 60-20

PEARLS

For the tension band wiring technique, active movement converts a distraction force into a compressive force owing to a flexion moment around the pivot point formed by the tension band, thereby promoting joint compression and union.

Figure 60-20 shows the postoperative appearance after fusion of the MCP joint of the right thumb and DIP joint of the index and long fingers. Thumb carpometacarpal joint arthroplasty was also done.

Postoperative Care and Expected Outcomes

- The finger is dressed in a soft bulky supportive dressing to prevent excessive postoperative motion. At the first dressing about 1 week after surgery, the finger is immobilized in a palmar trough splint. Supervised active motion to the proximal joint is allowed after the second week. The splint is worn for 6 weeks or until the radiographs show union, whichever is longer.
- Fusion of the joints should occur at about 6 to 8 weeks, after which the joint is stable enough for strengthening exercises and pinching activities.
- Function is significantly improved with well-aligned and stable joints (Fig. 60-20).

Evidence

Stern PJ, Gates NT, Jones TB. Tension band arthrodesis of small joints of the hand. *J Hand Surg [Am]*. 1993;18:194-197.

The authors discuss 290 arthrodesis procedures of the MCP and PIP joint in 203 patients. Complications include a 3% (9 patients) incidence of nonunion (4 with painless pseudarthroses, 1 requiring finger amputation), 10 superficial infections, and 3 malrotations. Twenty-five fusions (9%) required hardware removal. (Level V evidence)

Teoh LC, Yeo SJ, Singh I. Interphalangeal joint arthrodesis with oblique placement of an AO lag screw. *J Hand Surg [Br]*. 1994;19:208-211.

The paper described arthrodesis of the interphalangeal joint using a single interfragmentary screw placed laterally and obliquely across the joint. The technique offers better control of the desired angle of fusion. The fusion rate was 96% at an average of 8.2 weeks.

Uhl RL. Proximal interphalangeal joint arthrodesis using the tension band technique. *J Hand Surg [Am]*. 2007;32:914-917.

The author gives a detailed account of the tension band technique for arthrodesis of the PIP joint. (Level V evidence)

Uhl RL, Schneider LH. Tension band arthrodesis of finger joints: a retrospective review of 76 consecutive cases. *J Hand Surg [Am]*. 1992;17:518-522.

The authors present a series of 76 tension band arthrodesis procedures in 63 patients using parallel wire fixation with tension band technique. With a follow-up ranging from 6 to 38 months, radiographic fusion was achieved at a mean of 12 weeks, with a fusion rate of 99%. Technical problems included nonparallel pin placement and penetration of the wire tips, causing painful impingement of the soft tissues. (Level V evidence)

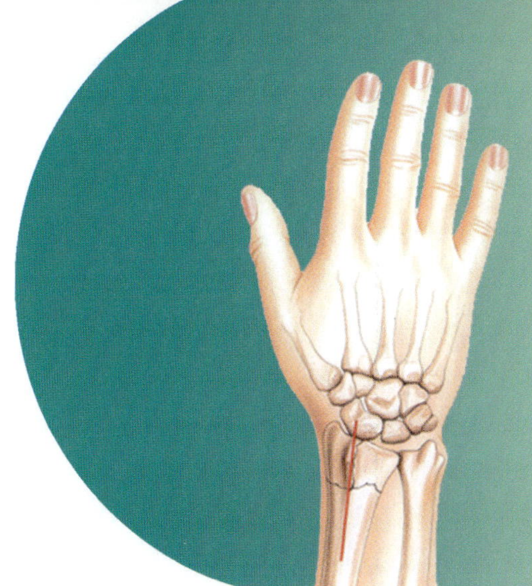

Section IX

THUMB CARPOMETACARPAL JOINT INSTABILITY AND ARTHRITIS

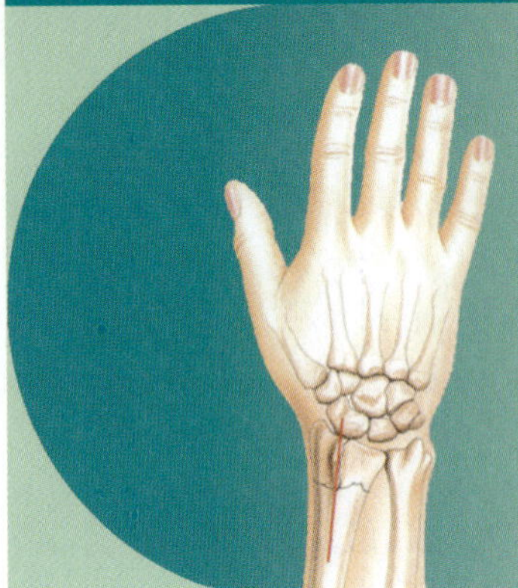

PROCEDURE 61

Trapeziometacarpal Ligament Reconstruction

Nathan S. Taylor and Kevin C. Chung

See Video 45: Thumb CMC Joint Beak Ligament Reconstruction Using the FCR Tendon

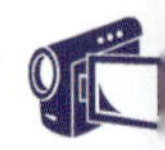

Indications

- Chronic posttraumatic instability of the thumb CMC joint
- Symptomatic laxity of the thumb CMC joint

Examination/Imaging

Clinical Examination

- The clinician should stress the trapeziometacarpal (TMC) joint and note any instability and laxity. The extent of ligament rupture (partial versus complete) allows varying degrees of hypermobility. Although hypermobility may be present bilaterally, greater excursion and symptomatic hypermobility should be evident on the affected side.

Imaging

- A lateral and pronated anteroposterior radiograph should be obtained to evaluate any existing joint disease and to identify the more commonly seen Bennett fracture-dislocation.
- A stressed anteroposterior radiograph of the bilateral thumbs with radial margins pressed together can help elucidate the degree of capsule laxity and presents both thumb joints for comparison (Fig. 61-1).

Surgical Anatomy

- The TMC joint is a biconcave saddle-shaped joint that provides motion in several planes to allow thumb flexion, extension, abduction, adduction, and opposition.
- The volar oblique (beak) ligament inserts volarly onto the trapezium from its confluence with articular cartilage on the beak of the thumb metacarpal and is considered the primary stabilizer of the TMC joint. It serves as the main restraint against dorsal translation of the metacarpal on the trapezium (Fig. 61-2).
- The thin and less well-defined dorsal ligament is reinforced by an expansion of the insertion of the abductor pollicis longus (APL) tendon onto the dorsal-radial aspect of the metacarpal.
- The radial artery traverses the anatomic snuffbox and overlies the dorsal capsule of the carpometacarpal (CMC) joint.
- The abductor pollicis longus (APL) and extensor pollicis brevis (EPB) tendons are within the first extensor compartment.

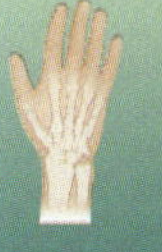

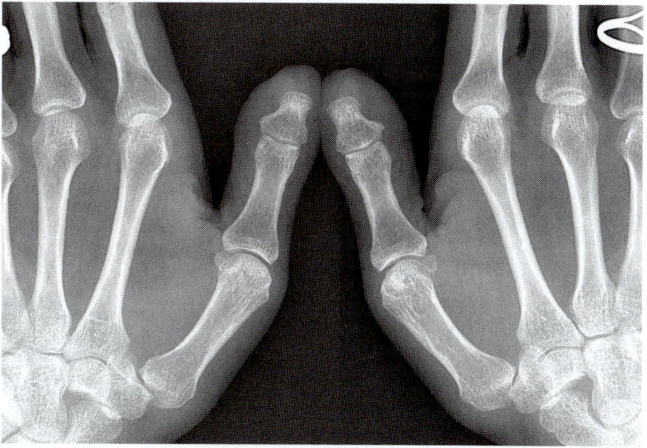

FIGURE 61-1

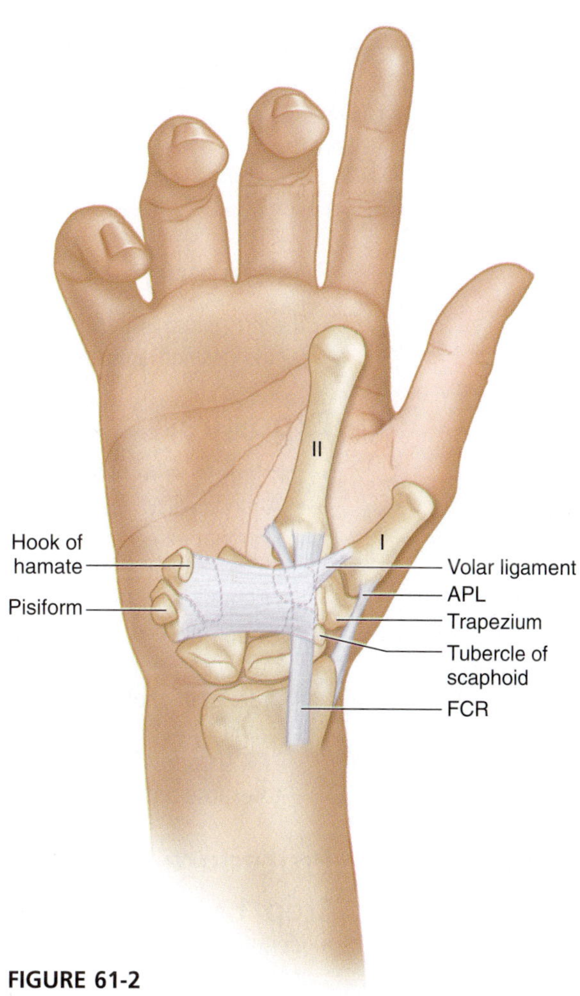

FIGURE 61-2

- The radial sensory nerve becomes subcutaneous after exiting through the interval between the brachioradialis and extensor carpi radialis longus (ECRL) muscles.
- The flexor carpi radialis (FCR) tendon is the most radial tendon palpable on the volar aspect of the wrist and is located just ulnar to the radial artery. The palmaris longus tendon, when present, is ulnar to the FCR tendon.
- The palmar cutaneous branch of the median nerve is located 1 mm ulnar to the FCR tendon.

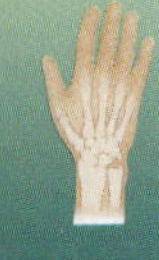

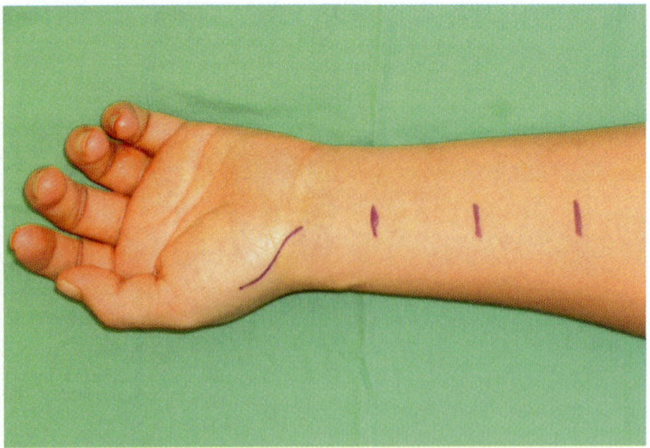

FIGURE 61-3

Positioning

- The procedure is performed under tourniquet control with the patient in the supine position and the extremity abducted with the hand on a hand table.

Exposures

- This procedure requires the following incisions.
  - A modified Wagner incision along the junction of glabrous and nonglabrous skin that extends from the distal extent of the thumb metacarpal in a curvilinear fashion along the border of the thenar eminence to just ulnar to the FCR tendon at the wrist crease. This exposes both the TMC joint and the FCR tendon deep to the subcutaneous fat. Skin flaps should be elevated sufficiently to visualize the dorsum of the metacarpal base.
  - A series of short volar transverse incisions centered over the FCR tendon at 3 and 6 cm proximal to the wrist crease for tendon harvest (Fig. 61-3). The FCR sheath is identified deep to the subcutaneous fat and sharply opened to expose and isolate the radial half of FCR.

PEARLS

One must identify and protect the radial sensory nerve branches, the radial artery, and the FCR tendon and avoid injury to the palmar cutaneous branch of the median nerve.

Procedure

Step 1

- Identify the radial edge of the thenar musculature at its insertion onto the metacarpal and elevate the muscle extraperiosteally to expose the metacarpal base, TMC joint, and trapezium (Fig. 61-4).
- The interval between the extensor pollicis longus and brevis is developed to expose the dorsal cortex of the metacarpal base.
- A hole is created at the base of the metacarpal from dorsal to volar 1 cm distal to the joint in a plane perpendicular to the axis of the thumbnail using a gouge or small bur. The volar hole should emerge at the apex of the volar beak of the metacarpal.

STEP 1 PEARLS

Although preoperative radiographs may appear normal, these can be deceiving, and degeneration of articular cartilage may be underappreciated. If there is clinical suspicion of articular degeneration, a transverse arthrotomy should be made to visualize the TMC joint surface. The arthrotomy is then closed with 3-0 braided absorbable suture.

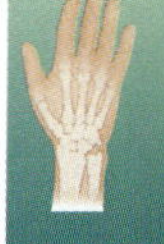

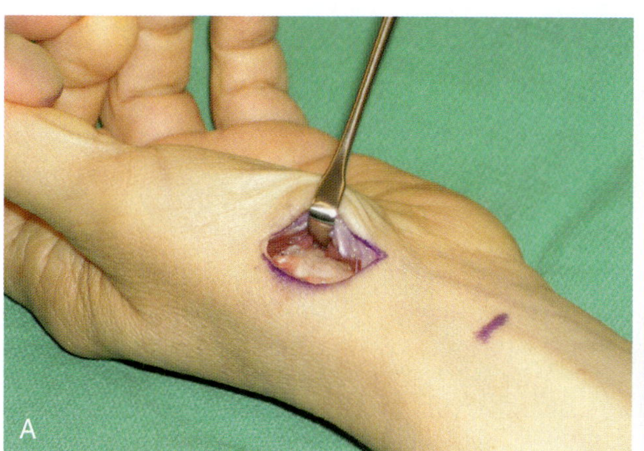

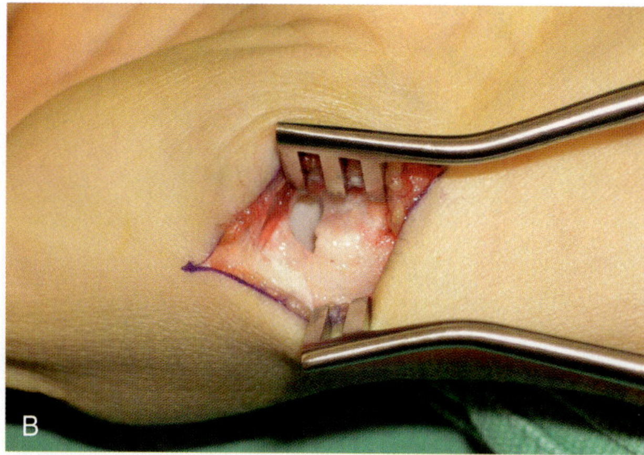

FIGURE 61-4

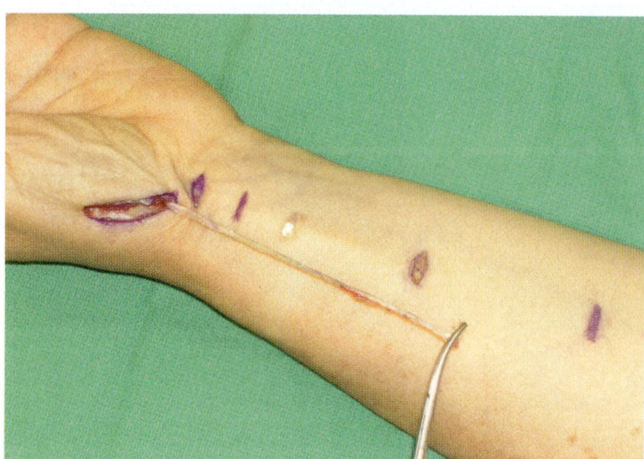

FIGURE 61-5

Step 2

- The FCR tendon is identified at the wrist crease, and the sheath is sharply opened proximally and distally.
- The radial half of the FCR tendon in the proximal forearm is transected proximally at 6 cm from the wrist crease and separated from the other half of the tendon using two small transverse incisions (Fig. 61-5). At the level of the wrist crease, the FCR is covered by a sheath that needs to be opened to trace the FCR slip close to its insertion at the base of the index metacarpal. The FCR rotates 90 degrees within the sheath; it is important to follow the fibers so that the tendon is not inadvertently transected. One should not slide the scissors through the tendon fibers but rather cut along the fibers to maintain the integrity of the tendon.

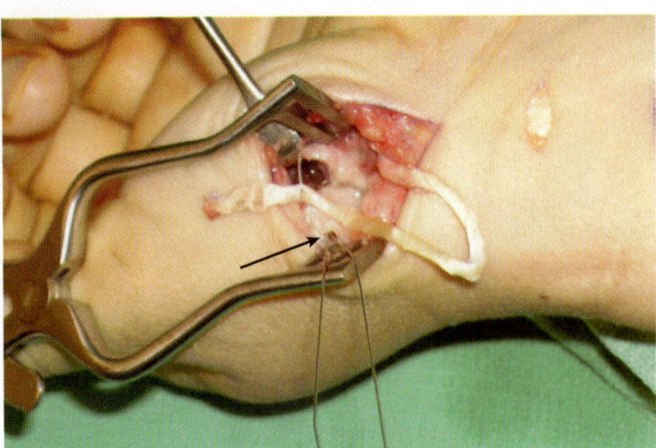

FIGURE 61-6

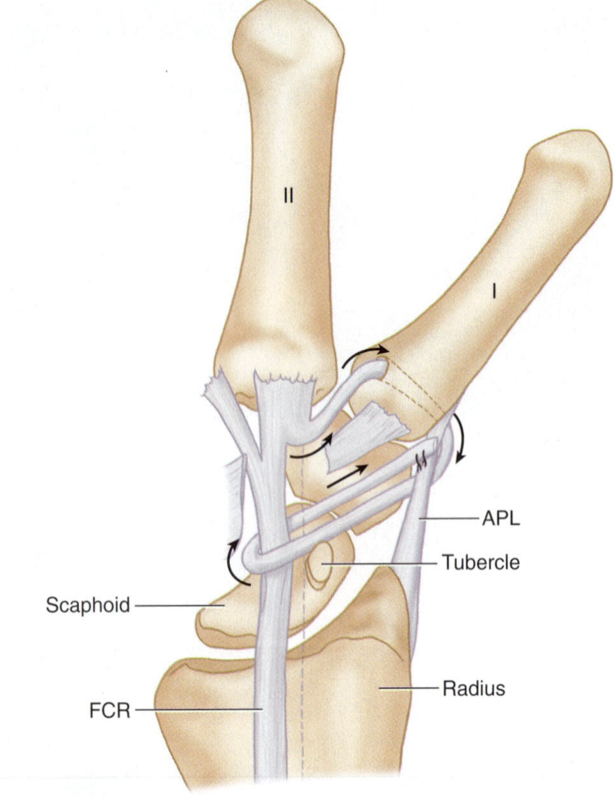

FIGURE 61-7

Step 3

- The free end of the FCR is redirected across the crest of the trapezium to enter the volar portion of the newly created hole at the beak of the thumb metacarpal and drawn dorsally through the metacarpal with the assistance of a wire suture (Figs. 61-6 and 61-7).
- The TMC joint is reduced under direct vision and held in extension and abduction to seat the metacarpal against the deep facet of the trapezium. It is unnecessary to pin the joint because the tendon is adequate to provide stability to the thumb CMC joint.
- The tendon is pulled taut and sutured to the dorsal periosteum using a 3-0 braided permanent suture. The tendon is then passed around the metacarpal base deep to the extensor pollicis brevis and APL, through a small split in the intact FCR tendon proximal to its insertion, and finally back across the joint and sutured to the APL tendon using 3-0 braided permanent suture (see Fig. 61-7). Additional 3-0 braided permanent sutures are placed at the junction through the FCR tendon (Fig. 61-8).

Step 4

- The thenar musculature is reattached using 3-0 braided absorbable suture.
- The tourniquet is released, and all bleeding points are cauterized.
- The skin is closed with 4-0 permanent monofilament horizontal mattress sutures, and the hand is placed in a thumb spica splint for 4 weeks.

Postoperative Care and Expected Outcomes

- The thumb spica splint is worn for 4 weeks followed by gentle active motion exercises for another 4 weeks. Strengthening is started 8 weeks after surgery.
- Thumb CMC joint stiffness typically lasts 4 to 6 weeks but may last as long as 4 months.

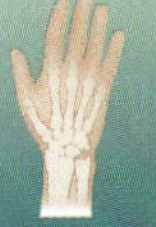

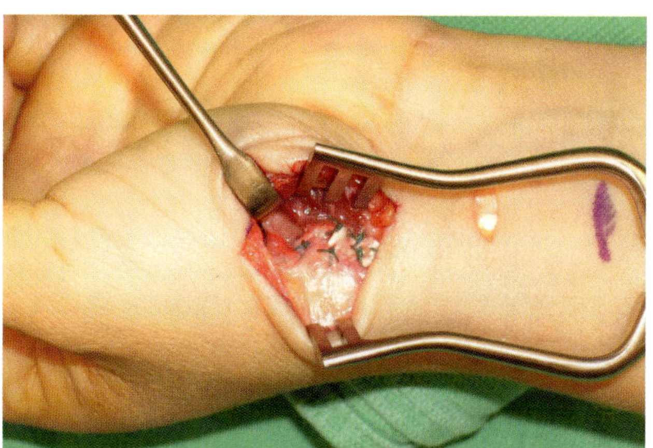

FIGURE 61-8

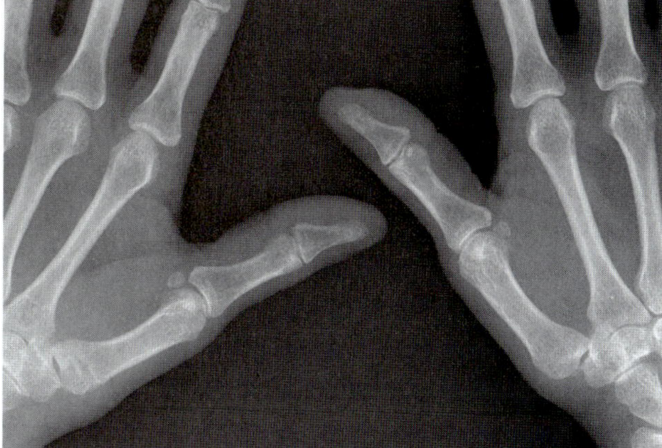

FIGURE 61-9

- The patient can expect complete or near-complete relief of pain with use of the thumb and minimal or no progression of degenerative arthritis when this surgery is performed before onset of significant articular cartilage degeneration. (Fig. 61-9 shows a late postoperative radiograph.)

Evidence

Eaton RG, Lane LB, Littler JW, Keyser JJ. Ligament reconstruction for the painful thumb carpometacarpal joint: a long-term assessment. *J Hand Surg [Am]*. 1984;9:692-699.

This study reviews the first 50 consecutive reconstructions, with an average follow-up of 7 years. Intractable pain was the primary indication for surgery. Each joint was examined both before and after surgery and rated as stage I through stage IV according to the radiographic appearance. Of the patients with zero or minimal articular changes (stages I and II), 95% achieved good or excellent results (little or no postoperative pain). Of the patients with moderate to advanced degenerative changes (stages III and IV), 74% achieved good or excellent results. All stage I cases and 82% of stage II cases were free of recognizable degeneration on follow-up radiographs up to 13 years postoperatively. These findings suggest that ligament reconstruction, which is now recommended only for stage I or stage II disease, will restore stability, reduce pain, and possibly even retard joint degeneration in a large proportion of patients with painful instability of the thumb CMC joint. (Level IV evidence)

Freedman DM, Eaton RG, Glickel SZ. Long-term results of volar ligament reconstruction for symptomatic basal joint laxity. *J Hand Surg [Am]*. 2000;25:297-304.

The long-term results of volar ligament reconstruction were assessed in 19 patients (24 thumbs). The average age at surgery was 33 years (range, 18 to 55 years). Twenty-three thumbs were radiographic stage I; a preoperative radiograph was not available in one. The follow-up period averaged 15 years (range, 10 to 23 years). At the final follow-up visit, 15 thumbs were stage I, 7 were stage II, and 2 were stage III. Fifteen patients were at least 90% satisfied with the results of the surgery. Only 8% of thumbs advanced to radiographic arthritic disease, which compares favorably with the 17% to 33% reported incidence of stage III/IV basal joint arthritis in the general population. (Level IV evidence)

Takwale VJ, Stanley JK, Shahane SA. Post-traumatic instability of the trapeziometacarpal joint of the thumb: diagnosis and the results of reconstruction of the beak ligament. *J Bone Joint Surg [Br]*. 2004;86:541-545.

The authors retrospectively reviewed reconstruction of the anterior oblique ligament using a slip of the flexor carpi radialis tendon in 26 patients with a mean age of 34.6 years and a mean follow-up of 55 months. They found that 87% obtained significant relief from pain, and mean grip strength recovered to 86% of the contralateral side. Eighty-one percent of patients noted a subjective improvement. The authors state that although their small sample size precludes statistical analysis, the trends noted in their study suggest that a better outcome may occur if surgery is performed early after a period of nonoperative management. (Level IV evidence)

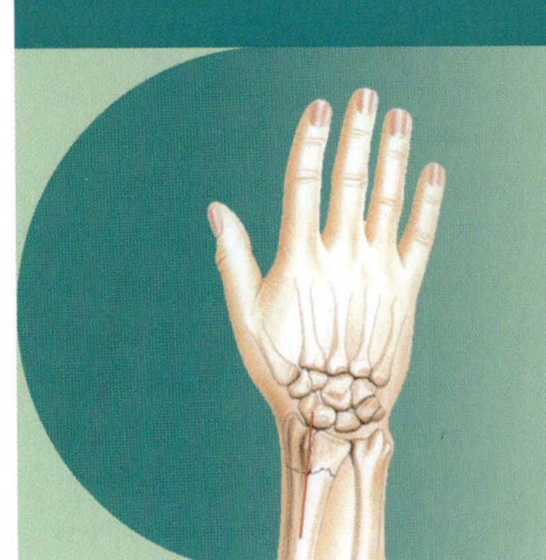

PROCEDURE 62

Trapeziectomy and Abductor Pollicis Longus Suspensionplasty

Nathan S. Taylor and Kevin C. Chung

See Video 46: Abductor Pollicis Longus Suspension Arthroplasty for Basal Joint Arthritis

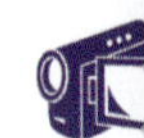

Indications

- Eaton stages II to IV disease (see later)
- Pain refractory to conservative treatment, including trapeziometacarpal (TMC) corticosteroid injection, thumb splinting, and isometric exercises

Examination/Imaging

Clinical Examination

- The patient's thumb metacarpal base may exhibit a dorsoradial prominence secondary to subluxation from ligamentous laxity (Fig. 62-1).
- The patient's thumb should be evaluated for tenderness along the TMC joint.
- The carpometacarpal (CMC) grind test is performed with axial compression, flexion, extension, and circumduction of the TMC joint, which should elicit crepitus and pain.
- The patient's thumb metacarpophalangeal (MCP) joint should be assessed during pinch for hyperextensibility. If unaddressed, the suspensionplasty will be stressed by obligatory metacarpal adduction. This hyperextensibility can be corrected with MCP joint capsulodesis or fusion if the deformity is severe.
- The patient should be evaluated for carpal tunnel syndrome, which may coexist in up to 43% of patients with TMC arthritis. Concomitant carpal tunnel release should be performed in these patients because trapeziectomy alone does not sufficiently increase carpal tunnel volume.
- An Allen test should be performed because the procedure typically requires mobilization of and potential injury to the radial artery.
- The patient should also be evaluated for concomitant trigger thumb.

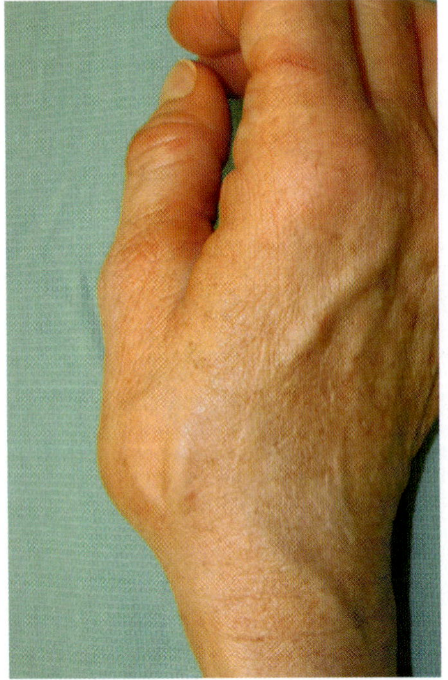

FIGURE 62-1

Imaging

- Posteroanterior, oblique, and lateral radiographs of the hand should be obtained to evaluate the extent of arthritis, osteophyte formation, joint loss, and joint subluxation (Fig. 62-2A to C).
- The Eaton classification is a staging system based on radiographic findings only and often does not correlate with the patient's symptoms. Some patients with severe arthritis may have minimal pain. Treatment should be based on the patient's symptoms and, most important, on the amount of pain in the arthritic joint.
  - *Stage I*—normal to slightly widened TMC joint secondary to ligamentous laxity or effusion, normal articular contours, and subluxation of less than one third of the joint space
  - *Stage II*—TMC joint narrowing and osteophytes less than 2 mm
  - *Stage III*—further TMC joint narrowing, subchondral cysts, sclerosis, osteophytes greater than 2 mm, subluxation greater than one third of the joint space
  - *Stage IV*—degenerative changes involving the scaphotrapezial joint

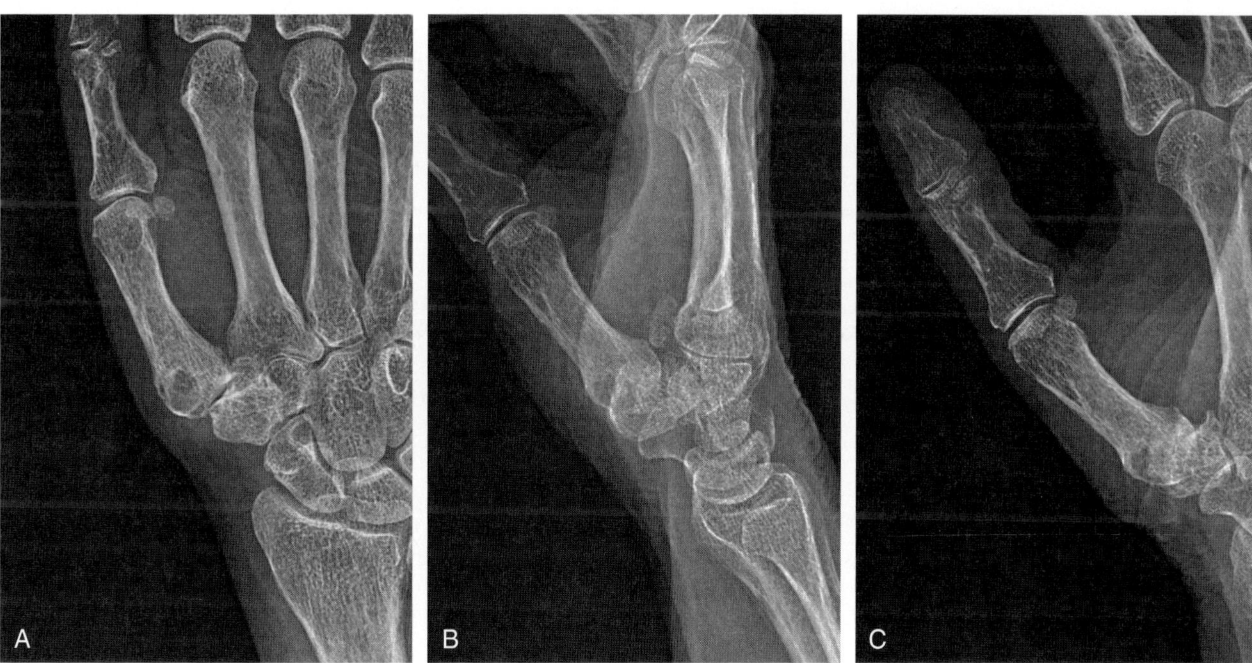

FIGURE 62-2

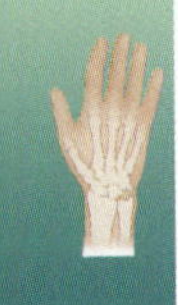

- A stress view of the TMC joint is obtained by having the patient press the thumb tips together while obtaining a 30-degree posteroanterior view centered on the thumbs to assess joint space loss and subluxation. Stress view is only obtained in stage I disease for patients with symptomatic joint laxity.
- Partial resection of the trapezoid should be performed if degenerative changes are present between the trapezoid and the scaphoid.

Surgical Anatomy

- The anterior oblique (beak) ligament inserts volarly onto the trapezium from its confluence with articular cartilage on the beak of the thumb metacarpal.
- The radial artery traverses the anatomic snuffbox and overlies the dorsal capsule of the CMC joint.
- The abductor pollicis longus (APL) and extensor pollicis brevis (EPB) tendons are within the first extensor compartment.
- The radial sensory nerve becomes subcutaneous after exiting through the interval between the brachioradialis and extensor carpi radialis longus (ECRL) muscles.
- The flexor carpi radialis (FCR) tendon traverses the volar and ulnar aspect of the trapezium.

PEARLS

The dorsal approach provides easy access to the trapezium.

For the trapeziectomy, one must identify and protect four structures: radial sensory nerve branches, radial artery, EPL tendon, and APL tendon.

Retract the EPL ulnarly and the APL radially and identify the radial artery, which will be located deep to the fatty tissue between these structures.

Positioning

- The procedure is performed under tourniquet control with the patient in the supine position and the extremity abducted with the hand on a hand table.

PITFALLS

If the distal incision is not centered on the metacarpal or the trapezium, the capsular elevation may be more challenging.

Exposures

- The APL suspensionplasty requires two incisions (Fig. 62-3).
  - A longitudinal incision centered over the anatomic snuffbox and TMC joint
  - A small chevron incision over the first extensor compartment about 5 cm proximal to the radial styloid

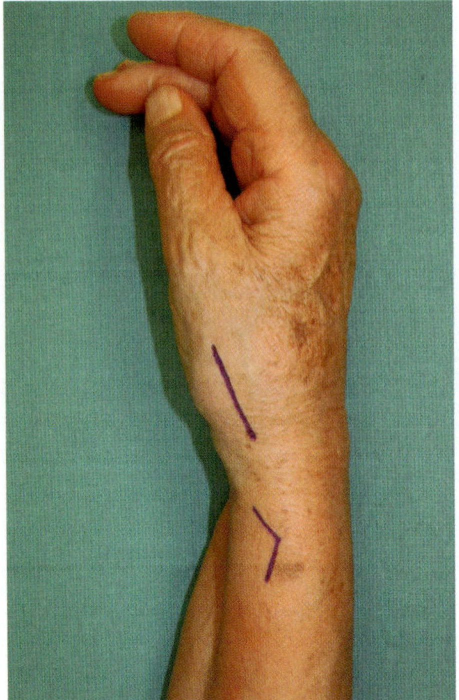

FIGURE 62-3

Procedure

Step 1

- The distal skin incision is made extending from 1 to 2 cm distal to the TMC joint to the radial styloid proximally.
- The proximal skin incision is made over the course of the first extensor compartment tendons after the trapeziectomy has been completed.

Step 2

- Sharply incise the TMC joint capsule and elevate the capsular flaps radially and ulnarly to expose the scaphotrapezial joint, the trapezium, and the thumb metacarpal base (Fig. 62-4).

Step 3

- An oscillating saw is used to cut the trapezium into three pieces (Figs. 62-5A and B), and an osteotome is then used to fracture the bone into separate pieces (Fig. 62-5C). Trapeziectomy is performed with a rongeur (Fig. 62-5D). If scapho-trapezoid arthritis is present, partial proximal trapezoidal resection is performed such that axial loading produces no contact between the scaphoid and trapezoid.

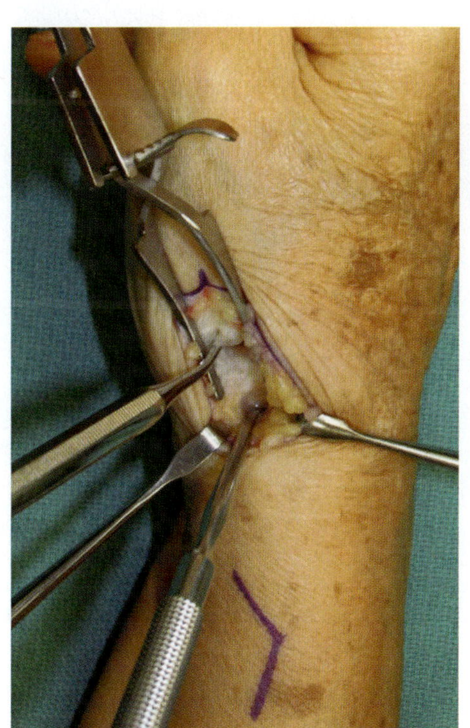

FIGURE 62-4

STEP 1 PEARLS

The EPL is identified at the ulnar aspect of the anatomic snuffbox.

The radial sensory nerve branches should be mobilized and retracted.

Perforating vessels from the radial artery to the dorsal capsule should be cauterized as the artery is mobilized and retracted ulnarly to gain access to the joint capsule.

STEP 1 PITFALLS

Failure to identify and adequately mobilize the radial artery can result in arterial injury.

STEP 2 PEARLS

The capsule should be sharply elevated to preserve these flaps for closure at the completion of the procedure.

STEP 2 PITFALLS

The radial artery is at risk for injury owing to its close proximity to the joint capsule.

STEP 3 PEARLS

The orientation of the saw cuts should be parallel to the course of the FCR tendon to avoid injury to this tendon as it passes volar to the trapezium at its proximal radial corner.

Traction on the thumb helps facilitate exposure of the trapezium.

There will be a substantial amount of osteophyte attaching to the volar joint capsule and the thenar muscle. All the osteophytes must be excised using both the scalpel and the rongeur.

In certain situations in which the interval between the trapezium and the scaphoid is blurred because of severe degenerative changes, it is useful to obtain a view using the fluoroscopy to be sure the correct bone is removed. It is conceivably possible to remove a portion of the distal scaphoid if not careful.

After trapeziectomy, traction should be exerted on the index and long fingers to assess the scaphotrapezoid joint.

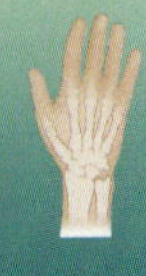

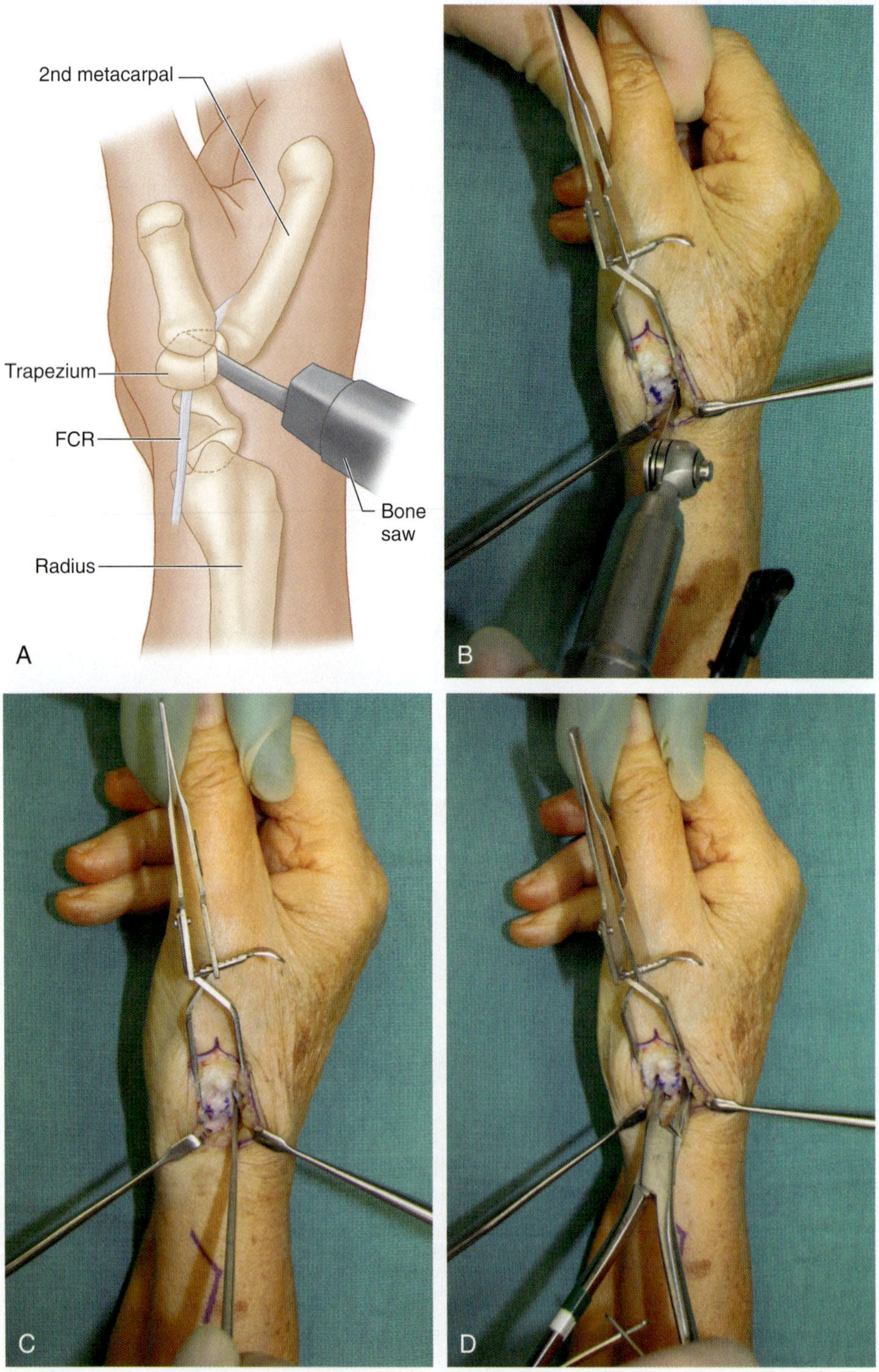

2nd metacarpal
Trapezium
FCR
Bone saw
Radius
A
B
C
D

FIGURE 62-5

Step 4

- Identify and release the first extensor compartment (Fig. 62-6). Identify the musculotendinous junction of the APL, divide the most radial slip of the APL at this junction (Fig. 62-7A), and begin to split it distally to its insertion on the base of the thumb metacarpal (Fig. 62-7B).

STEP 3 PITFALLS

If partial proximal trapezoidectomy is performed, one must be careful not to inadvertently resect some of the capitate.

STEP 4 PEARLS

One must take care to preserve the ulnar half of the APL tendon at its musculotendinous junction.

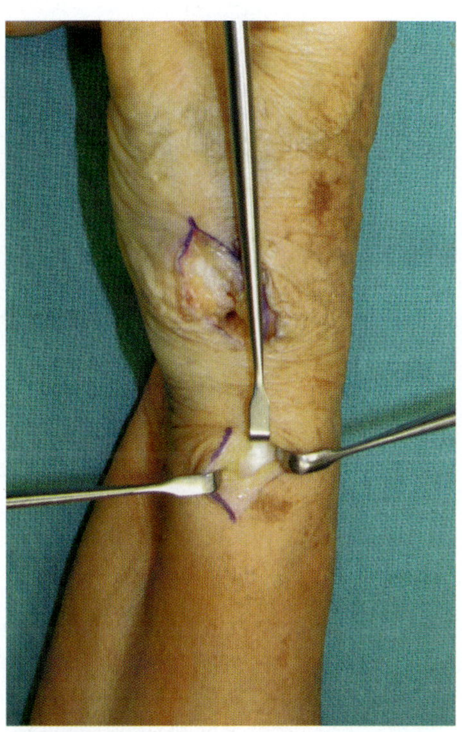

FIGURE 62-6

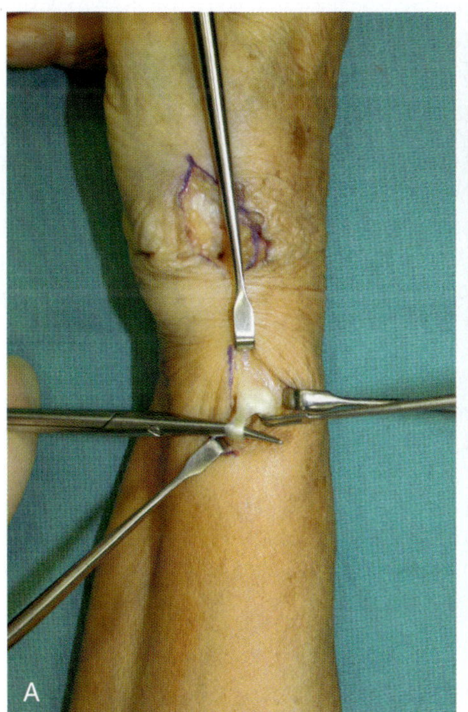

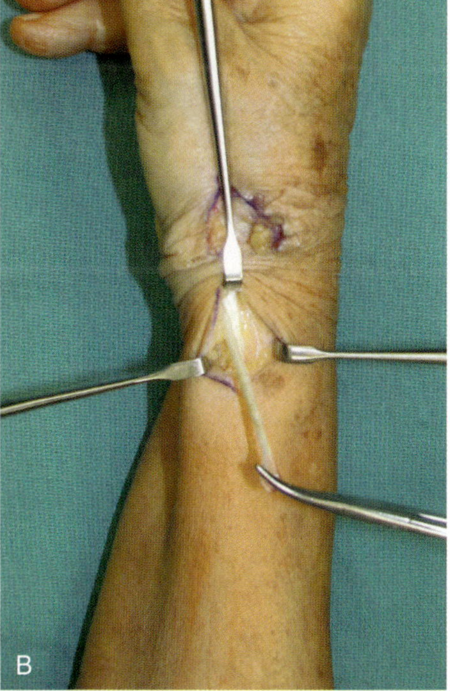

FIGURE 62-7

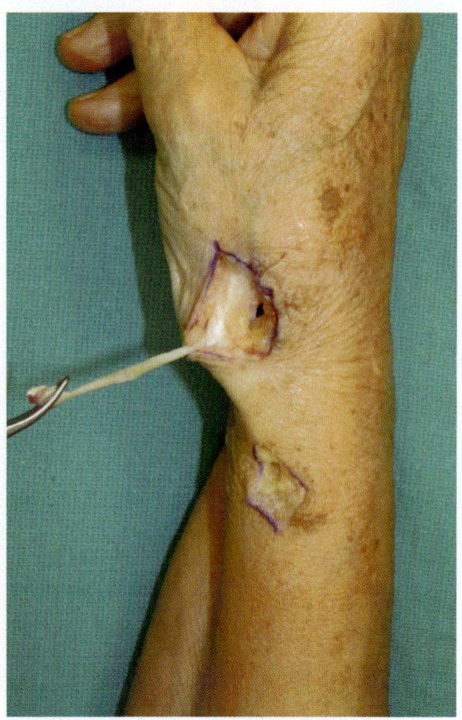

FIGURE 62-8

Step 5

- A hemostat is used to pass the APL tendon subcutaneously and into the arthroplasty space, and the remaining portion is split distally to its insertion at the base of the thumb metacarpal (Fig. 62-8). The ECRL tendon is then identified ulnar and deep to the EPL tendon, inserting into the base of the index metacarpal.

Step 6

- The APL tendon is passed volar to the EPL (Fig. 62-9A). A small incision is made in the ECRL tendon, and the APL slip is woven into the ECRL with a tendon passer (Figs. 62-9B and C).

Step 7

- Tension is set such that the thumb metacarpal base is suspended at the level of the index metacarpal base. The tendon weave is secured with two 3-0 braided permanent horizontal mattress sutures (Fig. 62-9D and E). The remaining tendon is cut, and a 4-0 braided absorbable suture is used to fashion the cut tendon into an accordion-like ball that is placed in the arthroplasty space (Fig. 62-10A and B).

Step 8

- Close the joint capsule with 4-0 braided absorbable suture. The tourniquet is then released, and all bleeding points are cauterized.

Step 9

- The skin is closed in layers with 4-0 absorbable monofilament dermal sutures and a 4-0 absorbable monofilament running subcuticular suture. The hand is placed in a thumb spica splint.

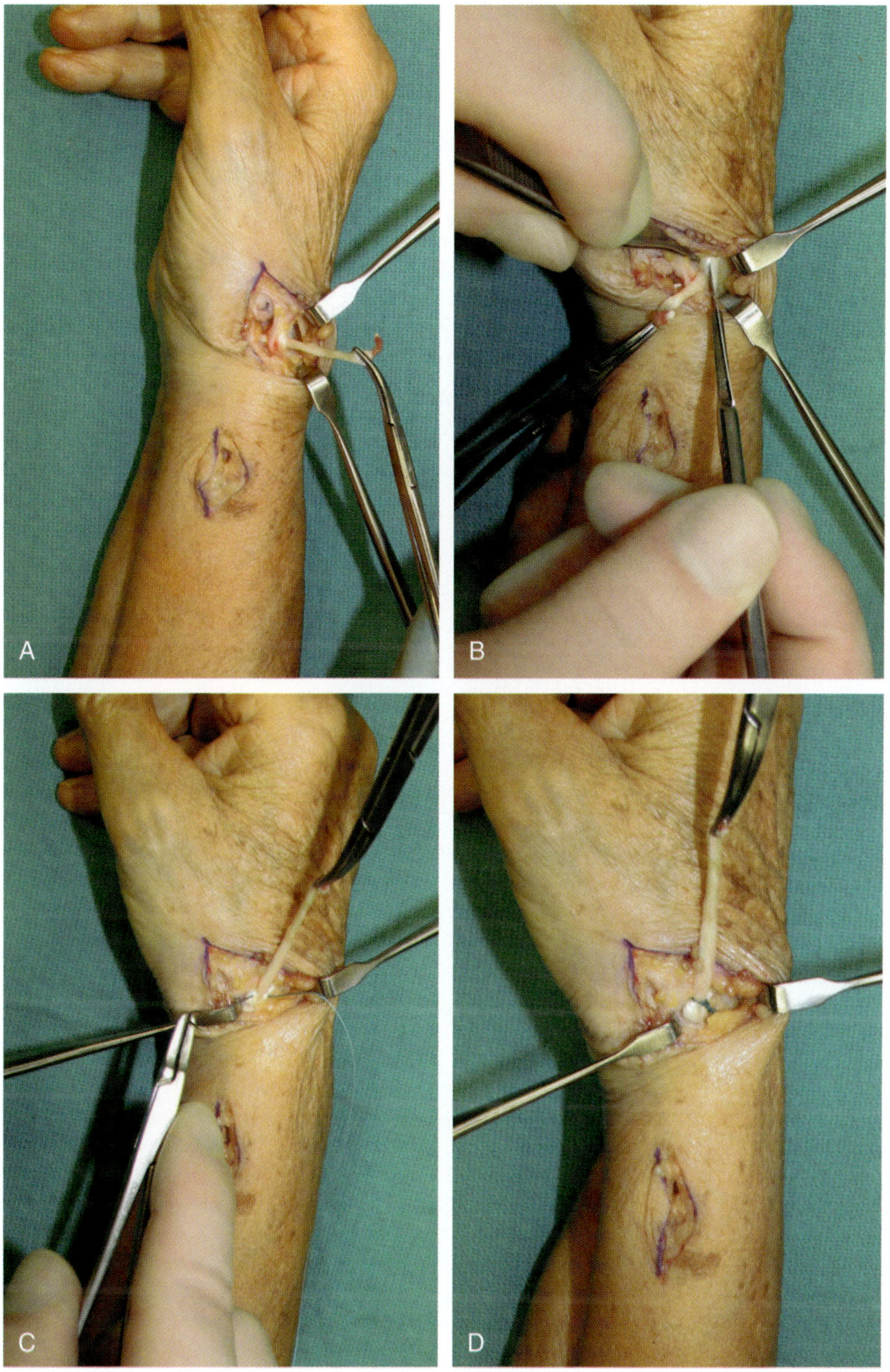

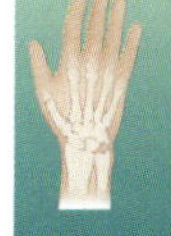

FIGURE 62-9 *Continued*

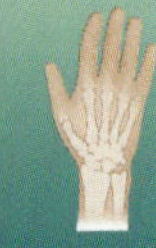

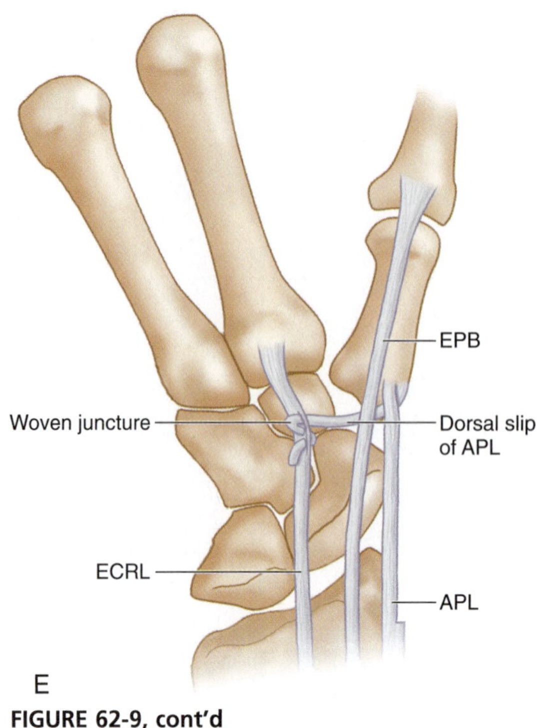

FIGURE 62-9, cont'd

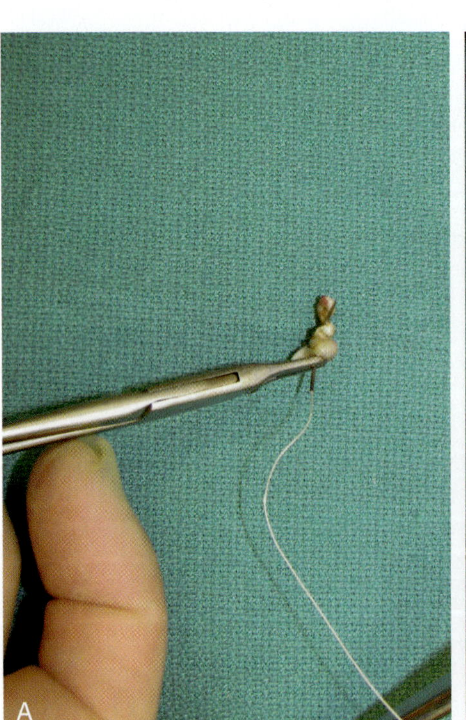

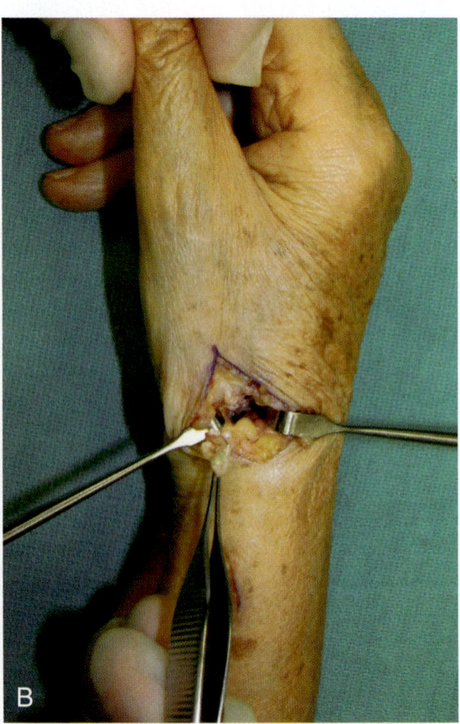

FIGURE 62-10

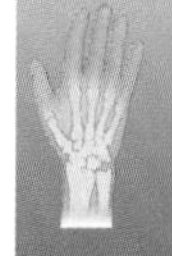

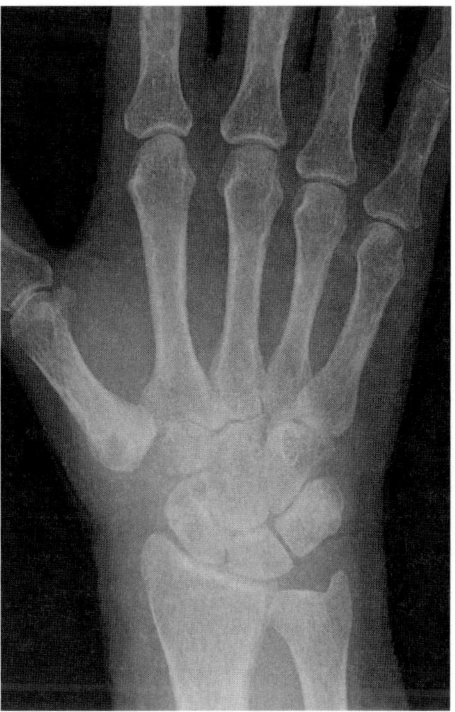

FIGURE 62-11

Postoperative Care and Expected Outcomes

- A postoperative thumb spica splint is worn for 4 weeks. Sutures are removed at the first postoperative visit (10 to 14 days after surgery) as needed, and scar massage techniques are taught to the patient. (Fig. 62-11 shows postoperative radiographic appearance.)
- Four weeks after surgery, hand therapy is begun for passive and active range-of-motion exercises. The splint is worn in between exercises.
- Six weeks after surgery, light strengthening exercises are begun, and unrestricted passive range of motion is allowed. Splint is worn in between exercises.
- Eight weeks after surgery, the splint is removed, and heavy strengthening is begun with grip and pinch exercises. Soft neoprene splint is worn as needed.

Evidence

Chang EY, Chung KC. Outcomes of trapeziectomy with a modified abductor pollicis suspension arthroplasty for the treatment of thumb carpometacarpal joint osteoarthritis. *Plast Reconstr Surg*. 2008;122:1-12.

The authors present the outcomes of 21 thumbs in 18 patients with thumb CMC arthritis treated with trapeziectomy and a variation of APL suspension arthroplasty. Prospective outcomes data were collected, and results were compared with the senior author's retrospective series of 35 flexor carpi radialis ligament reconstructive procedures and with the literature. The authors noted in their series a 32% loss of CMC joint height and 11% proximal migration of the metacarpal at 1 year. Results of improved grip strength were comparable to the literature, although this improvement was not statistically significant. Michigan Hand Outcomes Questionnaire results showed statistically significant improvements in activities of daily living, work, patient satisfaction, and pain. Shorter tourniquet times were reported for the APL suspensionplasty compared with the FCR ligament reconstruction procedure. The authors concluded that the APL suspension arthroplasty is a faster and technically easier technique that avoids any additional deficit by using an accessory tendon and produces acceptable patient-rated outcomes, especially in pain relief and satisfaction. (Level IV evidence)

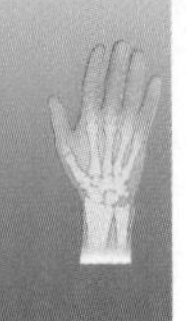

Sigfusson R, Lundborg G. Abductor pollicis longus tendon arthroplasty for treatment of arthrosis in the first carpometacarpal joint. *Scand J Plast Reconstr Hand Surg*. 1991;25:73-77.
The authors described a technique in which a portion of the APL was used in a figure-of-eight fashion around the FCR and remaining portion of the APL. Grip and pinch strengths more than 80% of the estimated normal hand were found. Scaphometacarpal height reduced to about 2 mm with pinch. Arthrosis of the scaphotrapezoid joint was a presumed potential cause of suboptimal results. (Level IV evidence)

Soejima O, Hanamura T, Kikuta T, et al. Suspensionplasty with the abductor pollicis longus tendon for osteoarthritis in the carpometacarpal joint of the thumb. *J Hand Surg [Am]*. 2006;31:425-428.
The authors report their experience with trapeziectomy and APL suspensionplasty without tendon interposition for painful trapeziometacarpal arthritis in 21 thumbs. Ten thumbs were classified as Eaton stage III, and 11 were classified as stage IV; all patients complained of pain with activity; and average follow-up was 33.3 months. Subjectively, 13 of the 21 thumbs were associated with no pain after surgery, 5 thumbs were associated with mild pain with strenuous activity, and 3 thumbs were associated with mild pain with light work. Objectively, radial and palmar abductions, grip strength, and key-pinch strength all improved postoperatively compared with preoperative assessment, although these findings were not statistically significant. The authors concluded that APL suspensionplasty has a favorable outcome in trapeziometacarpal osteoarthritis and that the APL tendon can be removed as a deforming force without any abduction weakness. They recognized the small sample size of their study as well as a short follow-up period and recommended additional prospective randomized studies of larger numbers with a longer follow-up. (Level IV evidence)

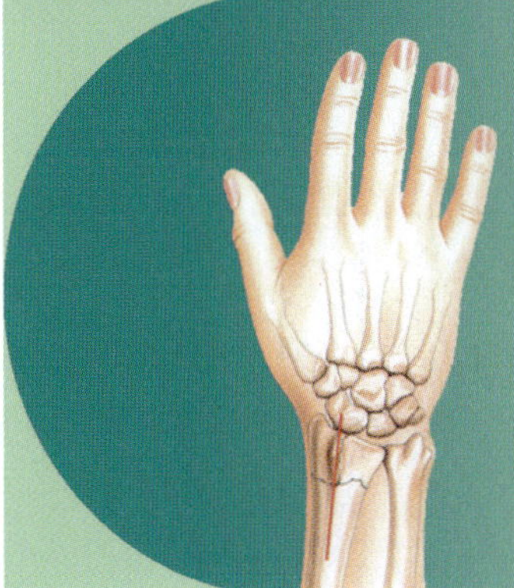

PROCEDURE 63

Trapeziometacarpal Fusion

Nathan S. Taylor and Kevin C. Chung

See Video 47: Fusion of Thumb Carpometacarpal Joint

Indications

- Posttraumatic degenerative osteoarthritis of the trapeziometacarpal (TMC) joint in manual workers who require great stability of the carpometacarpal (CMC) joint, which may not be achieved with trapezium excision and ligament reconstruction
- Patients with substantial joint laxity and severe thumb CMC joint deformity that cannot be treated with soft tissue reconstruction alone

The case presented subsequently is such a situation in a patient with lupus in which the ligaments are so lax and the thumb deformity so severe that thumb CMC fusion will provide a stable platform to achieve proper thumb posture and stability.

Examination/Imaging

Clinical Examination

- The patient's thumb should be evaluated for tenderness along the TMC joint.
- The grind test is performed with axial compression, flexion, extension, and circumduction of the TMC joint, which should elicit crepitus and pain.
- The patient's thumb metacarpophalangeal (MCP) joint should be assessed during pinch for hyperextensibility that can be corrected with MCP joint capsulodesis.
- The Allen test should be performed because the procedure typically requires mobilization of and potential injury to the radial artery.

Imaging

- Posteroanterior, oblique, and lateral radiographs of the hand should be obtained to evaluate extent of arthritis, osteophyte formation, and joint subluxation. Figure 63-1A and B demonstrates severe ligamentous laxity and subluxation of the TMC joint.

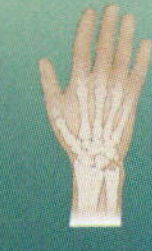

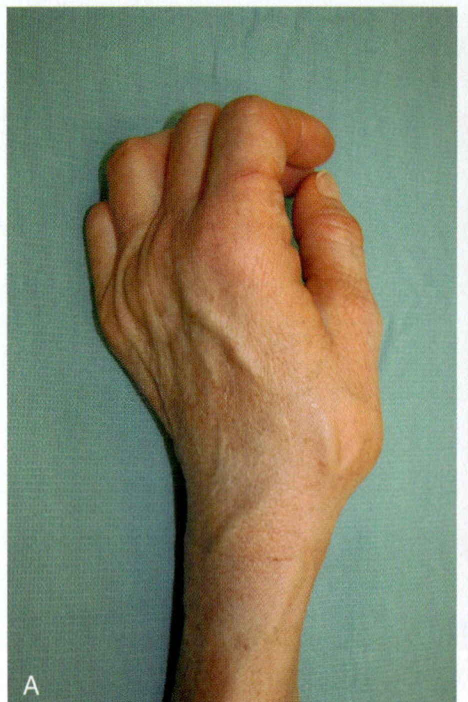

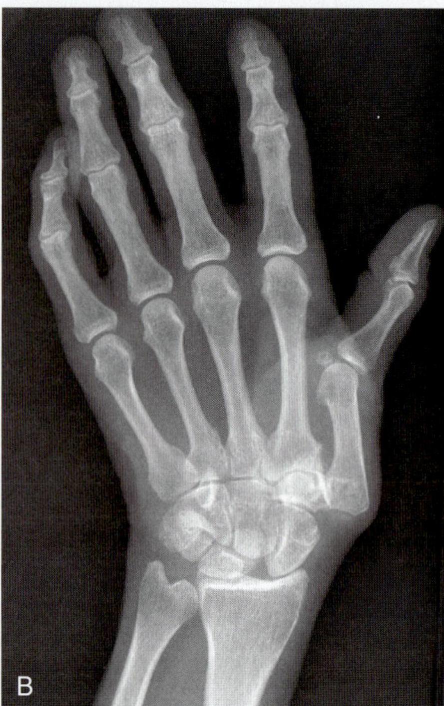

FIGURE 63-1

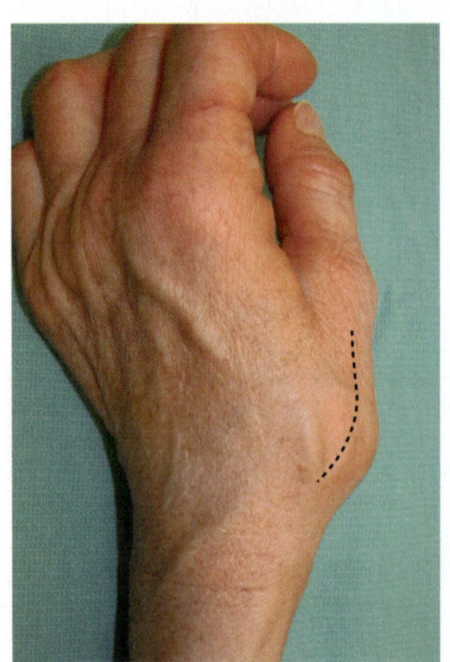

FIGURE 63-2

PEARLS

The radial sensory nerve branches are found within the subcutaneous tissue and should be protected. The radial artery is found in the interval between the EPL and EPB tendons deep to the subcutaneous fat and should be protected.

Surgical Anatomy

- The TMC joint is a biconcave saddle-shaped joint that provides motion in several planes to allow thumb flexion, extension, abduction, adduction, and opposition.
- The volar oblique (beak) ligament inserts volarly onto the trapezium from its confluence with articular cartilage on the beak of the thumb metacarpal and is considered the primary stabilizer of the TMC joint. It serves as the main restraint against dorsal translation of the metacarpal on the trapezium, and laxity of the beak ligament increases the risk for degenerative changes seen in the CMC joint due to loss of joint stabilization.
- The radial artery traverses the anatomic snuffbox and overlies the dorsal capsule of the CMC joint.
- The abductor pollicis longus (APL) and extensor pollicis brevis (EPB) tendons are within the first extensor compartment.
- The radial sensory nerve becomes subcutaneous after exiting through the interval between the brachioradialis and extensor carpi radialis longus (ECRL) muscles.

Positioning

- The procedure is performed under tourniquet control with the patient in the supine position and the extremity abducted with the hand on a hand table.

Exposures

- A 4-cm dorsal longitudinal incision overlying the TMC joint is made in the interval between the extensor pollicis longus (EPL) and EPB tendons to the level of the dorsal joint capsule (Fig. 63-2). The EPL tendon and radial artery should be retracted to expose the joint capsule.

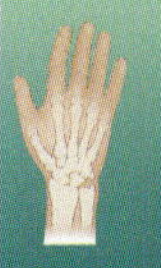

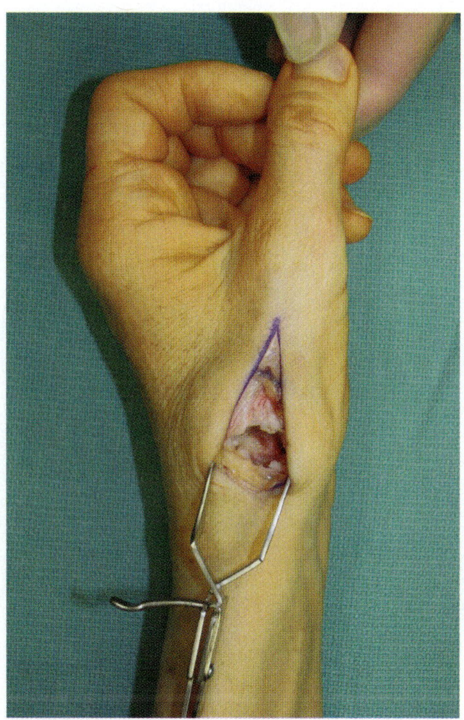

FIGURE 63-3

Procedure

Step 1

- Incise the TMC joint capsule followed by the periosteum longitudinally, and sharply elevate radial and ulnar periosteal flaps off the metacarpal and trapezium for later coverage of the implant (Fig. 63-3).

STEP 2 PEARLS

Longitudinal traction applied to the thumb helps expose the joint surfaces for articular resection.

Step 2

- Resect the articular cartilage and subchondral bone between the trapezium and metacarpal using a rongeur.

STEP 3 PEARLS

Intraoperative fluoroscopy is useful to confirm proper implant placement and screw fixation.

Cancellous bone graft (autologous or cadaveric) placed within any gaps can help augment bony union.

Step 3

- A 2.3-mm locking T-plate is applied for arthrodesis. The locking plate is particularly helpful for fusion of this joint because the trapezium may be devoid of strong cortical bone for secure screw purchase in the traditional plating system, which relies on the friction between the screw and the bone for stability. The locking plate system locks the screw to the plate, which adds additional stability to the fusion site. After confirming that the plate is in the center of the metacarpal and that the T portion is centered on the trapezium, a locking screw is placed to secure the plate to the metacarpal. The remaining screws are placed in a locking fashion to provide stable fixation.

Step 4

- The thumb is fixed in a position of function, typically 30 degrees of palmar abduction and 15 degrees of radial abduction (Fig. 63-4A and B).

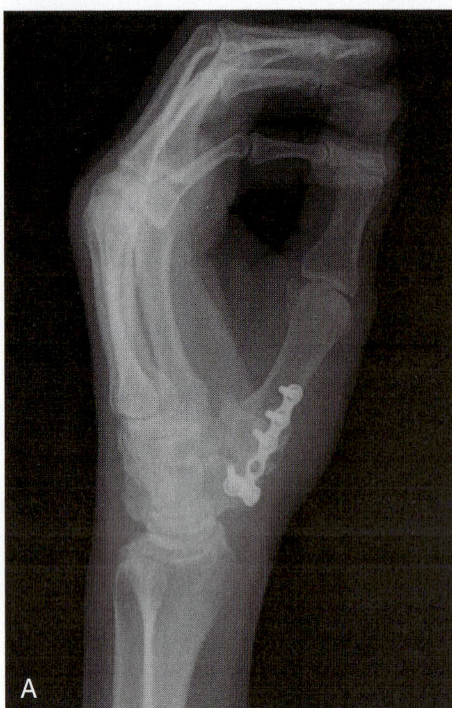

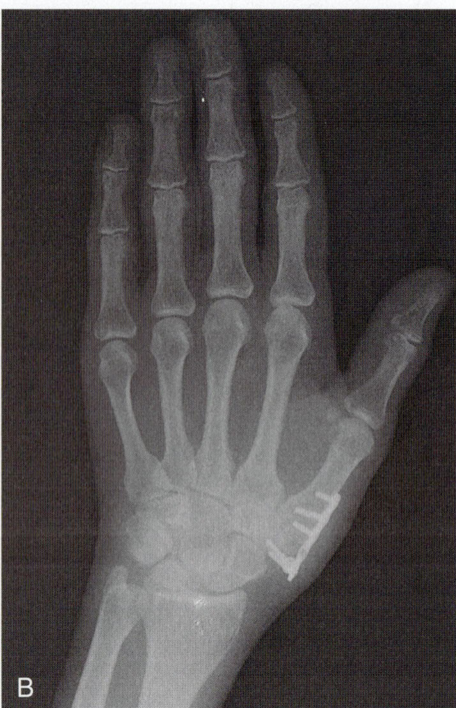

FIGURE 63-4

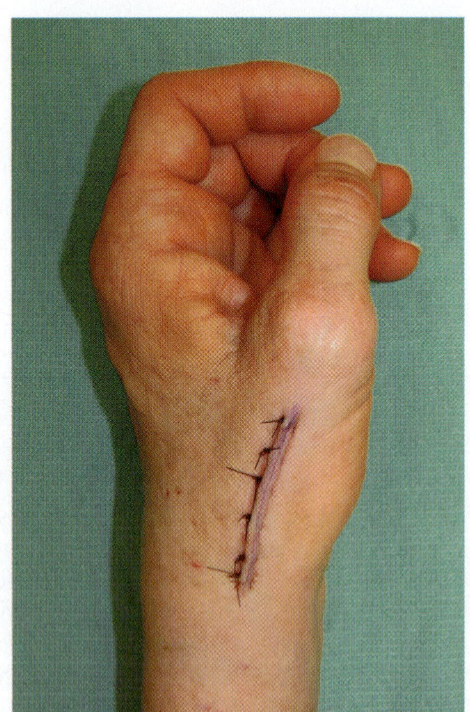

FIGURE 63-5

Step 5

- The periosteal flaps and joint capsule are closed in layers over the implant using 4-0 absorbable braided suture. The tourniquet is released, and all bleeding points are cauterized. Skin is closed using 4-0 permanent monofilament horizontal mattress sutures, and the hand is placed in a thumb spica splint (Fig. 63-5).

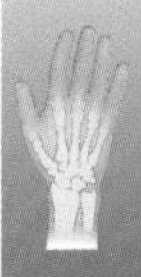

Postoperative Care and Expected Outcomes

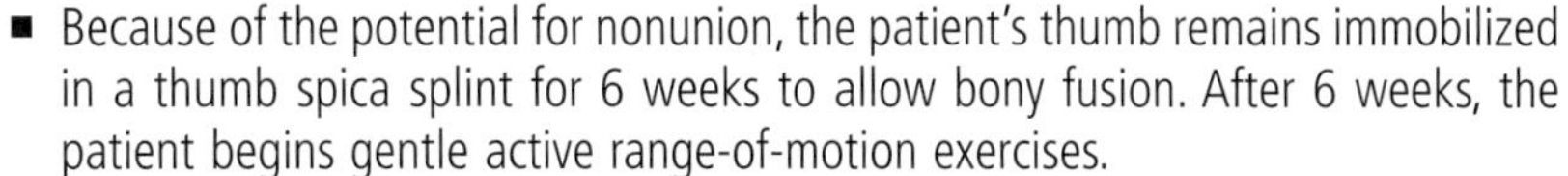

- Because of the potential for nonunion, the patient's thumb remains immobilized in a thumb spica splint for 6 weeks to allow bony fusion. After 6 weeks, the patient begins gentle active range-of-motion exercises.
- Expected outcomes include improved pain relief and improved hand function with insignificant change in strength despite loss of motion. Patients should be expected to return to their normal activities.

Evidence

Hartigan BJ, Stern PJ, Kiefhaber TR. Thumb carpometacarpal osteoarthritis: arthrodesis compared with ligament reconstruction and tendon interposition. *J Bone Joint Surg [Am]*. 2001;83:1470-1478.

The authors retrospectively reviewed 109 patients (141 thumbs) younger than 60 years who were treated with either trapeziometacarpal arthrodesis or trapeziectomy with ligament reconstruction and tendon interposition. Fifty-nine patients (82 thumbs) were available to complete a questionnaire and examination with an average follow-up of 69 months. The arthrodesis group available for follow-up included 29 patients (44 thumbs), whereas the trapeziectomy with LRTI group included 30 patients (38 thumbs). Both groups were similar with regard to age, gender, hand dominance, and duration of follow-up. Additional patients in both groups were available to complete a questionnaire. Their results showed no significant difference with regard to pain, function, and satisfaction. The arthrodesis group had significantly stronger lateral pinch and chuck pinch, although grip strength did not differ. The LRTI group had significantly better range of motion with opposition and the ability to flatten the hand. There was a higher complication rate in the arthrodesis group, with nonunion the most common complication. Despite this, pain improved in all nonunions, and all were satisfied with the outcome. The authors concluded that both procedures had similar results with regard to pain, function, and satisfaction despite minimal differences in strength and motion. (Level III evidence)

Kenniston JA, Bozentka DJ. Treatment of advanced carpometacarpal joint disease: arthrodesis. *Hand Clin.* 2008;24:285-294.

The authors present a review of carpometacarpal arthritis and its various treatment options, with special attention to arthrodesis. They include a detailed operative technique, discuss associated complications, and review the results reported in the literature over the past 40 years. They conclude that multiple surgical options are available for those patients who fail nonoperative management. These techniques are largely based on clinical symptoms, radiographic staging, and surgeon and patient preference. Arthrodesis remains an excellent option for patients with isolated CMC arthritis who require a pain-free and strong thumb. (Level III evidence)

Taylor EJ, Deari K, D'Arcy JC, Bonnici AV. A comparison of fusion, trapeziectomy and Silastic replacement for the treatment of osteoarthritis of the trapeziometacarpal joint. *J Hand Surg [Br]*. 2005;30:45-49.

The authors retrospectively reviewed the outcomes of three surgical treatments for osteoarthritis of the trapeziometacarpal joint. A total of 83 operations were performed (36 fusions, 25 trapeziectomies with [22] or without [3] ligament reconstruction, and 22 silicone trapezial replacements) with average follow-up between 33 and 42 months. The authors evaluated patient satisfaction, pain reduction, range of motion, tip and key pinch, and complication rates. They reported no significant difference in clinical outcomes among the three groups but noted a higher complication and reoperation rate in the fusion group. (Level III evidence)

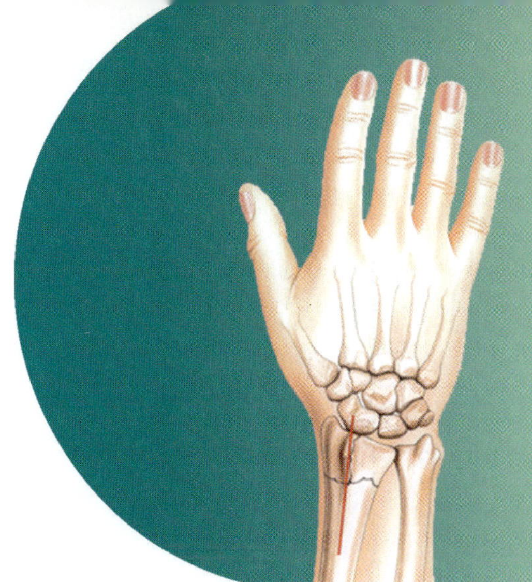

Section X
WRIST ARTHROSCOPY

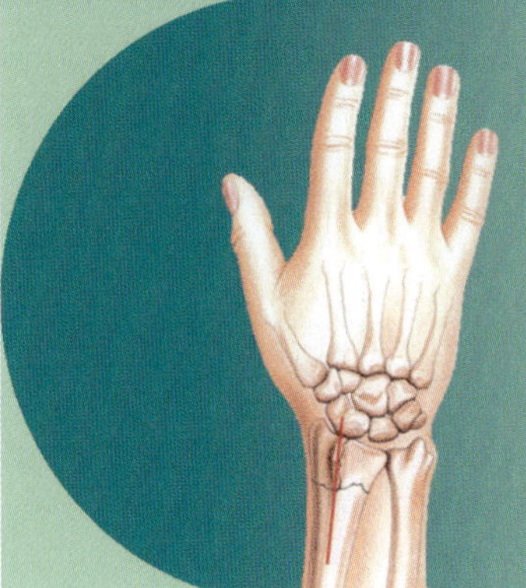

Diagnostic Wrist Arthroscopy

William B. Geissler and Daniel C. M. Williams

See Video 48: Diagnostic Wrist Arthroscopy

Indications

- Patients who have objective mechanical pathology of the wrist
- Diagnostic
  - To confirm diagnosis of intra-articular pathology determined by clinical examination or objective imaging studies
  - To establish a clinical diagnosis in patients with persistent mechanical wrist pain despite conservative treatment, with pain believed to originate from the wrist
  - To assess partial and complete tears of the interosseous ligaments, lesions of the triangular fibrocartilage complex (TFCC), cartilage defects in both the radiocarpal and midcarpal spaces, and chronic wrist pain of unknown etiology
- Therapeutic
  - Indications for operative intervention include treatment of fractures of both the scaphoid and distal radius, stabilization of acute interosseous ligament injuries, débridement and repair of tears of the TFCC, synovectomy, arthroscopic wafer ulnar shortening, detection and removal of loose bodies, radial styloidectomy, and wrist lavage.
  - Indications for wrist arthroscopy continue to expand as new techniques and instrumentation develop.

Examination/Imaging

Clinical Examination

- Arthroscopy has revolutionized the practice of hand surgery by providing the capability to examine and treat intra-articular abnormalities. Development of wrist arthroscopy is a natural transition from the successful application of arthroscopy of the larger joints. Wrist arthroscopy has seen considerable growth since Whipple reported the original description of the technique he developed for reviewing the intra-articular anatomy of the joints.

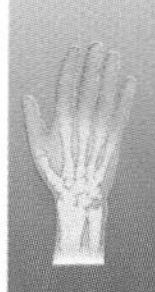

- A spectrum of injuries is seen in patients with interosseous ligament tears. The interosseous ligament stretches, partially tears, and develops into a full-thickness tear. Patients with scapholunate instability complain of point tenderness directly over the dorsum of the scapholunate ligament. Swelling may be seen localized in this area, and patients may have a positive Watson maneuver. The latter is performed by pushing the tubercle of the scaphoid dorsally with radial wrist deviation. Patients with lunotriquetral interosseous instability complain of point tenderness directly over the dorsum of the lunotriquetral interval. Patients may have a positive shuck test, in which anterior-posterior translation is felt between the lunate and triquetrum, causing point tenderness. A squeeze test consists of radial ulnar compression of the wrist between the thumb and index finger of the examiner. Patients with lunotriquetral instability will complain of pain at the lunotriquetral interval.
- Patients with injury to the TFCC complain of pain at the head of the ulna or the prestyloid recess.
- Patients with fractures of the scaphoid are tender in the snuffbox.
- Patients with fractures of the distal radius have generalized swelling around the wrist and are tender to palpation over the distal radius.

Imaging

- Multiview radiographs of the wrist on posterior-anterior and lateral planes are mandatory to evaluate for intra-articular pathology.
- Partial tears of the interosseous ligaments are rarely detected on plain radiographs, although dynamic instability may be identified on plain radiographs with dynamic views. Magnetic resonance imaging (MRI) has improved in detecting interosseous injuries. If interosseous ligament injuries are suspected, MRI arthrography is strongly recommended over MRI imaging alone to increase the accuracy of detecting interosseous ligament injuries.
- Patients with ulnar abutment and central tears of the TFCC can be identified on plain radiographs for patients with a markedly positive ulnar wrist in neutral rotation on radiography.

Surgical Anatomy

- The wrist is the labyrinth of eight carpal bones. Multiple articular surfaces with intrinsic and extrinsic ligaments and the TFCC form a perplexing joint that continuously challenges physicians with an array of diagnoses. Wrist arthroscopy allows direct visualization of the cartilage surfaces, carpal bones, and ligaments using bright light and magnification.
- The scapholunate interosseous ligament is best seen with the arthroscope in the 3-4 portal. The lunotriquetral interval is best seen with the arthroscope in the 4-5 or 6R portals owing to its more distal location. The scapholunate interval as seen from the midcarpal space should be tight and congruent. There should be no step-off or separation. The lunotriquetral interval may have slight play between the lunate and the triquetrum. An approximately 1-mm distal step-off of the triquetrum may be seen.

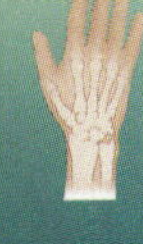

- Geissler defined an arthroscopic classification for interosseous ligament injury. A spectrum of injury is seen throughout this ligament. The ligament stretches and then tears, usually in a volar to dorsal direction. This arthroscopic classification is based on evaluation of the interosseous ligament from both the radiocarpal and midcarpal spaces. (Fig. 64-1 shows arthroscopic view of a normal scapholunate ligament.)
  - In Geissler grade I injuries, the normal concave appearance of the interosseous membrane as seen from the radiocarpal space becomes convex. There is attenuation of the interosseous ligament as seen from the radiocarpal space. The ligament changes from its normal concave appearance to convex. In the midcarpal space, there is no step-off. (Fig. 64-2 shows attenuation in the interosseous ligament.)
  - In Geissler grade II injuries, attenuation of the interosseous ligament from the radiocarpal space is found. In the midcarpal space, rotation of the carpal bones is seen, and a step-off is present. (Fig. 64-3 shows attenuation with a step-off in the interosseous ligament. S = scaphate; L = lunate.)

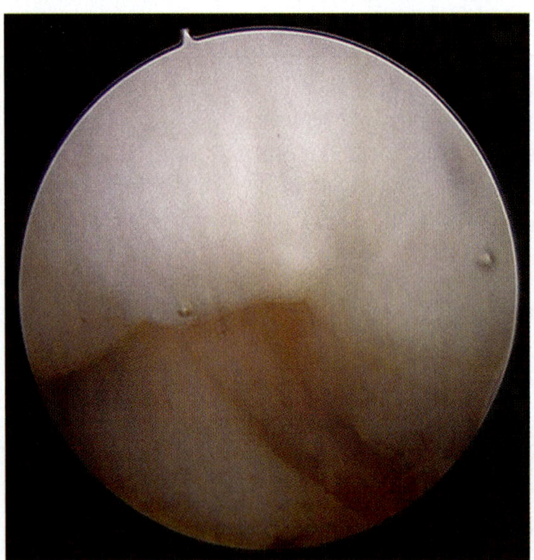

FIGURE 64-1

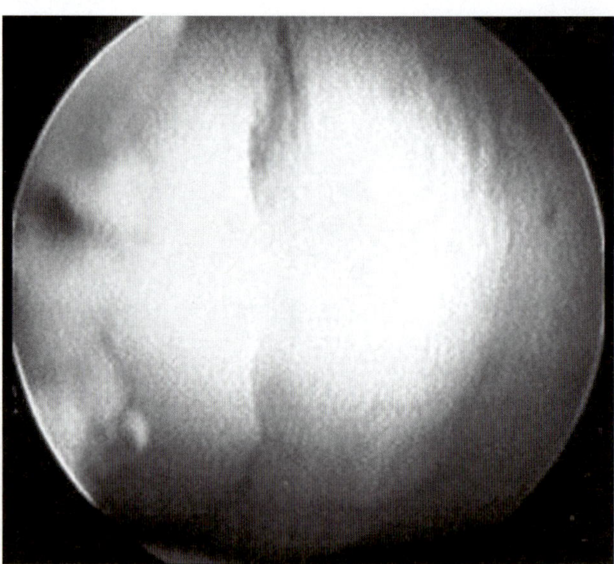

FIGURE 64-2

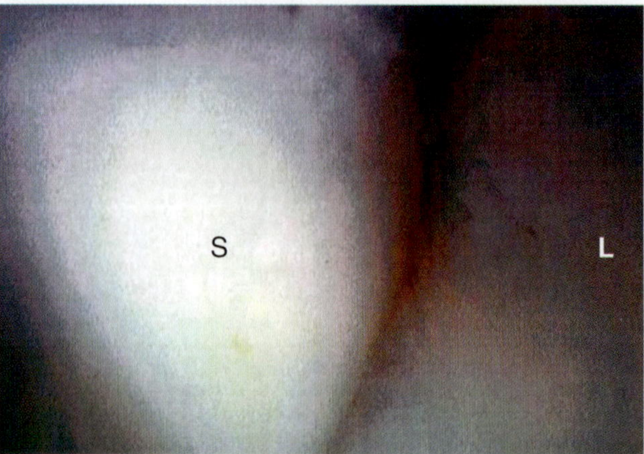

FIGURE 64-3

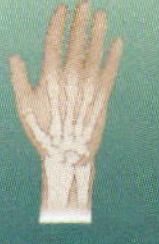

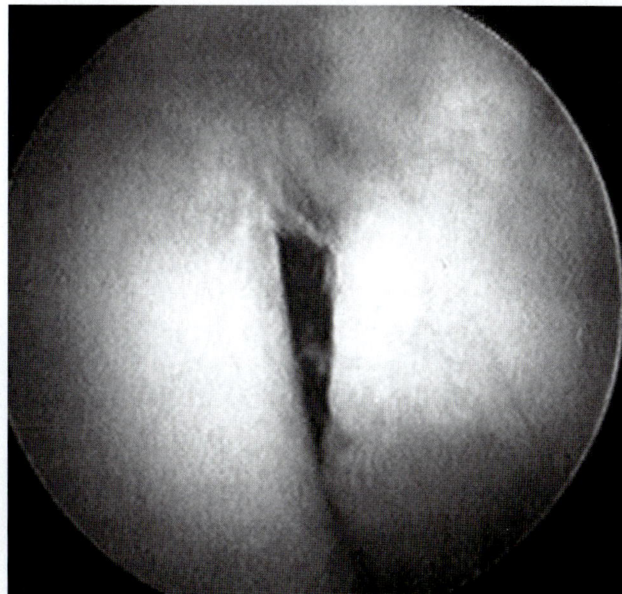

FIGURE 64-4

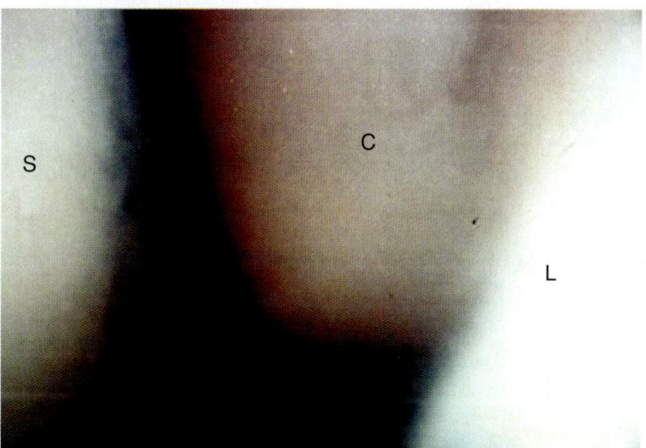

FIGURE 64-5

- In Geissler grade III injuries, the interosseous ligament tears in a volar to dorsal direction. A gap or separation between the carpal bones is seen from both the radiocarpal and midcarpal spaces. A probe will be placed between the separated carpal bones. (Fig. 64-4 shows a tear in the interosseous ligament.)
- In Geissler grade IV injuries, a complete tear of the interosseous ligament has occurred. The arthroscope may be freely passed between the involved carpal bones between the radiocarpal and midcarpal spaces. (Fig. 64-5 shows complete disruption of the interosseous ligament. The arthroscope passes freely between the carpal bones.)

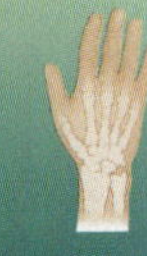

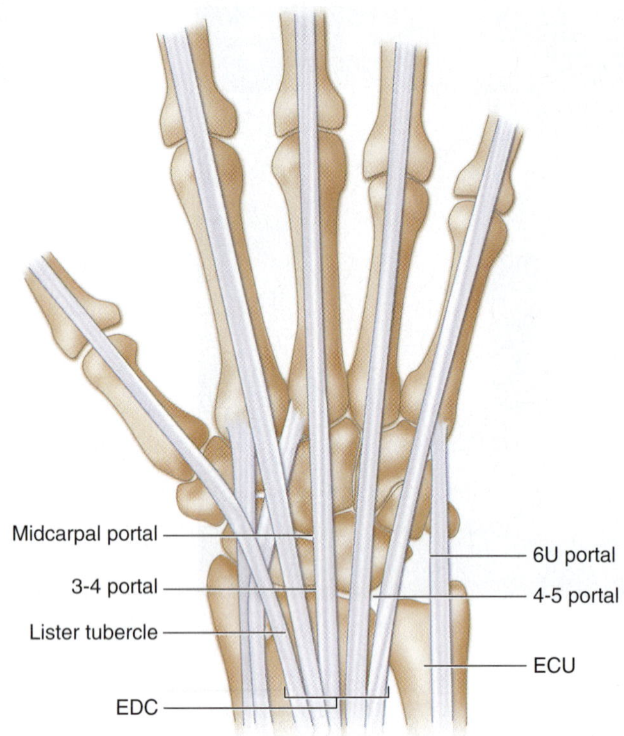

FIGURE 64-6

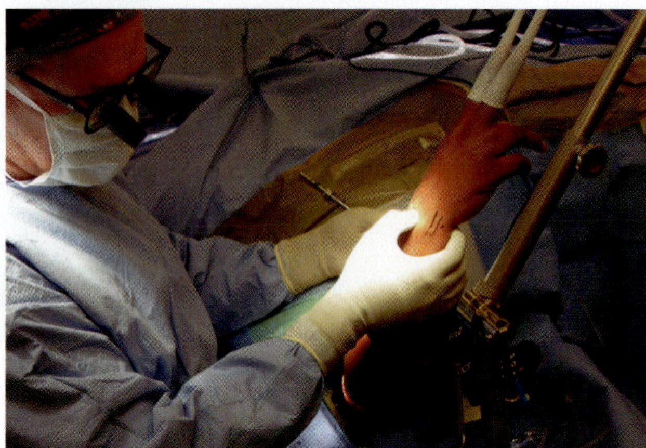

FIGURE 64-7

Exposures

- Wrist arthroscopy portals are made according to the space to which they correspond with respect to the extensor compartments (Fig. 64-6).
- The traditional portal is the 3-4 portal. This portal is made between the third and fourth dorsal compartments of the wrist. The 3-4 portal is located by palpating Lister tubercle by advancing the finger about 1 cm distal until the soft spot is noted over the dorsal lip of the radius. The 3-4 portal is in line with the radial border of the long finger. (Fig. 64-7 shows the thumb being used to palpate between the third and fourth dorsal compartments to identify the 3-4 portal space.) When the wrist is injected with arthroscopy fluid from the 6U portal, a bubble of swelling is typically noted over the 3-4 portal region. This further helps locate the 3-4 portal.
- The 4-5 portal is located by rolling the finger over the palpable fourth compartment and then finding the soft spot opposite the 3-4 portal on the ulnar aspect of the fourth compartment. As a general rule, the 4-5 portal lies slightly more proximal than the 3-4 portal because of the radial inclination of the distal radius. The 4-5 portal is a typical working portal that is in line with the midaxis of the ring metacarpal.
- The 6R and 6U portals are named according to their positions relative to the extensor carpi ulnaris tendon, with the 6R portal being radial and the 6U portal being ulnar to the tendon. The 6R portal is a typical working portal, and the 6U portal is typically used for inflow of fluid into the wrist. (Fig. 64-8 shows inflow through 6U, 6R being used as a working portal, and 3-4 being used as the arthroscope portal.)
- The 1-2 portal is made along the dorsal aspect of the snuffbox. By making this portal along the dorsal aspect, it prevents injury to the radial artery.

PEARLS

The key to making a wrist arthroscopy portal is to pull the skin against the tip of a no. 11 blade. Blunt dissection is then carried down to the level of the joint capsule. The arthroscope is introduced with a blunt trocar to avoid injury to the articular cartilage. (Fig. 64-9 shows blunt tip of arthroscope trocar.) Before committing to a skin incision, an 18-gauge needle is used to identify the exact location of the portal. If the portal location is too proximal or distal, the needle will not pass freely into the joint. (Fig. 64-10 shows an 18-gauge needle being used to help identify the correct place for the 3-4 portal.)

Keep in mind the slope of the distal radius and the radial inclination. The initial needle, as it is passed into the joint, should have about a 10-degree tilt from dorsal to volar to parallel the slope of the distal radius.

The 4-5 and 6R portals should be slightly proximal to the 3-4 portals following the inclination of the distal radius.

Both the radiocarpal and midcarpal spaces should be evaluated when wrist arthroscopy is performed.

Occasionally, dry arthroscopy is performed. In this manner, the arthroscope is introduced into the radiocarpal space without irrigation fluid. This is done to confirm a preoperative diagnosis in which the operative plan is eventually to open the wrist joint. In this manner, fluid extravasation into the soft tissues is limited, and the anatomy is not distorted.

PITFALLS

It is important to know the normal structures of the wrist and not to mistake them for pathologic changes.

Wrist arthroscopy portals must be precise. If a portal is off by just 1 to 2 mm, it can potentially cause intra-articular damage to the wrist and significantly impair visualization.

In fractures or in acute trauma, the wrist may be swollen. In this manner, it is important to palpate and identify the bony landmarks because the extensor tendons would not be palpable.

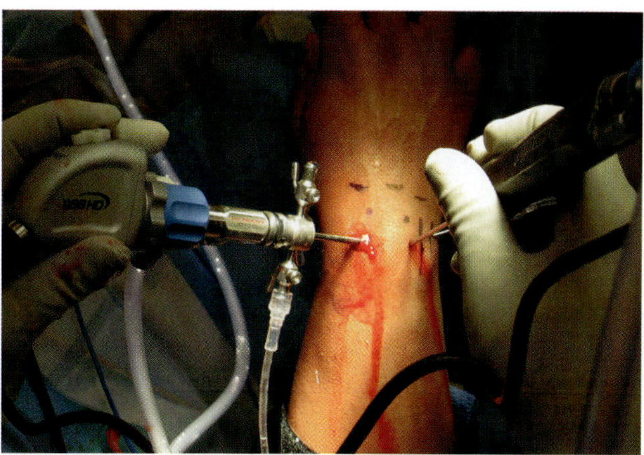

FIGURE 64-8

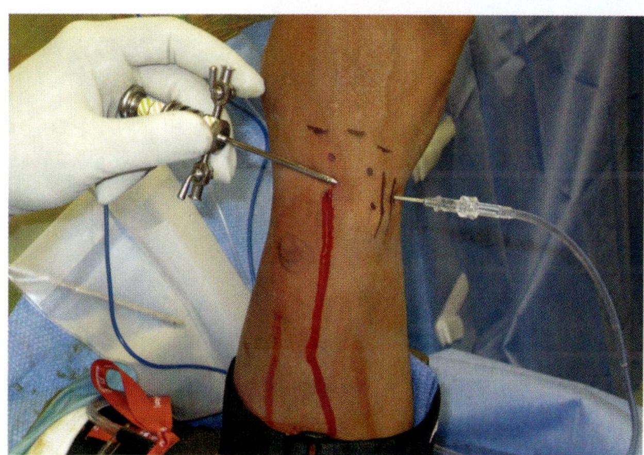

FIGURE 64-9

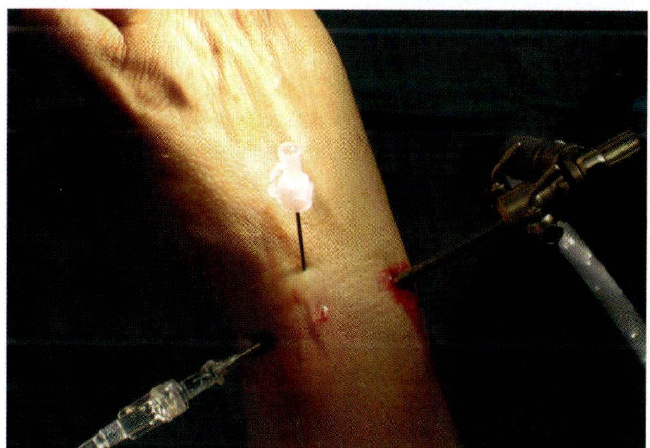

FIGURE 64-10

- The radial midcarpal portal is made 1 cm distal to the 3-4 portal. This portal gives good visualization of the midcarpal space. The ulnar midcarpal portal is made 1 cm distal to the 4-5 portal. Typically, there is more room in the ulnar midcarpal portal than the radial midcarpal portal. If the surgeon has difficulty entering the midcarpal space in the radial midcarpal portal, the ulnar midcarpal portal should be used because it has easier access.
- The STT portal is made just ulnar to the EPL tendon. This portal is best made with the arthroscope in the radial midcarpal portal, and a spinal needle is used to identify the exact location.

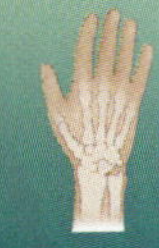

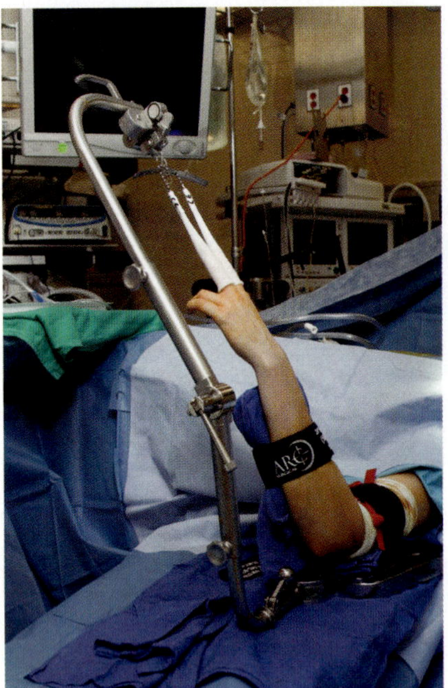

FIGURE 64-11

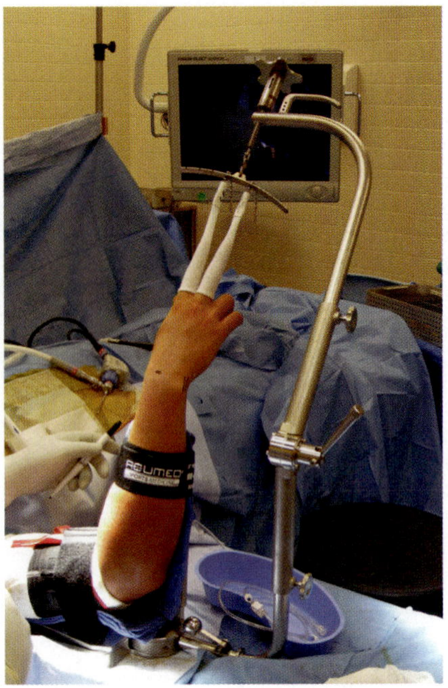

FIGURE 64-12

STEP 1 PEARLS

Towels are placed under the arm and forearm between the tower and the patient. This helps to avoid any potential abrasion of the skin from the metal traction tower (Fig. 64-12).

If a traction tower is not available, the wrist may be suspended overhead through finger traps and a shoulder traction apparatus.

If this is not available, the wrist may be placed in a horizontal position with finger traps and weights hanging over the end of the hand table.

STEP 1 PITFALLS

It is important to assess the temperature of the traction tower before wrist arthroscopy. If the tower has been used repeatedly, it may become very hot because it is sterilized and potentially can burn the patient.

If the traction tower apparatus is hot, it can be cooled off by placing it in a basin filled with irrigation fluid.

Procedure

Step 1

- The wrist is suspended with about 10 pounds of traction in a traction tower (Fig. 64-11).
- Slight flexion of the wrist makes it easier for entry for the arthroscopic instrumentation.
- Traction is provided through finger traps to the index and long fingers (see Fig. 64-12).

Step 2

- Inflow can be provided either through the 6U portal or through the arthroscopic cannula.
- Because of the small size of the arthroscopic cannula, it is recommended that inflow be provided through a separate inflow portal such as 6U.
- Outflow is provided through the arthroscopic cannula.
- An additional viewing portal is the 3-4 portal. The working portal is traditionally the 4-5 or 6R.

Step 3

- The radiocarpal space is evaluated in a radial to ulnar direction. The extrinsic radioscaphocapitate ligament is seen most radially along its insertion on the radial styloid, and the long radial lunate ligament, which is slightly wider, is just ulnar. (Fig. 64-13 shows the radioscaphocapitate and long radiolunate ligaments.)
- The radioscapholunate ligament (ligament of Testut) is next seen ulnarly. This is primarily a neurovascular structure (Fig. 64-14).
- The articular disk is identified ulnarly and palpated with a probe in the 6R portal.
- The ulnar triquetral and ulnar lunate ligaments are best seen with the arthroscope in the 6R portal. (Fig. 64-15 shows the ulnar triquetral ligament.)
- The lunotriquetral interosseous ligament is best identified with the arthroscope in the 6R portal.

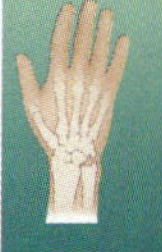

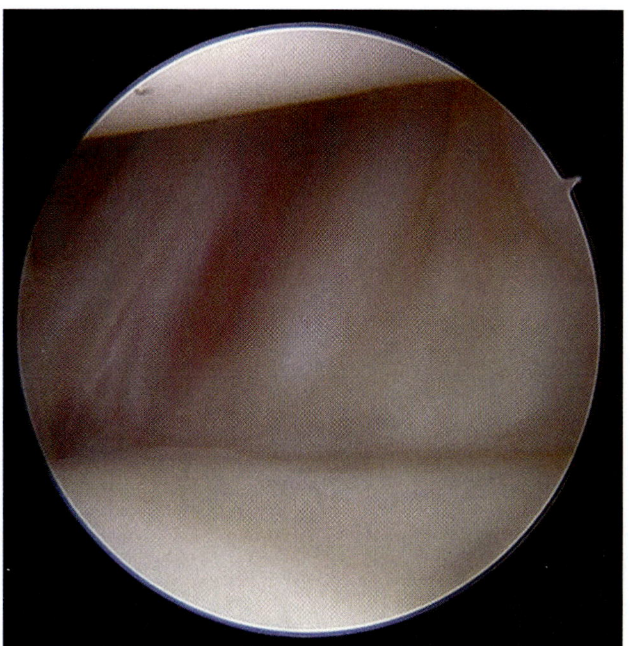

FIGURE 64-13

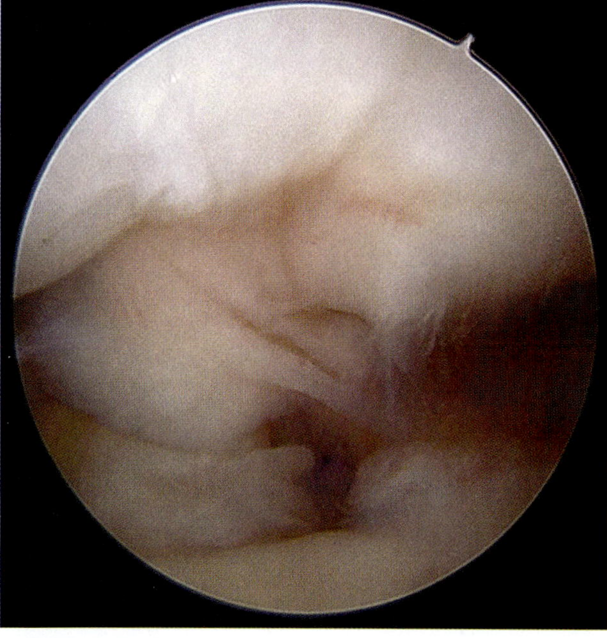

FIGURE 64-14

STEP 2 PEARLS

The 3-4 portal is most easily identified by rolling the tip of the thumb fingernail over the dorsal lip of the distal radius.

Arthroscopy portals may be made in the horizontal or longitudinal direction depending on the surgeon's preference. A horizontal incision may be potentially more cosmetic, although it may have a high risk for injury to the extensor tendons or dorsal cutaneous nerves. It is important not to insert the knife blade too deeply to avoid injury to these structures.

Outflow of fluid is through the irrigation tubing connected to the arthroscopic cannula. The irrigation tubing is placed into a basin so that the irrigation fluid does not run out on the operative field or into the surgeon's lap.

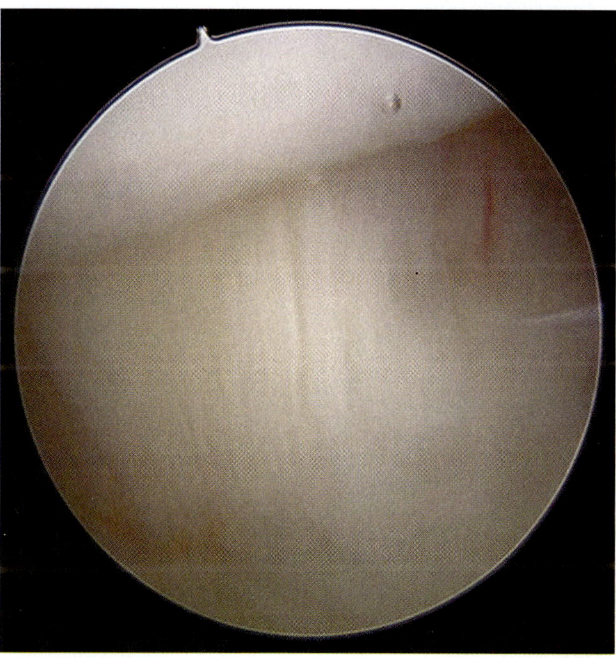

FIGURE 64-15

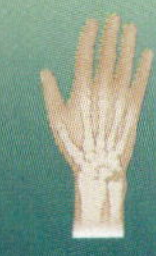

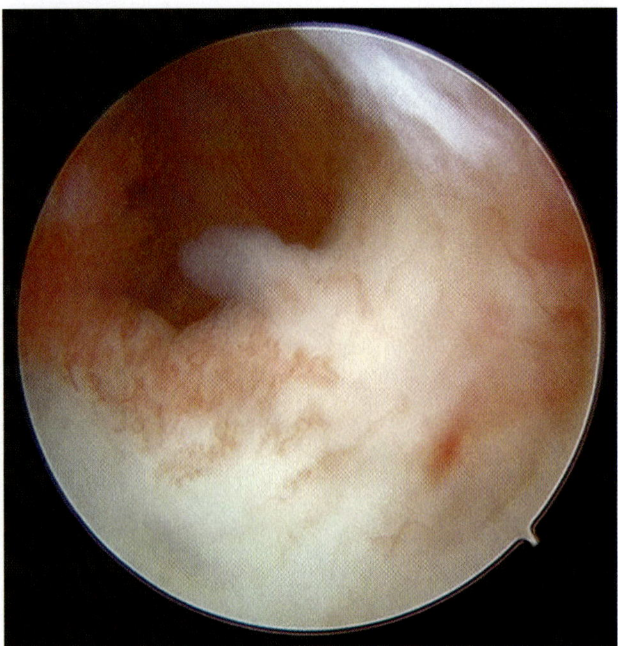

FIGURE 64-16

STEP 3 PITFALLS

The prestyloid recess is viewed arthroscopically as a normal fovea. Do not confuse a peripheral tear to the articular disk with this normal fovea. (Fig. 64-16 shows the prestyloid recess.) A peripheral tear of the TFCC disk usually is dorsal to the fovea.

The pisiform is seen about 60% of the time in normal wrist arthroscopy. This is a normal finding. Do not confuse a normal finding with pathologic changes of the wrist.

STEP 4 PEARLS

When inserting Kirschner wires for provisional fixation of a fracture or pinning acute interosseous ligament injuries, insert the wires in oscillation mode to minimize injury to the cutaneous nerves (Fig. 64-21).

If electrothermal shrinkage is being performed, it is important to monitor the temperature of the wrist arthroscopy fluid as it exits the wrist. The wrist is an extremely small joint, and the fluid can rapidly heat up with a thermal shrinkage probe causing potential burns to the wrist. (Fig. 64-22 shows use of electrothermal shrinkage.)

Step 4

- A needle is placed in the proposed ideal location for the radial midcarpal portal following diagnostic examination to the radiocarpal space.
- If a free flow of fluid is seen with the inflow through the 6U portal and the needle in the midcarpal space, one should be concerned about an interosseous ligament tear.
- The radial midcarpal portal is made after its ideal location is identified with a spinal needle.
- The ulnar midcarpal portal is made by placing a needle into the proposed location under direct visualization with the arthroscope in the radial midcarpal portal.
- Any widening or step-off of the scapholunate or lunotriquetral interosseous ligaments is best judged with the arthroscope in the midcarpal portal. (Fig. 64-17 shows midcarpal view of scapholunate ligament, Fig. 64-18 shows normal lunotriquetral interface, and Fig. 64-19 shows abnormal widening at lunotriquetral interface.)
- Articular cartilage defects, particularly of the capitate or hamate, are evaluated. (Fig. 64-20 shows arthroscopic view of the capitate and hamate interface.)
- These articular cartilage defects are more common in patients with a type II lunate.
- Fractures of the scaphoid are best seen with the arthroscope in the midcarpal space. Fractures of the proximal pole are best visualized with the arthroscope in the ulnar midcarpal portal, and fractures of the waist of the scaphoid are best seen with the arthroscope in the radial midcarpal portal.

Step 5

- Wrist arthroscopy portals are traditionally not closed. Depending on the procedure, usually a soft dressing is applied, and the patient can start range of motion.

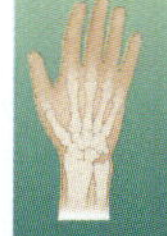

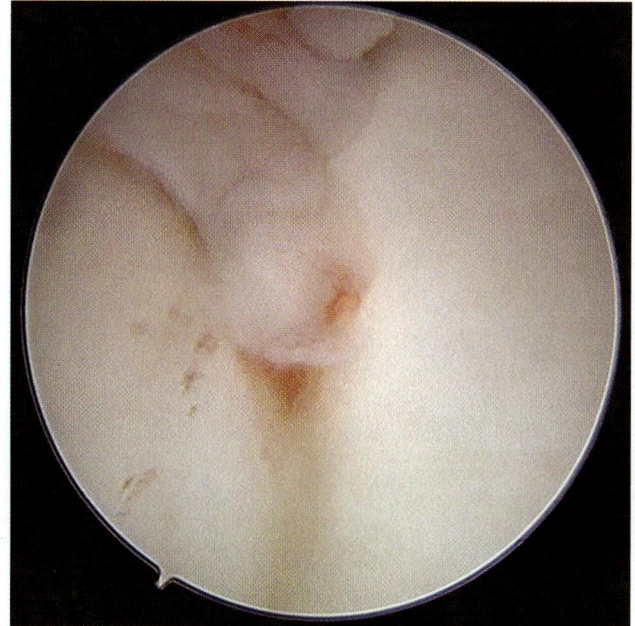

FIGURE 64-17

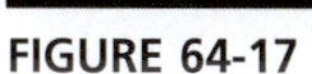

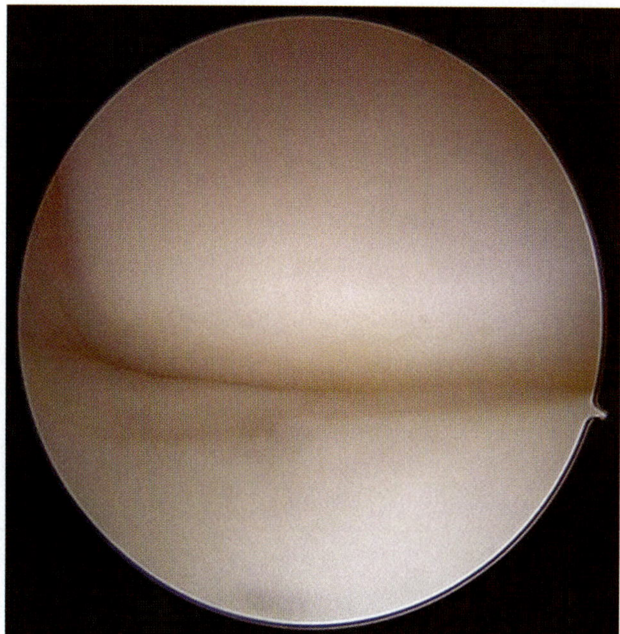

FIGURE 64-18

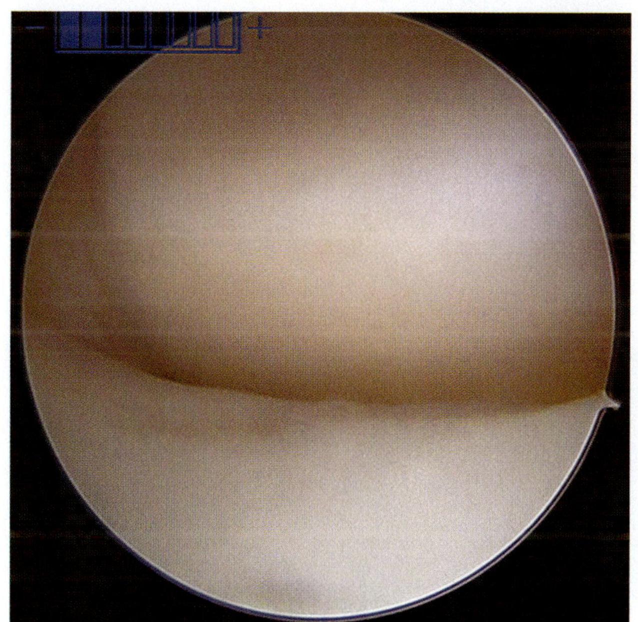

FIGURE 64-19

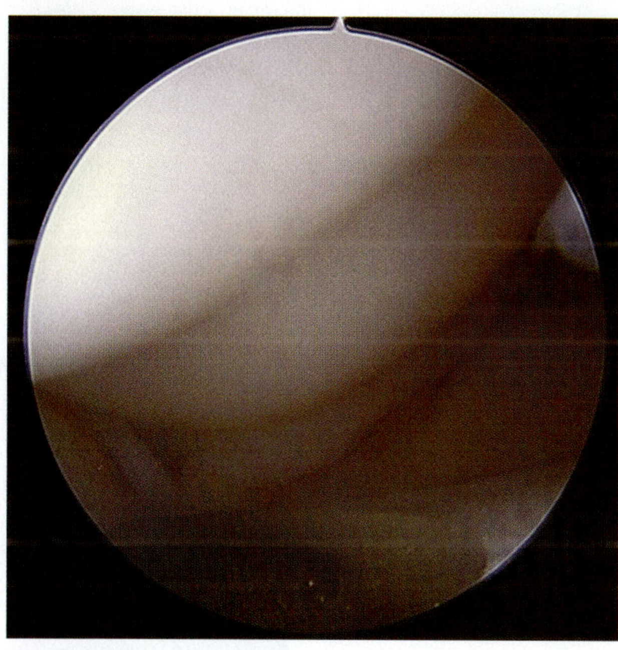

FIGURE 64-20

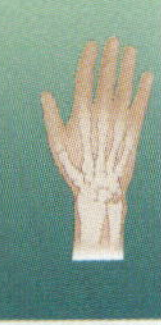

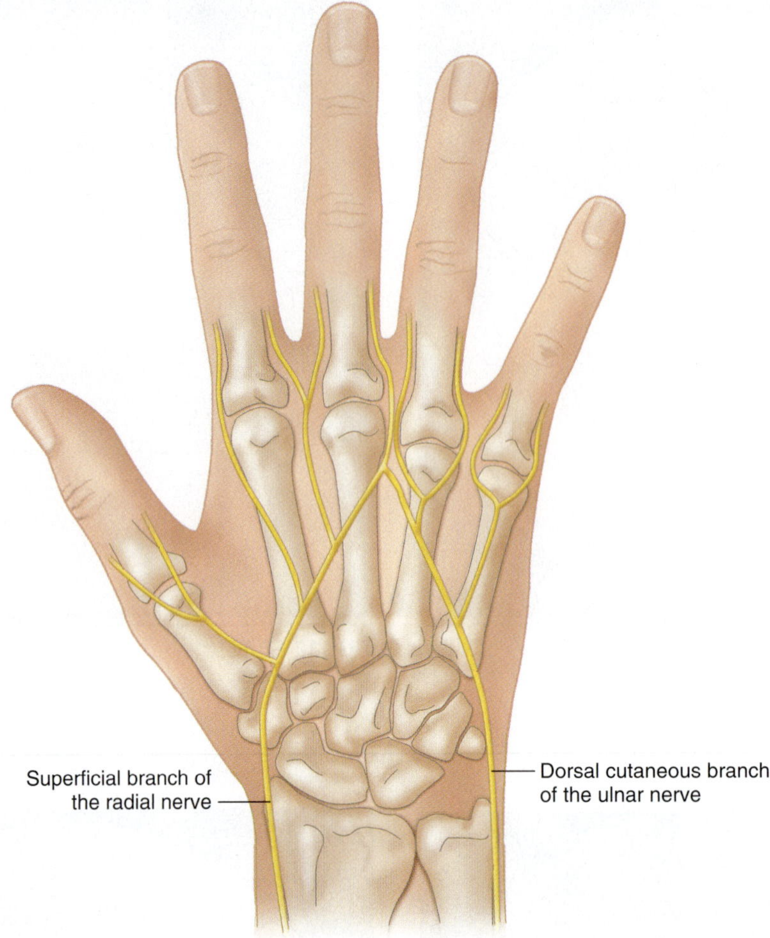

FIGURE 64-21

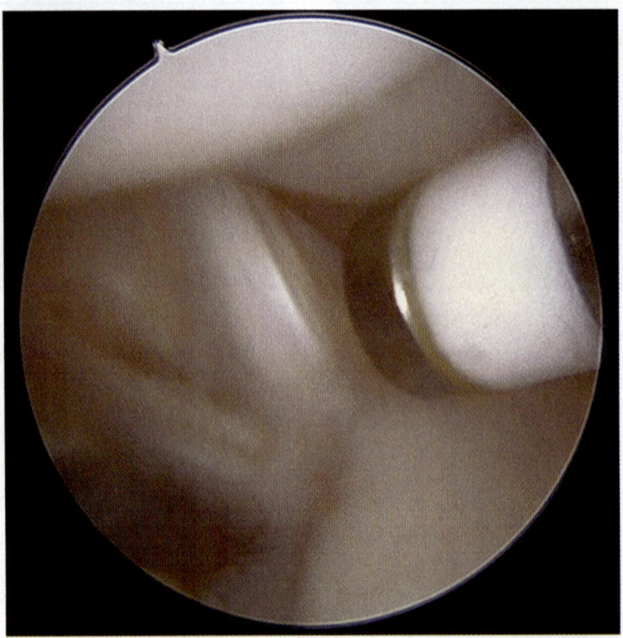

FIGURE 64-22

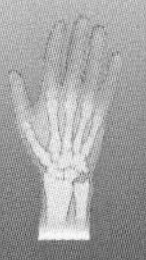

Postoperative Care and Expected Outcomes

- Postoperative care varies depending on the arthroscopic procedure performed. With traditional and diagnostic wrist arthroscopy, the patient keeps the wounds dry for about 3 days. Showers, not baths, are encouraged for the next 10 days to 2 weeks until the portals seal.
- Patients start range of motion of the fingers initially and progress to motion of the wrist and strengthening as tolerated.

Evidence

Chung KC, Zimmerman NB, Travis MT. Wrist arthrography versus arthroscopy: a comparative study of 150 cases. *J Hand Surg [Am]*. 1996;21:591-594.
The authors used triple-injection wrist arthrography and arthroscopy to evaluate 150 patients with suspected wrist ligamentous injuries. The diagnoses obtained by these two techniques were compared to determine the differences between the two modalities. All the patients in this study had both the clinical diagnosis of ligamentous injuries of the wrist and normal findings on x-ray films. Intercarpal abnormalities were found in 106 patients (71%) at wrist arthrography and in 136 patients (91%) at arthroscopy. There was only 42% agreement (63 patients) between the arthrographic and arthroscopic diagnoses. Eighty-seven patients (58%) had alterations of their arthrographic diagnoses following arthroscopy. For patients with normal arthrographic findings (44 patients), 88% underwent arthroscopy because there was insufficient correlation between the physical examination findings and the arthroscopic findings. Of the 44 patients with normal arthrographic findings, 35 patients (80% of the subgroup) had injuries found at arthroscopy. More than half of the patients had alterations in their arthrographic diagnoses following arthroscopy. The authors concluded that in a patient with suspected ligamentous injury of the wrist, wrist arthroscopy may be the most efficient method in arriving at a definitive diagnosis. (Level IV evidence)

Geissler WB, Freeland AE, Weiss APC, Chow JCY. Techniques of wrist arthroscopy. *J Bone Joint Surg [Am]*. 1999;81:1184-1197.
This paper presents the basic techniques of wrist arthroscopy and their application to common disorders of the wrist. (Level V evidence)

Johnstone DJ, Thorogood S, Smith WH, Scott TD. A comparison of magnetic resonance imaging and arthroscopy in the investigation of chronic wrist pain. *J Hand Surg [Br]*. 1997;22:714-718.
The authors conducted a prospective study wherein they evaluated 43 patients with chronic wrist pain using magnetic resonance imaging (MRI) and arthroscopy. Pathology within the wrist joint was detected in 30 cases with MRI and in 32 cases with arthroscopy. The sensitivity and specificity of MRI compared with arthroscopy were 0.8 and 0.7 for TFCC pathology, 0.37 and 1.0 for scapholunate ligament, and 0 and 0.97 for lunotriquetral ligament. They concluded that MRI is not helpful in the investigation of suspected carpal instability and that the results of MRI for TFCC injuries should be interpreted with caution. (Level IV evidence)

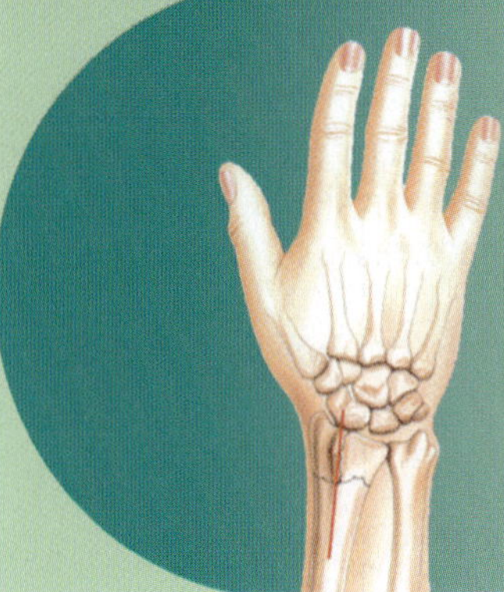

Arthroscopic Treatment for Septic Arthritis

William B. Geissler and Daniel C. M. Williams

Indications

- Arthroscopic synovectomy has been shown to be beneficial in patients with symptomatic, refractory reactive arthritis.
  - Arthroscopy will allow for diagnosis and treatment of suspected joint infection.
  - Arthroscopy assists in distinguishing between infectious and noninfectious inflammatory arthritis.
- Arthroscopy allows for not only continuous irrigation of joint space but also débridement of infected material.
  - Smaller incisions and quicker return to use of wrist are desired by the patient as well as the surgeon.

Examination/Imaging

Clinical Examination

- Examine the entire wrist for swelling, redness, warmth, and pain.
- The range-of-motion examination will produce exquisite pain with both active and passive motion.
- Hematogenous spread will manifest with systemic signs of infection, which may include fever, chills, tachycardia, and diaphoresis.
- Evaluation with laboratory tests should be done and should include white blood cell count (WBC), erythrocyte sedimentation rate, and C-reactive protein levels.
- Joint fluid can be obtained at the initiation of the procedure and should be evaluated with Gram staining, culture and sensitivity, WBC count, and crystal analysis.

Imaging

- Radiographs should be obtained and are useful for determining foreign bodies, soft tissue gas, and osteomyelitis.
- Magnetic resonance imaging can also be obtained and can give a better view of joint effusion, soft tissue fluid collections, and bone involvement.

Surgical Anatomy

- Structures to be identified and marked are Lister tubercle, articular margins, and the radius and ulna.
- Tendons that should be identified are the extensor digitorum communis (EDC), the extensor digiti minimi (EDM), and the extensor carpi ulnaris (ECU).
- Portal sites 3-4, 4-5, radial and ulna midcarpal, and 6U are marked before starting the procedure.

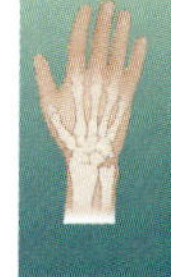

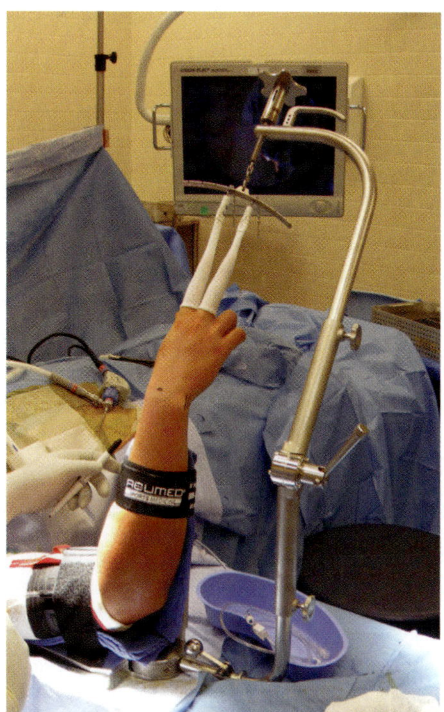

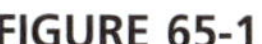

FIGURE 65-1

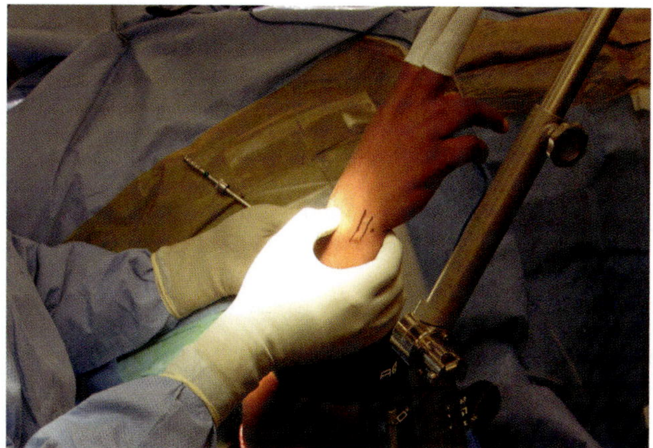

FIGURE 65-2

Positioning

- A sterile traction tower is used to suspend the elbow flexed at 90 degrees.
- The index and long finger are placed in finger traps, and a 10-lb weight is applied through the traction tower (Fig. 65-1).
- A gravity inflow system is used instead of the typical infusion pump system to help decrease the chance of disseminating infected fluid into the surrounding soft tissue structures.
- An arthroscope, 30-degree angled lens, camera, and full radius joint shaver setup are needed for this procedure.

Exposures

- Extremity exsanguination is generally contraindicated because of the joint infection. In some situations a tourniquet may be used to allow better visualization of the wrist joint. If a tourniquet is used, the arm is elevated to let the blood drain before tourniquet inflation.
- The anatomic landmarks are identified before starting the procedure. The portal sites are then marked, which are the radiocarpal, 3-4, 6R, 6U, and radial and ulna midcarpal portals.
- The 6R portal is located by palpating the ECU tendon. The portal is made just radial to the tendon.
- The 3-4 portal is located by palpating the concavity between the extensor pollicis longus and EDC tendons just distal to Lister tubercle in line with the radial border of the long finger (Fig. 65-2).
- The radial midcarpal portal is located about 1 cm distal to the 3-4 portal, and the ulna midcarpal portal is located about 1 cm distal to the 6R portal in line with the midaxis of the ring finger.

STEP 1 PEARLS

When introducing the blunt trocar, care must be taken not to plunge into the joint space. A controlled entrance is necessary to avoid injury to the internal structures.

The radioscaphocapitate, long radiolunate, triangular fibrocartilage complex, lunotriquetral interosseous ligament, ulnolunate ligament, and ulnotriquetral ligament can all be viewed from the 3-4 portal.

Inflow is provided through the 6U portal and outflow through the arthroscopic cannula. This allows for greater flow of fluid to irrigate the joint (Fig. 65-5).

Procedure

Step 1

- Inflow is initially placed through the 6U portal. The joint is inflated.
- A skin incision is made with a no. 11 blade scalpel at the 3-4 portal site. Only the skin should be incised, and the blade should be carried distally while the skin is retracted proximally with the thumb.
- A blunt curved hemostat should be used to dissect down to the wrist joint capsule using a spread and push technique. Care should be taken to avoid damaging the dorsal sensory nerves and the superficial veins that run in a longitudinal fashion (Fig. 65-3).
- To stay parallel to the articular surface, the trocar is angled 10 degrees proximally with respect to the volar inclination.
- Entry into the joint capsule should be done in a controlled fashion using gentle pressure on a blunt trocar (Fig. 65-4).
- The 3-4 portal will be used as the visualization portal.

Step 2

- An 18-gauge needle is inserted into the joint under visualization with the arthroscope in the 3-4 portal.

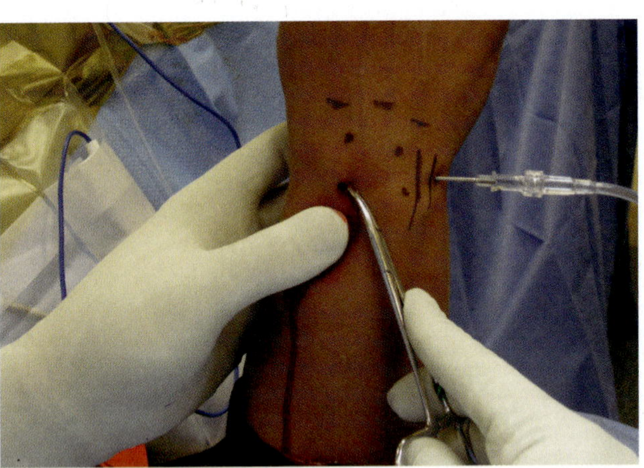

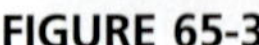

FIGURE 65-3

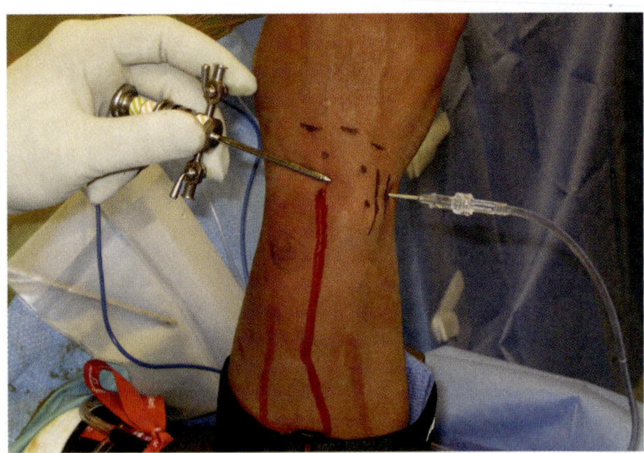

FIGURE 65-4

STEP 1 PITFALLS

Inflow through the arthroscope cannula does not provide sufficient irrigation of the joint because of the small space between the arthroscope and the cannula.

Visualization to the synovitis can be initially difficult. Be patient.

Visualization is key. Advance the arthroscope ulnarly near the 6R portal. Insert the shaver and start making room in the joint.

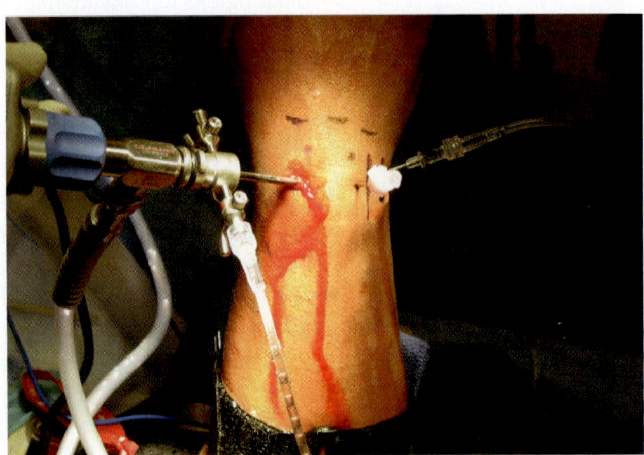

FIGURE 65-5

STEP 2 PEARLS

The ulnar half of the lunate, TFCC, and ulnocarpal ligaments are best viewed from the 6R portal.

STEP 2 PITFALLS

It is important to use a needle to identify the exact location of the 6R portal as viewed arthroscopically.

The TFCC and/or the articular cartilage of the lunate and triquetrum may be injured if the portal is too far distal or proximal.

STEP 3 PEARLS

When evaluating the TFCC, attention should be paid to any tears centrally or in the periphery or the articular disk, and these should be documented. The shaver can be used to help completely delineate the extent of the tear.

STEP 3 PITFALLS

It is important to know normal from abnormal.

Do not confuse the normal prestyloid recess with a peripheral tear of the TFCC.

The pisiform may be visualized about 60% of the time with the arthroscope in the 6R portal. This is a normal finding.

- A skin incision is made with a no. 11 blade scalpel at the 6R portal site. Only the skin should be incised, and the blade should be carried distally while the skin is retracted proximally.
- Once again, care should be taken to avoid damaging the superficial sensory nerves and veins when using a curved hemostat to dissect down to the joint capsule.
- Entry into the joint with a blunt trocar is made in a neutral position, instead of in an angled fashion.
- The 6R portal will be the working portal and will be used for the motorized shaver and suction.

Step 3: Radiocarpal Evaluation

- The radiocarpal joint should be examined in a systematic fashion.
- Beginning in a radial to ulnar fashion, the articular surfaces of the scaphoid, lunate, and triquetrum should be evaluated. Care should be taken to thoroughly examine the surfaces for cartilage erosion or wear.
- Next, the scapholunate, lunotriquetral, and radiocarpal ligaments should be examined. The ligaments should be carefully evaluated for laxity, step-offs, and tears.
- After evaluating those ligaments, the articular surface of the radius and the TFCC should be evaluated. Attention should be paid to any tears centrally or in the periphery or the articular disk.
- When synovitis, debris, or loculations are encountered, they should be débrided with the shaver as completely as possible (Fig. 65-6).
- It is easier to shave the reactive synovitis from the ulnar side of the wrist with the arthroscope in the 3-4 portal and the shaver in the 6R portal.
- The instruments are then reversed, and the radial synovitis is débrided with the shaver in the 3-4 portal and the arthroscope in the 6R portal.

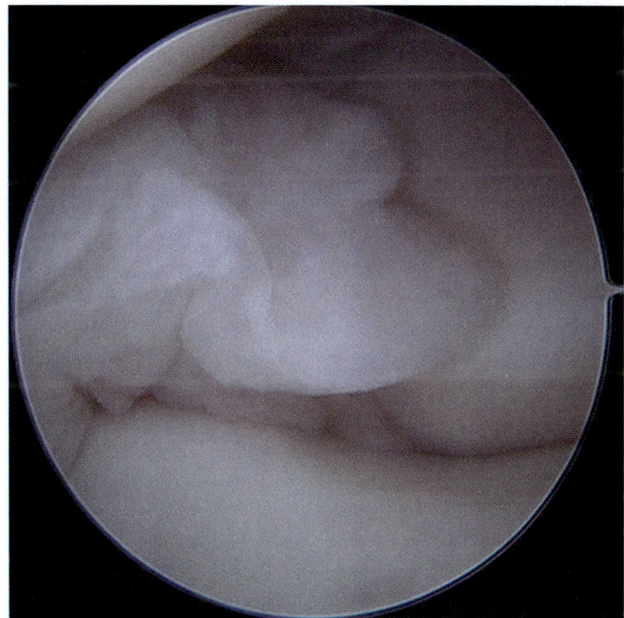

FIGURE 65-6

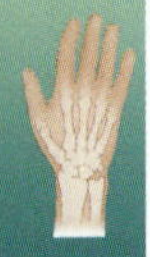

STEP 4 PEARLS

Both midcarpal and radiocarpal evaluations are needed to correctly use the Geissler classification system.

STEP 4 PITFALLS

It is easy to damage the articular cartilage of the midcarpal row when making the midcarpal portal.

Always use a needle to confirm the ideal location of the midcarpal portal before making an incision.

Always use a blunt trocar when placing the arthroscope in the midcarpal spaces.

Stop if resistance is felt.

Step 4: Midcarpal Evaluation

- After the proximal radiocarpal joint space has been thoroughly evaluated, the midcarpal space should be examined.
- The radial midcarpal and ulnar midcarpal portals are accessed in a fashion similar to that of the proximal portals.
- The radial midcarpal portal is used as the visualization portal, and the ulnar midcarpal portal is used as the working portal.
- The distal articular surface of the capitate is easily viewed and should be examined first.
- Next, the proximal row bones should be evaluated by inspecting the distal articular surfaces of the scaphoid, lunate, and triquetrum.
- The scapholunate and lunotriquetral ligaments and joints are evaluated for laxity, step-offs, tears, or widening.
- The Geissler classification system is useful in grading and describing any ligamentous injuries between the proximal row of carpal bones.
- The ulnar-sided synovitis is débrided with the arthroscope in the radial midcarpal portal and the shaver in the ulna midcarpal portal.
- The instruments are then reversed, and the radial synovitis is débrided with the shaver in the radial midcarpal portal and the arthroscope in the ulna midcarpal portal.

Postoperative Care and Expected Outcomes

- The skin incision can be either left open or loosely approximated with Steri-Strips.
- The wrist can be placed in a volar resting splint or can be placed in a soft dressing.
- Depending on the clinical scenario, postoperative intravenous antibiotics should be continued and tailored based on the Gram stain and culture and sensitivity results.
- Digital range-of-motion exercises are started immediately.
- Wrist range of motion and strengthening are initiated as tolerated.

Evidence

Birman MV, Strauch RJ. Management of the septic wrist. *J Hand Surg [Am]*. 2011;36:324-326.

This paper reviewed data on septic wrists treated with needle aspiration, open surgical technique, and arthroscopic management. Several retrospective studies were examined. Their review showed that all techniques were useful in some regard; however, there was no solid evidence to determine the relative effectiveness of the procedures. (Level IV evidence)

Goldenberg DL, Brandt KD, Cohen AS, Cathcart ES. Treatment of septic arthritis: comparison of needle aspiration and surgery as initial modes of joint drainage. *Arthritis Rheum*. 1975;18:83-90.

This paper compared needle aspiration of a septic joint with open surgical drainage. This is a retrospective study that compared data from 59 patients over an 8-year period. All of the patients had proven bacterial arthritis. Forty-two patients were treated with needle aspiration, and 17 were treated with open surgical drainage. Sixty-seven percent of patients treated with aspiration had complete recovery. Only 42% of patients treated with open surgery had complete recovery. Also, only 21% of patients in the aspiration group had poor results compared with 55% of in the open surgical group. Poor result was defined as flexion deformity of 10 degrees or greater, ankylosis, secondary osteomyelitis, or persistent effusion. This paper concluded that in initial management of a septic joint, needle aspiration is more favorable than open surgery. (Level IV evidence)

Sammer D, Shin A. Comparison of arthroscopic and open treatment of septic arthritis of the wrist. *J Bone Joint Surg [Am]*. 2010;92:107-113.

The authors used a retrospective comparison of patients treated with either arthroscopic or open surgical treatment of a septic wrist. The study looked at 11 years of data and involved a single institution. Their findings showed that arthroscopic treatment not only was effective but also led to fewer subsequent operations and shorter hospital stays. (Level IV evidence)

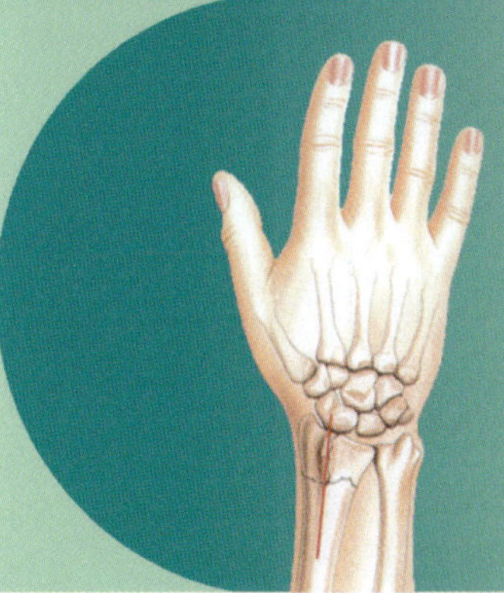

Arthroscopic Ganglionectomy

William B. Geissler and Daniel C. M. Williams

Indications

- Ideal indication
  - Symptomatic single dorsal wrist ganglion located between the third and fourth dorsal compartments with at least one failed aspiration
- Additional indications
  - Patient desiring rapid return to motion after surgery and early return to work and function
  - Suspicion of additional intra-articular pathology that needs evaluation

Examination/Imaging

Clinical Examination

- Ganglions are the most common tumors of the hand and represent about 50% to 70% of all soft-tissue hand tumors. Ganglions are more prevalent in females and usually appear between the second and fifth decades of life. Dorsal wrist ganglions are by far the most common cyst and account for 60% to 70% of all hand and wrist ganglions. The origin of the dorsal ganglion, with rare exception, arises over the junction of the dorsal capsule with the scapholunate intraosseous ligament. Angelides and Wallace stated that the transition between the dorsal capsule and the scapholunate interosseous ligament can serve as a duct with a one-way valve mechanism. The main cyst is usually located directly over the scapholunate ligament. However, the cyst may occur anywhere between the extensor tendons and can be connected to the ligament through a long pedicle. Palpation of the mass usually reveals the extent of the cyst in the direction of the pedicle. Transillumination or aspiration confirms the diagnosis preoperatively.
- Open excision of the dorsal ganglion is a time-proven procedure with a low recurrence rate. However, open excision of an occult ganglion frequently requires blunt dissection to identify the ganglion, which may lead to increased scarring and decreased range of motion. Arthroscopic excision allows precise identification of the stock and excision with potentially less scarring.

Imaging

- Radiographs of the involved region are usually unremarkable. Although plain radiographs are usually unremarkable, they may be helpful in evaluating additional pathologic changes to the wrist, including static wrist instability.
- Arthrograms may show communication of the wrist joint with the cyst via a one-way valve mechanism.
- Magnetic resonance imaging (MRI) may be helpful in detection of an occult dorsal ganglion. MRI evaluation is potentially helpful when additional intra-articular pathologic changes are suspected.

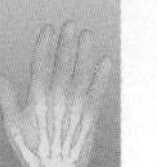

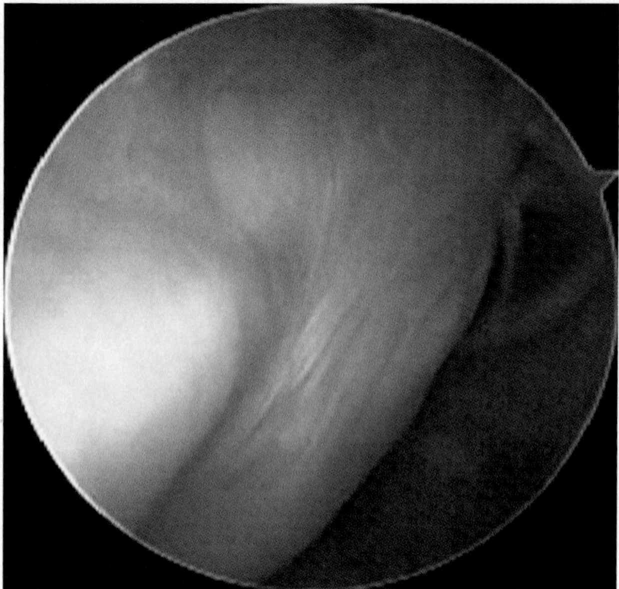

FIGURE 66-1

Surgical Anatomy

- Typically, the cyst appears between the extensor pollicis longus and the extensor digitorum communis tendons. Arthroscopically, the pearl or the origin of the ganglion stalk from the distal portion of the scapholunate interosseous ligament is identified with the arthroscope in the 4-5 or 6R portals. (Fig. 66-1 shows an arthroscopic view of the scapholunate ligament.) The cyst is seen about two thirds of the time.
- Attenuation or laxity of the scapholunate interosseous ligament may be seen with the arthroscope in the 3-4 portal and radiocarpal space, or widening of the scapholunate may be seen with the arthroscope in the radial midcarpal portal.

Positioning

- The patient is positioned in the traction tower with about 10 pounds of traction.
- The wrist is slightly flexed to make it easier to insert the arthroscope and arthroscopic instrumentation.
- Small joint instrumentation with a 2.7-mm or smaller arthroscope is used.
- Small joint shavers are used as well. Large joint instrumentation is not recommended for the wrist.
- A wrist traction tower helps provide traction to the wrist and stabilizes the forearm. If this is not available, the wrist can be suspended in a shoulder traction tower, although the forearm is not stabilized, and the wrist will be at neutral position.
- Another option, if the traction tower is not available, is to suspend the wrist horizontally over the hand table. Finger traps may be used with a weight placed at the end of the table to help suspend the wrist. This helps stabilize the forearm, but the wrist will be in neutral position for the procedure.

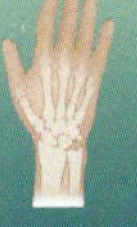

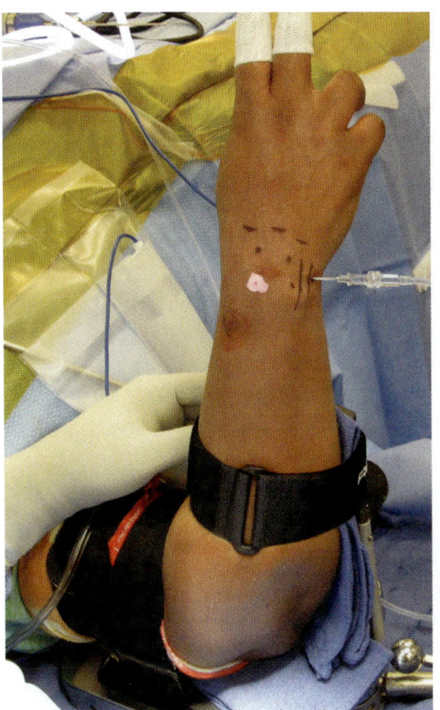

FIGURE 66-2

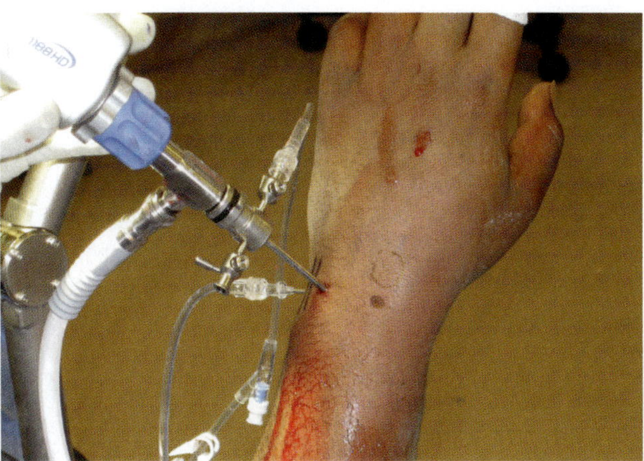

FIGURE 66-3

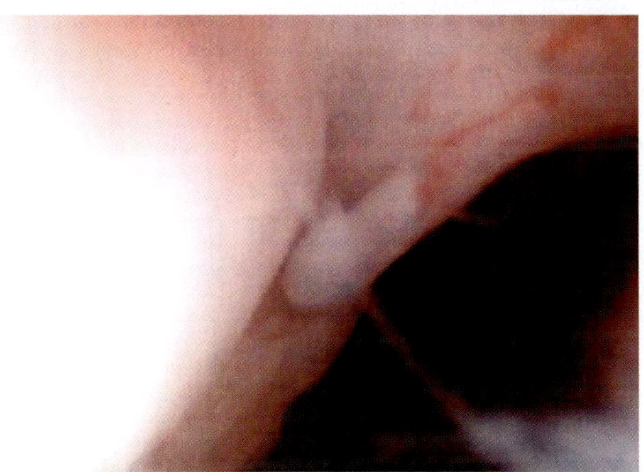

FIGURE 66-4

PEARLS

The ganglion cyst is usually located distal to the standard 3-4 portal. Because of this, the needle is at about a 45-degree angle to the dorsum of the hand, which allows it to enter through the cyst and then into the radiocarpal space.

It is occasionally helpful to turn the lights down in the operating room theater; the lights from the arthroscope will transilluminate the sack of the ganglion cyst. This can aid in placing the needle.

PITFALLS

It is important to know the normal structures of the wrist and not to mistake them for pathologic changes.

Wrist arthroscopy portals must be precise. If a portal is off by just 1 to 2 mm, it can potentially cause intra-articular damage to the wrist and significantly impair visualization.

In fractures or in acute trauma, the wrist may be swollen. In this case, it is important to palpate and identify the bony landmarks because the extensor tendons are not palpable.

Exposures

- Inflow is provided through a needle using the 6U portal (Fig. 66-2).
- The arthroscope is placed in the 4-5 or 6R portal to look across the wrist to identify the stalk of the ganglion. (Fig. 66-3 shows the arthroscope placed in the 6R portal, and inflow is maintained using the 6U portal.)
- The stalk of the ganglion will be identified at the junction of the scapholunate interosseous ligament to the dorsal capsule (Fig. 66-4).
- An 18-gauge needle is then inserted directly through the back of the ganglion into the radiocarpal space, as viewed arthroscopically with a scope in the 4-5 or 6R portal.

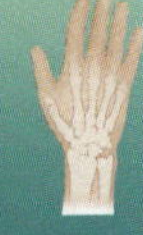

Procedure

Step 1

- The wrist is suspended in 10 pounds of traction in a traction tower. Inflow is provided through a needle using the 6U portal. (Fig. 66-5 shows the outline of the ganglion marked.) The arthroscope is placed in the 6R portal. A needle is placed through the sac of the ganglion to enter the radiocarpal space.
- The needle is seen entering the radiocarpal space through the sac of the ganglion with the arthroscope in the 6R portal.
- Notice the oblique path of the needle toward the more distally located ganglion to enter the radiocarpal space. The skin only is incised to make the portal.

Step 2

- The shaver is introduced through the distal 3-4 portal into the radiocarpal space (see Fig. 66-6).
- An approximately 1-cm full-thickness defect of the dorsal capsule is then created with the shaver (see Fig. 66-7).
- This defect is at the junction of the dorsal capsule and the scapholunate interosseous ligament.
- A small punch may also be used to create the capsular defect (see Fig. 66-8).

STEP 1 PEARLS

Make sure to incise the skin only by pulling the skin against the tip of a no. 11 blade. This is to avoid injury to the superficial cutaneous skin nerves and the dorsal extensor tendons.

STEP 1 PITFALLS

The sac of the ganglion cyst should be outlined with a marking pen before the reduction of the inflow through the 6U portal. This is to help note its location before the wrist becomes swollen from any fluid extravasation.

The shaver is introduced through the distal 3-4 portal into the radiocarpal space (Fig. 66-6).

An approximately 1-cm full-thickness defect of the dorsal capsule is then created with the shaver (Fig. 66-7).

This defect is at the junction of the dorsal capsule and the scapholunate interosseous ligament.

A small punch may also be used to create the capsular defect (Fig. 66-8).

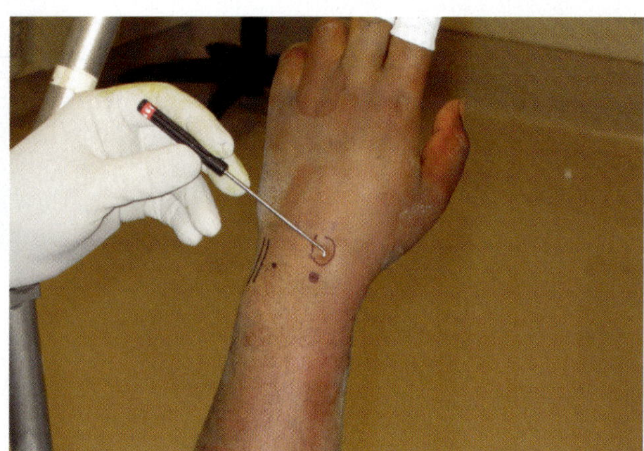

FIGURE 66-5

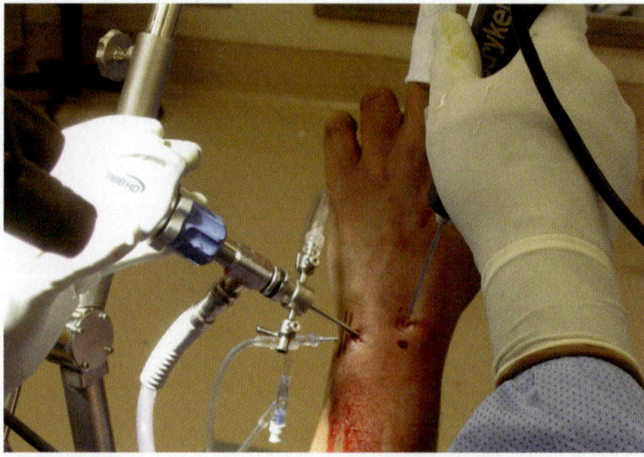

FIGURE 66-6

STEP 2 PEARLS

It is important to visualize the dorsal extensor tendons after the full-thickness defect has been created. Once the tendons are seen, this ensures that a full-thickness defect is made.

The tendon usually identified is the extensor carpi radialis brevis, although the tendons of the extensor digitorum communis may be identified as well (Fig. 66-9).

It is sometimes helpful to place the wrist at neutral or in slight extension if it is difficult to visualize in the dorsal capsule at its junction with the scapholunate interosseous ligament. This helps relax the dorsal capsule to improve visualization.

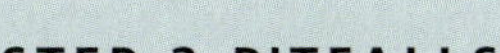

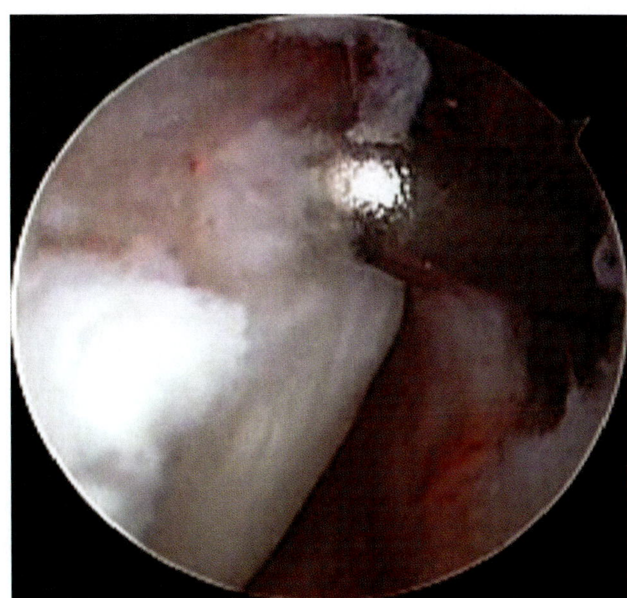

FIGURE 66-7

STEP 2 PITFALLS

Small joint instrumentation is used. A standard small shaver is not very aggressive compared with its larger counterparts, although it would be difficult, although not impossible, to shave through an entire extensor tendon. Caution is needed.

With a small joint punch, it would similarly be difficult to create a full-thickness defect in the overlying extensor tendons. However, it is important to visualize directly what the shaver or the punch contacts.

As one shaves the dorsal capsule, occasionally fluid from the cyst will be seen entering the joint. This will have a yellow, oily configuration.

Once the defect has been made, it is important to palpate the cyst to confirm that it has been decompressed.

After decompression of the ganglion cyst, the wrist is then evaluated for any additional disease through the radiocarpal and midcarpal portals.

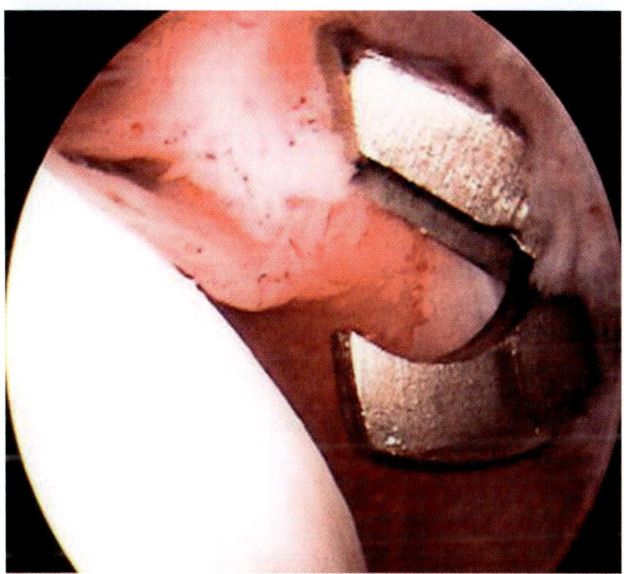

FIGURE 66-8

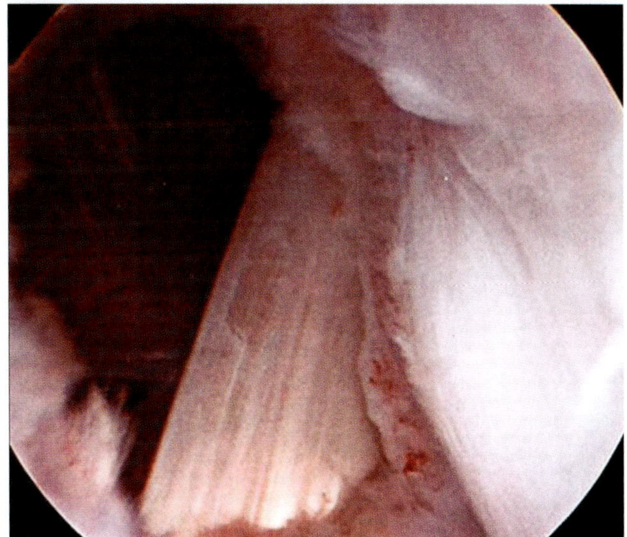

FIGURE 66-9

STEP 3 PITFALLS

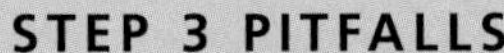

Similar to not injuring the extensor tendons, close attention is made not to débride the dorsal portion of the scapholunate interosseous ligament with either the shaver or the punch.

Step 3

- It is important to palpate the sac of the ganglion after resection of the dorsal capsule. It is particularly true in a multilobe ganglion. If a ganglion is not fully decompressed, further resection of the remaining ganglion will be required.

Step 4

- The wrist is placed in a soft dressing, and immediate digital range of motion is started.
- The dorsal 3-4 portal may require a single stitch depending on its size.

Postoperative Care and Expected Outcomes

- Immediate digital range of motion is initiated. The wound is kept dry for about 3 days to let the portals seal.
- Patients are able to return to work within 3 to 4 weeks, and recurrence rates are comparable to those following open excision.

Evidence

Geissler WB. Arthroscopic excision of dorsal wrist ganglia. *Tech Hand Upper Extremity Surg*. 1998;2:196-201.
The author reviewed arthroscopic excision of dorsal ganglions in 14 patients with a follow-up of more than 1 year. There was one recurrence in his study, for a 93% success rate. (Level V evidence)

Osterman AL, Raphael J. Arthroscopic resection of dorsal ganglions of the wrist. *Hand Clin*. 1995;11:7-12.
The authors reported no recurrences following arthroscopic dorsal ganglion excision with an average follow-up of 16 months (range, 9 to 23 months) and no patients lost to follow-up. The patients returned to work in 3.5 weeks. (Level V evidence)

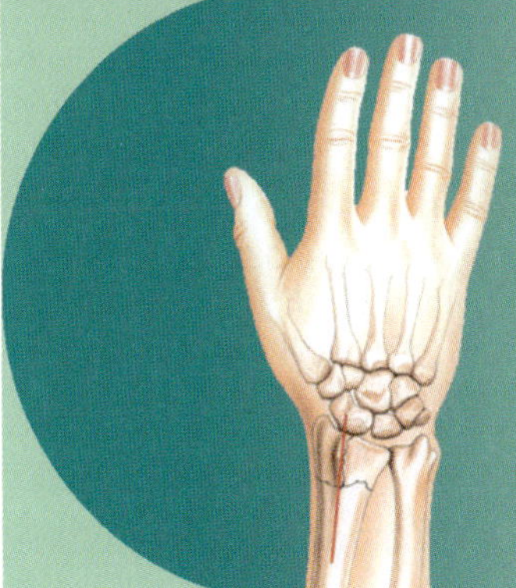

PROCEDURE 67

Arthroscopic Triangular Fibrocartilage Complex Repair

William B. Geissler and Daniel C. M. Williams

See Video 49: Arthroscopic TFCC Repair

Indications

- Traumatic peripheral ulnar tears of the triangular fibrocartilage complex (TFCC)

Examination/Imaging

Clinical Examination

- Patients complain of pain with twisting of the wrist, such as opening jars or doors.
- They may have pain over the prestyloid recess with hyperpronation and supination of the forearm and have point tenderness at the prestyloid recess.
- In more severe injuries to the TFCC, instability of the distal radial ulnar joint may be appreciated. The distal ulna may lie more dorsal in relation to the radius compared with the opposite side, and patients may have increased anterior and posterior translation of the distal ulna in relation to the radius.

Imaging

- Plain radiographs with the wrist in neutral position are mandatory to assess the relationship of the ulna to the radius. In patients who are markedly ulnar positive, the treating surgeon may consider repair, ulna shortening, or a combination of both.
- Wrist arthrograms frequently will yield false-negative results. This is because synovitis resulting from the tear will cover up the peripheral lesion.
- Magnetic resonance imaging is specific and sensitive for detection of peripheral ulnar tears to the TFCC.

Surgical Anatomy

- The TFCC is a complex soft tissue support system that stabilizes the ulnar side of the wrist and also serves to extend the articular surface of the radius to support the proximal carpal row. As described by Palmer, it is composed of the fibrocartilage articular disk, the volar and dorsal radioulnar ligaments, the meniscus homolog, and the floor of the ECU tendon sheath.
- The ulnar aspect of the articular disk has two main bundles. One bundle inserts on the ulnar styloid, and the second bundle inserts at its base. The deep bundle is called the ligamentum subcruentum. The deep bundle of the articular disk is not visible arthroscopically. With pronation and supination of the forearm, the superficial and deep layers lie opposite each other.

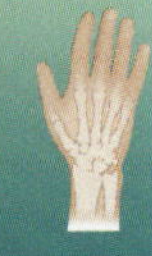

PEARLS

When incising the ECU tendon sheath for the outside-in technique, it is important to use sharp dissection through the sheath so that there will be a good layer to close to avoid instability to the ECU tendon.

Initial arthroscopic evaluation may not reveal a peripheral tear. It is important to palpate the articular disk with a probe to assess tension of the disk. If there is loss of normal tension, a peripheral tear is highly suspected.

Frequently, synovitis will cover up the peripheral tear. It is important to shave away the synovitis to evaluate for separation of the articular disk from the capsule.

- The arterial blood supply of the TFCC has been thoroughly studied. Thiru evaluated 12 cadaver specimens using latex injections. The ulnar artery supplies most of the blood to the ulnar portion of the TFCC through its dorsal and palmar radiocarpal branches. Thiru documented a complex of vessels that supplies the peripheral 15% to 20% of the articular disk. A similar study by Bedner and colleagues of 10 cadavers found penetration of vessels into the peripheral 10% to 40% of the articular disk. These studies confirm intact blood supply to the periphery of the articular disk with a potential to heal when repaired.

Positioning

- The wrist is suspended with about 10 pounds of traction in a traction tower (Fig. 67-1).
- The wrist is slightly flexed 10 to 20 degrees to allow easier access of the arthroscope and instrumentation. A small joint arthroscope (≤2.7 mm) is used. Small joint arthroscopy instrumentation is recommended. Large joint instrumentation is not appropriate for wrist arthroscopy.
- For the outside-in technique, an 18-gauge needle, 2-0 PDS suture, and a suture retriever are all that are needed.
- For the all-arthroscopic knotless technique, the Arthrex TFCC repair kit is required.

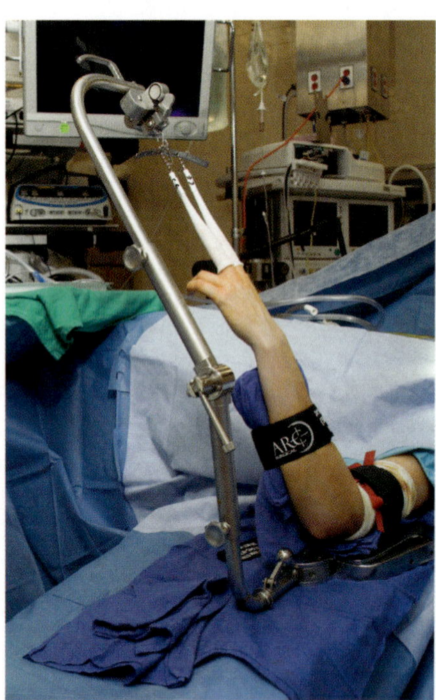

FIGURE 67-1

Exposures

- The arthroscope is in the 3-4 portal. A working 6R portal is made (Fig. 67-2).
- For the outside-in technique, following arthroscopic evaluation of the wrist, the 6R portal is elongated to about 2 cm in length along the radial border of the ECU tendon sheath. The tendon sheath is then opened, and the ECU tendon is retracted ulnarly.
- For the all-arthroscopic knotless technique, the arthroscope is in the standard 3-4 viewing portal, and the standard working 6R portal is made. An accessory 6-R portal is made about 1.5 cm distal to the 6R portal.
- The accessory 6R portal is made in line with the 6R portal and identified by using an 18-gauge needle to palpate the base of the ulna at the ulnar styloid.

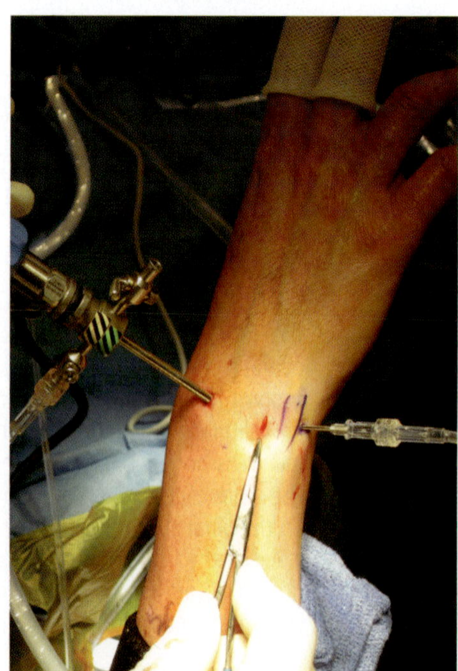

FIGURE 67-2

PITFALLS

When exposing the ECU tendon sheath, it is important to use blunt dissection to identify the transarticular branch of the dorsal sensory branch of the ulnar nerve. Frequently, this small nerve branch runs across the surgical field and should be retracted to avoid a potentially painful neuroma in this area.

It is important when making arthroscopy portals to incise the skin only by pulling the skin with the thumb against the tip of a no. 11 blade (Fig. 67-3). Blunt dissection is carried out with a hemostat to the joint capsule. The arthroscope is introduced with a blunt trocar in the 3-4 portal. In this manner, injury to the superficial cutaneous nerves and the articular cartilage can be avoided.

STEP 1 PEARLS

It is important to assess the entire wrist from both the radiocarpal and midcarpal portals. A portion of the greater injury to the ulnar side of the wrist involves the lunotriquetral interosseous ligament. The lunotriquetral interosseous ligament cannot be well visualized with the arthroscope in the 3-4 portal and needs to be visualized with the arthroscope in the 6R portal.

In addition, the midcarpal space should be further evaluated for midcarpal instability.

Subluxation of the ECU tendon is usually associated with a peripheral tear to the articular disk. If subluxation is suspected, the wrist is arthroscopically evaluated for a peripheral ulnar tear to the articular disk.

Procedure

Step 1

- Palmer type IB peripheral ulnar tears are amenable to arthroscopic repair. The tear usually presents on the dorsal ulnar aspect of the articular disk just ulnar to the 6R portal. The arthroscope is in the traditional 3-4 viewing portal, and a 6R portal is made just radial to the ECU tendon. Synovitis about the periphery of the articular disk is débrided to visualize the tear.
- The articular disk is palpated with a probe to verify loss of tension to the articular disk (Fig. 67-4).

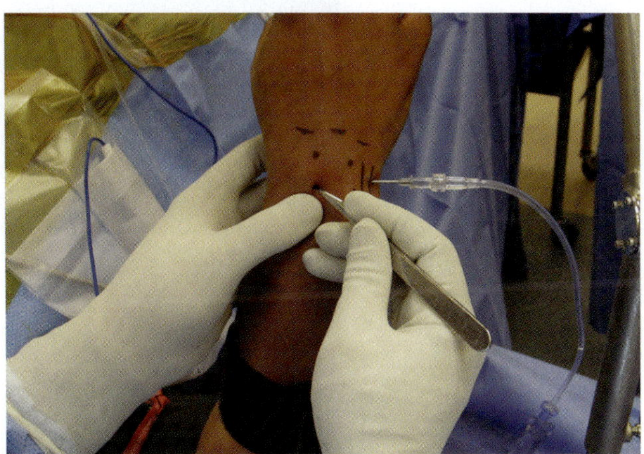

FIGURE 67-3

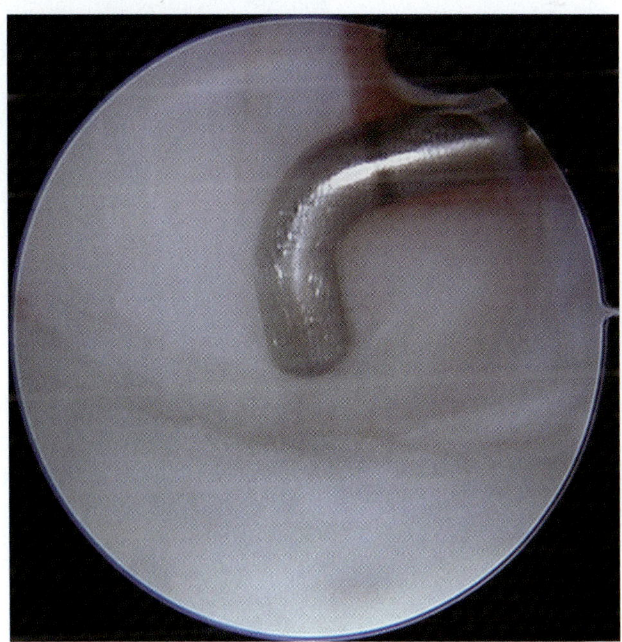

FIGURE 67-4

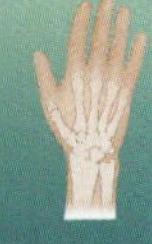

STEP 1 PITFALLS

It is important to débride arthroscopically any synovitis that may cover up a peripheral tear (Fig. 67-5).

It is important that blunt dissection be used to expose the tendon sheath of the ECU to avoid injury to the transarticular branch of the dorsal sensory branch of the ulnar nerve.

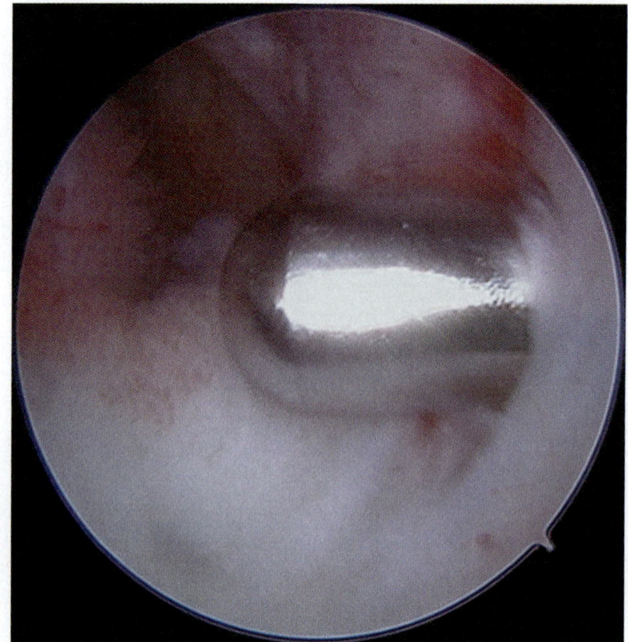

FIGURE 67-5

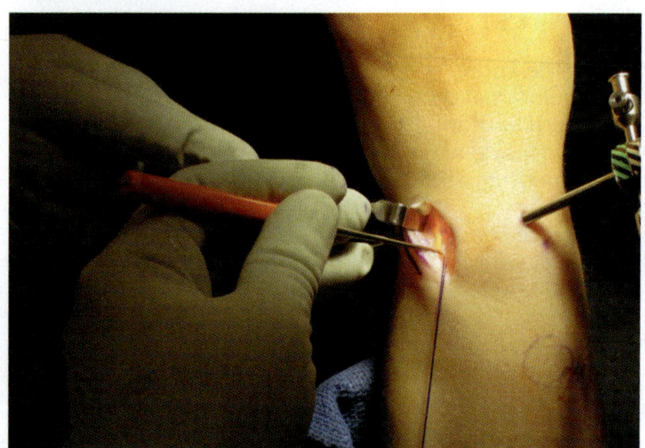

FIGURE 67-6

STEP 2 PEARLS

Sharp dissection is used to open up the tendon sheath of the ECU for repair following the procedure to avoid subluxation to the ECU tendon.

It is important to excise the sheath generously so that the tendon can easily be retracted to gain exposure to the sheath of the ECU.

STEP 2 PITFALLS

The transarticular branch of the dorsal sensory branch of the ulnar nerve should be identified by blunt dissection, when exposing the ECU tendon, to avoid neuroma formation.

Step 2

- The 6R portal is elongated to about 0.5 cm.
- Blunt dissection is used to expose the tendon sheath of the ECU and the transarticular branch of the dorsal sensory branch of the ulnar nerve. This is retracted and carefully protected.
- The tendon sheath is then opened along the radial aspect by blunt dissection. The tendon sheath of the extensor carpi ulnaris (ECU) is retracted ulnarly.
- The floor of the tendon sheath of the ECU is quite thick. This makes very good tissue for repair of the articular disk back to the tendon sheath of the ECU (Fig. 67-6).

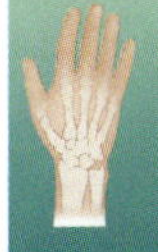

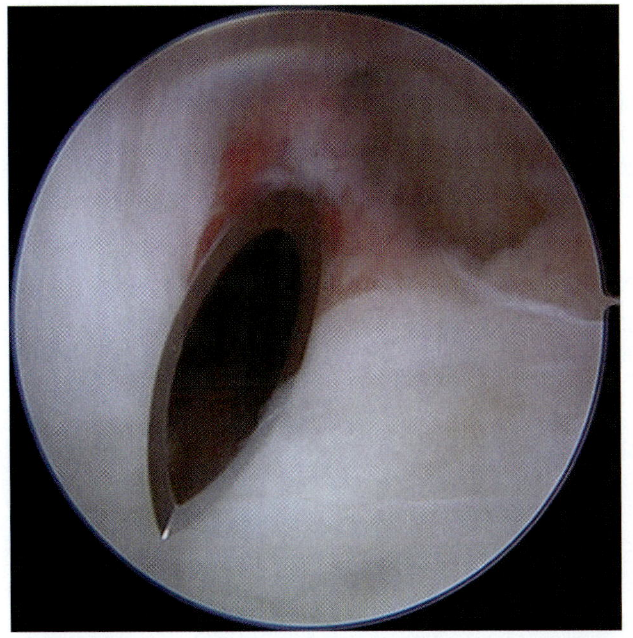

FIGURE 67-7

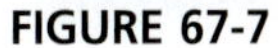

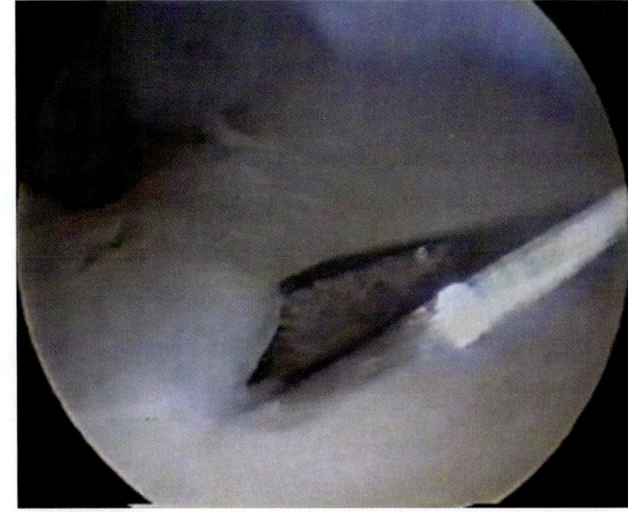

FIGURE 67-8

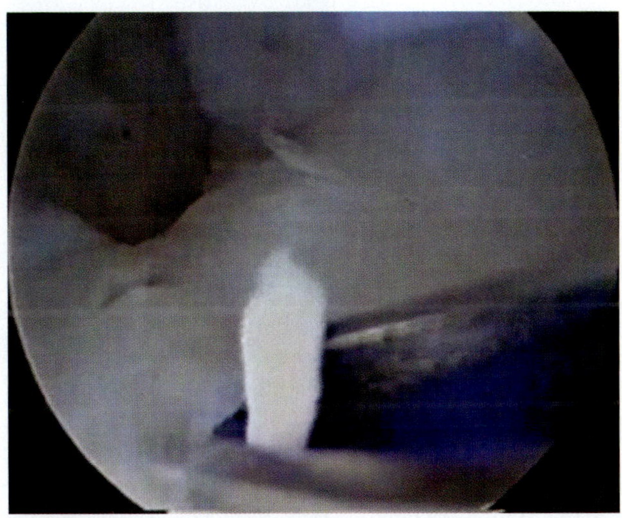

FIGURE 67-9

STEP 3 PEARLS

It may be difficult to insert the 2-0 PDS suture into the needle. It is frequently helpful to cut the plastic end from the needle to identify more easily the metal eyelet to the 18-gauge needle.

This makes the suture easier to thread through the 18-gauge needle into the joint.

STEP 3 PITFALLS

It is important to insert the needle as vertically as possible through the articular disk. The needle is as parallel to the ulna as possible.

In this manner, the needle and eventual suture will get good purchase onto the articular disk of the fibrocartilage complex.

If the needle is inserted too horizontally, it tends to shred through the articular disk with poor purchase, and the suture will pull through as it is tied.

Step 3

- An 18-gauge needle is inserted through the floor of the sheath of the ECU and through the peripheral tear as identified arthroscopically (Fig. 67-7).
- After the needle is identified through the peripheral tear, it is retracted and then inserted through the articular disk (Fig. 67-8).
- A 2-0 PDS suture is inserted through the needle into the joint as viewed arthroscopically (Fig. 67-9).
- Distal to the disk, a suture retriever is inserted into the joint to retrieve the suture.
- The suture then exits the tendon sheath of the ECU.

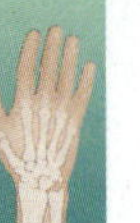

Step 4

- Three vertical simple sutures are placed using this technique (Fig. 67-10).
- Sutures are placed in a dorsal to volar direction. The wrist is then taken out of traction after the sutures are placed.
- With the wrist in supination, the sutures are tied on the floor of the tendon sheath of the ECU.
- The ECU tendon sheath is then closed to prevent subluxation to the tendon of the ECU.

STEP 4 PEARLS

It is difficult to achieve good tension on the suture knot when tying the knot through a small incision.

An arthroscopic-type sliding knot may be used, which makes it easier to tie the knot with good tension and to secure the articular disk back to the floor of the ECU tendon.

If an ulna-shortening osteotomy needs to be performed at the same sitting, the sutures are initially placed, and then the ulna is shortened. After the ulna is shortened, the sutures are tied.

STEP 4 PITFALLS

Dissolvable sutures should be used in this procedure. If permanent sutures are used, the suture knots may cause chronic irritation to the ECU tendon, and they are not recommended.

Step 5: Arthroscopic Knotless Technique

- In the all-arthroscopic knotless techniques, the arthroscope is in the 3-4 portal. A 6R working portal is made, and an accessory 6R portal is made about 1.5 cm distal to the 6R portal (Fig. 67-11).
- The accessory 6R portal is identified by using an 18-gauge needle to palpate the base of the ulna, and the portal is made.
- The synovitis is débrided as described earlier to expose the peripheral tear.

STEP 5 PEARLS

It is important to make the 6R portal in an ideal location for passage of a suture lasso. The accessory 6R portal is distal in line with the standard 6R portal.

The wrist should be slightly flexed in a traction tower. This makes identification of the accessory 6R portal easier for palpating the base of the ulna (Fig. 67-12).

STEP 5 PITFALLS

The tendency is to make the accessory 6R portal too volar.

If this happens, the suture anchor will not achieve good purchase into the ulna, and the articular disk will not be anatomically repaired back to its insertion onto the fovea of the ulna.

The arthroscopic knotless technique allows for anatomic repair of the deep layer of the articular disk back to the bone of the fovea of the ulna. This procedure may be indicated if greater instability of the distal radial ulnar joint is appreciated.

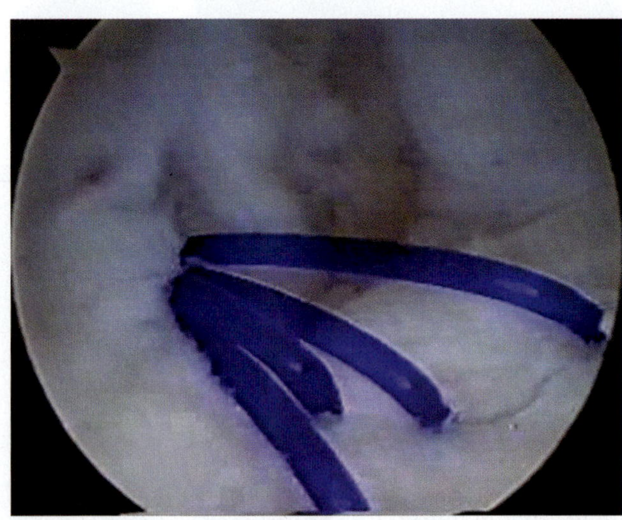

FIGURE 67-10

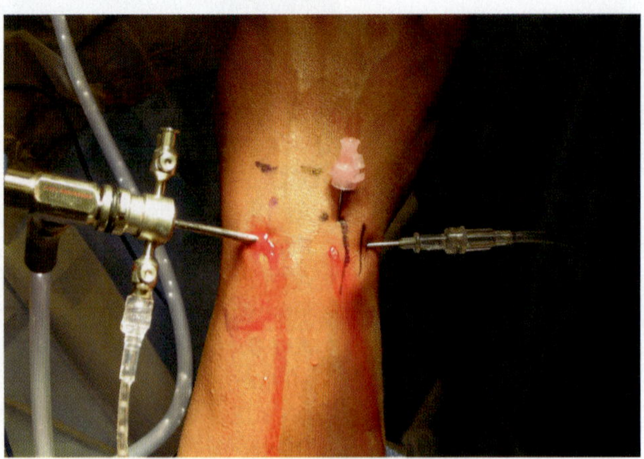

FIGURE 67-11

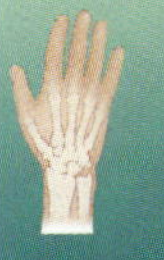

Step 6

- The suture lasso is inserted through the accessory 6R portal and then through the tear into the articular disk (Fig. 67-13).
- A suture retriever is inserted through the lasso, and the suture is pulled with a suture grasper out of the 6R portal (Figs. 67-14 and 67-15).

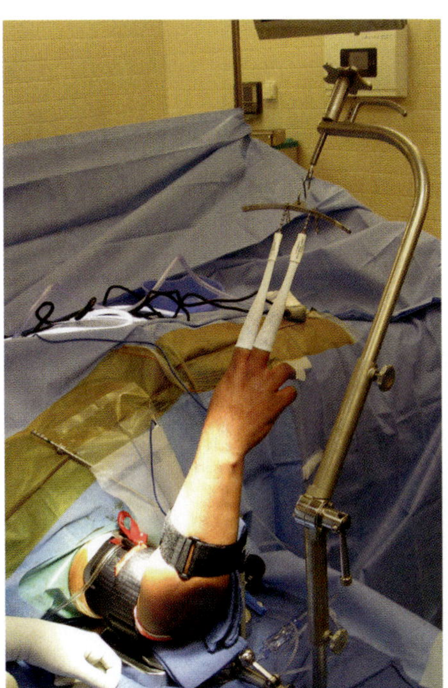

FIGURE 67-12

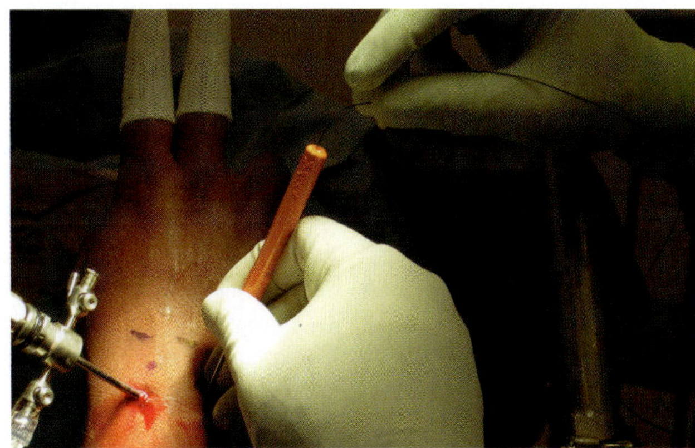

FIGURE 67-13

STEP 6 PEARLS

It is important to have a generous incision for the accessory 6R portal. This allows for easier passage of the suture lasso into the joint.

An alternative to passing a suture retriever through the suture lasso initially to pull the 2-0 fiber wire through the lasso is passing a 2-0 fiber wire stick (which is a stiffer suture) through the bend of the suture lasso.

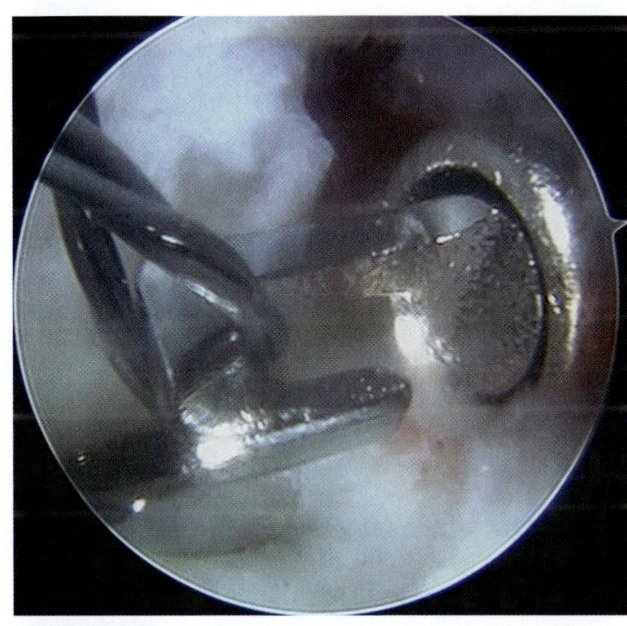

FIGURE 67-14

STEP 6 PITFALLS

It is important when retrieving the suture out of the 6R portal that no soft tissue is caught between the suture limbs.

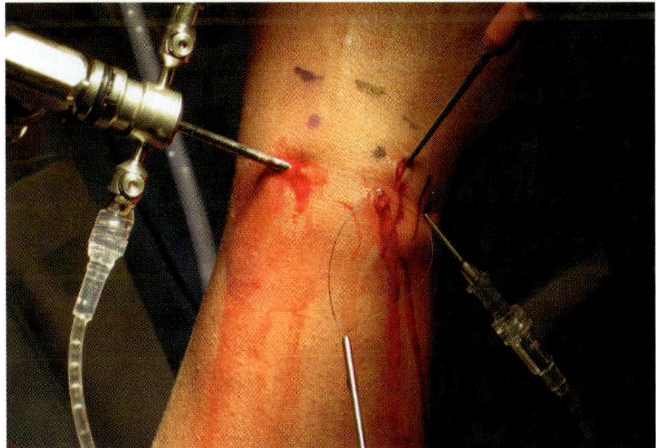

FIGURE 67-15

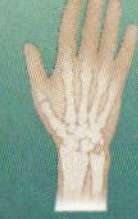

STEP 7 PEARLS

It is important to hold the cannula firmly against the bone of the ulna after the bone has been drilled. This will facilitate finding the hole with the anchor after it has been drilled.

STEP 7 PITFALLS

After the anchor has been placed with a suture, it is important to pull on it with the inserted handle. If the anchor is not fully inserted in the bone, the anchor will easily pull out.

The tendency is to slide off volarly from the ulna. Keeping the cannula in place can help to avoid this.

- A 2-0 fiber wire is then inserted through the suture retriever and pulled through the lasso in a proximal to distal direction, exiting the suture lasso distally (Fig. 67-16).
- The suture lasso is pulled back and reinserted through the articular disk, leaving a loop of suture in the radiocarpal space.
- A suture grasper is then inserted through the 6R portal, and the suture limb is pulled out of the 6R portal. In this manner, both suture limbs exit the 6R portal (Fig. 67-17).

Step 7

- An arthroscopic cannula is introduced into the accessory 6R portal in the radio-carpal space.
- The suture passer is then used to retrieve the suture limbs from the 6R portal out through the cannula in the accessory 6R portal (Fig. 67-18).
- The cannula is held firmly against the fovea of the ulna (Fig. 67-19).
- The ulna is then drilled with a cannulated drill.
- A guidewire is placed down the cannula.

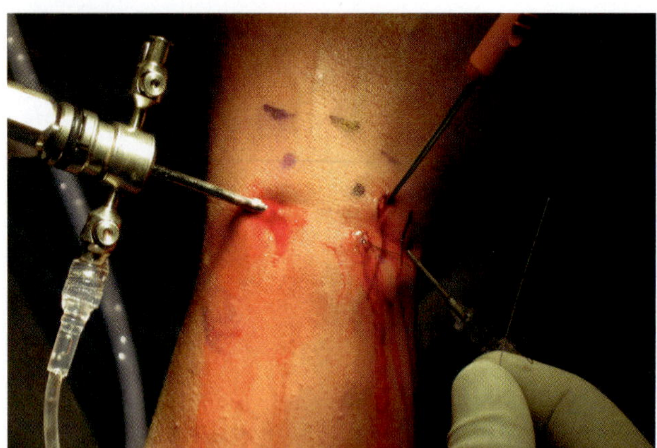

FIGURE 67-16

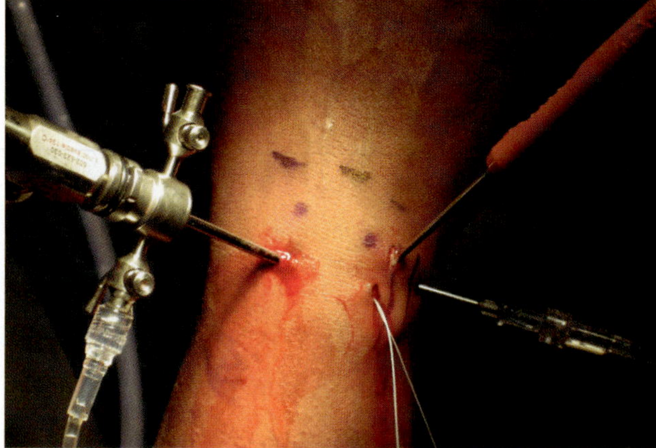

FIGURE 67-17

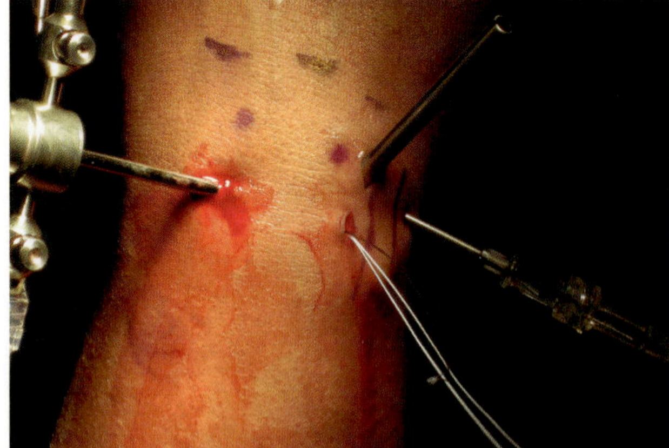

FIGURE 67-18

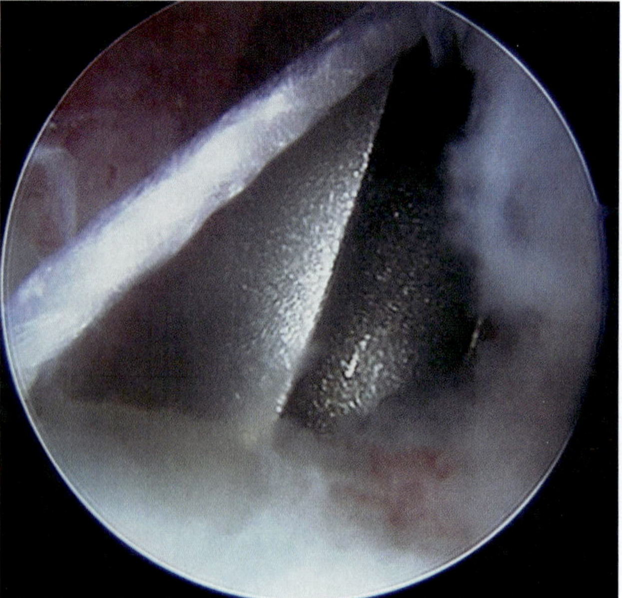

FIGURE 67-19

PEARLS

Patients are immobilized in about 45 degrees of supination, which seems to be most comfortable. Keeping the wrist at full supination for 4 weeks is harder for patients to tolerate.

Digital range-of-motion exercises can be performed while the patient is immobilized in the above-elbow splint.

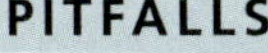

PITFALLS

It is important not to immobilize the patient in an above-elbow splint for more than 4 weeks. After 4 weeks of immobility, the patient starts to develop flexion contracture of the elbow.

- If necessary, a fluoroscopic picture can be used to confirm position of the guidewire in the base of the ulna.
- The ulna is then drilled with a cannulated drill.
- While the cannula is held firmly onto the ulna to avoid losing location of the drill hole, the suture limbs are inserted into the anchor, and the anchor is impacted into the ulna, securing the articular disk back down to bone (Figs. 67-20 through 67-22).
- The sutures limbs are then clipped.

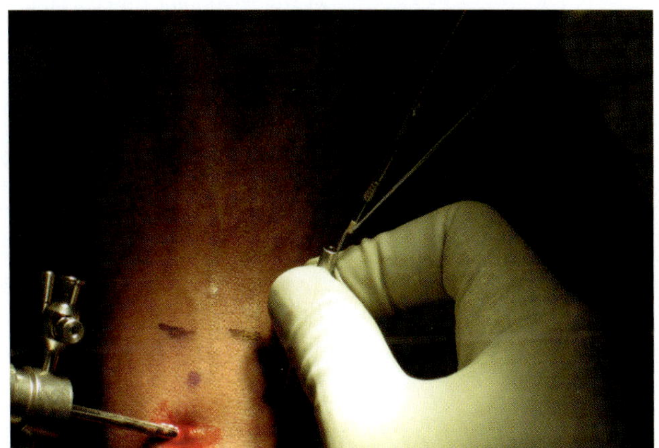

FIGURE 67-20

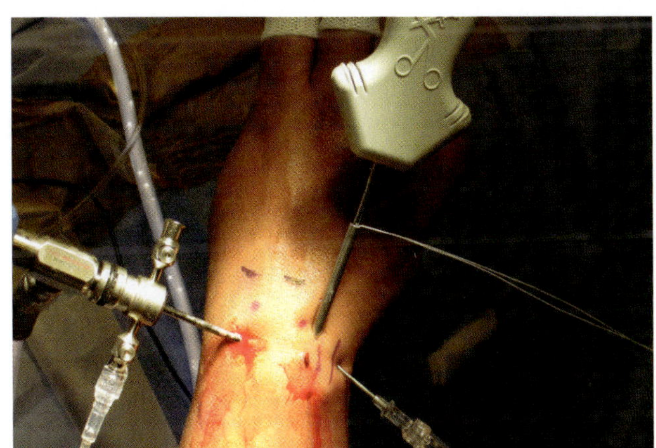

FIGURE 67-21

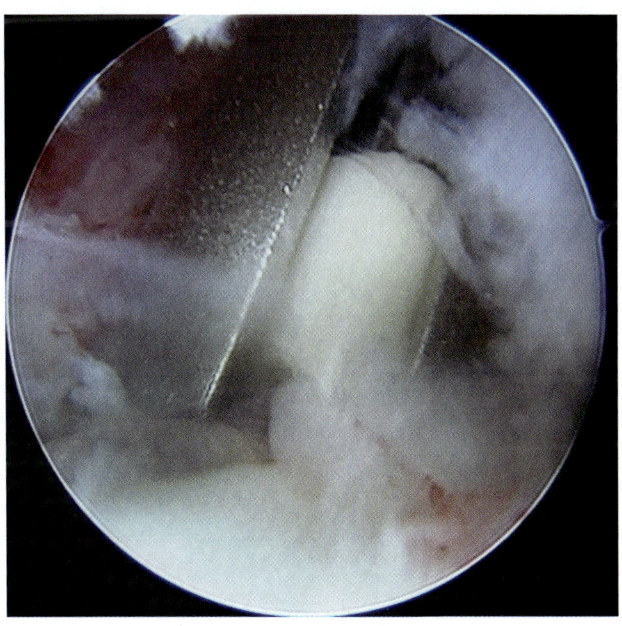

FIGURE 67-22

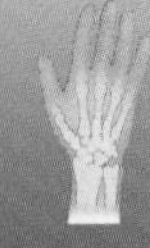

Postoperative Care and Expected Outcomes

- The wrist is placed in a sugar-tong splint in about 45 degrees of supination.
- The wrist is immobilized in an above-elbow splint for 4 weeks.
- After 4 weeks, the patient is then placed in a removable cock-up wrist brace for 3 weeks.
- Physical therapy exercises for range of motion and strengthening are initiated about 7 weeks after surgery.

Evidence

Corso SJ, Savoie FH, Geissler WB, et al. Arthroscopic repair of peripheral avulsion of the triangular fibrocartilage complex of the wrist: a multicenter study. *Arthroscopy.* 1997;13:78-84.

The authors conducted a multicenter study to assess arthroscopic repair of the TFCC. A total of 44 patients (45 wrists) from three institutions were reviewed. Twenty-seven of the 45 wrists had associated injuries, including distal radius fracture (4) and partial or complete rupture of the scapholunate (7), lunotriquetral (9), ulnocarpal (2), or radiocarpal (2) ligaments. There were two fractured ulnar styloids and one scapholunate accelerated collapse (SLAC) wrist deformity. The peripheral tears were repaired using a zone-specific repair kit. The patients were immobilized in a Munster cast, allowing elbow flexion and extension but no pronation or supination for 4 weeks, followed by 2 to 4 weeks in a short-arm cast or VersaWrist splint. All patients were reexamined independently 1 to 3 years postoperatively by a physician, therapist, and registered nurse. The results were graded according to the Mayo modified wrist score. Twenty-nine of the 45 wrists were rated excellent, 12 good, 1 fair, and 3 poor. Overall, results in 42 of the 45 patients (93%) were rated as satisfactory, and these patients returned to sports or work activities. One patient had chronic pain, and two patients had ulnar nerve symptoms, although motion was normal in all, and their grip strength was at least 75% of the opposite hand. The authors concluded that arthroscopic repair of peripheral tears of the TFCC was a satisfactory method of repairing these injuries. (Level IV evidence)

Trumble TE, Gilbert M, Vedder N. Isolated tears of the triangular fibrocartilage: management by early arthroscopic repair. *J Hand Surg [Am].* 1997;22:57-65.

The authors evaluated functional outcomes of arthroscopic repair of TFCC tears treated within 4 months of injury in 24 patients. The patients' average age was 31 years (range, 22 to 38 years); the average follow-up period was 34 months (range, 26 to 48 months). All patients had wrist pain limiting their participation in work before surgery. Patients with central attrition tears identified by arthroscopy were excluded from the study. Twenty-three patients had a preoperative arthrogram. Twelve of the patients with positive arthrogram findings had an avulsion of the TFCC from the sigmoid notch (Palmer type 1D tears). Of the 11 patients with negative arthrograms, 10 had ulnar tears in capsular attachments of the TFCC. The ulna variance averaged 0.2 mm $\pm$ 0.6 mm. Separate arthroscopic techniques were developed for reattaching the TFCC to the radius (9 patients) versus attaching it to the peripheral capsule on the volar or ulnar side of the wrist (8 patients). Postoperatively, there was significant relief of pain ($P < .01$). Postoperative range of motion averaged 89% $\pm$ 9% SD of the contralateral side, and grip strength averaged 85% $\pm$ 20% SD of the contralateral side. Thirteen of the 19 patients returning to work did so in their original jobs. (Level IV evidence)

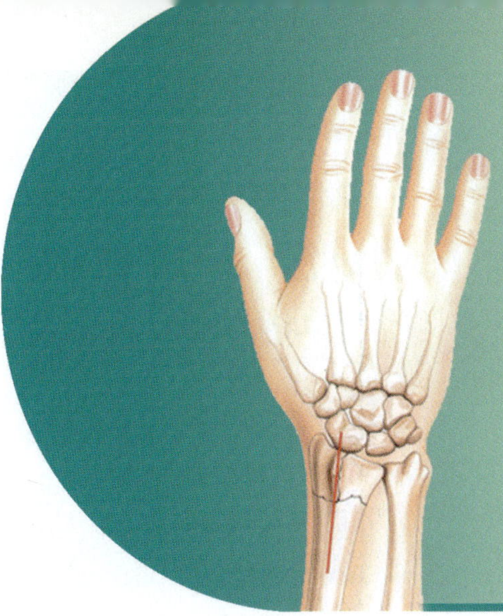

Section XI

CARPAL FRACTURES AND LIGAMENTOUS INSTABILITY

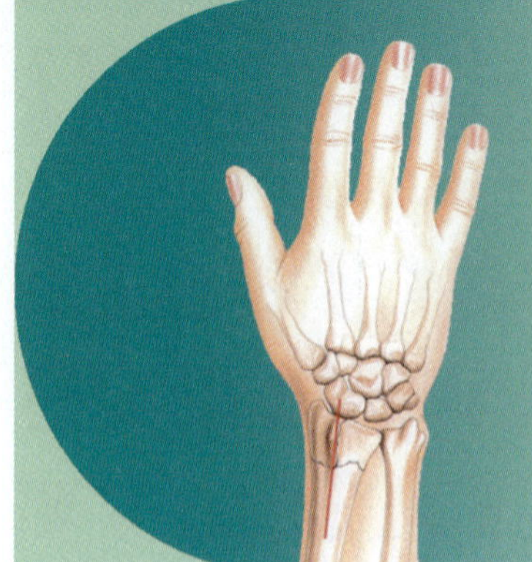

PROCEDURE 68

Percutaneous Screw Fixation of Scaphoid Fractures

Louis W. Catalano III and Christopher M. Jones

See Video 50: Screw Fixation of Scaphoid Fracture

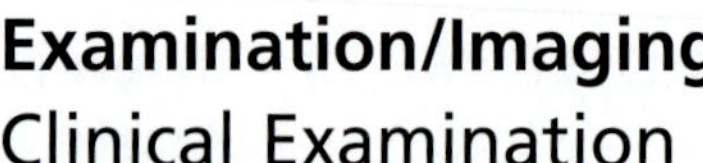

Indications

- Nondisplaced scaphoid fractures
- Displaced scaphoid fractures for which a closed reduction or K-wire-assisted reduction can be performed
- If anatomic reduction of the fracture is not possible by closed means, percutaneous fixation should not be attempted. Instead, open reduction is preferred.

Examination/Imaging

Clinical Examination

- Fractures of scaphoid are frequently missed in the emergency room or dismissed by the patient as a wrist sprain. Thus, the physician must have a high suspicion in young and middle-aged patients who present with wrist pain after a fall on an outstretched hand.
- General dorsoradial edema and focal snuffbox tenderness are highly suggestive of an acute scaphoid fracture (Fig. 68-1).
- The distal pole of scaphoid may be tender to palpation (Fig. 68-2).
- Axial compression of thumb may also produce pain.

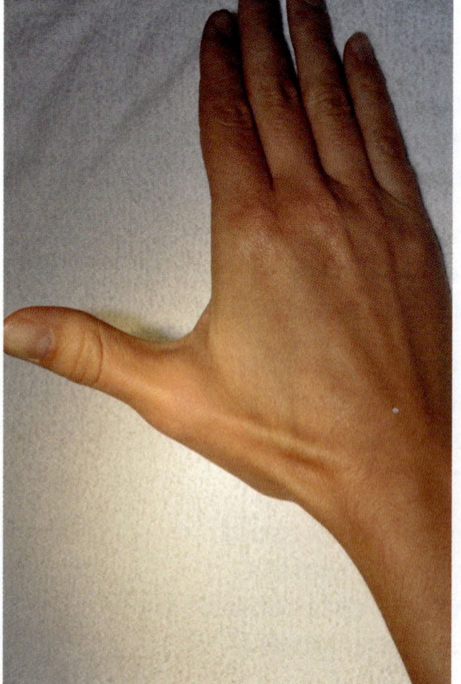

FIGURE 68-1

Imaging

- The initial posteroanterior (PA) and lateral radiographs may fail to demonstrate a scaphoid fracture (Fig. 68-3). The incidence of false-negative radiographs for acute fractures has been shown to be up to 25%.
- Additional helpful radiographic views include (1) clenched-fist PA, which can exaggerate a fracture deformity and help make a diagnosis; (2) ulnar-deviated PA that positions the scaphoid in extension showing the waist more clearly (Fig. 68-4); and (3) pronated oblique view.
- Magnetic resonance imaging (MRI) is highly sensitive for making the diagnosis—cortical disruption with bone marrow edema is diagnostic. For chronic injuries, MRI is valuable in assessing proximal pole vascularity (Fig. 68-5).
- Although radiographs are usually sufficient for preoperative planning, computed tomography (CT) can be helpful in further delineating the fracture pattern.

Surgical Anatomy

- The scaphoid is the largest bone in the proximal carpal row, and its axis lies about 45 degrees to the longitudinal axis of the wrist.
- Eighty percent of the scaphoid surface is covered by articular cartilage, leaving limited space for vascular supply.

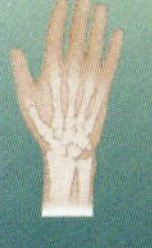

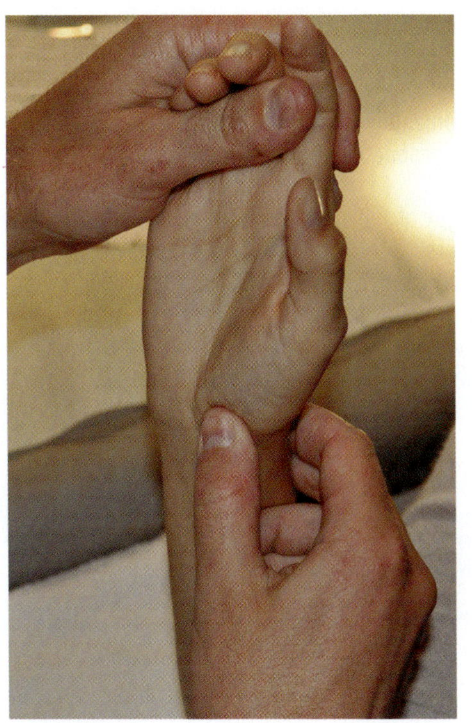

FIGURE 68-2

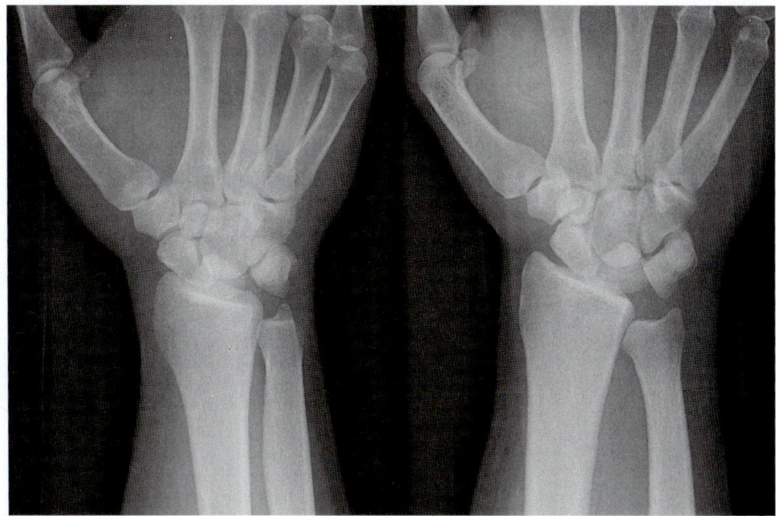

FIGURE 68-3

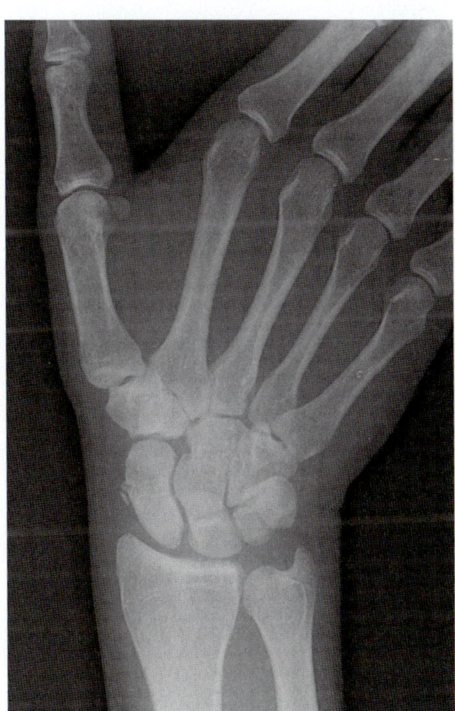

FIGURE 68-4

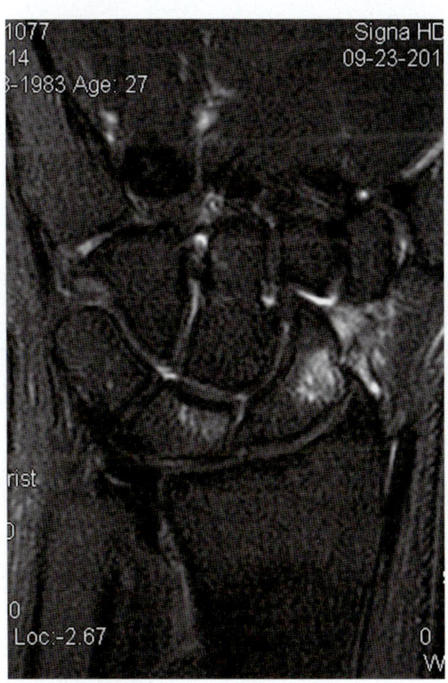

FIGURE 68-5

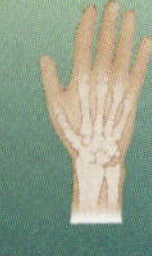

- The scaphoid articulates with the trapezoid, trapezium, capitate, lunate, and radius and serves as a mechanical link between the proximal and distal carpal rows.
- Multiple intrinsic and extrinsic ligaments attach to the scaphoid (Fig. 68-6). The most important is the radioscaphocapitate, which provides an axis on which the scaphoid flexes.
- A dorsal groove courses the length of the scaphoid and provides attachment points for ligaments and blood vessels.
- A dorsal branch of the radial artery provides 70% to 80% of the blood supply (Fig. 68-7).
- A second nutrient artery enters volarly and supplies only the distal pole.
- There is no nutrient artery to the proximal pole; thus, it is susceptible to avascular necrosis when fractured.

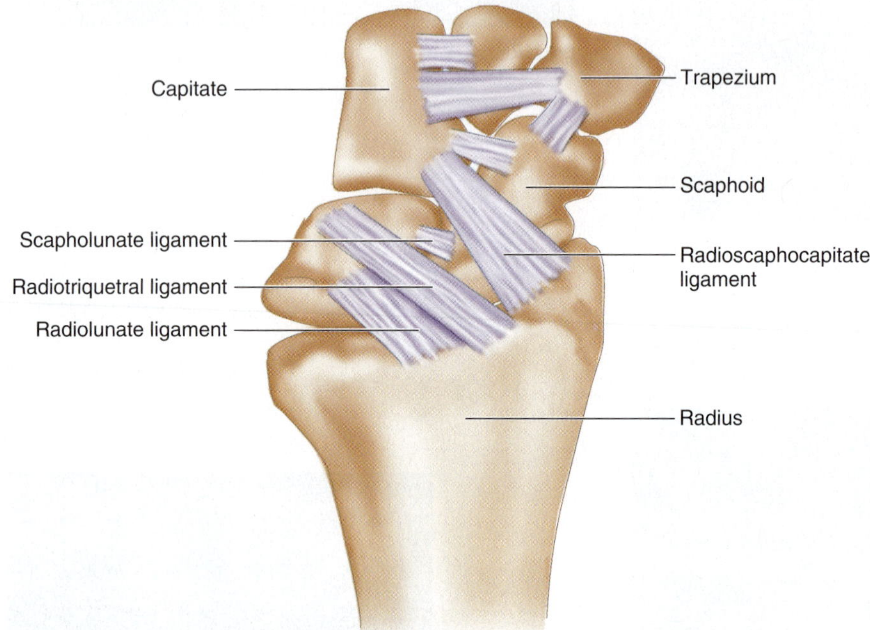

FIGURE 68-6

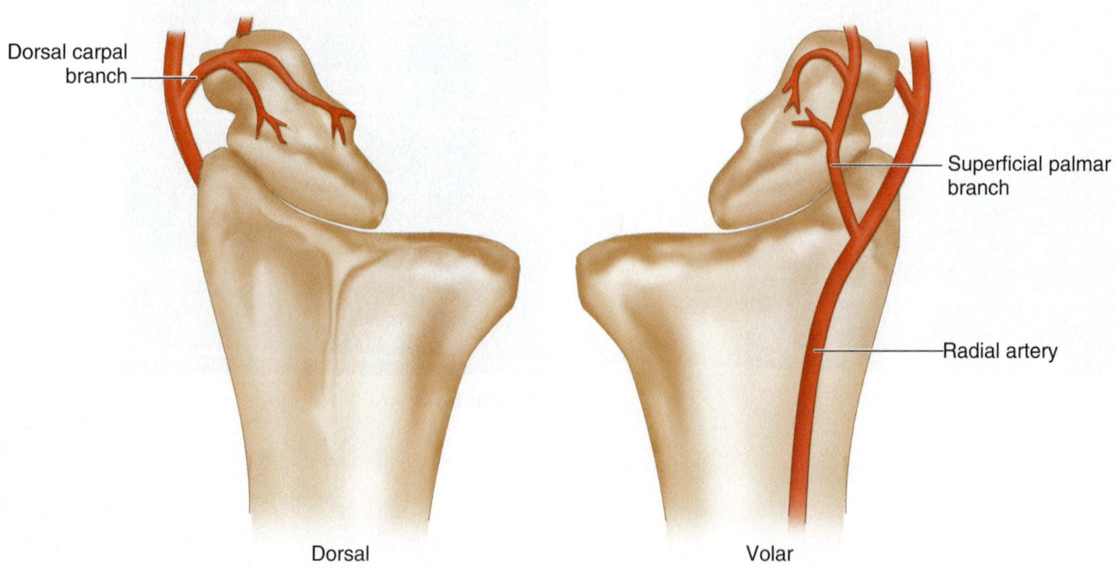

FIGURE 68-7

POSITIONING EQUIPMENT

- A towel roll can be used to position the wrist in extension for a volar approach or in flexion for a dorsal approach.

Positioning

- The patient is positioned supine on the operating room table with the arm abducted on a radiolucent hand table.
- A minifluoroscope is positioned vertically at the end of the hand table with the image intensifier under the table.

Exposures

- Either a volar or dorsal approach can be used. We find the dorsal approach easier for most fractures because the starting point is easier to find. For the volar approach, the guidewire also usually has to pass through the trapezium or around the trapezium, making screw placement difficult.
- For extreme proximal pole fractures, a dorsal approach is preferred because it is easier to optimize the screw position in the smaller fragment for maximal thread purchase.

Procedure

Step 1: Dorsal Approach—Finding the Starting Point

- The wrist is flexed 60 degrees over a rolled towel bump.
- To find the starting point, the guidewire is introduced through the skin about 1 cm distal to the Lister tubercle and advanced to just over the lip of the dorsal distal radius (Fig. 68-8).
- The starting position at the proximal ulnar edge of the scaphoid is found fluoroscopically (Fig. 68-9).
- A lateral fluoroscopic view should show the tip of the guidewire aligned down the central axis of the scaphoid.

STEP 1 PEARLS

Use the minifluoroscope and a K-wire to determine the alignment of the scaphoid axis on PA and lateral views. Draw out the anticipated trajectory of the screw on the skin with a marking pen as a guide for the wire placement.

It is sometimes helpful to first use a 22-gauge needle to find the appropriate starting point and trajectory.

STEP 1 PITFALLS

If the wrist is not flexed enough, the starting point will be too dorsal on the proximal pole.

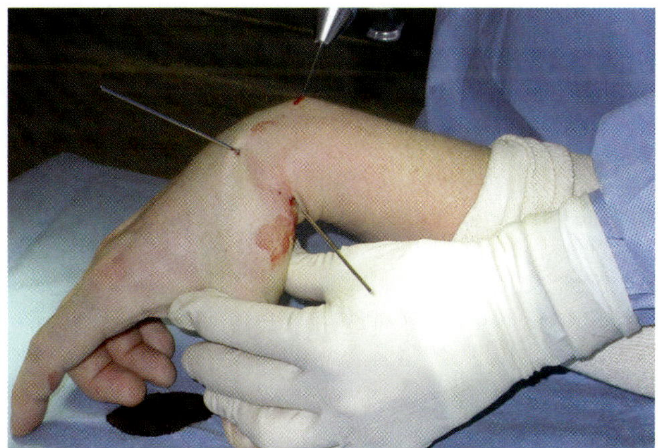

FIGURE 68-8

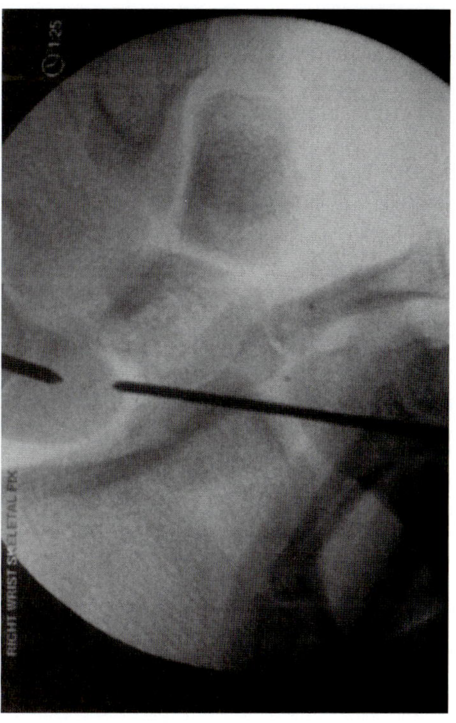

FIGURE 68-9

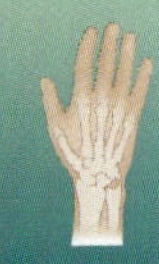

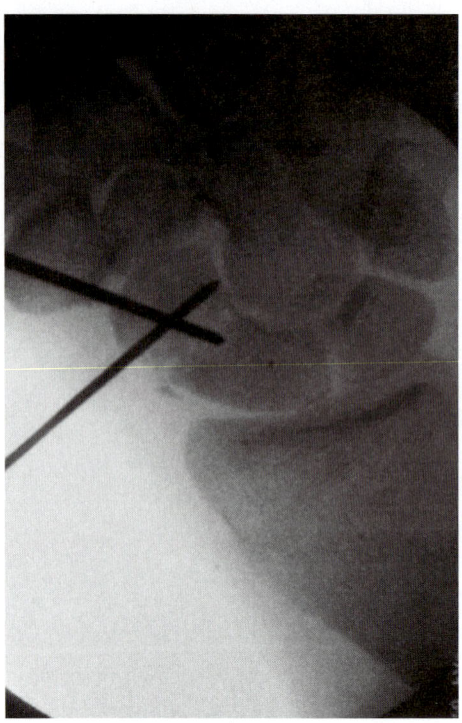

FIGURE 68-10

STEP 2 PEARLS

For scaphoid waist fractures, the distal fragment typically needs to be both extended and rotated on its axis for an anatomic reduction.

STEP 2 PITFALLS

Scrutinize the fluoroscopic images to ensure that the fracture is reduced on multiple views. Slight incongruity on one view might represent marked displacement on another view.

Be wary of the radial artery when placing the percutaneous reduction wires because the radial artery passes through the snuffbox.

STEP 3 PEARLS

Imperfect guidewires can be left in place and used as a reference for placement of a new wire.

Too many attempts at passing the wire will create multiple pathways through the bone, making it challenging to develop the right path. So get your first shot right!

STEP 3 PITFALLS

Resist temptation to extend the wrist with the guidewire in place. This will bend the wire and make it impossible to ream over it. Even worse, the wire could break, requiring a difficult open extrication.

Step 2: Reducing the Fracture (if Necessary)

- If the fracture is displaced, 0.062-inch K-wires can be inserted dorsally into each fragment and used as joysticks to facilitate the reduction.
- Alternatively, the two K-wires can be inserted in the distal fragment—one dorsally and one radially—to reduce the fracture (Fig. 68-10).

Step 3: Placing the Guidewire

- With the fracture reduced, carefully advance the guidewire through the scaphoid and evaluate its placement with the minifluoroscope. To obtain a true PA view, flex the elbow until the hand is parallel to the table. Keep the wrist flexed to avoid bending the wire.
- Alternatively, the wire can be fully advanced out of the thenar eminence so that the proximal tip just clears the radioscaphoid joint. It is now possible to freely flex and extend the wrist without bending the guidewire.
- If you plan on placing just one screw, the goal is to have the wire perfectly centered down the axis of the scaphoid on both views (Figs. 68-11 and 68-12).
- With the guidewire tip just in subchondral bone, measure the interosseous length by placing another guidewire of equal length parallel to it at the entry point (either distal or proximal) and measuring the difference (Fig. 68-13). The headless screw should be 3 to 5 mm shorter than this measured length to ensure that all of the threads are buried.
- Before reaming, advance the wire so that it is partially through the skin volarly. This will prevent it from loosening when reaming over the wire. Additionally, if the wire were to break when drilling, it could then be removed easily.

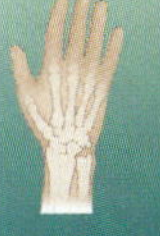

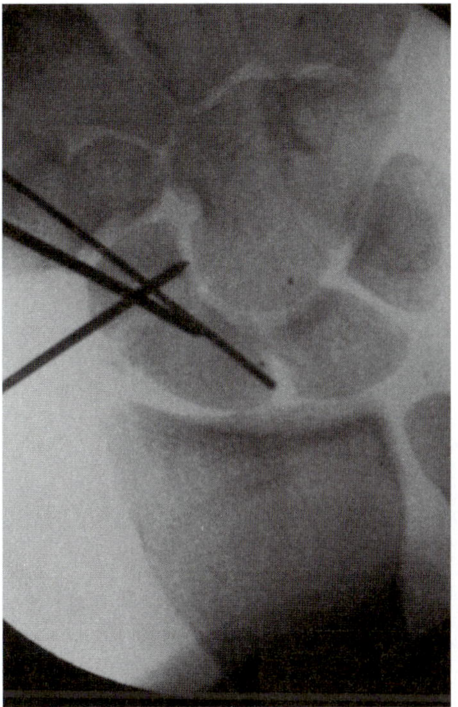

FIGURE 68-11

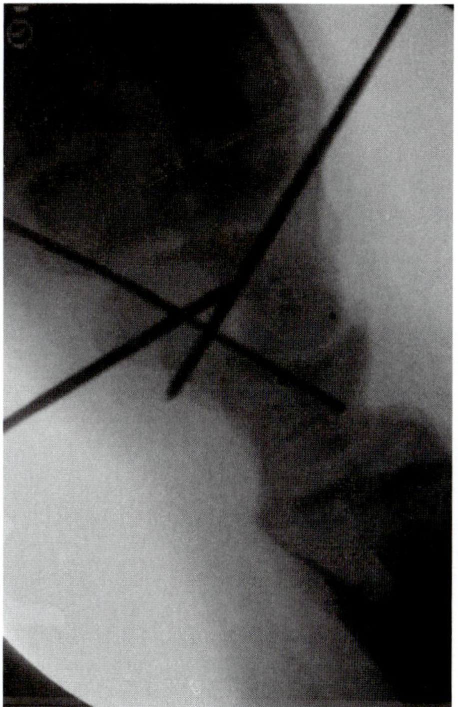

FIGURE 68-12

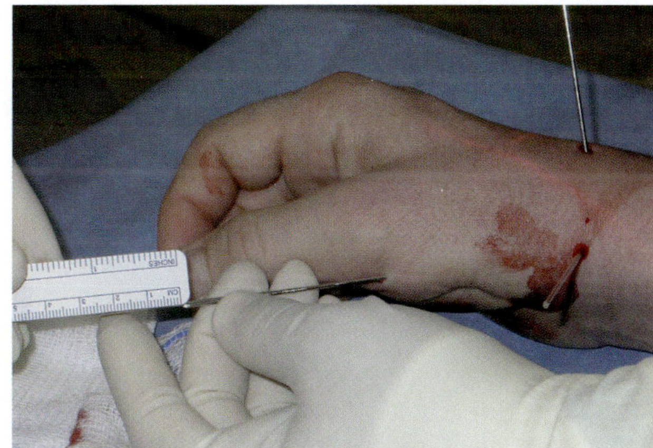

FIGURE 68-13

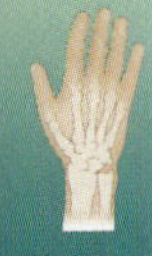

STEP 4 PEARLS

Maintain reduction with the K-wire joysticks when reaming, placing the screw into the distal fragment. This is particularly important in young patients with dense bone.

STEP 4 PITFALLS

If you do not ream exactly collinear with the guidewire, you risk shearing the wire. Headless screws with guidewires less than 0.045 inches in diameter are particularly susceptible.

Step 4: Reaming

- Before reaming, an antirotation wire should be placed parallel and 3 to 4 mm away from the first. This wire serves both to maintain reduction once the guidewire has been overdrilled and to oppose the rotational forces exerted when twisting in the headless screw.
- A 5-mm incision is made at the wire entry site, and blunt dissection is performed down to the capsule to ensure that the extensor tendons are not pierced by the wire (Fig. 68-14).
- By means of a power or hand reamer, carefully ream over the guidewire up to the subchondral bone of the distal fragment (Fig. 68-15).

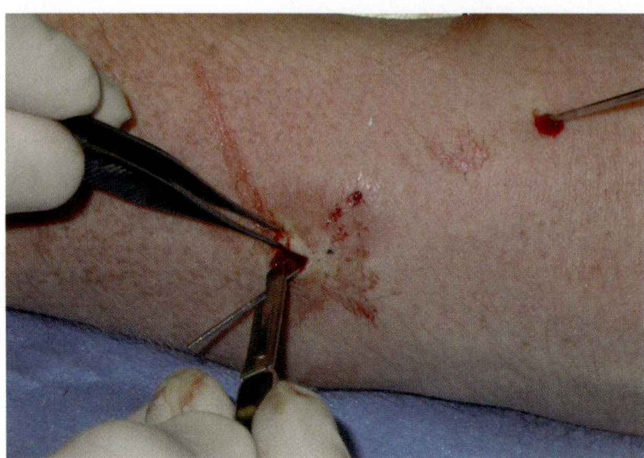

FIGURE 68-14

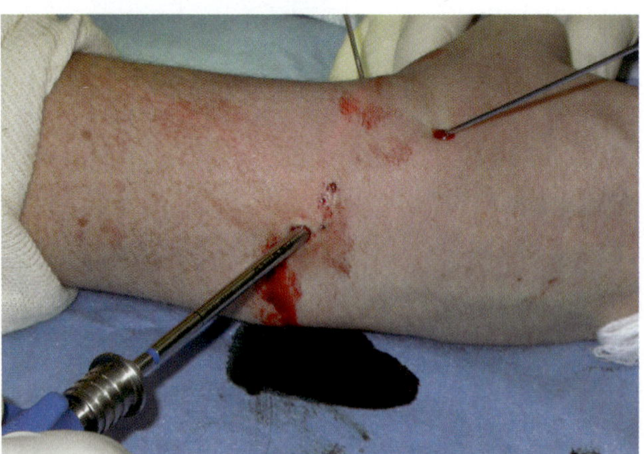

FIGURE 68-15

STEP 5 PEARLS

We prefer a "mini" headless screw (e.g., Acutrak Mini) over a standard-sized screw because it is more appropriately sized to the dimension of the scaphoid in most patients. Standard-sized screws fill nearly the entire medullary canal and could theoretically inhibit bony fusion.

For more comminuted fractures, it might be advantageous to place two smaller headless screws side by side.

STEP 5 PITFALLS

If the fracture is not well stabilized or the reamer hole is not aligned as the screw is driven across the fracture site, it can actually distract the fracture.

Step 5: Screw Insertion

- Insert a headless screw under fluoroscopic guidance until it is just short of the distal cortex (Fig. 68-16).
- Remove the guidewires. Verify fluoroscopically that the fracture is well reduced and that the screw is fully contained in the bone (Fig. 68-17).

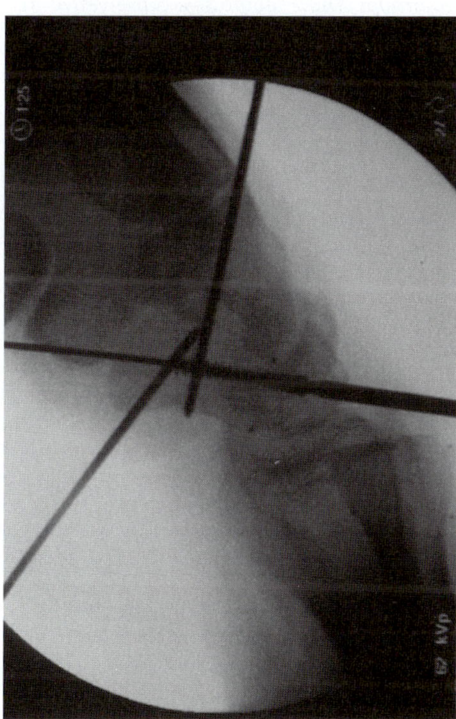

FIGURE 68-16

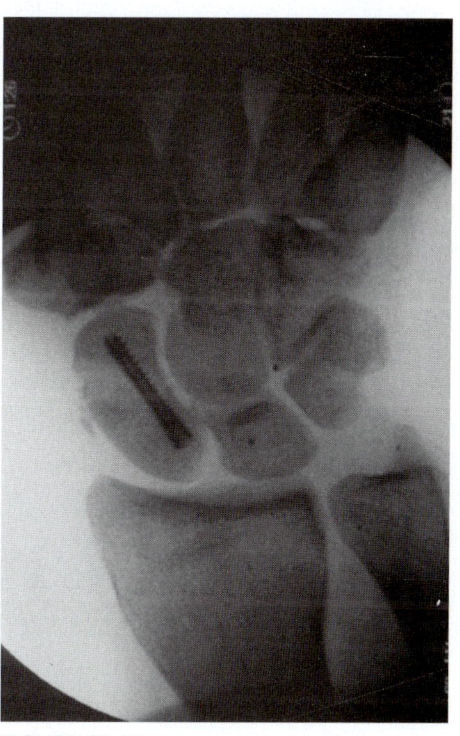

FIGURE 68-17

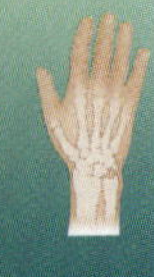

PEARLS

Proximal pole fractures generally should be immobilized longer because healing occurs more slowly.

It is difficult to assess fracture healing on plain radiographs. CT is the best tool to confirm bridging bony union.

PITFALLS

Patients should be cautioned that it could take up to 3 months for the fracture to unite and that they need to protect the wrist until that time.

Postoperative Care and Expected Outcomes

- A postoperative volar and dorsal thumb spica splint is removed at the 2-week postoperative visit. This is replaced with a removable Orthoplast thumb spica splint, constructed by the occupational therapist, which is worn at all times until healing is confirmed radiographically.

Evidence

Bond CD, Shin AY, McBride MT, Dao KD. Percutaneous screw fixation or cast immobilization for nondisplaced scaphoid fractures. *J Bone Joint Surg [Am].* 2001;83:483-488.

Twenty-five full-time military personnel with an acute nondisplaced fracture of the scaphoid were randomized to either cast immobilization or fixation with a percutaneous cannulated Acutrak screw (Acumed, Beaverton, Ore). Screw fixation resulted in faster radiographic union (7 vs. 12 weeks) and return to military duty (8 vs. 15 weeks) compared with cast immobilization. There was no significant difference in the range of motion of the wrist or in grip strength at the 2-year follow-up evaluation. Overall patient satisfaction was high in both groups. (Level III evidence)

Dias JJ, Wildin CJ, Bhowal B, Thompson JR. Should acute scaphoid fractures be fixed? A randomized controlled trial. *J Bone Joint Surg [Am].* 2005;87: 2160-2168.

This randomized prospective trial evaluated cast treatment versus internal fixation with a headless screw for nondisplaced and minimally displaced scaphoid waist fractures. Ten of the 44 fractures treated nonoperatively had not healed radiographically at 12 weeks, and, as a consequence, their management was altered. (Seven had screw fixation.) Complications occurred in 13 patients who had been managed operatively, but all were minor, and 10 were related to the scar. At 26 weeks, there was no difference in any functional outcome measured between the two groups. Thus, "aggressive conservative treatment" is recommended whereby fracture healing is assessed with plain radiographs or CT scans after 6 to 8 weeks of cast immobilization. Surgical fixation with or without bone grafting is advised if a gap is identified at the fracture site. (Level III evidence)

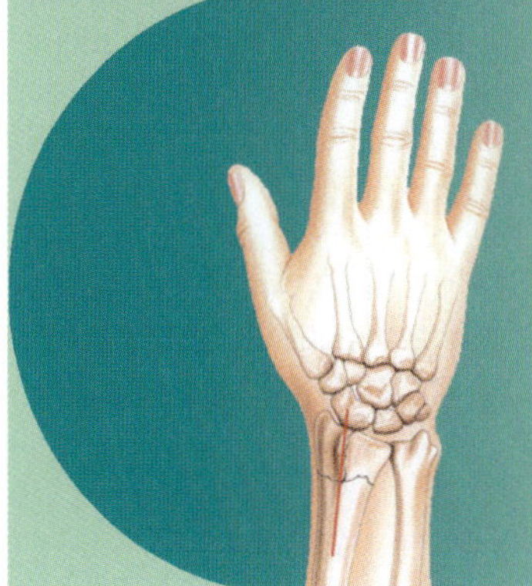

PROCEDURE 69

Vascularized Bone Grafting for Scaphoid Nonunion

Louis W. Catalano III and Christopher M. Jones

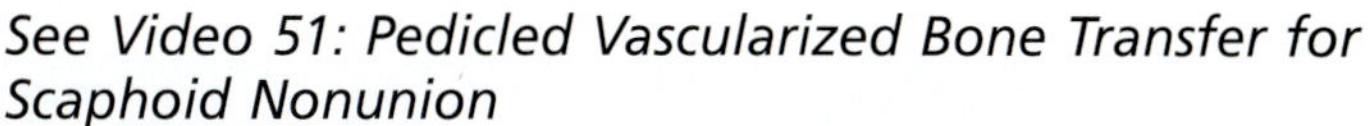

See Video 51: Pedicled Vascularized Bone Transfer for Scaphoid Nonunion

Indications

- Scaphoid fracture nonunions are seen that have developed avascular necrosis (AVN).
- Vascularized bone grafting is contraindicated in fracture nonunions associated with significant degenerative changes in the radioscaphoid or midcarpal joint. These wrists require a salvage procedure.
- A scaphoid nonunion humpback deformity cannot be corrected unless a structural graft is used.

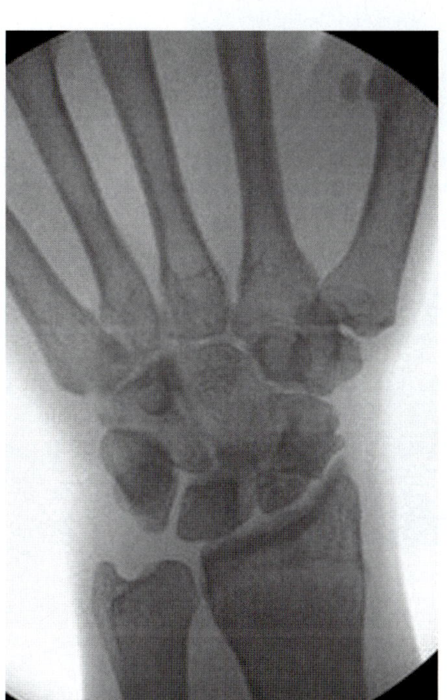

FIGURE 69-1

Examination/Imaging

Clinical Examination

- General dorsoradial edema and focal snuffbox tenderness are highly suggestive of a scaphoid fracture.
- The distal pole of the scaphoid may also be tender to palpation, and axial compression of the thumb may reproduce the pain.
- Decreased wrist motion and grip strength are common findings in patients with a scaphoid nonunion.

Imaging

- Wrist radiographs including scaphoid views should be obtained to evaluate the overall fracture pattern, carpal alignment, and degree of radiocarpal and midcarpal arthritis. Chronic scaphoid nonunions display a characteristic pattern of wrist arthritis and carpal instability—scaphoid nonunion advanced collapse (SNAC), as described by Watson and Ballet. The hallmark of AVN on radiographs is increased bone density, fragmentation, and collapse (Fig. 69-1).

- A thin-cut computed tomography (CT) scan with reconstructions carefully aligned in the axis of the scaphoid is helpful to elucidate scaphoid angular deformity (as measured by intrascaphoid angles), translation, comminution, and degenerative changes. This study best quantifies the deformity and necessary reconstruction.
- Magnetic resonance imaging (MRI) is the only noninvasive study able to assess vascularity of the scaphoid and identify AVN (Fig. 69-2). An MRI should be obtained in every patient for whom there is a concern about the viability of the proximal pole. Contrast-enhanced imaging has a sensitivity of 66%, a specificity of 88%, and an accuracy of 83%.

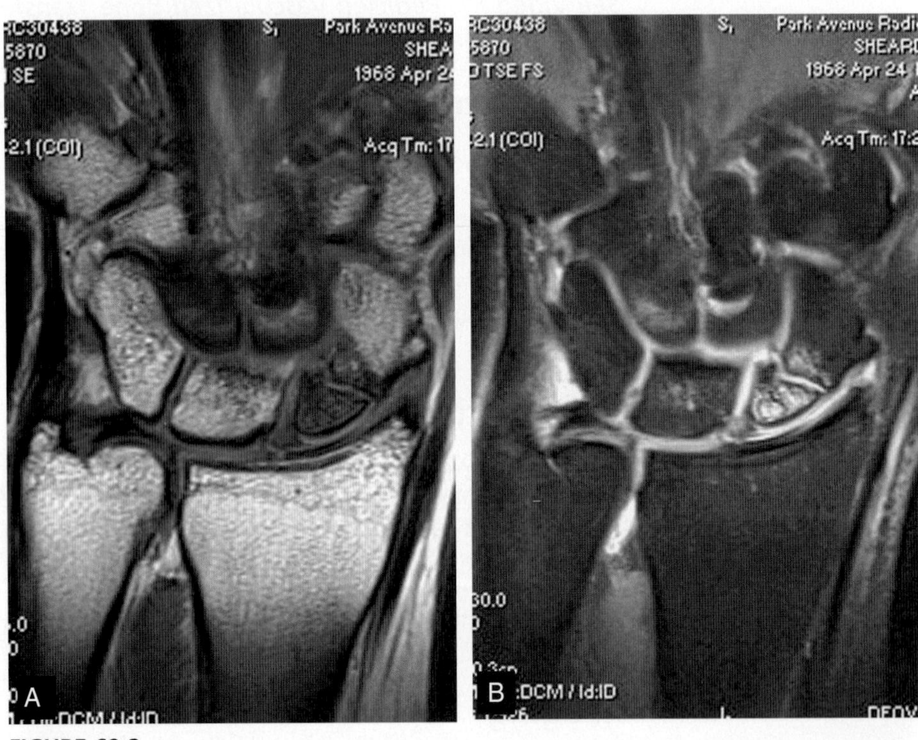

FIGURE 69-2

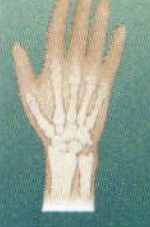

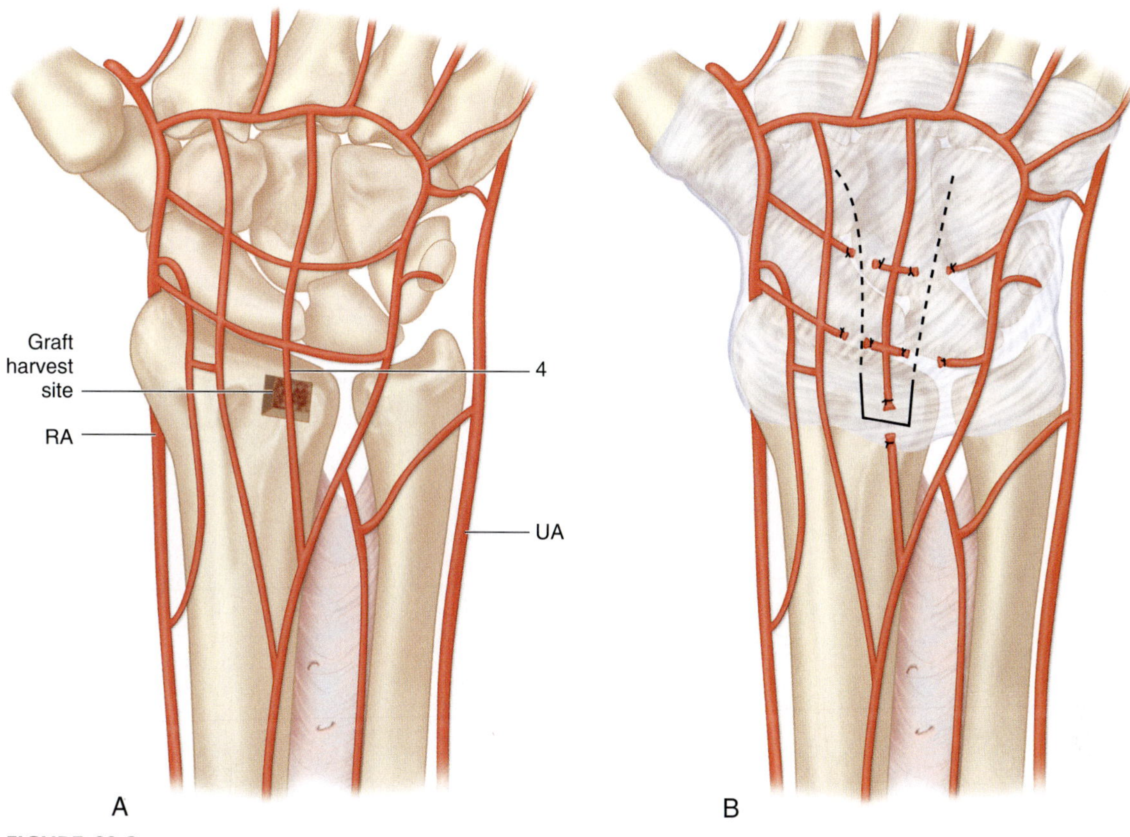

FIGURE 69-3

Surgical Anatomy

- Eighty percent of the scaphoid surface is covered by articular cartilage, leaving limited space for vascular supply.
- A dorsal branch of the radial artery provides 70% to 80% of the blood supply.
- A second nutrient artery enters volarly and supplies only the distal pole.
- There is no nutrient artery to the proximal pole; thus, it is susceptible to AVN when fractured.
- Dorsal distal-radius vascularized bone grafts have been shown to be based on consistent vascular anatomy (Fig. 69-3A).
- The pedicled graft described in this chapter is based on the artery of the fourth extensor compartment. The fourth extensor compartment artery is less than 1 mm in diameter and between 1 and 2 cm in length (see Fig. 69-3A and B).
- Rotation of the graft on the capsular pedicle of only 10 to 30 degrees allows placement of the graft on the proximal scaphoid.

Positioning

- The patient is positioned supine on the operating room table with the arm abducted on a radiolucent hand table.
- A minifluoroscope is positioned vertically at the end of the hand table with the image intensifier under the table.

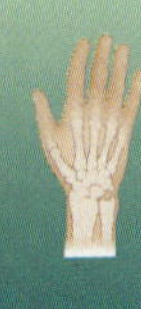

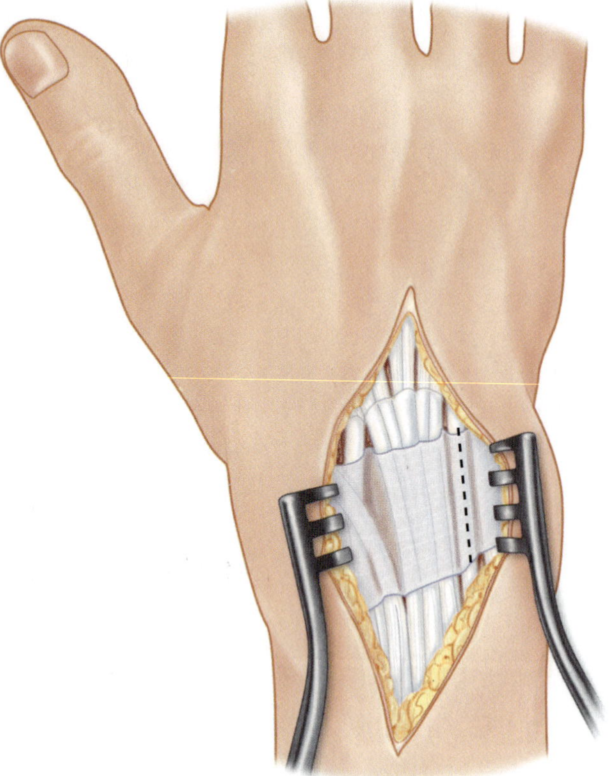

FIGURE 69-4

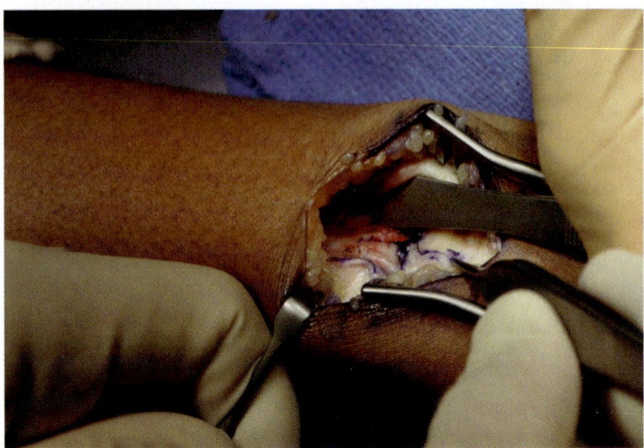

FIGURE 69-5

PITFALLS

Be mindful to not elevate any portion of the capsule off the distal radius when dissecting the extensor retinaculum off the capsule for exposure.

Exposures

- Multiple vascularized grafts have been described. One of the more popular grafts is that based on the 1,2 intercompartmental supraretinacular artery (1,2 ICSRA) as described by Zaidemberg. We prefer to use a dorsal capsular distal-radius graft as described by Sotereanos and coworkers because it does not involve dissection of tiny vessels, is less technically demanding, and is more durable during flap rotation.
- A 4-cm dorsal incision is made centered over the radiocarpal joint, ulnar to the Lister tubercle (Fig. 69-4).
- The extensor retinaculum over the third and fourth dorsal compartments is released. The extensor pollicis longus (EPL) tendon is retracted radially and the extensor digitorum communis (EDC) tendons ulnarly, exposing the dorsal wrist capsule (Fig. 69-5).
- Carefully elevate the extensor sheaths off the capsule at the medial and lateral borders to increase exposure of the graft.

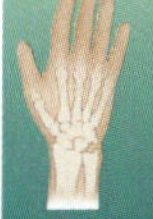

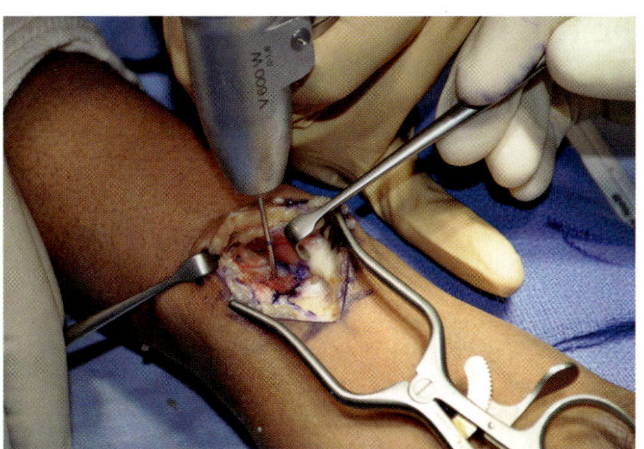

FIGURE 69-6

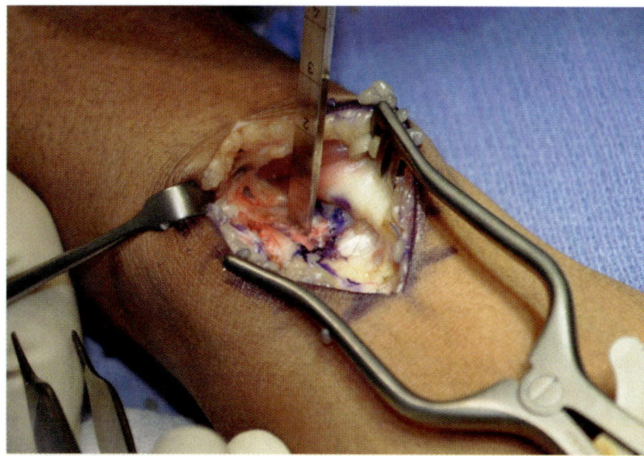

FIGURE 69-7

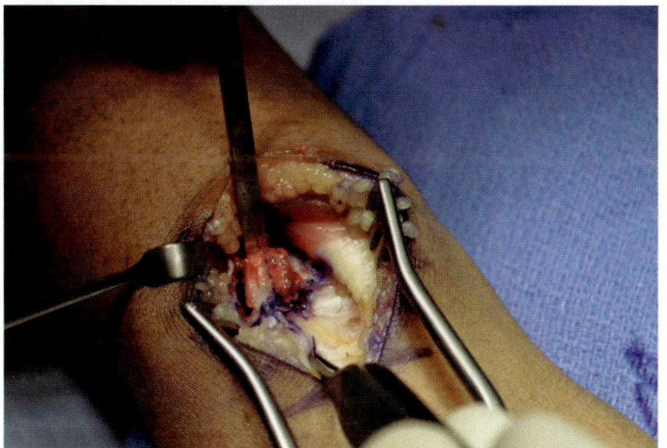

FIGURE 69-8

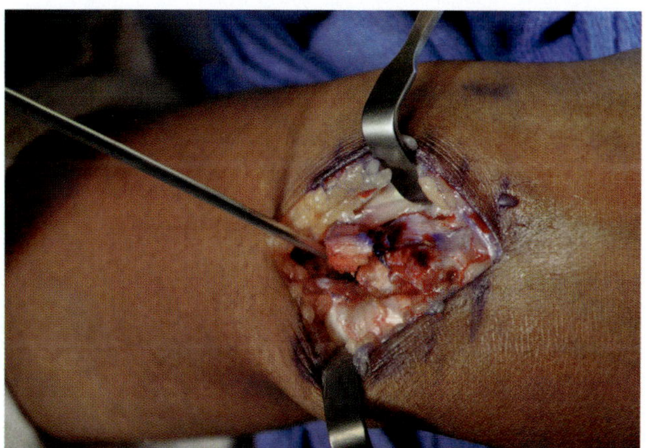

FIGURE 69-9

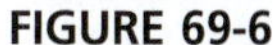

STEP 1 PEARLS

There is a longitudinal ridge of bone a few millimeters ulnar to the Lister tubercle where the capsular attachment is thickest and likely contains the fourth extensor compartment artery. Center the bone block over this ridge to maximize blood supply to the graft.

STEP 2 PEARLS

To ensure the integrity of the pedicle, release the portion of the capsule attached to the distal edge of the radius subperiosteally, going from proximal to distal.

Procedure

Step 1: Cutting the Graft

- A capsular-based pedicle about 1.5 cm wide is outlined on the dorsal surface of the wrist capsule, narrowing down to a 1 × 1 cm distal-radius bone block (see Fig. 69-3B).
- The bone block is situated at the dorsal ridge of the distal radius, just ulnar to the Lister tubercle, and should be about 7 mm in depth.
- The outline of the graft is "postage-stamped" using a 0.045-inch K-wire or similarly sized drill bit (Fig. 69-6).

Step 2: Elevate the Graft and Pedicle

- The proximal, medial, and lateral edge osteotomies are completed with a straight osteotome (Fig. 69-7).
- The graft is then carefully elevated with a curved osteotome, leaving 2 to 3 mm of distal radius cortex intact (Fig. 69-8).
- Full-thickness dorsal capsular incisions are made, and the capsular flap is dissected away from the underlying tissues. The capsular attachment to the portion of the distal radius cortex left intact is carefully released with a scalpel. Be particularly mindful not to disturb the capsular attachment to the bone graft (Fig. 69-9).

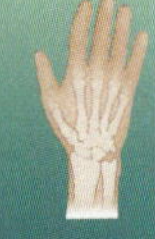

STEP 2 PITFALLS

If you do not leave a 2- to 3-mm distal edge of radial cortex intact, a fracture can propagate into the radiocarpal joint on elevation of the bone block.

The dorsal scapholunate ligament is just deep to the capsular flap and can be injured with an overzealous capsular incision.

Step 3: Scaphoid Preparation and Fixation

- After the flap has been elevated, the proximal half of scaphoid is visible.
- Identify the nonunion site and débride it of nonviable tissue with small curets and rongeurs, preserving bone stock and intact cartilage.
- If there is pseudoarthrosis with a cartilage shell primarily intact, it is not débrided but rather is left intact.
- The scaphoid is then fixed using a headless screw as described in Procedure 68, although using an open technique (Fig. 69-10).

STEP 3 PEARLS

Aim for placing the headless screw volar to the central axis of the scaphoid to allow room for the graft to be inset dorsally.

Step 4: Insetting the Graft

- The tourniquet is now deflated to check the viability of the graft. It may take several minutes to see punctate bleeding from the graft.
- A trough, slightly smaller than the bone block, is created on the dorsal aspect of the scaphoid with a high-speed bur. The trough should be centered over the nonunion site and deep enough to hold the bone block securely (Fig. 69-11).
- The bone block, attached to its capsular pedicle, is then press-fit into the trough (Fig. 69-12).
- Final fluoroscopic posteroanterior and lateral images after the graft was inset are shown in Figure 69-13.

STEP 4 PEARLS

If the graft does not exhibit punctate bleeding or if the pedicle was compromised when harvesting the graft, the 1,2 ICSRA vascularized bone graft can still be used.

STEP 4 PITFALLS

There is usually very little rotation required of the graft to inset it (10 to 30 degrees). However, be sure to release enough capsule distally so that there is no tension on the capsular pedicle that might compromise its blood flow.

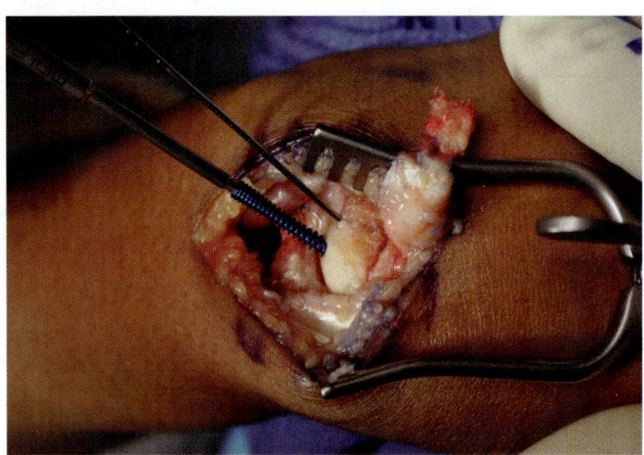

FIGURE 69-10

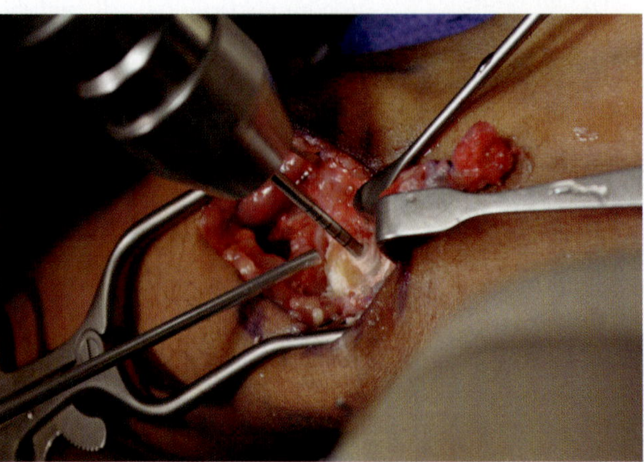

FIGURE 69-11

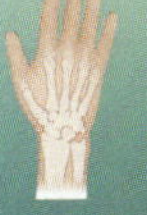

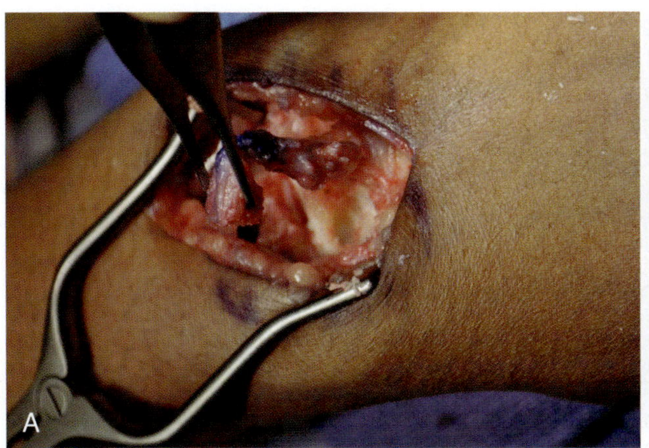

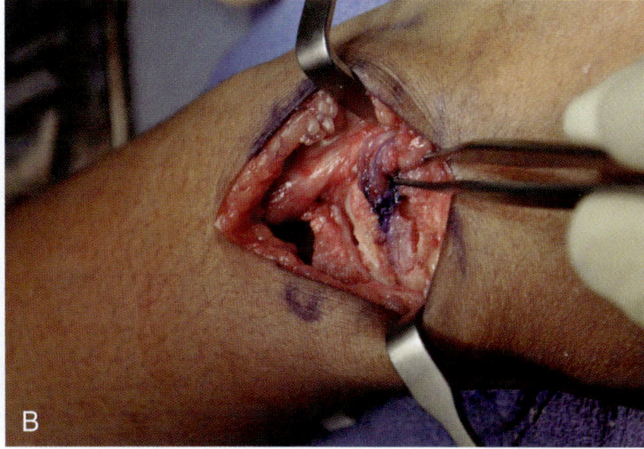

FIGURE 69-12

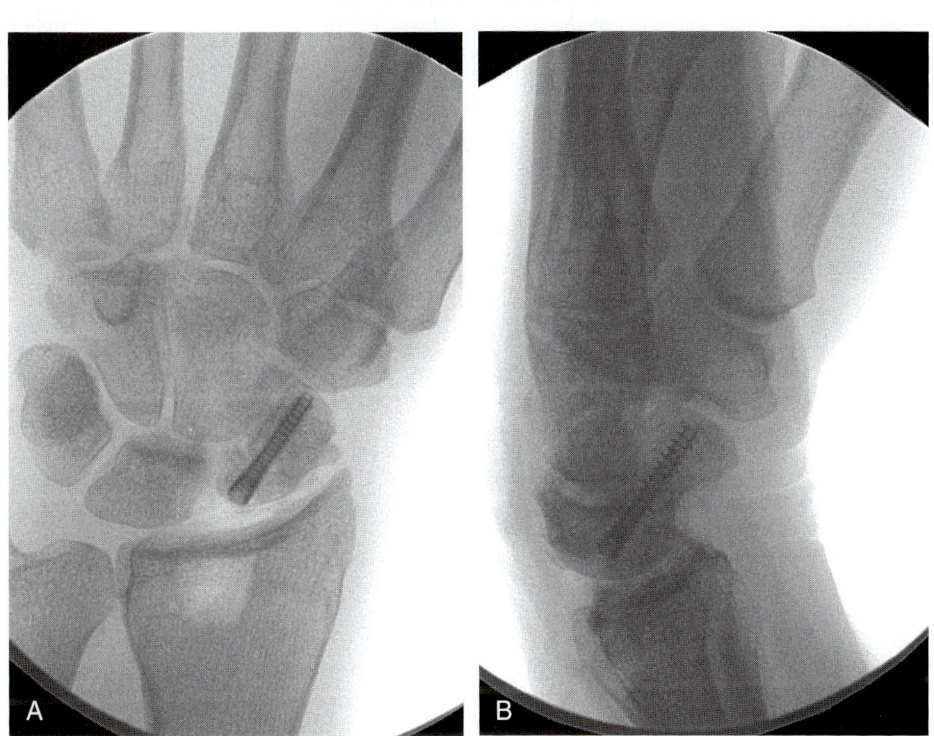

FIGURE 69-13

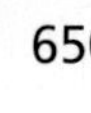

Step 5: Closure

- The wound is irrigated and closed in layers.
- The extensor retinaculum can be repaired; however, the EPL tendon should be placed radial to the Lister tubercle to minimize the risk for tendon irritation at the bone graft donor site.
- A volar and dorsal short-arm splint with a thumb component is applied in the operating room.

Postoperative Care and Expected Outcomes

- At the first office visit 2 weeks after surgery, the patient is fitted with a short-arm thumb spica cast to wear for an additional 4 weeks.
- When the cast is taken off, a removable Orthoplast thumb spica splint, constructed by an occupational therapist, is worn at all times until healing is confirmed by radiograph or CT scan.

Evidence

Sotereanos DG, Darlis NA, Dailiana ZH, et al. A capsular-based vascularized distal radius graft for proximal pole scaphoid pseudarthrosis. *J Hand Surg [Am]*. 2006;31:580-587.
This paper describes in detail the technique for a capsular-based distal radius graft for scaphoid avascular necrosis. The authors also present a case series of 13 patients in whom this graft was used. At a mean follow-up of 19 months, 10 of the patients achieved bony union. There were no complications other than the three persistent nonunions. This union rate compares favorably with the results of other free or pedicled grafts. (Level V evidence)

Sunagawa T, Bishop AT, Muramatsu K. Role of conventional and vascularized bone grafts in scaphoid nonunion with avascular necrosis: a canine experimental study. *J Hand Surg [Am]*. 2000;25:849-859.
The effectiveness of vascularized and conventional bone grafts in the treatment of scaphoid fracture nonunion with avascular necrosis was evaluated in 12 adult dogs. A dorsal radius inlay graft was placed at a simulated nonunion site—conventional on one side, and vascularized with a reverse-flow arteriovenous pedicle on the other. They found that 73% of the vascularized grafts and none of the conventional grafts healed. Also, at 6 weeks, bone blood flow in the proximal pole was significantly higher on the side of the vascularized graft. This study reinforces the healing potential vascularized grafts can provide and supports their use for the treatment of scaphoid nonunions. (Level IV evidence)

PROCEDURE 70

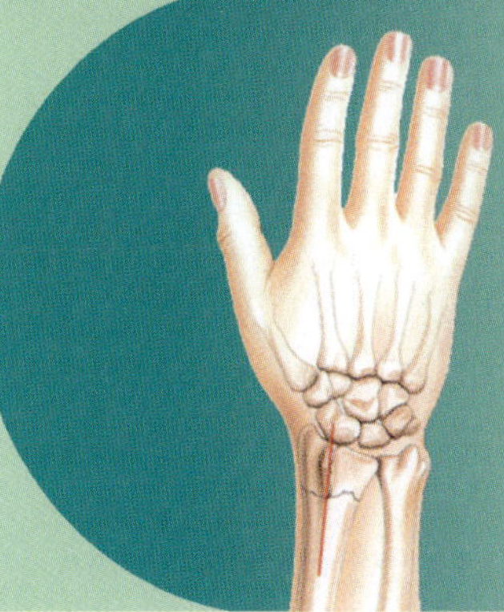

Medial Femoral Condyle Vascularized Bone Flap for Scaphoid Nonunion

Pao-Yuan Lin, Sandeep J. Sebastin, and Kevin C. Chung

See Video 52: Free Medial Femoral Condyle Vascularized Bone Transfer for Scaphoid Nonunion

Indications

- The main indication is a history of previously failed bone grafting, with plain radiographic and magnetic resonance imaging (MRI) evidence of avascular necrosis associated with scaphoid foreshortening.
- If there are intraoperative findings showing no bleeding from the proximal and distal scaphoid, it is appropriate to reconstruct the defect with vascularized bone flap.
- Another indication of medial femoral condyle vascularized bone flap is atrophic nonunion of a long bone with a small bone defect that is surrounded by poorly vascularized bed.
- If the nonunion site has punctate bleeding after débridement, corticocancellous wedge bone grafting through the dorsal approach for proximal pole nonunion and through the volar approach for waist nonunion with humpback deformity should be attempted.

Examination/Imaging

Clinical Examination

- Patients present with radial-sided wrist or anatomic snuffbox tenderness.
- Patients may show decreased grip strength and wrist motion, particularly during extension.

Imaging

- Posteroanterior (PA), lateral, and oblique radiographs of the hand should be taken to assess any dorsal intercalated segment instability (DISI) deformities or scaphoid foreshortening.
- Bone scans are useful in visualizing the fracture 4 hours after injury, but not for detection of a nonunion.
- Computed tomography (CT) scans are useful in assessing pseudoarthrosis and show the extent of bone loss. Furthermore, they can pinpoint the exact position of the fractured fragments and determine whether there is any necrosis of the proximal pole. Humpback deformity may be revealed in sagittal views.
- An MRI with intravenous contrast (gadolinium) will help determine proximal pole vascularity. Cartilage erosions and osseous avascular necrosis are evaluated mainly in T1-weighted sequences.

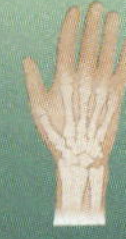

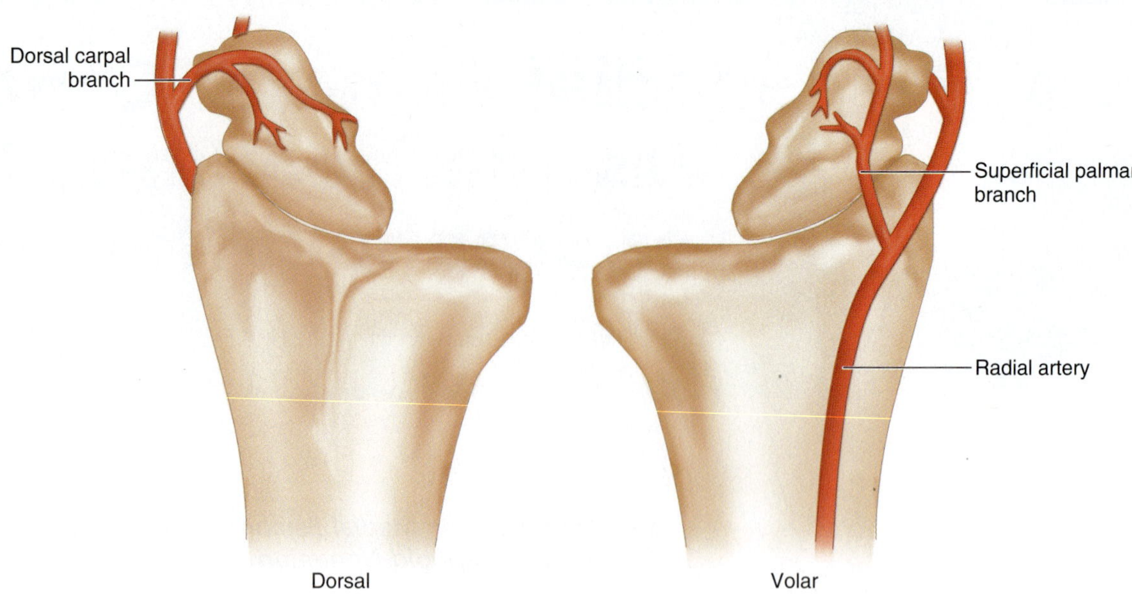

FIGURE 70-1

Surgical Anatomy

Recipient Site: Vascular Anatomy of Scaphoid

- The major blood supply to the scaphoid is through the radial artery, which enters through the dorsal ridge and supplies 70% to 80% of the intraosseous vascularity to the entire proximal pole. This vessel and its branches enter distally and dorsally in retrograde fashion to the scaphoid. The dorsal vessels travel proximally along the dorsal scaphoid ridge, and the majority of vessels enter the scaphoid waist and continue as intraosseous vessels. The scaphoid proximal pole is uniquely susceptible to avascular necrosis following fracture owing to high dependence on a single dominant retrograde traveling intraosseous vessel (Fig. 70-1).
- Volar radial artery branches provide the blood supply to 20% to 30% of the bone in the region of the distal tuberosity.

Donor Site: Medial Femoral Condyle

- The superficial femoral artery gives off the descending genicular artery branch just proximal to the adductor hiatus. The descending genicular artery travels distally and gives off a saphenous branch proximally and musculare branches distally. The superior medial genicular artery arises from the superficial femoral artery more distally.
- The descending genicular artery and superior medial genicular artery continue distally, penetrate the bone, and provide the blood supply to the medial femoral condyle as intraosseous nutrient vessels.
- The saphenous branch of the descending genicular artery supplies the medial femoral condyle skin flap (Fig. 70-2).

Positioning

- The procedure is performed under general anesthesia and tourniquet control for the affected upper limb. The patient is positioned supine with the arm on a hand table. The ipsilateral knee is maintained in the position of slight flexion and abduction.

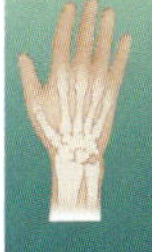

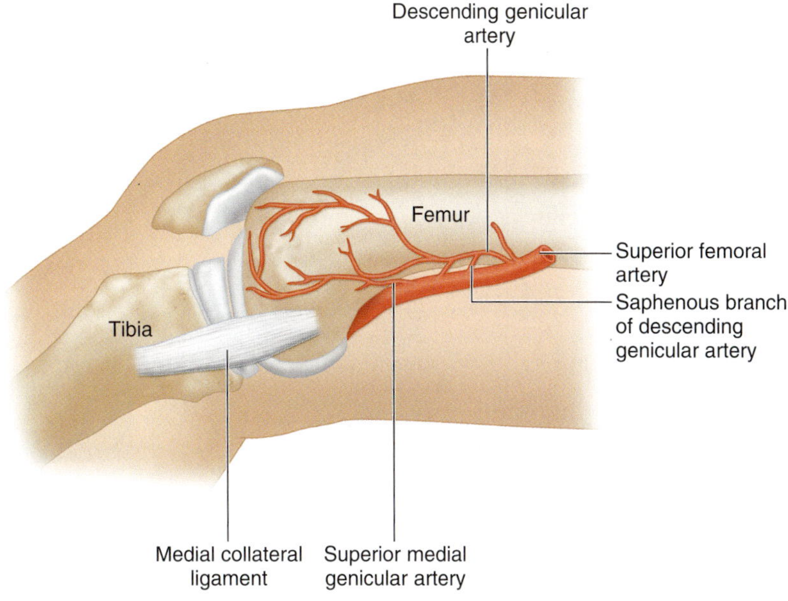

FIGURE 70-2

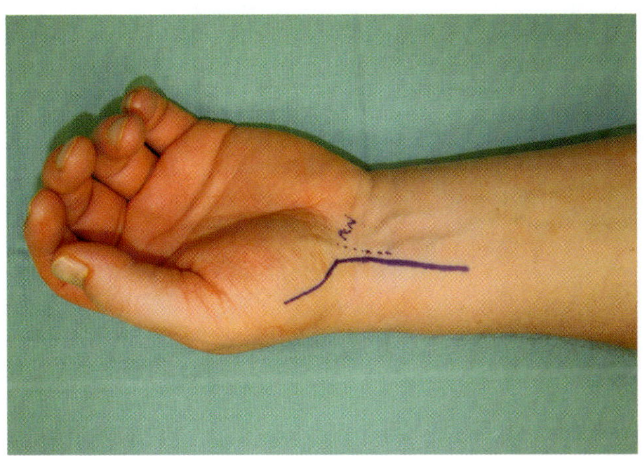

FIGURE 70-3

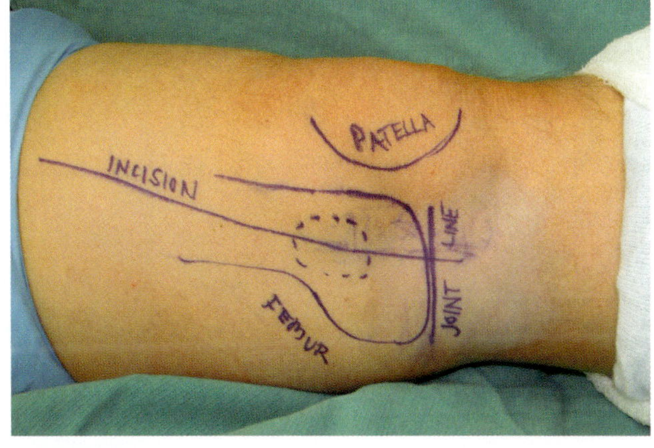

FIGURE 70-4

Exposures

- The scaphoid and radial artery are exposed by a palmar incision. This curvilinear incision extends proximally from the radial aspect of the thenar eminence parallel and radial to the flexor carpi radialis (Fig. 70-3).
- The medial femoral condyle of the ipsilateral medial knee and its nutrient vessels are exposed using a longitudinal lower medial thigh incision (Fig. 70-4).

Procedure

Team 1: Donor Site (Bone Graft Harvest)

Step 1

- The femur, patella, and femoral-tibial joint line at the ipsilateral lower medial thigh are marked. A skin incision line centered on the femur from the femoral-tibial joint to the proximal femur is drawn (see Fig. 70-4).

STEP 1 PEARLS

The incision line should be long enough (about 20 cm) to sufficiently expose the pedicle of the bone flap.

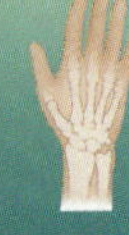

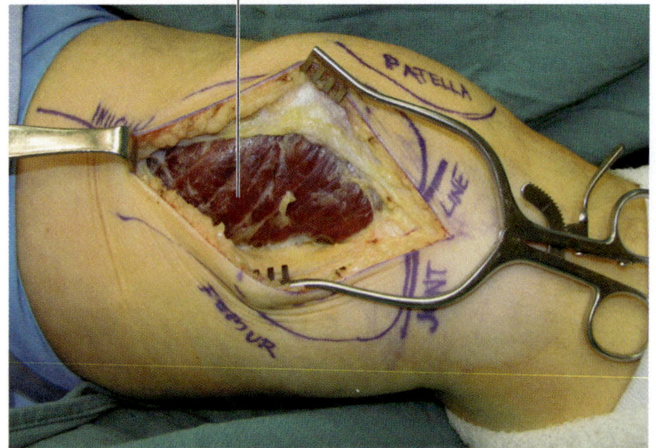

FIGURE 70-5

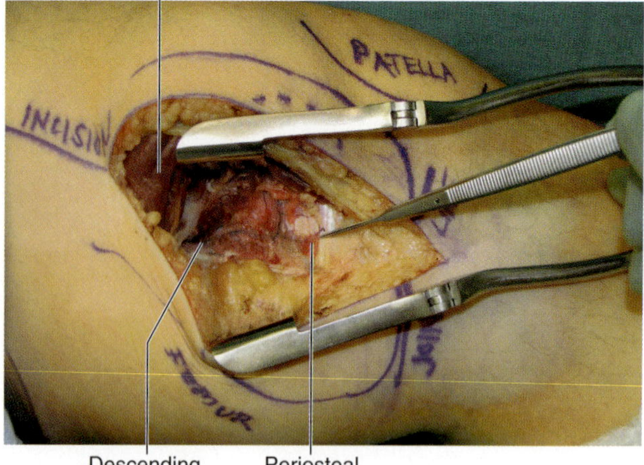

FIGURE 70-6

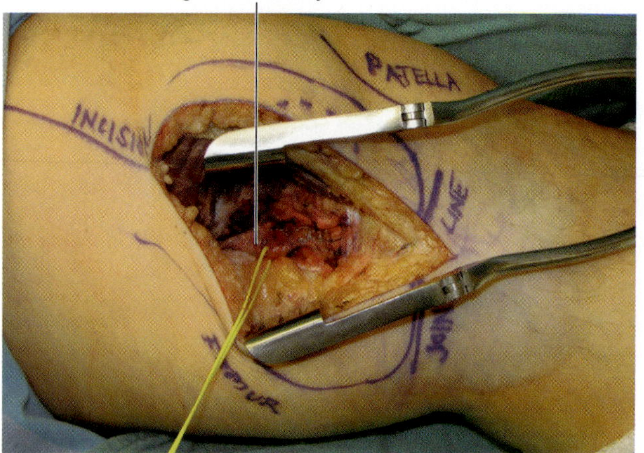

FIGURE 70-7

Step 2

- Skin is incised in longitudinal fashion, and the underlying subcutaneous tissues are dissected until the vastus medialis (VM) muscle fascia is exposed (Fig. 70-5).
- Hemostasis is adequately obtained with Bovie cautery during the soft tissue dissection.

Step 3

- The VM muscle is elevated and retracted to the anterior side of the thigh, and the nutrient vessel of the medial femoral condyle bone graft is identified (Fig. 70-6).

STEP 3 PEARLS

It is easy to elevate the VM muscle from the distal-posterior aspect of the muscle in the loose areolar tissue plane between the VM muscle and medial femoral condyle.

Step 4

- Determine the sizable nutrient pedicle (usually the descending genicular artery) of the medial femoral condyle bone graft and dissect the pedicle proximally until an adequate length (5 cm) of vascular pedicle is mobilized (Fig. 70-7).

STEP 4 PEARLS

The pedicle length of the descending genicular artery is about 13.7 cm, and of the superior medial genicular artery, 5.2 cm. If anastomoses are planned at the radial artery in the wrist, a 5-cm pedicle length should suffice.

Step 5

- Based on the size of the defect, a rectangular medial femoral condyle bone graft is selected at the area where the distal nutrient branches of the descending genicular artery penetrate into the bone.

STEP 5 PEARLS

The medial collateral ligament of the knee is near the area of the bone graft and should be identified and protected.

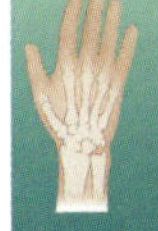

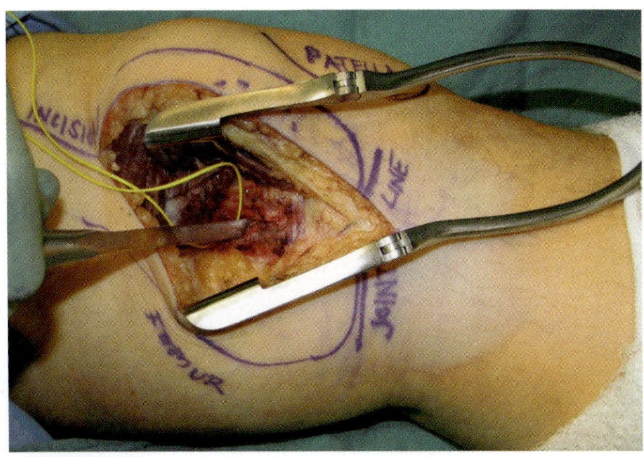

FIGURE 70-8

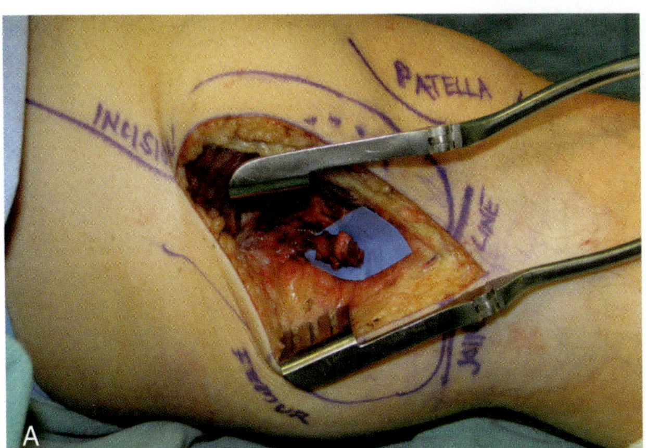

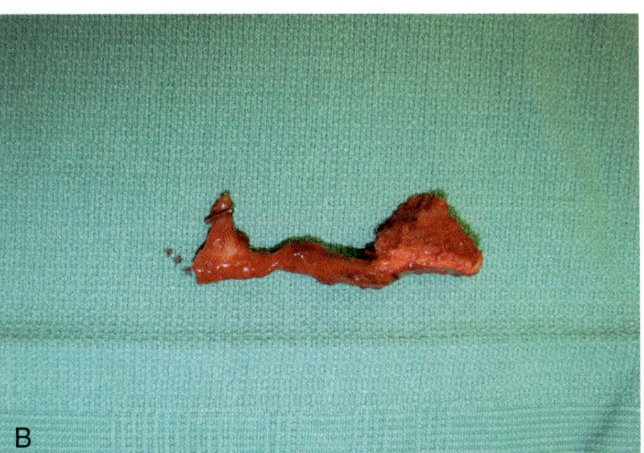

FIGURE 70-9

STEP 6 PEARLS

It is effective to elevate the pedicle from the more proximal bone with meticulous dissection before making the bone cuts.

To assist removal of the bone graft with less risk for fracture, an additional cut is made, angled 45 degrees just distal to the bone graft.

STEP 6 PITFALLS

Care should be taken to protect the nutrient vessels while cutting the bone.

STEP 7 PEARLS

The length of the pedicle depends on the need of recipient site; usually 5 cm is enough.

Additional cancellous bone graft can be harvested to fill any defect in the proximal pole.

- The size of the bone graft should be sufficient to fill the defect. Bone graft from this location has sufficient cortical bone to provide a strong strut to correct the humpback deformity of the scaphoid. The distal radius bone graft typically does not have sufficient cortical bone strong enough to buttress the bone defect. The bone graft is usually 10 to 12 mm in thickness.

Step 6

- The periosteum is sharply incised using a no. 15 blade, and the bone is cut with a small osteotome along the marking line (Fig. 70-8).

Step 7

- The vascular pedicle is ligated and divided.
- The bone graft is prepared and transferred to the recipient site for filling the scaphoid defect and performing microvascular anastomosis (Fig. 70-9A and B).

Step 8

- The defect created in the medial femoral condyle is filled with artificial bone graft.
- A suction drain is inserted, and the wound is closed in a layered fashion with absorbable sutures.

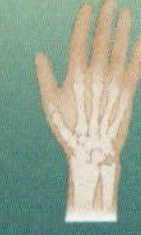

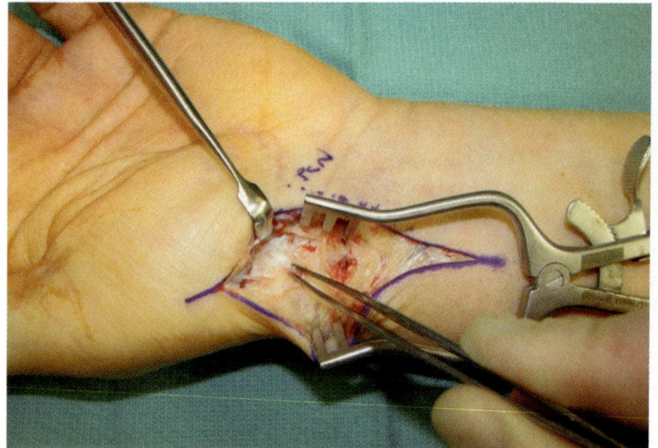

FIGURE 70-10

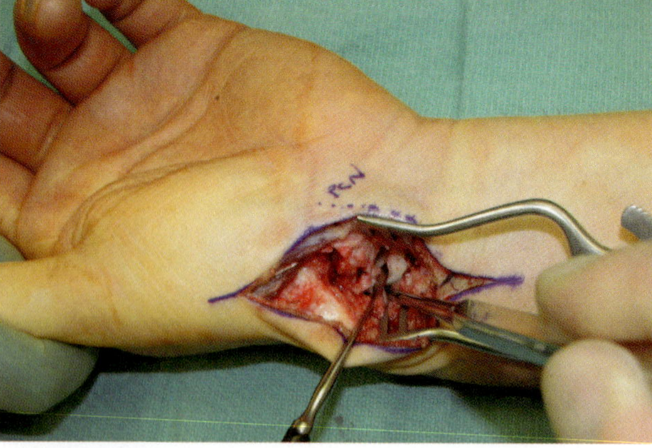

FIGURE 70-11

STEP 1 PITFALLS

If the incision is too close to the thenar crease, it is easy to injure the palmar cutaneous branch of the median nerve.

STEP 2 PEARLS

The radioscaphocapitate (RSC) and long radiolunate (LRL) ligaments are identified and incised. Much of the LRL and a portion of the RSC are left intact to help stabilize the proximal pole.

Preserving this ligamentous support also helps maintain fracture reduction.

Volar capsulotomy in the scaphotrapezial joint is performed to improve the visualization of the scaphoid.

STEP 3 PITFALLS

The articulation between the scaphoid and capitate is carefully exposed to facilitate visualization during reduction.

Step 9

- The patient's knee is protected with a soft bulky dressing.
- A knee immobilizer is typically useful for patient comfort in the immediate postoperative period.

Team 2: Recipient Site Preparation and Microanastomosis

Step 1

- The skin and subcutaneous tissue are dissected along the incision line.

Step 2

- The FCR sheath is opened, the tendon retracted ulnarly, and the floor of the FCR tunnel sharply incised longitudinally to expose the radiocarpal joint at the level of the scaphoid (Fig. 70-10).

Step 3

- The scaphoid is then examined, paying attention to the articular cartilage of the radioscaphoid and midcarpal joints.
- A Freer elevator is used to define the location of the nonunion and the borders of the scaphoid.
- Fibrous and/or necrotic tissues at the proximal and distal poles are examined carefully. A small curet or rongeur is used for débridement and removal of intervening fibrotic tissue (Fig. 70-11).

Step 4

- The tourniquet is deflated to assess punctate bleeding from the nonunion site.
- The absence of punctate bleeding suggests avascularity, and further débridement is performed until punctate bleeding is confirmed (Fig. 70-12).
- The size of the bony defect is measured after débridement.
- A slow-speed bur is helpful to débride the fibrous nonunion, but the scaphoid must be constantly irrigated during burring to prevent additional bone necrosis.

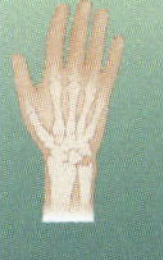

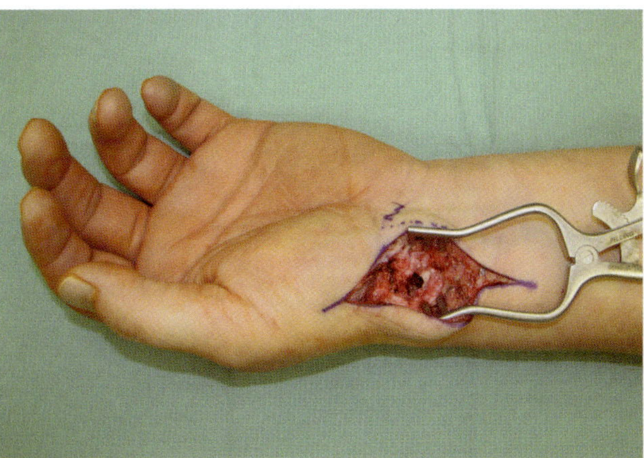

FIGURE 70-12

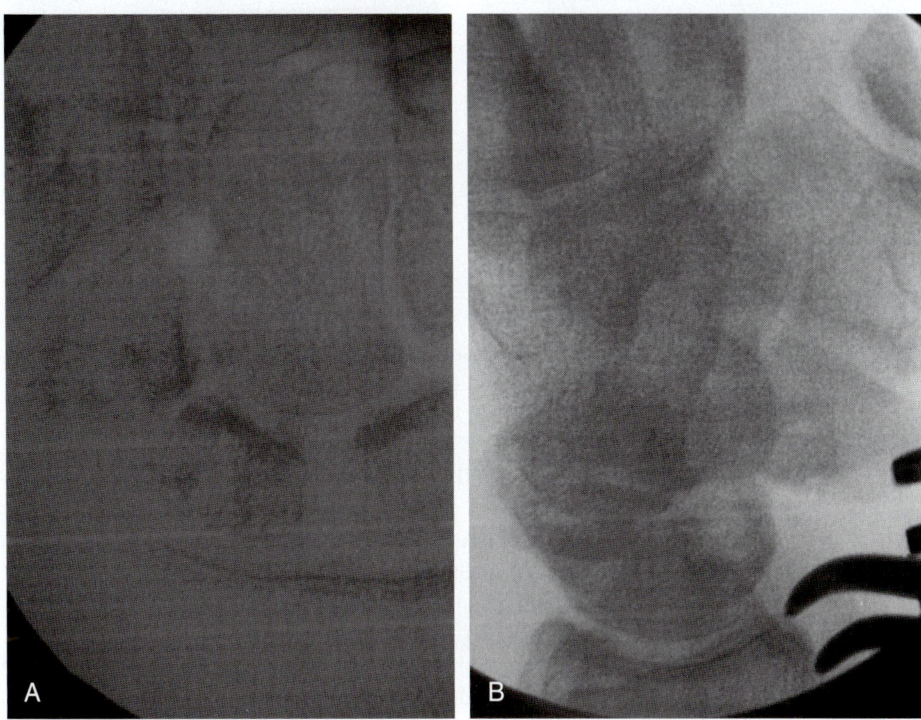

FIGURE 70-13

Step 5

- The DISI deformity is corrected by flexing the wrist under fluoroscopic imaging until the radiolunate angle is neutral (Fig. 70-13A and B).
- The scaphoid is then prepared to accept the graft.

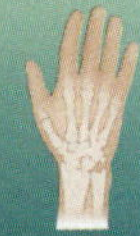

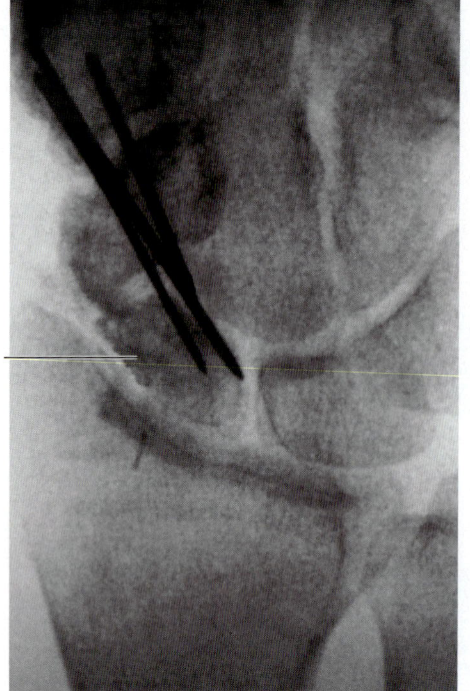

FIGURE 70-14

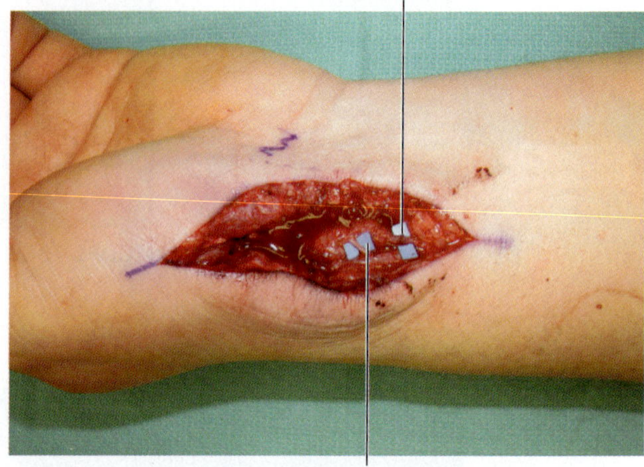

FIGURE 70-15

Step 6

- Recipient vessels (radial artery, concomitant vein, or cephalic vein) are dissected and prepared for anastomosis.

Step 7

- The bone graft harvested from the medial femoral condyle is further shaped to fit the defect.
- The flap is inserted into the defect, and Kirschner wires (or headless cannulated screws) are passed through the scaphoid and bone flap for fixation under fluoroscopic imaging to confirm correction of the scaphoid shortening and DISI deformity (Fig. 70-14).
- The K-wires should be left under the skin and removed when the bone has healed, typically 3 months after surgery.

STEP 7 PEARLS

It is better to place the periosteal surface (cortical surface) palmarly to preserve the vascularity of the bone flap, allowing the cortical bone to correct the humpback deformity.

Step 8

- The recipient artery (descending genicular artery or superior medial genicular artery) is anastomosed to the radial artery in an end-to-side fashion using 9-0 nylon sutures under microscopic magnification.
- The venae comitantes of the descending genicular artery or superior medial genicular artery is anastomosed to the venae comitantes of the radial artery or to the cephalic vein in an end-to-end fashion by 9-0 nylon sutures (Fig. 70-15).

Step 9

- After microanastomosis, the wound is closed with 4-0 nylon sutures (Fig. 70-16).
- A hand-held Doppler is used to detect the signal of arterial anastomosis, and the location is marked for postoperative monitoring.
- A thumb spica dorsal short-arm splint is applied to keep the thumb abducted and the wrist in slight flexion.

STEP 9 PITFALLS

If the wound is closed too tightly, it is possible to compress the vessels.

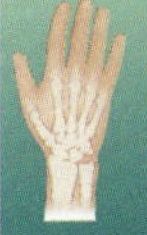

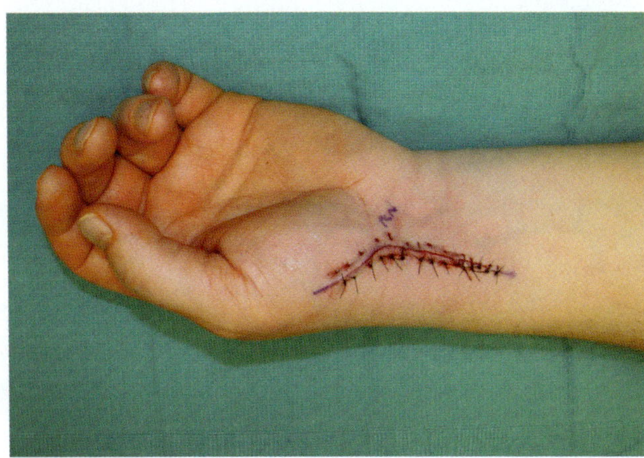

FIGURE 70-16

Postoperative Care and Expected Outcomes

- The splint maintains the thumb in abduction and the wrist in slight flexion for 2 weeks.
- The stitches are removed 2 weeks after surgery, and thumb spica short-arm cast or splint (for a reliable patient) is applied for 8 to 12 weeks until the vascularized bone graft is united. CT scan can confirm healing of the scaphoid before allowing the patient to initiate unrestricted activities.
- The thigh is immobilized for a few days postoperatively until the patient feels comfortable.

Evidence

Doi K, Hattori Y. Vascularized bone graft from the supracondylar region of the femur. *Microsurgery*. 2009;29:379-384.
Thirty-three patients received medial femoral condyle vascularized bone grafts. Thirty-one of theses patients had achieved bony union. Eleven of the 33 patients were treated for scaphoid nonunions. In this study, the authors mentioned that this flap can achieve good results when used to treat the long bone with small bone defects, avascular necrosis of the talus, and scaphoid nonunions. (Level IV evidence)

Jones DB Jr, Burger H, Shin AY, et al. Treatment of scaphoid waist nonunions with an avascular proximal pole and carpal collapse: a comparison of two vascularized bone grafts. *J Bone Joint Surg [Am]*. 2008;90:2616-2625.
Retrospective review of two vascularized bone graft (medial femoral condyle and distal radial pedicle graft) reconstructive groups from two different institutions. For distal radial pedicle grafts, 6 of the 10 cases failed, and the mean union time of success for the remaining 4 cases was 19 weeks. There was no significant change in the revised carpal height ratio or the carpal angles between preoperative and postoperative radiographs. In the medial femoral condyle bone graft group, all 12 cases united. The mean union time was 13 weeks. Comparing the preoperative and postoperative radiographs showed that the average decrease of lateral intrascaphoid angle and scapholunate angle was 25 degrees and 5 degrees, respectively, showing marked improvement. However, all medial femoral condyle graft group patients reported knee pain that persisted about 6 weeks postoperatively. (Level III evidence)

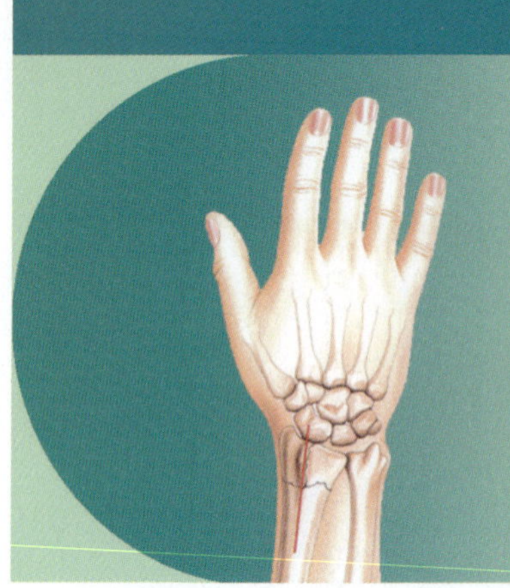

PROCEDURE 71

Open Reduction and Acute Repair of Perilunate Fracture-Dislocations

Louis W. Catalano III and Christopher M. Jones

Indications

- Acute and subacute (<6 weeks old) perilunate dislocations are seen.
- Chronic perilunate dislocations (>7 weeks old) may be best treated with salvage procedures such as proximal row carpectomy or wrist fusion.

Examination/Imaging

Clinical Examination

- Severe wrist edema, tenderness, and ecchymosis may accompany the extreme pain that the patient is experiencing.
- Passive wrist motion is usually limited, painful, and disjointed (not smooth).
- It is essential that a thorough neurovascular examination be performed to rule out acute carpal tunnel syndrome.
- If numbness, tingling, and two-point discrimination worsen after closed reduction, immediate carpal tunnel release should be performed (along with open reduction and fixation).
- If the neurovascular examination is improving or normal and a good reduction is achieved, the surgery can be performed electively.

Imaging

- Lunate and perilunate dislocations are occasionally missed in the emergency room and dismissed as a severe wrist sprain despite having adequate imaging. Therefore, it is essential to obtain a thorough radiographic examination and scrutinize the images to prevent missing an acute injury.
- A standard radiographic series of the wrist must be obtained to evaluate for dislocation. Assess for disruption of Gilula arc lines on the posteroanterior image. On a lateral radiograph, the radial shaft, lunate, capitate, and metacarpal shafts should be collinear (Fig. 71-1).
- Radiographs should also be inspected to rule out associated radial styloid, scaphoid, capitate, or triquetral fractures (Fig. 71-2).
- Computed tomography can help better define any questionable fractures of the carpal bones.
- Magnetic resonance imaging is rarely used.

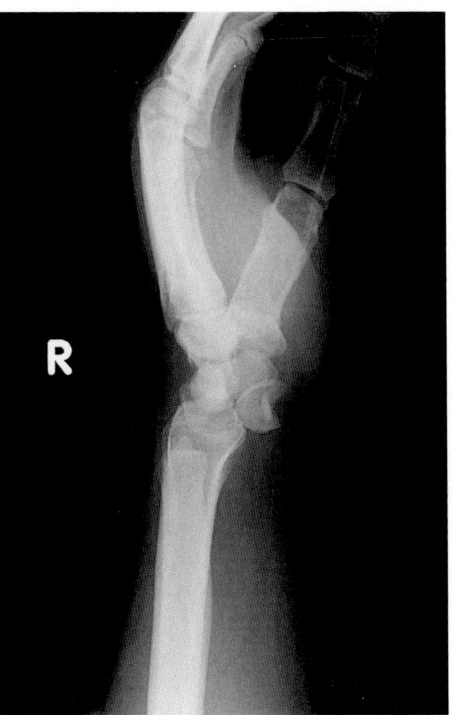

FIGURE 71-1

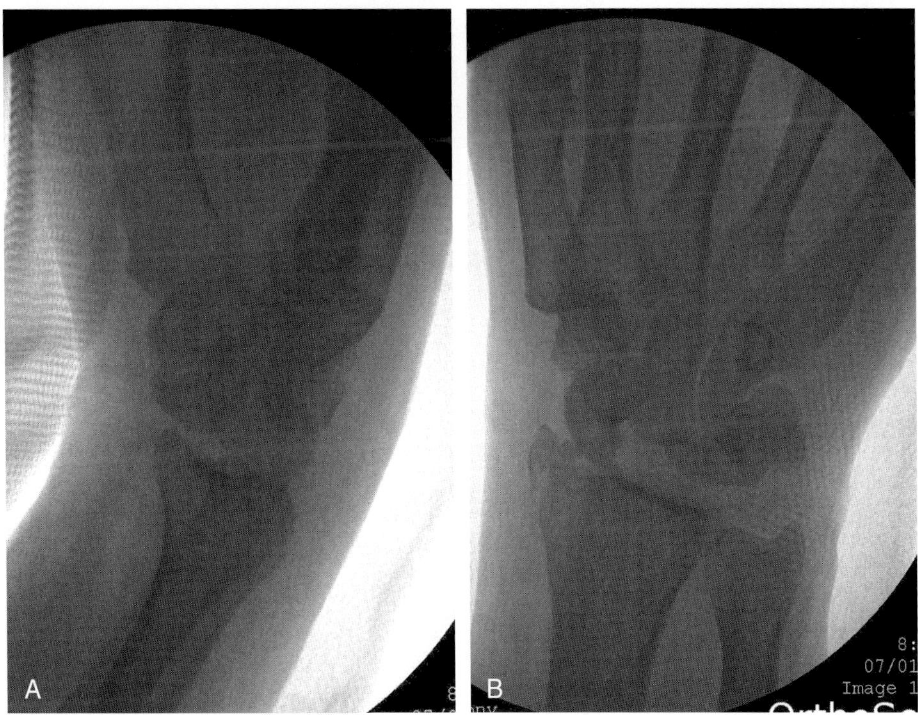

FIGURE 71-2

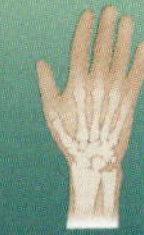

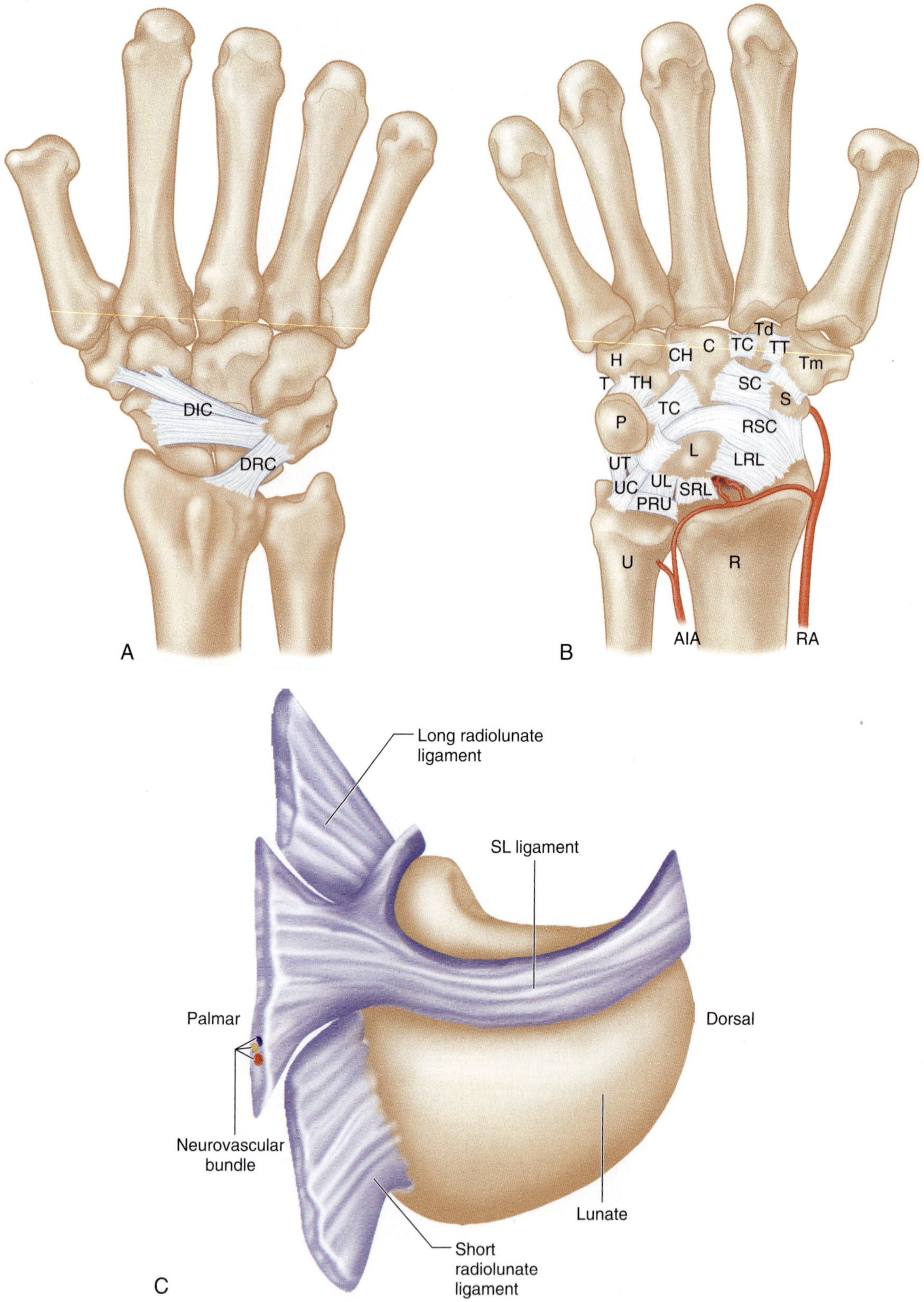

FIGURE 71-3

Surgical Anatomy

- The dorsal radiocarpal and intercarpal ligaments are frequently ruptured in these severe injuries (Fig 71-3A).
- The strong volar ligaments have a characteristic transverse rent that is repaired through the volar approach (Fig. 71-3B).

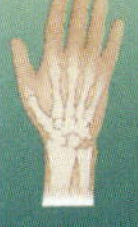

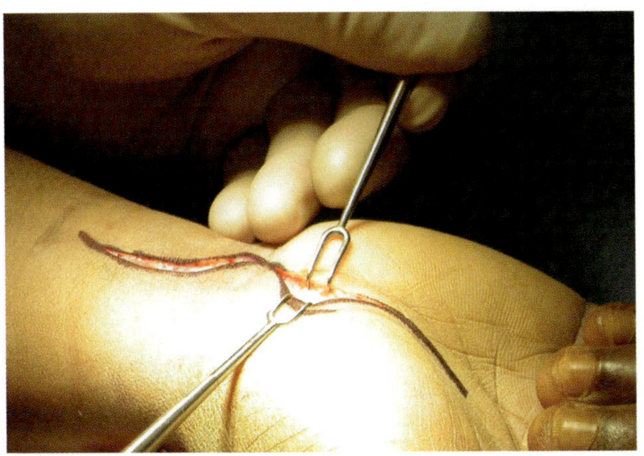

FIGURE 71-4

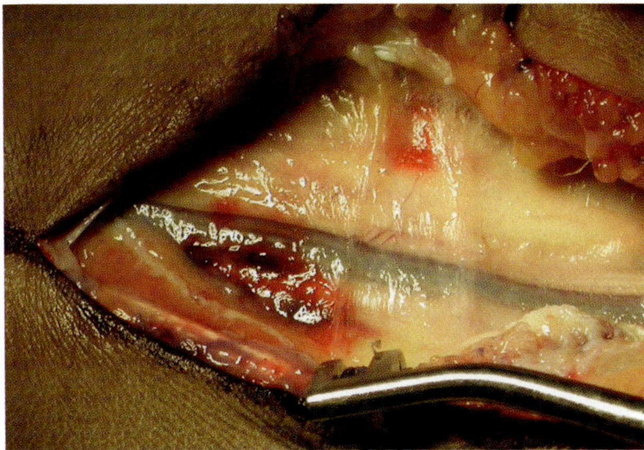

FIGURE 71-5

- The lunate dislocates through the space of Poirier, a relatively weak region of the volar capsule just below the arc of the radioscaphocapitate and ulnocapitate ligaments (see Fig. 71-3B).
- The dorsal portion of the scapholunate ligament is the thickest and strongest portion of the C-shaped ligament and should be repaired if adequate ligament tissue is present (Fig. 71-3C).
- The short radiolunate ligament serves as the pivot for the lunate when it dislocates into the carpal tunnel. It also provides blood supply to the dislocated lunate to prevent avascular necrosis.

Positioning

- The patient is positioned supine on the operating room table with the arm abducted on a radiolucent hand table.
- A minifluoroscope is positioned vertically at the end of the hand table with the image intensifier under the table.
- Five to 10 pounds of longitudinal traction using finger traps may be helpful to obtain and maintain lunate reduction and proper position of the carpal bones.

PITFALLS

A 90-degree angle should be made at the wrist flexion crease to prevent the longitudinal scar from creating a flexion contracture postoperatively.

Exposures

- A 7- to 8-cm longitudinal dorsal incision centered over the wrist is made, with exposure of the carpus through the third dorsal compartment (extensor pollicis longus [EPL] sheath).
- An extended carpal tunnel release incision is also made at the wrist. This extends from the Kaplan cardinal line distally to 3 to 4 cm proximal to the distal wrist flexion crease (Fig. 71-4).

STEP 1 PEARLS

Frequently, osteochondral fractures of the lunate, scaphoid, capitate, and triquetrum are found and must be removed.

Exposure must extend ulnarly to the triquetrum to visualize the lunotriquetral (LT) joint.

Procedure

Step 1: Volar Approach

- After the extended carpal tunnel incision, dissection is carried down through the transverse carpal ligament and distal antebrachial fascia to completely decompress the median nerve (Fig. 71-5).

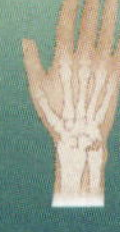

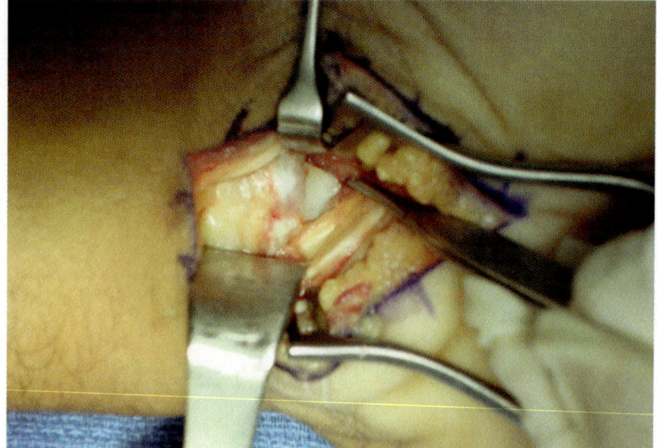

FIGURE 71-6

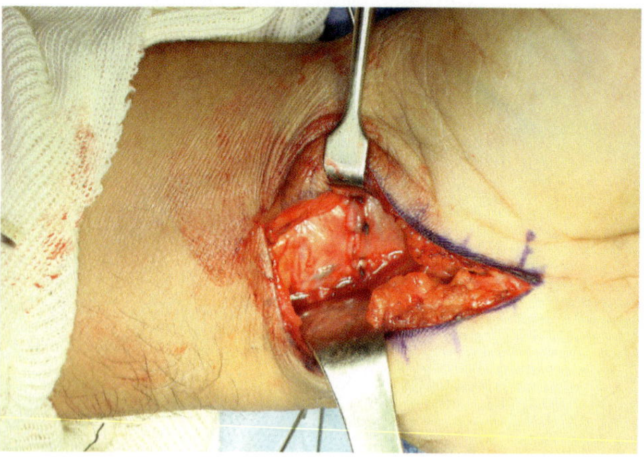

FIGURE 71-7

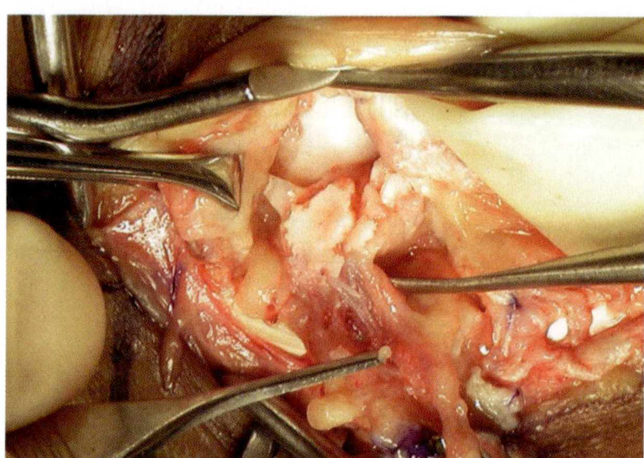

FIGURE 71-8

- The nerve and all flexor tendons are retracted to expose the floor of the carpal tunnel, the transverse ligamentous rent, and lunate within the carpal tunnel if it had not been previously reduced (Fig. 71-6).
- The lunate can be manually reduced with dorsal pressure and some longitudinal traction.
- The transverse ligamentous rent is repaired using multiple 3-0 braided non-absorbable sutures (Fig. 71-7).

Step 2: Dorsal Approach

- After elevation and retraction of the EPL, deeper capsular exposure reveals the severe dorsal radiocarpal and intercarpal ligamentous damage (Fig. 71-8).
- The ligament disruption often provides adequate exposure of the carpal bones; if not, a longitudinal capsulotomy is performed.
- A 0.062-inch K-wire is inserted into the lunate to use as a joystick for reduction.
- By means of the joystick, the lunate is made to be collinear with the longitudinal axis of the radius (as verified on the radiographs) and then held reduced with a temporary 0.062-inch dorsal radioulnate K-wire.
- Alternatively, a K-wire can be placed retrograde from the capitate through the lunate to hold the lunate reduction. Unlike the radiolunate wire, this wire does not need to be removed at the completion of the surgery.

STEP 2 PEARLS

Perfect reduction of the lunate in the fossa and collinear with the radius shaft is the foundation on which the remainder of the carpus will be attached.

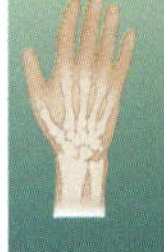

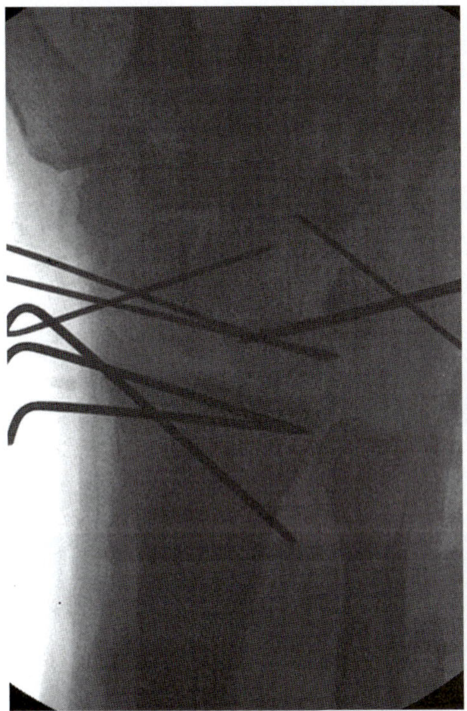

FIGURE 71-9

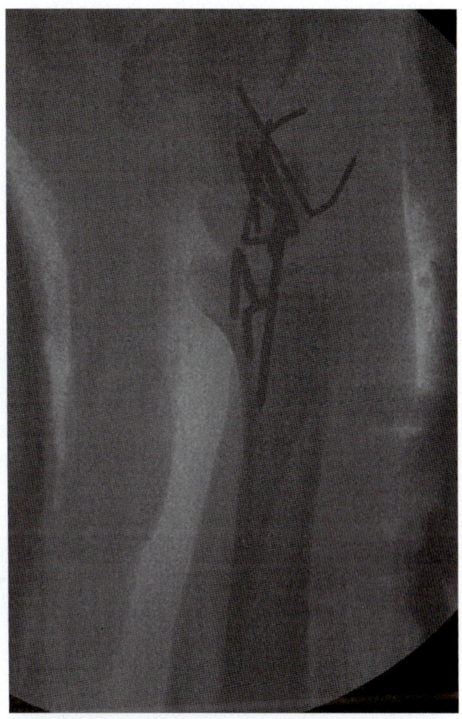

FIGURE 71-10

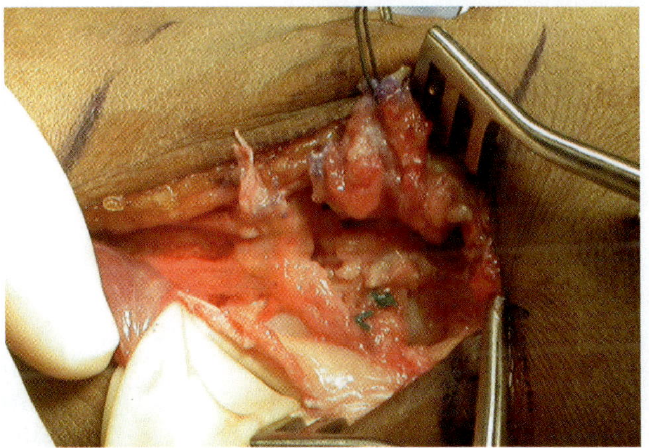

FIGURE 71-11

Step 3

- A 0.062-inch K-wire is inserted into the scaphoid and used as a joystick to extend the scaphoid out of the flexed position.
- Once a scapholunate angle of about 45 degrees is achieved, the scaphoid is pinned to the lunate and capitate using two to three 0.045-inch K-wires (Figs. 71-9 and 71-10).

STEP 4 PEARLS

Adequate reduction and fixation of the LT joint is often overlooked. Recall that this joint is completely disrupted (as is the scapholunate [SL] joint) and should be treated similarly.

Step 4

- The LT joint is reduced with a fracture reduction clamp, and the reduction is verified on radiographs.
- The LT joint is held with two 0.045-inch K-wires, and the triquetrum can be pinned to the hamate/capitate using another 0.045-inch K-wire (see Figs. 71-9 and 71-10).

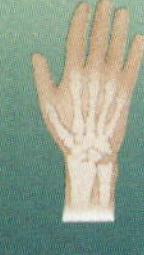

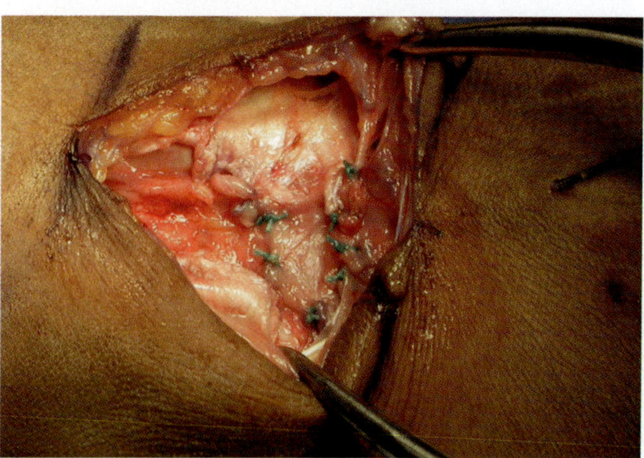

FIGURE 71-12

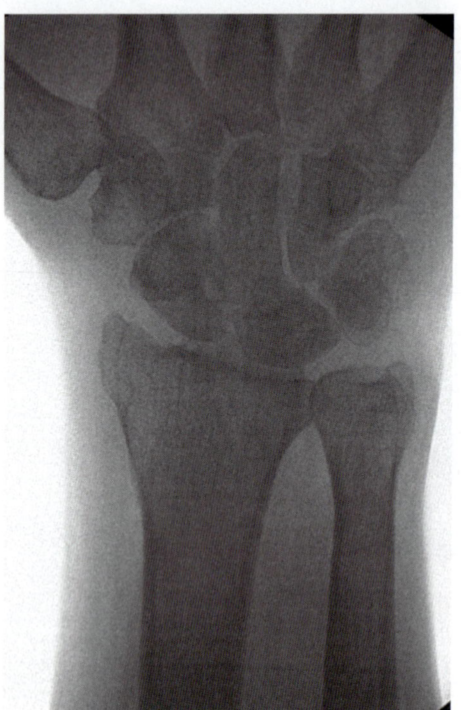

FIGURE 71-13

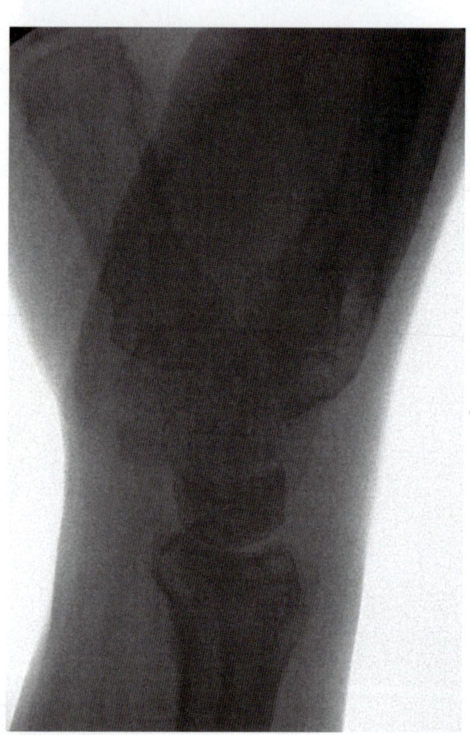

FIGURE 71-14

STEP 5 PEARLS

Every attempt should be made to repair these vital ligaments to maintain joint reduction after pin removal.

PEARLS

No formal pin site care is needed.

The cast and pins are removed 9 to 10 weeks after surgery (Figs. 71-13 and 71-14).

Formal occupational therapy is started immediately after pin removal and continues for 2 to 4 months.

Step 5

- Inspection of the SL and LT ligaments will determine the feasibility of ligamentous repair.
- The ligaments may be avulsed from the scaphoid, lunate, or triquetrum or may be torn in midsubstance.
- If midsubstance tears are noted, repair is completed with 3-0 nonabsorbable sutures (Fig. 71-11).
- If bony avulsions are found, repair is completed with mini-suture anchors.

Additional Steps

- A tight dorsal capsular/ligament repair is performed using 3-0 nonabsorbable sutures to help fortify the intrinsic ligament repairs (Fig. 71-12).
- *Closure:* Volar skin closure is achieved with 5-0 nylon sutures, and dorsal skin closure is achieved with 5-0 plain catgut sutures.

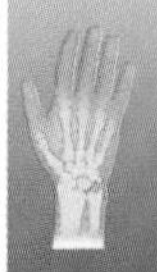

Postoperative Care and Expected Outcomes

- A bulky short arm thumb spica splint is applied postoperatively.
- The patient is seen at 2- to 3-week intervals for assessment of pin sites, and radiographs are taken to verify the reduction.
- Severe injuries such as this often lead to restricted wrist range of motion and development of early wrist arthritis.

Evidence

Hildebrand KA, Ross DC, Patterson SD, et al. Dorsal perilunate dislocations and fracture-dislocations: questionnaire, clinical, and radiographic evaluation. *J Hand Surg [Am]*. 2000;25:1069-1079.
These authors reviewed 22 consecutive patients (23 wrists) who underwent open reduction and internal fixation of dorsal perilunate dislocations and fracture-dislocations through combined dorsal and volar approaches using intercarpal fixation only within the proximal carpal row. The follow-up period averaged 37 months. Motion was instituted an average of 10 weeks after injury. Average flexion-extension motion arc and grip strength in the injured wrist were 57% and 73%, respectively. The authors found that the scapholunate angle increased and the revised carpal height ratio decreased over time. Three patients (3 wrists) required wrist arthrodesis, and a fourth patient had an immediate scaphoid excision and four-corner arthrodesis secondary to an irreparable scaphoid fracture. One patient required a proximal row carpectomy to treat septic arthritis. Nine of the remaining 18 wrists had radiographic evidence of arthritis, most often at the capitolunate or scaphocapitate articulations. Short form-36 mental summary scores were significantly greater than age- and gender-matched United States population values. The disabilities of arm, shoulder, and hand evaluation, Mayo wrist score, and patient-rated wrist evaluation all reflected loss of function. Despite this, 73% of all patients had returned to full duties in their usual occupations, and 82% were employed. (Level V evidence)

Trumble T, Verheyden J. Treatment of isolated perilunate and lunate dislocations with combined dorsal and volar approach and intraosseous cerclage wire. *J Hand Surg [Am]*. 2004;29:412-417.
In this study, 22 patients were treated with a combined dorsal and volar approach with intraosseous wiring and pinning for isolated perilunate and lunate dislocations. Outcomes were assessed after an average of 49 months. The authors found that patient satisfaction was high in 15 of 22 patients, and 7 patients stated that they had problems with activities of daily living. Sixteen of the patients said that they were able to return to their previous level of activity. The wrist flexion-extension arc and grip strength averaged 80% and 77%, respectively, and follow-up radiographs showed no significant change in scapholunate angle or gap. The cerclage wire had to be removed in 16 patients. This study demonstrates a reasonable return to function and pain relief, given the magnitude of the injury, using a combined dorsal and volar approach with intraosseous cerclage wire. (Level V evidence)

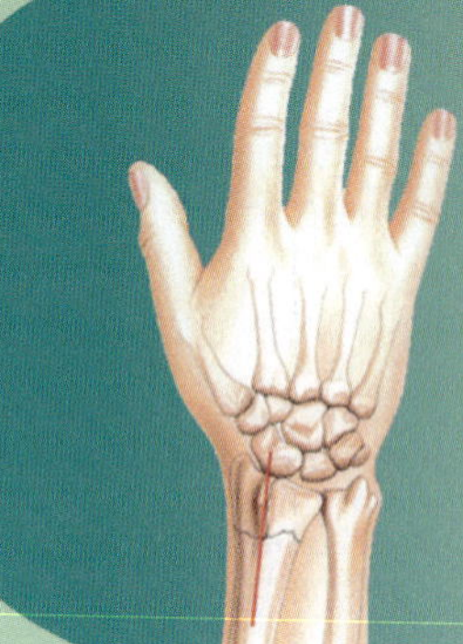

Dorsal Capsulodesis for Scapholunate Instability Using Suture Anchors

Shimpei Ono, Sandeep J. Sebastin, and Kevin C. Chung

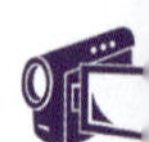

See Video 53: Dorsal Capsulodesis for Scapholunate Ligament Injury

Indications

- Static or dynamic dorsal intercalated segmental instability (DISI) deformity is found without a wide scapholunate (SL) gap.
- We determine the treatment for SL instability based on clinical presentation, radiographic appearance, and arthroscopic and intraoperative findings. Our current algorithm for selection of appropriate procedure for SL instability is indicated in Table 72-1.

Table 72-1 Selection of Treatment

	Radiograph (Posteroanterior and Lateral Views)				Arthroscopy		
	Static		*Clenched Fist*				
Stage	*SL gap*	*DISI*	*SL gap*	*DISI*	*Geissler Grading*	**Intraoperative**	**Treatment**
I (Pre-dynamic)	–	–	–	–	Grade I	–	Arthroscopic synovectomy Pinning of SL joint × 4-6 wk Wrist splint × 8-10 wk
II (Dynamic)	–	–	+	+	Grade II	Partial tear of SL ligament (usually dorsal part is intact)	Dorsal capsulodesis Pinning of SL joint × 4-6 wk Wrist splint × 8-10 wk
III (Static)	+	+	+	+	Grade III	Complete tear of SL ligament Scaphoid and lunate can be reduced	FCR ligament reconstruction Pinning of SL joint × 4-6 wk Wrist splint × 8-10 wk
					Grade IV	Complete tear of SL ligament Scaphoid and lunate cannot be reduced	Four-corner fusion/PRC

Table 72-2 Arthroscopic Grading of Scapholunate Ligament Injuries (Geissler)

	Appearance of ligament	Appearance of Joint	
Grade	*Radiocarpal Scope*	*Radiocarpal Scope*	*Midcarpal Scope*
I	Attenuated (Normal concave ligament appears convex)	No gap	No step-off
II	Attenuated, partial tear	No gap	Step-off + (Probe [~2 mm] cannot be passed through joint)
III	Complete tear	Gap +	Step-off + (Probe [~2 mm] can be passed through joint)
IV	Complete tear	Gap +	Step off + (2.7-mm arthroscope can be passed through joint)

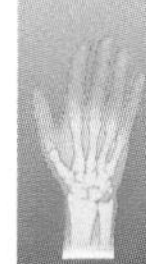

Examination/Imaging

Clinical Examination

- Patients complain of radial-sided wrist pain especially with loading activities, weakness of grip, and swelling, along with discomfort at extremes of wrist extension and radial deviation.
- Tenderness is found in the radial snuffbox or over the SL interval just distal to the Lister tubercle.
- The following two provocative tests have been described for global assessment of wrist pain. These tests are useful in patients when the history and findings of examination do not match. However, they do not indicate the location or nature of the pathology.
  - *Carpal shake test:* This involves grasping the patient's distal forearm and passively shaking or passively extending and flexing the wrist. Lack of patient resistance or complaints suggests a low level of carpal disease.
  - *Sitting hand test:* The patient is asked to support his or her weight off the chair while seated. This maneuver produces stress across the wrist, and patients with wrist disease find it difficult to perform this.
- One or more of the following provocative tests may be positive depending on the degree of injury to the SL ligament and integrity of the secondary stabilizers.
  - *Scaphoid shift test (Watson):* The examiner places four fingers behind the radius. The thumb is placed on the scaphoid tuberosity, and the other hand is used to move the wrist passively from ulnar to radial deviation. In ulnar deviation, the scaphoid is extended, whereas in radial deviation, the scaphoid is flexed. Pressure on the tuberosity while the wrist is moved from ulnar deviation to radial deviation prevents the scaphoid from flexing. In such circumstances, if the SL ligaments are completely insufficient or torn, the proximal pole subluxates dorsally out of the scaphoid fossa, inducing pain on the dorsoradial aspect of the wrist. When pressure is released, a typical clunk may occur, indicating an abrupt self-reduction of the scaphoid back into its normal position.
  - *Resisted long finger extension test:* The patient is asked to extend the long finger against resistance with the wrist partially flexed. This compresses any areas of synovitis under the tendon and causes pain. If the pain occurs over the SL joint, it is suggestive of SL disease. This maneuver is very sensitive but not specific.
  - *SL ballottement test (shear test/lift test) (Dobyns):* The lunate is firmly stabilized with the thumb and index finger of one hand, while the scaphoid, held with the other hand (thumb on the palmar tuberosity and index on the dorsal proximal pole), is displaced dorsally and palmarly with the other hand. A positive result elicits pain, crepitus, and excessive mobility of the scaphoid.

Imaging

- Stress views, including the clenched-fist view, posteroanterior maximal radial deviation, and posteroanterior maximal ulnar deviation, are useful in the diagnosis of dynamic SL instability.
- Arthroscopic examination has become the standard method of evaluation of interosseous ligamentous injuries. The arthroscopic classification of ligament injuries proposed by Geissler (Table 72-2) is useful in determining treatment options.

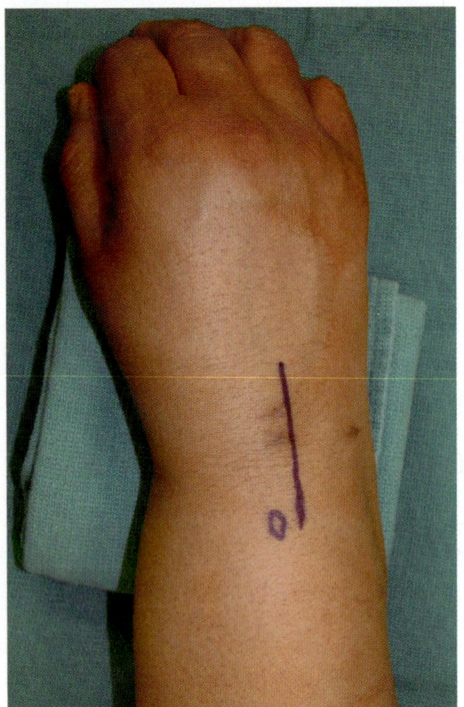

FIGURE 72-1

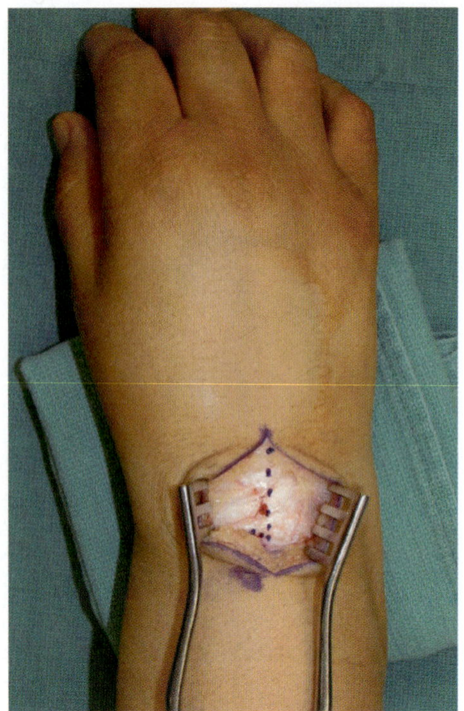

FIGURE 72-2

Surgical Anatomy

- The SL ligament is a C-shaped structure that connects the dorsal, proximal, and volar surfaces of the scaphoid and lunate. Partial SL ligament tears most often involve only the proximal and volar components of the SL interosseous ligament complex. The dorsal ligament is much stronger than its volar counterpart and may resist substantial traumatic torques without yielding.
- The normal kinematics of the SL joint is governed by the SL ligament, a primary stabilizer, and by an envelope of surrounding extrinsic ligaments that act as secondary stabilizers, namely the radioscaphocapitate (RSC), the long and short radiolunate (LRL and SRL) ligaments on the volar side, and the dorsal radiocarpal (DRC) and dorsal intercarpal (DIC) ligaments on the dorsal side.
- When the scaphoid has lost its connections to the lunate, the role of secondary stabilizers is particularly important. Their failure results in the static carpal malalignment.

Exposures

- A 6-cm dorsal longitudinal incision centered over the radiocarpal joint in line with the long finger metacarpal is made (Fig. 72-1). Sharp dissection is carried down to the extensor retinaculum. Skin and subcutaneous tissue flaps are raised on both sides. The third dorsal compartment is identified and does not need to be opened along its entire length. The wrist capsule is opened longitudinally and dissection performed to elevate the second and fourth compartments, such that the second and fourth compartment tendons are maintained within the compartment (Fig. 72-2). This exposes the scaphoid and lunate.
- Figure 72-3 shows a Freer elevator within the SL interval demonstrating a partial rupture of the SL dorsal ligament.

PITFALLS

Care is taken not to injure both branches of the radial sensory nerve.

Avoid dissection along the dorsal ridge portion of the scaphoid to prevent compromise to the blood supply to the proximal pole of the scaphoid.

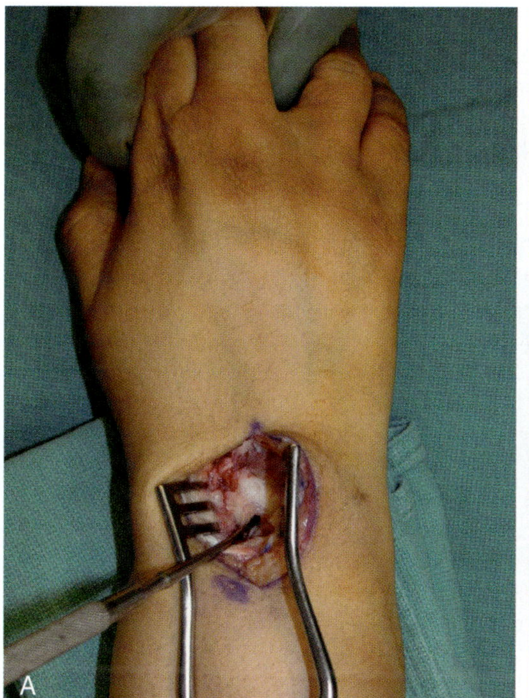

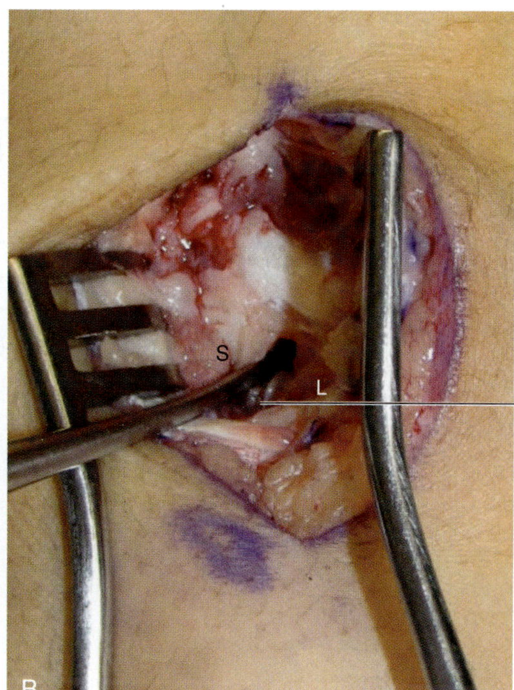

FIGURE 72-3

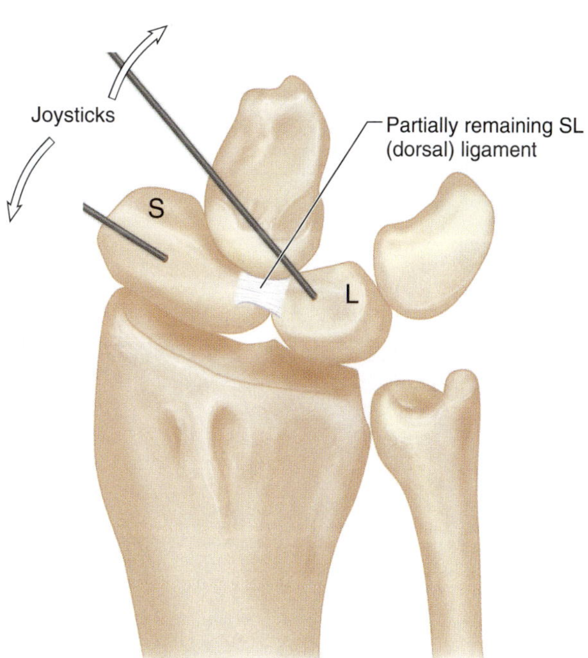

FIGURE 72-4

STEP 1 PEARLS

The scaphoid needs to be extended, and the lunate needs to be flexed. This is done using the joystick K-wires. Directing the scaphoid K-wire proximally and the lunate K-wire distally makes correction of the deformity easier.

Procedure

Step 1: Reduction of Scaphoid and Lunate

- Two 0.045-inch K-wires are placed dorsally into the scaphoid and lunate, respectively, to act as joysticks for reduction of these two bones (Fig. 72-4).

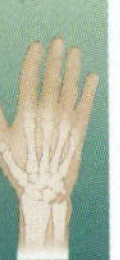

STEP 2 PEARLS

Anatomic reduction should be confirmed fluoroscopically and by direct inspection, with careful evaluation of the SL angle as well as the contours of the radioscaphoid and midcarpal articulations.

STEP 3 PEARLS

A drill hole should be prepared on the dorsal surface of the distal pole of the scaphoid, adjacent to the scaphotrapezial joint, well distal to the scaphoid axis of rotation.

STEP 3 PITFALLS

Care is taken not to injure the vascular pedicle entering the scaphoid at its dorsal ridge (Fig. 72-7).

Step 2: Maintenance of SL Reduction

- While an assistant maintains the scaphoid and lunate in their corrected positions, two K-wires are drilled percutaneously from the radial side of the wrist through the scaphoid into the lunate.
- Remove the joystick K-wires.

Step 3: Make a Drill Hole in the Scaphoid, and Insert a Bone Anchor

- Make a drill hole at the most distal part of the scaphoid (Fig. 72-5).
- A 1.8-mm bone anchor suture (Mitek Mini QuickAnchor or similar) is placed in the drill hole (Fig. 72-6).

Step 4: Secure the Dorsal Capsule to the Scaphoid

- The anchor suture is passed through the dorsal capsule and tied securely to prevent the scaphoid from flexing (Fig. 72-8).

Step 5: Assess Final Fixation

- A final fluoroscopic examination is done to confirm that the lunate is in neutral position and the carpal bones are aligned correctly (Fig. 72-9).

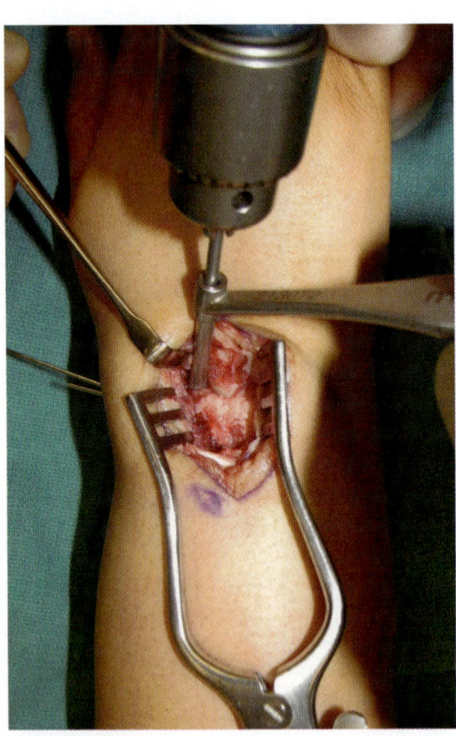

FIGURE 72-5

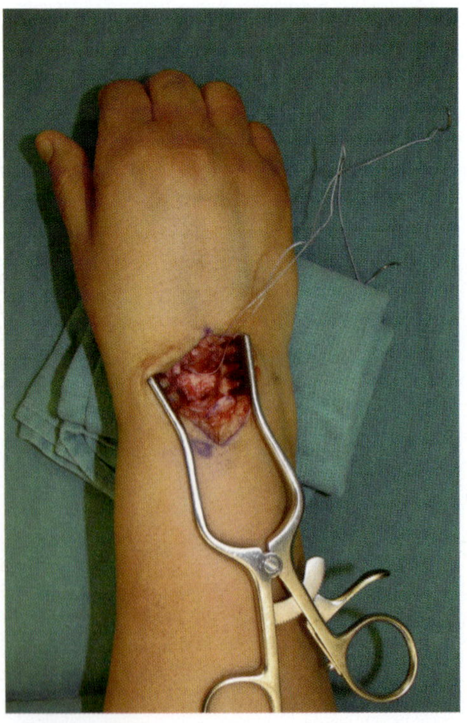

FIGURE 72-6

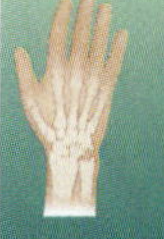

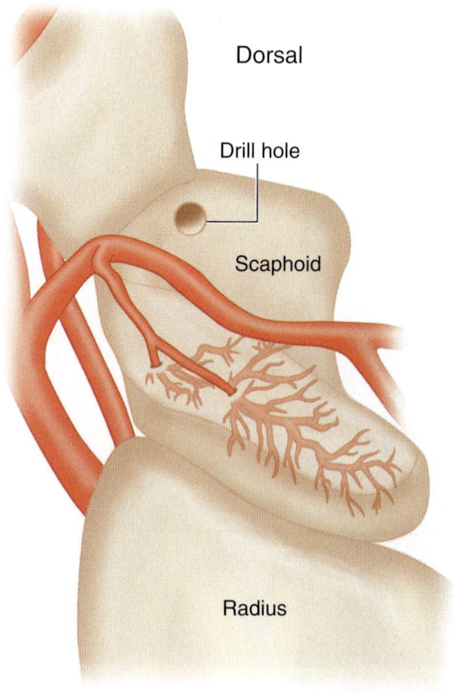

FIGURE 72-7

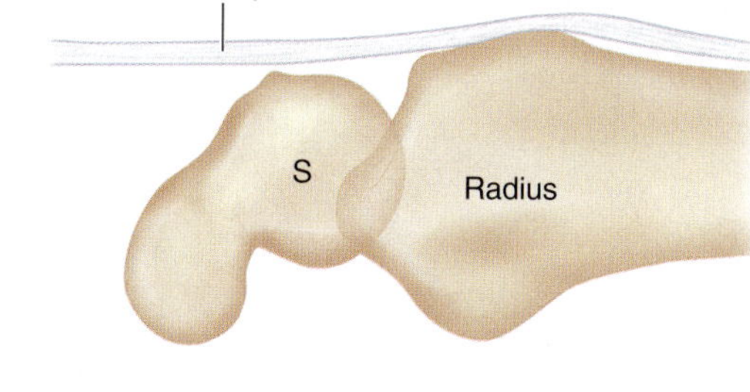

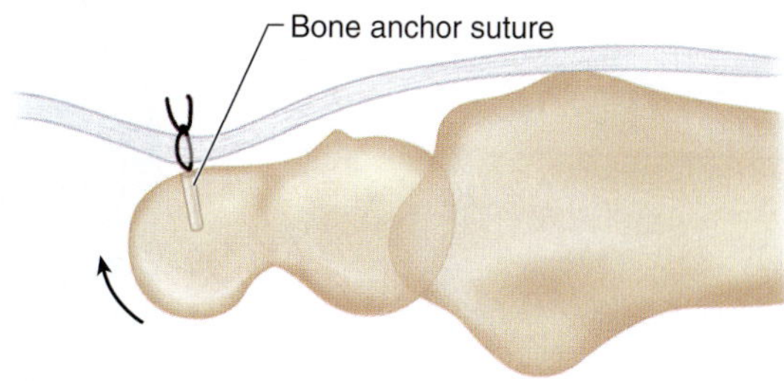

FIGURE 72-8

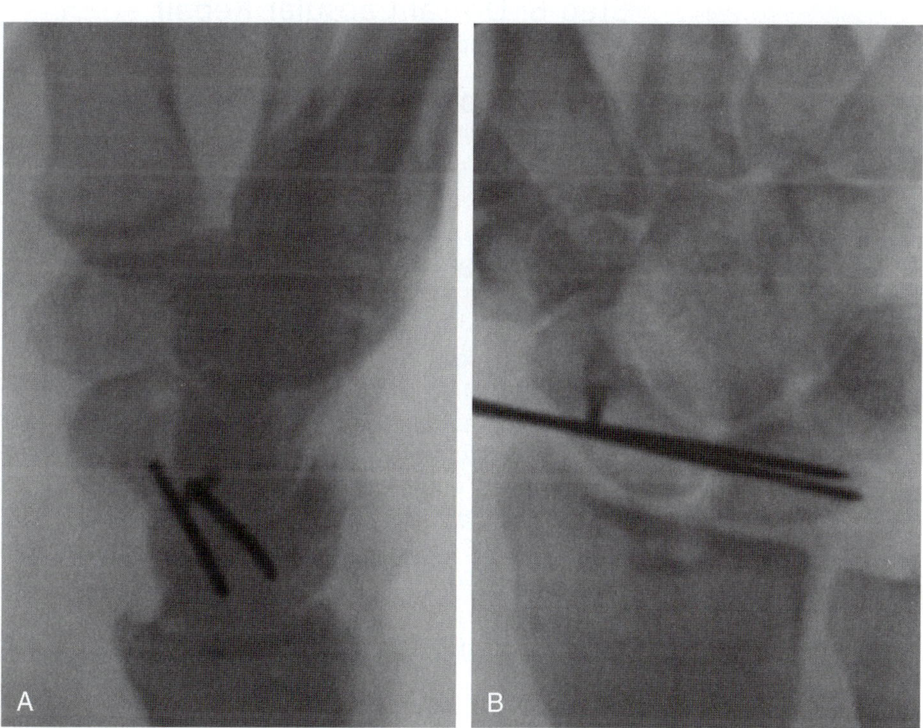

FIGURE 72-9

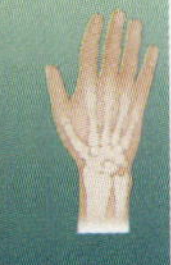

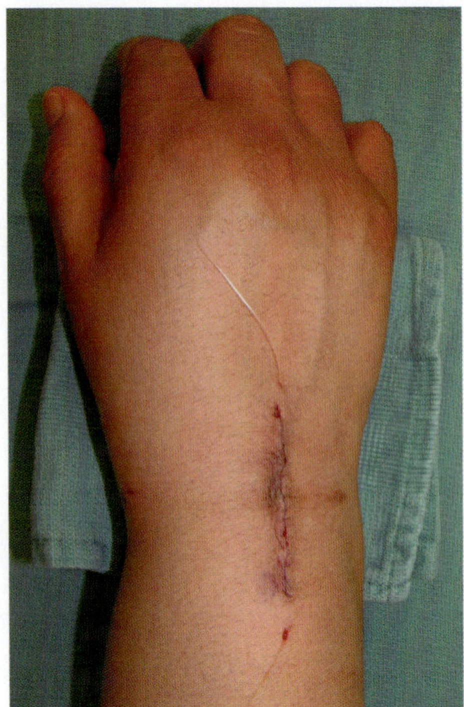

FIGURE 72-10

Step 6: Dorsal Capsular Repair

- The dorsal capsule is repaired using 3-0 Ethibond suture.

Step 7: Closure

- The tourniquet is released, and hemostasis is obtained.
- The extensor retinaculum is then closed using 3-0 Ethibond suture.
- Finally, the skin is closed using 4-0 monocryl suture (Fig. 72-10).

Postoperative Care and Expected Outcomes

- Following surgery, the patient is placed in a volar wrist splint for 8 weeks.
- Ten days after the operation, the wound is examined and sutures are removed.
- The K-wires are removed 6 to 8 weeks after the surgery. The K-wires are often cut under the skin to avoid pin tract infection, which is common when the K-wires are left outside the skin for more than 3 weeks.
- Eight weeks after the surgery, the patient is transitioned to a removable volar splint for an additional 4 weeks, and gentle active wrist range of motion commences.
- Although the wrist's range of motion decreases about 20%, most patients have significant improvement in pain after this procedure.

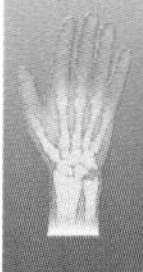

Evidence

Gajendran VK, Peterson B, Slater Jr RR, Szabo RM. Long-term outcomes of dorsal intercarpal ligament capsulodesis for chronic scapholunate dissociation. *J Hand Surg [Am]*. 2007;32:1323-1333.

The authors reviewed the patients undergoing dorsal intercarpal ligament capsulodesis (DILC) for chronic (>6 weeks), flexible, static SLD. Only patients with follow-up evaluation of greater than 60 months were included. Physical examination, radiographs, and validated outcome instruments were used to evaluate the patients. Twenty-one patients (22 wrists) met the inclusion criteria. Fifteen of 21 patients (16 wrists) were available for follow-up evaluation. Average follow-up period was 86 months. Physical examination revealed average wrist flexion and extension of 50 degrees and 55 degrees, respectively; radial and ulnar deviation of 17 degrees and 36 degrees, respectively; and grip strength of 43 kg. Disabilities of the Arm, Shoulder and Hand; Short Form-12; and Mayo wrist scores averaged 19, 78, and 78, respectively. Radiographs revealed an average SL angle and gap of 62 degrees and 3.5 mm, respectively. Eight of the 16 wrists in the study demonstrated arthritic changes on radiographs. The authors concluded that the DILC does not consistently prevent radiographic deterioration and the development of arthrosis in the long term; however, the level of functionality and patient satisfaction remained relatively high in 58% of their patients, suggesting a lack of correlation between the radiographic findings and development of arthrosis and the functional outcomes and patient satisfaction. (Level IV evidence)

Moran SL, Cooney WP, Berger RA, Strickland J. Capsulodesis for the treatment of chronic scapholunate instability. *J Hand Surg [Am]*. 2005;30:16-23.

The authors reviewed retrospectively the intermediate-term results of dorsal capsulodesis for cases of chronic SLD. Patients had to have a minimum follow-up period of 2 years for inclusion in the study. Thirty-one patients were identified with isolated chronic SLD. Of the 31 patients, 18 had dynamic carpal instability, and 13 had static carpal instability. The time from injury to surgery averaged 20 months. The follow-up period averaged 54 months (range, 24 to 96). All patients underwent a dorsal capsulodesis procedure using either a Blatt or Mayo technique. Results were reviewed clinically and radiologically. Static and dynamic groups were compared with a Student t *test. Results showed a 20% decrease in wrist motion after capsulodesis and no improvement in grip strength after surgery. Most patients had improvement in pain, but only two patients were completely pain free. Radiographically, the SL gap and SL angle increased over time. There was no statistical difference in overall wrist motion, grip strength, or wrist score between the dynamic and static groups. The time to surgery and age had no significant effect on overall outcome. The authors concluded that the dorsal capsulodesis provided pain relief for patients with both dynamic and static SL instability. Although pain was improved, it was not completely resolved in most cases. From a radiographic perspective, dorsal capsulodesis did not provide maintenance of carpal alignment in cases of chronic SL dissociation. (Level IV evidence)*

Wintman BI, Gelberman RH, Katz JN. Dynamic scapholunate instability: results of operative treatment with dorsal capsulodesis. *J Hand Surg [Am]*. 1995;20:971-979.

The authors presented 19 patients who underwent 20 dorsal capsulodesis procedures for dynamic SL instability. Seventeen patients (18 wrists) were evaluated by a questionnaire and physical examination after a mean postoperative follow-up period of 34 months. The diagnosis was based on a combination of characteristic symptoms of SL instability and physical findings consisting of dorsal wrist tenderness at the SL interval and a positive scaphoid shift test. Following surgery, a significant decrease was noted in symptoms of pain and clunking. Functional status was improved postoperatively; the most significant gains were seen in opening jars, sweeping, shoveling, and throwing. Fifteen of 17 patients returned to their original occupations, although 7 of those who returned to their original occupations did so with some restrictions. Objective evaluation by physical examination revealed a significant improvement in wrist stability as determined by the scaphoid shift test, and an average loss of 12 degrees of flexion. Fifteen of 17 patients (16 of 18 wrists) stated that they would undergo the surgery again if faced with the same choice. The authors concluded that dorsal radioscaphoid capsulodesis of the wrist in patients with dynamic SL instability provides substantial improvement over preoperative status. (Level IV evidence)

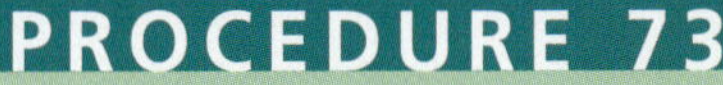
PROCEDURE 73

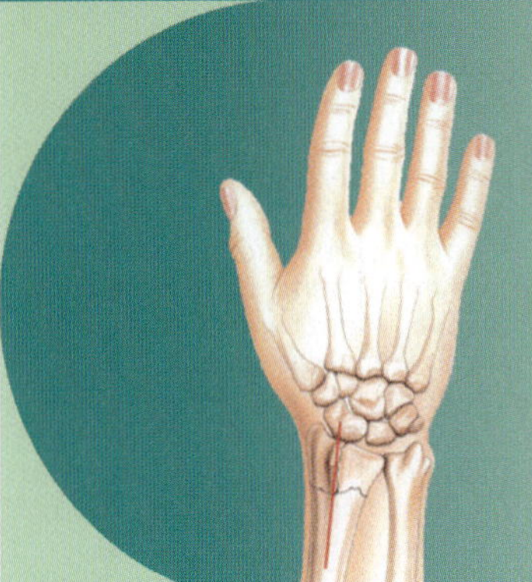

Scapholunate Ligament Reconstruction Using a Flexor Carpi Radialis Tendon Graft

Shimpei Ono, Sandeep J. Sebastin, and Kevin C. Chung

See Video 54: Scapholunate Ligament Reconstruction Using the Flexor Carpi Radialis Tendon

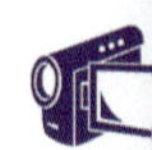

Indications

- Scapholunate (SL) dissociation associated with carpal malalignment (dorsal intercalated segmental instability [DISI]) without osteoarthritic change, particularly in radioscaphoid joint.

Examination/Imaging

Clinical Examination

- Patients complain of radial-sided wrist pain especially with loading activities, weakness of grip, and swelling.
- Tenderness is found in the radial snuffbox or over the SL interval just distal to the Lister tubercle.
- Discomfort is reported at extremes of wrist extension and radial deviation.
- The scaphoid shift test (Watson test) may be positive in SL dissociation. The examiner places four fingers behind the radius. The thumb is placed on the scaphoid tuberosity, and the other hand is used to move the wrist passively from ulnar to radial deviation. In ulnar deviation, the scaphoid is extended, whereas in radial deviation, the scaphoid is flexed. Pressure on the tuberosity while the wrist is moved from ulnar deviation to radial deviation prevents the scaphoid from flexing. In such circumstances, if the SL ligaments are completely insufficient or torn, the proximal pole subluxates dorsally out of the scaphoid fossa, inducing pain on the dorsoradial aspect of the wrist. When pressure is released, a typical clunk may occur, indicating an abrupt self-reduction of the scaphoid back into its normal position (Fig. 73-1). This test is painful for the patient and should be done selectively, when obvious SL separation is not seen on radiograph.
- A positive SL ballottement test may be elicited. The examiner holds the patient's scaphoid between the thumb (placed over the scaphoid tuberosity on the palmar side) and index finger (placed over the proximal pole of the scaphoid on the dorsum) of one hand, while holding the lunate between the thumb and index of the other hand. The examiner then attempts to move the scaphoid and lunate in opposite directions. If the test induces pain, this test is positive, and the patient may have SL instability (Fig. 73-2).

Imaging

- A gap greater than 3 mm between the scaphoid and lunate on a standard posteroanterior (PA) view indicates SL dissociation. The presence of a flexed scaphoid on a PA view (signet ring sign) (Fig. 73-3A) and an extended lunate on a lateral view is suggestive of SL dissociation with associated carpal malalignment (DISI) (Fig. 73-3B).

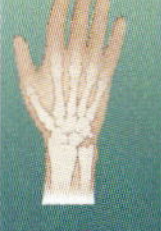

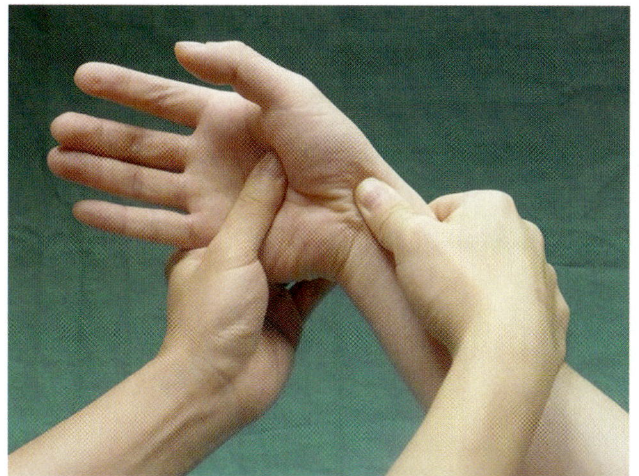

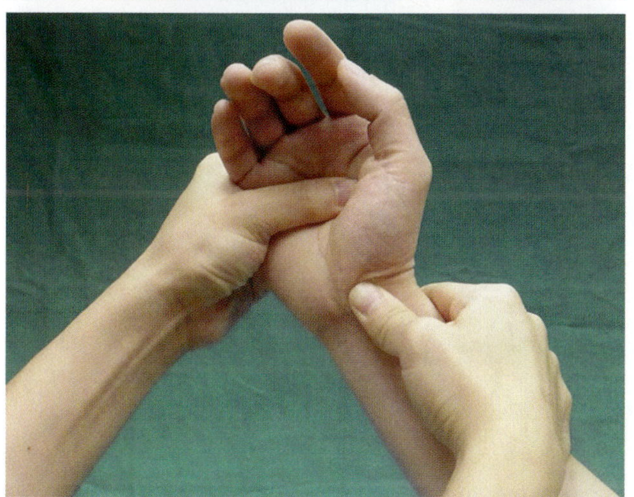

FIGURE 73-1

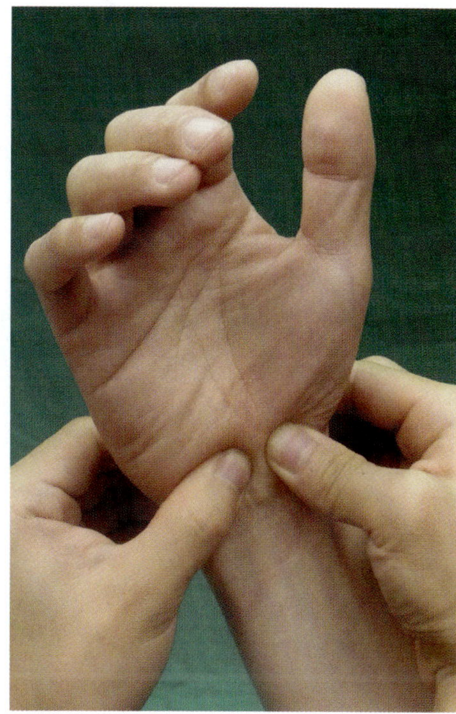

FIGURE 73-2

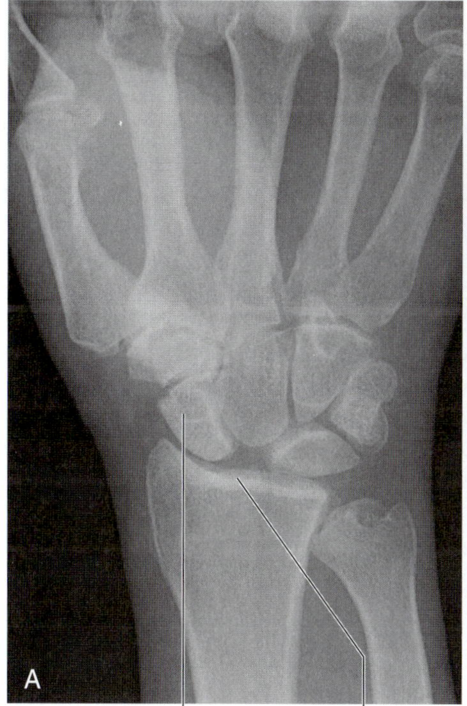

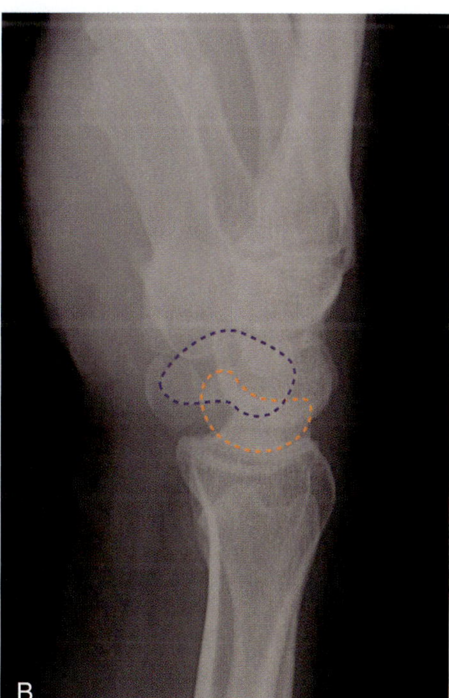

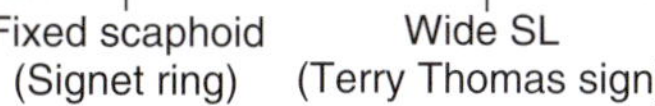

FIGURE 73-3

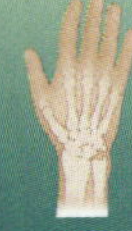

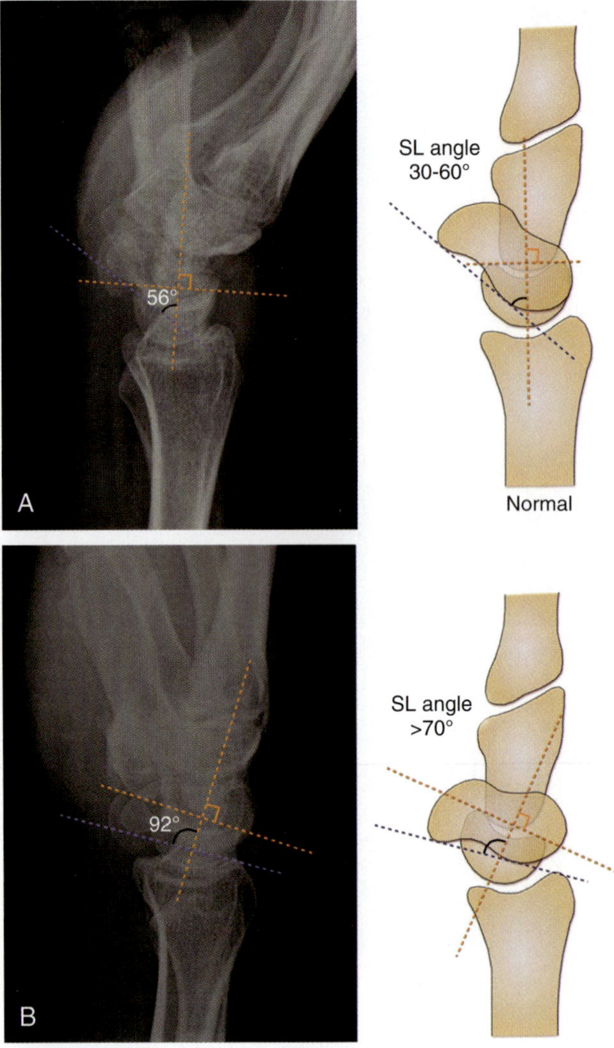

FIGURE 73-4

- The normal SL angle ranges from 30 to 60 degrees (Fig. 73-4A). An SL angle greater than 70° indicates DISI (Fig. 73-4B). The SL angle is formed by intersection of the scaphoid axis (a line joining the most palmar point on the distal pole with the most palmar point on the proximal pole of the scaphoid) and lunate axis (a line drawn perpendicular to the line joining the most distal palmar and dorsal points of the lunate).
- The presence of osteoarthritic changes involving the radiocarpal or midcarpal joints is a contraindication for ligament reconstruction. Figure 73-5 shows radiographs of a patient with bilateral SL dissociation. He has osteoarthritic changes involving the radial styloid and radioscaphoid joint on the left side.
- Magnetic resonance imaging is often valuable to define other injuries and disorders that may affect the surgical outcome.
- Arthroscopy can be used to determine the extent of SL ligament disruption and the presence of arthritis.

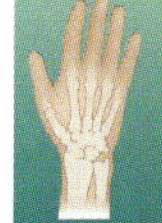

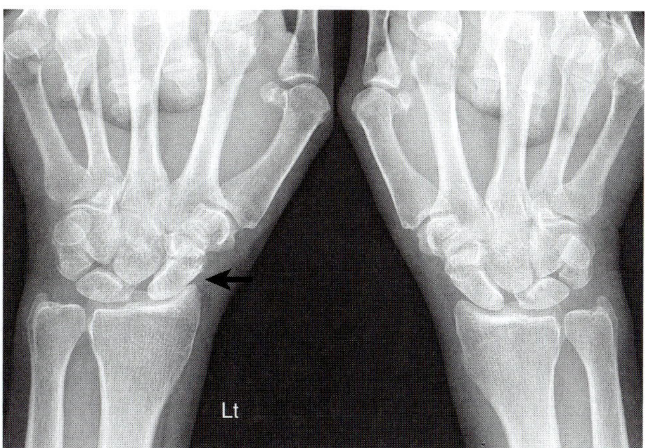

FIGURE 73-5

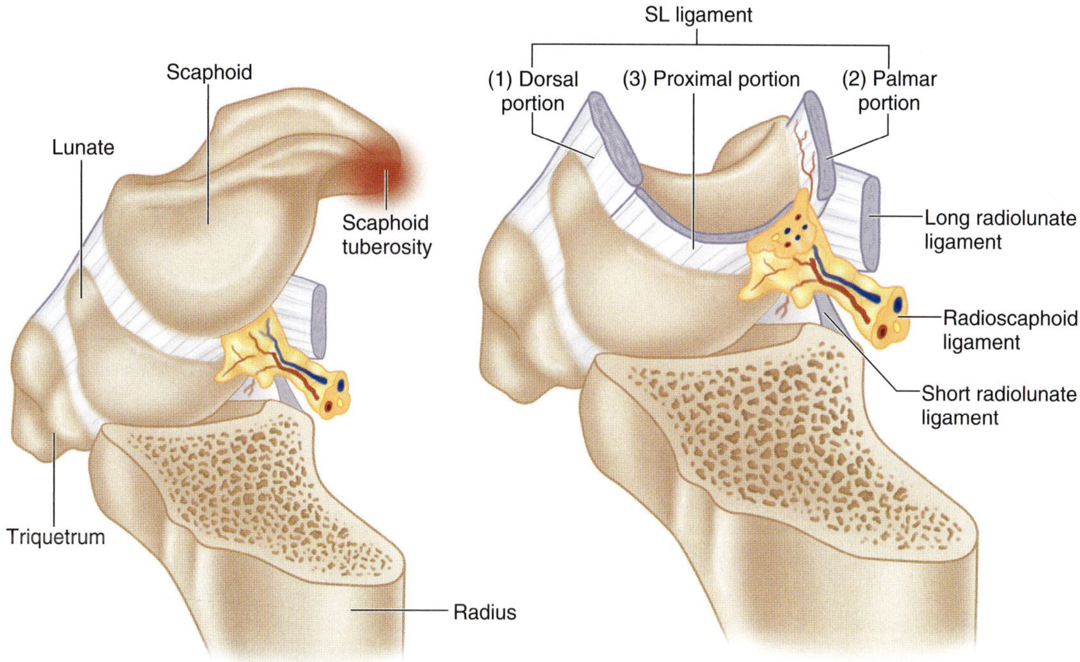

FIGURE 73-6

Surgical Anatomy

- The SL ligament is a C-shaped structure that connects the dorsal, proximal, and volar surfaces of the scaphoid and lunate. It has three portions: (1) the dorsal portion, which has the highest rupture strength and is responsible for rotational and translational restraint; (2) the proximal membranous portion; and (3) the volar portion (Fig. 73-6).

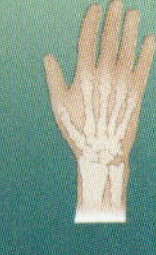

Exposures

Dorsal

- An 8-cm longitudinal dorsal wrist incision centered over the Lister tubercle is made (Fig. 73-7).
- The extensor retinaculum over the third compartment is opened, and the extensor pollicis longus (EPL) is retracted radially to expose the dorsal wrist capsule.
- The dorsal capsule is then opened through a longitudinal incision to visualize the SL interval (Fig. 73-8).

Volar

- Three 1-cm incisions along the course of flexor carpi radialis (FCR) are made. Another oblique incision is made over the scaphoid tuberosity (Fig. 73-9).

PEARLS

Some authors recommend a ligament-sparing capsulotomy to expose the carpal bones. Here the incision is made in line with the fibers of the dorsal intercarpal and radiocarpal ligaments, and a trapezoid capsular flap is raised (Fig. 73-10).

PITFALLS

The branches of the superficial radial nerve and the palmar cutaneous branch of the median nerve should be identified and protected.

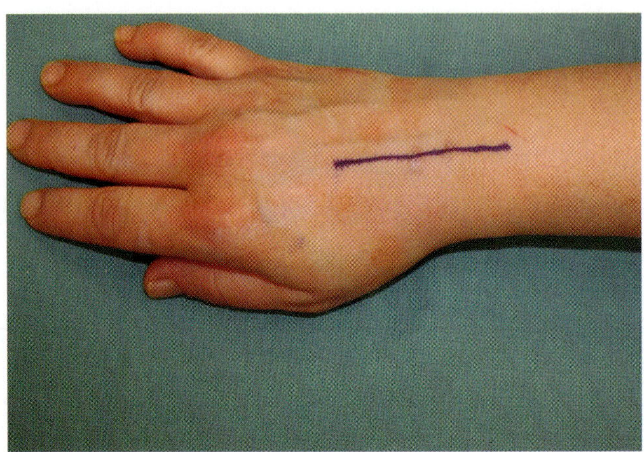

FIGURE 73-7

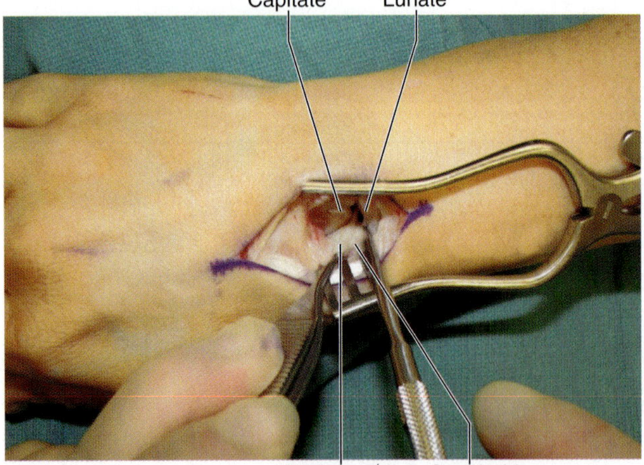

FIGURE 73-8

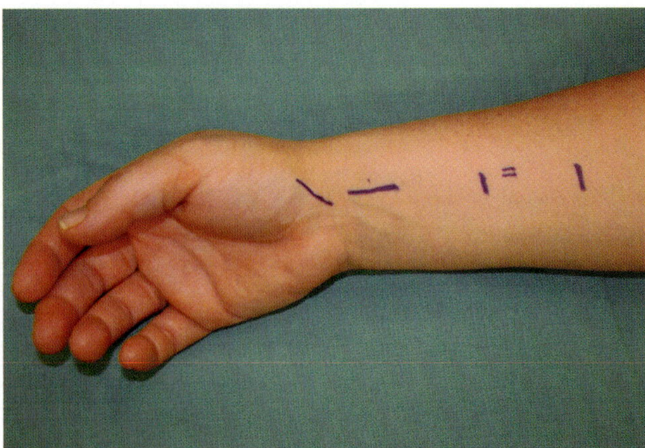

FIGURE 73-9

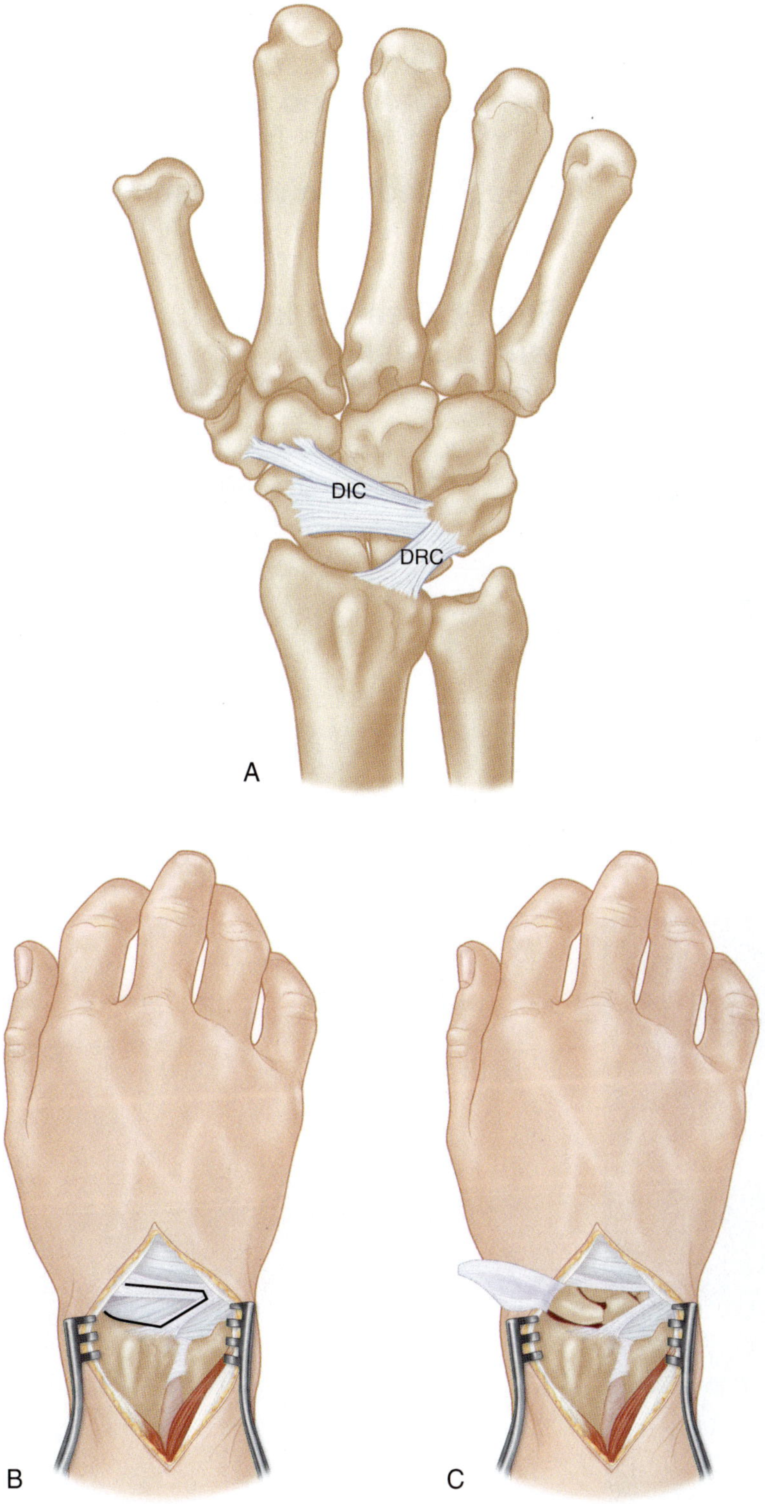

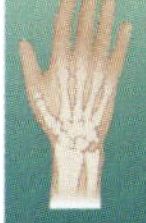

FIGURE 73-10

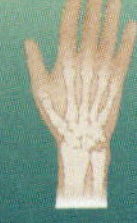

Procedure

Step 1: Excise Scar Tissue between the Scaphoid and Lunate

- The scar tissue between the scaphoid and lunate is excised.

Step 2: Reduction of Scaphoid and Lunate

- Two 0.045-inch K-wires are placed dorsally into the scaphoid and lunate, respectively, to act as joysticks for reduction of these two bones (Fig. 73-11).

STEP 2 PEARLS

Make certain that the joystick K-wires engage the bone well and do not pull out. Sometimes using threaded wires may ensure more secure purchase of the carpal bones. The wires must be drilled away from the anticipated tunnel that will contain the FCR tendon slip.

The scaphoid is flexed, and the lunate is extended. To correct the DISI, one needs to extend the scaphoid and flex the lunate. This is done using the joystick K-wires. Directing the scaphoid K-wire proximally and the lunate K-wire distally makes correction of the deformity easier.

Step 3: Create a Bone Tunnel within Scaphoid

- A K-wire is passed from the scaphoid tuberosity and exits on the dorsum of the scaphoid.
- This K-wire is used to guide a 2.7-mm cannulated drill from the dorsum to the palmar side, and a hole is made in the scaphoid (Fig. 73-12).

STEP 4 PEARLS

The FCR rotates 90 degrees within the sheath; it is important to follow the fibers so that the tendon is not inadvertently transected. One should not slide the scissors through the tendon fibers but rather cut along the fibers to maintain the integrity of the tendon.

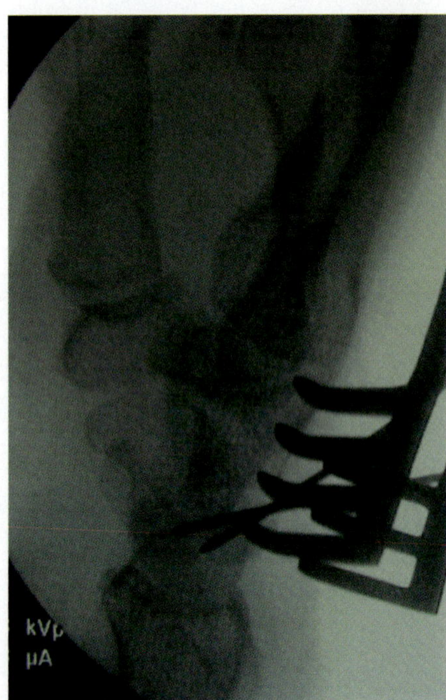

FIGURE 73-11

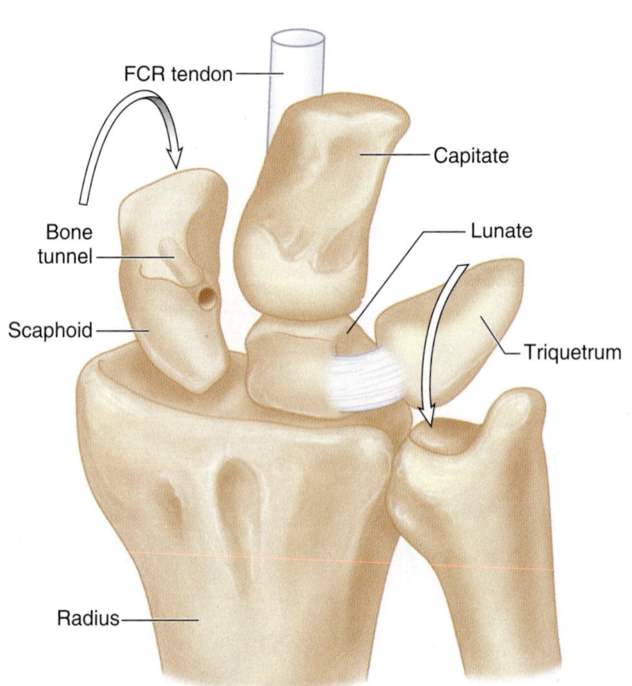

FIGURE 73-12

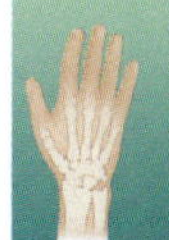

Step 4: Harvest a Strip of Distally Based FCR

- A distally based 3-mm wide and 8- to 10-cm long strip of FCR is harvested from the radial aspect of the tendon (Figs. 73-13 and 73-14).

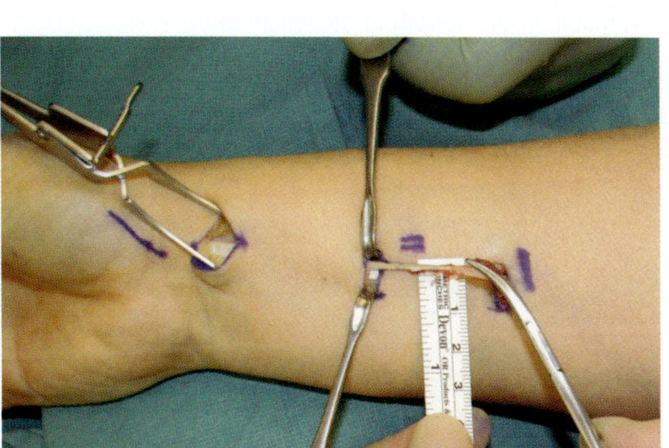

FIGURE 73-13

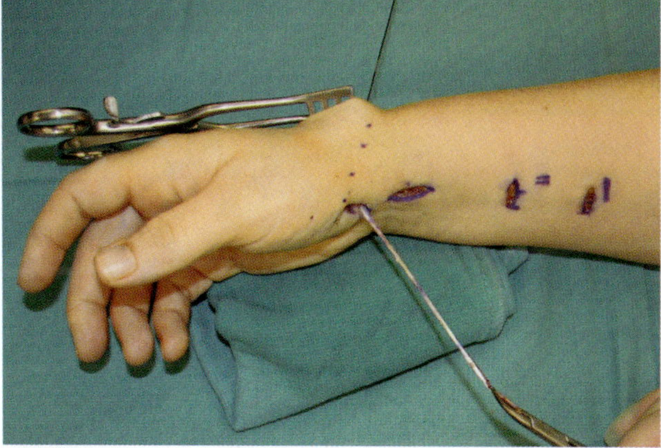

FIGURE 73-14

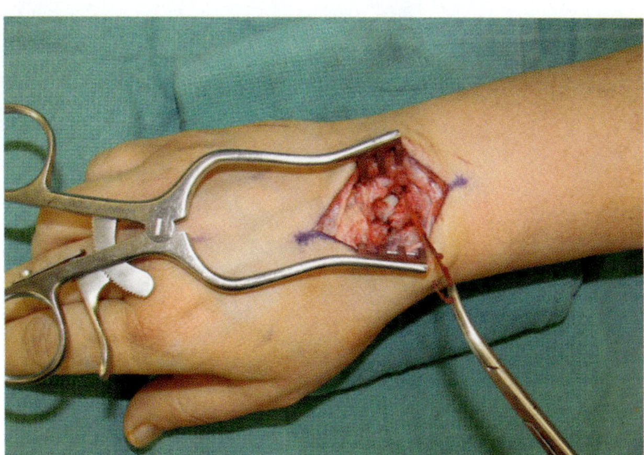

FIGURE 73-15

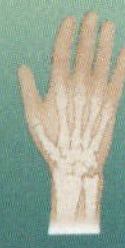

Step 5: Pass the FCR through the Scaphoid Tunnel

- A grasping suture is placed at the cut end of the distally based FCR and passed through the scaphoid tunnel from volar to dorsal (Fig. 73-15).

Step 6: Reduce SL Interval

- The scaphoid and lunate are now reduced using the previously placed joystick K-wires, and the reduction is maintained by passing fresh K-wires across the SL and scaphocapitate joints (Fig. 73-16).
- The reduction of the SL joint is confirmed using fluoroscopy, and the joystick K-wires are removed.

Step 7: Secure the FCR to the Lunate

- A shallow trough is made on the dorsum of the lunate using a bur.
- The FCR graft is secured in the midportion of this trough using a 1.8-mm bone anchor suture (Mitek Mini QuickAnchor or similar) (Fig. 73-17).
- The remaining portion of the FCR graft is passed through a slit in the distal portion of the dorsal radiotriquetral ligament and sutured back to itself over the lunate (Fig. 73-18).

STEP 5 PEARLS

A fine 25-gauge wire can be passed through the tunnel, and the suture placed at the end of the tendon graft is tied to the bent tip of the wire to retrieve the suture through the tunnel. Then the suture can be pulled gently through the tunnel, taking the tendon graft along with it.

STEP 5 PITFALLS

It is better to harvest a narrow strip of FCR. Forcing a wide strip through the scaphoid bone tunnel is risky and may fracture the scaphoid.

STEP 6 PEARLS

The joystick K-wires can only correct the flexion-extension deformity of the scaphoid and lunate. To reduce the gap between these two bones, we use a bone reduction clamp or towel clip applied on the dorsal surface of these two bones to bring them together (see Fig. 73-16).

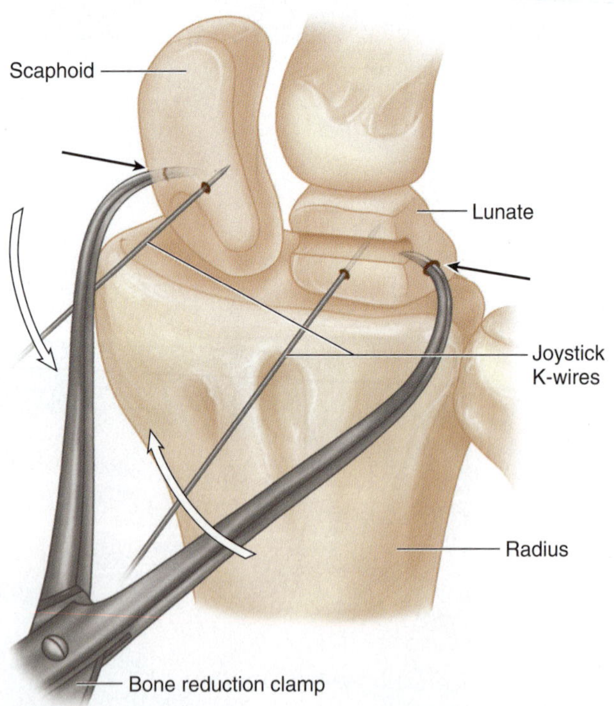

FIGURE 73-16

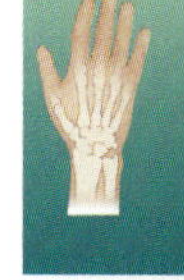

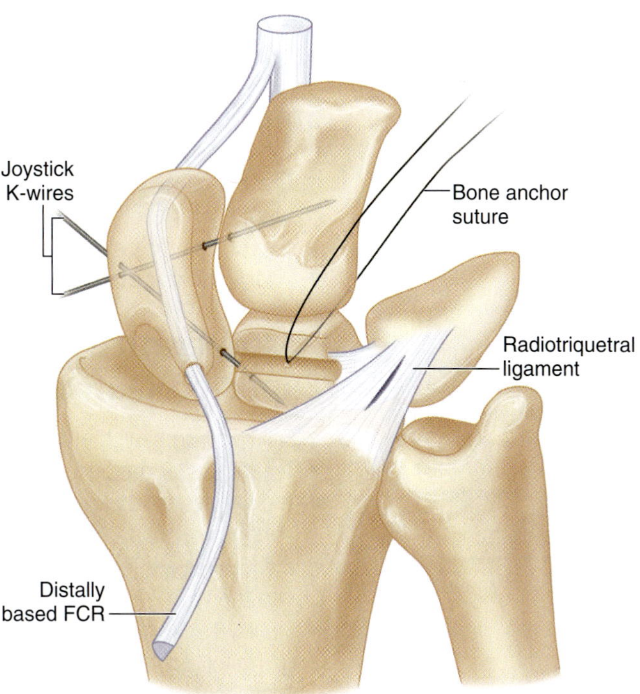

FIGURE 73-17

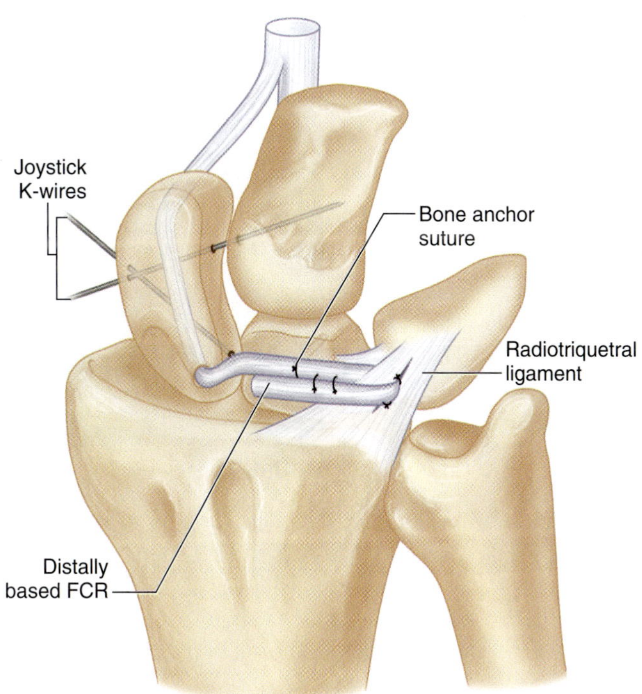

FIGURE 73-18

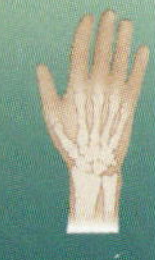

Step 8: Repair of Dorsal Wrist Capsule

- The dorsal capsule is repaired using 3-0 Ethibond suture.

Step 9: Closure

- The tourniquet is released, and hemostasis is obtained.
- The EPL is transposed dorsal to the extensor retinaculum to avoid ischemic rupture of the EPL, which may occur with postoperative swelling in the EPL sheath. The extensor retinaculum is then closed using 3-0 Ethibond suture.
- Finally, the skin is closed using 4-0 PDS suture.

PEARLS

In therapy, initial restriction of radial and ulnar deviation and concentration on the dart thrower's motion lessens the force on the reconstructed SL ligament.

Postoperative Care and Expected Outcomes

- Following surgery, the patient is placed in a volar wrist splint for 8 weeks.
- Ten days after the operation, the wound is examined and sutures are removed.
- The K-wires are removed 6 to 8 weeks after the surgery (Fig. 73-19). The K-wires are often cut under the skin to avoid pin tract infection, which is common when the K-wires are left outside the skin for more than 3 weeks. Pin tract infection into the wrist is a disastrous complication.
- Eight weeks after the surgery, the patient is transitioned to a removable volar splint for an additional 4 weeks, and gentle active wrist range of motion commences.

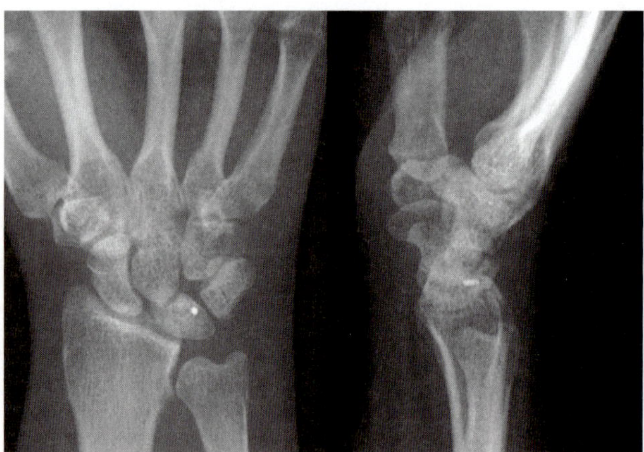

FIGURE 73-19

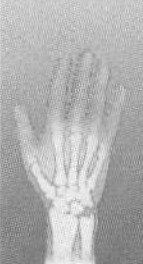

Evidence

Chabas JF, Gay A, Valenti D, et al. Results of the modified Brunelli tenodesis for treatment of scapholunate instability: a retrospective study of 19 patients. *J Hand Surg [Am]*. 2008;33:1469-1477.

The authors conducted a retrospective analysis of 19 patients who underwent a modified Brunelli tenodesis. After surgery, 15 patients had no to mild pain with a mean visual analogue scale score of 3 out of 10. The average wrist motion was 50 degrees of extension, 41 degrees of flexion, 24 degrees of radial deviation, and 29 degrees of ulnar deviation (75%, 73%, 68%, and 86% of the uninvolved wrists, respectively). The grip strength was 78% of the uninvolved wrists. One patient progressed to stage 2 scapholunate advanced collapse. Ligament reconstruction using the FCR gave satisfactory results to correct reducible chronic SL instability without osteoarthritis. This repair technique achieved a relatively pain-free wrist, with acceptable grip strength and normal SL distance but with a loss in the arc of motion and a loss of correction of SL angle. (Level IV evidence)

van den Abbeele KLS, Loh YC, Stanley JK, Trail IA. Early results of a modified Brunelli procedure for scapholunate instability. *J Hand Surg [Br]*. 1998;23:258-261.

The authors introduced a modification of the Brunelli procedure. Instead of anchoring the tendon to the dorsum of the radius, which restricted radiocarpal motion, they anchored the distal end of the tendon graft to the dorsal lunotriquetral ligament. Twenty-two patients with a diagnosis of SL instability underwent this procedure. The authors followed the patients for an average of 9 months. Seventeen patients had relief of pain with an improvement in grip strength. The range of motion was reduced in extension and flexion, remained unchanged for radial deviation, and improved for ulnar deviation. The radiologic appearance of dynamic or static SL instability did not change after the procedure. Most patients (17 of 22) felt subjective improvement and stated that they would have the operation again. The short-term results were encouraging for most patients, and the authors felt that more long-term follow-up was needed before recommending the procedure. (Level IV evidence)

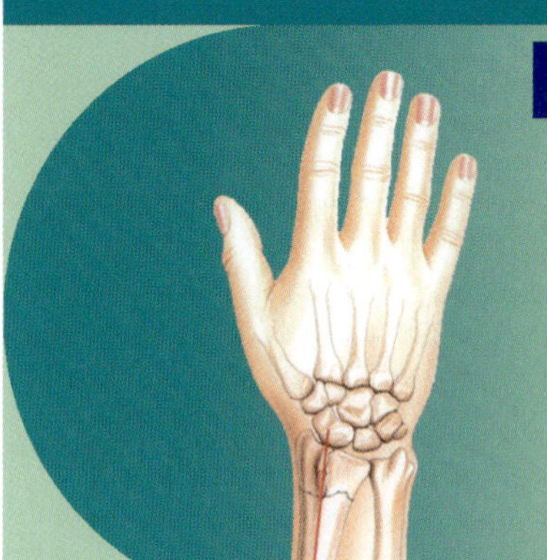

PROCEDURE 74

Lunotriquetral Ligament Reconstruction Using a Slip of the Extensor Carpi Ulnaris Tendon

Shimpei Ono, Sandeep J. Sebastin, and Kevin C. Chung

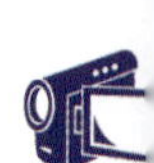

See Video 55: Lunotriquetral Ligament Reconstruction Using the Extensor Carpi Ulnaris Tendon

Indications

- Symptomatic lunotriquetral (LT) dissociation without arthritis

Examination/Imaging

Clinical Examination

- Patients with LT instability present with ulnar-sided wrist pain. Other causes of ulnar-sided wrist pain include ulnar impaction syndrome, extensor carpi ulnaris (ECU) subluxation, distal radioulnar joint (DRUJ) instability, triangular fibrocartilage complex (TFCC) injuries, pisotriquetral arthritis, and hook of hamate fractures.
- The following clinical tests can help differentiate LT instability from other causes of ulnar-sided wrist pain.
  - *LT compression test:* A radially directed pressure over the triquetrum often elicits pain in patients with LT ligament instability (Fig. 74-1).
  - *LT ballottement test:* The lunate is stabilized with the thumb and index finger of one hand, whereas the triquetrum and pisiform are displaced dorsally and palmarly with the other hand. A positive result elicits pain, crepitus, and excessive displaceability of the joint (Fig. 74-2).

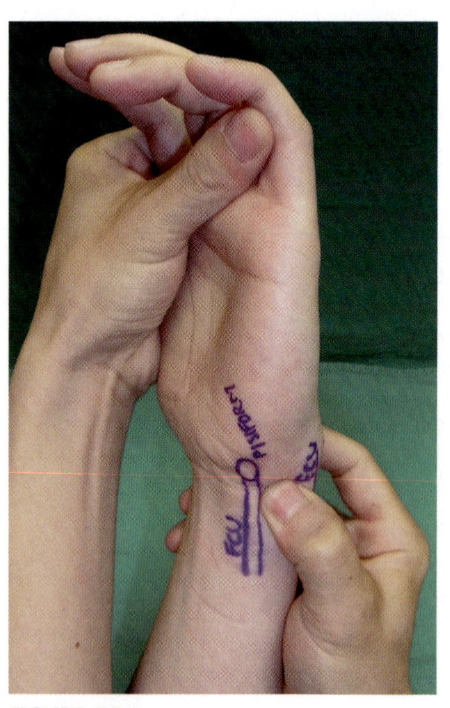

FIGURE 74-1

Imaging

- A posteroanterior radiograph may show a step-off between the lunate and triquetrum and the disruption of the normal convex arc of the proximal carpal row (Gilula line). Unlike the scapholunate dissociation, a gap in the LT interval is rarely seen in patients with LT instability.
- Plain radiographs may show a volar intercalated segment instability (VISI) deformity, marked by volar tilting of the lunate (Fig. 74-3).
- Wrist arthroscopy is useful to diagnose an LT ligament tear when plain radiographs are normal (Fig. 74-4). The LT interosseous space is tightly closed in normal subjects, whereas in LT dissociations, the space can be opened with the probe, and a gap can be seen between the involved carpals from the midcarpal portal.

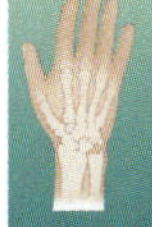

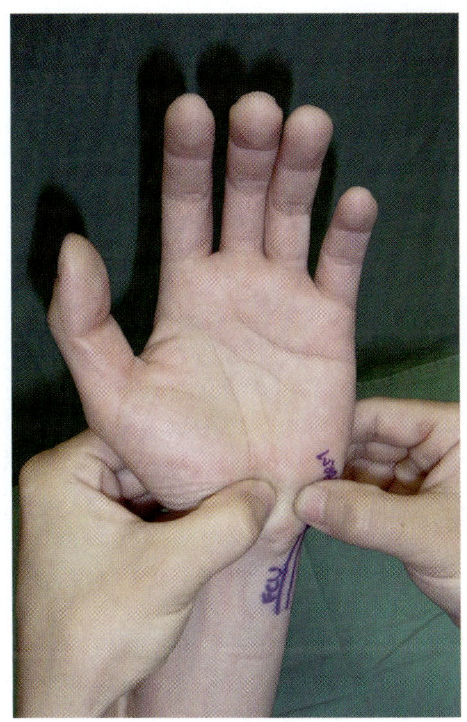

FIGURE 74-2

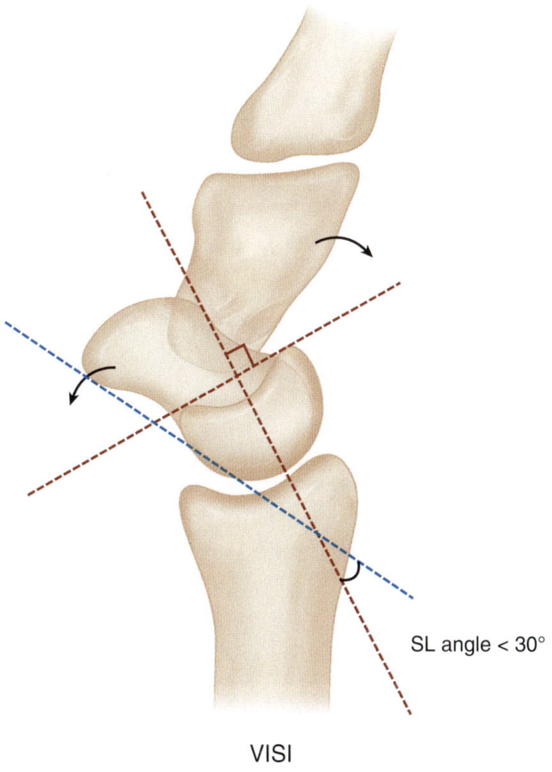

FIGURE 74-3

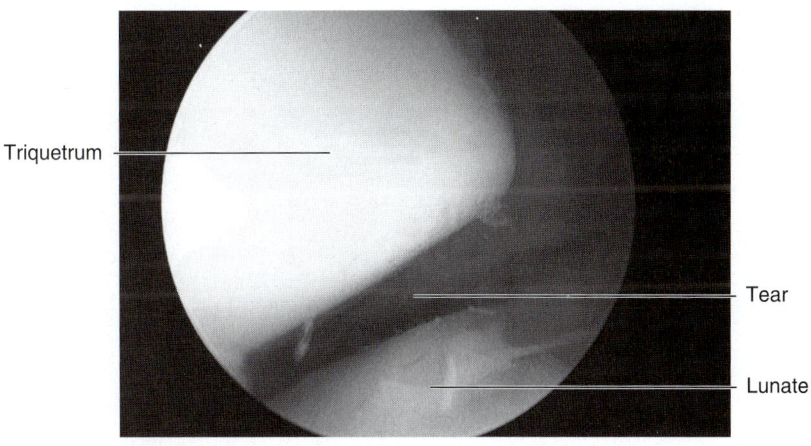

FIGURE 74-4

Surgical Anatomy

- The LT ligament is C shaped, spanning the (1) dorsal, (2) proximal, and (3) palmar edges of the joint surfaces. The palmar region is the thickest and strongest. It is the primary stabilizer of the LT joint. Additional supports of the LT joint include the ulnocarpal (ulnolunate, ulnocapitate, and ulnotriquetral ligaments), midcarpal (triquetrohamate and triquetrocapitate ligaments), and dorsal carpal (dorsal intercarpal and radiotriquetral) ligaments (Figs. 74-5 and 74-6).

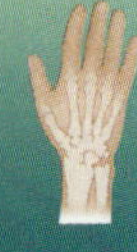

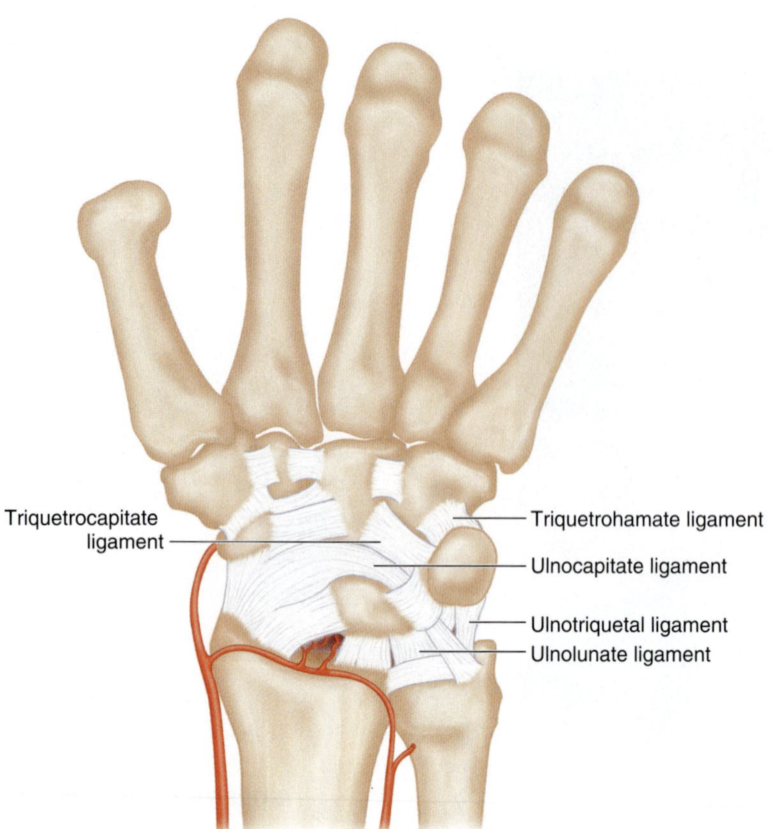

FIGURE 74-5

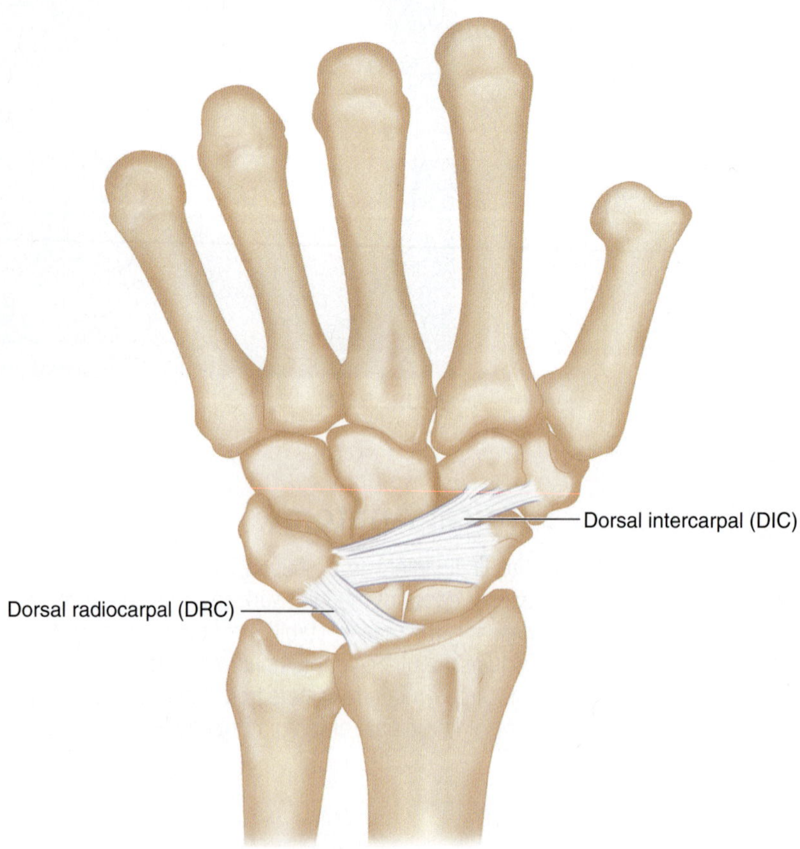

FIGURE 74-6

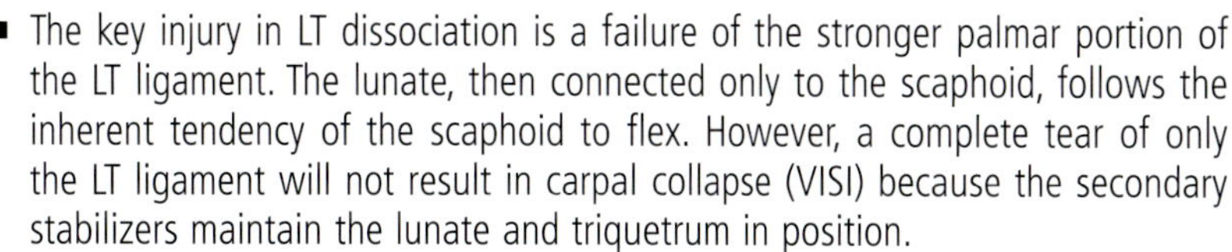

- The key injury in LT dissociation is a failure of the stronger palmar portion of the LT ligament. The lunate, then connected only to the scaphoid, follows the inherent tendency of the scaphoid to flex. However, a complete tear of only the LT ligament will not result in carpal collapse (VISI) because the secondary stabilizers maintain the lunate and triquetrum in position.

Exposures

Dorsal

- A 6-cm longitudinal incision centered over the radiocarpal joint is made over the dorsal wrist between the fourth and fifth compartments (Fig. 74-7).
- The wrist capsule is opened through a longitudinal incision. A longitudinal incision is also quite suitable for later imbrication of the ulnar wrist capsule over the LT ligament repair.
- Figure 74-8 shows a Freer elevator in the LT interval demonstrating a complete rupture of the LT ligament.
- The ECU tendon is identified in the proximal portion of this incision.

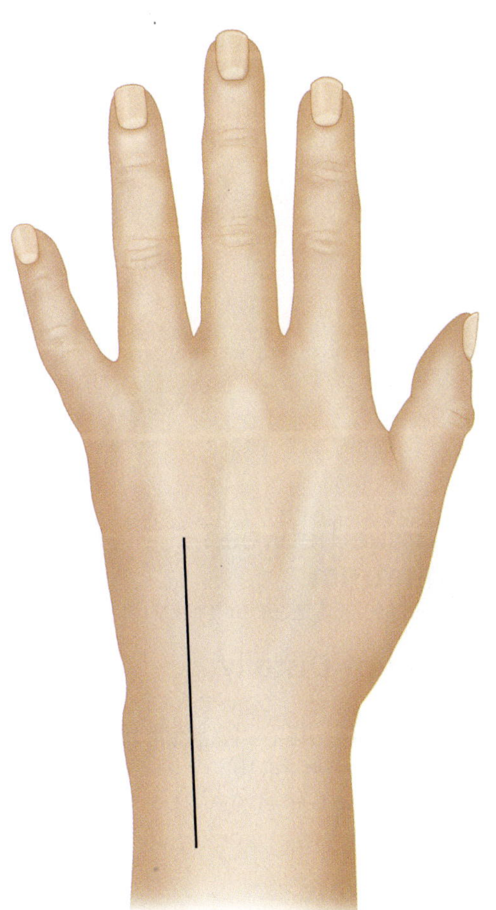

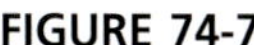

FIGURE 74-7

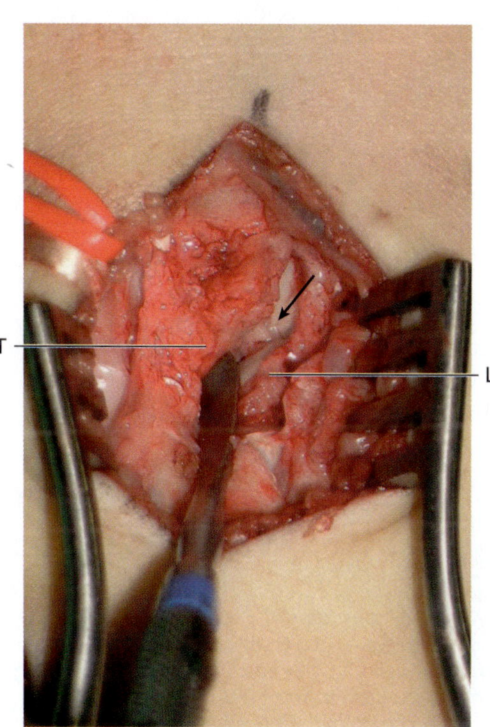

FIGURE 74-8

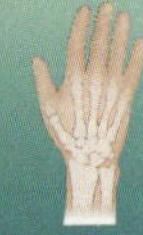

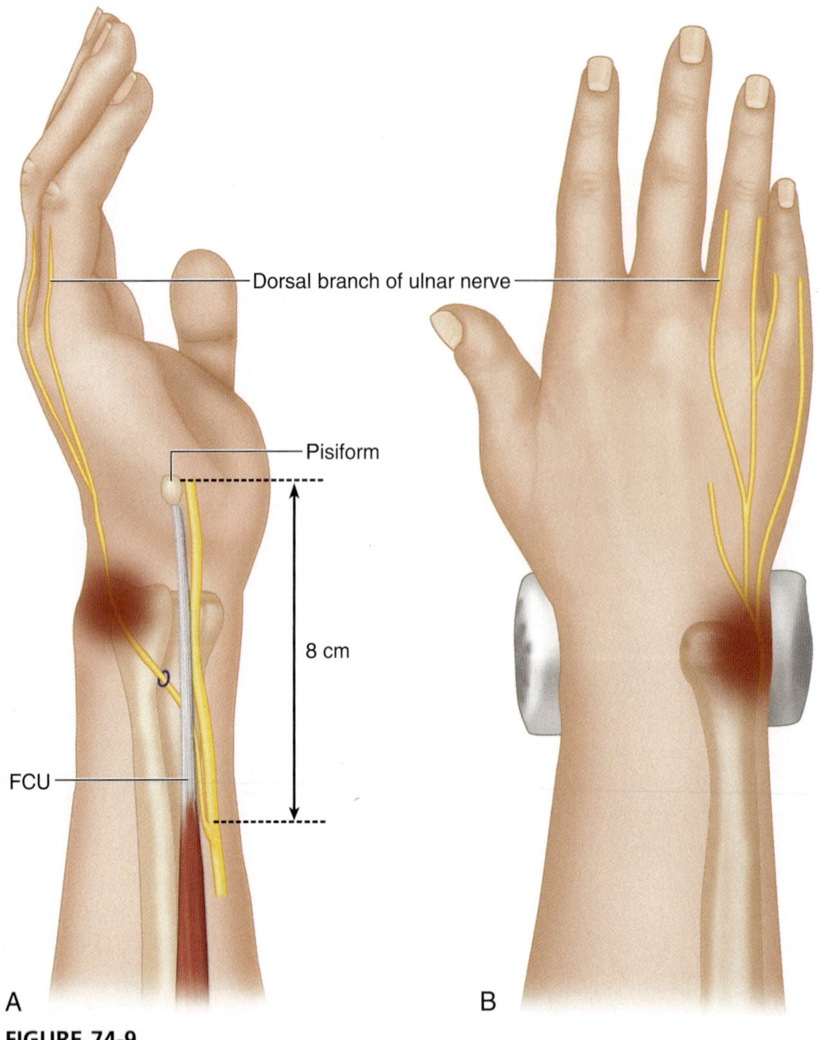

FIGURE 74-9

PITFALLS

Branches of the ulnar dorsal sensory nerve should be protected. This nerve arises from the ulnar aspect of the ulnar nerve about 8 cm proximal to the pisiform. It then passes dorsal to the flexor carpi ulnaris (FCU) and pierces the deep fascia about 5 cm from the pisiform. It reaches the dorsum of the hand after coursing in close relation to the ulnar styloid process (Fig. 74-9).

STEP 2 PEARLS

A narrow strip of tendon is easier to pass in the drill holes placed within the lunate and the triquetrum.

Procedure

Step 1: Excise Scar Tissue between the Lunate and Triquetrum

- The scar tissue between the lunate and triquetrum is excised.

Step 2: Harvest a Strip of Distally Based ECU

- A distally based 3-mm wide and 8- to 10-cm long strip of ECU is harvested from the radial aspect of the tendon (Fig. 74-10).
- The tendon is dissected to its insertion at the base of the small finger metacarpal.

Step 3: Reduction of Lunate and Triquetrum

- Two 0.045-inch Kirschner wires (K-wires) are inserted into the lunate and the triquetrum to act as joysticks to reduce the carpal bones (Fig. 74-11).

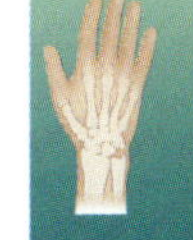

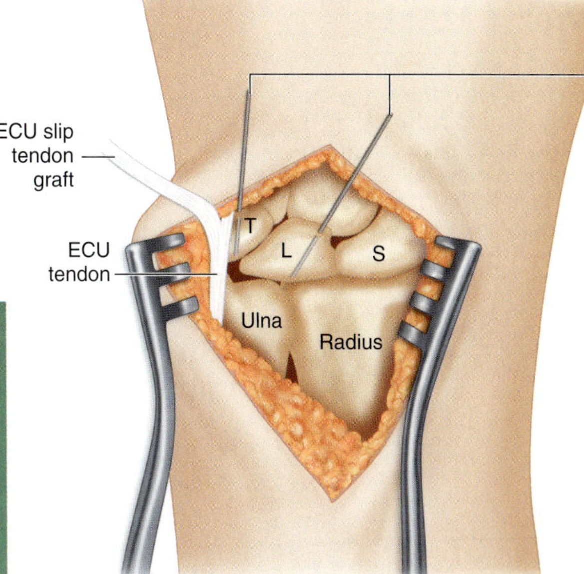

FIGURE 74-11

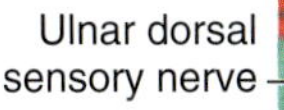

FIGURE 74-10

STEP 3 PEARLS

The joystick K-wires are used to correct the VISI deformity. The lunate is flexed and the triquetrum extended (Fig. 74-12). The lunate K-wire should be inserted in an oblique distal to proximal direction, whereas the triquetral K-wire should be inserted in an oblique proximal to distal direction. The VISI deformity can be corrected by making both K-wires perpendicular to the axis of the forearm.

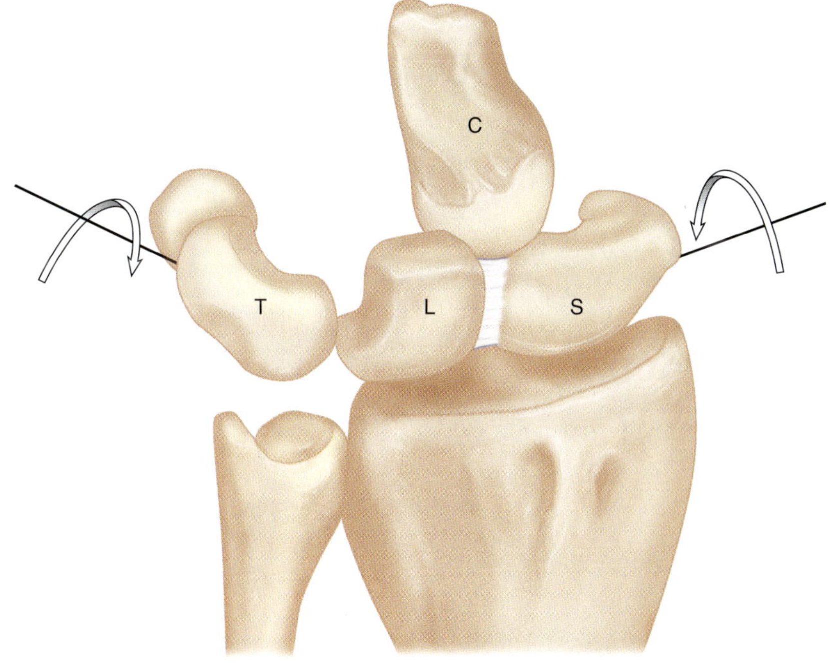

FIGURE 74-12

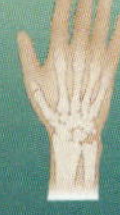

STEP 4 PEARLS

The most difficult part of the operation is to avoid fracturing the carpal bones during bone tunnel drilling. An alternative technique is to use a curved sharp awl to create the bone tunnel. This is less traumatic than using the drill.

Step 4: Create a Bone Tunnel within Triquetrum and Lunate

- A K-wire is passed from the distal, dorsal, and ulnar aspect of the triquetrum to exit at the proximal, palmar, and radial corner of triquetrum. Once acceptable placement of the K-wire is confirmed, a 2.5-mm cannulated drill is inserted over the K-wire to create a bone tunnel within the triquetrum.
- A similar bone tunnel is created from the distal, dorsal, and radial corner of the lunate to exit at the proximal, palmar, and ulnar aspect of the lunate (Fig. 74-13). A microcurette is used to remove the cartilage remnants at the exit sites of the drill holes.

Step 5: Pass the ECU through the Lunate and Triquetrum Tunnel

- The tendon is passed through the drill holes by pulling the sutures on the tendon through the bone tunnel. The tendon should be passed from the dorsum of the triquetrum to the LT interval and then from the LT interval over to the dorsum of the lunate (Fig. 74-14).

STEP 6 PEARLS

It is important to maintain the lunate in neutral position.

Step 6: Secure the ECU Graft to Itself and over the Remnant of the LT Ligament

- The VISI deformity is corrected using the previously placed joystick wires, and the corrected position is maintained by a 0.045-inch K-wire passed between the lunate and triquetrum (Fig. 74-15).
- The end of the tendon graft is sutured back to itself and to any remnants of the LT ligament over the triquetrum using 3-0 Ethibond sutures (Fig. 74-16). This will tighten the triquetrum against the lunate (Fig. 74-17).

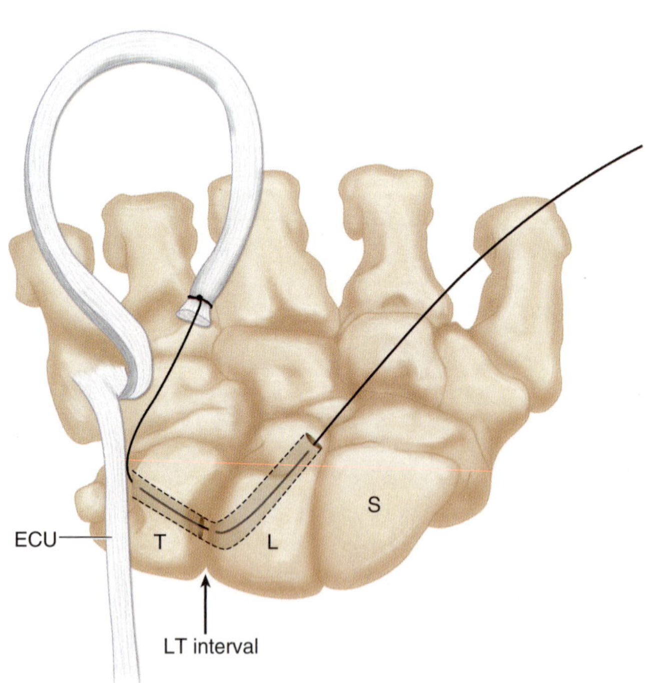

FIGURE 74-13

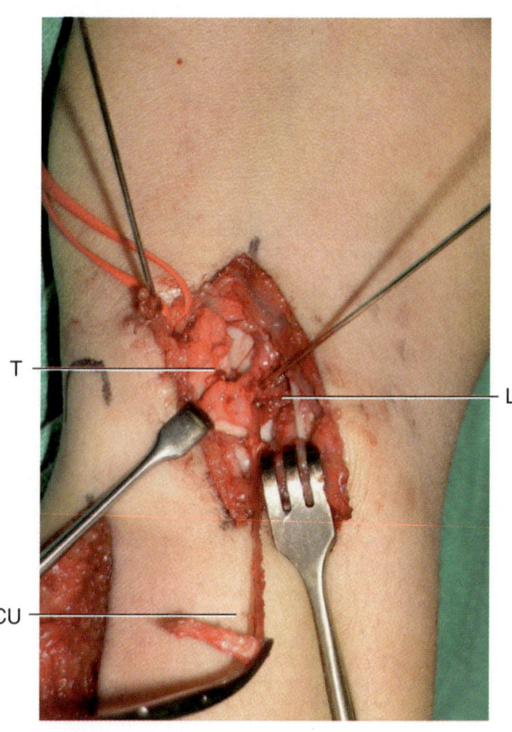

FIGURE 74-14

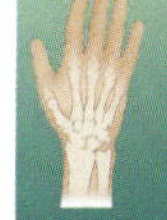

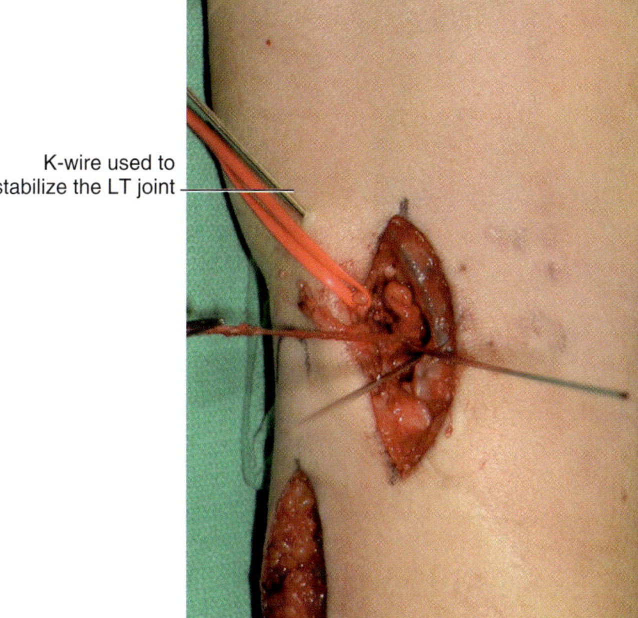

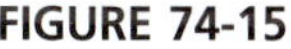

FIGURE 74-15

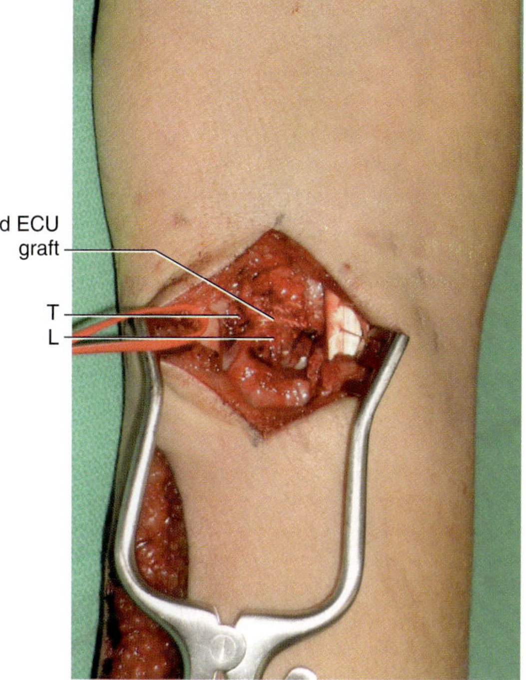

FIGURE 74-16

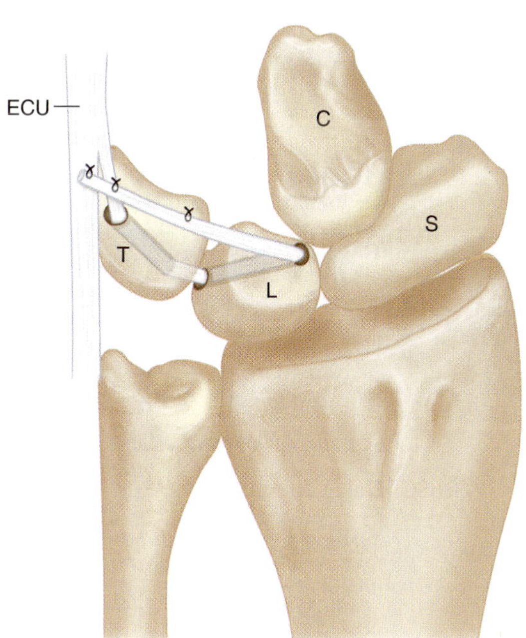

FIGURE 74-17

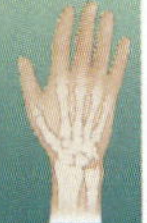

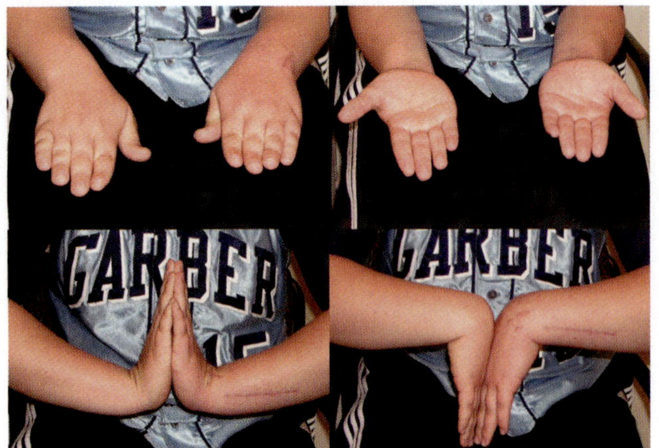

FIGURE 74-18

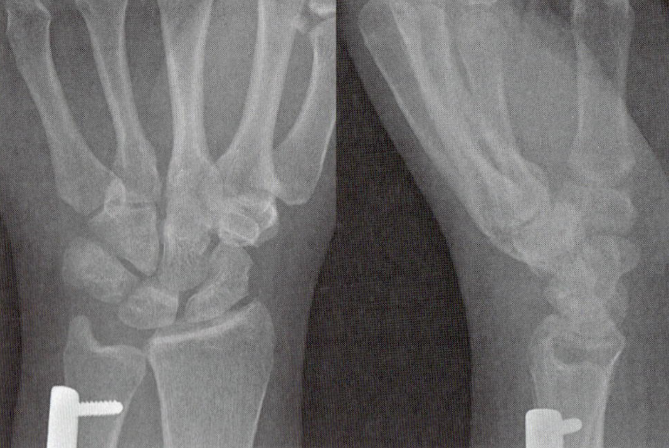

FIGURE 74-19

Step 7: Closure

- The extensor retinaculum over the fourth and fifth compartments is closed using 3-0 Ethibond sutures.
- The two joystick K-wires are removed, and the K-wire stabilizing the lunate and triquetrum is cut under the skin.
- The wrist capsule is closed tightly. The tourniquet is deflated, and all bleeding areas are cauterized.

Postoperative Care and Expected Outcomes

- The patient is kept in a wrist volar splint for 8 weeks.
- After 8 weeks, the K-wires are removed, and the patient starts gentle range-of-motion exercises (Figs. 74-18 and 74-19).
- Pain is generally significantly improved in about 90% of patients after this procedure. The postoperative grip strength and range of wrist motion are usually increased, and the patient's satisfaction at long-term follow-up is also high (about 90%).

Evidence

Shin AY, Weinstein LP, Berger RA, Bishop AT. Treatment of isolated injuries of the lunotriquetral ligament in comparison of arthrodesis, ligament reconstruction, and ligament repair. *J Bone Joint Surg [Br]*. 2001;83:1023-1028.

This is a retrospective review of 57 patients with LT ligament injury treated with arthrodesis, direct ligament repair, or ligament reconstruction using a slip of the ECU tendon. The outcomes were compared by using the following: written questionnaires; the Disabilities of the Arm, Shoulder, and Hand (DASH) score; range of movement; strength; morbidity; and rates of reoperation. Isolated LT injury was confirmed by arthroscopy or arthrotomy. The mean age of the patients was 30.7 years, and the injuries were subacute or chronic in 98.2%. Eight patients underwent LT reconstruction using a distally based strip of the tendon of ECU, 27 had LT repair, and 22 had LT arthrodesis. The mean follow-up was 9.5 years. The probability of remaining free from complications at 5 years was 68.6% for reconstruction, 13.5% for repair, and less than 1% for arthrodesis. Of the LT arthrodeses, 40.9% developed nonunion, and 22.7% developed ulnocarpal impaction. The probabilities of not requiring further surgery at 5 years were 68.6% for reconstruction, 23.3% for repair, and 21.8% for arthrodesis. The DASH scores for each group were not significantly different. Objective improvements in strength and movement and subjective indicators of pain relief and satisfaction were significantly higher in the LT repair and reconstruction groups than in those undergoing arthrodesis. (Level III evidence)

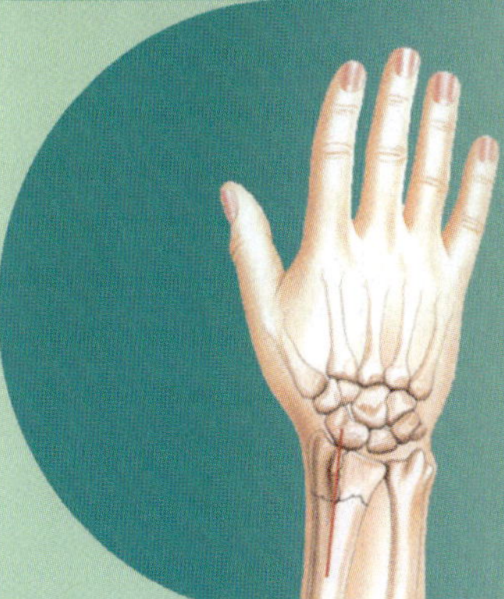

PROCEDURE 75

Scaphotrapeziotrapezoid Arthrodesis and Lunate Excision with Replacement by Palmaris Longus Tendon

Akio Minami

Indications

- Advanced avascular necrosis of the lunate from late stage IIIA to early stage IV according to the Lichtman preoperative 5-stage classification.
- This procedure is mainly indicated for stage IIIB Kienböck disease, which is associated with carpal collapse with a fixed palmar scaphoid flexion.
- A radiograph showing generalized arthrosis is not suitable for scaphotrapeziotrapezoid (STT) arthrodesis and lunate excision with replacement by the palmaris longus tendon.
- This procedure is contraindicated in patients with preoperative advanced osteoarthrosis between the radius and scaphoid because of the risk for further progression of osteoarthrosis at the radioscaphoid joint.

Examination/Imaging

Clinical Examination

- A complete examination of the involved and contralateral extremity is indicated, especially if the patient has a history of autoimmune disease or infection.
- Documentation of baseline pinch and grip strength is helpful.
- Attention to soft tissue swelling must be given because some patients have associated capsular inflammation, thickening, and synovitis.
- Pain can be elicited in all directions of motion, and frequently there is a notable decrease in the arc of motion, particularly in extension.
- Degree of pain, range of motion of the wrist, and grip strength of both wrists should be meticulously measured preoperatively to evaluate postoperative results.

Imaging

Plain Radiographs

- *Staging:* Lichtman modification of Stahl staging
  - *Stage 0:* Radiographs are normal, and magnetic resonance imaging (MRI) may show lunate density changes, edema, or fracture (according to the Amadio modified Lichtman staging based on MRI findings).

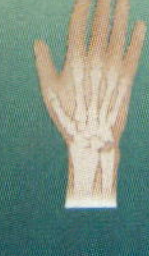

- *Stage I:* Radiographs are normal, but bone scan or tomograms may reveal a sclerotic line representative of a lunate fracture. Occasionally, an indistinct line consistent with the fracture may be visible on plain films (Fig. 75-1A).
- *Stage II:* Lunate density changes are apparent, but carpal alignment remains normal, and lunate size is preserved (Fig. 75-1B).
- *Stage IIIA:* Plain films demonstrate lunate collapse, fragmentation, and displacement; on anteroposterior and lateral views, lunate elongation may be seen without static carpal collapse (Fig. 75-1C).

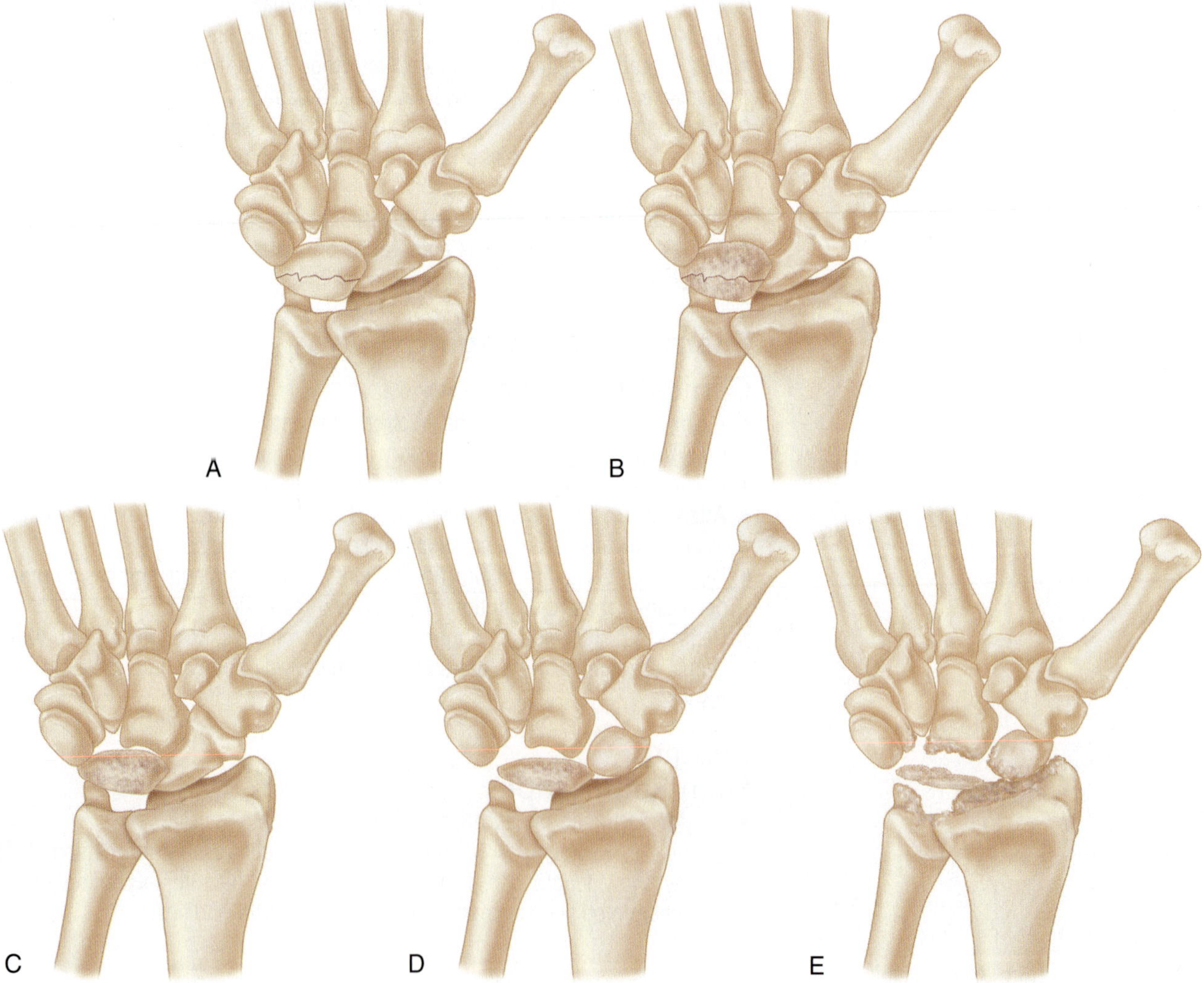

FIGURE 75-1

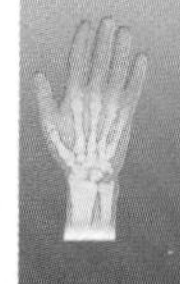

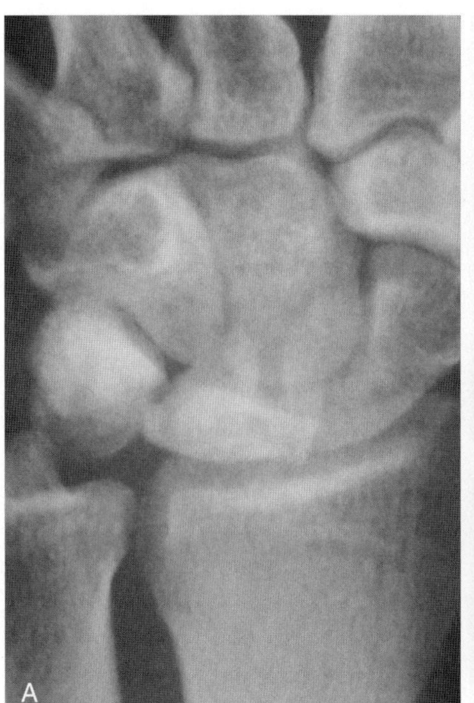

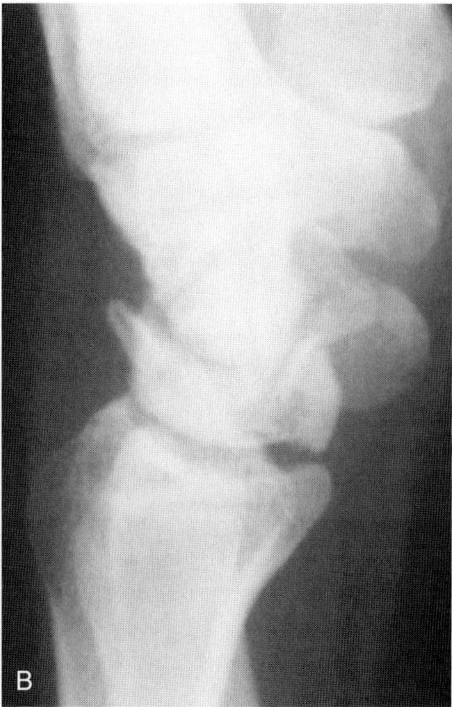

FIGURE 75-2

- *Stage IIIB:* Lunate collapse is accompanied by carpal collapse with a fixed palmar scaphoid flexion (Fig. 75-1D).
- *Stage IV:* All stage III findings are present plus generalized arthritis (Fig. 75-1E).

- Posteroanterior (PA) and lateral radiographs with the wrist in neutral rotation and neutral flexion-extension (Fig. 75-2).
- Ulnar variance radiographic views with the wrist in full pronation and full supination. The carpal height ratio is measured from PA view with the wrist in neutral position. The Stahl index is also measured from lateral view.
- Lunate sclerosis, carpal instability patterns, and fragmentation are seen.
- Shortened scaphoid in the long axis and cortical ring sign of the scaphoid are seen in stage IIIB, which indicates scaphoid in flexed position.
- Evaluation of relationship among scaphoid, trapezium, and trapezoid.

Computed Tomography

- Computed tomography (CT) is needed to evaluate precisely the bony architecture of the lunate and the remainder of the carpus to determine which procedure is indicated and to determine whether arthritic changes of the midcarpal and radiocarpal joints are present.
- A CT scan is useful for evaluation of fragmentation or fracture patterns and associated collapse.

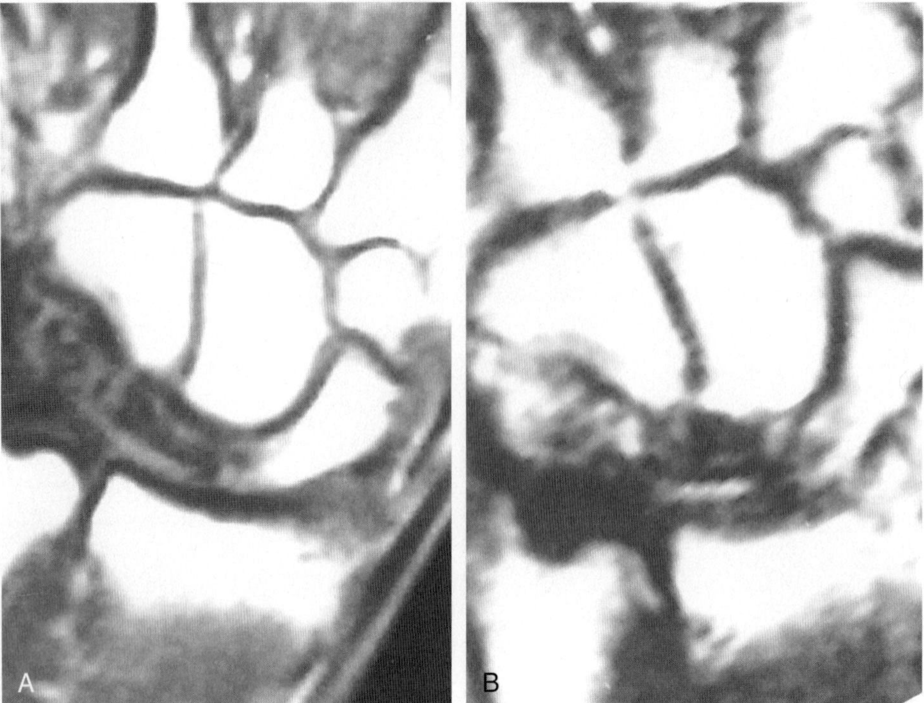

FIGURE 75-3

Magnetic Resonance Imaging

- MRI will show decreased uptake in both T1- and T2-weighted images. Gadolinium contrast has improved diagnosis and evaluation of lunate vascularity (Fig. 75-3).
- It is important to differentiate between ulnar impaction of the lunate and true Kienböck disease.
- Stage 0 has been proposed when lunate edema is visible on MRI only. MRI can show the degree of devascularization or revascularization.

Bone Scan

- A three-phase bone scan is useful to determine the blood flow to the lunate. This scan is highly sensitive, but specificity is low.

TREATMENT OPTIONS

Radial shortening osteotomy and capitate shortening may also unload the lunate.

Instead of STT arthrodesis, some surgeons prefer to perform scaphocapitate (SC) arthrodesis.

Revascularization with a vascularized bone graft has been advocated in early stages, and successes have been reported in late stages as well.

Core decompression of the lunate has also been described.

Salvage procedures for painful wrists that have not responded to the STT arthrodesis include total wrist arthrodesis, partial or total wrist arthroplasty, or proximal row carpectomy.

Controversies

- Pain relief is reliable but may not completely alleviate the pain.

Positioning

- The patient is placed in supine position with the involved extremity on a hand table.
- A pneumatic tourniquet is placed high on the operative arm.
- The table is oriented to allow for intraoperative fluoroscopy.

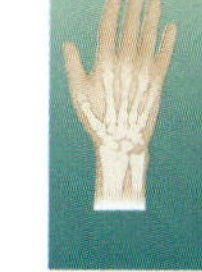

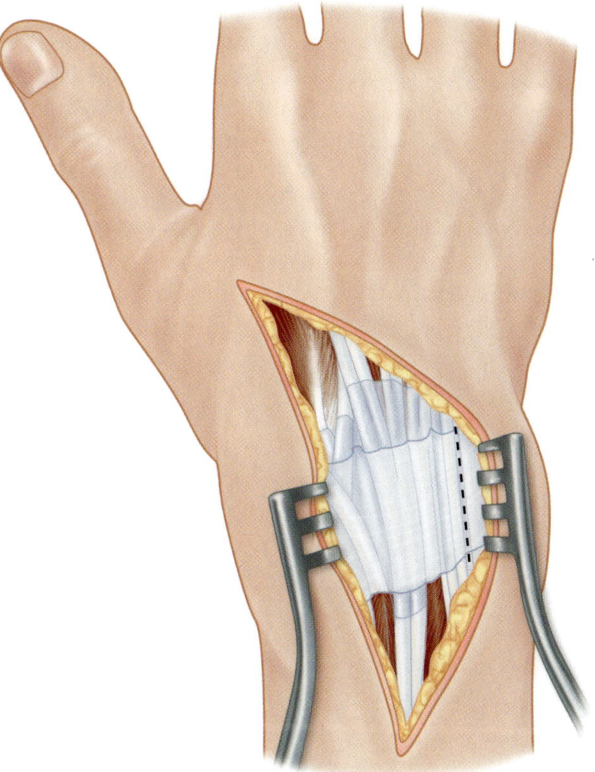

FIGURE 75-4

PEARLS

The radial superficial branches and radial artery are protected during the entire procedure.

PITFALLS

The superficial branches of the radial nerve on the dorsoradial aspect of the hand and the dorsal radial artery and veins between the first and second metacarpal bases are identified and carefully protected during the procedure.

INSTRUMENTATION/ IMPLANTATION

Various types of small osteotomes and chisels are useful to remove the cortex of scaphoid, trapezium, and trapezoid. A low-powered surgical bur is also convenient to expose cancellous bones between the scaphoid, trapezium, and trapezoid.

A hand-held drill is necessary to insert K-wires between the scaphoid, trapezium, and trapezoid.

STEP 1 PEARLS

Consider excision of a 1-cm segment of the posterior interosseous nerve to denervate the dorsal wrist capsule to decrease pain.

Exposures

- A dorsal long oblique incision is made from the space between the first and second carpometacarpal joints, passing the Lister tubercle, to 3 cm proximal to the radiocarpal joint to expose the lunate and three joints (scaphotrapezium, scaphotrapezoid, trapeziotrapezoid joints) (Fig. 75-4).

Procedure

- Superficial branches of the radial nerve are retracted during the procedure.

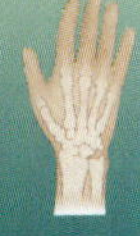

STEP 1 PITFALLS

The lunate is ideally removed as one bone, although this is not easy. Therefore, we prefer to remove the lunate piecemeal.

The palmar wrist capsule and ligaments are protected during removal of the lunate.

If the palmaris longus tendon is absent, the plantaris tendon or a half slip of the extensor carpi radialis longus tendon is harvested.

- Through the proximal half of the incision, the extensor retinaculum is exposed. The capsular flap is incised between the third and fourth dorsal compartments to expose the lunate (Fig. 75-5).
- The lunate is removed piecemeal or entirely in one piece, with great care to avoid injury to the palmar wrist ligaments (Fig. 75-6).
- An ipsilateral palmaris longus tendon is removed with a tendon stripper.
- The tendon strip is rolled into a "rugby ball," sutured to itself, and inserted into the defect of the excised lunate.
- The dorsal capsule is closed securely (Fig. 75-7).

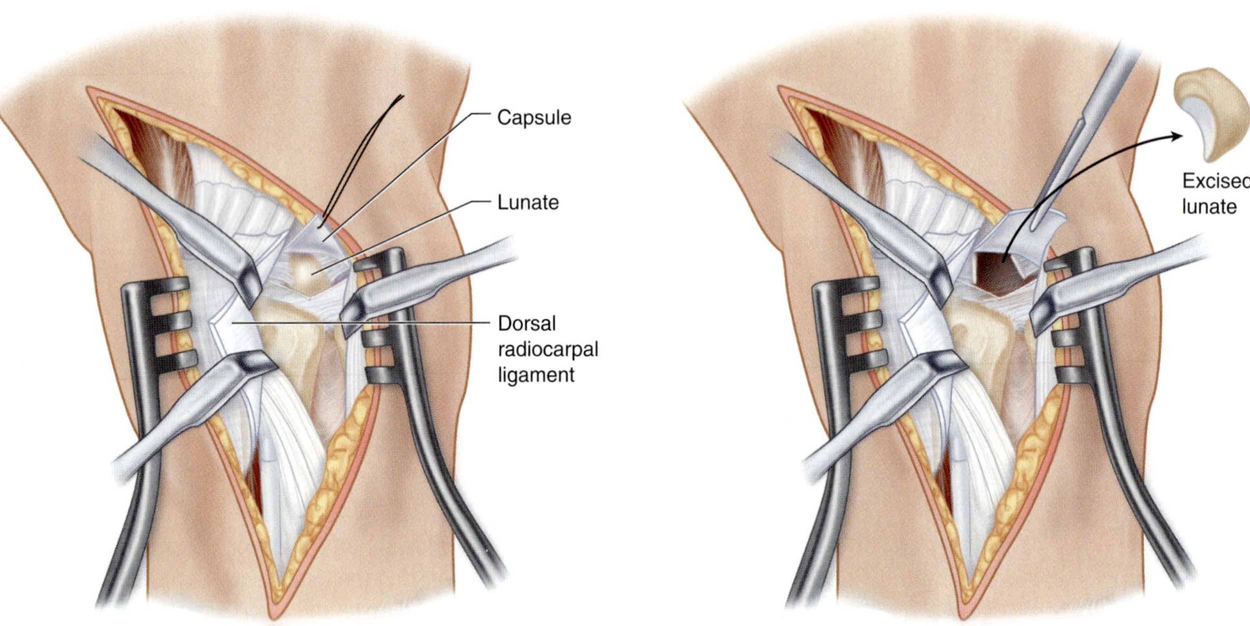

FIGURE 75-5

FIGURE 75-6

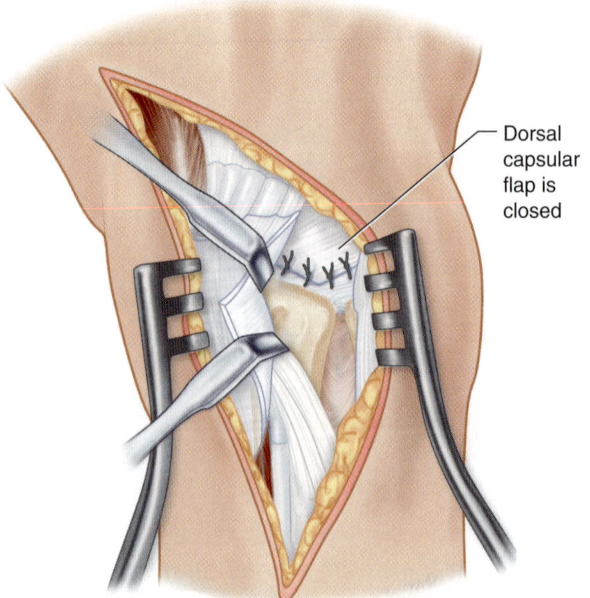

FIGURE 75-7

STEP 2 PEARLS

Removal of the cortex between the scaphoid, trapezium, and trapezoid and packing of the cancellous bone graft from the iliac crest into the three joint spaces should be performed to obtain solid fusion.

STEP 2 PITFALLS

Care should be taken to avoid injury to the flexor carpi radialis and flexor pollicis longus tendons when the three points are being prepared for arthrodesis.

K-wires should be inserted with care to avoid injury to the branches of the superficial radial nerve.

Step 2

- Through the distal half of the incision, the wrist and thumb extensors are exposed.
- Wrist and thumb extensors are retracted.
- The articular surfaces between the scaphoid, trapezium, and trapezoid are exposed.
- The articular cartilage and subchondral bone of the three joints are removed to expose the cancellous bone (Fig. 75-8).
- Cancellous bone from the iliac crest is grafted into the joint spaces to prevent shortening of the carpus (Fig. 75-9).

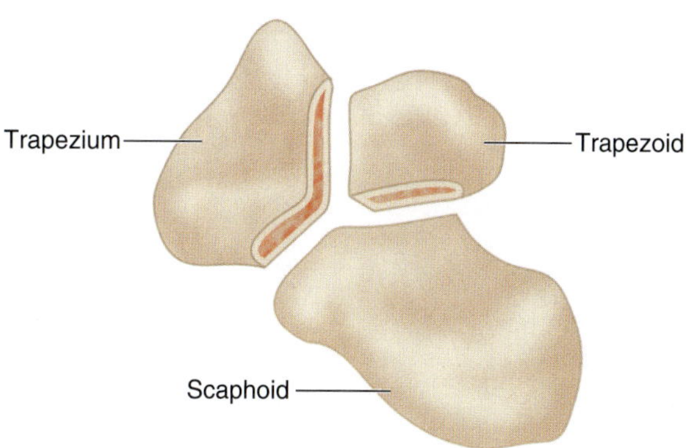

FIGURE 75-8

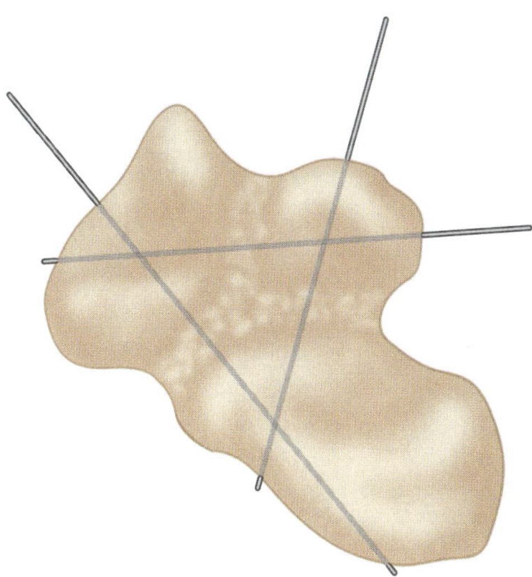

FIGURE 75-9

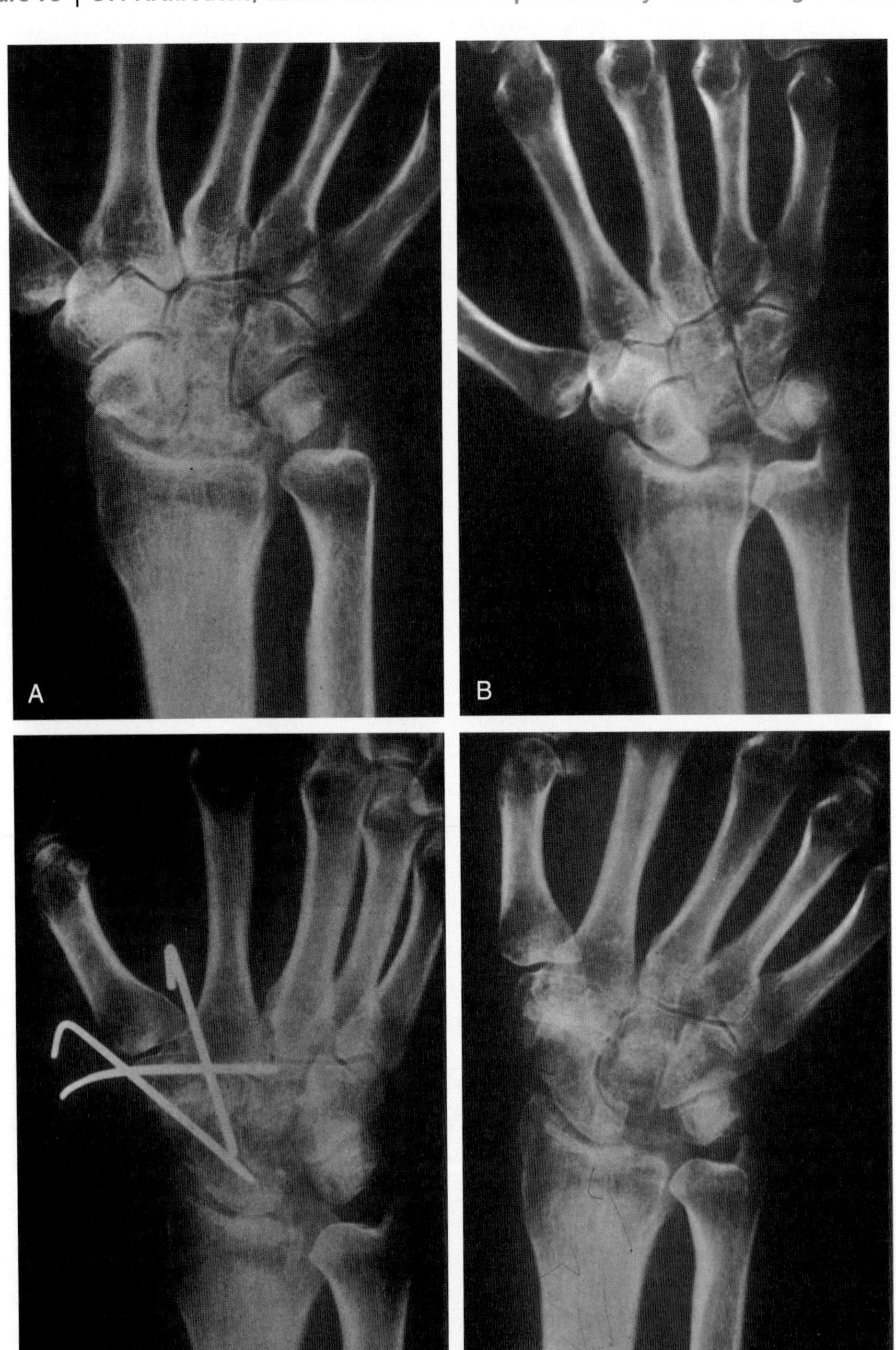

FIGURE 75-10

Step 3

- The proximal pole of the scaphoid is depressed until it is under the dorsal surface of the lunate fossa on the radius to reduce the flexed posture of the scaphoid. This distal pole is pulled dorsally, if necessary, and K-wires are then driven percutaneously through the scaphoid into the capitate to maintain reduction (see Fig. 75-9).
- The position of the scaphoid is confirmed by intraoperative imaging (Fig. 75-10).
- Figure 75-10A shows a preoperative radiograph of Kienböck disease classified by stage IIIB.

STEP 3 PITFALLS

K-wire fixation of the proximal scaphoid to the radius must be avoided because this can greatly decrease motion in the radiocarpal joint and increase the stress at the site of the arthrodesis.

STEP 4 PEARLS

Watson emphasized that the scaphoid should lie about 45 degrees to the long axis of the forearm in the lateral projection. We emphasize the importance of the radioscaphoid angle in STT arthrodesis to prevent late postoperative arthrosis at the radioscaphoid joint.

- Figure 75-10B shows a radiograph of the excision of the lunate.
- Figure 75-10C shows a radiograph of an STT arthrodesis after the removal of the lunate.
- Figure 75-10D shows a radiograph 3 years after excision of the lunate and STT arthrodesis.

Step 4

- Insertion of K-wires (size: 1.2 mm) only into the scaphoid, trapezium, and trapezoid.

Step 5

- The tourniquet is released, and meticulous hemostasis is achieved by using a bipolar coagulator. The dorsal capsule is closed.
- The wound is irrigated, and skin closure of the surgeon's choice is performed.

Postoperative Care and Expected Outcomes

- The patient is placed in a well-padded short-arm thumb spica splint with the thumb in maximal opposed position and the wrist and forearm in neutral positions.
- The patient is given instructions on routine splint care, told to maintain a non–weight-bearing status for the upper extremity, and encouraged to work on gentle finger range-of-motion exercises.
- The postoperative splint is removed about 2 weeks after surgery. The wound is examined, and sutures are moved. The patient is then placed in a short-arm thumb spica cast. Finger range of motion is assessed to determine whether stiffness of the interphalangeal or metacarpophalangeal joints has developed.
- Six weeks after surgery, the patient's cast is removed, and unions among three bones are evaluated by plain radiographs or CT. A short-arm thumb spica cast is applied until arthrodesis is obtained.
- The patient is re-evaluated 10 or 12 weeks after surgery. Union should be achieved at this point. If so, the patient is not placed in a cast but rather is given a removable splint for comfort and to protect the surgical site. Wrist range of motion is emphasized.

Evidence

Minami A, Kato H, Suenaga N, et al. Scaphotrapezio-trapezoid fusion: long-term follow-up study. *J Orthop Sci.* 2003;8:319-322.

The authors evaluated clinical and radiologic results of 30 STT fusions in 30 patients (23 with Kienböck disease, 6 with isolated STT osteoarthroses, and 1 dislocation of the trapezium) with mean follow-up of 84 months. Twenty-six patients returned to their previous activities. STT fusion is an effective procedure for Kienböck disease and isolated STT arthrosis, although radioscaphoid arthrosis occurred in 23% of this series. (Level III evidence)

Minami A, Kimura T, Suzuki K. Long-term results of Kienböck's disease treated by triscaphe arthrodesis and excisional arthroplasty with a coiled palmaris longus tendon. *J Hand Surg [Am].* 1994;19:219-228.

Fifteen patients with Kienböck disease (stages IIIA:1, IIIB:11, and IV:3) were treated with STT arthrodesis and lunate excisional arthroplasty and a coiled palmaris longus tendon replacement, with average follow-up period of 57 months. Five patients revealed postoperative progress of osteoarthritic changes at the radioscaphoid joint. The authors concluded that stage IIIB is a specific indication for STT arthrodesis. (Level IV evidence)

Watson HK, Ryu J, DiBella A. An approach to Kienböck's disease: Triscaphe arthrodesis. *J Hand Surg [Am].* 1985;10:17-87.

Sixteen patients with Kienböck disease were treated with STT arthrodesis (fusion of the scaphoid, trapezium. and trapezoid) with or without silicone rubber lunate arthroplasty. After an average follow-up of 20.5 months, relief of pain was satisfactory in all 16 patients. (Level IV evidence)

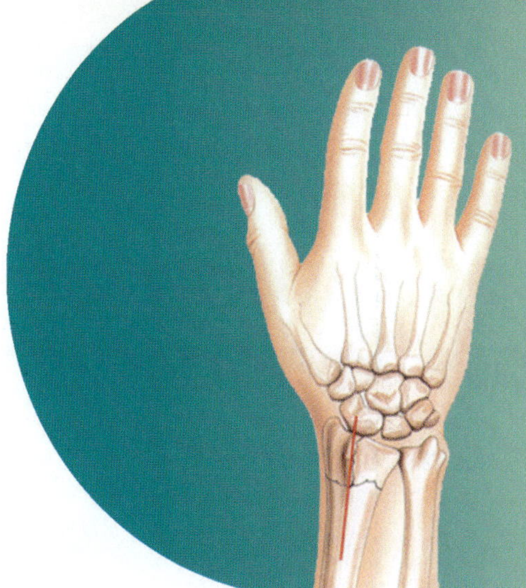

Section XII

DISTAL RADIUS FRACTURES AND DISTAL RADIOULNAR JOINT REPAIR AND RECONSTRUCTION

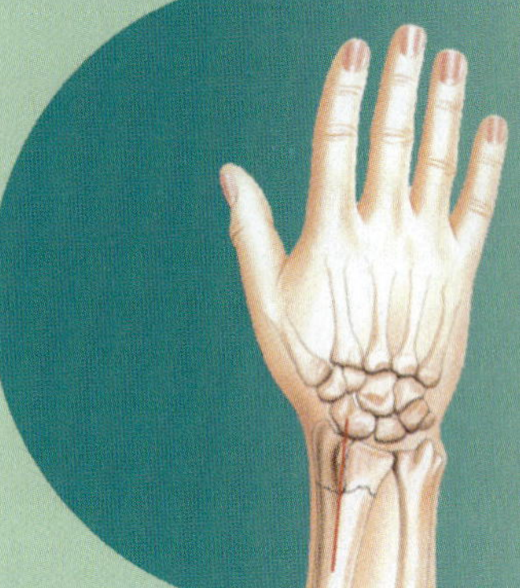

Percutaneous Pinning of Distal Radius Fractures

John T. Capo and Naveen K. Ahuja

See Video 57: Percutaneous Pinning of Distal Radius Fractures

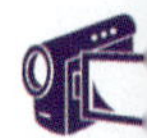

Indications

- Unstable displaced extra-articular distal radius fractures
- Simple two- or three-part intra-articular distal radius fractures
- Displaced distal radius fractures in children and adolescents

Examination/Imaging

Clinical Examination

- The extremity of the patient should be examined for open injuries and neurovascular status, particularly median nerve function.
- The distal ulna should be examined for dorsal prominence or instability.
- The elbow should be examined for tenderness at the radial head and collateral ligaments.

Imaging

- Anteroposterior and lateral images of the wrist should be obtained. These will demonstrate the specific fracture pattern of the injury. (Fig. 76-1A and B shows a 47-year-old woman who sustained an intra-articular distal radius fracture with some angulation and displacement.)
- If there is significant intra-articular comminution, a computed tomography scan will provide more information on the location and displacement of the fracture fragments.

Surgical Anatomy

- The pins are placed dorsoradially in the radial styloid and dorsoulnarly in the intermediate column of the radius.
- The surgical interval is between the first and second dorsal compartments for the radial-sided pins and between the fourth and fifth compartment for the ulnar-sided pins.

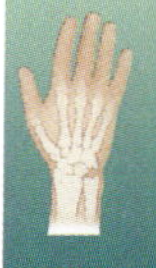

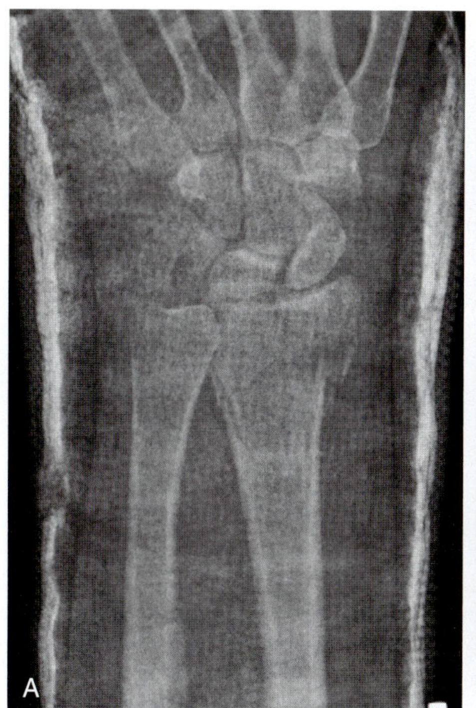

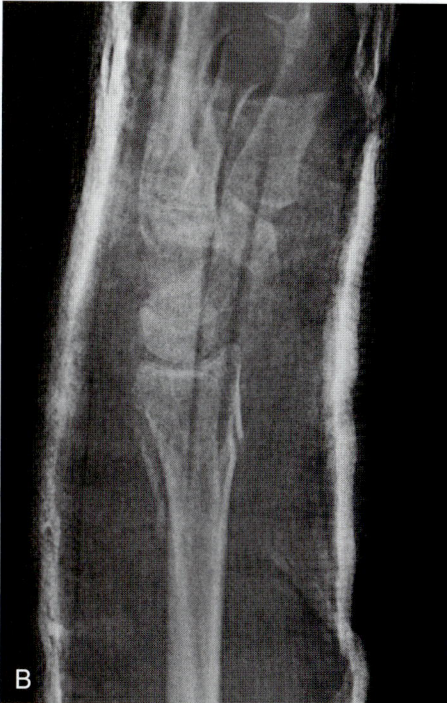

FIGURE 76-1

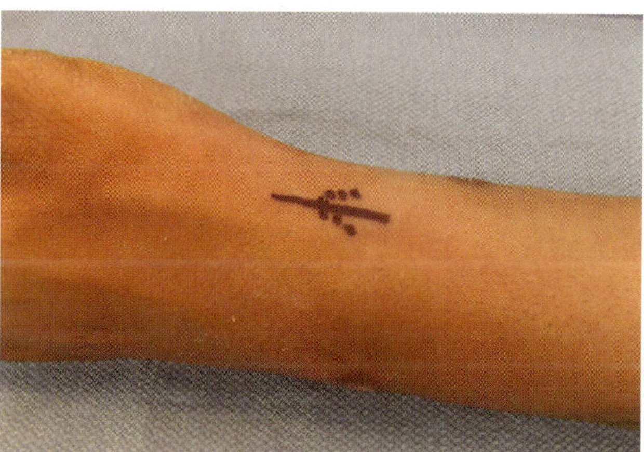

FIGURE 76-2

Positioning

- The procedure is done on a hand table with the forearm pronated.
- A tourniquet is placed on the upper arm but is usually not needed.

Exposures

- The radial-sided pins are placed first. A 2-cm incision is made over the radial styloid (Fig. 76-2).

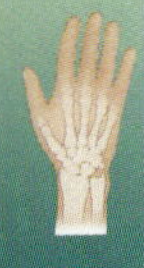

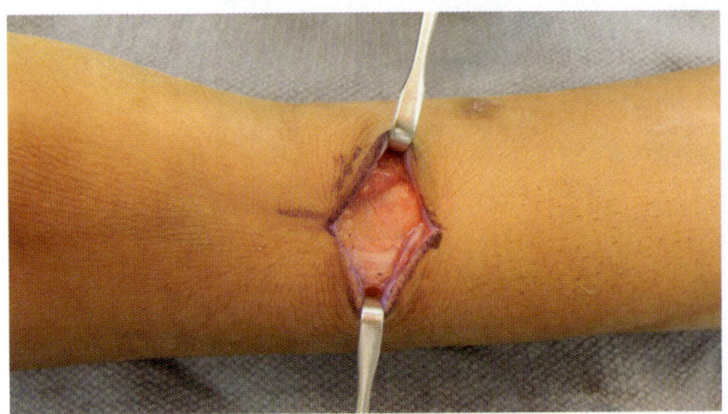

FIGURE 76-3

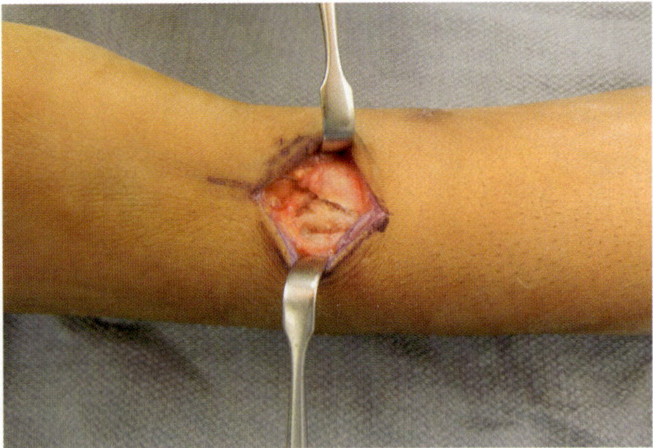

FIGURE 76-4

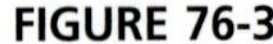

PEARLS

The branches of the superficial nerve are identified and retracted with the skin flaps.

- The soft tissue flaps are elevated, and the skin is retracted. Branches of the superficial nerve are identified and carefully protected (Fig. 76-3).
- The tip of the radial styloid is identified, and the periosteum is elevated. The tendons of the first and second dorsal compartments are reflected off the radius enough to safely insert two pins. The tendons are left within the compartments and are elevated subperiosteally (Fig. 76-4).

STEP 1 PEARLS

The radial styloid can be easily fragmented, and multiple passes of the K-wires should be avoided.

If there is difficulty in reducing the fracture, a blunt elevator can be placed percutaneously. This can be inserted into the fracture site dorsally and used to lever the fracture into a reduced position.

STEP 1 PITFALLS

Caution should be taken if the radial-sided pins are placed percutaneously. The tendons of the first compartment and superficial radial nerve can easily be damaged.

Procedure

Step 1

- The radial styloid pins are inserted using a soft tissue protector. The first pin is placed into the distal fragment only. The pins are typically 0.062-inch Kirschner wires (Fig. 76-5).
- The wrist and distal fragment are flexed over a towel bump to reduce the displacement or angulation of the fracture. With the fracture reduced, a dorsoulnar pin is placed percutaneously. This pin is placed at the dorsoulnar corner of the distal radius (Fig. 76-6).

Step 2

- With the wrist flexed and the fracture reduced, the pins in the distal fragment are driven across the fracture and into and through the cortex of the proximal shaft.
- An additional pin is placed from the radial styloid and across the fracture.
- Anteroposterior and lateral images should show good alignment of the fracture with restoration of volar tilt and ulnar inclination (Fig. 76-7A and B).

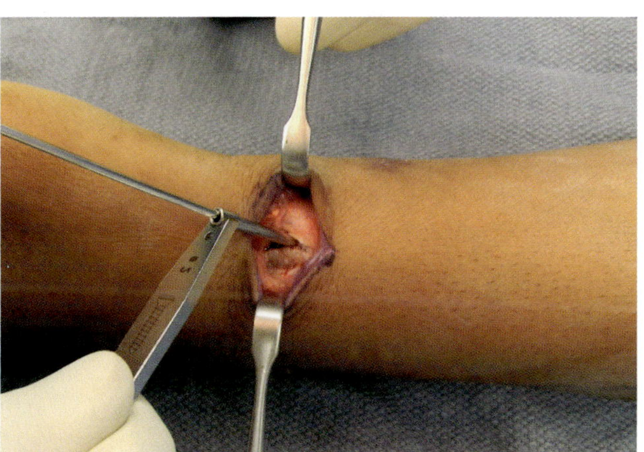

FIGURE 76-5

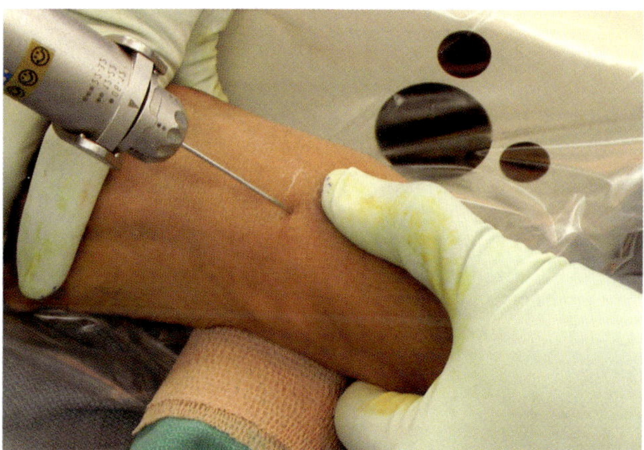

FIGURE 76-6

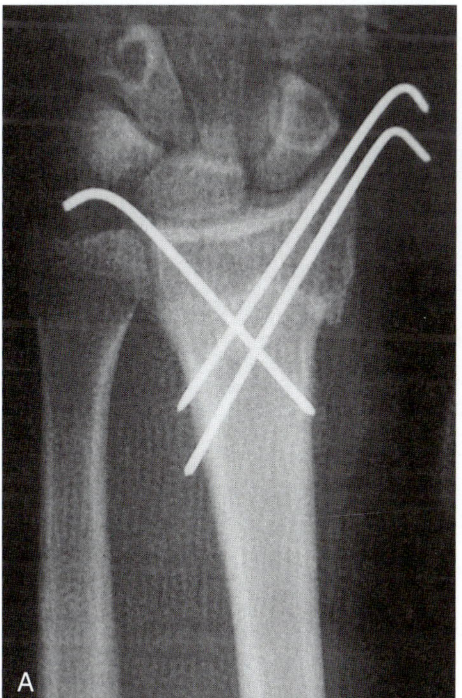

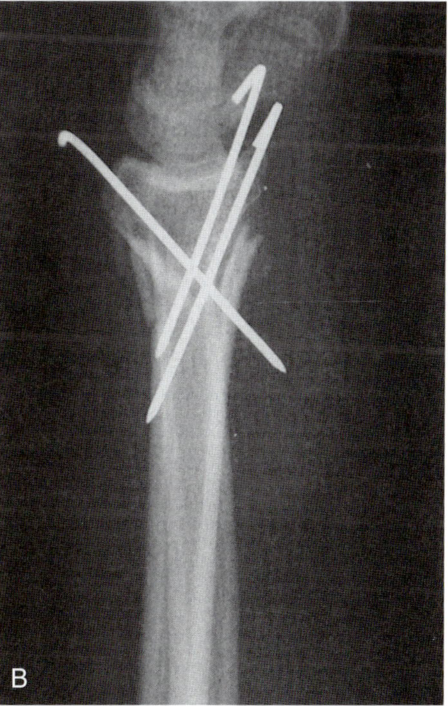

FIGURE 76-7

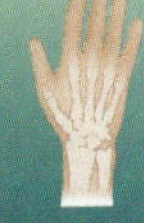

STEP 2 PEARLS

If the bone is very osteopenic and is not held by the pins well, then an intrafocal Kapandji technique can be used. The pins are placed through the fracture site on the dorsoradial and dorsoulnar side of the distal fragment and thereby buttress the fragment in place.

The fracture is first elevated with an osteotome and levered volarly to restore the volar tilt (Fig. 76-8A). A K-wire is then placed at the same level but driven into the intact volar cortex to hold the buttressed fragment. Additional wires can be driven along the dorsal fracture, and the radial edge of the fracture can also be elevated to restore the radial inclination (Fig. 76-8B).

At times, a combination of intrafocal pinning and pinning through the fracture fragments can be used (Fig. 76-9A and B).

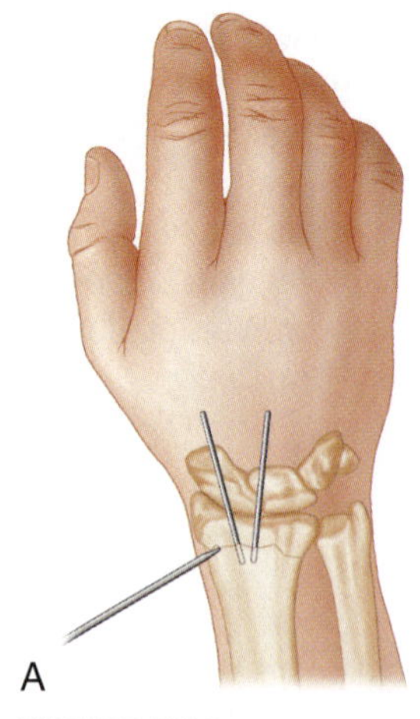

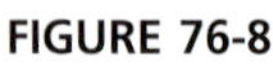

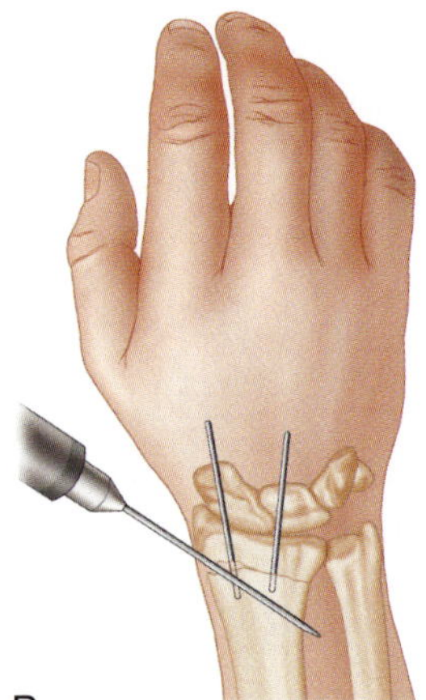

FIGURE 76-8

STEP 2 PITFALLS

Care should be taken not to over-reduce the fragment. Excessive volar flexion can displace the fragment volarly.

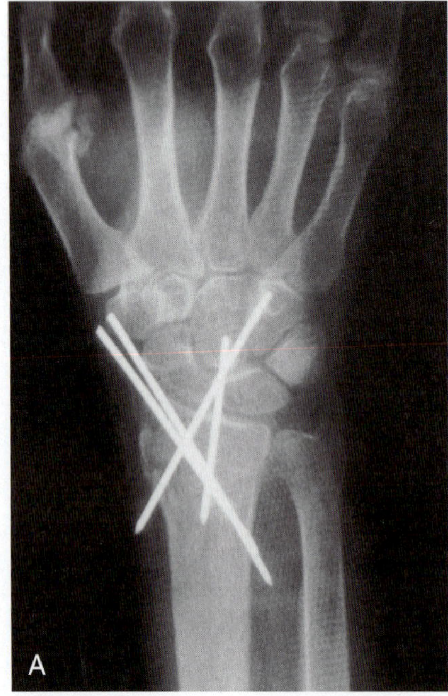

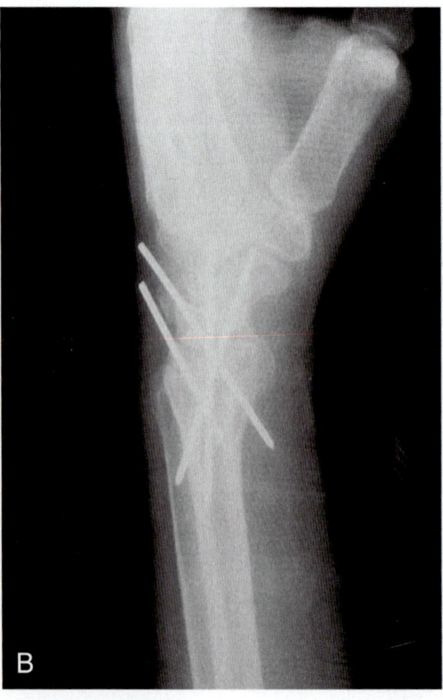

FIGURE 76-9

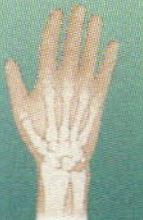

STEP 4 PEARLS

Pediatric fractures can often be stabilized with a single smooth K-wire.

PEARLS

Early ROM can begin with the pins in and be increased after the pins are removed. The final clinical result is usually functional wrist flexion and extension as well as forearm rotation (Fig. 76-14A and B).

Step 3

- The radial-sided wound is closed with 4-0 nylon sutures, with care taken to avoid the branches of the superficial radial nerve.
- The pins are bent at an angle to avoid skin impingement and covered with a plastic pin cap.
- The pin sites are covered with a nonadherent dressing and then a bulky gauze dressing to push the skin down off the pins.
- A volar or sugar tong splint is placed for added support.

Step 4

- The technique is also useful for displaced pediatric fractures. Appropriate fractures are transphyseal or metaphyseal. Radiographs demonstrate a displaced, nonreducible physeal fracture in a 15-year-old boy (Fig. 76-10A and B).
- Closed reduction and percutaneous pinning are usually easily achieved with general anesthesia and muscular paralysis (Fig. 76-11A and B).
- Pins are removed after 4 to 5 weeks in the clinic. Final radiographs should show a healed fracture with good alignment of the articular surface (Fig. 76-12A and B).

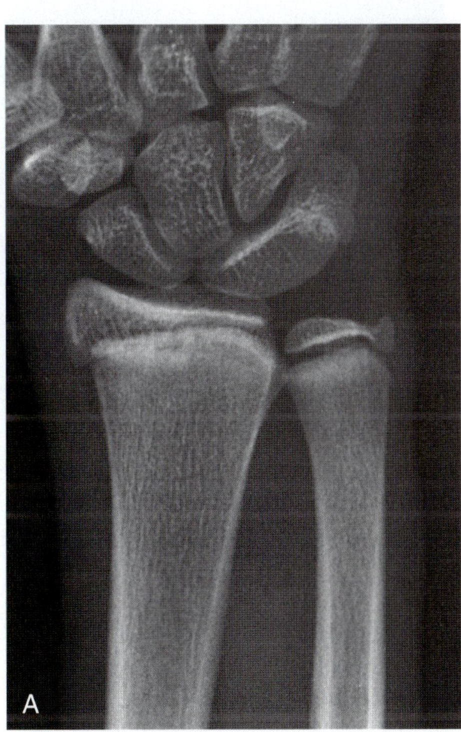

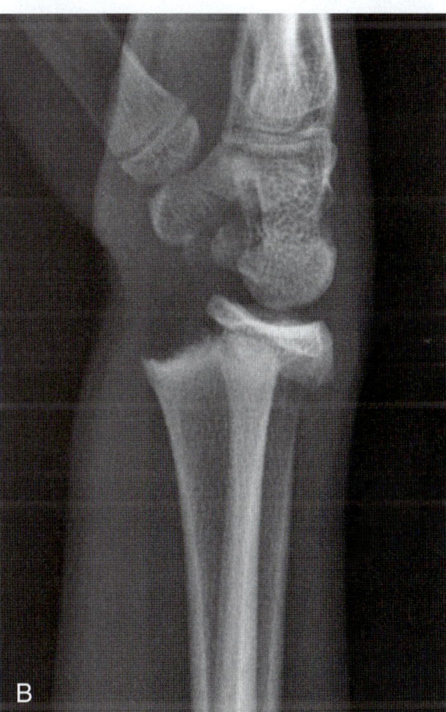

FIGURE 76-10

Postoperative Care and Expected Outcomes

- Patients are seen after 2 weeks for a dressing change and suture removal.
- Finger and elbow range of motion (ROM) is allowed after 2 weeks.
- In adults, the K-wires are removed in the office 5 to 6 weeks after surgery.
- Final radiographs at healing should show good alignment of the articular surface. After the pins are removed, there may be some settling of the distal fragment (Fig. 76-13A and B).

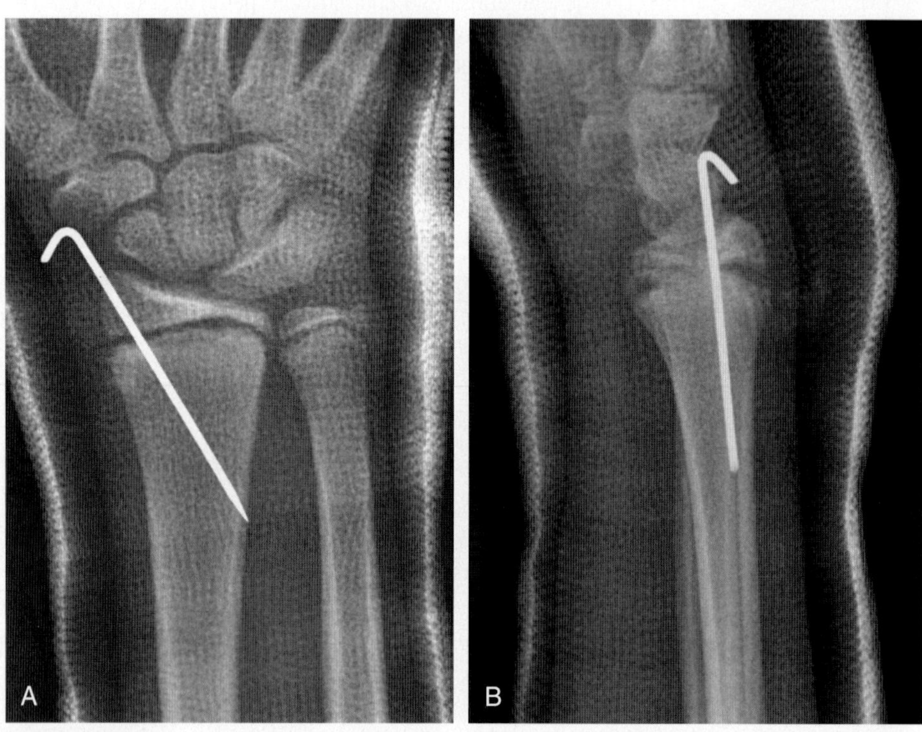

FIGURE 76-11

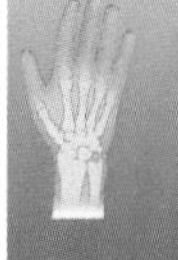

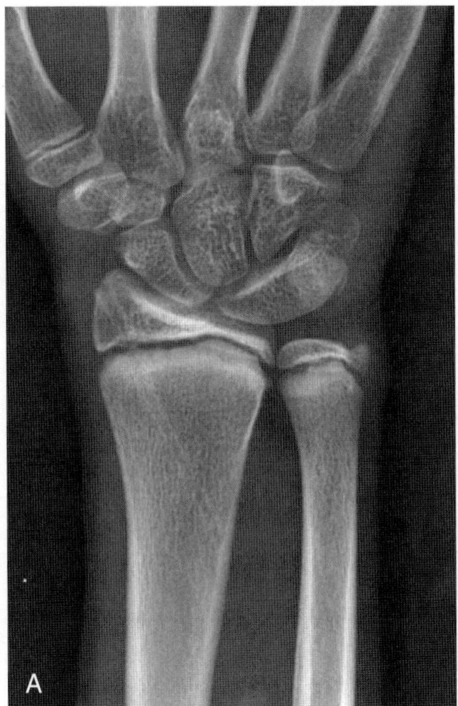

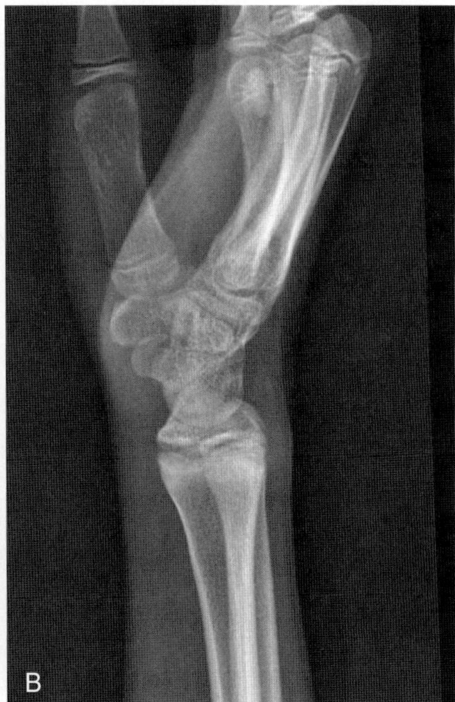

FIGURE 76-12

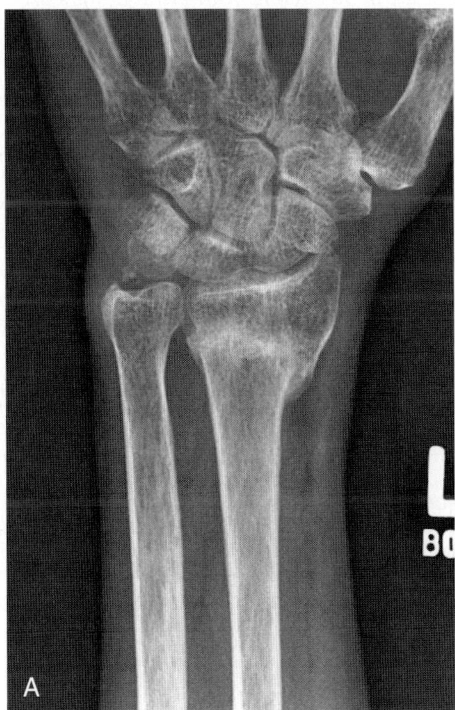

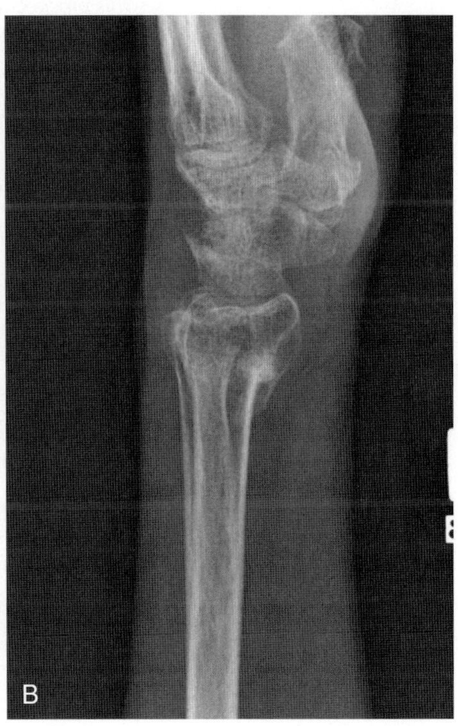

FIGURE 76-13

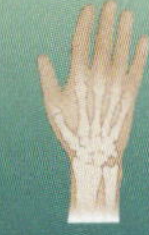

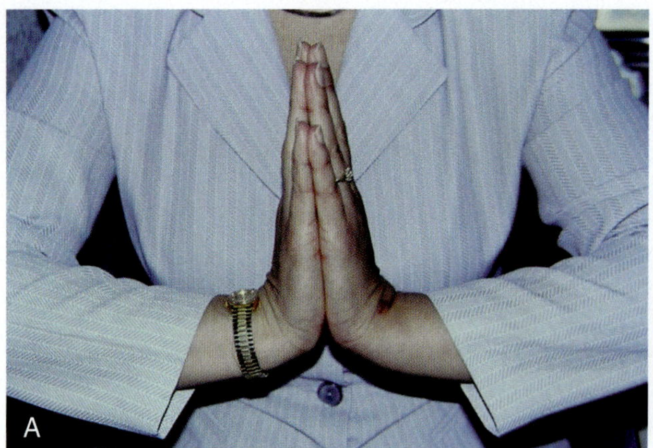

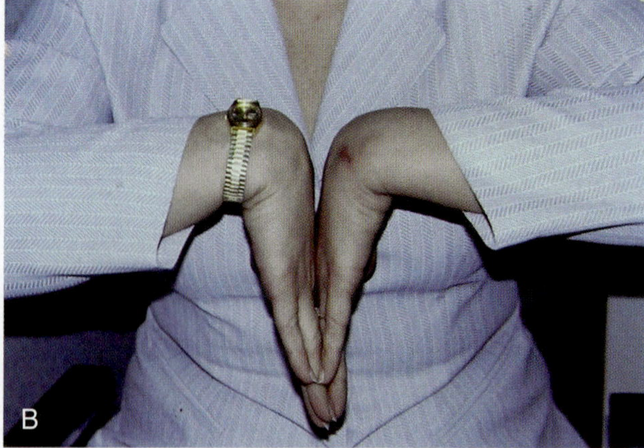

FIGURE 76-14

Evidence

Harley BJ, Schargenberger A, Beaupre LA, et al. Augmented external fixation versus percutaneous pinning and casting for unstable fractures of the distal radius—a prospective randomized trial. *J Hand Surg [Am]*. 2004;29:815-824.

This prospective, randomized study showed that in patients younger than 65 years, percutaneous pinning and casting were equivalent to augmented external fixation. Fifty-five patients were enrolled and followed for 1 year both clinically and radiographically. Both groups were similar in terms of fracture type and AO-ASIF class. Specifically, there was no significant difference in radial length, radial angulation, volar tilt, DASH scores, total ROM, or grip strength. (Level II-3 evidence)

Lenoble E, Dumontier C, Goutallier D, Apoil A. Fracture of the distal radius: a prospective comparison between trans-styloid and Kapandji fixations. *J Bone Joint Surg [Br]*. 1995;77:562-567.

This prospective study of 96 patients with extra- or intra-articular distal radius fractures with a dorsally displaced posteromedial fragment were treated with either trans-styloid or Kapandji (intrafocal) fixation. Patients were followed at 6 weeks and 3, 6, 12 and 24 months. Although there was some improvement in range of motion in early follow-up with Kapandji fixation, at 24 months the results were similar in both groups. (Level III evidence)

Naidu SH, Capo JT, Moulton M, et al. Percutaneous pinning of distal radius fractures: a biomechanical study. *J Hand Surg [Am]*. 1997;22:252-257.

This cadaveric study used 12 fresh-frozen radii with a dorsally comminuted osteotomy 2.5 cm proximal to the radial styloid to test 12 different pin combinations: 4 pin configurations were used with 3 different pin sizes. Rigidity was greatest with respect to cantilever bending and torsion with two radial styloid pins and one pin from the ulnar corner of the radius. Additionally, a minimum pin size of 0.62 inch was required to discern differences in rigidity among different pin configurations. (Level II-3 evidence)

Trumble TE, Wagner W, Hanel DP, et al. Intrafocal (Kapandji) pinning of distal radius fractures with and without external fixation. *J Hand Surg [Am]*. 1998:23:381-394.

This study subdivided 73 patients into groups according to age, degree of comminution, and whether external fixators were used in combination with percutaneous pinning. In older patients (55 years), the use of external fixators resulted in better range of motion, grip strength, and pain relief. In younger patients, external fixation only resulted in superior results if two sides of the radial metaphysis were comminuted. Additionally, functional results were improved by restoration of palmar and radial tilt as well as radial length. (Level III evidence)

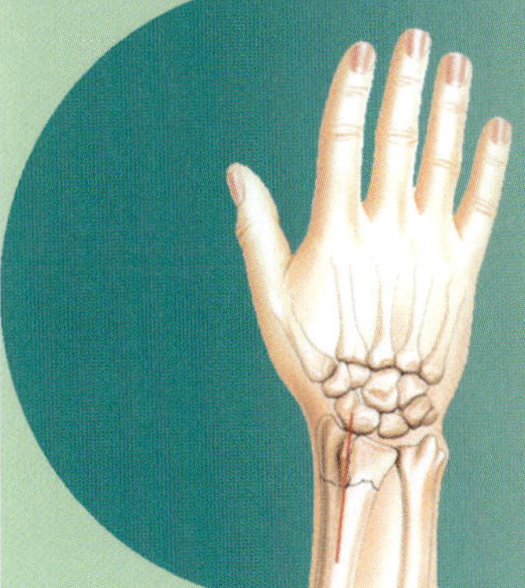

PROCEDURE 77

Volar Plating of Distal Radius Fractures

John T. Capo

See Video 58: Volar Locking Plate Fixation for Distal Radius Fractures

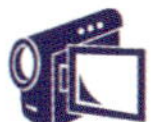

Indications

- Unstable displaced extra-articular fractures
- Displaced intra-articular fractures
- Volar shearing fractures

Examination/Imaging

Clinical Examination

- The extremity of the patient should be examined for open injuries and neurovascular status, particularly median nerve function.
- The distal ulna should be examined for dorsal prominence or instability.
- The elbow should be examined for tenderness at the radial head and collateral ligaments.

Imaging

- Anteroposterior view of a right distal radius fracture in 32-year-old male laborer (Fig. 77-1A)
- Lateral view of fracture demonstrating intra-articular extension of fracture and dorsal angulation and displacement (Fig. 77-1B)

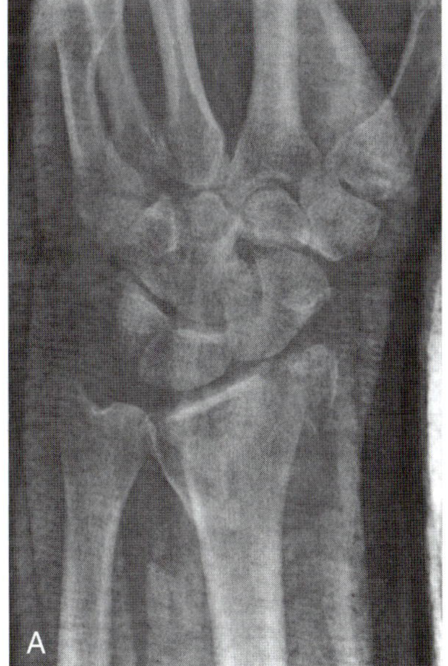

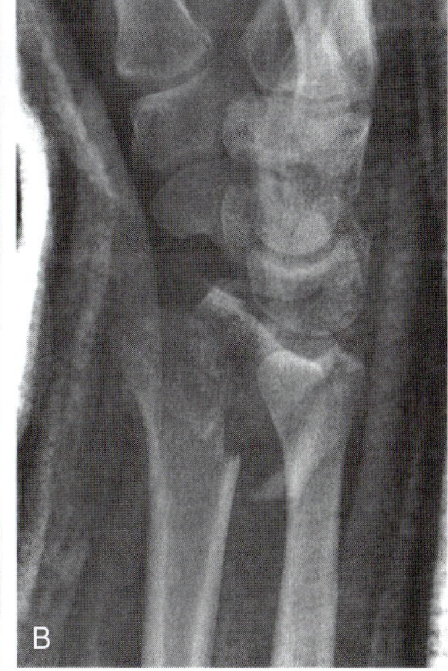

FIGURE 77-1

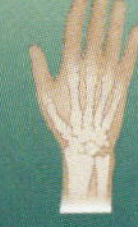

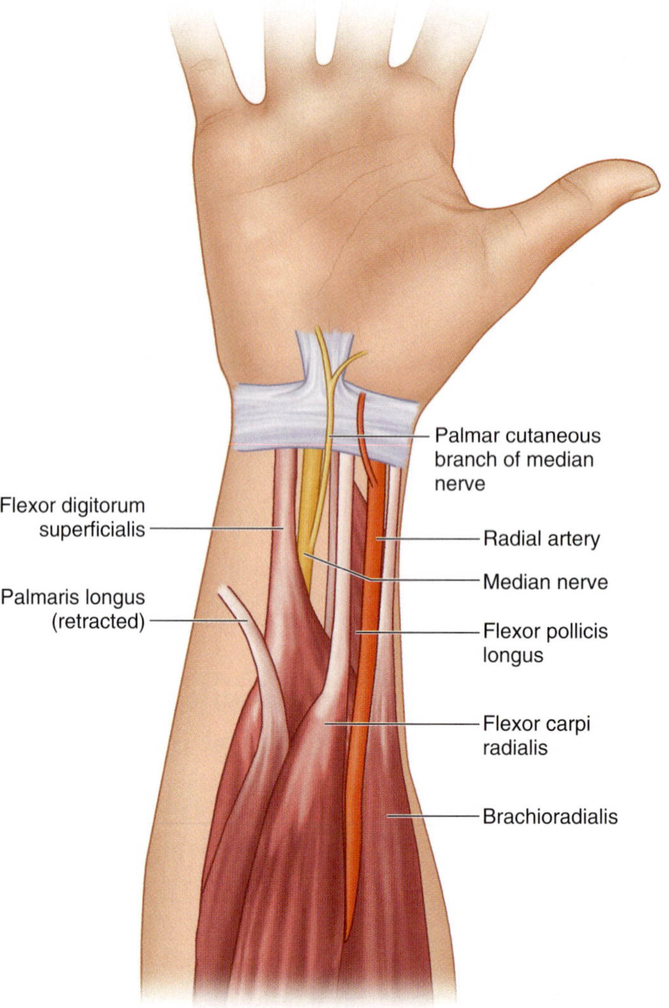

FIGURE 77-2

Surgical Anatomy

- Drawing of volar anatomy of forearm and wrist. The surgical interval is between the flexor carpi radialis (FCR) tendon and radial artery and brachioradialis (BR) insertion (Fig. 77-2).
- The palmar cutaneous branch of the median nerve arises 5 cm proximal to the radial styloid between the palmaris longus and the FCR.
- The flexor pollicis longus (FPL) muscle belly covers the pronator quadratus (PQ) and must be reflected from radial to ulnar.
- The PQ muscle is sharply divided radially and is elevated from the distal radius to expose the fracture.
- The BR inserts into the distal radius and may be detached to decrease the deforming forces on the distal fragment.

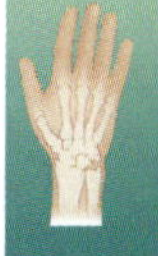

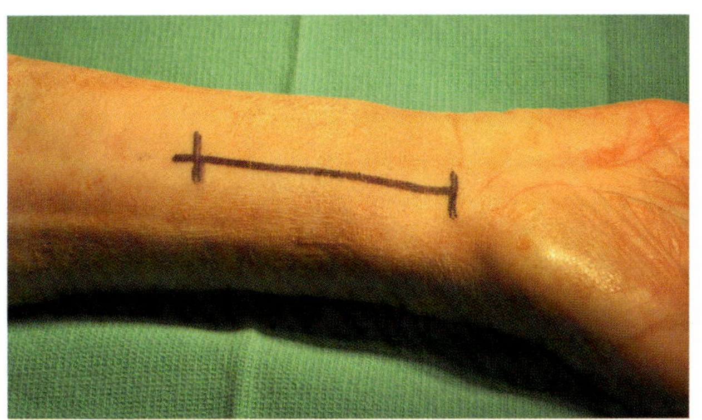
FIGURE 77-3

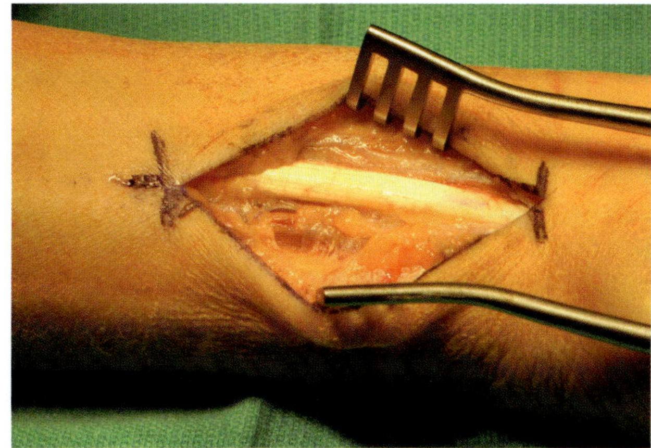
FIGURE 77-4

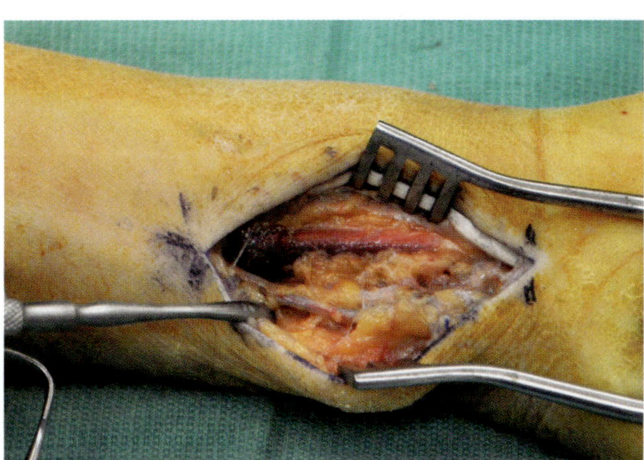
FIGURE 77-5

PEARLS

It is helpful to mobilize the radial artery and ligate its small crossing branches during the exposure. This minimizes bleeding and also allows for better exposure of the BR for release.

Do not take the reflection of the soft tissue too far distally on the radius. This may result in release of the volar carpal ligaments from the distal radius and induce carpal instability.

Positioning

- The operation is performed with the arm supinated on a hand table under tourniquet control.

Exposures

- An incision about 7 cm in length is made over the forearm between the radial artery and the FCR. The distal aspect of the incision stops at the volar wrist crease (Fig. 77-3). If the incision needs to be extended more distally, a V-shaped zigzag extension should be made.
- The FCR tendon is exposed and released from its sheath. The dissection should remain on the radial aspect of the FCR (Fig. 77-4).
- The radial artery and its accompanying venae comitantes are exposed and retracted radially. All ulnar crossing vessels are coagulated (Fig. 77-5).

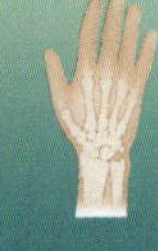

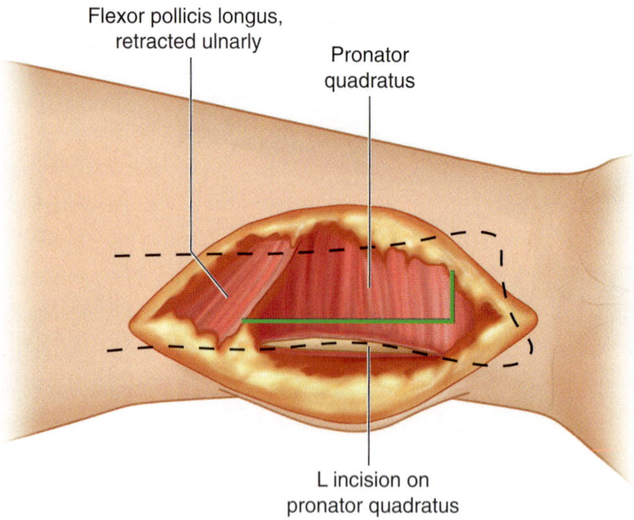

FIGURE 77-6

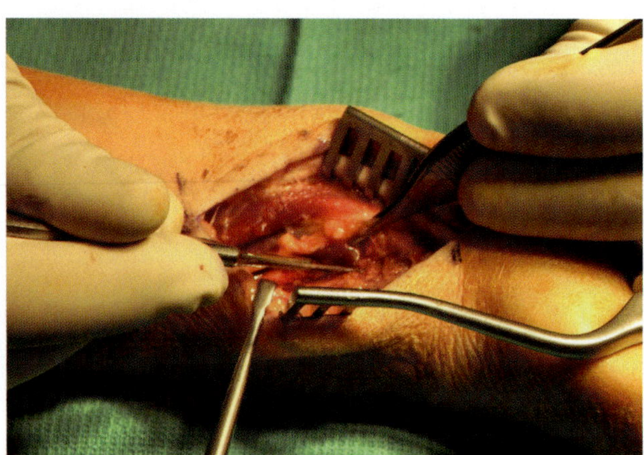

FIGURE 77-7

PITFALLS

Dissection should not be performed ulnar to the FCR tendon because the palmar cutaneous branch of the median nerve may be damaged.

During release of the BR tendon, the dissection must remain entirely on bone, or the tendons of the first dorsal compartment tendons may be damaged.

- The PQ is elevated from the distal radius by making an L-shaped incision and releasing it radially and distally (Fig. 77-6). The PQ is sharply released from the radius to expose the fracture (Fig. 77-7).

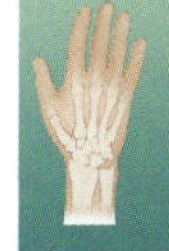

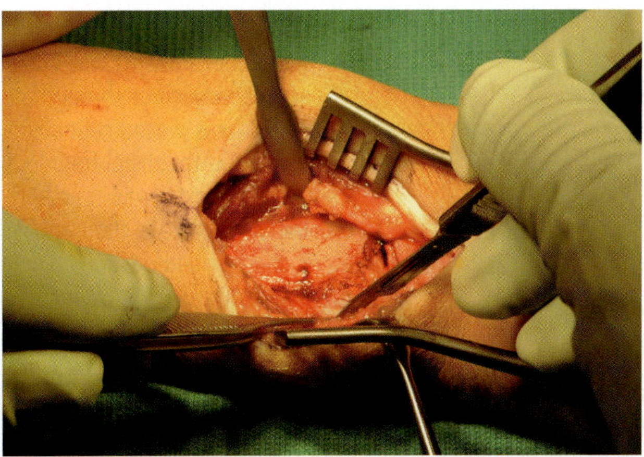

FIGURE 77-8

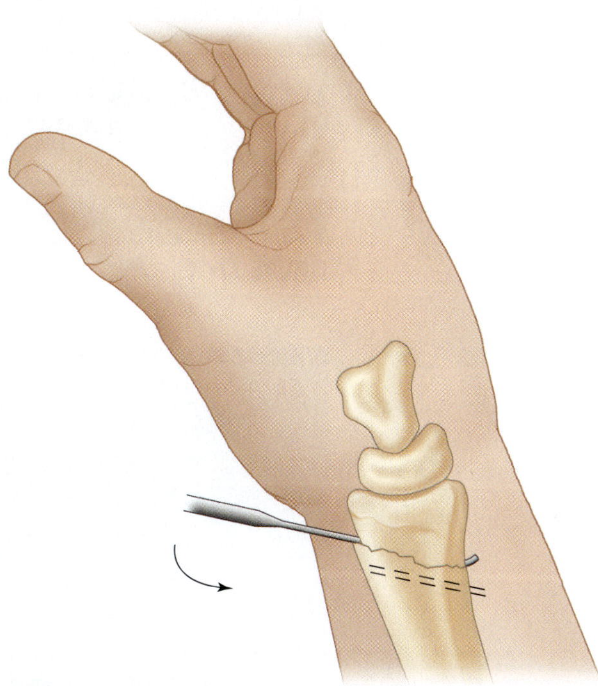

FIGURE 77-9

Procedure

Step 1

- The volar radius is exposed, and the distal fragment is exposed by releasing the BR tendon. The distal fragment is usually displaced dorsally (Fig. 77-8).
- A Freer elevator may be used to lever the distal fragment for fracture reduction (Fig. 77-9). The elevator should be inserted to the dorsal cortex to completely disimpact the distal fragment to aid in reduction.
- Alternatively, the distal fragment can be reduced to the radial shaft by flexing the hand and wrist, thereby realigning the distal fragment and promoting reduction.

STEP 1 PEARLS

The hand and distal fragment may be placed on a large towel-bump to aid in reducing the fragment.

STEP 1 PITFALLS

Care should be taken not to over-reduce the fracture, thus creating increased volar displacement.

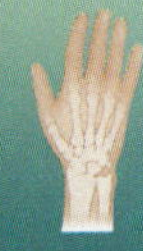

STEP 2 PEARLS

During radiographic assessment of plate placement, the anteroposterior view confirms proper radioulnar placement, whereas the lateral view is critical in determining proper proximal-distal placement.

STEP 2 PITFALLS

Do not place the plate too distal because this may result in radiocarpal screw penetration.

Step 2

- The reduced fracture may be provisionally held with K-wires placed through the open approach or through a small separate radial styloid incision (Fig. 77-10).
- The plate is placed centrally on the radial shaft and as far distally as necessary to capture the distal fragment. It is crucial to be familiar with the specific plate distal locking screw trajectory for proper plate placement (Fig. 77-11).
- The volar plate is then applied to the radial shaft, and a screw is inserted first in the elongated elliptical hole. A 2.0-mm drill bit is drilled in the center of the hole, and a 2.7-mm screw is then placed (Fig. 77-12).

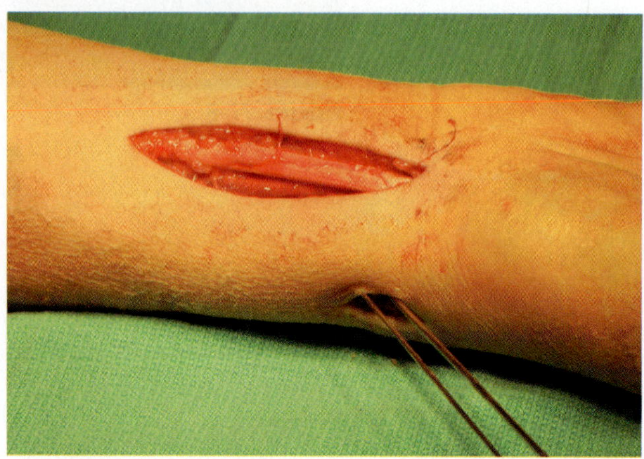

FIGURE 77-10

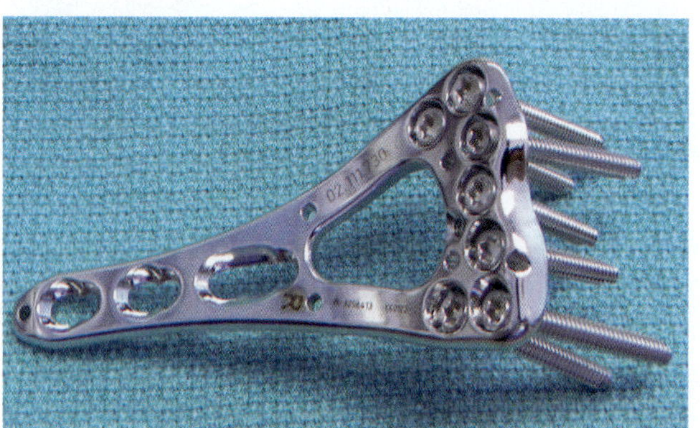

FIGURE 77-11

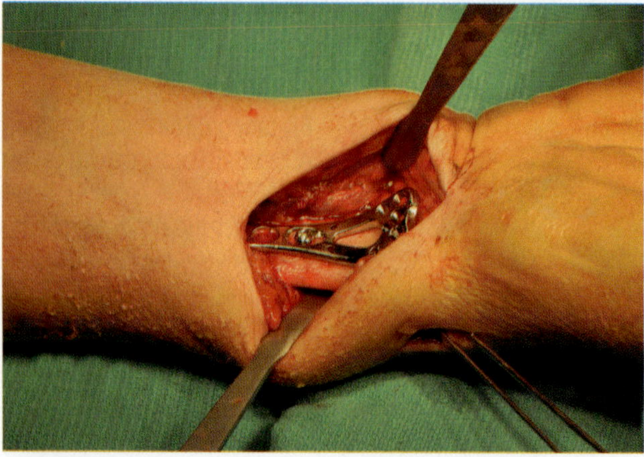

FIGURE 77-12

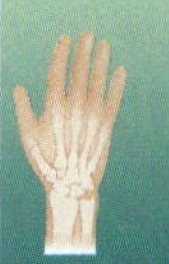

- The plate placement is checked with fluoroscopy. The plate may be shifted distally or proximally by loosening and then retightening the shaft screw.
- Once plate placement is confirmed as ideal, a second 2.7-mm screw is placed in the shaft to fix the plate placement.

STEP 3 PEARLS

A fossa lateral view of the distal radius should be taken to ensure no joint penetration of the screws. A fossa lateral view is taken by holding the forearm at about 22 degrees of inclination with regard to the hand table. This corrects the overlap of the articular surface caused by the radial inclination on a standard lateral view (Fig. 77-15).

The designed purpose of the distal screw row is for subchondral support, whereas the proximal screw row provides distal-dorsal fixation.

Step 3

- The distal screws are next placed in the plate with the wrist in a flexed position. These screws are 2.4 mm in size and are drilled with a 1.8-mm drill bit. If the fracture is properly reduced, a locking screw may be placed (Fig. 77-13).
- If there is some separation between the distal fragment and the plate, a non-locking screw may be placed first to draw the bone to the plate and thus improve the reduction. This screw may be later exchanged for a locked screw if desired.
- A sufficient number of screws should be placed in the distal aspect of the plate to ensure adequate purchase of all the fracture fragments (Fig. 77-14).
- The provisional K-wires can be removed, or left in place for 3 weeks if added support of the fracture is required.

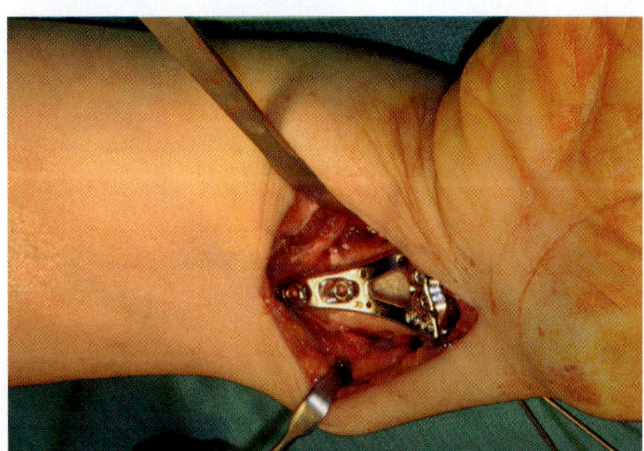

FIGURE 77-13

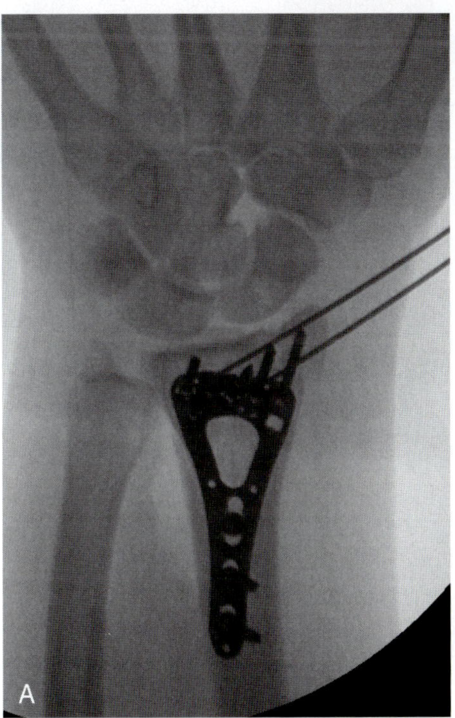

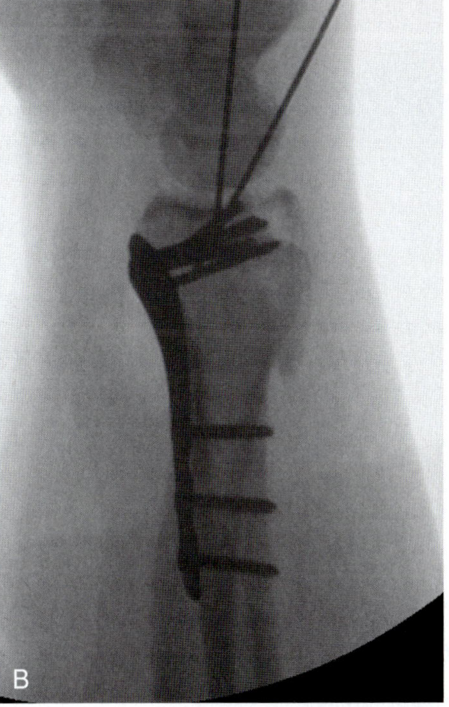

FIGURE 77-14

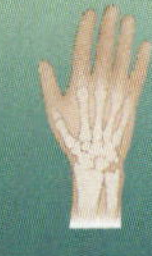

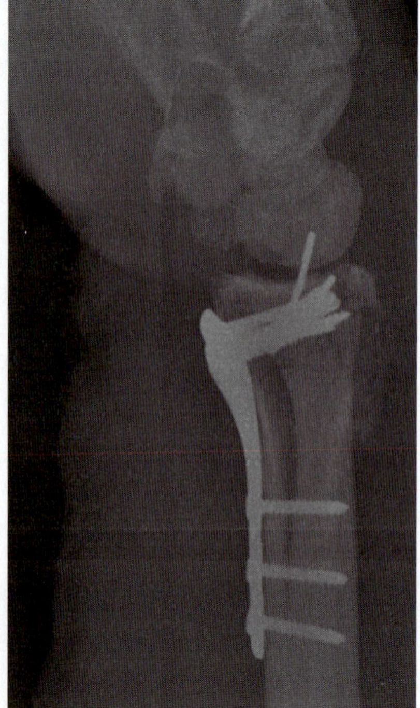

FIGURE 77-15

STEP 3 PITFALLS

The screws should not be placed too long because their self-tapping design makes the tips sharp and may cause an attritional tendon rupture.

Care should be taken to avoid joint penetration with the screws in both the radiocarpal and distal-radial ulnar joints.

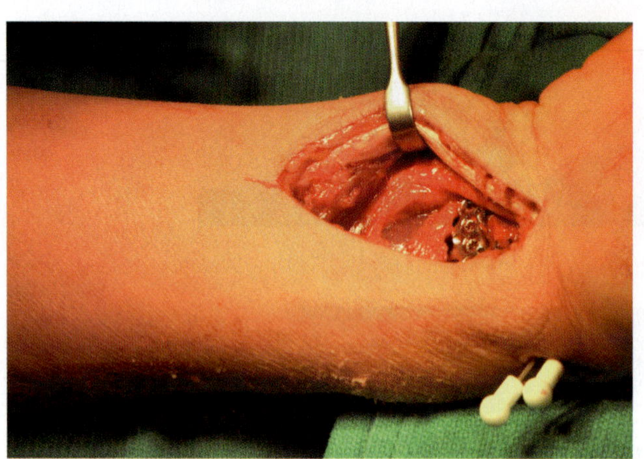

FIGURE 77-16

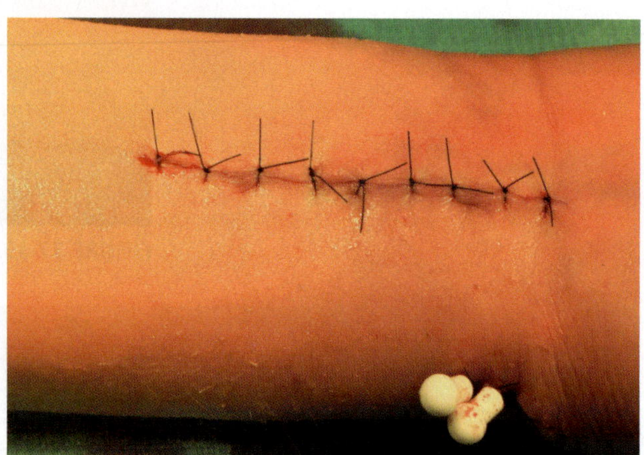

FIGURE 77-17

Step 4

- The PQ is replaced over the plate and sutured to its radial attachment and periosteum (Fig. 77-16).
- The wound is closed with 3-0 Vicryl sutures in the subcutaneous tissue and interrupted 3-0 nylon sutures in the skin (Fig. 77-17).
- The patient is placed in a short-arm volar splint at the end of the surgical procedure.

STEP 4 PEARLS

- The PQ often cannot be completely reattached, but even a partial closure provides some soft tissue coverage of the plate.
- If the BR was released, it may be reattached in a step-cut lengthening fashion.

STEP 4 PITFALLS

When reattaching the PQ, ensure that no sutures are placed in the first dorsal compartment tendons.

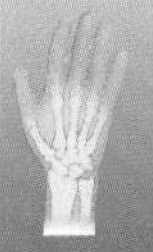

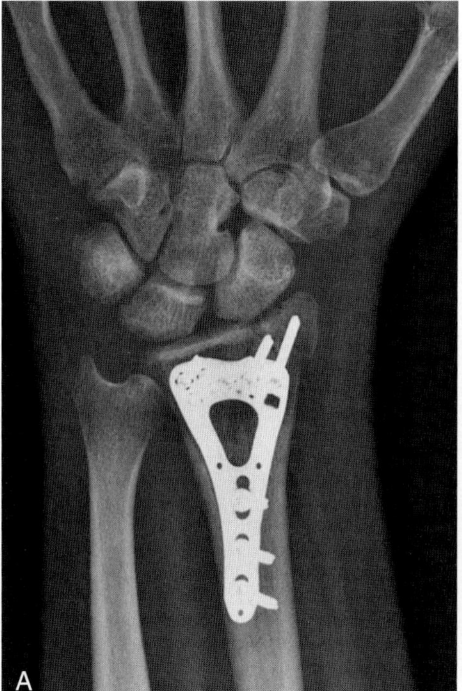

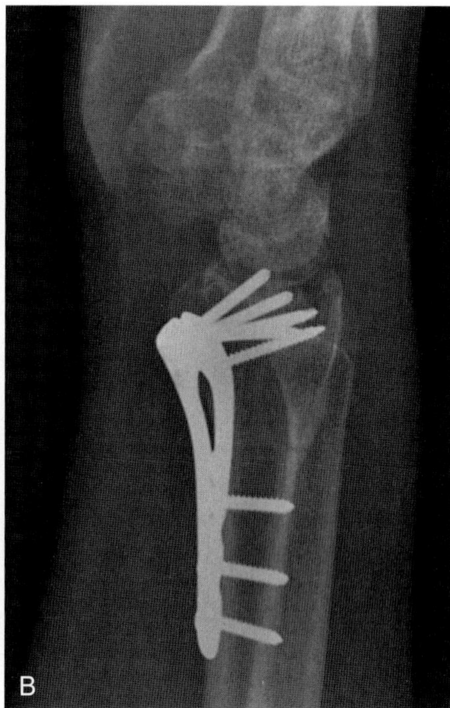

FIGURE 77-18

Postoperative Care and Expected Outcomes

- The patient is seen 10 to 14 days after surgery, and the sutures are removed.
- Gentle range of motion (ROM) of the wrist is begun at that time.
- Aggressive finger ROM is begun immediately after surgery to decrease edema and avoid digital stiffness.
- Final postoperative radiographs should show a well-reduced fracture with a congruent joint surface (Fig. 77-18).

Evidence

Orbay J, Badia A, Khoury RK, et al: Volar fixed-angle fixation of distal radius fractures: the DVR plate. *Tech Hand Up Extrem Surg*. 2004;8:142-148.

This article reviews the technique for volar fixed-angle fixation of distal radius fractures, which provides the advantage of stable internal fixation without incurring the complications of the dorsal approach. This fixed-angle plate was introduced specifically for the purpose of managing both dorsal and volar displaced fractures from the volar aspect. The surgical approach is an extended form of the flexor carpi radialis exposure, which allows improved dorsal access by mobilizing the proximal radius out of the way, allowing access to the fracture fragments. This approach addressed the need for reducing fractures with significant articular displacement that also needed débridement of the dorsal organized hematoma or callus (in old fractures). The plate's ability to stabilize the distal radius by taking full advantage of the principles of subchondral support and buttress fixation enabled the use of this implant in severely osteoporotic bone and in fractures with severe articular fragmentation or displacement. (Level V evidence)

Orbay JL, Fernandez DL. Volar fixed-angle plate fixation for unstable distal radius fractures in the elderly patient. *J Hand Surg [Am]*. 2004;29:96-102.

This is a retrospective study that reviewed the outcome of distal radius fractures in the elderly population treated with a volar fixed-angle internal fixation plate. Postoperative regimen included immediate finger motion, early functional use of the hand, and application of wrist splint for an average of 3 weeks. Standard radiographic fracture parameters were measured, and final functional results were evaluated by documenting finger motion, wrist motion, and grip strength. Twenty-four unstable distal radius fractures in 23 patients

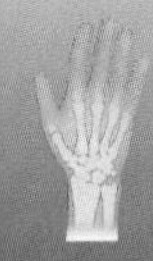

were evaluated. Average follow-up was 63 weeks. Average volar tilt was 6 degrees, and radial tilt was 20 degrees. Radial shortening averaged less than 1 mm. Final extension was 58 degrees, flexion 55 degrees, pronation 80 degrees, and supination 76 degrees. Grip strength was 77% of the contralateral side. No plate failures or significant loss of reduction were documented, although there was settling of the distal fragment (1 to 3 mm) in 3 patients. The authors concluded that volar fixed-angle plate for unstable distal radius fractures in the elderly patient provided stable internal fixation and allowed early return to function. This technique minimized morbidity by successfully stabilizing osteopenic bone and was associated with a low complication rate. (Level V evidence)

Rizzo M, Katt BA, Carothers JT. Comparison of locked volar plating versus pinning and external fixation in the treatment of unstable intraarticular distal radius fractures. *Hand*. 2008;3:111-117.
This is a retrospective study that compared volar locking plate with external fixation with percutaneous pinning for treatment of unstable distal radius fractures. There were 41 patients reviewed for the ORIF group and 14 patients for the external fixation group. Clinical and functional outcomes were measured by the DASH score. Pain scores and radiographic measurements were also documented. Two years after the surgery, range of motion and grip strengths were similar in the two groups. Pain scores using the VAS showed no significant difference. DASH scores were better for the volar locking plate group. For radiographic analysis, significantly better outcome was observed with volar plating in terms of volar tilt, articular step-off, and ulnar variance. Significant difference was also documented in the number of hand therapy visits required, which favored the ORIF group. Two pin tract infections were documented in the external fixation group, whereas no complications were observed in the volar plate group. Overall, the study favors the use of locked volar plate over external fixation based on the parameters examined. (Level IV evidence)

Souer JS, Ring D, Matschke S, et al. Comparison of functional outcome after volar plate fixation with 2.4-mm titanium versus 3.5-mm stainless-steel plate for extra-articular fracture of distal radius. *J Hand Surg [Am]*. 2010;35:398-405.
This is a level III therapeutic study comparing the functional outcome of use of a titanium 2.4-mm precontoured plate with that of a stainless-steel oblique 3.5-mm T-shaped plate to test. Twenty-four patients treated with a 2.4-mm titanium plate and 38 patients treated with a 3.5-mm stainless-steel plate for an extra-articular and dorsally angulated distal radius fracture were retrospectively analyzed. The two groups were evaluated for differences in motion, grip strength, pain, Gartland and Werley score, DASH score, and Short Form-36 score at 6, 12, and 24 months of follow-up. Regression analysis and the likelihood ratio test were used to determine the group differences and their change over time. There were no significant differences in wrist function and arm-specific health status between patients treated with a 2.4-mm plate and those treated with a 3.5-mm plate at 6, 12, or 24 months of follow-up. However, in patients treated with a 2.4-mm plate, there was an observed trend toward greater wrist flexion at 1 year (66 degrees vs. 55 degrees; P = .07) and greater flexion-extension arc (137 degrees vs. 123 degrees; P = .08) and pronation-supination arc (172 degrees vs. 160 degrees; P = .07) 24 months after surgery. They concluded that similar results can be expected in patients treated with either a precontoured 2.4-mm titanium plate or a 3.5-mm stainless-steel T-shaped plate for a dorsally angulated extra-articular distal radius facture. (Level III evidence)

Wei DH, Raizman NM, Bottino CJ, et al. Unstable distal radial fractures treated with external fixation, a radial column plate, or a volar plate: a prospective randomized trial. *J Bone Joint Surg [Am]*. 2009;91:1568-1577.
This is a therapeutic level I study that compared the functional outcomes of treatment of unstable distal radial fractures with external fixation, a radial column plate, and a volar plate. Follow-up conducted at varying intervals postoperatively demonstrated that at 6 weeks, the DASH score was better with volar plate than with external fixation, but the score was similar between volar plate and radial column plate use. At 3 months, DASH scores are significantly better with volar plate use than with external fixation and radial column plate use. At 6 months and 1 year, DASH scores for the three groups were comparable with those for the normal population. Grip strength was similar for the three groups at 1 year. Significantly better lateral pinch strength was observed with volar plate use compared with radial column plate use at 3 months and 1 year, but no significant difference was observed at subsequent intervals. The range of motion of the wrist was not significantly different among the three groups from 12 weeks postoperatively. At 1 year, radial inclination and radial length were significantly better in the radial column plate group than in the other two groups. In conclusion, unstable distal radial fractures treated with locked volar plate recovered more quickly compared with external fixation and radial column plate use. However, 1 year after surgery, all three techniques provided good subjective and objective functional outcomes. (Level I evidence)

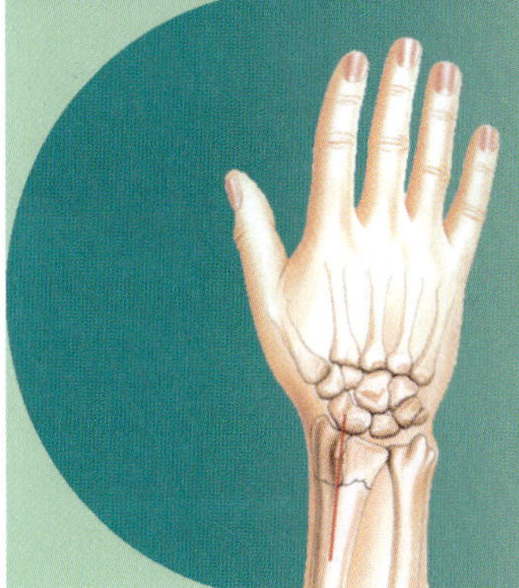

PROCEDURE 78

Dorsal Plate Fixation and Dorsal Distraction (Bridge) Plating for Distal Radius Fractures

Safi R. Faruqui and Peter J. Stern

Dorsal Plating of Distal Radius Fractures

Indications

- Highly comminuted, articular distal radius fractures
- Dorsal shearing fractures
- Die-punch lunate facet fractures
- Dorsal radiocarpal fracture dislocations

Examination/Imaging

Clinical Examination

- Initial examination is usually performed in the emergency department and needs to include mechanism and time of injury, hand dominance, medical comorbidities that may alter treatment, and occupation.
- Assess whether the fracture is an open or closed injury.
- Thorough musculoskeletal examination, especially the ipsilateral extremity, is necessary to rule out concomitant injuries.
- Identify any associated neurovascular and soft tissue injuries.
- Identify whether patient has any sign or symptoms of acute median or ulnar nerve injury.

Imaging

- Initial radiographic evaluation must include posteroanterior, lateral, and oblique views (Fig. 78-1).

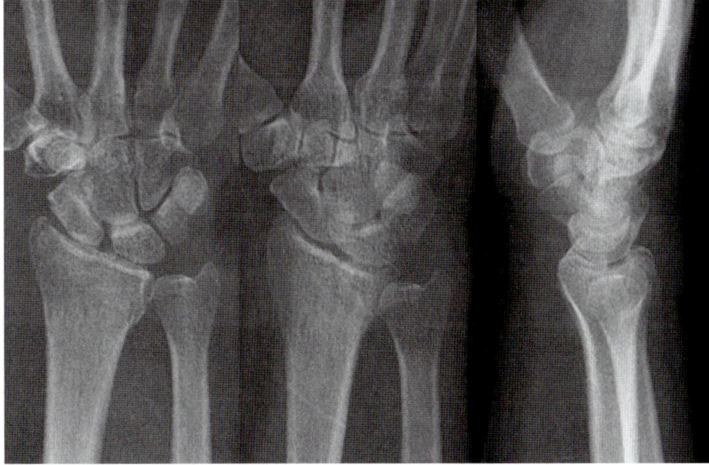

FIGURE 78-1

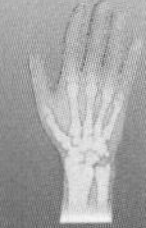

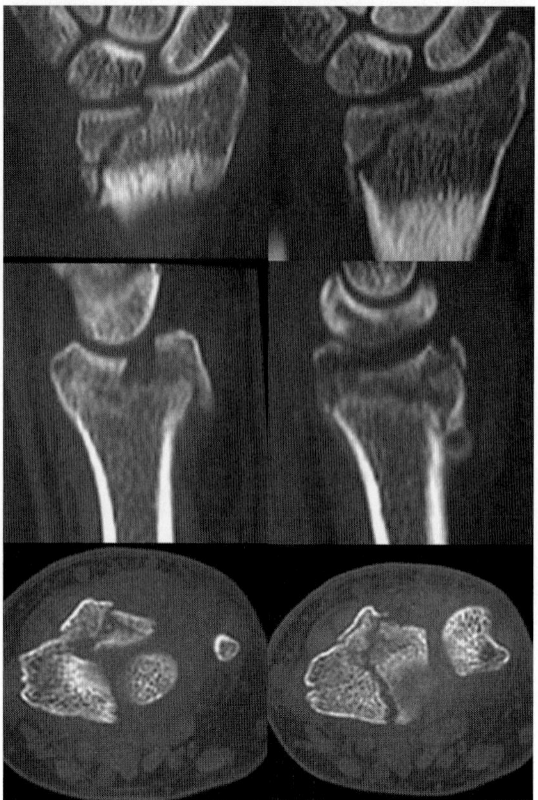

FIGURE 78-2

- Assessment must include fracture angulation, displacement, radial shortening, comminution, intra-articular extension, and any ulnar-sided injuries.
- Combined lesion of a radial styloid with a dorsal marginal or facet fracture (AO type B2.2) is common and can be misdiagnosed as a Colles fracture on lateral radiographs.
- The lunate facet often has a coronal fracture line that separates this facet into dorsal and volar fragments.
- Computed tomography scan provides excellent delineation of intra-articular extension as well as characterization of fracture comminution for preoperative planning (Fig. 78-2).
- There is also typically subchondral collapse of the lunate facet that must be addressed to ensure articular reduction.
- Proximal injuries must be ruled out by physical examination and radiographs of the elbow.

Surgical Anatomy

- Knowledge of the anatomic relationships of the extensor retinaculum, six dorsal extensor compartments, and convex dorsoradial cortex is essential for understanding surgical approaches as well as placement of implants on the dorsum of the radius (Fig. 78-3).
- Extensor retinaculum prevents the extensor tendons from dorsal displacement (bowstringing) and divides the tendons into six extensor compartments by vertical septae.

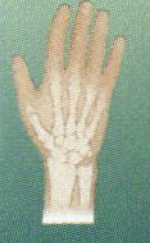

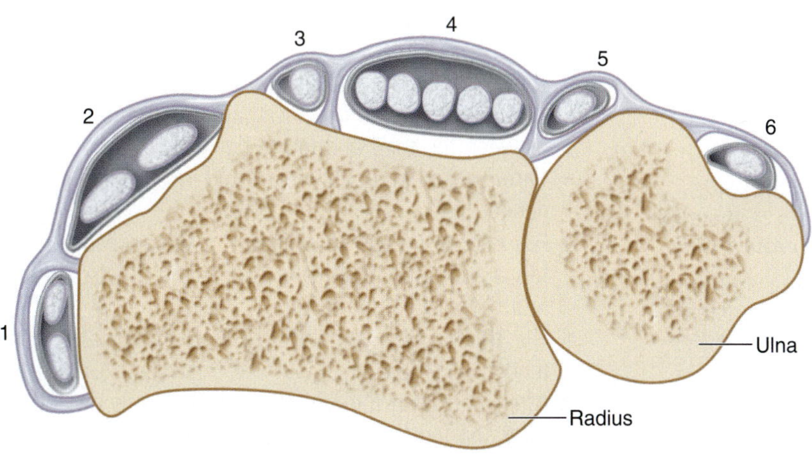

FIGURE 78-3

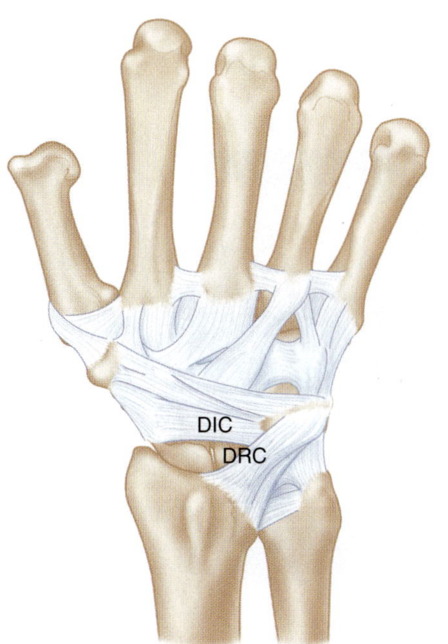

FIGURE 78-4

- The extensor pollicis longus (EPL) tendon, which lies in the third dorsal compartment, passes ulnar to the Lister tubercle and is mobilized during exposure of the dorsal distal radius.
- The extensor indicis proprius tendon and the extensor digitorum communis tendon lie in the fourth dorsal compartment and are elevated subperiosteally to minimize tendon contact with dorsally placed implants.
- Elevation of the second dorsal compartment, which contains the radial wrist extensors, puts the dorsal sensory branch of the radial nerve and the dorsal radial artery at risk, particularly if the dissection is extended distally.
- The terminal branch of the posterior interosseous nerve lies on the floor of the fourth dorsal compartment along its radial side; it can be sacrificed, if necessary, without clinical consequence.
- The articular surface of the distal radius is biconcave and triangular, with the surface divided into two hyaline covered, concave facets for articulation with the scaphoid and lunate.
- There are two dorsal ligaments that are intimately associated with the dorsal capsule: the dorsal radiocarpal (DRC) (radiotriquetral) and dorsal intercarpal (DIC) (scaphotriquetral) ligaments (Fig. 78-4).

PEARLS

Large, longitudinal veins should be preserved if possible, but crossing veins may be divided.

Full-thickness flaps will contain the dorsal sensory branches of the ulnar and radial nerve and protect them.

Subperiosteal elevation of the fourth compartment minimizes implant contact with the extensor tendons.

Exposures

- The dorsal distal radius is approached through a straight, longitudinal incision in line with the third metacarpal and centered just ulnar to the Lister tubercle, between the third and fourth dorsal compartments (Fig. 78-5).
- Care is taken to identify and avoid injury to the superficial branch of the radial nerve.
- Full-thickness flaps containing the skin, subcutaneous tissues, and superficial fascia are raised together to expose the extensor retinaculum and the third and fourth dorsal compartments.
- The third dorsal compartment is longitudinally incised to mobilize the EPL tendon (Fig. 78-6).
- After mobilizing the EPL, the retinaculum is divided between the septa of the third and fourth dorsal compartments.
- Using a periosteal elevator or sharp dissection, the fourth compartment is then elevated subperiosteally from the dorsum of the distal radius, keeping the deep surface of the compartment intact.
- The distal radius is exposed sharply by elevation of the periosteum.
- Exposure of the intermediate column requires dissection to continue in an ulnar direction to the distal radioulnar joint (DRUJ).
- A longitudinal capsulotomy may be needed to expose the distal radius articular surface, which requires detaching the dorsal capsular insertions on the distal nonarticular lunate.

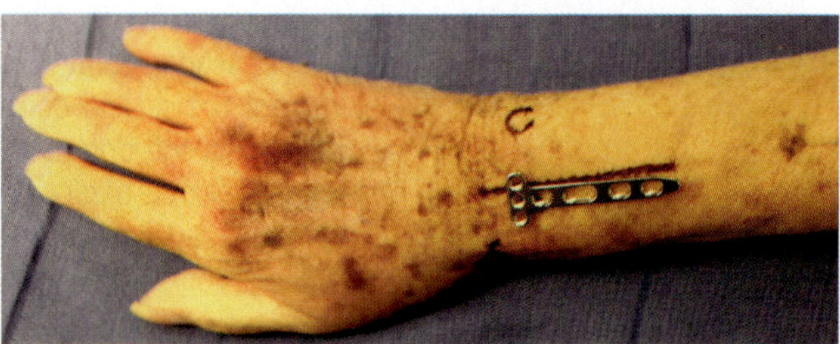

FIGURE 78-5

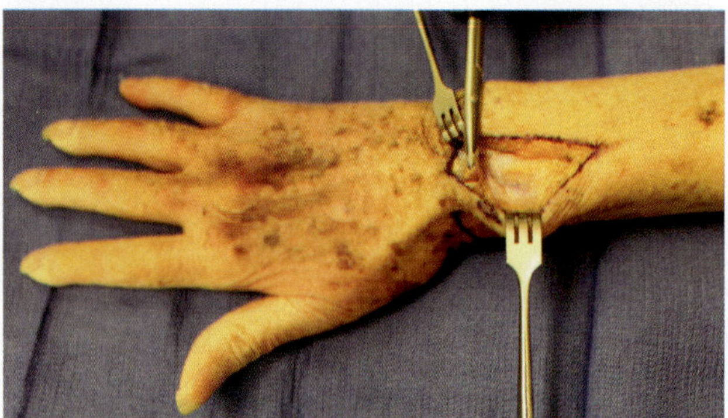

FIGURE 78-6

PITFALLS

If the distal extension of the incision is past the base of the third metacarpal, the dorsal sensory branches of both the radial and ulnar nerves are at risk.

The EPL tendon is left above the retinaculum at closure to minimize the risk for tendon injury by ischemia or direct contact with an implant.

Care must be exercised not to enter the DRUJ. If the dorsal radioulnar ligament is divided during ulnar dissection, radioulnar instability can result.

The intercarpal ligaments must be protected during capsulotomy.

STEP 1 PEARLS

Removal of the Lister tubercle will allow the plate to sit flush with the dorsal cortex and hence be less prominent.

STEP 1 PITFALLS

Failure to reduce articular fragments may lead to symptomatic radiocarpal arthrosis.

Use of the nick-and-spread method to insert percutaneous K-wire fixation is imperative to prevent injury to the branches of the superficial radial nerve.

STEP 2 PEARLS

Allograft or bone graft substitute may be utilized to fill in metaphyseal defects to enhance stability.

STEP 2 PITFALLS

Care must be taken not to insert screws into the radiocarpal joint. Rotational fluoroscopy and direct visualization are critical to avoid this error.

Procedure

Dorsal Plate Fixation for Distal Radius Fractures

Step 1: Reduction of Dorsally Angulated Fractures

- Once the proximal fracture lines and articular surface are exposed and assessed, all hematoma is evacuated.
- Lister tubercle is removed with a rongeur or small osteotome (Fig. 78-7).
- Reduction of the dorsal angulation can be performed with the use of narrow-angled Homan retractors along the proximal fragment.
- With gentle traction and lifting of the bone retractors, reduction of the dorsal angulation can be achieved.
- Provisional fixation with Kirschner wires (0.045-in.) can be used to hold the reduction and is checked fluoroscopically.

Step 2: Fixation of Dorsally Angulated Fractures

- After satisfactory reduction is performed, a 2.4-mm low-profile dorsal T-plate (Fig. 78-8) can be placed directly over the dorsal surface of the distal radius.
- Preliminary fixation of the plate with a single, bicortical compression screw placed in the oblong hole of the plate will allow for proximal-distal adjustments in plate position as determined clinically and fluoroscopically.

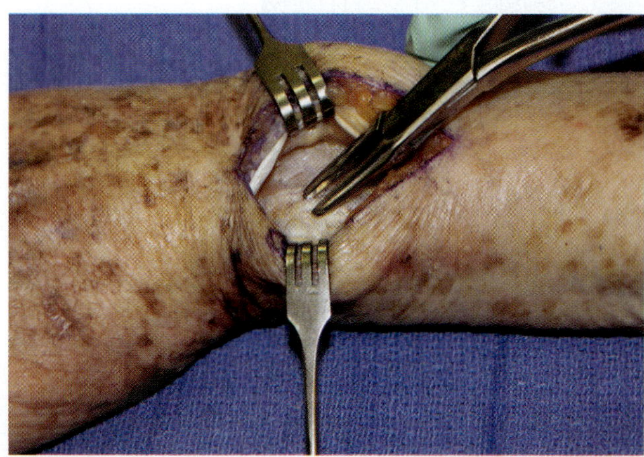

FIGURE 78-7

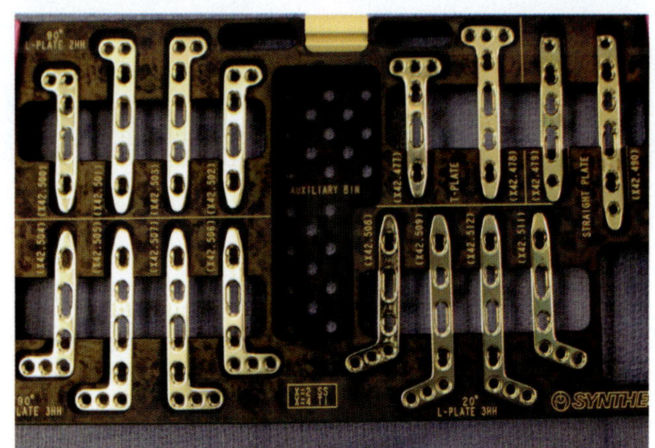

FIGURE 78-8

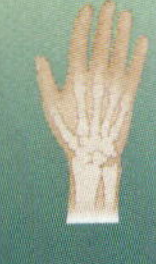

- It is important to provisionally bend the plate to fit the contour of the dorsal radial cortex so that the plate lies flush with the dorsal cortex.
- Although several options for plating are available, including locking and non-locking plates, one must consider contouring a fixed-angle plate by threading a locking guide into the plate before contouring; this will avoid damage to the threads of the locking mechanism.
- The final placement is checked by fluoroscopy in anteroposterior and lateral views to confirm proper positioning of the plate.
- Three to five 2.7-mm screws are then placed bicortically along the distal row of the plate, using fluoroscopy to confirm placement.
- Two additional proximal screws are then inserted bicortically, and final fluoroscopic assessment is performed.

STEP 3 PEARLS

Having small and mini-implants as well as external fixation available can be invaluable to address difficult fracture patterns.

Metaphyseal bone defects should be addressed with cancellous bone grafting to help support the articular anatomy.

Step 3: Reduction and Fixation of Dorsal Marginal Fractures

- It is important to assess carpal subluxation and initially restore the radial styloid fragment if present (Fig. 78-9A).
- This reduction is usually accomplished with traction and ulnar deviation of the hand and wrist, and then provisional K-wire fixation (Figs. 78-9B and 78-10).
- Once the appropriate-sized 2.4-mm plate has been contoured, the locking screw guide is placed in the proximal screw hole and is used to hold and contour the plate.

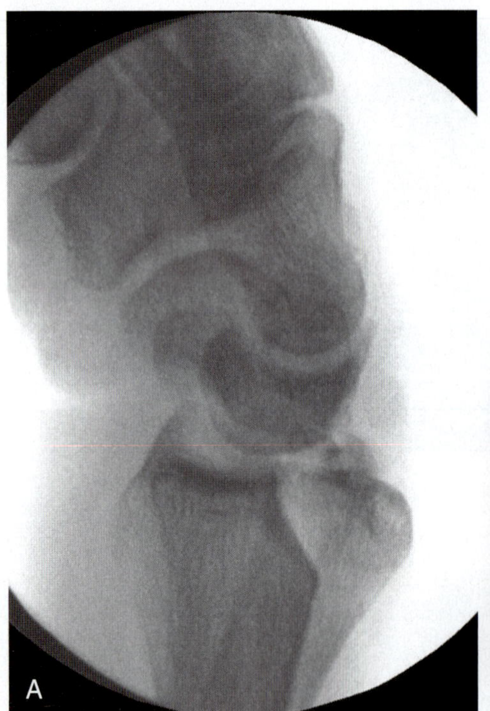

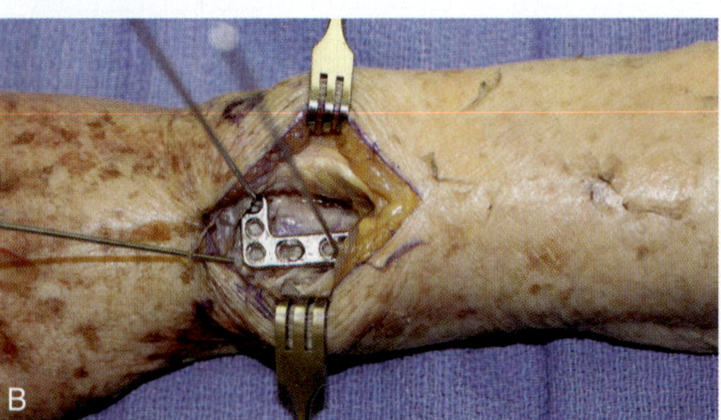

FIGURE 78-9

- Preliminary fixation of the plate with a single, bicortical screw placed in the oblong hole will allow for proximal-distal plate adjustments as determined clinically and fluoroscopically (Fig. 78-11).
- A provisional K-wire is then placed through the threaded locking guide at the distal end of the plate but not into the radius to facilitate quick placement after reduction of the carpus.
- The dorsal lip or marginal fracture can be reduced now against the scaphoid and lunate, which will correct any associated dorsal carpal subluxation.
- The marginal fracture will then be provisionally fixed into the volar cortex through the provisional K-wire that had been previously placed into the threaded locking guide at the distal end of the plate.
- Congruity of the articular surface must be confirmed with direct visualization as well as fluoroscopically.
- If the plate is acting purely as a buttress, distal locking screws are not necessary.

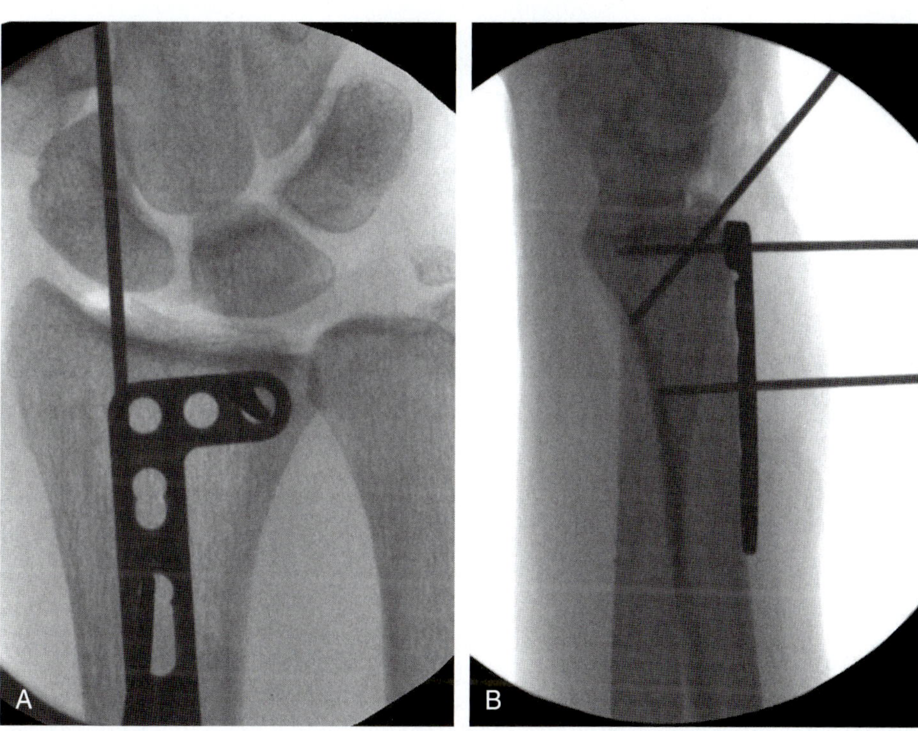

FIGURE 78-10

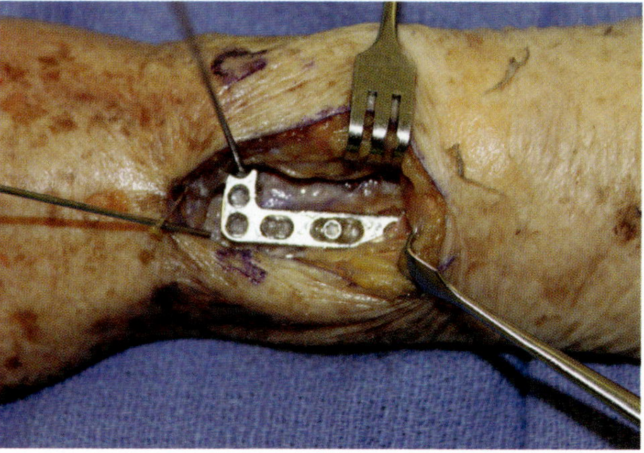

FIGURE 78-11

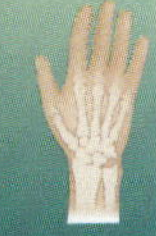

STEP 3 PITFALLS

Failure to recognize styloid component or any volar-ulnar fragments will lead to incongruity of articular surface and radiocarpal arthrosis.

These fractures may be associated with dorsal radiocarpal subluxation, volar ligament injuries, articular surface impaction, and avulsion fractures.

All bicortical fixations should be checked radiographically to ensure that they are not prominent volarly.

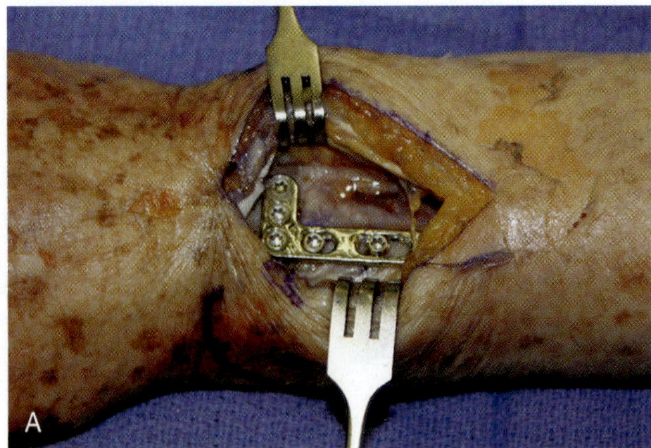

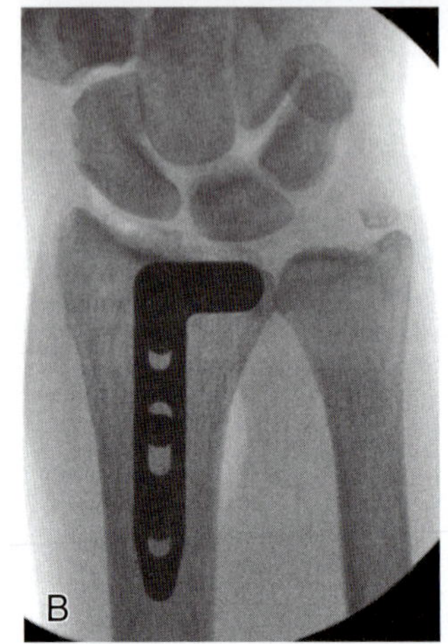

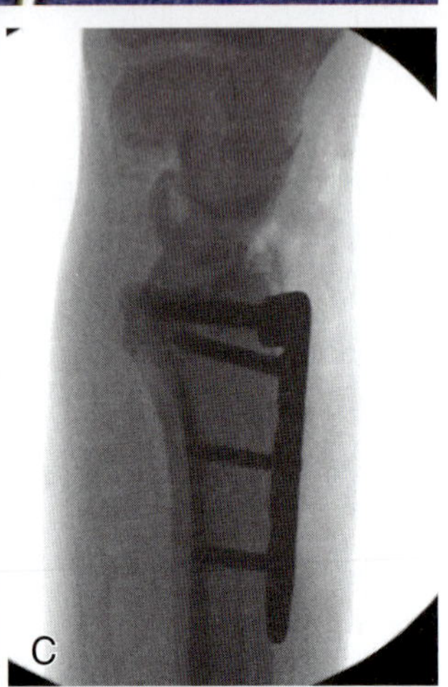

FIGURE 78-12

- If additional fixation for stability is necessary, 2.4-mm screws are then placed bicortically along the distal row of the plate, using fluoroscopy to confirm placement.
- One or two additional bicortical screws are placed proximally to the proximal extent of the fracture to finalize construct (Figure 78-12).

Step 4: Reduction and Fixation of Lunate Facet Fractures

- Subchondral collapse of the lunate facet can be addressed with the use of a Freer elevator or dental pick placed into the facet fracture line in the metaphysic.
- The lunate facet fragment is then manually reduced by elevating the depressed surface and checked both by fluoroscopy and directly if an arthrotomy has been made to ensure adequate reduction.
- A provisional K-wire can be placed along the subchondral surface from the radial styloid to the sigmoid notch to act as a buttress for the reduced lunate facet fracture.
- For provisional reduction of coronal facet fractures, temporary K-wires can also be placed to stabilize the coronal fracture line.
- For sagittal splits, intrafragmentary compression is possible using a large bone reduction clamp.
- One point of the clamp is placed along the ulnar border of the lunate facet, one point is placed along the radial styloid, and after compression of the clamp, a transverse provisional K-wire is placed to hold reduction.

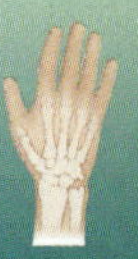

STEP 4 PEARLS

If there are nonarticular fragments seen along the dorsal aspects of the scaphoid and lunate facet that still have capsular attachments, an effort should be made to save them with their attachments.

Bone grafting metaphyseal defects after elevation of depressed articular fragments is essential to maintain reduction.

STEP 4 PITFALLS

Failure to appreciate the volar-ulnar fragment may lead to displacement and insufficient buttressing of the fracture.

- When an impacted fragment is elevated, there will often be a metaphyseal void that must be filled with cancellous allograft or bone graft substitute to support the articular surface.
- After preliminary reduction is confirmed both by direct visualization and fluoroscopy, an L-shaped 2.4-mm plate is typically used for buttress fixation of the intermediate column and articular surface (see Fig. 78-8).
- The dorsoulnar plate usually needs to be contoured to allow placement along the dorsoulnar aspect of the distal part of the radius.
- The plate is then fixed proximally to the shaft well distally along the L-portion of the plate.
- It is especially important to obtain bicortical screw fixation along the ulnar side of the radius if there is a coronal split in the facet because it is vital to obtain compression of the volar ulnar fragment.
- If stable fixation cannot be obtained with only a dorsal approach, a volar approach between the FCR and radial artery may be used to stabilize the volar cortex.
- If this fails, an external fixator can be applied.
- The wrist is taken through a range of motion, including flexion, extension, supination, and pronation, to ensure clinical stability.

Step 5: Assessment of DRUJ Stability and Wound Closure

- After stabilization of the radius, any instability of the DRUJ should be assessed (defined as greater than 8 mm of palmar to dorsal translation of the ulna relative to the radius).
- Large fractures of the ulnar styloid, as well as displaced ulnar head fractures, should raise suspicions of instability.
- If instability is noted, consideration should be given to a closed reduction and percutaneous pinning of the DRUJ with the forearm maintained in supination.
- If no instability is noted, no immobilization is necessary.
- If an arthrotomy has been made, the dorsal capsule should be closed with 3-0 nonabsorbable suture.
- The extensor retinaculum should be repaired with interrupted 2-0 absorbable suture, making sure the EPL tendon remains in its transposed position superficial to the retinaculum.
- After wound irrigation, the skin should be closed with either nylon or Prolene sutures in an interrupted fashion.

Postoperative Care and Expected Outcomes

- A bulky sterile dressing and volar splint, leaving the thumb and fingers free, is applied for postoperative comfort for 7 to 10 days (except in those with DRUJ instability).
- After removal of dressing, active and passive digital range-of-motion exercises are initiated.
- A custom, short-arm volar splint is applied in neutral position, which can be removed five to seven times daily to perform active wrist range-of-motion exercises.
- An elastic garment should be used to control postoperative edema.
- Weaning of splint for activities of daily living can be started at 4 weeks.
- After clinical and radiographic evidence of fracture healing is seen (6 to 8 weeks), the splint is discontinued completely.

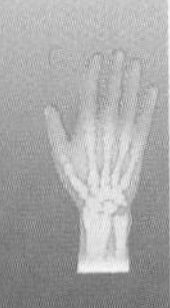

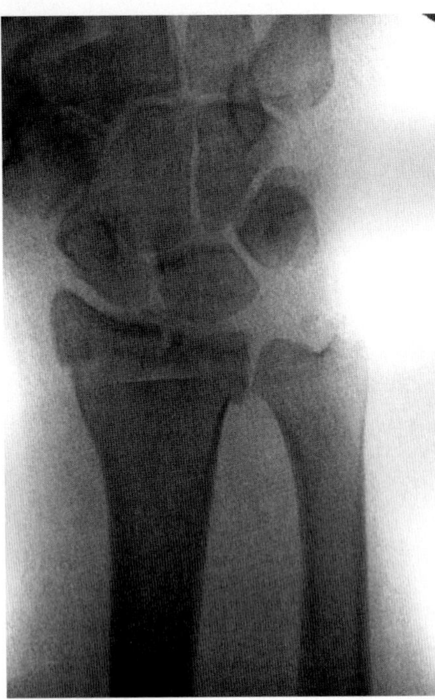

FIGURE 78-13

Dorsal Distraction (Bridge) Plating

Indications

- Highly comminuted, articular distal radius fractures as well as those associated with significant metaphyseal and diaphyseal comminution
- Polytrauma patients to facilitate activities of daily living
- Extensive tendon injuries that may require multiple procedures and an extended period of time for soft tissue and osseous healing
- Severe osteoporosis in which fracture fixation is expected to be poor
- Patients who refuse external fixation for psychological or aesthetic concerns

Examination/Imaging

Clinical Examination

- The likelihood for additional traumatic injuries in the polytrauma patient remains high and must be identified preoperatively.

Imaging

- Initial plain radiographic evaluation must include posteroanterior, lateral, and oblique views (Figs. 78-13 and 78-14).
- Ulnar deviation views can be used in patients with suspected scaphoid fractures.
- Proximal injuries must be ruled out with radiographs of the elbow and forearm.
- Computed tomography scan provides excellent delineation of intra-articular extension as well as characterization of fracture comminution for operative planning (Fig. 78-15).

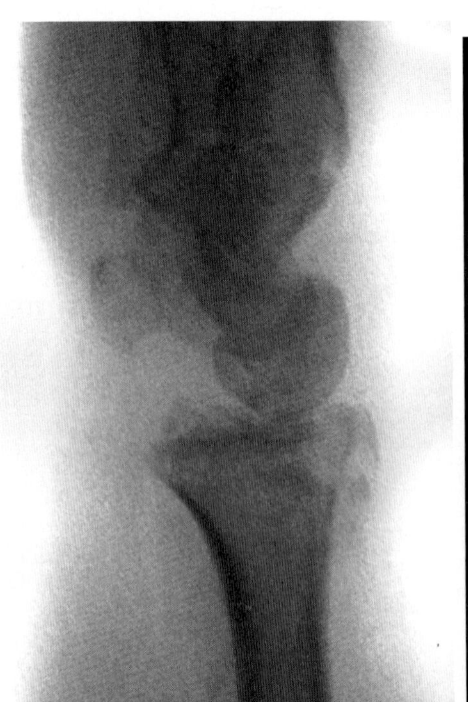

FIGURE 78-14

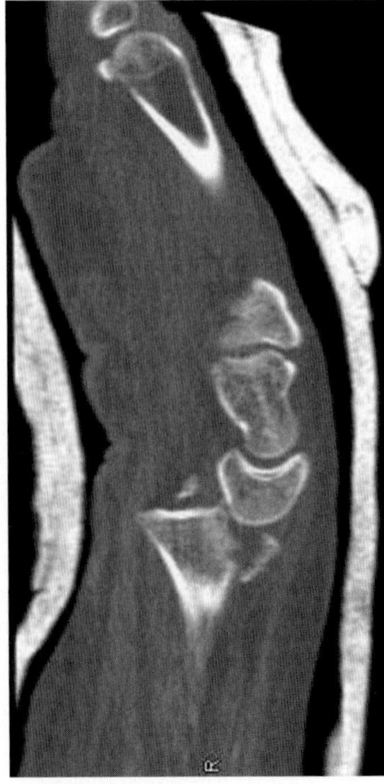

FIGURE 78-15

Surgical Anatomy

- The EPL tendon should be released from its compartment and freed from its groove to prevent injury or impingement of the plate onto the tendon if an open articular reduction is necessary.
- The plate should pass superficial to the joint capsule and periosteum and within the second dorsal compartment, occupied by the extensor carpi radialis longus (ECRL) and extensor carpi radialis brevis (ECRB).
- The extensor tendons over the index finger metacarpal must be identified and retracted to facilitate distal fixation.
- The proximal portion of the plate will be placed along the dorsoradial aspect of the radial shaft adjacent to the brachioradialis and outcropping muscles.
- The superficial branch of the radial nerve is at risk during the proximal dissection of the radial shaft.

PEARLS

Placement of incisions is facilitated with fluoroscopic guidance.

The surgeon holds the distal end of the plate at the index metacarpal neck-shaft junction and identifies the proximal extent of the plate over the radial shaft to ensure placement of three screws proximal to the fracture.

The third incision also allows for exposure of the fracture when necessary, permitting metaphyseal bone grafting and articular reduction.

PITFALLS

The superficial branch of the radial nerve must be identified and protected.

Exposures

- The exposure involves two or three dorsal incisions and is performed under tourniquet control (Fig. 78-16).
- A 4-cm incision is made dorsally over the midpart of the shaft of the index finger metacarpal, with the extensor tendons identified and retracted.
- A second 4- to 6-cm incision is made on the dorsoradial aspect of the radial shaft, just proximal to the outcropping muscle bellies (extensor pollicis brevis and abductor pollicis longus).
- The interval between the ECRL and ECRB is used to expose the radial diaphysis.
- The surgeon must expose enough radial shaft to secure three screws proximal to the fracture site, no less than 4 cm proximal to the most proximal comminuted segment.
- A third incision, about 3 cm in length over the Lister tubercle, can be made if an articular reduction or bone graft is necessary; the EPL is mobilized to facilitate reduction.

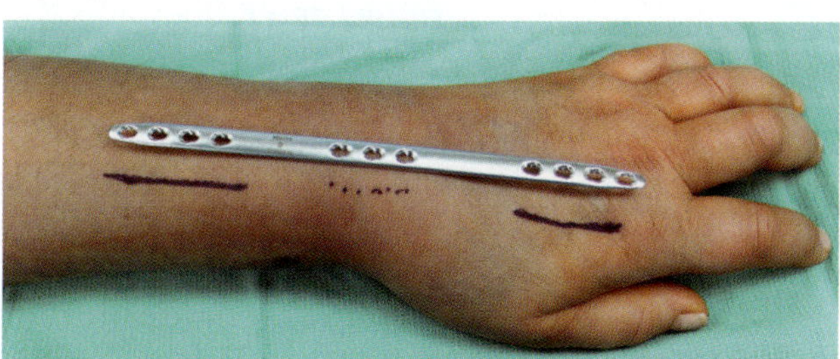

FIGURE 78-16

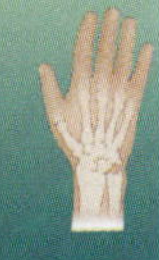

STEP 1 PEARLS

The Distal Radius Bridge Plate is a 2.4-mm combination plate with tapered ends and smooth, beveled edges.

STEP 1 PITFALLS

Do not place the plate too distally on the metacarpal; it should extend no farther distally than the index metacarpal neck.

Procedure

Dorsal Distraction (Bridge) Plating

Step 1: Selection of an Appropriate-Length Plate

- A 20-hole, 2.4-mm Distal Radius Bridge Plate (Synthes, Paoli, PA) is used (Fig. 78-17).
- If this custom plate is not available, a 2.7- or 3.5-mm limited contact dynamic compression plate (LC-DCP) can be substituted.
- Under fluoroscopic guidance, hold the distal end of the plate at the metacarpal neck and identify the proximal extent of the plate over the radial shaft to allow the placement of three screws proximal to the fracture.

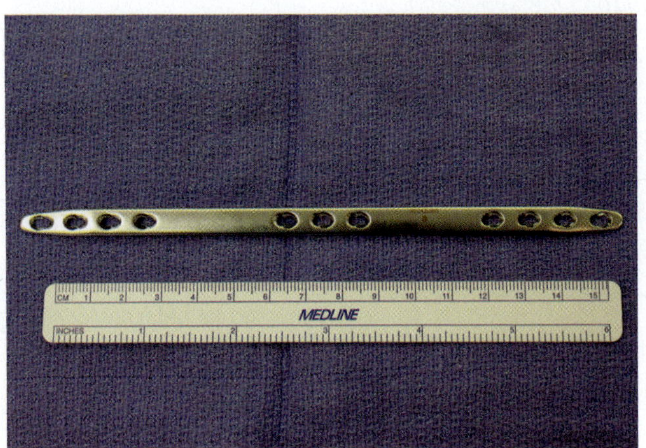

FIGURE 78-17

Step 2: Retrograde Passage of the Plate

- After exposures have been made, a periosteal elevator or long Metzenbaum scissors is carefully inserted proximal to distal along the floor of the second compartment to create a tunnel between the extensor tendons and the periosteum and joint capsule (Fig. 78-18).
- The plate should lie superficial to the periosteum and along the floor of the second dorsal compartment.
- The plate is then passed from the distal to proximal incision under the index finger extensor tendons (Fig. 78-19).

STEP 2 PEARLS

Retraction of the ECRB and ECRL in the proximal wound will allow for visualization of the radial shaft and the periosteal elevator so that long scissors can be passed subperiosteally.

The trajectory of the plate is parallel to the radial aspect of the undersurface of the extensor tendons to the index finger.

STEP 2 PITFALLS

Evaluate the position of the plate to ensure that it does not impinge on the ECRB or ECRL.

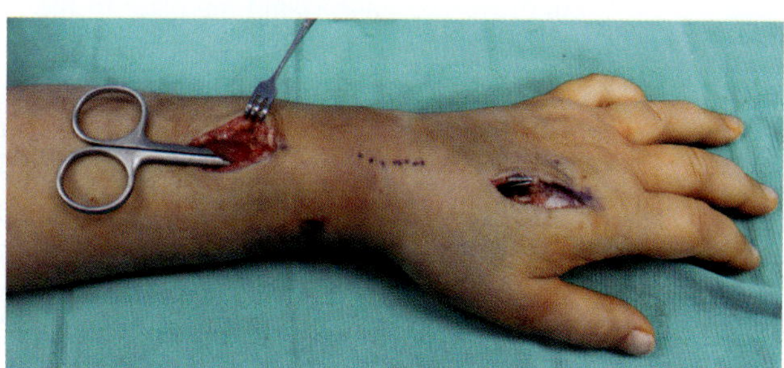

FIGURE 78-18

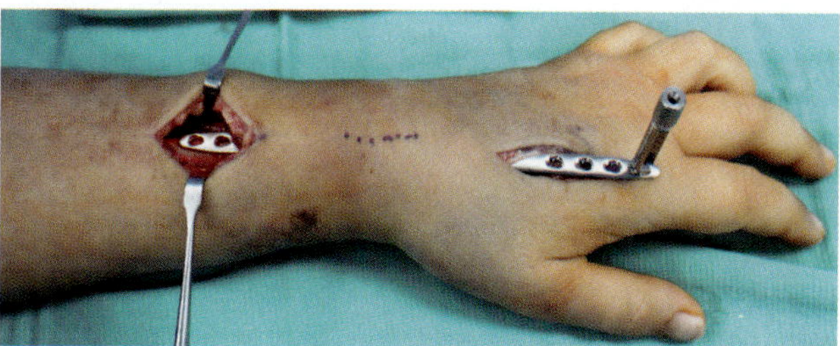

FIGURE 78-19

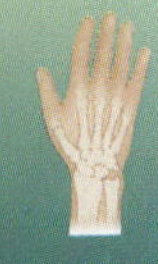

Step 3: Initial Plate Fixation to the Index Metacarpal

- The fracture is initially reduced with manual traction of the wrist.
- Using fluoroscopy, the plate is then aligned centrally over the index metacarpal distally and the radial shaft proximally.
- A bicortical screw is placed in the second-to-last hole in the center of the metacarpal shaft.

STEP 3 PEARLS

Using only a single screw will allow, if necessary, slight adjustments of the plate position for fracture reduction and plate alignment.

To avoid possible rotary displacement of the hand in relation to the shaft, it is important to obtain provisional reduction of both radial inclination and length before securing the plate to the metacarpal shaft.

STEP 3 PITFALLS

Rotary displacement of the fracture will occur if the distal screw is not in the midline of the metacarpal shaft.

Step 4: Plate Fixation to the Radial Shaft

- Reapply traction to the arm to restore radial length and confirm alignment with fluoroscopy.
- Maintain traction, centralize the proximal portion of plate over the radial shaft, and clamp the plate to the proximal radial shaft using serrated bone-holding clamps.
- Reassess the fracture alignment using fluoroscopy to ensure restoration of radial length, inclination, and palmar tilt.
- Perform a clinical as well as a fluoroscopic assessment to ensure proper fracture alignment and absence of rotational abnormalities.
- Three bicortical proximal screws are placed in the shaft to secure the plate.
- Two additional bicortical screws are applied to the metacarpal shaft to ensure three distal points of fixation (Fig. 78-20).
- Final radiographic assessment is repeated to ensure maintenance of reduction (Fig. 78-21).

STEP 4 PEARLS

Assess supination and pronation of the forearm with the plate clamped proximally to the radial shaft to confirm a full range of motion.

It is very helpful to maintain the arm in 45 to 60 degrees of supination while maintaining distraction before the serrated clamp is applied proximally to avoid pronation of the distal fragment.

Once plate placement has been determined with at least one proximal and distal screw, locking screws can be used, particularly in osteopenic bone.

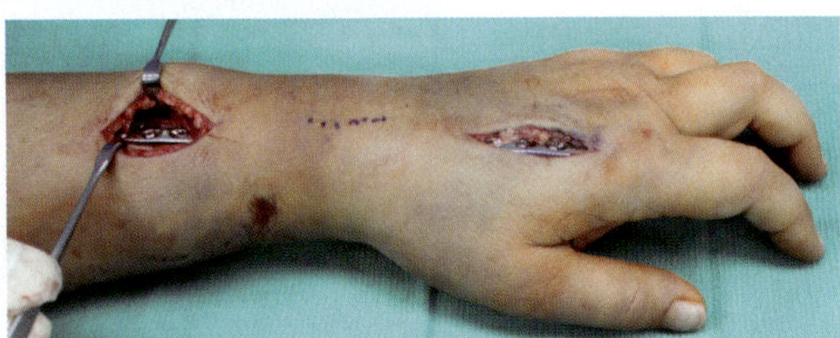

FIGURE 78-20

STEP 4 PITFALLS

Overdistraction (defined as a radiocarpal space greater than 5 mm) must be avoided to prevent possible permanent loss of finger range of motion as well as the potential development of complex regional pain syndrome.

Extrinsic extensor tightness can also develop with overdistraction; it is vital to ensure full passive digital range of motion after plate fixation.

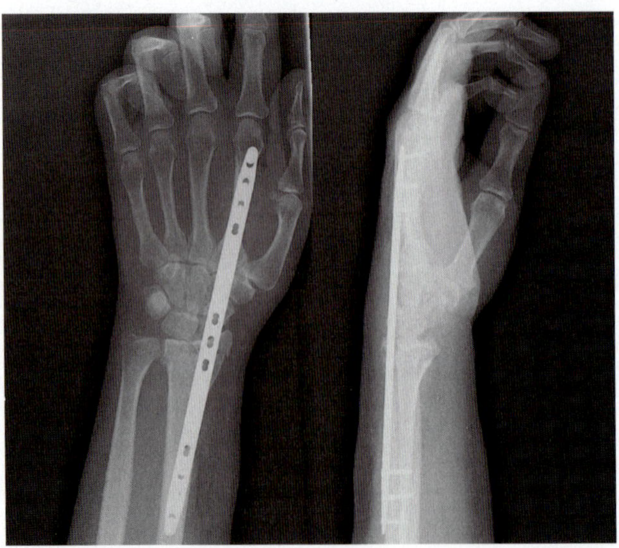

FIGURE 78-21

STEP 5 PEARLS

It is absolutely essential to address any depressed articular fragments that do not reduce with ligamentotaxis.

Bone grafting for both subchondral and metaphyseal defects that are magnified or created by the distraction is an essential component for long-term maintenance of articular reduction and fracture healing.

K-wires should be left outside or deep to the skin and removed at 6 weeks.

STEP 5 PITFALLS

Failure to reduce articular fragments may lead to symptomatic radiocarpal arthrosis.

Use of the nick-and-spread method to insert percutaneous K-wire fixation is imperative to prevent injury to the branches of the superficial radial nerve.

Contraindications to bone grafting include grade III open fractures with gross contamination and soft tissue defects that preclude primary wound closure.

After stabilization of the radius, any instability of the DRUJ should be assessed (defined as greater than 8 mm of palmar to dorsal translation of the ulna relative to the radius).

Large fractures of the ulnar styloid as well as displaced ulnar head fractures should raise suspicions of instability.

If instability is noted, the forearm should be maintained in supination for 3 to 4 weeks.

If no instability is noted, immobilization is unnecessary.

If an arthrotomy has been made, the dorsal capsule should be closed with 3-0 nonabsorbable suture.

Step 5: Fixation of the Articular Surface and Diaphyseal Fragments (if Necessary)

- If there are any diaphyseal fragments that are amenable to lag screw fixation to the shaft, this can be performed at this time.
- Reduction of the articular surface can be performed through the third incision used to free the EPL tendon and pass the plate proximally.
- Using a dental pick or Freer elevator, the articular incongruity can be reduced through an empty hole in the plate or adjacent to the plate.
- Subchondral and metaphyseal support for maintaining articular reduction can be achieved with allograft or bone graft substitute.
- When feasible, a 2.7-mm cortical screw is then inserted through the plate directly under the lunate fossa to act as a buttress against subchondral collapse.
- K-wires (0.45 or 0.62 inch) can also be placed percutaneously to hold small articular fragments reduced.
- *Case series:* Posteroanterior radiograph of another case (Fig. 78-22A)
- *Case series:* Radiographs of the plate bridging the fracture (Fig. 78-22B).

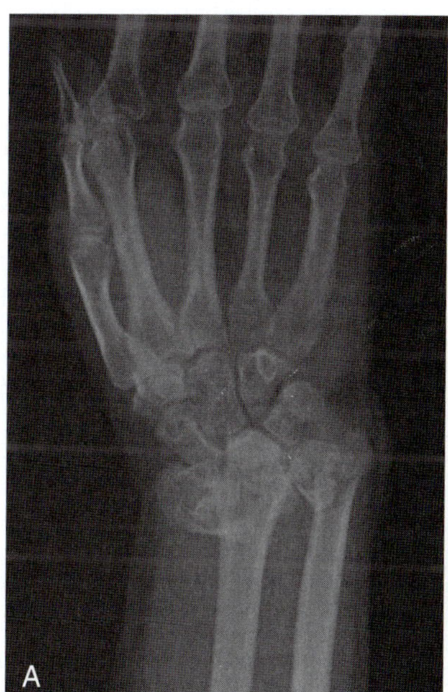

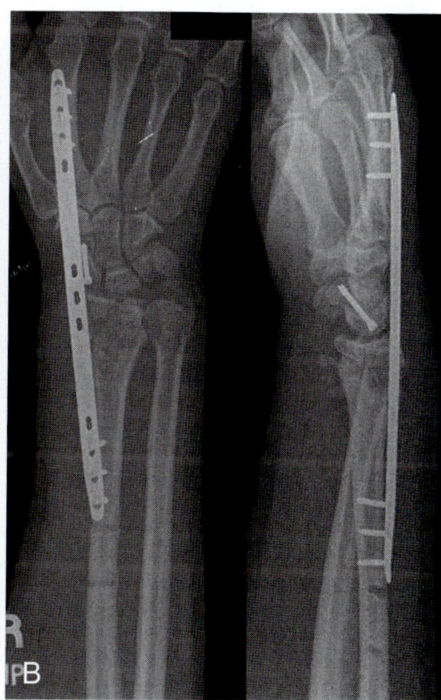

FIGURE 78-22

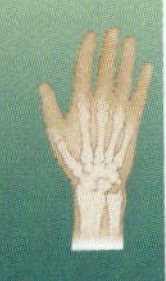

PEARLS

Patients may return to work with distraction in place if they can maintain their restrictions.

A platform walker for mobilization may be used in polytrauma patients if the fixation is deemed stable enough intraoperatively.

Hardware removal can electively be scheduled for about 8 to 12 weeks after surgery depending on the nature of the fracture and documentation of radiographic union.

Range-of-motion exercises of the wrist and fingers are started immediately after plate removal, and no splinting is required.

PITFALLS

Maintain distraction plate until radiographic osseous healing has occurred (bridging callous seen in both the coronal and sagittal plane).

Judging osseous healing may be difficult to visualize with the 3.5-mm plate.

Early removal may lead to late fracture collapse.

Late removal can lead to possible extensor tendon attrition and rupture and permanent wrist stiffness.

Postoperative Care and Expected Outcomes

- A bulky dressing and splint are used postoperatively for pain control for a few days (except in those with DRUJ instability).
- Active and passive digital range-of-motion exercises are started immediately and maintained throughout the distraction period.
- After the first postoperative visit at 7 to 10 days, a thermoplastic short-arm splint is applied, and an elastic garment is applied to control edema.
- Pronation and supination are encouraged.
- Patients may use the affected extremity for activities of daily living.
- Patients may not lift greater than 5 pounds.
- As noted by Hanel and colleagues (2006), the duration of plate immobilization does not correlate with the range of motion of the wrist or with the DASH score at 1 year.

Evidence

Burke EF, Singer RM. Treatment of comminuted distal radius with the use of an internal distraction plate. *Tech Hand Upper Extrem Surg*. 1998;2:248-252.
The authors describe the original technique of dorsal distraction plating using a 3.5-mm plate. They provide the rationale behind use of this plating as well as an example case. (Level V evidence)

Carter PR, Frederick HA, Georgiann FL. Open reduction and internal fixation of unstable distal radius fractures with a low-profile plate: a multicenter study of 73 fractures. *J Hand Surg [Am]*. 1998;23:300-307.
This was a multicenter, prospective study with excellent follow-up that was used to determine the safety and efficacy of a new low-profile plate for unstable distal radius fractures. Seventy-one patients were followed for a minimum of 1 year. Autologous bone graft was used in 64 fractures. After fixation, active wrist motion was begun at an average of 14 days, and satisfactory open reduction was obtained in 93% of the fractures and maintained in 88%. Ninety-five percent of the fractures demonstrated good or excellent outcomes using a standardized evaluation. Eighty-one percent of the outcomes were rated as excellent. (Level IV evidence)

Ginn TA, Ruch DS, Yang CC, Hanel DP. Use of a distraction plate for distal radial fractures with metaphyseal and diaphyseal comminution: surgical technique. *J Bone Joint Surg [Am]*. 2006;88:29-36.
An updated surgical technique is presented by the authors in excellent detail. They describe their method with updated pitfalls and pearls that they have learned from their experience in distraction plating. This is a follow-up to their prospective review of distraction plating, which demonstrated good results for this difficult problem. (Level V evidence)

Hanel DP, Lu TS, Weil WM. Bridge plating of distal radius fractures: the Harborview method. *Clin Orthop Relat Res*. 2006;445:91-99.
This article, as well as the article by Ginn and colleagues, is the basis of the technique described in this chapter. The authors performed a retrospective chart review of 62 consecutive patients treated with dorsal distraction plating. Inclusion criterion included patients with high-energy injuries that had fracture extension into the radius and ulna diaphysis and patients with multiple injuries that required load bearing through the injured wrist to assist with mobilization. The authors describe their technique in detail and review their experience. Fracture healing occurred in all 62 patients. There were no articular gaps or step-offs greater than 2 mm, and the distal radioulnar joint was stable. There were no cases of excessive postoperative finger stiffness or reflex sympathetic dystrophy. There was one broken fixation plate and one ruptured ECRL tendon in a patient who did not follow the author's recommendation for time frame of removal. (Level V evidence)

Kamath AF, Zurakowski D, Day CS. Low-profile dorsal plating for dorsally angulated distal radius fractures: an outcomes study. *J Hand Surg [Am]*. 2006;31:1061-1067.
This study evaluated the functional outcome of dorsal plating for dorsally angulated distal radius fractures at a single institution. Thirty patients, with a median age of 59 years, had fixation performed with low-profile, stainless-steel dorsal plates and were then followed for an average of 18 months. Four patients had AO type A fractures, 5 had type B fractures, and 21 had type C fractures. Radiographic parameters, range of motion, and strength compared with the uninjured side were recorded. The functional outcome was evaluated by the Disabilities of the Arm, Shoulder, and Hand (DASH) questionnaire and

the Gartland-Werley scoring system. Outcomes found that compared with the contralateral side, the mean extension and flexion were 88% and 81%, respectively; pronation and supination were 89% and 87%, respectively; and grip strength and thumb pinch were 78% and 94%, respectively. The mean postoperative DASH questionnaire score was 15 points, and 28 patients had Gartland-Werley scores of good or excellent. No patients needed to have their plates removed, and no extensor tendon rupture was reported. The authors found that on average, patients can expect to have 80% of their range of motion and strength after dorsal plating for distal radius fractures. In addition, about 93% of the patients can expect to have good to excellent functional outcomes. (Level IV evidence)

Lozano-Calderón SA, Doornberg J, Ring D. Fractures of the dorsal articular margin of the distal part of the radius with dorsal radiocarpal subluxation. *J Bone Joint Surg [Am]*. 2006;88:1486-1493.
The authors retrospectively reviewed 20 patients with a fracture of the dorsal articular margin of the distal part of the radius with dorsal radiocarpal subluxation. They found a wide spectrum of associated injuries, including torn volar ligaments, displaced and rotated volar marginal lip fractures, and impaction of the volar and central articular surface. Eighteen patients underwent surgical reconstruction of the articular surface and application of dorsal buttress plates with use of a variety of surgical approaches. Outcomes were assessed radiographically and with use of the modified Mayo wrist score and the DASH questionnaire. Average follow-up was 30 months postoperatively. Nineteen fractures had healed without substantial loss of alignment, and 1 patient had recurrent dorsal subluxation after plate removal. The final average amounts of wrist and forearm motion were 59 degrees of flexion, 56 degrees of extension, 87 degrees of pronation, and 85 degrees of supination. The average grip strength was 85% of that of the contralateral, uninjured hand. The final functional results using Mayo and DASH scores were overall good despite the complex nature of the fracture and associated injuries. (Level V evidence)

Papadonikolakis A, Ruch DS. Internal distraction plating of distal radius fractures. *Tech Hand Upper Extrem Surg*. 2005;9:2-6.
The authors describe their method for internal distraction plating for highly comminuted distal radius fractures, especially in elderly patients. Their technique involves the use of 3.5, 2.7, or 2.5 dynamic compression plates. An excellent step-by-step description of their techniques, as well as a thorough historical perspective, is included their manuscript. Their indications, contraindications, complications, and expected rehabilitation are also well described. They conclude that their current approach represents an alternative that provides union of the fracture with excellent alignment, functional range of motion, and minimal functional disability. (Level V evidence)

Rozental TD, Beredjiklian PK, Bozentka DJ. Functional outcome and complications following two types of dorsal plating for unstable fractures of the distal part of the radius. *J Bone Joint Surg [Am]*. 2003;85:1956-1960.
This excellent study reviewed the functional outcome and complications after dorsal plating for dorsally displaced, unstable fractures of the distal part of the radius. Twenty-eight patients with a mean age of 42 years were followed for 21 months. Nineteen patients had been treated with a Synthes titanium pi plate, and 9 had been treated with a low-profile stainless steel plate. There were no instances of loss of reduction, malunion, or nonunion. The mean score on the DASH questionnaire was 14.5 points. All patients had an excellent (19 patients) or good (9 patients) result according to the scoring system of Gartland and Werley. Nine patients had postoperative complications requiring repeat surgical treatment for hardware removal or extensor tendon reconstruction. All nine reoperations were performed in patients who had been treated with a Synthes plate, whereas none was performed in patients who had been treated with a low-profile plate. Regardless of the type of plate used, all of the patients in the study had a good or excellent long-term functional outcome. (Level IV evidence)

Ruch DS, Ginn TA, Yang CC, et al. Use of a distraction plate for distal radial fractures. *J Bone Joint Surg [Am]*. 2005;87:945-954.
This is a prospective review of 22 patients treated with a distraction plate for a comminuted distal radial fracture. All patients were followed prospectively with use of radiographs, physical examination, and DASH scores. All fractures united by an average of 110 days. Radiographs showed good restoration of palmar tilt (average of 4.6 degrees) and neutral ulnar variance. Flexion and extension averaged 57 degrees and 65 degrees, respectively, and pronation and supination averaged 77 degrees and 76 degrees, respectively. Both DASH scores as well as Gartland-Werley ratings were mostly "excellent" and "good." The duration of plate immobilization did not correlate with the range of motion of the wrist or with the DASH score at 1 year. (Level IV evidence)

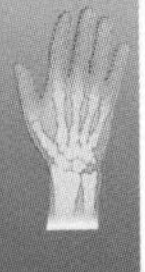

Simic PM, Robison J, Gardner MJ, et al. Treatment of distal radius fractures with a low-profile dorsal plating system: an outcomes assessment. *J Hand Surg [Am]*. 2006;31:382-386.

Functional and radiographic outcomes after internal fixation of acute, displaced, and unstable distal radius fractures were reviewed by the authors. Sixty consecutive unstable fractures were treated using a low-profile dorsal plating system. There were 29 type A, 14 type B, and 8 type C fractures (AO classification system). Fifty patients with 51 fractures returned for outcomes assessment by physical examination, plain radiographs, and completion of a validated musculoskeletal function assessment questionnaire. Minimum follow-up was set at 1 year, and the mean follow-up period was 24 months. Objective functional assessment was obtained through the DASH questionnaire. Outcomes analysis showed no cases of extensor tendon irritation or rupture. Hardware removal was performed in 1 patient, but no extensor tendon irritation or rupture was evidenced. The mean DASH score was 11.9; implant-related discomfort was minimal. All patients had an excellent (31 patients) or good (19 patients) result according to the scoring system of Gartland and Werley. All patients were found to have full extensor tendon glide and metacarpophalangeal joint motion and uniformly good to excellent recovery of wrist and hand function. (Level IV evidence)

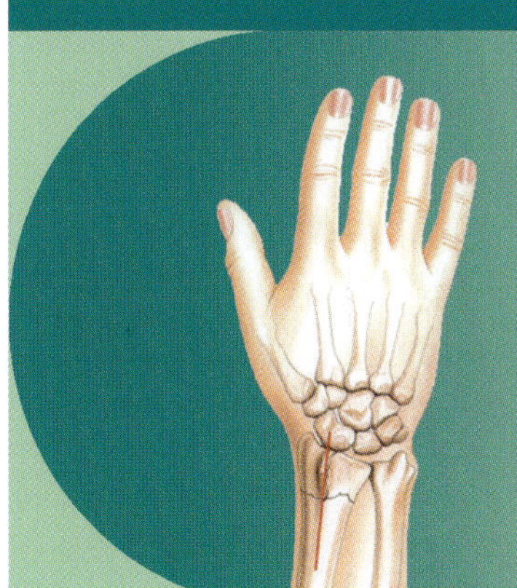

PROCEDURE 79

External Fixation of Comminuted Intra-articular Distal Radius Fractures

John T. Capo and Ramces Francisco

Indications

- Unstable unreducible extra-articular distal radius fractures
- Displaced intra-articular distal radius fractures that can be reduced by closed or percutaneous means
- Highly comminuted distal radius fractures that are reduced openly and fixed with plates or pins that require unloading of the carpus to allow healing

Examination/Imaging

Clinical Examination

- The extremity of the patient should be examined for open injuries and neurovascular status, particularly median nerve function.
- The distal ulna should be examined for dorsal prominence or instability.
- The elbow should be examined for tenderness at the radial head and collateral ligaments.

Imaging

- Anteroposterior and lateral images of the wrist should be taken; these will demonstrate the nature of the fracture (Fig. 79-1).

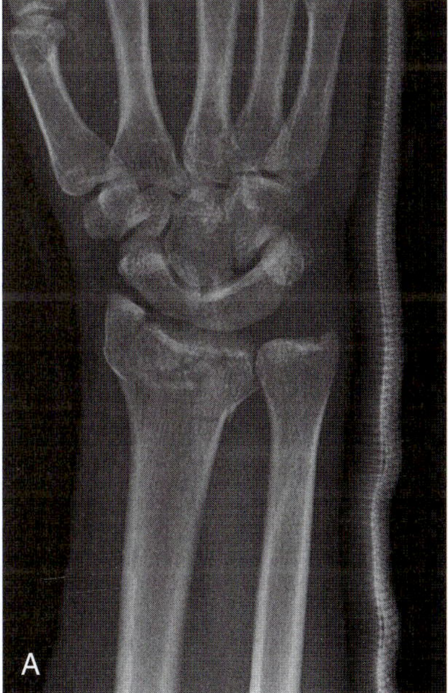

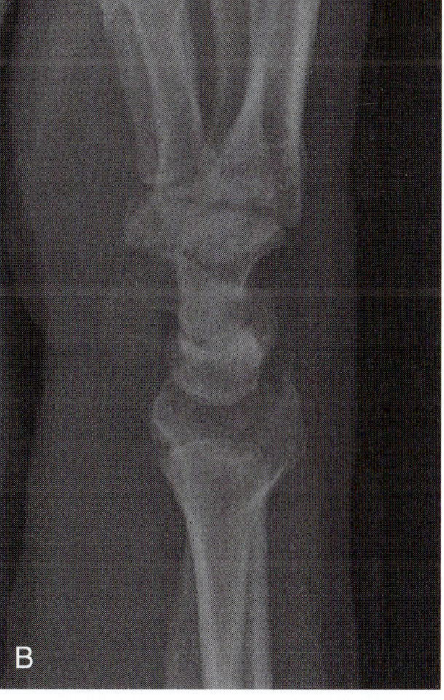

FIGURE 79-1

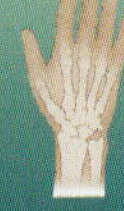

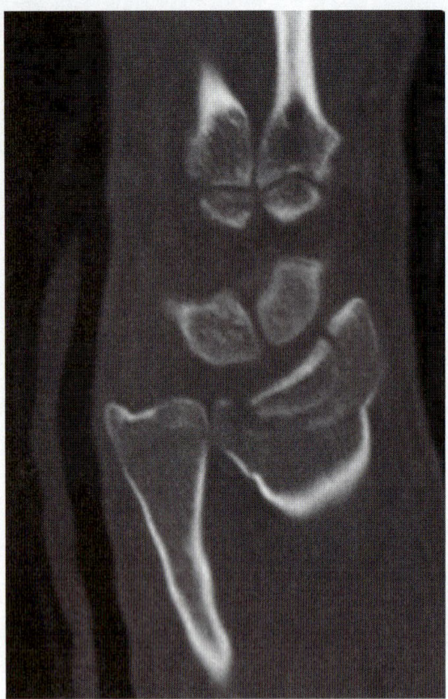

FIGURE 79-2

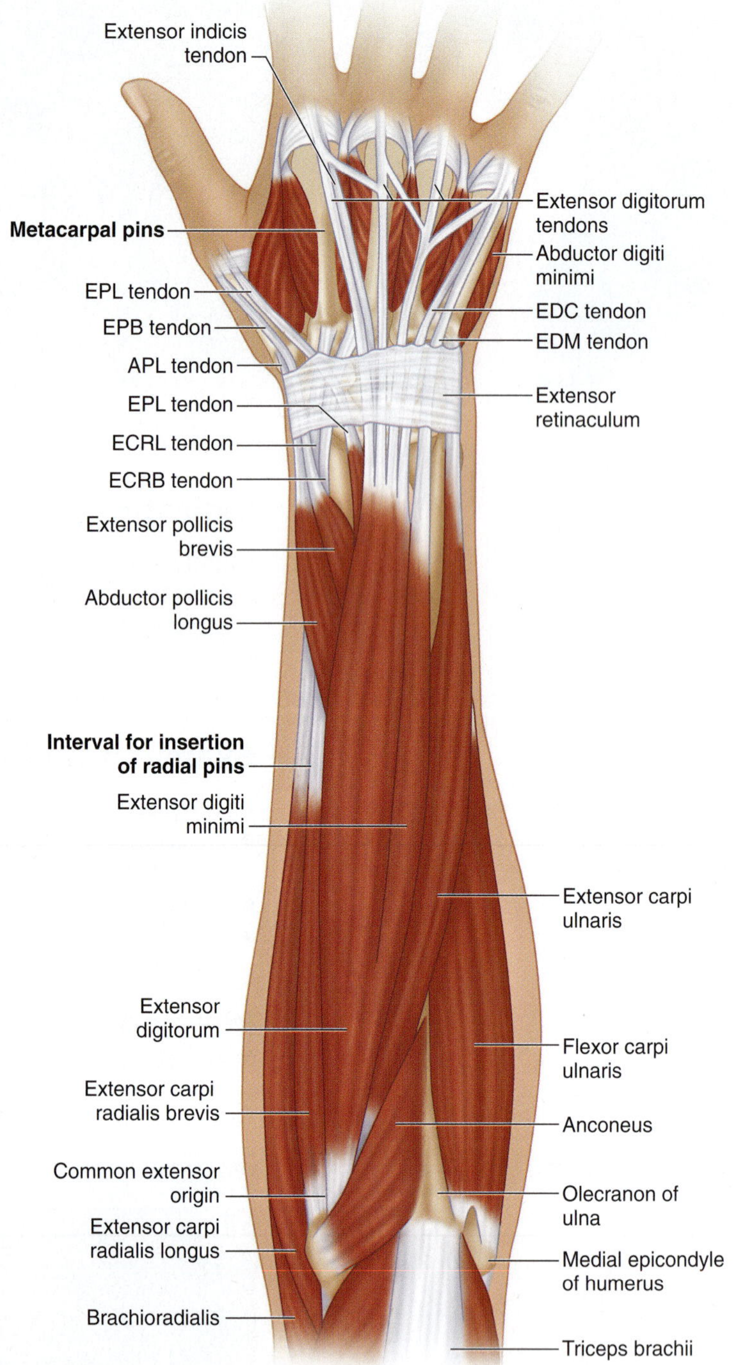

FIGURE 79-3

- If there is significant intra-articular comminution, a computed tomography scan will provide more information on the location and displacement of the fracture fragments (Fig. 79-2).

Surgical Anatomy

- The external fixator is placed dorsoradially across the wrist. The distal pins are placed in the second metacarpal, the proximal pins are placed in the radial shaft about a hand's breadth proximal to the radial styloid. This position is just proximal to the "outrigger" muscles—abductor pollicis longus (APL) and extensor pollicis brevis (EPB)—as they cross the radial shaft (Fig. 79-3).

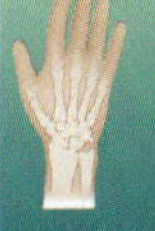

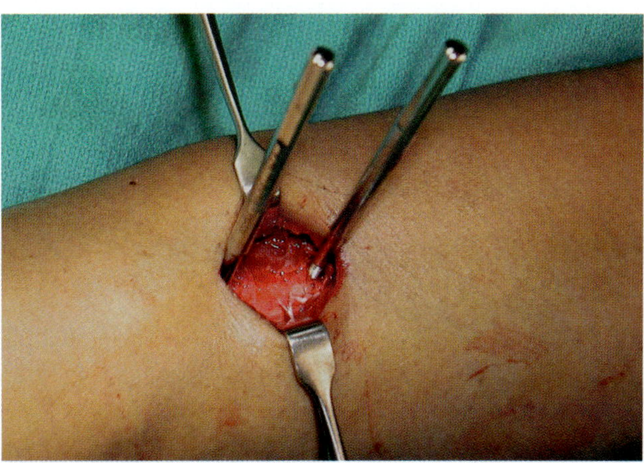

FIGURE 79-4

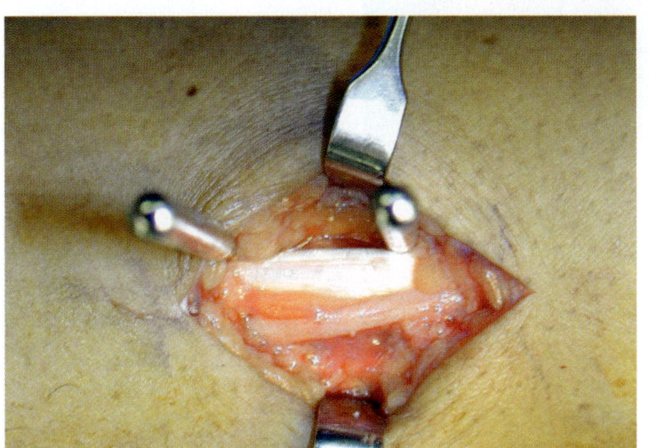

FIGURE 79-5

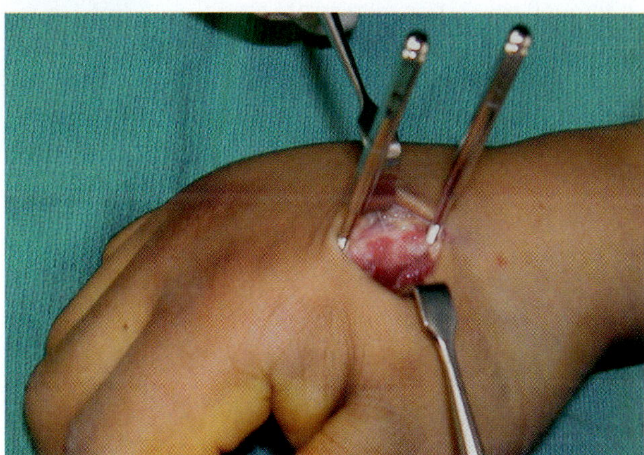

FIGURE 79-6

Positioning

- The procedure is done on a hand table with the forearm pronated.

Exposures

- The first pin of the external fixator is placed in the radial shaft, and the second pin is placed in the second metacarpal. After alignment of the wrist is established, the external fixation bar slides over these two pins. The remaining pins for the metacarpal and the radius can be inserted by marking the appropriate position on the arm to permit smooth fitting of all the pin slots on the external fixator.
- The radial shaft pins are placed through a 3-cm incision on the "bare area" of the radius, proximal to the first compartment tendons in a dorsoradial position. The deep interval is between the extensor carpi radialis longus (ECRL) and the brachioradialis (BR) tendons. The radius should be directly visualized as the pins are placed into the bone (Fig. 79-4)
- The superficial radial nerve (SRN) needs to be visualized and protected in the proximal exposure (Fig. 79-5).
- The second metacarpal pins are placed on the dorsoradial aspect. The extensor tendons and first dorsal interosseus (FDI) muscle need to be retracted and protected (Fig. 79-6).

PEARLS

By placing the pins between the ECRL and extensor carpi radialis brevis (ECRB), the tendons act as a barrier between the SRN and the pins.

PITFALLS

The superficial radial nerve can be injured if either the radial shaft or metacarpal pins are placed percutaneously.

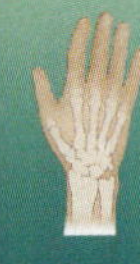

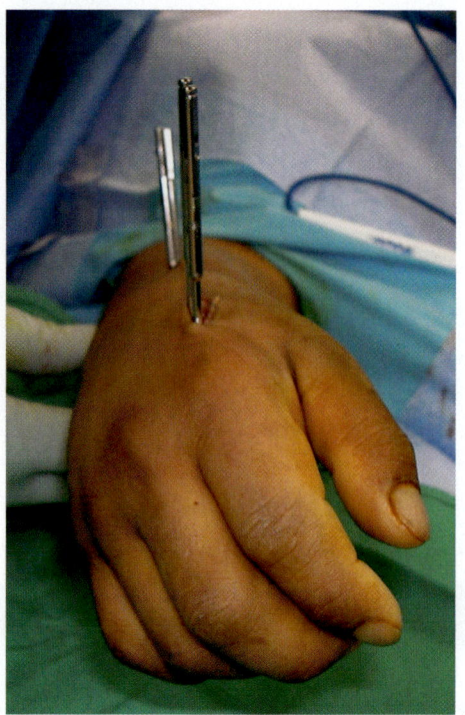

FIGURE 79-7

STEP 1 PEARLS

The pins should be bicortical and assessed for stability before the fixator is placed.

If the bone is osteopenic, the proximal metacarpal pin may be placed through the second metacarpal base into the third metacarpal base.

STEP 1 PITFALLS

If the metacarpal pins are placed too long, the motor branch of the ulnar nerve may be at risk for injury.

STEP 2 PEARLS

The frame should not be overdistracted, which may induce carpal stiffness or the inability to allow finger flexion owing to tightening of the finger extensors.

After the distal radius is stabilized, the distal ulna is checked for stability. If the distal radioulnar joint is unstable, the distal ulna is reduced and pinned to the radius. Alternatively the triangular fibrocartilage complex may be repaired, or a large ulnar styloid fracture fixed.

STEP 2 PITFALLS

If the external fixator is placed in excessive volar flexion and ulnar deviation, postoperative finger motion will be limited, and carpal tunnel symptoms may occur.

Procedure

Step 1

- The pins for the external fixator are placed in a dorsoradial position, about 45 degrees from radial midlateral. This position prevents the fixator from obstructing postoperative radiographs and allows the thumb full range of motion (ROM), particularly extension (Fig. 79-7).
- The position of the pins should be confirmed by fluoroscopy to be within the respective bone and of appropriate length. The images should be saved for documentation of the case (Fig. 79-8).
- The incisions that were used for pin placement are then closed with interrupted 3-0 nylon sutures. This closure should not be overly tight because the skin tension may change after distraction of the fixator.

Step 2

- The fixator bar is placed across the fractures and attached to the half-pins through clamps.
- Distraction and ulnar deviation are imparted to the fracture to induce a provisional reduction. A single 0.062-inch K-wire may be placed percutaneously dorsally to assist in holding the reduction (Fig. 79-9).

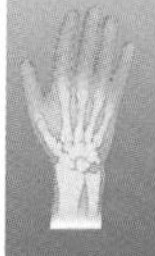

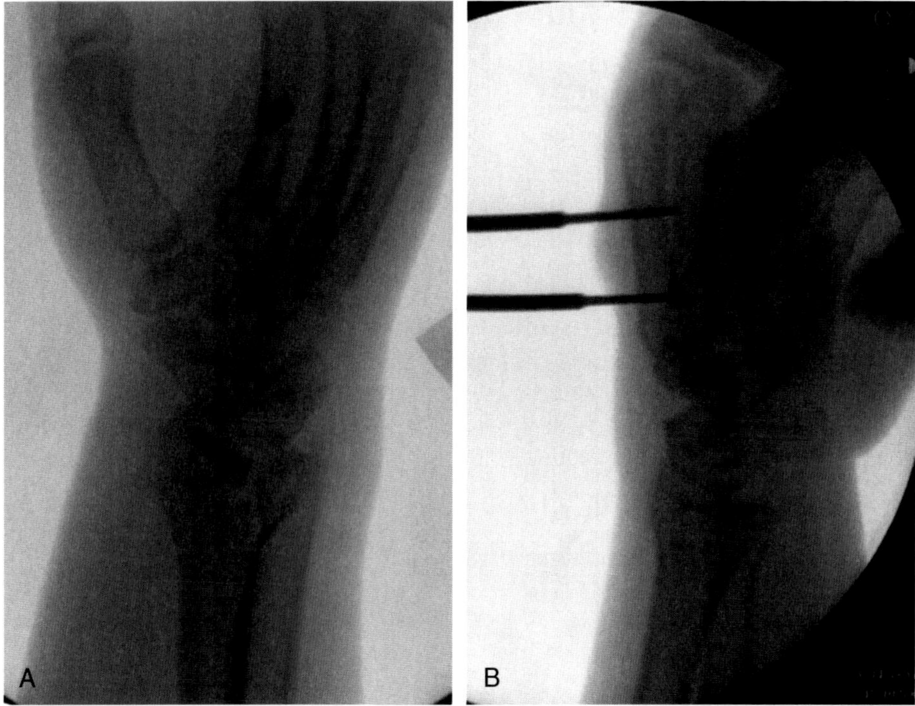

FIGURE 79-8

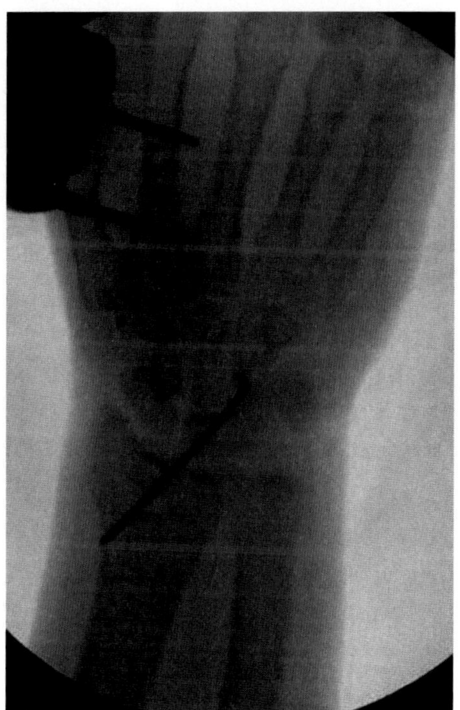

FIGURE 79-9

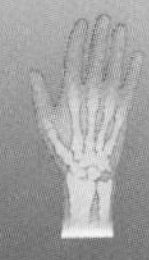

- A second K-wire can be placed through the radial styloid to stabilize the fracture fragments. The distal radius alignment should be checked with anteroposterior and lateral images to ensure that the joint surface is congruent, has no step-off, and possesses the proper inclination and tilt (Fig. 79-10).
- The frame should be tightened and ensured to be stable and not impede finger motion.
- At the close of the procedure, the fingers should have full passive flexion and extension, and the hand should not be placed in excessive flexion or ulnar deviation.

Step 3

- The pin sites are dressed with a nonadherent dressing, and a thick layer of gauze is used to push the skin away from the pins.
- A volar splint may be applied for postoperative pain control and soft tissue stabilization.

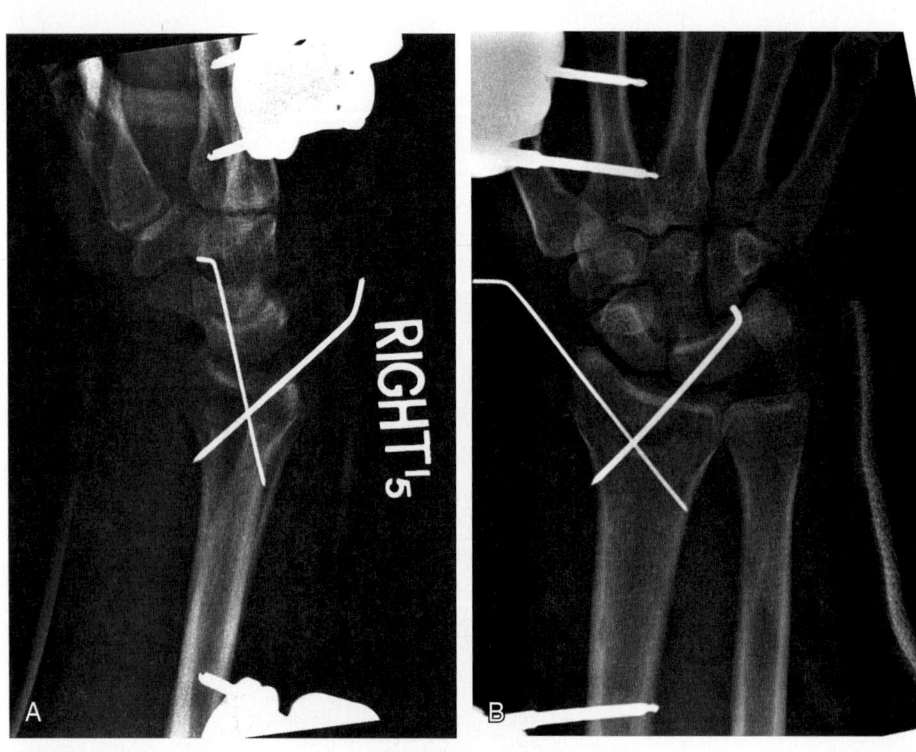

FIGURE 79-10

Postoperative Care and Expected Outcomes

- The dressings are removed after 7 to 10 days, and the pin sites and wounds are evaluated.
- The pin sites are dressed for the first 3 weeks. If there is any discharge, half-strength peroxide is used to clean them daily.
- The percutaneous pins may be removed in the office after 3 to 4 weeks. The external fixator is left in place, and finger ROM is encouraged (Fig. 79-11).
- After the sutures are removed, the incisions are dry, and the percutaneous pins are removed, the patients may shower with the fixator in place.
- The fixator is removed in the office after 4 to 6 weeks, and the pin sites are dressed sterilely.
- Final radiographs should demonstrate a healed fracture with an anatomic articular surface and a reduced carpus (Fig. 79-12).

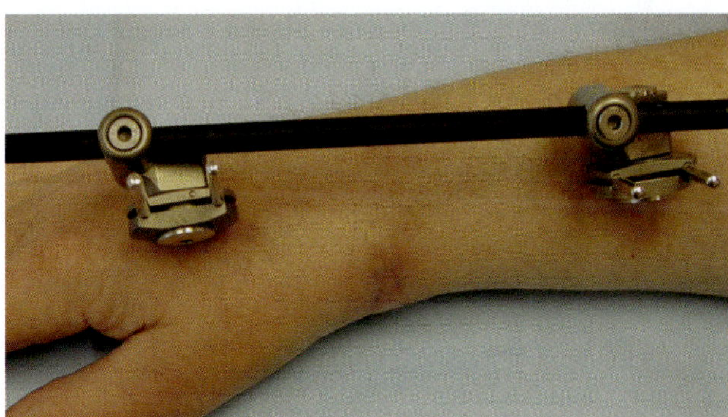

FIGURE 79-11

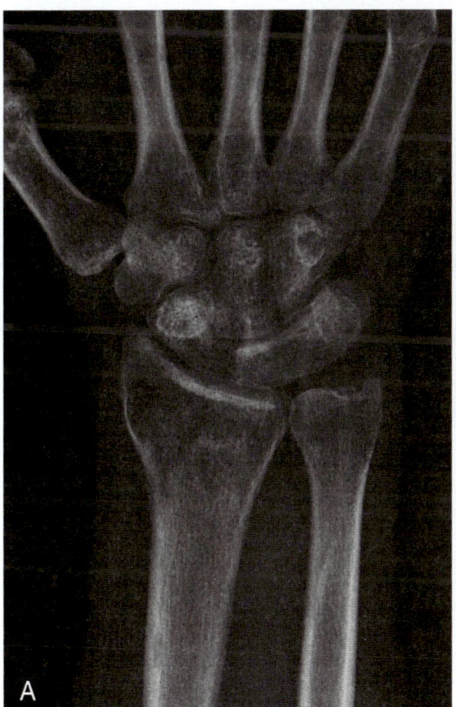

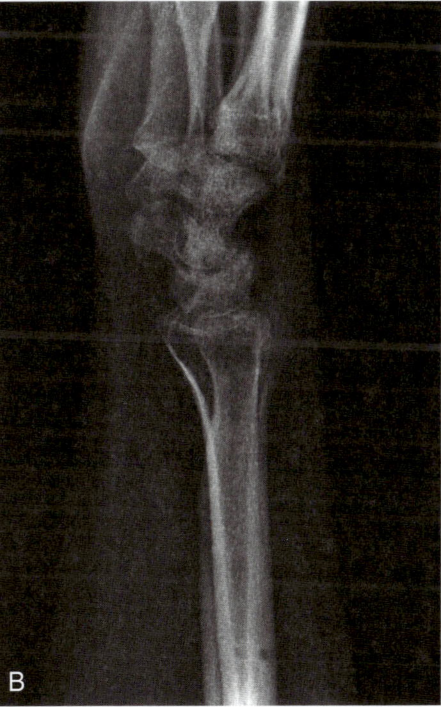

FIGURE 79-12

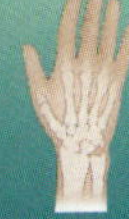

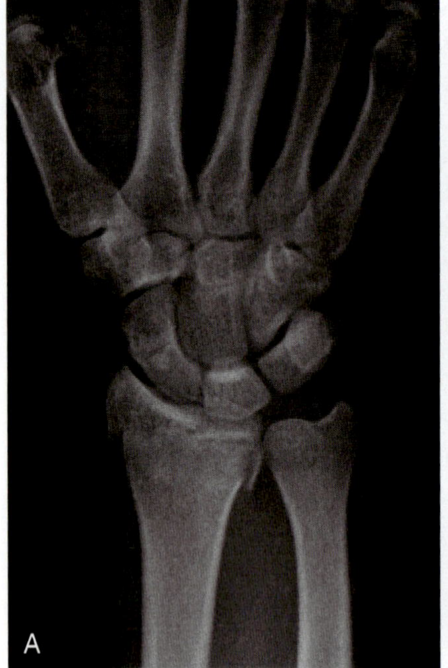

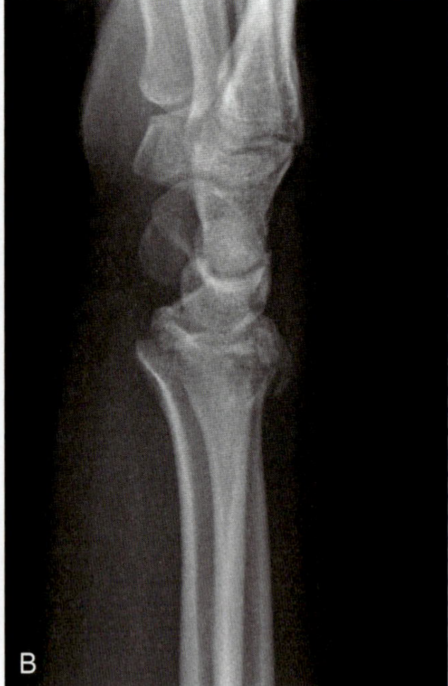

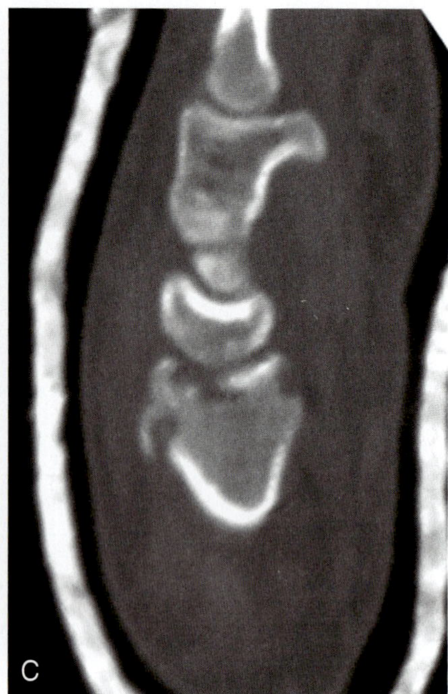

FIGURE 79-13

PEARLS

In a comminuted fracture, the reduction achieved with external fixation and percutaneous pins alone may be inadequate (Fig. 79-13).

Persistent articular displacement (die-punch fragment) can be reduced through a limited open approach and fixation with small plates (Fig. 79-14).

The fixator is left in place to unload the joint until early fracture healing.

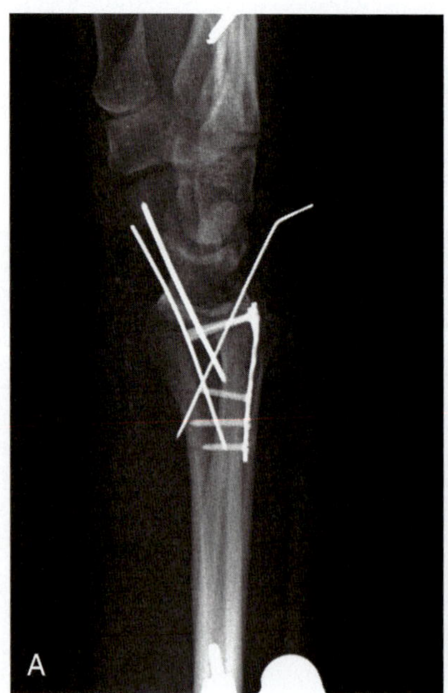

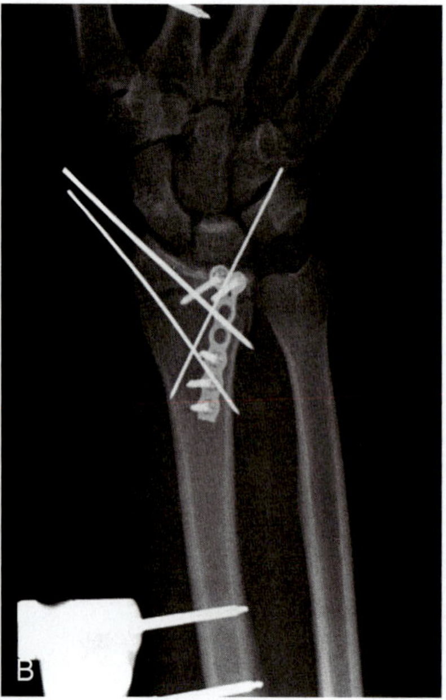

FIGURE 79-14

Evidence

Capo JT, Rossy W, Henry P, et al. External fixation of distal radius fractures: effect of distraction and duration. *J Hand Surg [Am]*. 2009;34:1605-1611.

Twenty-four patients with closed distal radius fractures treated with a spanning external fixator plus supplementary percutaneous K-wires were evaluated at an average follow-up time of 22 months. All fractures were extra-articular (A type) or simple intra-articular (C type). The amount of distraction attained by the fixator was determined by measuring the carpal height ratio on plain radiographs. Using the Gartland-Werley classification, there were 11 excellent, 10 good, and 3 fair results. Statistical analysis indicated that a higher carpal height ratio at the initial reduction positively correlated (P = .041) with an excellent outcome. Duration of external fixation did not have a significant impact on the final outcome within the parameters studied (P = .891). Average wrist range of motion at follow-up was as follows: flexion, 54.1 degrees (75% of the contralateral side); extension, 59.0 degrees (78%); radial deviation, 18.0 degrees (85%); ulnar deviation, 22 degrees (73%); pronation, 79.0 degrees (95%); and supination, 76.6 degrees (93%). None of the individual components of range of motion correlated negatively with increasing distraction at fixator application or duration of fixation. (Level V evidence)

Kreder HJ, Hanel DP, Agel J, et al. Indirect reduction and percutaneous fixation versus open reduction and internal fixation for displaced intra-articular fractures of the distal radius: a randomized, controlled trial. *J Bone Joint Surg [Br]*. 2005;87:829-836.

A total of 179 adult patients with displaced intra-articular fractures of the distal radius were randomized to receive indirect percutaneous reduction and external fixation (n = 88) or open reduction and internal fixation (n = 91). Patients were followed for 2 years. During the first year, the upper limb musculoskeletal function assessment score, the SF-36 bodily pain sub-scale score, the overall Jebsen score, and pinch strength and grip strength improved significantly in all patients. There was no statistically significant difference in the radiologic restoration of anatomic features or the range of movement between the groups. During the 2-year period, patients who underwent indirect reduction and percutaneous fixation had a more rapid return of function and a better functional outcome than those who underwent open reduction and internal fixation, provided that the intra-articular step and gap deformity were minimized. (Level III evidence)

Leung F, Tu YK, Chew WY, Chow SP. Comparison of external and percutaneous pin fixation with plate fixation for intra-articular distal radial fractures: a randomized study. *J Bone Joint Surg [Am]*. 2008;90:16-22.

This is a therapeutic level I study that compared the outcomes for external fixation combined with percutaneous pin fixation versus plate fixation. At 1 and 2 years after surgery, results of plate fixation were better than external fixation according to both the Gartland-Werley point system and the Modified Green-O'Brien system. The study also showed continuous clinical improvement for at least 24 months. Another finding in this study was that both types of fixation were similarly effective for managing AO group C1 fractures, but better clinical and radiographic results were observed with plate fixation for AO group C2 fractures. However, for group C3 fractures, both plating and external fixation had difficulty achieving accurate reduction and maintaining stable fixation. In terms of arthritis grade, plate fixation demonstrated significantly better results both at 1 and 2 years after surgery. Some of the limitations present in this study include the heterogenous fixation in both groups and the inability to use a validated patient-assessed scoring system. (Level I evidence)

Margaliot Z, Haase SC, Kotsis SV, et al. A meta-analysis of outcomes of external fixation versus plate osteosynthesis for unstable distal radius fractures. *J Hand Surg [Am]*. 2005;30:1185-1199.

The study is a systemic review and meta-analysis of literature on external and internal fixation of distal radius fracture. MEDLINE and EMBASE database were searched for articles published between 1980 and 2004. In the 46 articles that were included, meta-analysis did not demonstrate any statistical or clinical differences in grip strength, wrist range of motion, radiographic alignment, pain, and physician-rated outcome between these two groups. Although higher rates of infection, hardware failure, and neuritis were documented with external fixation, tendon complications and early hardware removal were more apparent with the internal fixation group. The drawback in this review is the considerable heterogeneity in all the studies, which affects the precision of meta-analysis. The review shows that in contrast to external fixation, plate osteosynthesis provides rigid fixation and allows for immediate motion. However, both techniques may achieve similar outcome in the long-term. (Level II evidence)

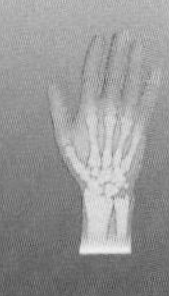

Wei DH, Raizman NM, Bottino CJ, et al. Unstable distal radial fractures treated with external fixation, a radial column plate, or a volar plate: a prospective randomized trial. *J Bone Joint Surg [Am]*. 2009;91:1568-1577.
This is a therapeutic level I study that compared the functional outcomes of treatment of unstable distal radial fractures with external fixation, a radial column plate, and a volar plate. Follow-up conducted at varying intervals postoperatively demonstrated that at 6 weeks, the DASH score was better with volar plate than with external fixation but similar with use of volar plate and radial column plate. At 3 months, DASH scores were significantly better with volar plate than with external fixation and radial column plate. At 6 months and 1 year, DASH scores for the three groups were comparable with those for the normal population. Grip strength was similar for the three groups at 1 year. The range of motion of the wrist was not significantly different among the three groups from 12 weeks postoperatively. At 1 year, radial inclination and radial length were significantly better in the radial column plate than the other two groups. In conclusion, unstable distal radial fractures treated with locked volar plate recovered more quickly compared with external fixation and radial column plate. However, 1 year after surgery, all three techniques provided good subjective and objective functional outcomes. (Level I evidence)

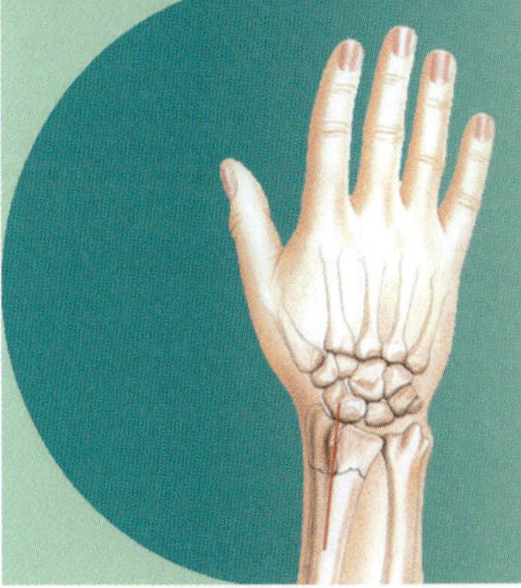

PROCEDURE 80

Corrective Osteotomy of Malunited Distal Radius Fractures

Jesse B. Jupiter

Indications

- Deformity by itself may or may not be symptomatic. A decision for surgery should be based on functional impairment, pain, loss of motion, and limitation of grip strength.
- Alteration of radiocarpal alignment will affect normal carpal kinematics and changes in the vectors of the extensor and flexor tendons (Fig. 80-1).
- Dorsally malunited fracture can result in a midcarpal instability (Figs. 80-2 and 80-3).
- Although there is no fixed radiographic criteria for correction of deformity, the lower limits of deformity at which symptoms are likely to be present include radial deviation of 20 to 30 degrees, sagittal tilt of 10 to 20 degrees dorsally, and radial shortening of 0 to 2 mm. Articular incongruity greater than 2 to 3 mm may also require osteotomy.

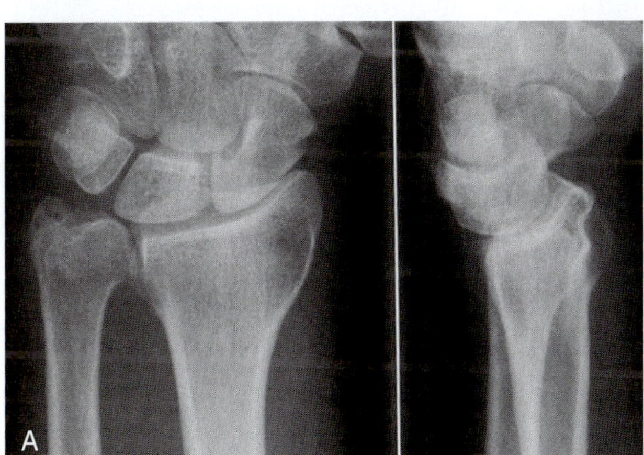

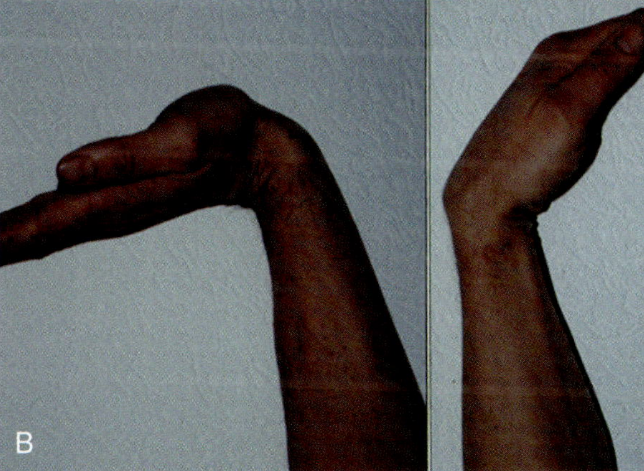

FIGURE 80-1

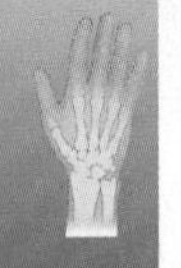

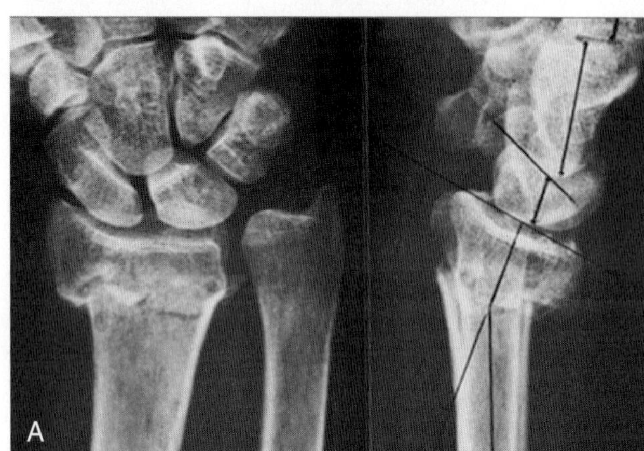

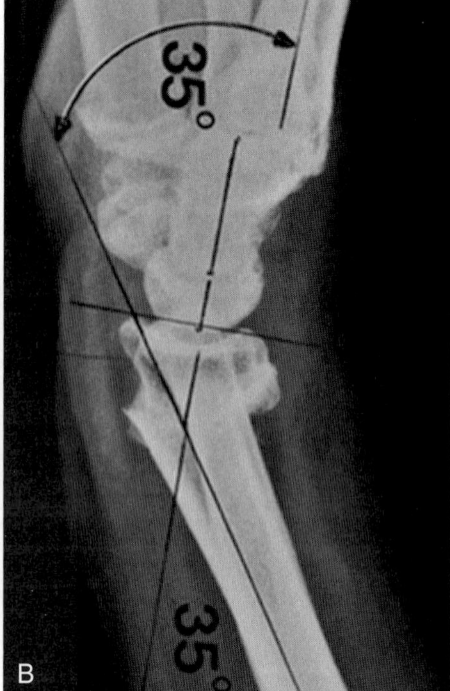

FIGURE 80-2

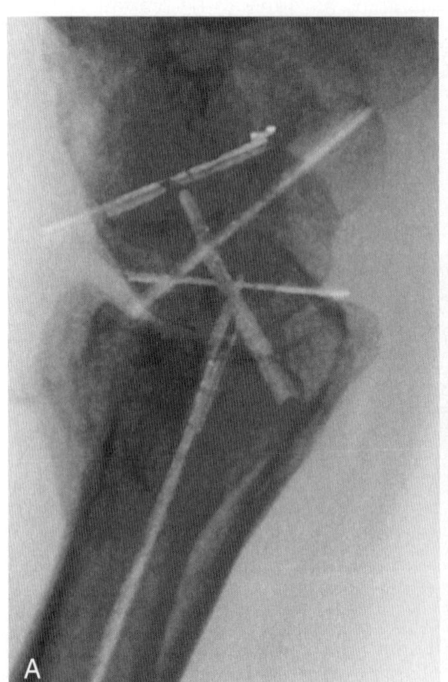

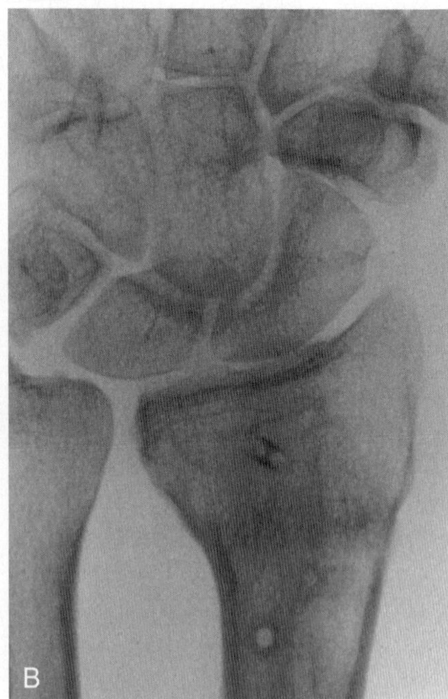

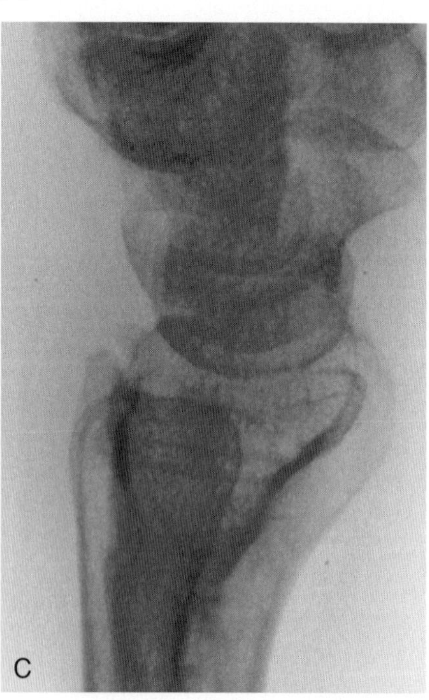

FIGURE 80-3

Relative Indications for Osteotomy

- Limited function
- Pain
- Midcarpal instability
- Distal radioulnar joint incongruity
- Prearthritic articular incongruity

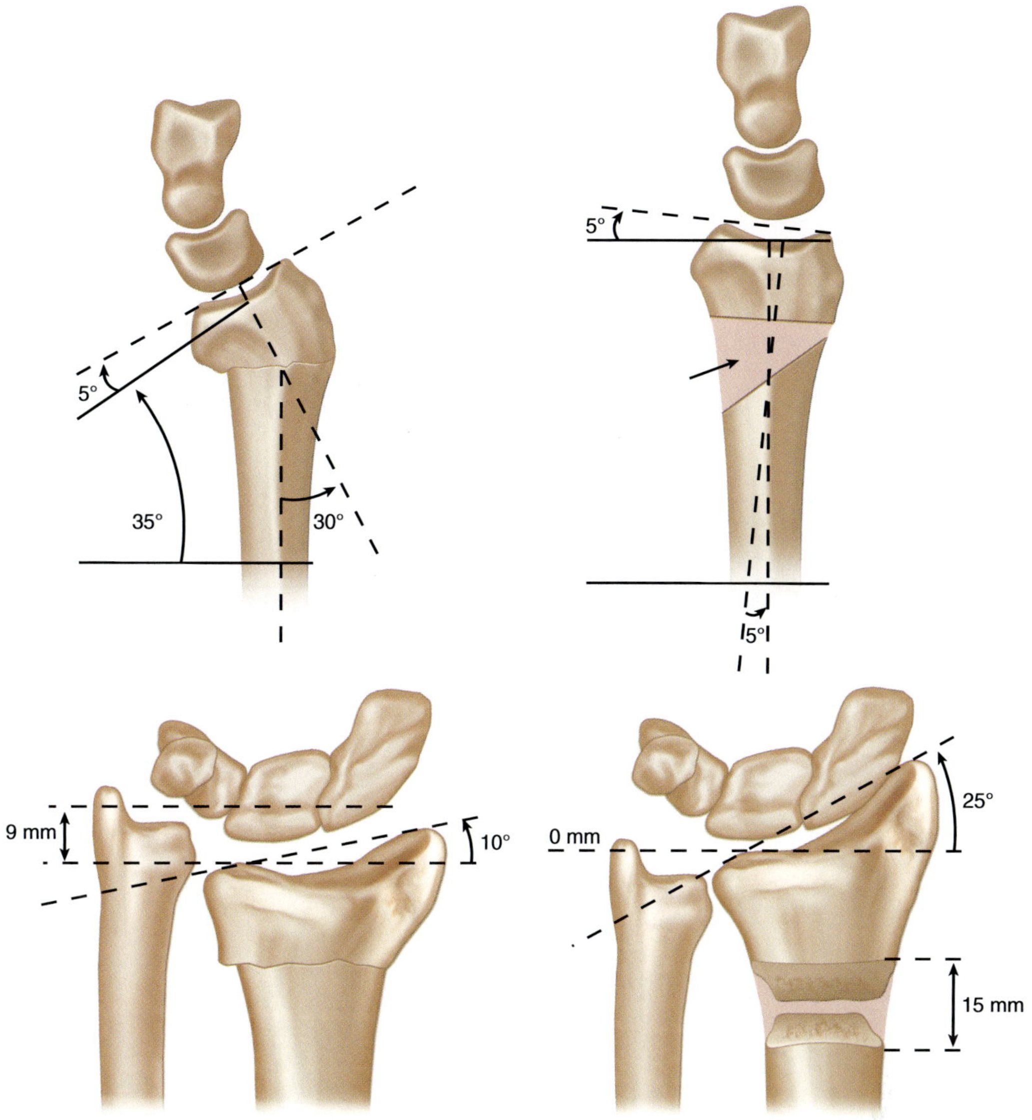

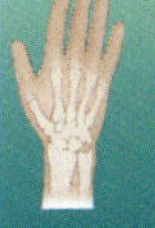

FIGURE 80-4

Relative Contraindications for Osteotomy

- Advanced degenerative arthritis
- Fixed carpal malalignment
- Limited functional capabilities
- Extensive osteoporosis

Examination/Imaging

Clinical Examination

- Along with standard examination of wrist and forearm mobility, examination should include digital mobility, grip strength, and neurovascular function. Trophic changes or soft tissue edema would preclude surgical intervention.

Imaging

- Standard anteroposterior, lateral, and oblique radiographs of *both* wrists are essential for preoperative planning.
- For most deformities, tracings can be made from the anteroposterior and lateral radiographs and superimposed on each other. The angle and precise location of the deformity can be identified in the frontal and sagittal planes (Fig. 80-4).

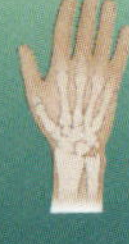

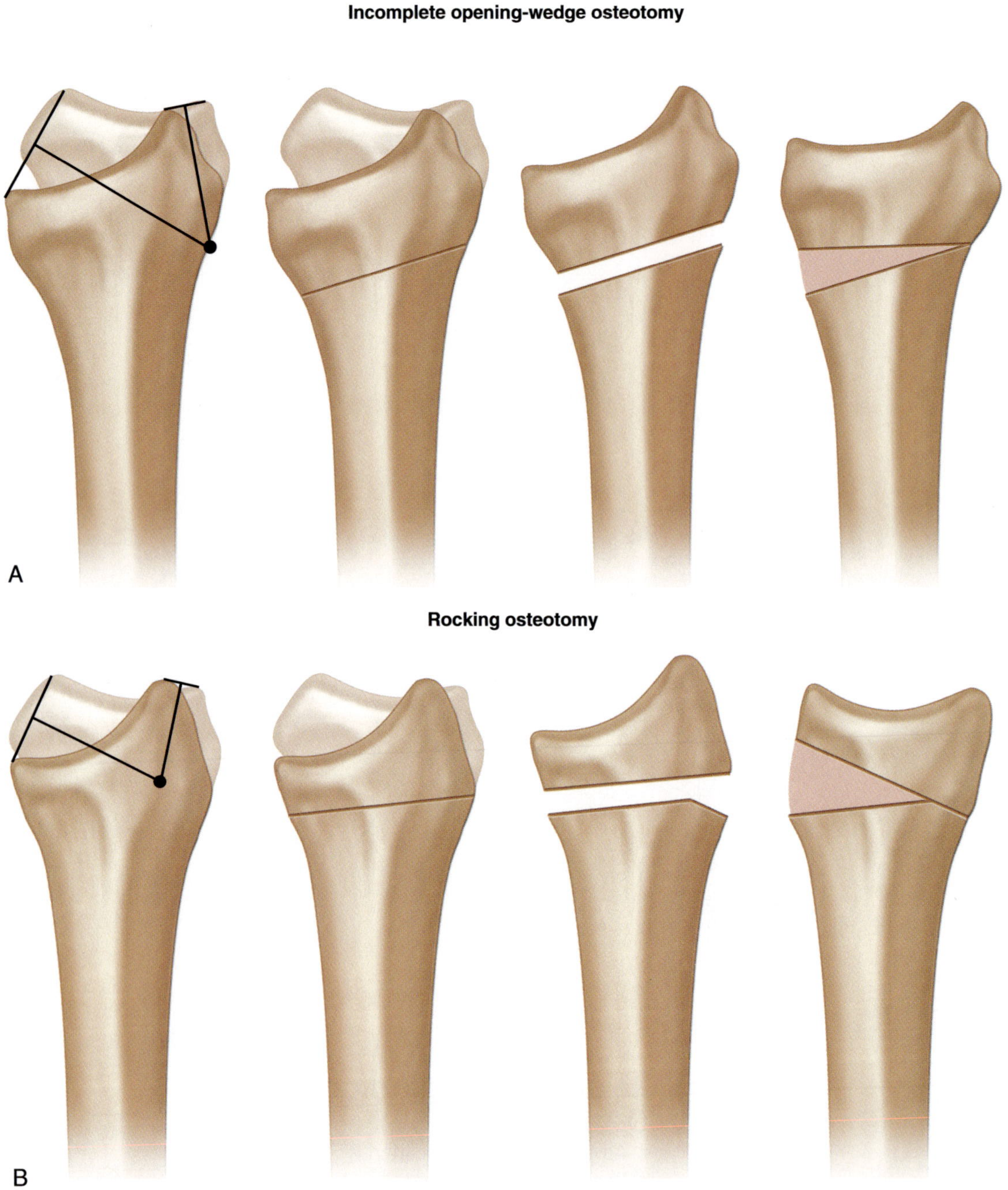

Incomplete opening-wedge osteotomy

A

Rocking osteotomy

B

FIGURE 80-5

- By superimposing the tracings in the sagittal and frontal planes and drawing a line from the most volar and dorsal lips, a perpendicular line can be drawn midpoint on each line. Where these two intersect will define the type of osteotomy required and the need for lengthening of the distal fragment (Fig. 80-5).

Timing

- Osteotomy can be considered when no soft tissue trophic changes or swelling exist, radiographs show limited disuse osteopenia, and digital motion is recovered.
- In the absence of trophic changes, early surgical intervention (6 to 12 weeks postinjury) can facilitate correction through incompletely ossified fracture callous, minimize the development of soft tissue contracture and distal radioulnar joint stiffness, and limit the duration of economic and psychological impact on the patient.

Complete full-thickness interpositional osteotomy

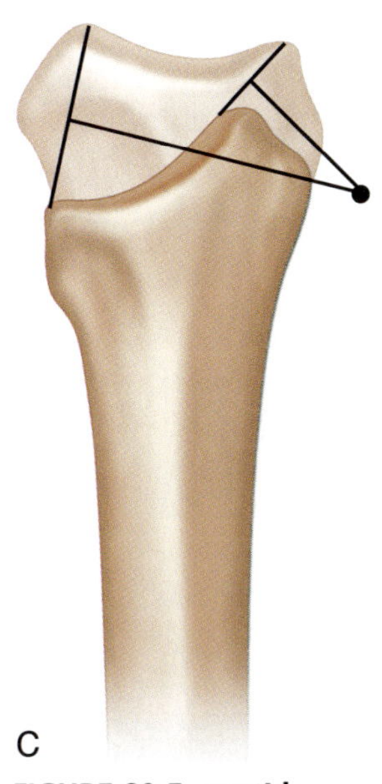
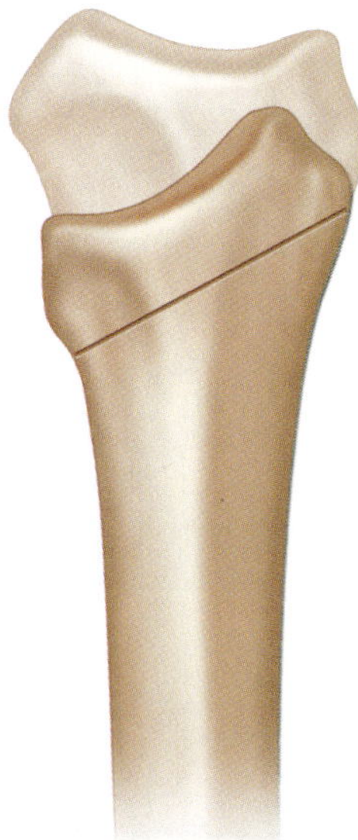
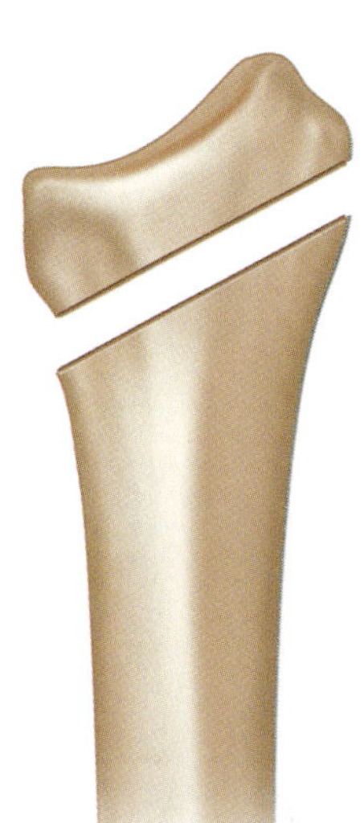
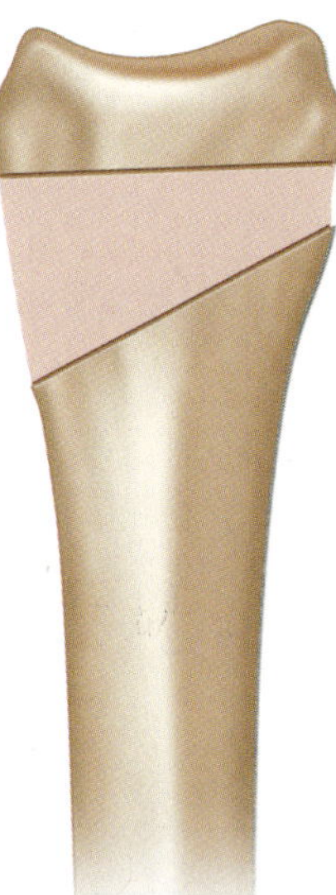

C

FIGURE 80-5, cont'd

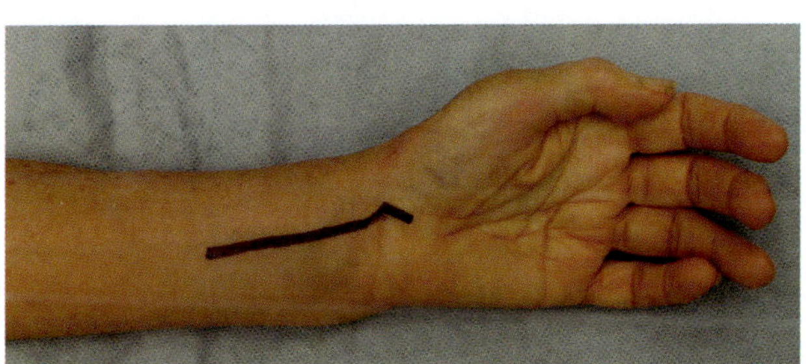
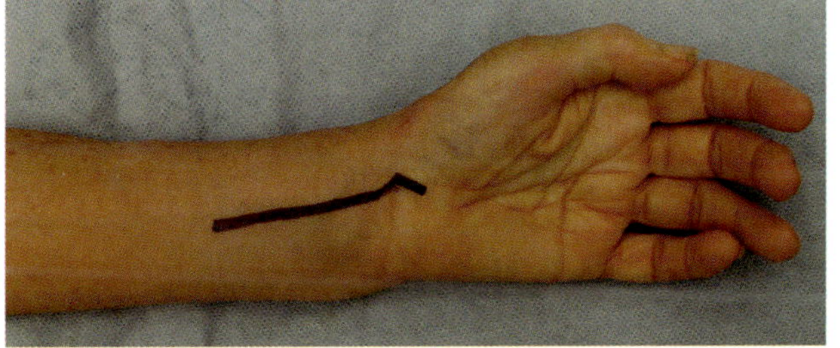

FIGURE 80-6

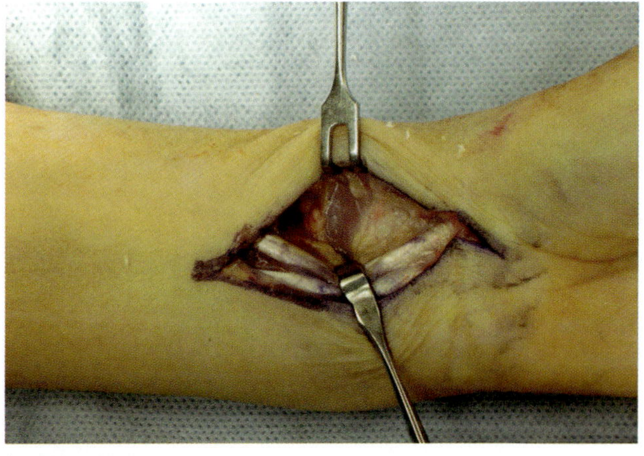

FIGURE 80-7

PEARLS

The site of the deformity must be exposed completely before osteotomy.

Intraoperative imaging will confirm the location and direction of the deformity.

Additional exposure is aided by release of the proximal sheath of the flexor carpi radialis as it enters the proximal palm.

PITFALLS

Avoid injury to the palmar cutaneous branch from the median nerve.

Positioning

- The patient is supine with the involved arm on a standard hand table and upper arm tourniquet in place.
- The ipsilateral iliac crest may be prepared if autogenous bone graft is to be used.
- Image intensification is essential.

Exposures

Volar

- The distal part of the anterior Henry approach involves exposure between the flexor carpi radialis and radial artery (Fig. 80-6).
- The muscle belly of the flexor pollicis longus is retracted ulnarly to expose the pronator quadratus, which is elevated from its insertion on the radius (Fig. 80-7).

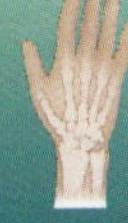

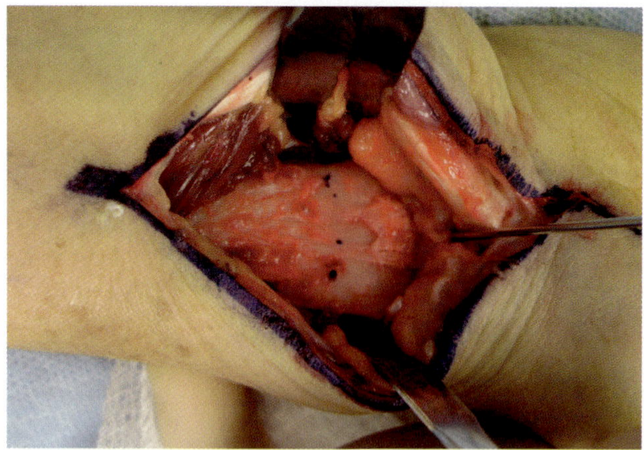

FIGURE 80-8

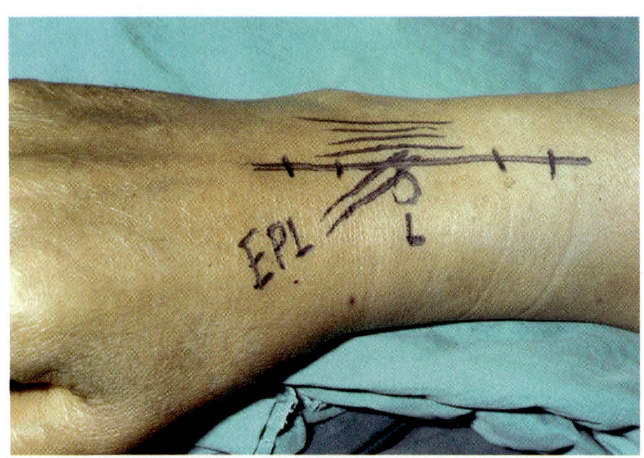

FIGURE 80-9

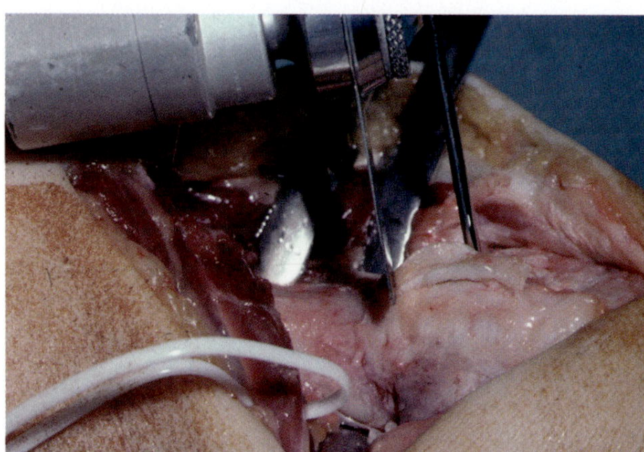

FIGURE 80-10

PEARLS

The entire metaphysis should be visualized to help judge rotational malalignment.

PITFALLS

Disruption of the retinacular coverage of the second and fourth extensor compartments will expose the extensor tendons to the underlying plate.

Branches of the radial sensory nerve are at risk with dissection along the radial column.

- Exposure and realignment of the distal fragment are improved by Z-lengthening of the tendon of the brachioradialis.
- Small Hohmann retractors are placed along the borders of the distal radius at the site of the deformity (Fig. 80-8).

Dorsal

- The skin incision is between 6 and 8 cm extending 2 to 3 cm distal to the Lister tubercle (Fig. 80-9).
- Opening the extensor retinaculum can be done either between the second and third or between the third and fourth extensor compartments.
- The extensor pollicis longus (EPL) is elevated out of the compartment, whereas the second and fourth extensor compartments are elevated between the volar sheaths of the compartments.
- Small Hohmann retractors are placed on both sides of the distal radius metaphysis at the level of the malunion (Fig. 80-10).

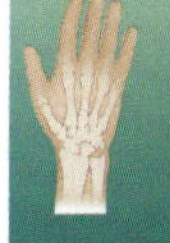

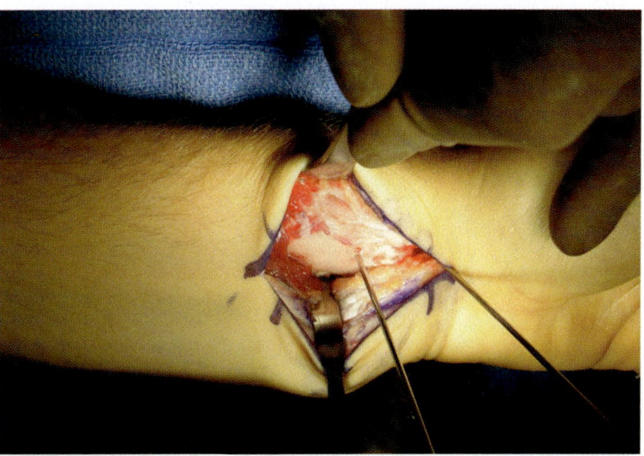

FIGURE 80-11

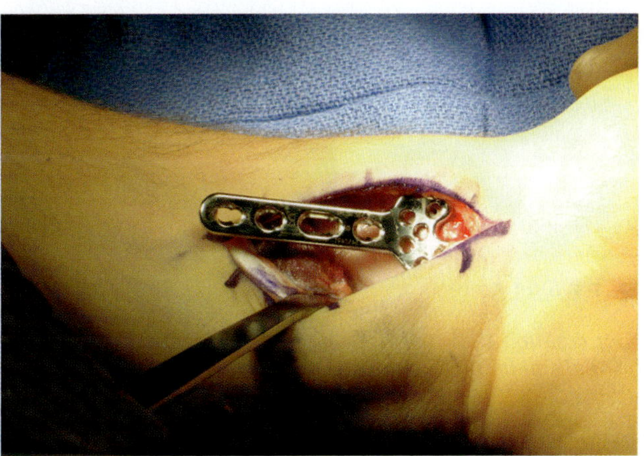

FIGURE 80-12

Procedure

Volar Approach—Dorsal Malunion

Step 1

- The radiocarpal joint is located, and a smooth K-wire is placed parallel to the articular surface.
- Two additional K-wires are placed perpendicular to both the distal fragment and radial shaft (Fig. 80-11).
- The distal limb of the volar plate is temporarily screwed to the distal fragment with the proximal limb of the plate subtending the deformity angle in the sagittal and frontal planes (Fig. 80-12).

STEP 1 PEARLS

Careful preoperative planning will define the deformity in all planes in order to place the implant in a manner in which it will facilitate correction of the deformity.

STEP 1 PITFALLS

The application of the distal limb of the plate must put the distal screws in the subchondral bone to provide optimal support of the distal fragment.

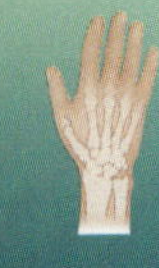

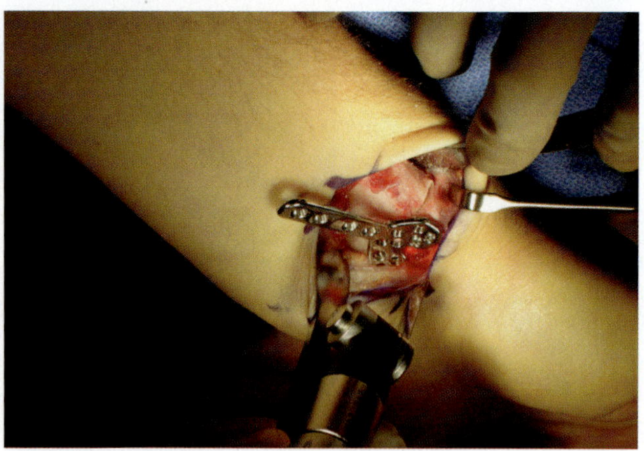

FIGURE 80-13

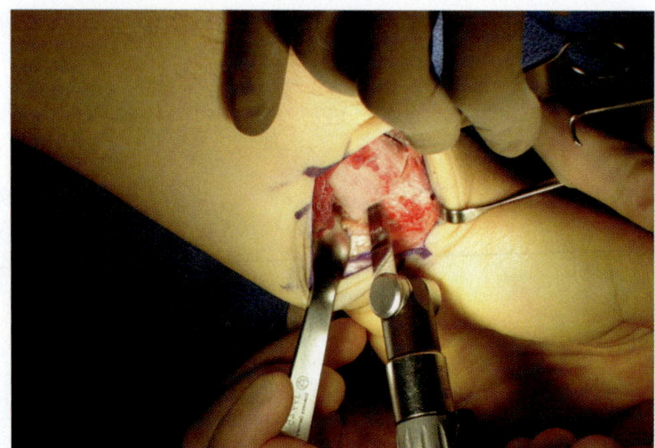

FIGURE 80-14

STEP 2 PEARLS

One should consider creating the osteotomy with the distal limb of the plate still attached.

Complete the osteotomy with a thin osteotome to avoid risk for injury to the extensor tendons.

STEP 2 PITFALLS

Failure to create the osteotomy parallel to the articular surface can lead to translation during realignment.

STEP 3 PEARLS

If the distal fragment has disuse osteoporosis, caution must be taken when trying to use the plate to help in the reduction.

The small laminar spreader is most useful in reduction and lengthening.

STEP 3 PITFALLS

Failure to release the dorsal callous and periosteum will make it very difficult to achieve reduction.

Step 2

- The osteotomy cut is made parallel to the articular surface in the sagittal plane (Figs. 80-13 and 80-14).
- The plate is reattached to the distal fragment (Fig. 80-15).

Step 3

- By supinating the distal fragment while pronating the radial shaft, the dorsal callous and periosteum are released (Fig. 80-16).
- A laminar spreader is placed in the osteotomy to help regain some length and help reduce the distal fragment (Fig. 80-17).

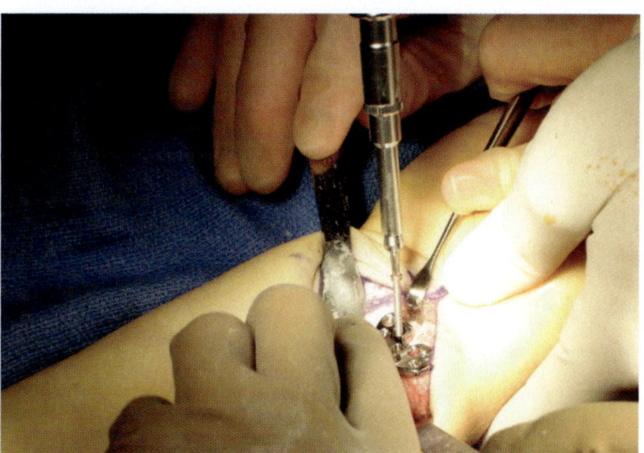

FIGURE 80-15

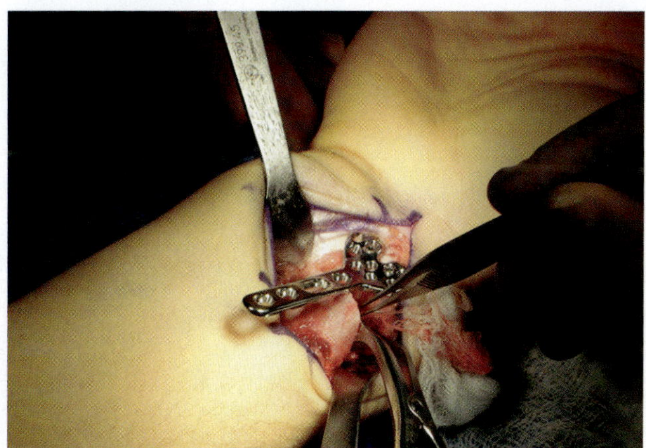

FIGURE 80-16

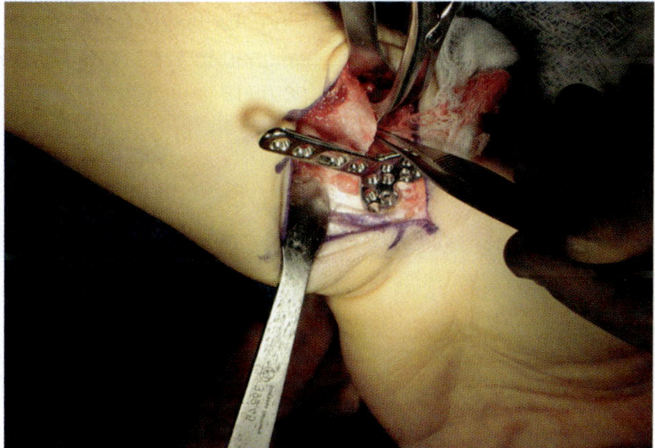

FIGURE 80-17

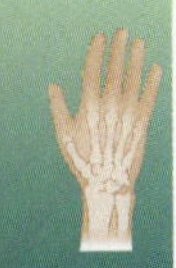

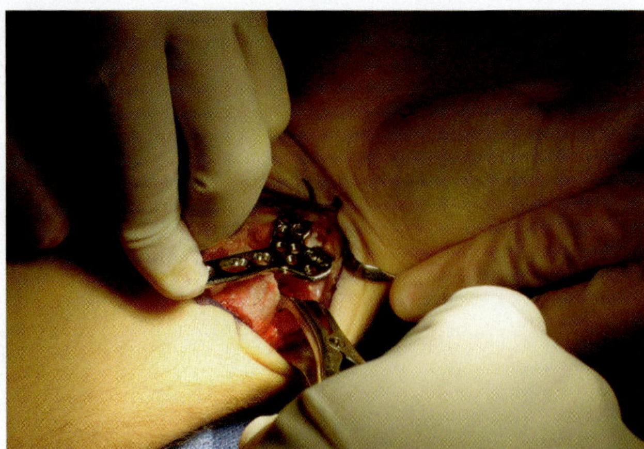

FIGURE 80-18

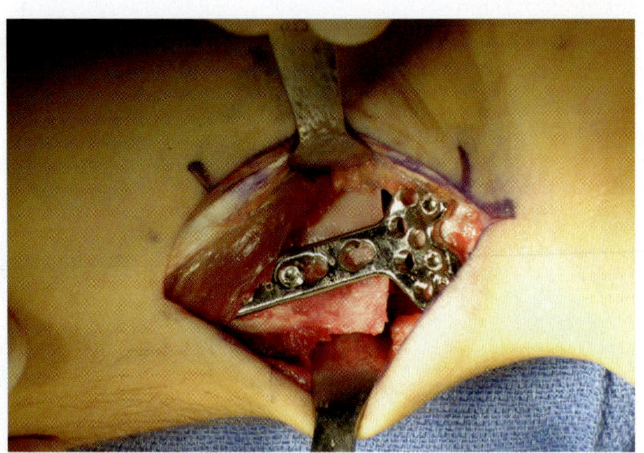

FIGURE 80-19

STEP 4 PEARLS

The use of a bone clamp will help bring the proximal limb of the plate onto the radius shaft.

Bone substitutes will be effective with less morbidity than iliac crest graft.

STEP 4 PITFALLS

Poor preoperative planning will make it difficult to use the implant and to perform the reduction.

Screw penetration through the dorsal cortex can produce tendon irritation or rupture.

PITFALLS

Care should be taken not to overcorrect the physiologic palmar tilt when manipulating the distal fragment into extension.

Screw penetration through the dorsal cortex risks attrition tendinitis and rupture.

Step 4

- Using the laminar spreader, the length is gained while the proximal limb is realigned to the radius shaft (Fig. 80-18).
- The plate is attached to the shaft with screws (Fig. 80-19).
- Bone graft or bone substitute is packed into the defect from the radial side.

Postoperative Care and Expected Outcomes

- A volar splint and bulky dressing remain for 7 to 10 days, after which time active motion is started.
- The adjuvant use of a splint will depend on the patient's needs.
- The ultimate outcome regarding strength and motion may take up to 12 to 18 months to reach (Fig. 80-20).

Procedure

Correction of Volar Malunions

- The surgical approach is similar to that already described.
- Volarly angulated malunions require a palmar open wedge osteotomy.
- Volarly displaced malunions tend to heal with a pronation deformity of the distal radius (Fig. 80-21).

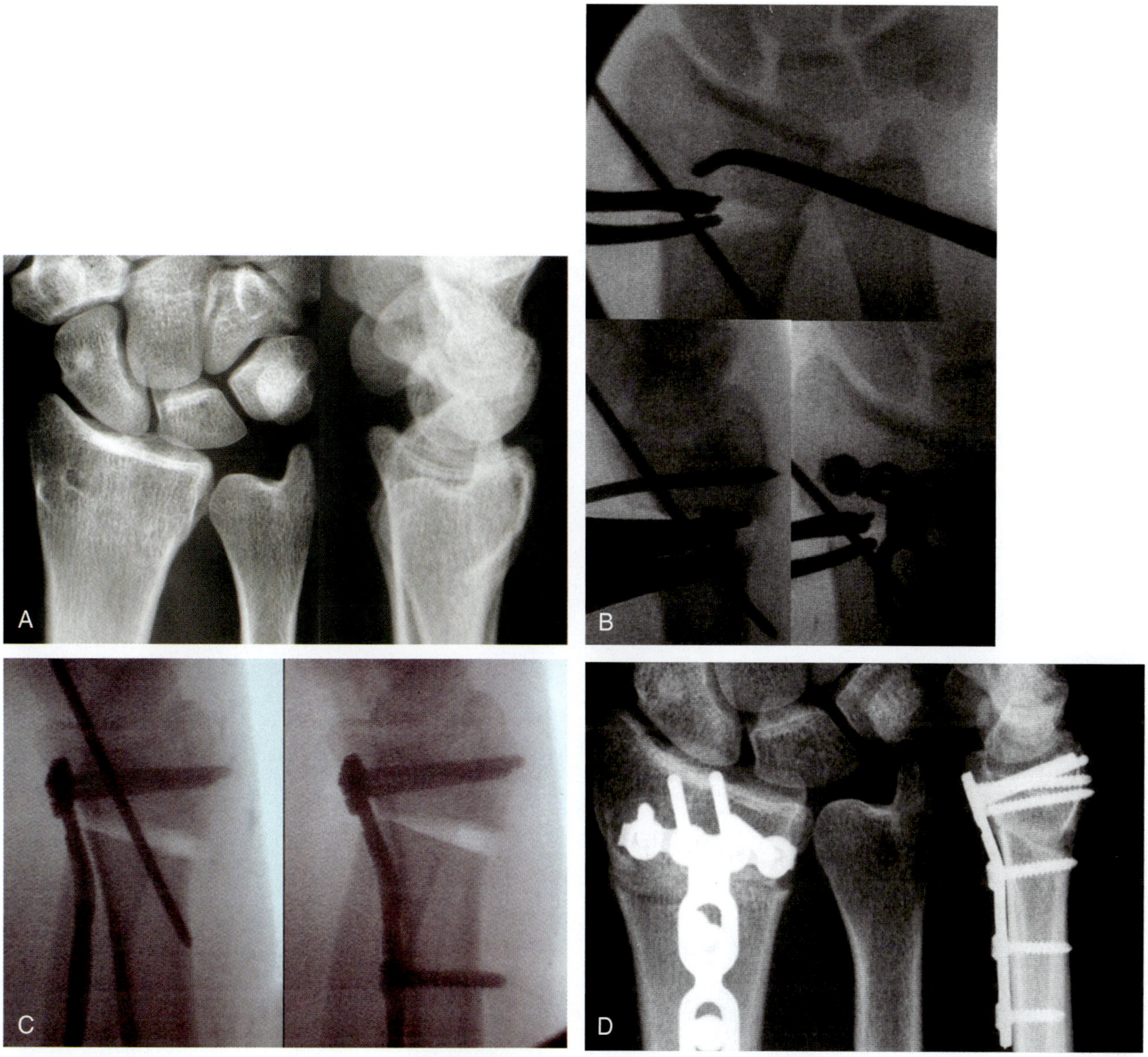

FIGURE 80-20

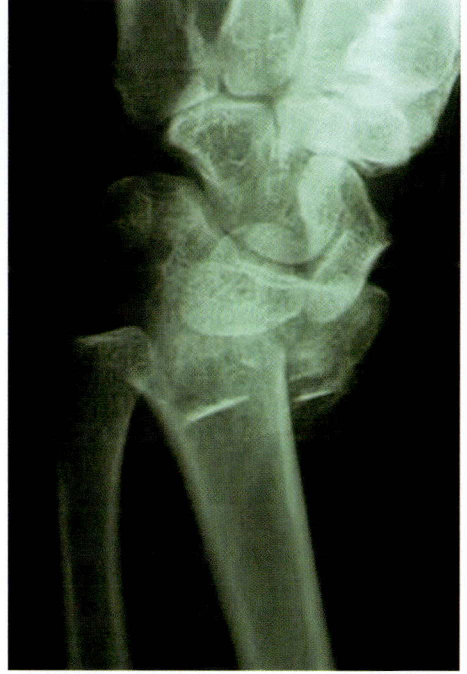

FIGURE 80-21

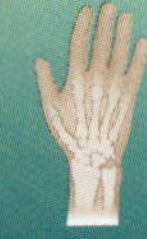

Procedure

Dorsal Approach

Step 1

- A smooth Kirschner wire is inserted through the dorsal wrist capsule parallel to the articular surface.
- Two threaded 2.5-mm Kirschner wires are inserted on both sides of the deformity to subtend the angle of correction (Fig. 80-22).
- A distractor can be attached to the pins to help gain length and maintain the corrected alignment (Fig. 80-23).

STEP 1 PEARLS

A small distractor is helpful to slowly gain length and realign the distal fragment (Fig. 80-23).

Placement of the K-wires follows the orientation determined by the preoperative plan.

If angular correction alone is required, the osteotomy is made parallel to the joint surface (Fig. 80-24).

If rotational correction is also required, the osteotomy should be made perpendicular to the distal fragment in both the frontal and sagittal planes.

STEP 1 PITFALLS

Incorrect placement of the osteotomy may create a secondary deformity.

Failure to release the brachioradialis tendon will inhibit lengthening of the distal fragment.

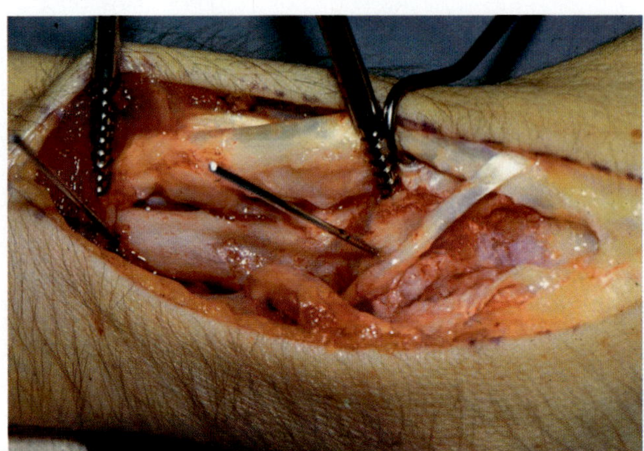

FIGURE 80-22

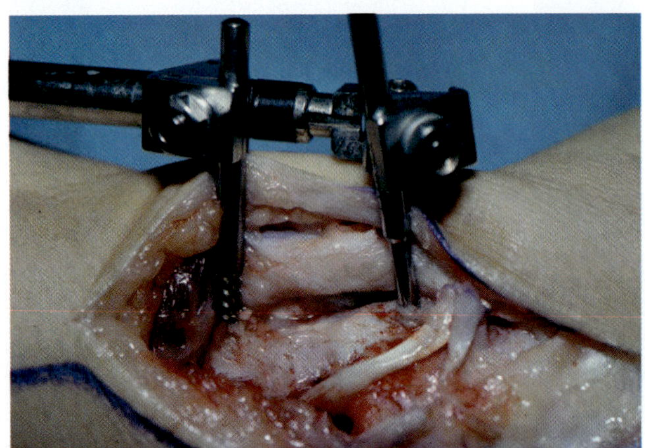

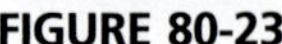

FIGURE 80-23

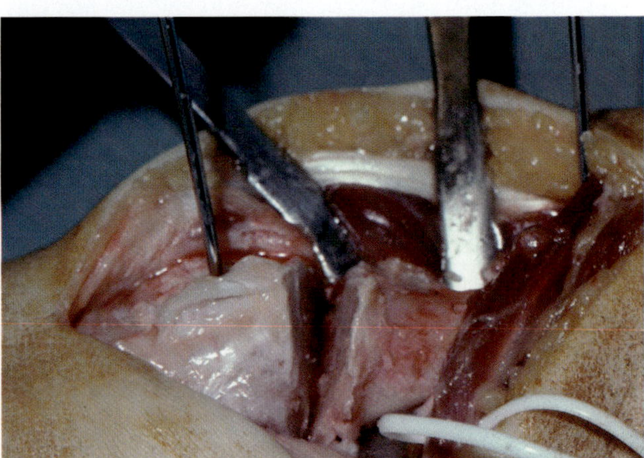

FIGURE 80-24

Step 2

- Using a thin blade, the osteotomy is made parallel to the distal K-wires.
- The distractor can facilitate slow lengthening (Fig. 80-25).

Step 3

- Implant selection can be either two small 2.4-mm plates, one dorsally on the intermediate column and one between the first and second extensor compartments or, alternatively, an implant shaped to the dorsal anatomy of the distal radius.

STEP 2 PEARLS

When creating the osteotomy, the volar cortex can be left intact if an opening wedge without lengthening has been planned.

Temporary stabilization of the osteotomy can be done by placing smooth K-wires obliquely across the osteotomy.

STEP 2 PITFALLS

Avoid the osteotomy cut entering the sigmoid notch!

STEP 3 PEARLS

Careful image control is needed to confirm the alignment correction and position of the proposed implant.

If two small 2.4-mm plates are to be used, the dorsal plate on the intermediate column is placed first to check position of the distal screws (Fig. 80-26).

STEP 3 PITFALLS

The distal locking screws can penetrate the radiocarpal joint unless the distal part of the plate is bent slightly to direct the screws in a proximal direction.

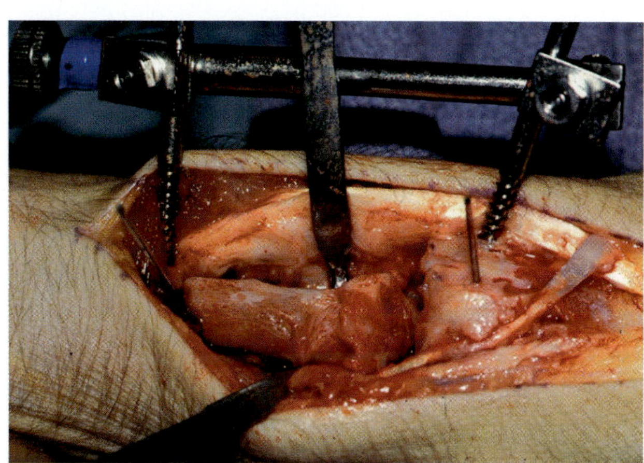

FIGURE 80-25

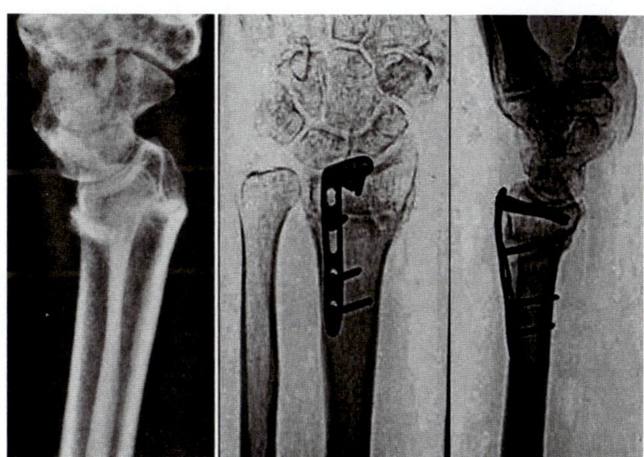

FIGURE 80-26

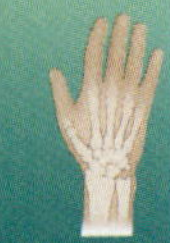

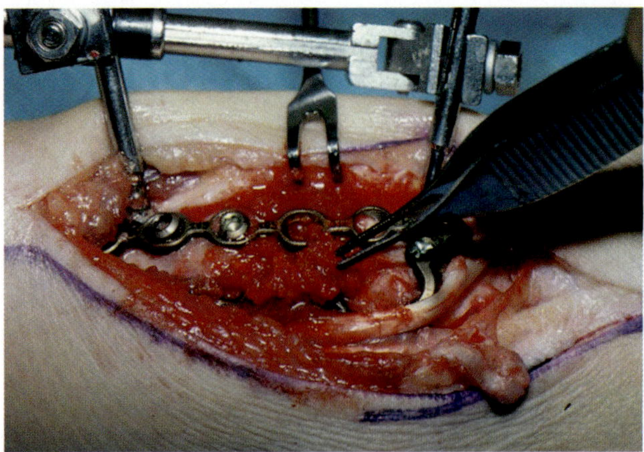

FIGURE 80-27

Step 4

- The three-dimensional defect created by the osteotomy is filled with either cancellous iliac crest graft or a bone substitute (Fig. 80-27).
- Closure of the extensor retinaculum is done with the EPL tendon outside the closure to prevent ischemic rupture of the avascular portion of the EPL at the Lister tubercle.

STEP 4 PEARLS

Applying the internal fixation before placing the bone graft allows cancellous graft or bone substitute to be used.

Angular stable locking plates have avoided the need for structural support with corticocancellous bone graft.

STEP 4 PITFALLS

Overcorrection of the distal fragment can result in volar displacement of the distal fragment.

Closure of the extensor retinaculum without transposition of the thumb extensor risks tendon rupture.

Postoperative Care and Expected Outcomes

- See volar approach.

Evidence

Jupiter JB, Ring D. A comparison of early and late reconstruction of malunited fractures of the distal end of the radius. *J Bone Joint Surg [Am].* 1996;78:739-748.
The authors retrospectively compared 10 malunited distal radius fractures that had been corrected early (6 to 14 weeks after injury) against 10 malunited distal radius fractures that were corrected late (30 to 48 weeks) and found that the results were similar. However, they preferred an earlier correction because it was technically easier and reduced the overall period of disability. (Level IV evidence)

Prommersberger KJ, van Schoonhaven J, Lanz UB. Outcome after corrective osteotomy for malunited fractures of the distal end of the radius. *J Hand Surg [Br].* 2002;27:55-60.
A large series of corrective osteotomies for dorsal (n = 29) and palmar (n = 20) malunited distal radius fractures is presented, together with objective follow-up data at 18 months. The authors conclude that function is correlated with restoration of alignment, and patients with multiplanar deformities fare less well after surgical correction. (Level V evidence)

Ring D, Roberge C, Morgan T, et al. Osteotomy for malunited fractures of the distal radius: a comparison of structural and nonstructural autogenous bone grafts. *J Hand Surg [Am].* 2002;27:216-222.
This retrospective study compared the use of cancellous bone graft versus a corticocancellous bone graft after corrective osteotomy of malunited distal radius fractures. Radiographic and functional results were comparable between both groups, and the authors preferred cancellous bone grafting because it was simpler. (Level IV evidence)

PROCEDURE 81

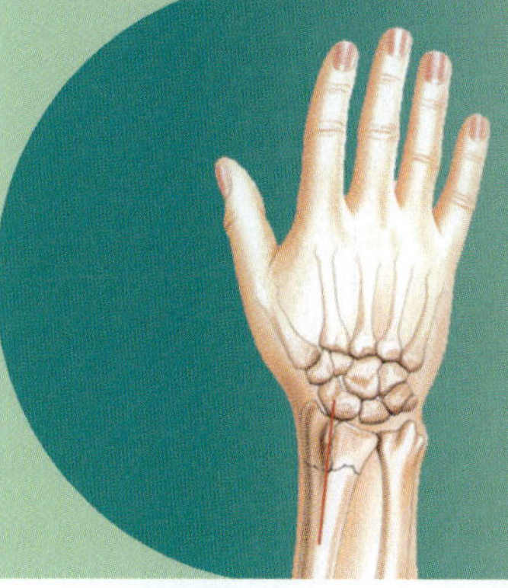

Ulnar Shortening Osteotomy

Jennifer Waljee, Sandeep J. Sebastin, and Kevin C. Chung

See Video 59: Ulnar Shortening Osteotomy

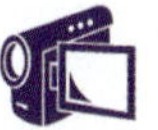

Indications

- Ulnar impaction syndrome (ulnocarpal abutment)
- Malunited distal radius fractures with loss of radial height
- Madelung deformity
- Longitudinal instability of the forearm after radial head resection
- Premature distal radial physeal closure (e.g., gymnast wrist)

Examination/Imaging

Clinical Examination

- Patients with ulnar impaction syndrome present with ulnar-sided wrist pain, swelling, and limitation of motion. This may coexist with other causes of ulnar-sided wrist pain, including triangular fibrocartilage complex (TFCC) injuries, distal radioulnar (DRU) joint instability, and lunotriquetral ligament injuries, among others. It is important to consider these conditions before attributing the symptoms to ulnar impaction syndrome, particularly among patients with negative ulnar variance.
- The following provocative clinical tests are helpful in the diagnosis of ulnocarpal impaction syndrome.
  - *Ulnocarpal stress test (TFCC grind test):* The wrist is maintained in maximal ulnar deviation, and the examiner axially loads it while passively pronosupinating the wrist. The test is positive when patient has ulnar-sided wrist pain during this maneuver. This test is positive in patients with ulnocarpal abutment syndrome and TFCC injuries (Fig. 81-1).
  - *Ulnar foveal sign:* This test is performed with the elbow flexed and the examiner supporting the patient's wrist and hand by maintaining the forearm in neutral rotation and the wrist in neutral position. The examiner then presses the thumb distally and deep into the interval soft spot between ulnar styloid and pisiform. The foveal sign is positive when there is exquisite tenderness compared with the contralateral side and replicates the pain felt by the patient. This test is sensitive in the diagnosis of foveal detachment of the TFCC and ulnotriquetral ligamentous injuries (Fig. 81-2).

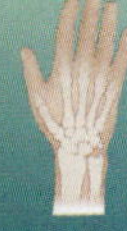

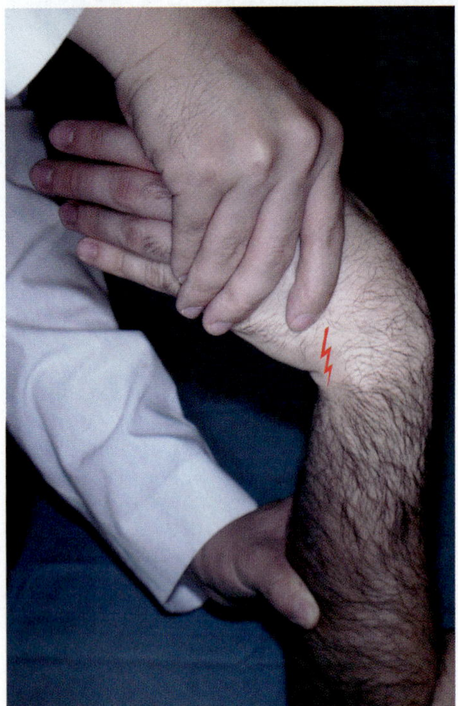

FIGURE 81-1

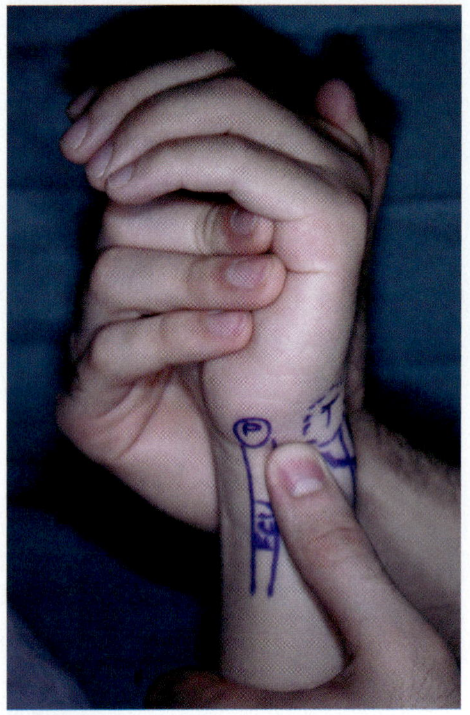

FIGURE 81-2

Imaging

- A neutral rotation posteroanterior view will help determine ulnar variance. Ulnar variance describes the relative positions of the distal articular surface of the radius and ulna. When both the distal radius and the distal ulna are at the same level, it is called neutral variance (12%). If the distal ulna is distal to the radius, it is called positive ulnar variance (55%), and if the distal ulna is proximal to the radius, it is called negative ulnar variance (33%). A variance of −2 mm to +2 mm is considered normal (Fig. 81-3). Ulnar variance increases with pronation (up to 1 mm) and with forceful grip (up to 2 mm) (Fig. 81-4).
- A positive ulnar variance is associated with ulnar impaction syndrome. Other radiological features include cystic changes and sclerosis in the ulnar corner of the lunate, triquetrum, and radial portion of the distal ulnar head (Fig. 81-5).
- Magnetic resonance imaging can identify degenerative changes related to ulnar impaction syndrome earlier than plain radiographs because it can reveal subchondral bone marrow edema and early chondromalacia on fat-suppressed, T2-weighted and short T1-weighted inversion recovery images (Fig. 81-6).
- Wrist arthroscopy is the most accurate modality for diagnosis of ulnar impaction syndrome. Any other associated pathology of the wrist can also be evaluated and the condition of the TFCC noted. Palmer has proposed a classification of degenerative TFCC tears (Table 81-1).

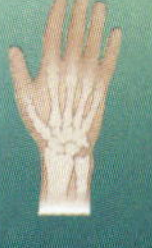

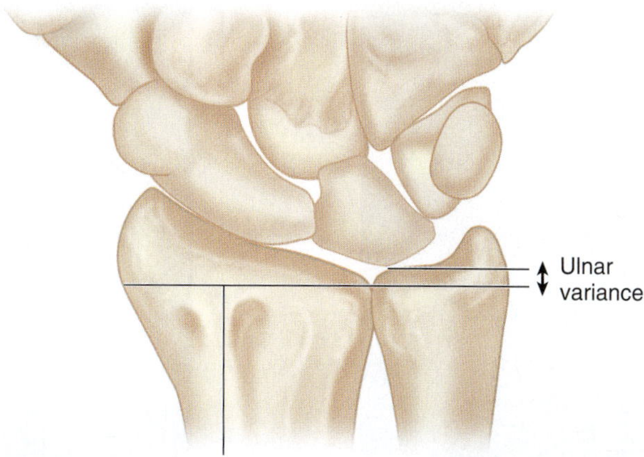

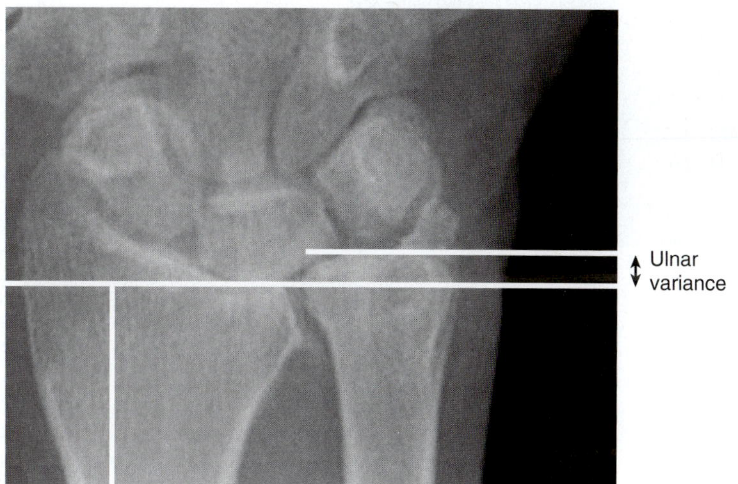

FIGURE 81-3

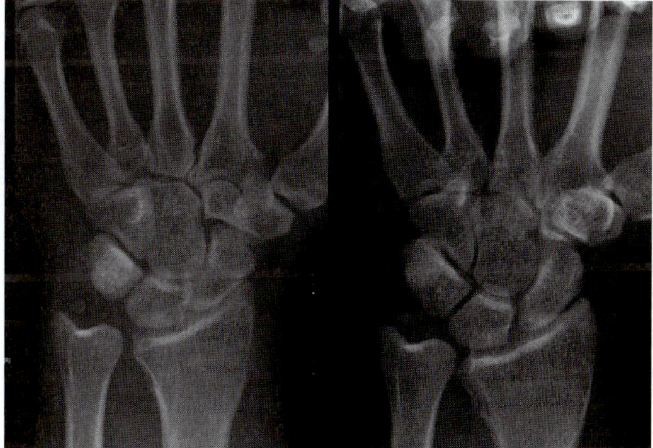

FIGURE 81-4

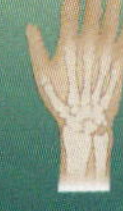

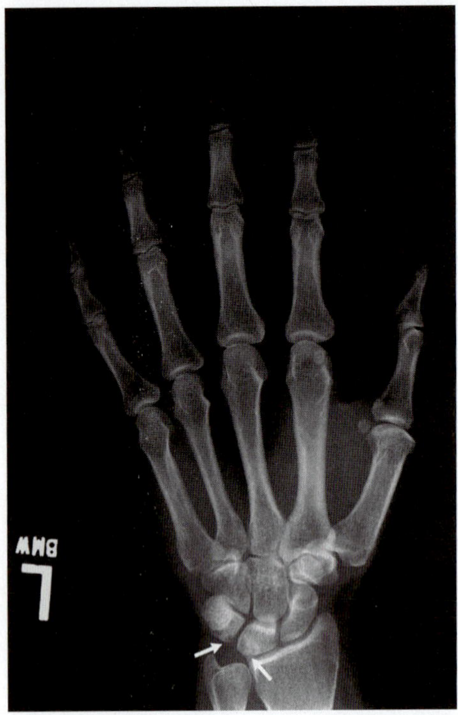

FIGURE 81-5

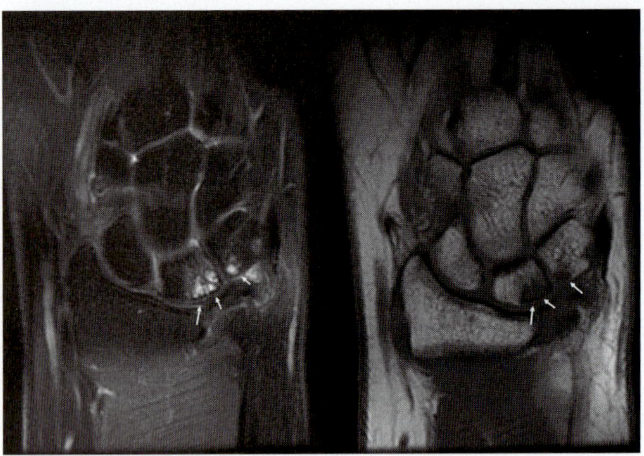

FIGURE 81-6

Table 81-1 Palmar Classification of TFCC Injuries

Type 1	Traumatic Lesions
1a	Isolated central disk perforation
1b	Peripheral ulnar-sided tear of TFCC (with or without ulnar styloid fracture)
1c	Distal TFCC disruption from distal ulnocarpal ligaments
1d	Radial TFCC disruption ± sigmoid notch fracture
Type 2	**Degenerative Lesions**
2a	TFCC wear
2b	2a with lunate and/or ulnar chondromalacia
2c	TFCC perforation with lunate and/or ulnar chondromalacia
2d	2c + lunotriquetral ligament perforation
2e	2d + ulnocarpal arthritis

Surgical Anatomy

- The radiocarpal joint transmits 82% of the load across the wrist, whereas the ulnocarpal joint transmits the remaining 18% in a neutral ulnar wrist. In subjects with a 2.5-mm positive ulnar variance, the load transmission across the ulna increases to 42%. This substantial increase in load in a positive ulnar wrist puts it at a high risk for ligamentous and articular degeneration. Increased dorsal tilt of the radius can further exacerbate loading onto the ulnar wrist. On the contrary, in a 2.5-mm negative ulnar variance wrist, the load transmission decreases to 4.3%. This is the basis for the ulnar shortening osteotomy.

Positioning

- The patient is positioned supine with the affected extremity on a hand table. The procedure is performed under tourniquet control.
- Intraoperative fluoroscopy will be required, and the table should be placed such that the C-arm can be positioned with ease.

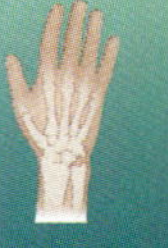

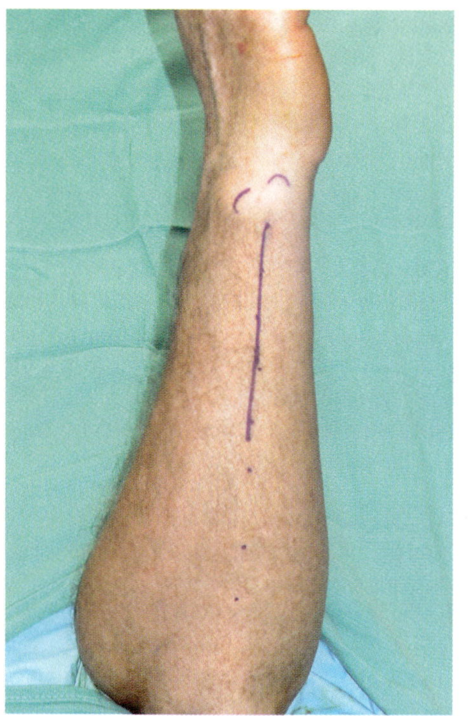

FIGURE 81-7

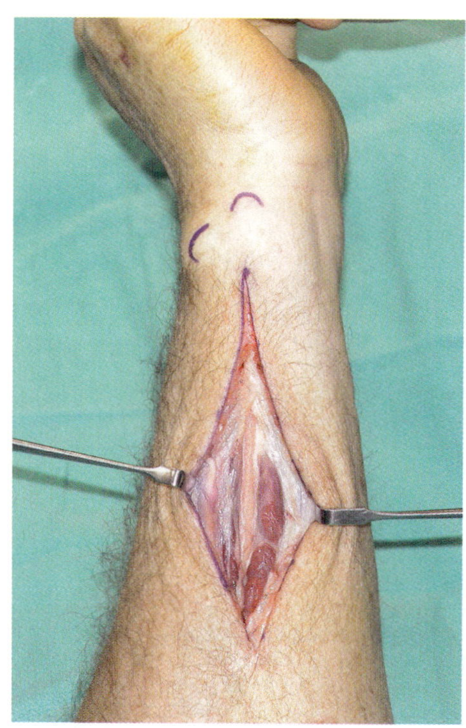

FIGURE 81-8

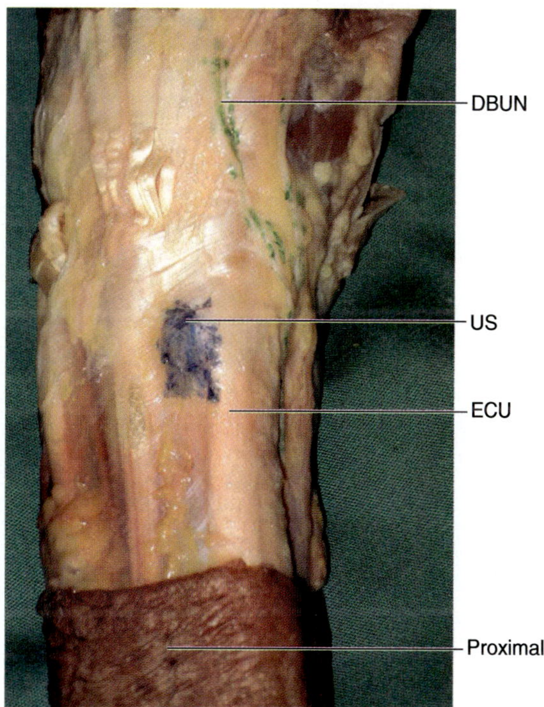

FIGURE 81-9

PITFALLS

Care should be taken to avoid the dorsal cutaneous branch of the ulnar nerve. It arises about 8 cm proximal to the ulnar styloid, passes below the FCU, and runs in an oblique course toward the ulnar styloid (Fig. 81-9).

Exposures

- A 10-cm longitudinal incision is made on the subcutaneous border of the ulna beginning 1 to 2 cm proximal to the ulnar styloid (Fig. 81-7). The flexor carpi ulnaris (FCU) and extensor carpi ulnaris (ECU) are identified, and the interval between them is developed to expose the subcutaneous border of the ulna (Fig. 81-8).

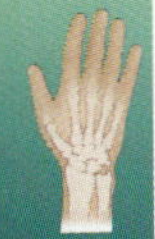

The compression plate can be placed on the volar surface or the subcutaneous dorsal surface of the ulna. Placement on the subcutaneous dorsal surface is easier, but the plate is palpable, can cause soft tissue irritation, and usually requires removal at a later date. Placement on the volar surface avoids these complications but requires more dissection and soft tissue stripping, which may result in a higher incidence of nonunion. The senior author prefers to place the plate on the subcutaneous dorsal surface of the ulna.

STEP 2 PEARLS

It is important to prebend the ulnar plate before applying it to bone. This will ensure that the volar cortex does not open up when the compression screws are tightened.

- A Rayhack device (Generation I) is used to create a precision oblique osteotomy. A six-hole low-profile locking plate or a six-hole limited contact dynamic compression plate can be used. The use of the newer lower-profile locking plates can be used to reduce the incidence of soft tissue irritation that require plate removal.

Procedure

Step 1: Preparation of Osteotomy Site

- The soft tissues are retracted with a self-retaining retractor, and the site of the osteotomy is selected. This is usually 5 to 7 cm from the ulnar styloid, 2 to 3 cm from the proximal end of the sigmoid fossa, and distal to the origin of the interosseous membrane on the ulnar shaft (Fig. 81-10).
- The periosteum is divided sharply with a scalpel, and a periosteal elevator is used to expose the site of the osteotomy circumferentially for 1 to 2 cm.

Step 2: Placement of Saw Guide

- The selected plate is placed on the exposed dorsal subcutaneous surface of the ulna. The distal end of the plate should be 3 to 4 cm from the ulnar styloid, and the long elliptical hole on the plate should be distal to the proposed osteotomy site. The position of the second plate hole (from proximal) is marked on the bone. The plate is then removed.
- The saw guide is placed such that the second hole on the guide (from proximal) is lined up with the previously marked second hole on the plate (Fig. 81-11).

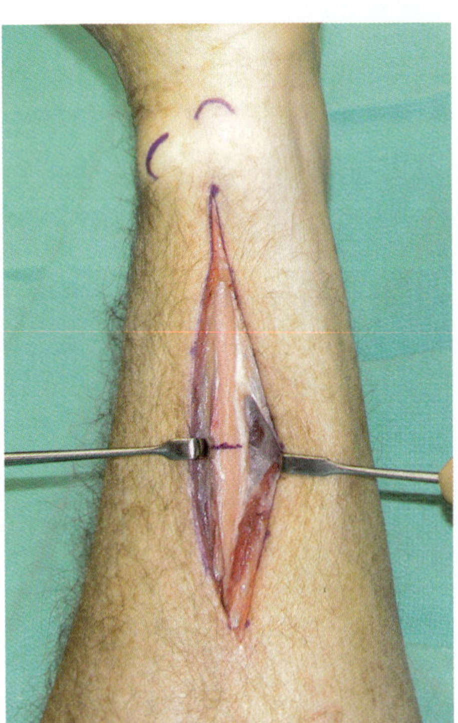

FIGURE 81-10

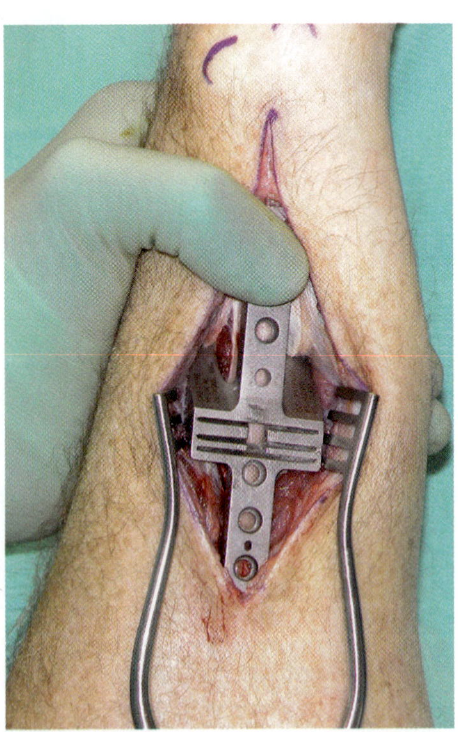

FIGURE 81-11

STEP 2 PITFALLS

The first hole of the saw guide is not drilled if a low profile locking plate is being used. This hole represents the site where a 2.7-mm locking screw will be placed.

- The saw guide is held manually and using a straight drill guide, a 2.5-mm drill is used to make a hole through the second hole on the guide. The depth of the hole is measured, the hole is tapped with a 3.5-mm tap, and a 3.5-mm cortical screw is inserted (Fig. 81-12). This procedure is repeated for the fourth and then the third holes on the saw guide (Fig. 81-13).

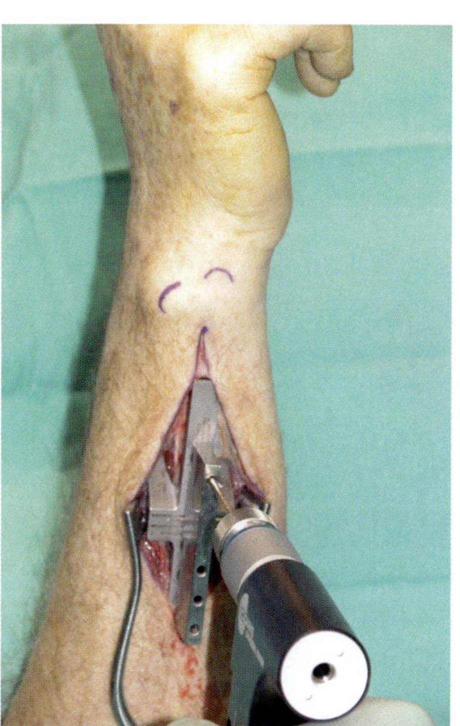

FIGURE 81-12

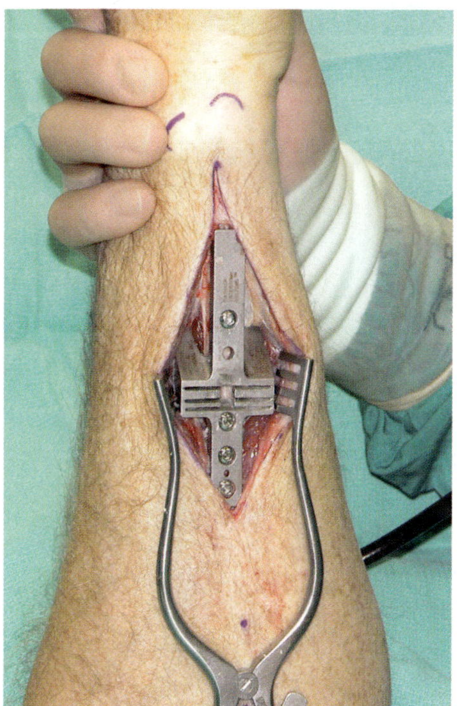

FIGURE 81-13

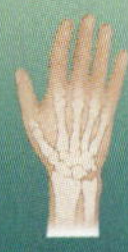

STEP 3 PEARLS

Continuous saline irrigation should be used during the osteotomy to minimize thermal necrosis.

These 3.5-mm screws will be reused. Place these screws in order so that they can be used in the same hole again.

Step 3: Performing Oblique Osteotomy

- The amount of bone removed should equal the amount of positive ulnar variance plus the amount of negative ulnar variance desired as measured on the neutral posteroanterior view. In general, about 2 to 2.5 mm of negative ulnar variance is desired, and typically a 3- to 5-mm segment of bone is resected. The anticipated shortening in a Rayhack system depends on the slots that are used to make the parallel oblique osteotomy cuts (slots 1 and 2 = 3.5 mm; slots 2 and 3 = 4.9 mm; and slots 1 and 3 = 7.4 mm) (Fig. 81-14).
- The saw is used to make the distal cut first, followed by the proximal cut.
- The 3.5-mm screws holding the saw guide, and the saw guide and the segment of excised bone are removed in sequence (Fig. 81-15).

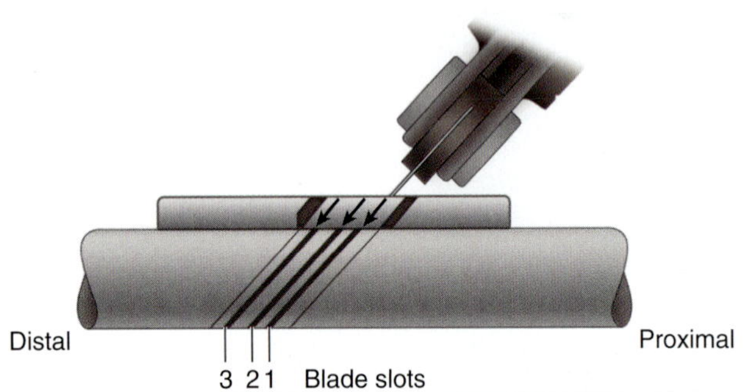

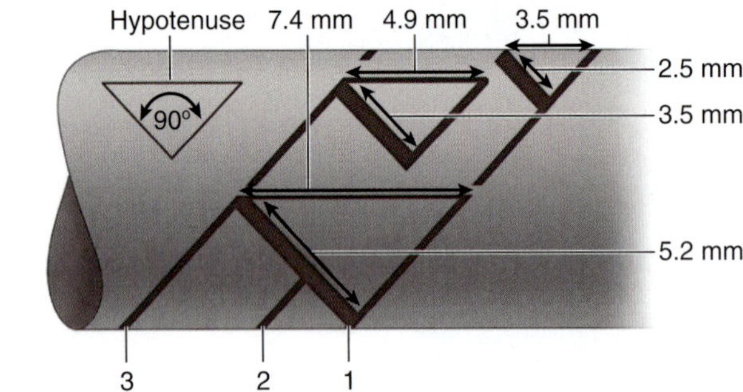

FIGURE 81-14

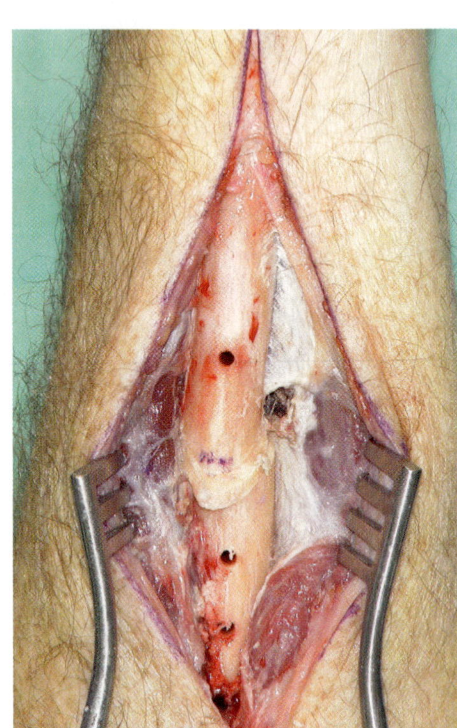

FIGURE 81-15

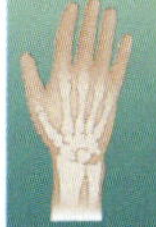

STEP 4 PEARLS

Even compression is achieved by alternating between both the compression screws.

Even compression is confirmed by intraoperative fluoroscopy.

STEP 4 PITFALLS

Overcompression should be avoided because visual compression alone is adequate. Further compression will be achieved by the interfragmentary lag screw.

Step 4: Application of Plate, Compression Device, and Compression of Osteotomy

- The previously selected prebent six-hole low-profile plate (or a six-hole LC-DCP) is placed over the ulna, and a 3.5-mm screw is passed into the second hole of the plate (first hole on the ulna) to fix the plate to the ulna.
- The compression device is then placed over the plate and secured in position to the plate and the ulna by passing a screw through the third hole of the plate (first hole of compression device and second hole on ulna). This screw should be 4 mm longer than the previously passed screw (Fig. 81-16).
- Another screw is passed through the sliding block of the compression device onto the elliptical hole on the plate and the third hole on the bone. This screw is not tightened fully (Fig. 81-17).
- The compression device is compressed horizontally by using the horizontal compression screws until the osteotomy surfaces appear to be compressed.

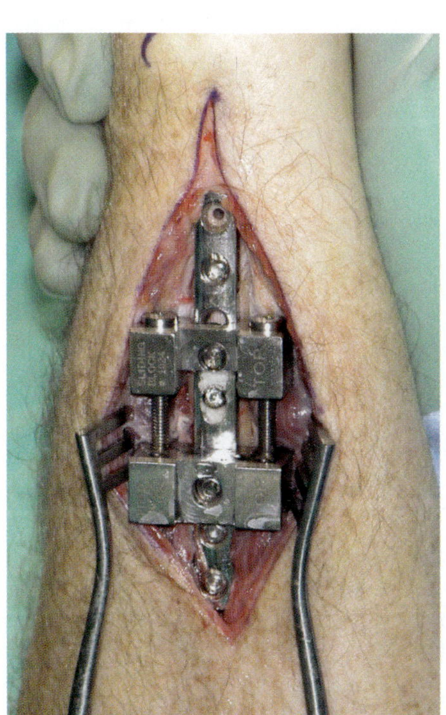

FIGURE 81-16

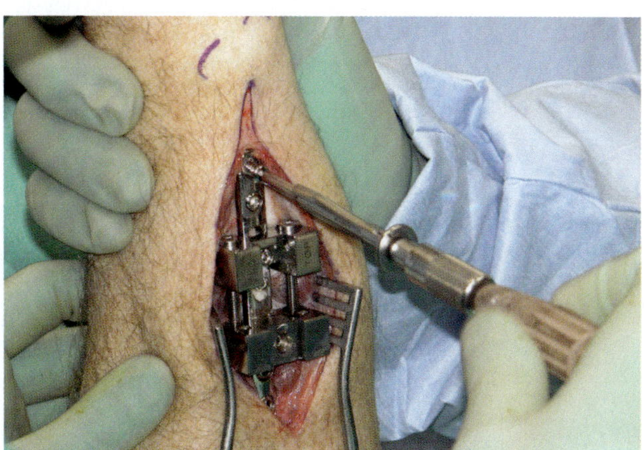

FIGURE 81-17

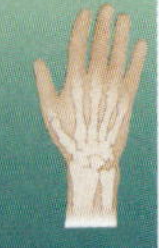

STEP 5 PITFALLS

The 2.7-mm drill bit should be used only for the near cortex. Care should be taken to prevent inadvertent drilling of both cortices.

Step 5: Placement of Interfragmentary Lag Screw

- The 22-degree angled drill guide is placed into the round hole of the compression block.
- A 2.7-mm drill bit is used to drill the near cortex. A 2.7-mm drill bushing is placed into the drill guide, and the far cortex is drilled with a 2.0-mm drill bit.
- The angled drill guide is removed, and the depth of the hole is measured. The drill guide is reapplied, and the far cortex is tapped with a 2.7-mm tap. The drill guide is removed, and the 2.7-mm cortical lag screw is inserted to provide additional compression.

STEP 6 PEARLS

True posteroanterior and lateral views are best obtained by doing an anteroposterior view with the forearm in supination or 30 degrees short of full supination and a posteroanterior view with the forearm in pronation. Any screws deemed to be excessively long or too short may be replaced.

Step 6: Final Fixation of Plate

- A hand-held drill guide and a 2.5-mm drill bit are used to make a hole through the fifth hole of the plate. This hole is measured and tapped, and 3.5-mm cortical screw is placed.
- A locking screw drill guide is inserted into the sixth hole, and a 2.3-mm drill bit is used to make a hole. This hole is measured, and a 2.7-mm locking screw is placed.
- The compression device is removed, and the original screws for holes 3 and 4 are reinserted (Fig. 81-18).
- Intraoperative fluoroscopy is used to confirm the position of the plate and screws (Fig. 81-19).

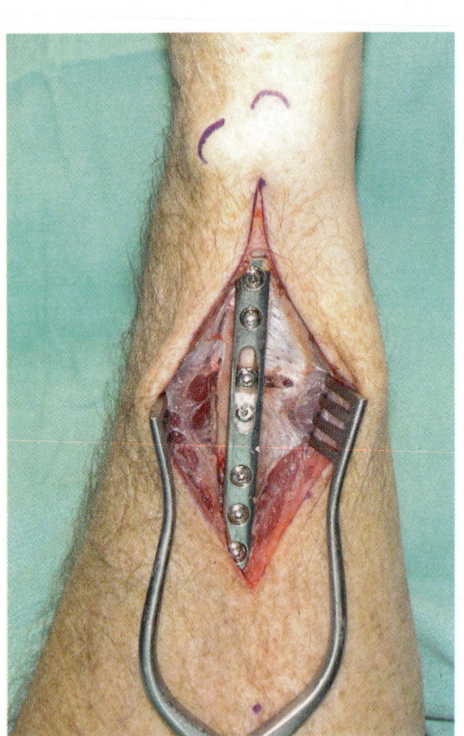

FIGURE 81-18

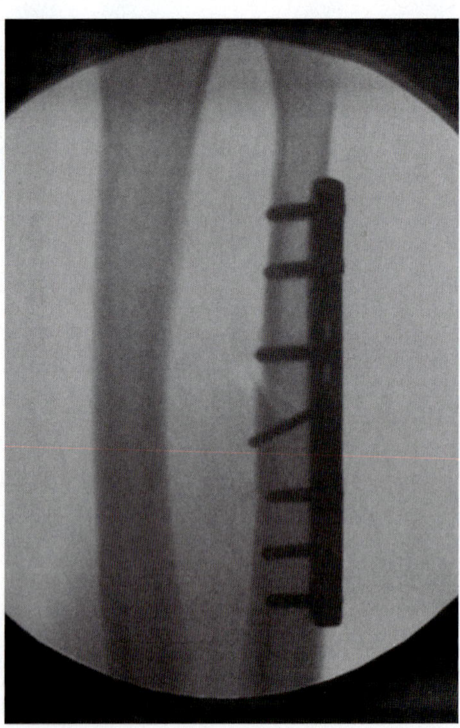

FIGURE 81-19

Step 7: Wound Closure

- The tourniquet is released and hemostasis secured. The wound is irrigated and closed in layers, and a sterile dressing is applied. An ulnar gutter splint is placed over the forearm and wrist.

Postoperative Care and Expected Outcomes

- The wrist is maintained in an ulnar-sided splint for 4 weeks, with early range-of-motion exercises initiated. Splinting can be discontinued and progressive strengthening exercises started once bony union is evident (Figs. 81-20 and 81-21).
- Complications following ulnar shortening osteotomy include bony nonunion (5%), chronic pain, DRU joint stiffness, hardware prominence requiring removal, and injury to the dorsal sensory branch of the ulnar nerve.

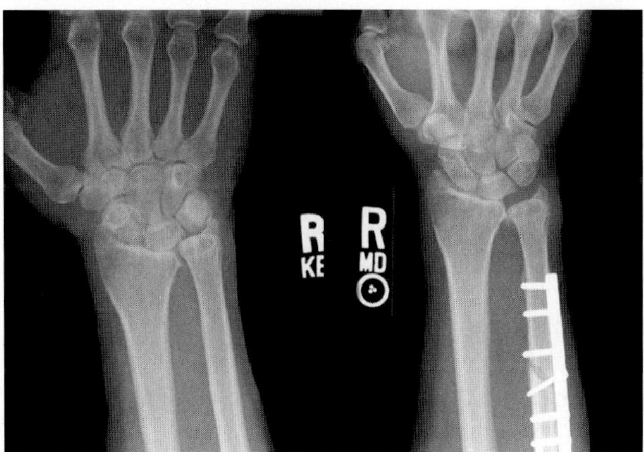

FIGURE 81-20

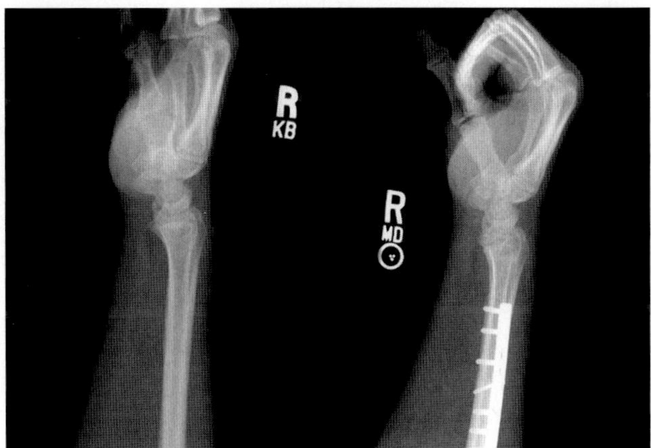

FIGURE 81-21

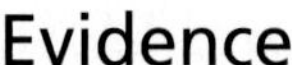

Evidence

Baek GH, Chung MS, Lee YH, et al. Ulnar shortening osteotomy in idiopathic ulnar impaction syndrome. *J Bone Joint Surg [Am]*. 2006;88:212-220.
The authors describe the outcomes following 31 ulnar shortening osteotomy procedures in 29 patients who were followed for about 3 years postoperatively. The authors report a significant improvement in patient-reported outcome, a reduction in dorsal subluxation, and resolution of degenerative cystic carpal changes within 2 years of the operation. (Level IV evidence)

Chen NC, Wolfe SE. Ulna shortening osteotomy using a compression device. *J Hand Surg [Am]*. 2003;28:88-93.
This article examines 18 patients over a 10-year period with ulnar impaction syndrome who underwent ulnar shortening osteotomy with a compression device technique, and outcomes were assessed using the Chun and Palmer wrist grading system. Overall, favorable outcomes were achieved with respect to function and pain. However, 8 patients required plate removal for hardware prominence and discomfort. (Level IV evidence)

Kitzinger HB, Karle B, Low S, Krimmer H. Ulnar shortening osteotomy with a premounted sliding-hole plate. *Ann Plast Surg*. 2007;58:636-639.
This article examines 27 patients who underwent ulnar shortening osteotomy over a 2-year period. They report an improvement in patient-reported function, as measured by DASH scores, and in pain, measured along a visual analog scale. Although grip strength and range of motion improved significantly following the procedure, 6 patients complained of discomfort related to hardware. (Level IV evidence)

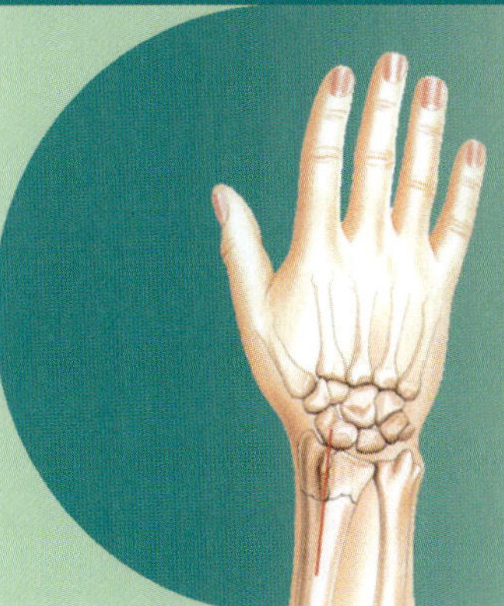

PROCEDURE 82

Radioulnar Ligament Reconstruction for Chronic Distal Radioulnar Joint Instability

Jennifer Waljee, Sandeep J. Sebastin, and Kevin C. Chung

See Video 60: Reconstruction for Chronic Volar Subluxation of the Ulna

See Video 61: Distal Radioulnar Joint Ligament Reconstruction for Ligamentous Instability

Indications

- Distal radioulnar (DRU) joint reconstruction is indicated for symptomatic chronic DRU joint instability, typically caused by distal radius fracture malunion, basilar ulnar styloid fracture nonunion, and isolated DRU joint dislocation or subluxation.

Examination/Imaging

Clinical Examination

- DRU joint instability may coexist with other causes of ulnar-sided wrist pain. These include extensor carpi ulnaris (ECU) tendinitis, flexor carpi ulnaris (FCU) tendonitis, ECU subluxation, ulnar impaction syndrome, lunotriquetral (LT) instability, and pisotriquetral arthritis. It is important to consider these conditions before attributing the symptoms to DRU joint instability. The following clinical tests are suggestive of DRU joint instability:
    - *The piano key sign:* The forearm is pronated and rested on a table surface, and the ulnar head is depressed. If the DRU joint is unstable, the ulnar head can be depressed easily and springs back into position like a piano key (Fig. 82-1).

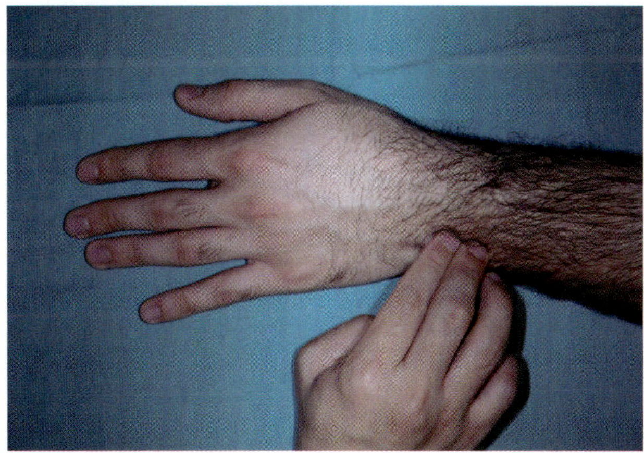

FIGURE 82-1

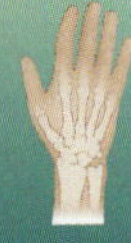

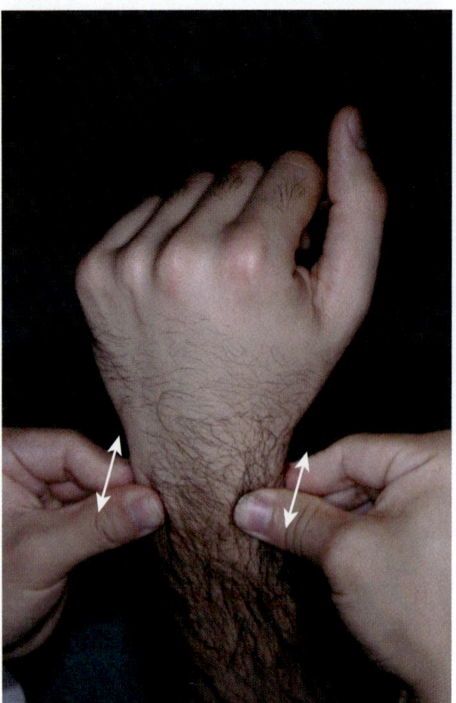

FIGURE 82-2

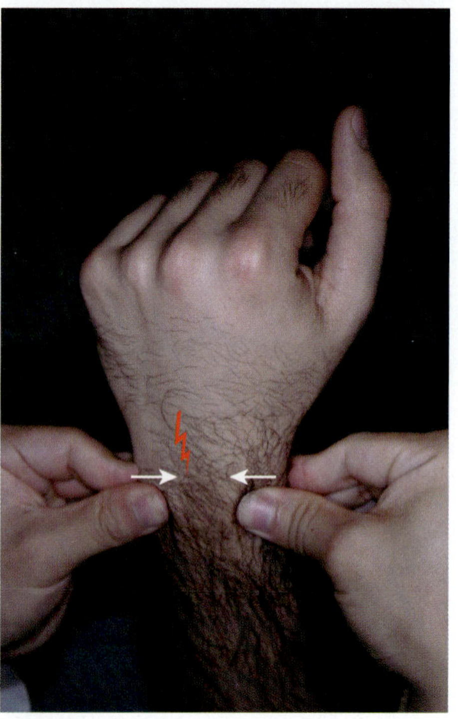

FIGURE 82-3

- *The radioulnar ballottement test:* The distal radius is stabilized between the thumb and fingers of one hand, and the distal ulna is grasped and moved in a volar to dorsal direction with the other hand. Excessive motion or pain in comparison to the other wrist is indicative of DRU joint instability. This maneuver is performed with the forearm in neutral, supinated, and pronated positions. More laxity normally occurs in the neutral position than in either pronation or supination because the joint capsule tightens as the limits of both motions are approached. It is essential to compare to the contralateral extremity because the normal range of motion and laxity of the DRU joint vary considerably among individuals (Fig. 82-2).
- *The press test:* The patient rises from a chair using his or her hands for assistance by pushing against a tabletop located in front of him or her. DRU joint instability is shown by greater "depression" of the ulnar head on the affected side and is often associated with pain.

■ It is also important to rule out the presence of DRU joint arthritis because it represents a contraindication to ligament reconstruction. The following clinical test is useful in determining the presence of DRU joint arthritis.
  - *Ulnar compression test:* This test is performed with the elbow in flexion and the forearm in neutral position. A radially directed force is applied to the ulnar head to compress it against the sigmoid notch. Patients with DRU joint synovitis or arthritis will complain of pain over the joint (Fig. 82-3).

■ The patient should be examined for the presence of the palmaris longus (PL) to be used as a tendon graft.

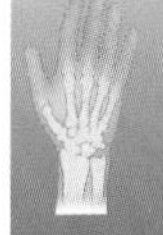

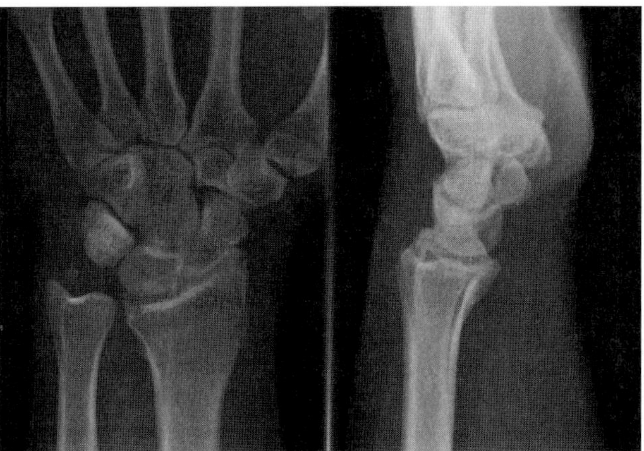

FIGURE 82-4

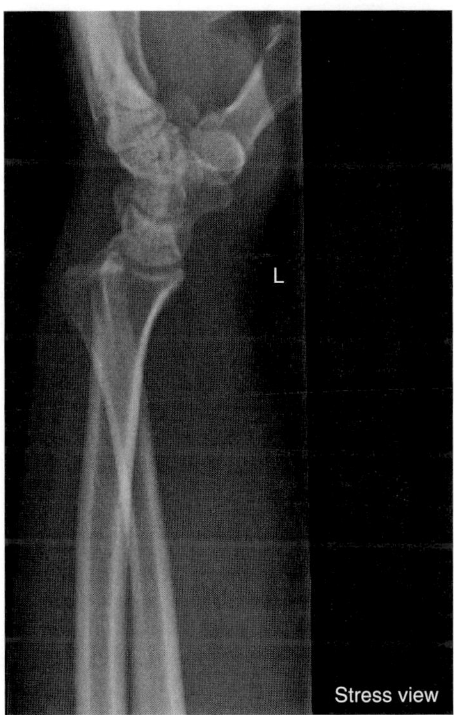

FIGURE 82-5

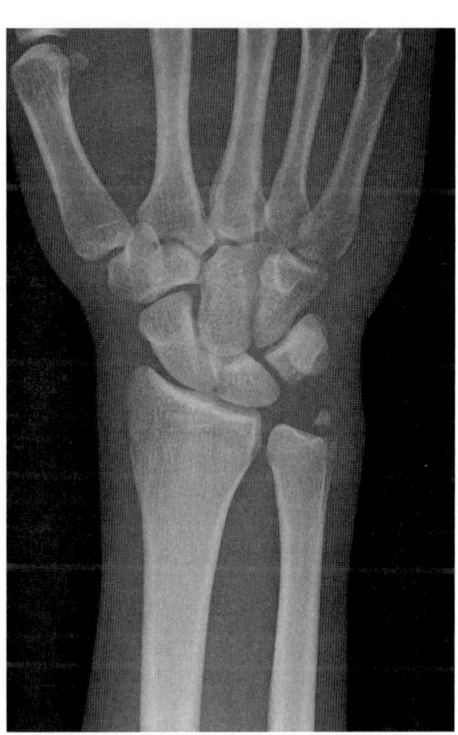

FIGURE 82-6

Imaging

- A posteroanterior view radiograph may show widening of the DRU joint, and the lateral view demonstrates the ulnar head dorsal or volar to the radius (Fig. 82-4). A weighted lateral view (taken with patient holding 5 to 8 pounds of weight) can be used to demonstrate the instability that occurs only on loading (Fig. 82-5). Other indirect signs of instability include a basal ulnar styloid fracture (Fig. 82-6) and a displaced fleck fracture from the fovea.

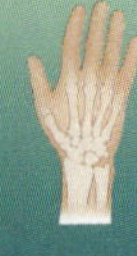

PEARLS

To ensure that the lateral radiograph is adequate, the index, long, and ring metacarpals; the proximal pole of the scaphoid on the lunate; and the radial styloid in the center of the lunate should all be superimposed on one another. Additionally, the palmar surface of the pisiform should be visible midway between the palmar surfaces of the distal pole of the scaphoid and the capitate (Fig. 82-8).

- A computed tomography (CT) scan is useful in determining subtle degrees of DRU joint instability. CT scans of both wrists in identical forearm positions should be done. It is also useful in ruling out DRU joint arthritis and in assessing the comptenecy of the sigmoid notch, especially in patients with joint instability following distal radius fractures.
- Magnetic resonance imaging (Fig. 82-7) and arthroscopy are useful in assessment of the triangular fibrocartilage complex (TFCC) and in ruling out other causes of ulnar-sided wrist pain.

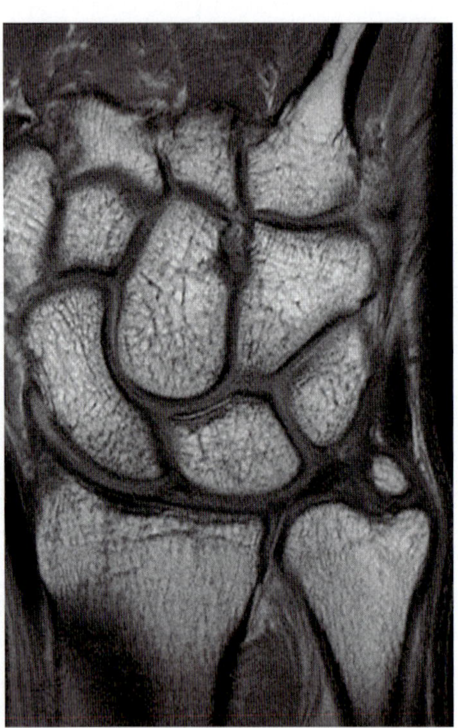

FIGURE 82-7

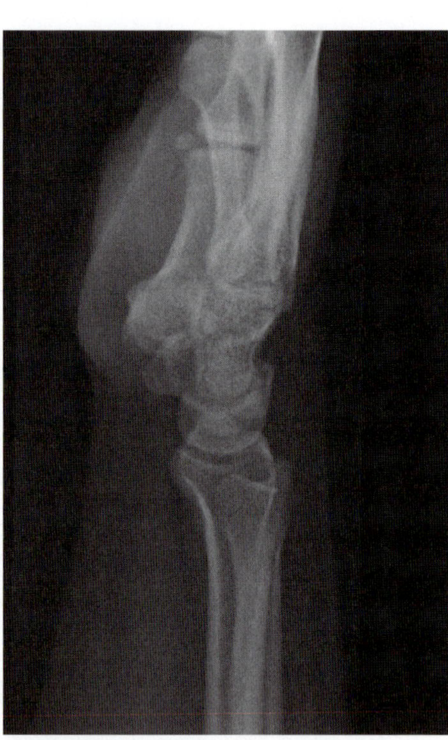

FIGURE 82-8

Surgical Anatomy

- The DRU joint is formed by the sigmoid notch of the radius and the ulnar head. It is the distal pivot for pronosupination. This joint is stabilized predominantly by ligaments, the fibrocartilaginous lips at the rim of the sigmoid notch, and the shape of the sigmoid notch in the coronal plane.
- The stabilizers of the DRU joint include the TFCC, pronator quadratus (PQ), ECU, and interosseous membrane (Fig. 82-9).
- The TFCC refers to all the soft tissues that span and support the DRU joint and ulnocarpal joints. The TFCC includes the triangular fibrocartilage (TFC, or articular disk), meniscus homologue, palmar and dorsal radioulnar ligaments, ulnar collateral ligament, ulnotriquetral ligament, ulnolunate ligament, ECU subsheath, and prestyloid recess.
- The palmar and dorsal radiolulnar ligaments are the main stabilizers of the DRU joint. These ligaments extend from the palmar and dorsal distal margins of the sigmoid notch and converge in a triangular configuration to attach to the ulna. Each radioulnar ligament divides in the coronal plane into a deep limb that inserts into the fovea and a superficial limb that inserts into the midportion of the ulnar styloid (Fig. 82-10).

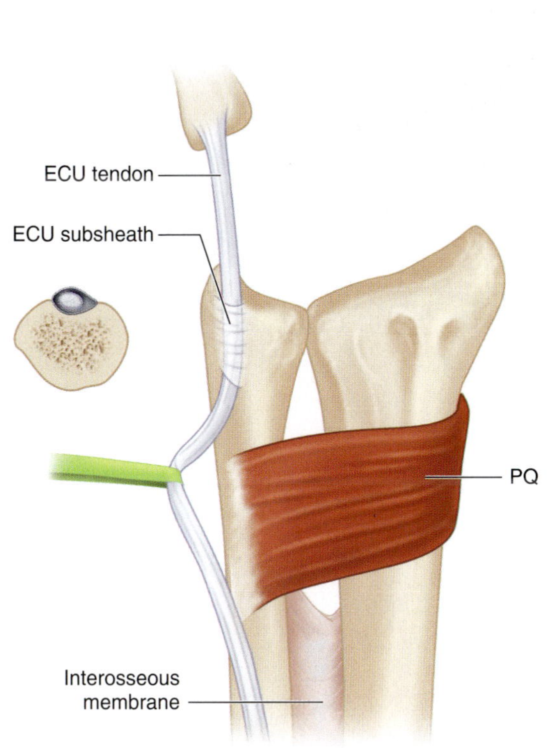
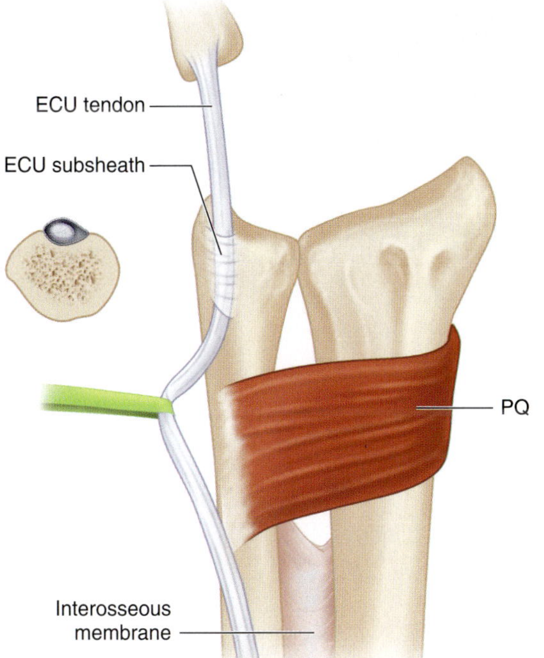

FIGURE 82-9

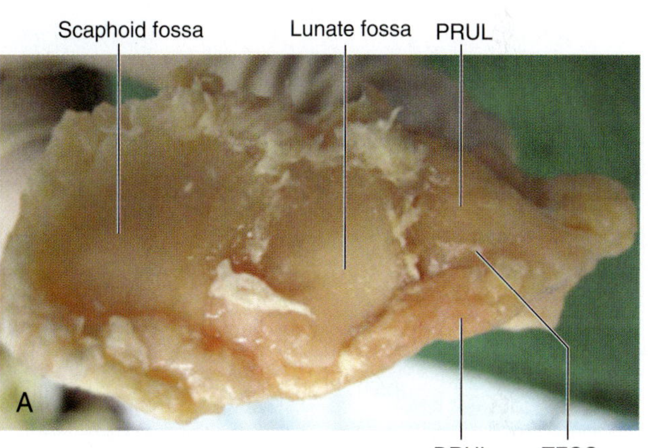

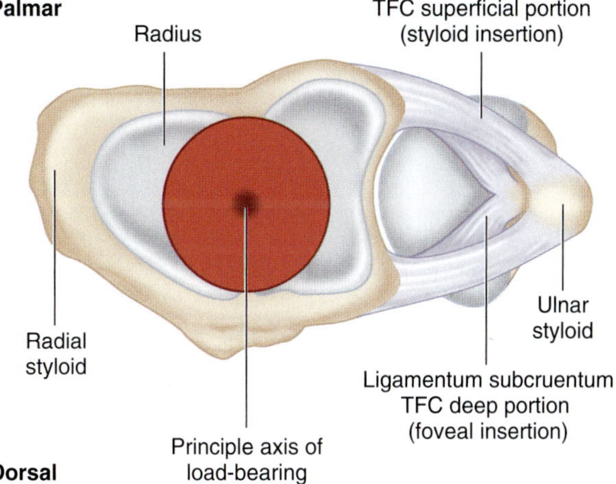
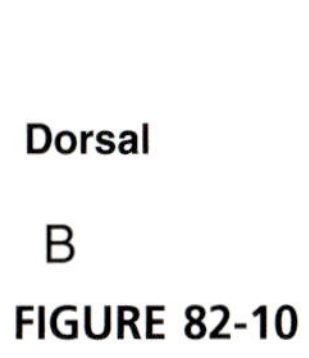

FIGURE 82-10

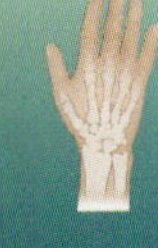

Positioning

- The patient is positioned supine with the affected extremity on a hand table. The procedure is performed under tourniquet control.
- The arm is strapped to the arm board using a soft roll and secured with tape. The forearm is held vertical and in neutral alignment using "Chinese finger traps" similar to the position used in wrist arthroscopy. This position is maintained by a traction tower using a 5-lb weight (Fig. 82-11)
- Intraoperative fluoroscopy will be required, and the table should be placed such that the C-arm can be positioned with ease.

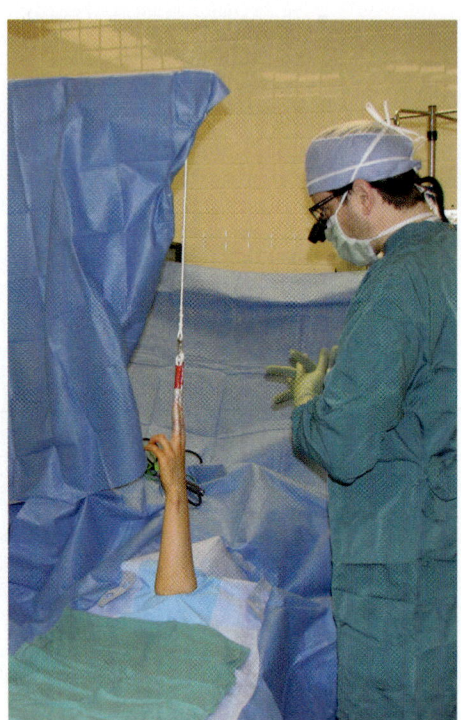

FIGURE 82-11

PITFALLS

The dorsal cutaneous branch of the ulnar nerve should be identified, mobilized, and protected.

Exposures

- A Y-shaped incision centered over the ulnar head is made on the ulnar border of the distal forearm. The vertical limb extends 5 cm proximal to the ulnar head along the ulnar border of the forearm. The volar limb extends to the pisiform, and the dorsal limb extends to the Lister tubercle (Fig. 82-12).
- Three skin flaps (distal, volar, and dorsal) are raised in a plane superficial to the tendons and extensor retinaculum (Fig. 82-13).

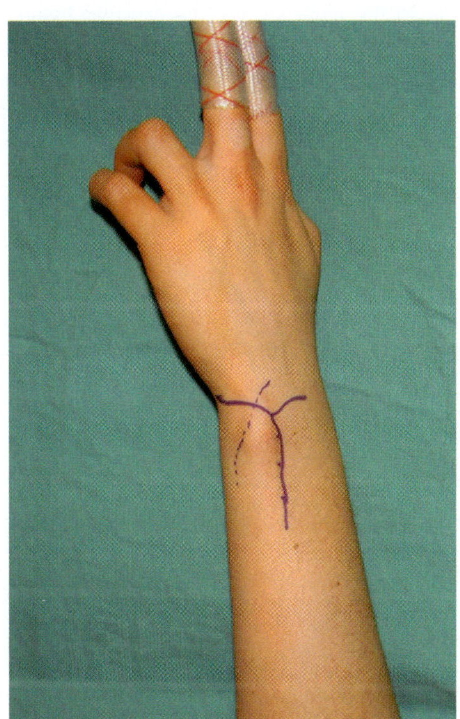

FIGURE 82-12

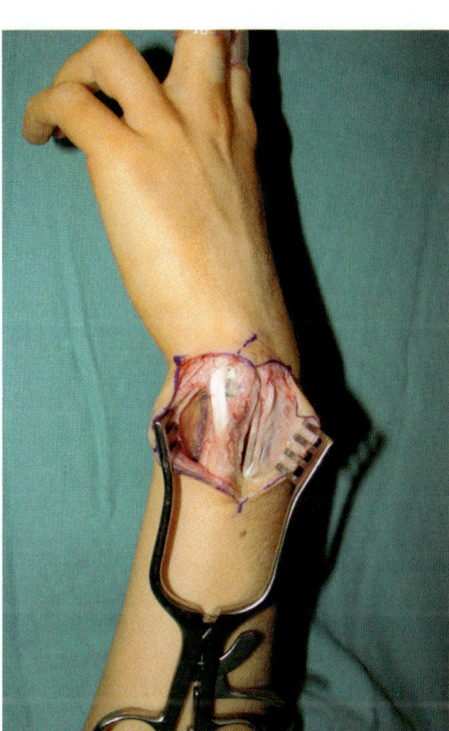

FIGURE 82-13

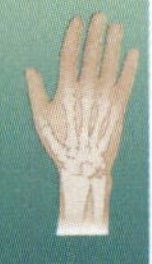

STEP 1 PEARLS

The articular surface of the sigmoid notch and ulnar head are examined for arthritic changes. Ligament reconstruction can be performed only if there is no evidence of DRU joint arthritis. If arthritis is present, a salvage procedure, such as the Sauve-Kapandji or Darrach procedure, or a hemiresection should be considered.

Procedure

Step 1: Development of Volar Plane

- The FCU and the ulnar neurovascular bundle are identified. A plane is developed deep to these structures to expose the ulnar styloid, palmar surface of the ulnar head, and palmar rim of the sigmoid fossa (Fig. 82-14)
- The capsular tissue immediately radial to the ulnar styloid is divided, and subperiosteal dissection is done to expose the palmar surface of the ulnar fovea.

Step 2: Development of Dorsal Plane

- The extensor retinaculum is divided longitudinally over the sixth compartment, and the ECU subsheath is identified. The sheath is divided along the ulnar border of the ECU, and the ECU is retracted ulnarly. This exposes the dorsal capsular tissues immediately radial to the ulnar styloid. The capsular tissue is divided longitudinally to expose the dorsal surface of the ulnar fovea (Fig. 82-15).
- The extensor retinaculum is divided between the fourth and fifth compartments. The tendons are retracted, and the floor of this compartment is incised to expose the dorsal rim of the sigmoid notch.

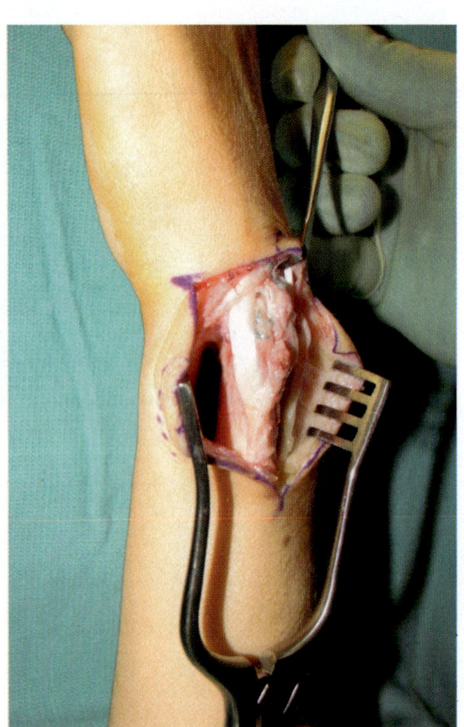

FIGURE 82-14

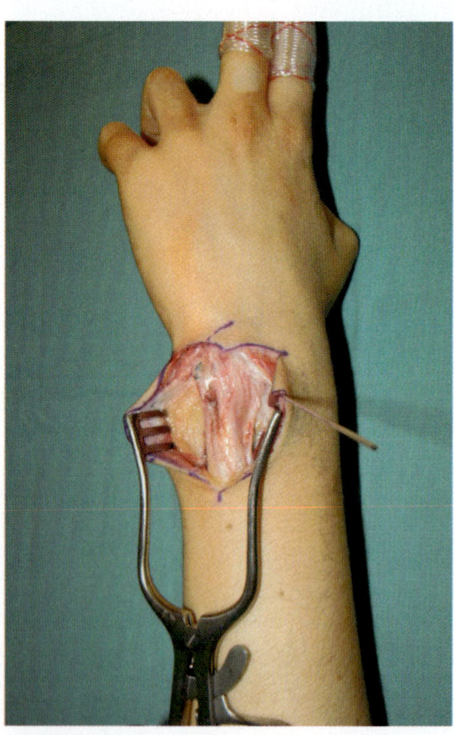

FIGURE 82-15

Step 3: Harvest of Palmaris Longus Tendon Graft

- A PL tendon graft is harvested by three separate 1-cm transverse incisions in the forearm (Fig. 82-16).

STEP 3 PITFALLS

One should take care to avoid injury to the palmar cutaneous branch of the median nerve. The nerve runs on the radial aspect of the PL.

A long tendon graft (at least 10 cm) makes ligament reconstruction easier. If required, a few centimeters of intramuscular tendon should also be harvested.

Step 4: Creation of Bone Tunnel in the Radius

- A K-wire is passed about 1 cm from volar edge of the sigmoid fossa to a similar position on the dorsal edge of the sigmoid fossa. This is done under fluoroscopic guidance to ensure that the wire is not within the radiocarpal or the radioulnar joints.
- A 2.3- to 3-mm cannulated drill is passed over the K-wire to make a bone tunnel within the radius, and the K-wire is removed.

STEP 4 PEARLS

The tunnel should be made at a sufficient distance (1 cm) from both the distal and the ulnar articular surface of the radius to avoid a fracture of the bone during creation of the tunnel or passage of the tendon graft.

It is better to make the tunnel from volar to dorsal because the entry point can be controlled and inadvertent injury to the median nerve prevented.

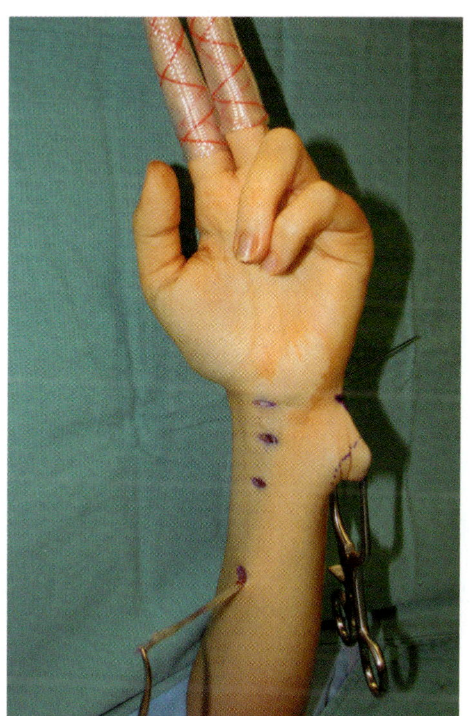

FIGURE 82-16

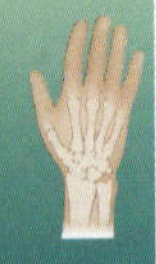

STEP 5 PEARLS

Moistening the tendon graft will prevent it from desiccating and make passage through the bone tunnels easier.

A hemostat should be attached to the free end of the tendon graft before pulling on the wire loop to pass the tendon through the bone tunnel in the radius. This will prevent the entire tendon from coming out through the bone tunnel.

Step 5: Passage of Tendon Graft

- A 25-gauge stainless steel wire loop is fashioned and passed from dorsum to the volar surface through the bone tunnel in the radius. One end of the PL tendon graft is fixed to the wire by twisting the loop. The wire is pulled back to bring the tendon out of the dorsal portion of the tunnel (Fig. 82-17).
- A pointed tendon passer is passed from the previously exposed dorsal surface of the fovea, through any remnants of the dorsal radioulnar ligament, deep to the extensor tendons to emerge at the dorsal portion of the tunnel in the distal radius. This grabs the tendon graft and brings it out at the fovea. Similarly, the tendon passer is passed from the palmar surface of the fovea, through any remnants of the palmar radioulnar ligament, deep to the flexor tendons to bring the palmar end of the tendon graft to the fovea.

Step 6: Creation of Bone Tunnel in Ulna

- A K-wire is passed obliquely from the fovea to exit at the ulnar border of the ulna about 1.5 cm proximal. The position of the wire is confirmed by intraoperative fluoroscopy. A 2.3- to 3-mm cannulated drill is passed over the above K-wire to make a bone tunnel within the ulna, and the K-wire is removed (Fig. 82-18).
- The ulnar tunnel needs to be wider compared with the distal radius tunnel because both ends of the tendon graft need to pass through it. If the diameter of the ulna seems narrow, the senior author prefers not to make a bone tunnel in the ulna to avoid the risk for a fracture. In such cases, the author anchors the ends of the tendon graft to the fovea and the ulna using bone anchors.

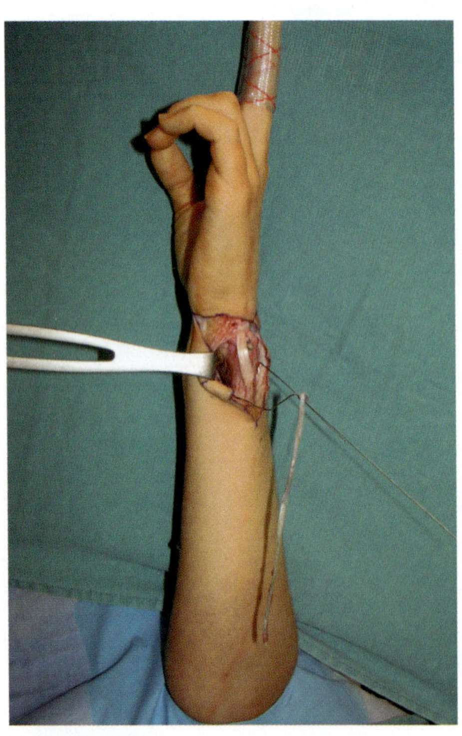

FIGURE 82-17

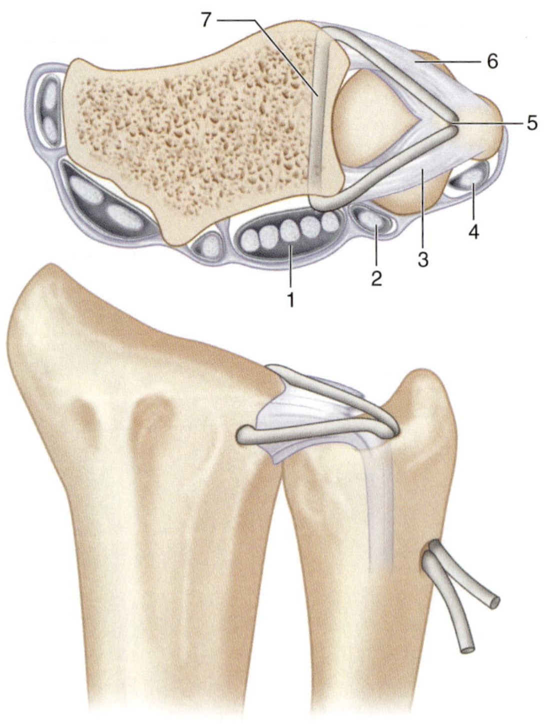

1. Extensor digitorum communis tendons
2. Extensor digiti minimi tendon
3. Extensor carpi ulnaris tendon
4. Dorsal radioulnar ligament
5. Tunnel through ulnar fovea
6. Palmar radioulnar ligament
7. Palmaris longus graft in distal radius tunnel

FIGURE 82-18

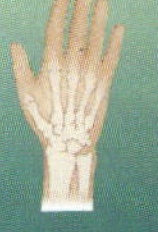

Step 7: Passage of Tendon Graft through Ulna

- Both ends of the tendon graft are passed through the bone tunnel in the ulna using a 25-gauge stainless steel wire loop as described previously. The wire loop is passed from outside-in to emerge at the fovea, both tendon ends are grasped, and the wire is pulled out to bring the tendon ends at ulnar border of the ulna.
- This step can be omitted, if a bone tunnel has been not been made in the ulna.

STEP 8 PEARLS

The K-wires should catch four cortices (two of ulna and two of radius). They should protrude slightly (5 mm) outside the radius and ulna, but buried under the skin. If the K-wires break during the healing phase, it will be easier to retrieve them if they are palpable on both sides.

Step 8: Reduction and Pinning of DRU Joint

- The forearm is held in neutral rotation, the ulnar head is reduced into the sigmoid fossa, and the reduction is maintained with one or two 0.045-inch K-wires passed from the ulna to the radius about 4 to 5 cm proximal to the ulnar styloid.
- The position of the wires is confirmed by intraoperative fluoroscopy (Figs. 82-19 and 82-20).

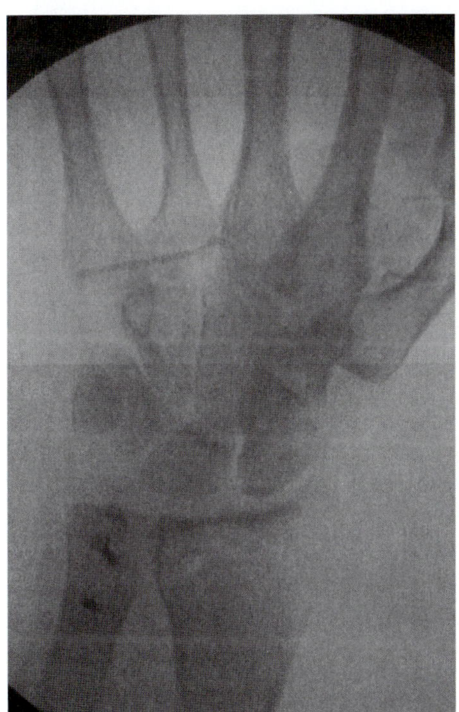

FIGURE 82-19

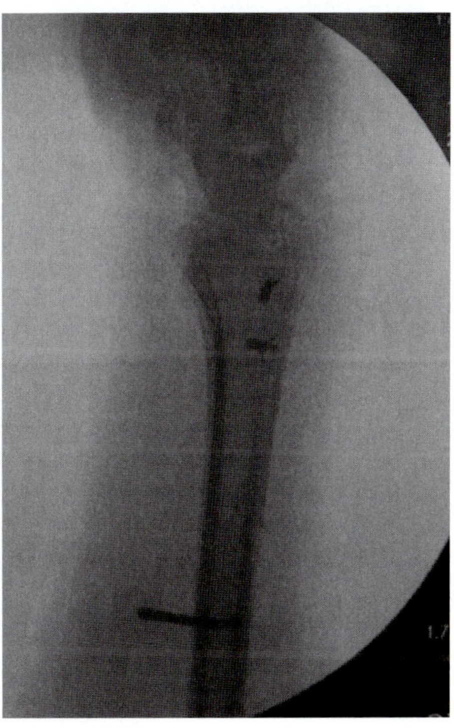

FIGURE 82-20

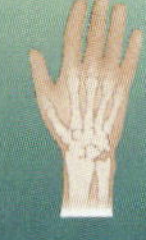

Step 9: Suture Fixation of Reconstructed Ligaments

- If both ends of the tendon graft are passed through a bone tunnel in the ulna, they are looped around the shaft of the ulna and sutured to each other, and a bone anchor placed proximal to the ulnar exit hole, as tightly as possible.
- If an ulnar bone tunnel has not been used, two or more bone anchors are passed at the fovea and on either side of the ulnar styloid. The tendon graft is looped around the shaft of the ulna and sutured to each other and to the bone anchors as tightly as possible (Fig. 82-21).

Step 10: Closure

- The ECU sheath is reapproximated over the DRU joint, and the sheath is then closed using nonabsorbable, braided sutures.
- The extensor retinaculum is closed with absorbable suture. The tourniquet is released and hemostasis secured.
- The subcutaneous tissue and skin are closed in layers (Fig. 82-22).
- A sugar tong splint is provided to keep the forearm and wrist in neutral position.

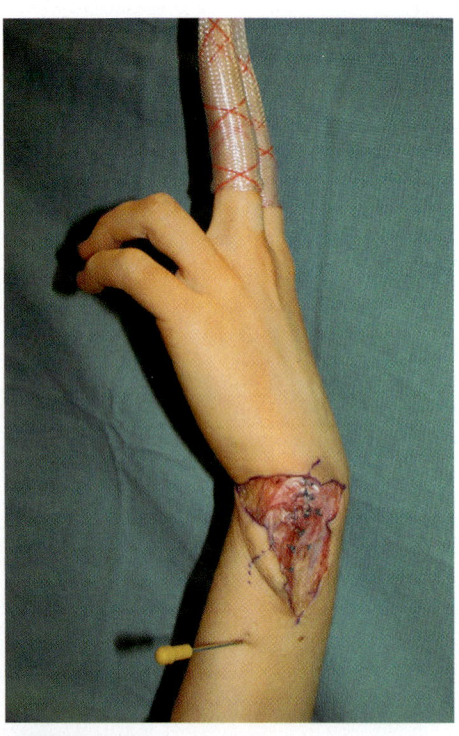

FIGURE 82-21

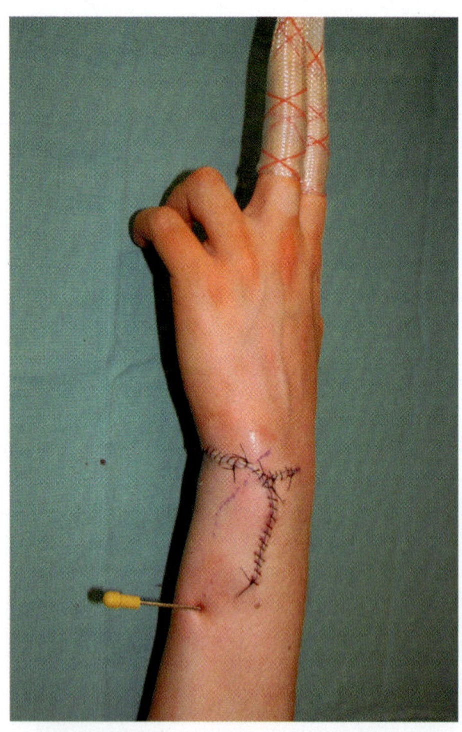

FIGURE 82-22

Postoperative Care and Expected Outcomes

- The wound is inspected 2 weeks after surgery, and all sutures are removed. A thermoplastic Muenster-type splint that keeps the forearm and wrist in neutral position is provided. The patient is allowed active finger motion only.
- At 6 weeks the K-wires are removed, and the patient is encouraged to start wrist flexion and extension exercises, but pronation and supination are restricted for another 2 weeks. The splint is discontinued after 8 weeks, and gentle pronation and supination range-of-motion and strengthening exercises are initiated.
- Up to 80% to 90% of patients have reported resolution of pain and restoration of DRU joint stability after ligament reconstruction. However, an average of 10 to 20 degrees of pronation and supination range of motion is lost (Figs. 82-23 and 82-24).

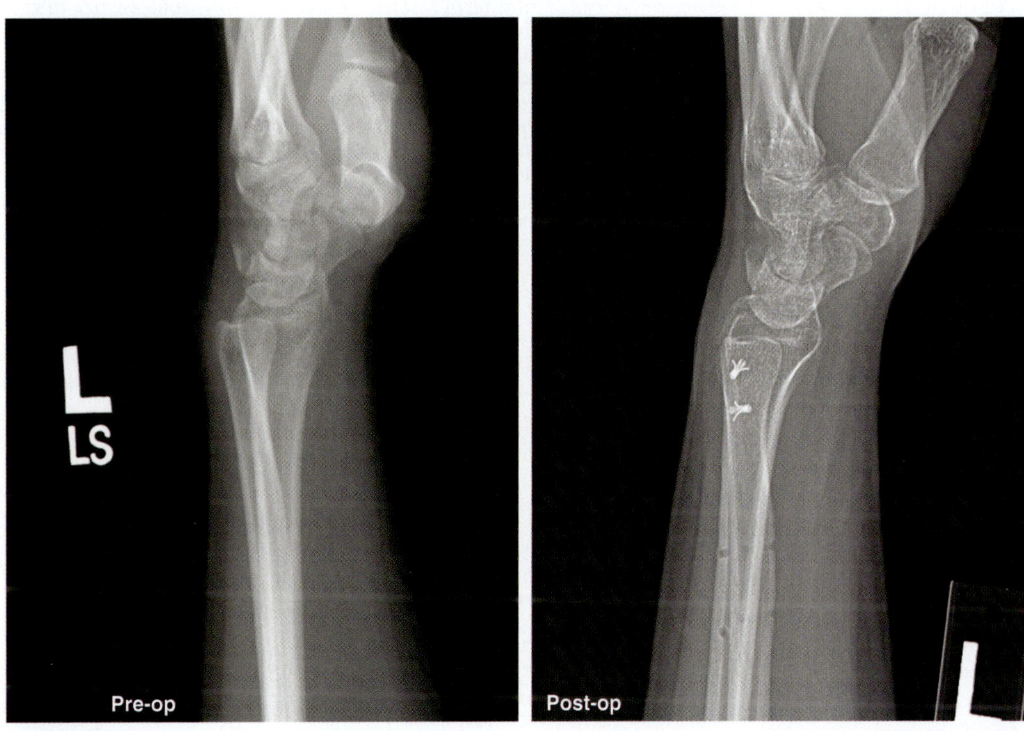

FIGURE 82-23

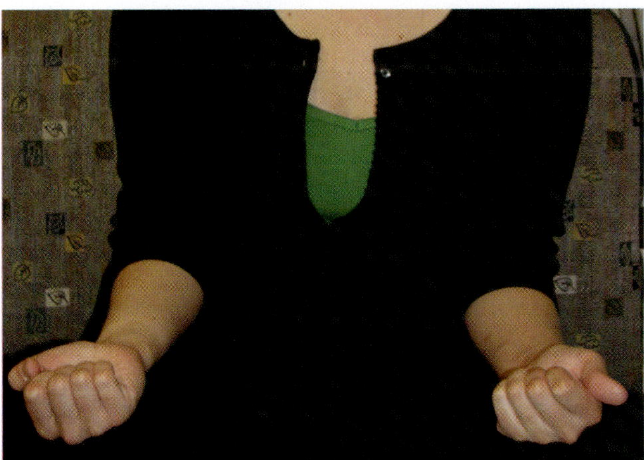

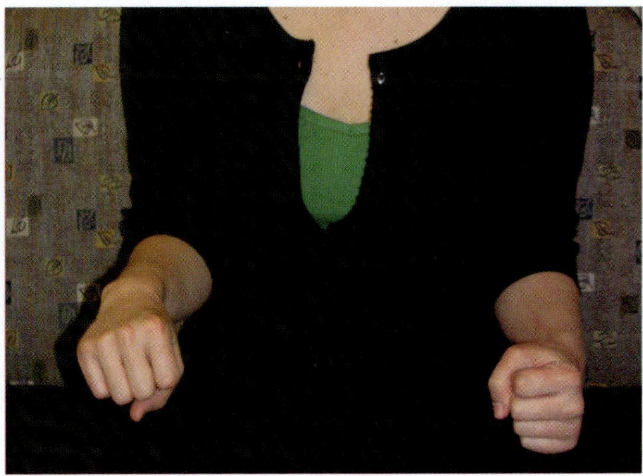

FIGURE 82-24

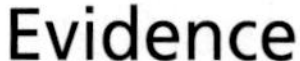

Evidence

Adams BD, Berger RA. An anatomic reconstruction of the distal radioulnar ligaments for posttraumatic distal radioulnar joint instability. *J Hand Surg [Am]*. 2002;27:243-251.
This article describes a commonly used technique of distal radioulnar ligament reconstruction for posttraumatic DRU joint instability in 14 patients with 4 years' follow-up. This technique restored stability and range of motion with pronation and supination for all patients except for those with associated ulnocarpal ligament injury and sigmoid notch deficiency. (Level V evidence)

Gofton WT, Gordon KD, Dunning CE, et al. Comparison of distal radioulnar joint reconstructions using an active joint motion simulator. *J Hand Surg [Am]*. 2005;30:733-742.
This report compares the joint kinematics after four types of DRU joint reconstruction (capsular repair, two radioulnar ligament reconstructions, and radioulnar tethering) in 11 cadaveric upper extremities. The authors report that all reconstructions improved stability, with capsule repair and radioligament reconstructions being superior to radioulnar tethering procedures in restoring DRU joint motion. (Level V evidence)

Teoh LC, Yam AKT. Anatomic reconstruction of the distal radioulnar ligaments: long-term results. *J Hand Surg [Br]*. 2005;30:185-193.
The authors describe outcomes after open ligamentous repair for chronic DRU joint instability in nine patients with an average of 9 years of follow-up. Patient outcomes were assessed using the Mayo Wrist Score, and the authors report significant improvement in wrist scores following the repair that extended throughout the postoperative period. At follow-up, arthritis did not develop in any patients, but two patients developed recurrent instability. (Level IV evidence)

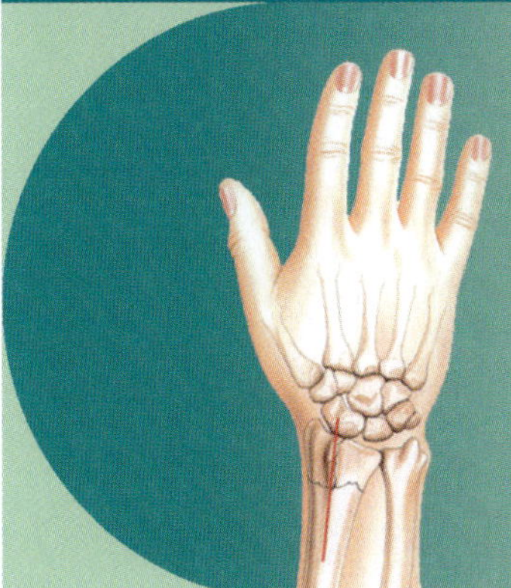

Darrach Procedure

Nathan S. Taylor and Kevin C. Chung

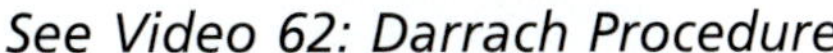

See Video 62: Darrach Procedure

Indications

- Older, sedentary patients with posttraumatic distal radioulnar (DRU) joint arthritis, rheumatoid arthritis, and osteoarthritis without preexisting radiocarpal instability.
- Destruction of the triangular fibrocartilage complex with caput ulna syndrome and painful pronation and supination of the DRU joint.
- The Darrach procedure (distal ulna head excision) is preferred in patients with no ulnar translation of the carpus and low chance of translation in the future.
- In the setting of radiocarpal instability, the Darrach procedure can be performed concomitantly with a partial or total wrist fusion.

Examination/Imaging

Clinical Examination

- Evaluate active and passive wrist and DRU joint motion and compare with the opposite side. The affected wrist should be taken through full wrist motions of flexion-extension, pronation-supination, and radioulnar deviation with axial loading to assess stability and pain.
- Painful crepitus with pronation and supination indicate DRU joint arthritis that can be accentuated with manual compression of the joint.
- Dorsal wrist swelling can indicate extensor tendon synovitis. Palpation of the inflamed wrist is painful, and wrist mobility may be limited.
- Caput ulna syndrome is diagnosed as dorsal prominence of the ulnar head with accompanying ulnopalmar subluxation and supination of the carpus. The DRU joint will be swollen and painful on palpation. There may be painful limitation of pronation and supination.
- ECU subluxation and tendonitis should be distinguished from DRU joint arthritis by noting ECU subluxation with supination and ulnar deviation.
- Lunotriquetral (LT) instability from ligamentous tears should be distinguished from DRU joint arthritis by performing the LT shear test. The lunate is stabilized between the examiner's thumb and index finger, and the triquetrum is sheared against the lunate in a dorsopalmar direction with the examiner's other hand.
- The prominent caput ulna can cause extensor tendon ruptures, primarily at the fourth and fifth extensor compartments.

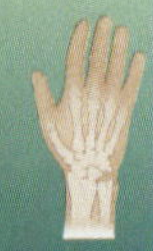

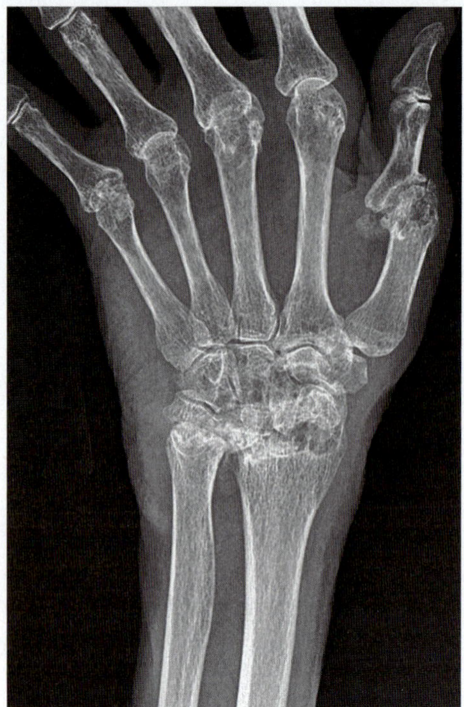

FIGURE 83-1

Imaging

- Standard three views of the wrist are useful to assess extent of arthritis and wrist stability. Changes associated with arthritis include osteophytes, joint space narrowing, erosive changes, cystic lesions, and disuse osteopenia (Fig. 83-1).
- For differentiation of extensor tendon from joint synovitis, ultrasonography is the diagnostic tool of choice.
- Computed tomography and magnetic resonance imaging are typically not necessary in the evaluation of the DRU joint in rheumatoid arthritis.

Surgical Anatomy

- The dorsal sensory branch of the ulnar nerve lies in the subcutaneous tissue of the dorsal ulnar wrist.
- In the presence of caput ulna syndrome, the sixth dorsal compartment with the ECU is subluxed palmarly. The fifth dorsal compartment with the extensor digiti minimi (EDM) crosses the ulnar head.
- The pronator quadratus originates at the distal radius and inserts on the distal ulna and is an important dynamic stabilizer of the distal ulna. The distal ulna should be excised to the level of the sigmoid notch to preserve the attachments of the pronator quadratus on the distal ulna.

Positioning

- The procedure is performed under tourniquet control with the patient in the supine position and the extremity abducted with the hand on a hand table.
- Support of the wrist in slight flexion is helpful.

Exposures

- A dorsal longitudinal incision over the distal ulna with a zigzag at the wrist is used for wide exposure to the level of the extensor retinaculum (Fig. 83-2A and B).
- Approach the ulna between the EDM and ECU and incise the periosteum to raise radial and ulnar periosteal flaps for later closure (Fig. 83-3A and B).

PEARLS

Make certain to identify and protect the dorsal ulnar sensory nerve.

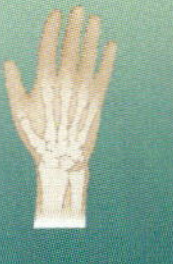

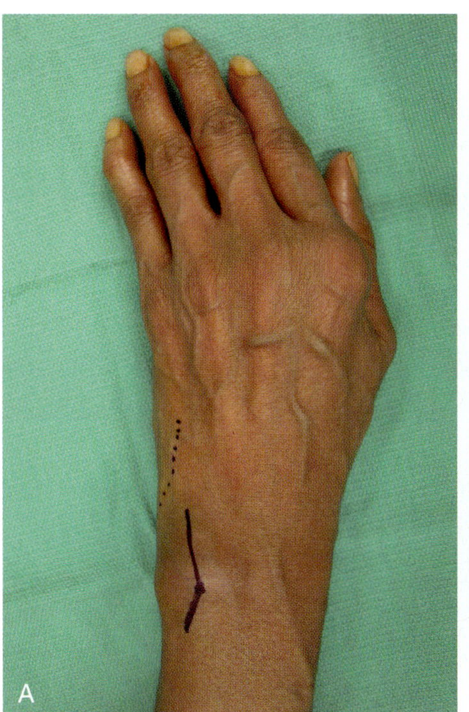

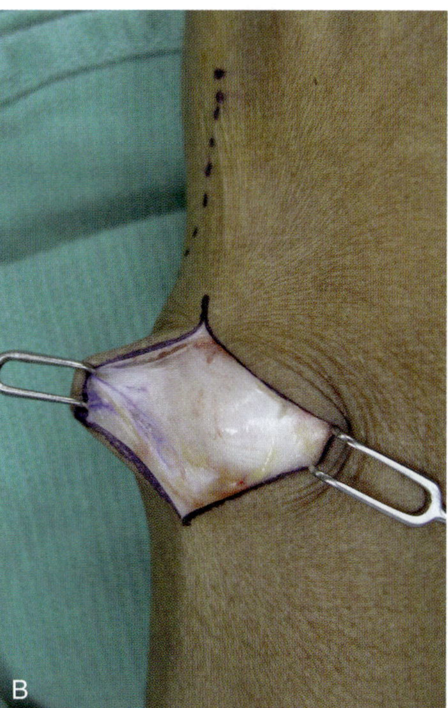

FIGURE 83-2

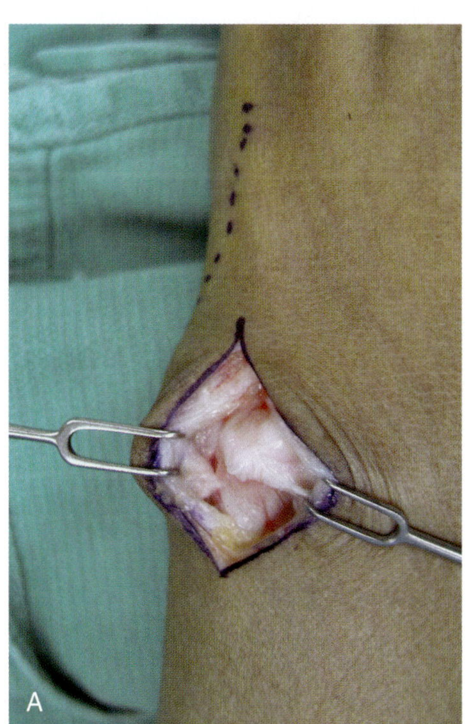

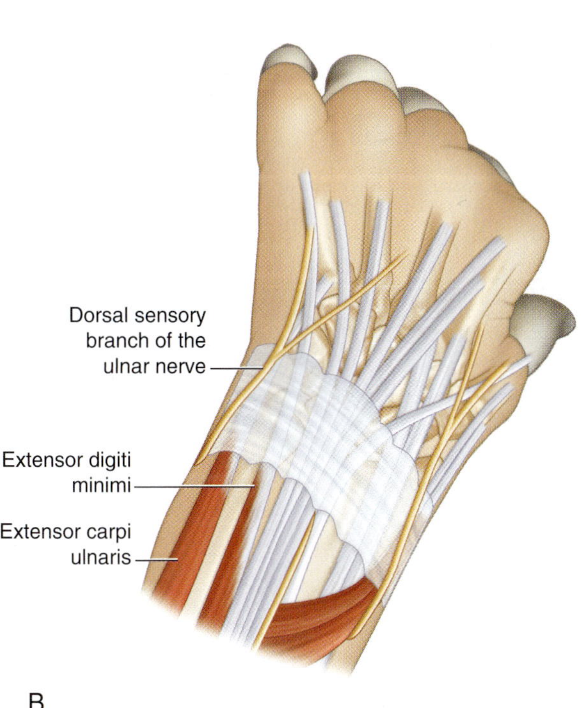

FIGURE 83-3

Procedure

Step 1

- Use an oscillating saw to resect 20 mm of distal ulna at 45 degrees so that the long end of the oblique cut is along the ulnar border to minimize ulnar impingement against the radius (Fig. 83-4).

Step 2

- Sharply excise the ulnar head from the surrounding soft tissue with a no. 15 blade (Fig. 83-5).
- Remove any sharp edges with a rongeur.
- Synovitis within the sigmoid notch is removed with a rongeur.

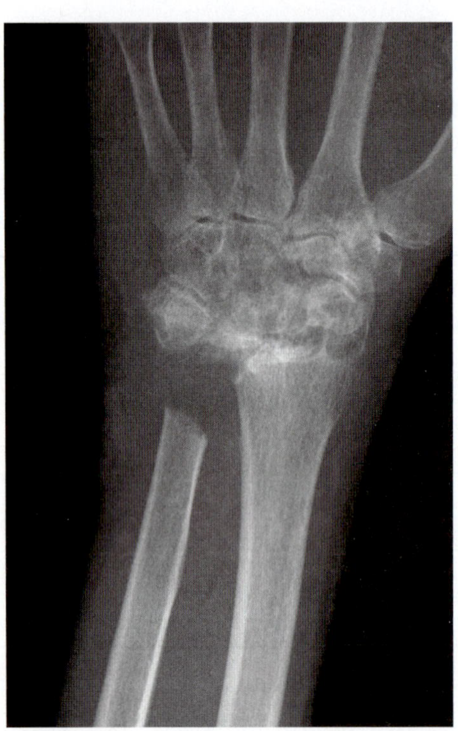

FIGURE 83-4

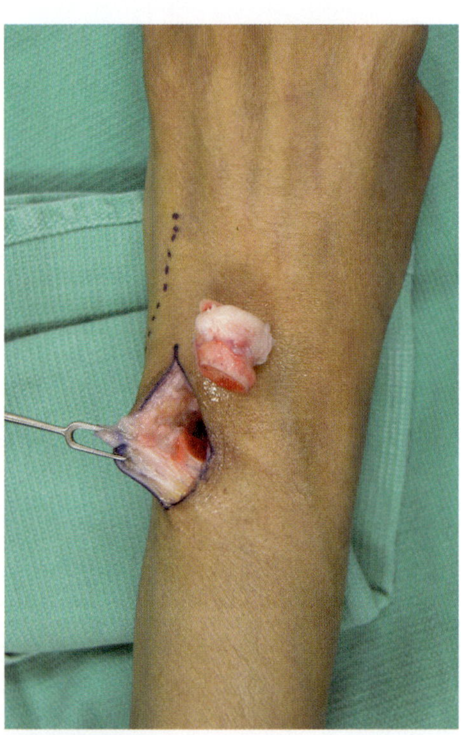

FIGURE 83-5

Step 3

- The dorsal wrist capsule is imbricated with 2-0 or 3-0 braided permanent horizontal mattress sutures with the wrist fully supinated, taking care to note that the ulna is not dorsally prominent in this position (Fig. 83-6). If the distal ulna stump is unstable with pronation-supination, an ulna-stabilizing procedure can be performed using a distally based ulnar half ECU tenodesis to correct prominence of the ulnar stump. This is performed as follows:
  - Drill a hole in the dorsal cortex of the distal ulna stump using a 3-mm bur.
  - The distally based ulnar half of the ECU is woven from inside the ulnar canal and out the hole dorsally and sutured to itself with the ulna stump reduced palmarly and the wrist extended 15 degrees and ulnarly deviated 15 degrees.
  - The dorsal wrist capsule is then imbricated as described previously.
- The tourniquet is released, and all bleeding points are cauterized.
- The skin is closed with 3-0 absorbable monofilament dermal sutures and 4-0 absorbable monofilament running subcuticular suture.

Postoperative Care and Expected Outcomes

- The wrist is immobilized in a sugar tong splint with the forearm fully supinated for 4 weeks, keeping the fingers free for movement.
- Gentle active range of motion is begun at 4 weeks. If an ulnar stump–stabilizing procedure has been performed, pronation and supination should be limited until 6 weeks postoperatively.
- The patient should be expected to return to full activities as tolerated at 6 to 8 weeks.

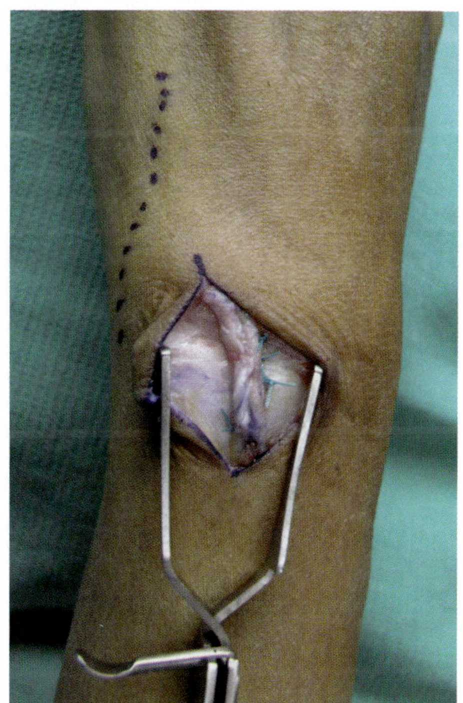

FIGURE 83-6

Evidence

De Witte PB, Wijffels M, Jupiter JB, Ring D. The Darrach procedure for post-traumatic reconstruction. *Acta Orthop Belg.* 2009;75:316-322.

The authors report their experience with the Darrach procedure in 26 patients with a mean age of 53 years to address posttraumatic stiffness, instability, nonunion, and radioulnar length discrepancy. With an average follow-up of 21 months, the authors note an average improvement in total arc of forearm rotation of 87 degrees, from 49 to 136 degrees ($P < .001$*), and pain reduction (*$P = .04$*), with only two patients requiring reoperation related to the residual ulna. They conclude that the Darrach procedure significantly improves forearm rotation and reduces pain in patients with posttraumatic problems of the DRU joint with a low complication and reoperation rate. (Level IV evidence)*

George MS, Kiefhaber TR, Stern PJ. The Sauve-Kapandji procedure and the Darrach procedure for distal radio-ulnar joint dysfunction after Colles' fracture. *J Hand Surg [Br].* 2004;29:608-613.

The authors retrospectively evaluated the results of 30 Darrach procedures and 18 Sauve-Kapandji procedures for the treatment of distal radioulnar joint derangement following malunion of displaced intraarticular distal radius fractures in patients younger than 50 years. In the Sauve-Kapandji group, 12 patients completed the Disabilities of the Arm, Shoulder, and Hand (DASH) survey at a mean of 4 years postoperatively, and 9 patients were available for follow-up examination at a mean of 2 years postoperatively. In the Darrach group, 21 patients completed the DASH survey at a mean of 6 years postoperatively, and 13 patients were available for follow-up examination at a mean of 4 years postoperatively. There were no significant differences between the two groups with regard to forearm or wrist range of motion, grip strength, Modified Mayo Wrist scores, or DASH scores. All patients in the Sauve-Kapandji group showed radiographic fusion of the DRU joint, and one patient was revised to a Darrach procedure for a painful click with complete resolution of symptoms. Six patients in the Darrach group showed evidence of significant regrowth of the ulnar stump, and one patient showed significant ulnar carpal translation. The authors conclude that both procedures yield comparable and unpredictable results following Colles fracture in patients younger than 50 years. The Sauve-Kapandji procedure is better in younger patients because it maintains the ulnocarpal buttress, preserves the triangular fibrocartilage complex and ulnocarpal ligaments, provides a more physiologic pattern of force transmission from the hand to the forearm, and maintains the extensor carpi ulnaris tendon in its compartment. (Level III evidence)

Minami A, Iwasaki N, Ishikawa J, et al. Treatments of osteoarthritis of the distal radioulnar joint: long-term results of three procedures. *Hand Surg.* 2005;10:243-248.

The authors retrospectively evaluated 61 wrists in 61 patients with an average age of 59.8 years with osteoarthritis of the distal radioulnar joint treated by three consecutive procedures (20 Darrach, 25 Sauve-Kapandji, and 16 hemiresection-interposition arthroplasty procedures). Postoperative pain, range of motion, grip strength, return to work status, and radiographic results were evaluated over an average follow-up of 10 years (range 5 to 14 years). The authors found that pain relief was superior with the Sauve-Kapandji and hemiresection-interposition arthroplasty procedures compared with the Darrach procedure, although this was not statistically significant. Both the Sauve-Kapandji and hemiresection-interposition arthroplasty procedures had statistically significant improvements in wrist flexion and extension, grip strength, and return to original work status compared with the Darrach procedure. All procedures showed statistically significant improvements in forearm supination and pronation. The authors conclude that the Darrach procedure is better indicated for severe osteoarthritic changes of the distal radioulnar joint in elderly patients; the Sauve-Kapandji procedure is indicated when the triangular fibrocartilage complex cannot be reconstructed or with positive ulnar variance greater than 5 mm even with intact triangular fibrocartilage complex; and the hemiresection-interposition arthroplasty procedure is indicated when the triangular fibrocartilage complex is intact or could be reconstructed. (Level III evidence)

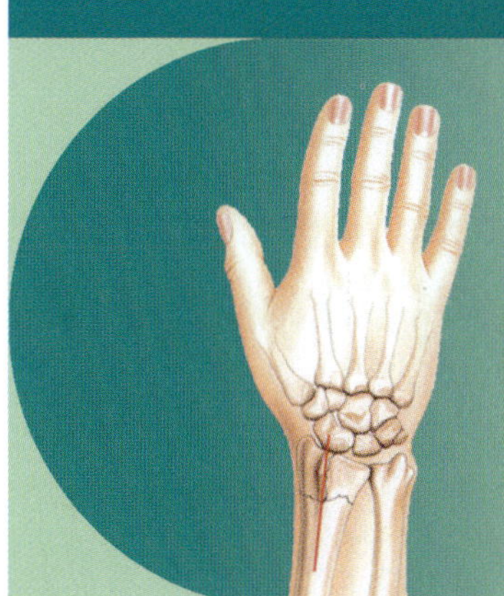

PROCEDURE 84

Sauve-Kapandji Arthrodesis for Distal Radioulnar Joint Arthritis

Nathan S. Taylor and Kevin C. Chung

See Video 63: Shelf Arthroplasty for Rheumatoid DRUJ Arthritis

Indications

- Arthritis of the distal radioulnar (DRU) joint in young (<45 years of age) active patients with stable radiocarpal ligaments. This procedure maintains the ulnocarpal buttress and retains the triangular fibrocartilage complex (TFCC) to provide a more physiologic pattern of force transmission from the hand to the forearm and offers improved strength and function.
- Malunited distal radius fractures with DRU joint arthritis.
- Early presentation of rheumatoid arthritis with intact wrist ligaments.
- Chronic DRU joint instability without arthritis.
- In the setting of radiocarpal instability, the Sauve-Kapandji procedure can be performed to stabilize the ulnar wrist, which may obviate the immediate need for a partial or total wrist fusion.

Examination/Imaging

Clinical Examination

- Differentiating DRU joint arthritis and ulnocarpal impaction syndrome is important in treating degenerative conditions of the ulnar wrist. Both can present with pain and swelling, decreased grip strength, and stiffness. Moreover, both may coexist and require treatment to relieve symptoms. This distinction should be made in order to proceed with the appropriate surgery.
- Visible subluxation of the DRU joint indicating instability due to ligamentous laxity or injury.
- Marked tenderness with stressing of the DRU joint.
- Forearm range of motion focusing on the DRU joint.

Imaging

- Posteroanterior, oblique, and lateral radiographs of the wrist are useful to identify signs of degenerative arthritis. Findings include joint space narrowing, volar subluxation of the radius, and osteophyte formation along the proximal margin of the ulnar head, typically sparing the sigmoid notch (Fig. 84-1A and B).
- Assess for ulnar carpus translation present preoperatively because this may indicate a need for a wrist-stabilizing procedure such as a radiolunate, radioscapholunate, or total wrist arthrodesis.
- Computed tomography (CT) or magnetic resonance imaging (MRI) of the DRU joint will better define the articular surface and joint congruity.

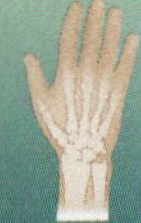

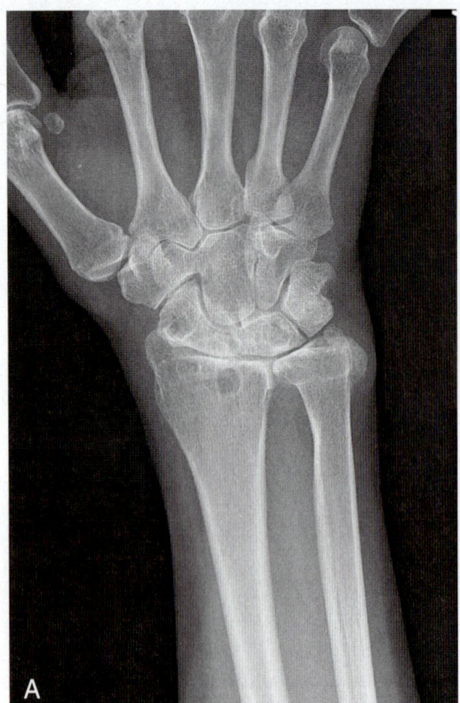

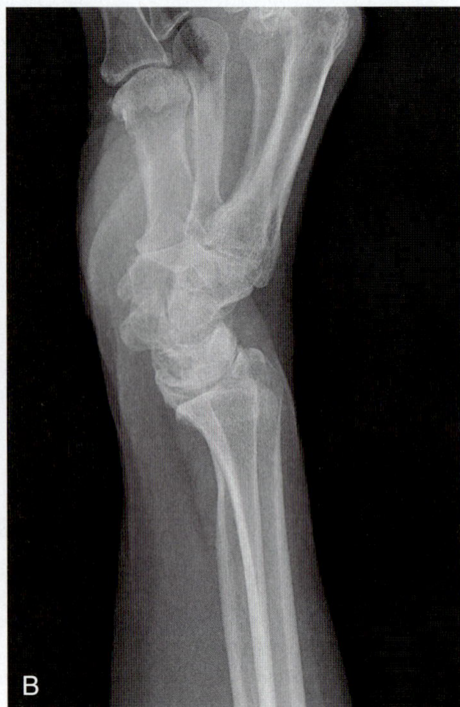

FIGURE 84-1

Surgical Anatomy

- DRU joint fit can be affected by changes in the position of the sigmoid notch. A common cause of poor fit of the DRU joint is injuries affecting the length of the radius relative to the ulna. Although the shape of this joint and the relative bone length are variable, joint congruency is required for normal function. Clear changes in congruency are usually evident on plain radiographs, but CT or MRI can give better anatomic definition of the bone and joint shape, in addition to the TFCC attachment to the ulnar head fovea.
- The dorsal branch of the ulnar nerve is at risk during incision. Along the ulnar head lies the stabilizing sheath of the extensor carpi ulnaris (ECU) tendon. This sheath must be opened, and the ECU tendon must be displaced when repairing the TFCC.

Positioning

- The procedure is performed under tourniquet control with the patient in the supine position and the extremity abducted with the hand on a hand table.

PEARLS

Make certain to identify and protect the dorsal ulnar sensory nerve.

The DRU joint capsule is incised longitudinally just ulnar to the fifth dorsal compartment.

Exposures

- A dorsal midline incision with a zigzag at the wrist is used for wide exposure to the level of the extensor retinaculum (Fig. 84-2A and B).
- Approach the ulna between the extensor digiti minimi (EDM) and ECU and incise the periosteum to raise radial and ulnar periosteal flaps for later closure (Fig. 84-3).

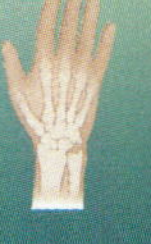

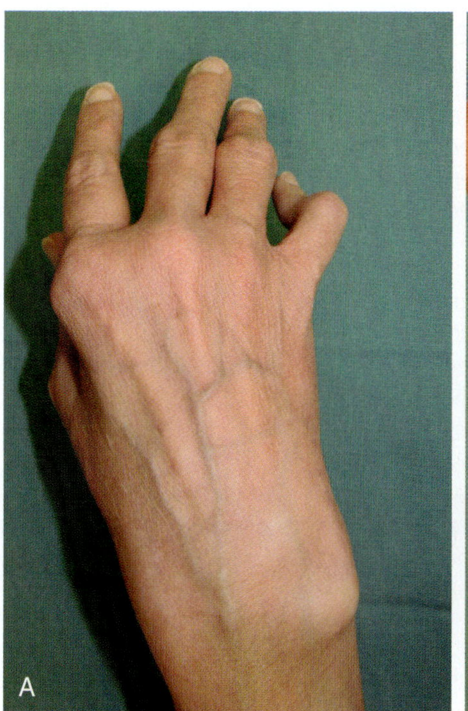

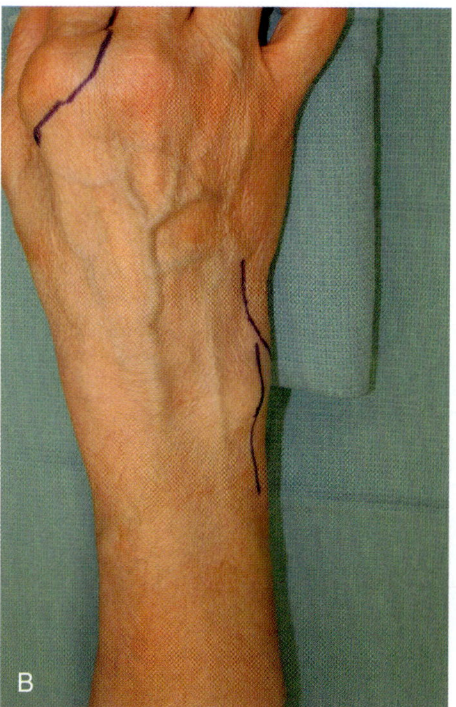

FIGURE 84-2

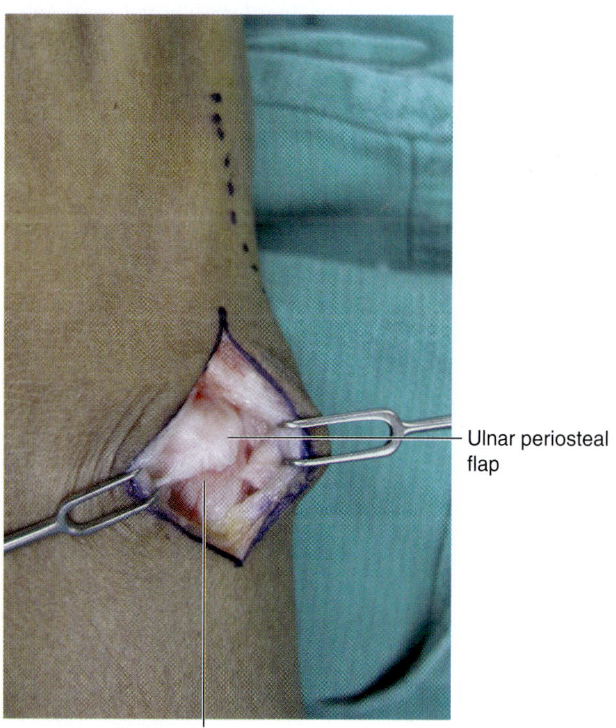

FIGURE 84-3

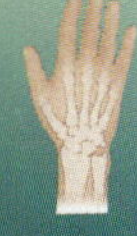

STEP 1 PEARLS

Obtain the best possible fit of the DRU joint.

Preoperative ulnar positive variance should be corrected at the time of the arthrodesis.

Some surgeons argue that it is not necessary to prepare the joint in any patient with rheumatoid arthritis because it will likely fuse with immobilization alone. However, the authors recommend visualization and surface preparation of the DRU joint in all cases to ensure fusion.

STEP 1 PITFALLS

Failure to obtain a level joint between the radius and ulna

STEP 2 PEARLS

Confirm with radiographs that axial alignment of the distal ulnar segment and the radius is colinear.

Procedure

Step 1

- A 1-cm segment of ulna bone is removed proximal to the sigmoid notch. The cartilage is removed from the DRU joint bone surfaces with a 3-mm bur until punctate bleeding is seen. A temporary K-wire is placed to stabilize the distal ulna to the radius, and angular positioning is checked by fluoroscopy.

Step 2

- The resected bone is morselized and used as bone graft around the compressed DRU joint. Placement of bone graft within the DRU joint is avoided by the senior author because it will impede reduction and possibly slow healing by increasing the distance between bone surfaces.
- Stabilization by K-wires is certainly acceptable, but the senior author prefers to use a compression screw to provide more rigid fixation. A 3.5-mm cannulated screw, or a headless screw, is used for internal fixation that is placed over the K-wire. If necessary, a temporary K-wire is placed percutaneously to prevent rotation of the distal ulna fragment. This K-wire can be removed in clinic 3 weeks after the operation.

Step 3

- The goal of the Sauve-Kapandji arthrodesis is to regain painless and stable forearm rotation. The new fibrous pseudarthrosis at the junction between the two ulnar sections can be unstable. During the operation, the position of the two ulnar stumps should be assessed during rotation in a pushing-pulling manner. If the ends are unstable because of soft tissue attenuation, the senior author prefers the ulnar half of the ECU as a tenodesis:
- Drill a hole in the dorsal cortex of the distal ulna stump using a 3-mm bur.
- The distally based ulnar half of the ECU is woven from inside the ulnar canal and out the hole dorsally and sutured to itself, stabilizing the proximal ulnar stump (Fig. 84-4).

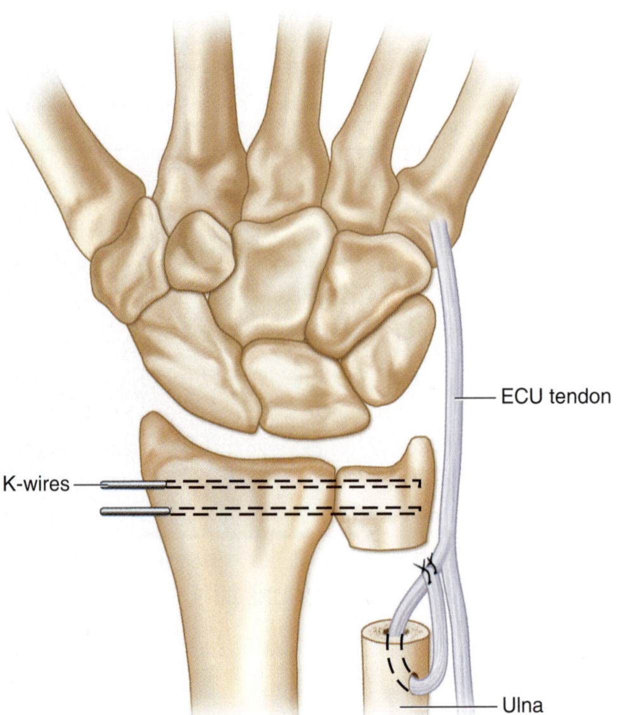

FIGURE 84-4

Step 4

- The dorsal wrist capsule is imbricated with 2-0 or 3-0 braided permanent horizontal mattress sutures.
- The tourniquet is released, and all bleeding points are cauterized.
- The skin is closed with 3-0 absorbable monofilament dermal sutures and 4-0 absorbable monofilament running subcuticular suture.

Procedure

Modified Sauve-Kapandji Procedure

Step 1

- The senior author prefers the shelf arthroplasty procedure proposed by Fujita and colleagues when there is poor bone quality in the distal part of the ulna. In such situations a routine Sauve-Kapandji procedure would provide insufficient osseous support for the ulnar aspect of the carpus. An oblique osteotomy is made 30 mm proximal to the end of the ulna (Fig. 84-5A and B). The distal ulna is removed and turned 90 degrees with the proximal bone facing the sigmoid notch.

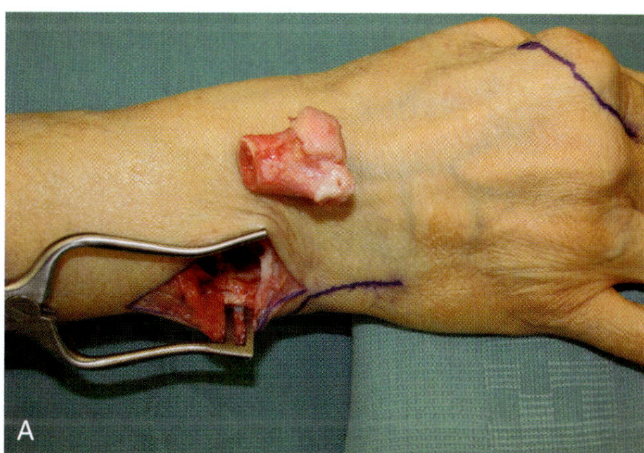

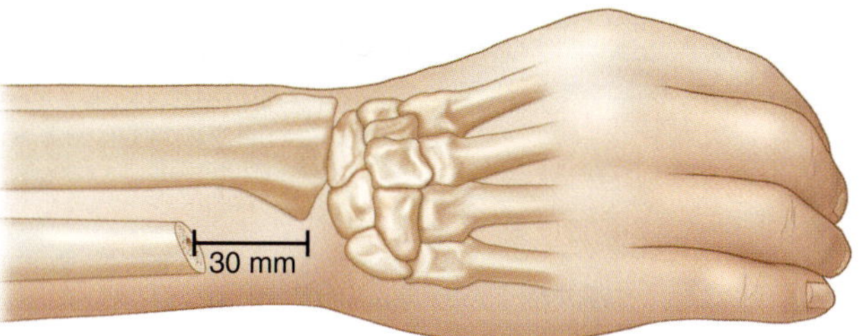

FIGURE 84-5

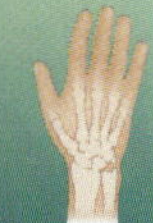

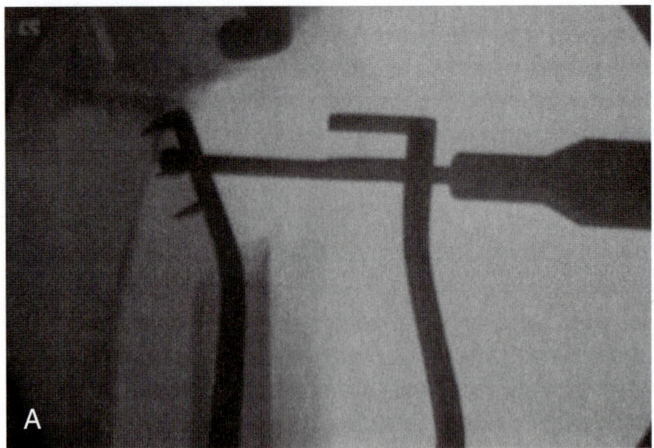

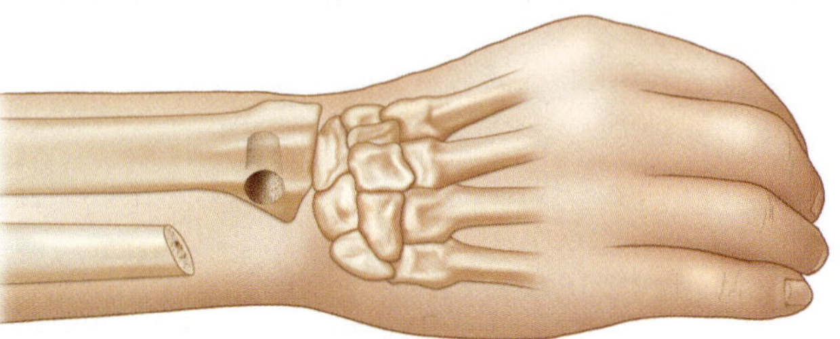

FIGURE 84-6

Step 2

- A slot is made with a bur over the sigmoid notch to fit the ulna (Fig. 84-6A and B). This ensures greater bone contact to enhance fusion, particularly in situations in which the distal ulna bone quality is poor. It also theoretically gives better ulna-sided support to the ulnar wrist, analogous to a bookshelf construct.

STEP 3 PEARLS

About 12 to 15 mm of distal ulna should protrude to provide support to the ulnar wrist.

Step 3

- The proximal end of the cut distal ulna is inserted into the slot in the sigmoid notch for a press fit. A headless screw is placed through the distal ulna and into the radius to provide rigid fixation (Fig. 84-7A to C). Contouring of the head of the distal ulna is necessary to avoid a large bump over the ulnar wrist.

Step 4

- The dorsal wrist capsule is imbricated with 2-0 or 3-0 braided permanent horizontal mattress sutures.
- The tourniquet is released, and all bleeding points are cauterized.
- The skin is closed with 3-0 absorbable monofilament dermal sutures and 4-0 absorbable monofilament running subcuticular suture.

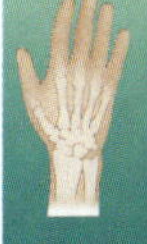

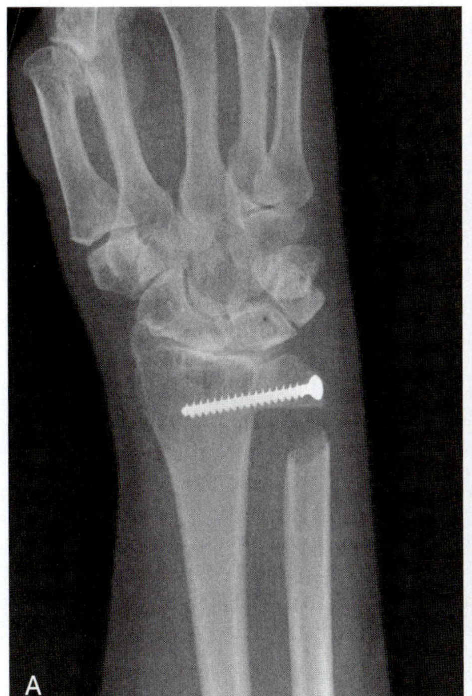

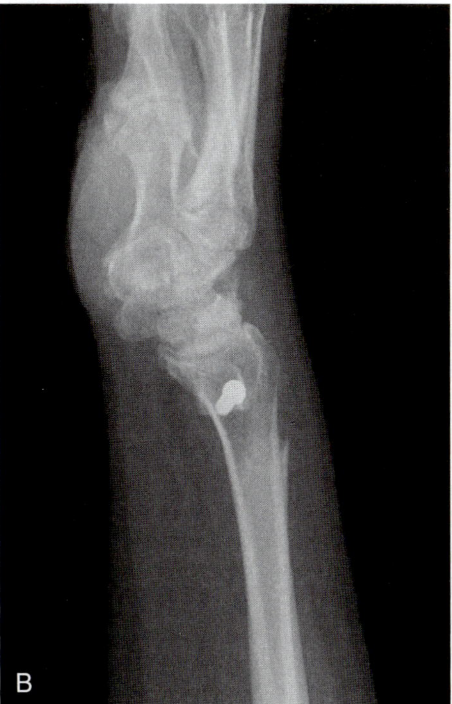

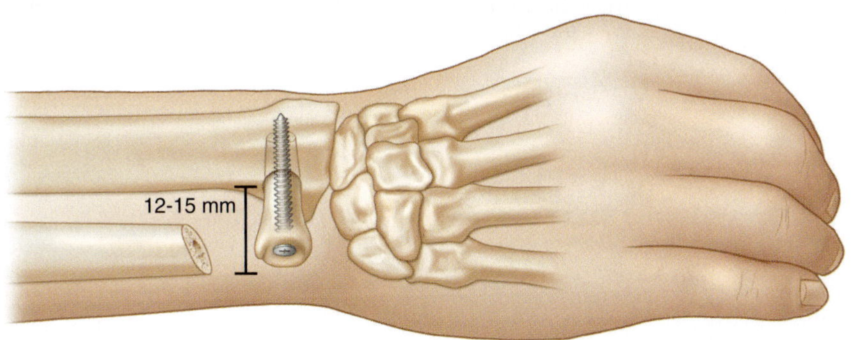

C

FIGURE 84-7

Postoperative Care and Expected Outcomes

- Postoperative positioning and early exercises
  - Immediately after surgery, the authors position the forearm in neutral rotation with an above-elbow splint. This is maintained for 7 to 10 days. The fingers and shoulder can be moved during this time.
  - At 7 to 10 days, the compliant patient will be fitted with a removable splint. The patient is splinted for a total of 4 weeks before initiation of forearm rotation exercises (active and active-assisted) four times a day. The exercises probably reduce the chance of heterotrophic bone formation that can limit motion.
- Intermediate exercises (6 to 8 weeks after surgery)
  - When the incision has healed and the tissues are minimally swollen, the patient may begin grip strengthening. No effort to resist rotation is begun earlier than 12 weeks.

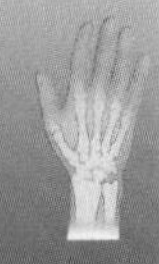

- Grip strengthening is often begun without complete bone healing apparent on radiographs. However, the surgeon should be certain that fixation is secure.
- Late exercise
  - Rotational strengthening is initiated when radiographic bone healing is apparent and grip strength has maximized.
- Patients can reasonably expect the following outcomes:
  - Fifty percent recovery of forearm rotation
  - Sufficient strength for use in sports (including, e.g., golf, basketball)
  - Less pain (it is hard to achieve no pain)
  - Durability of result

Evidence

Fujita S, Masada K, Takeuchi E, et al. Modified Sauve-Kapandji procedure for disorders of the distal radioulnar joint in patients with rheumatoid arthritis. *J Bone Joint Surg [Am]*. 2006;88:24-28.

This paper describes the innovative procedure mentioned in this chapter to perform a DRU joint arthrodesis. The shelf is provided by turning the excised distal ulna to insert into a slot made in the radius. Fusion is assured because of greater bone contact. (Level IV evidence)

Kobayashi A, Futami T, Tadano I, et al. Radiographic comparative evaluation of the Sauve-Kapandji procedure and the Darrach procedure for rheumatoid wrist reconstruction. *Mod Rheumatol*. 2005;15:187-190.

This is a retrospective study comparing radiographic outcomes of the Sauve-Kapandji and Darrach procedures. Each group contained 13 wrists. There was no significant difference between the two groups in mean carpal height ratio. The authors concluded that radiographic outcomes were no different between the two groups. (Level III evidence)

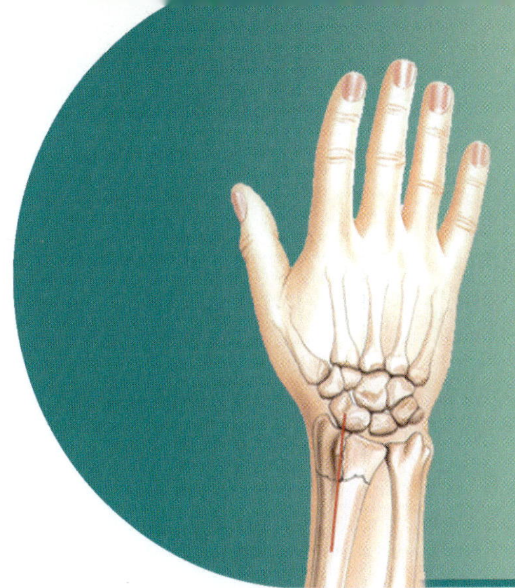

Section XIII

WRIST OSTEOARTHRITIS

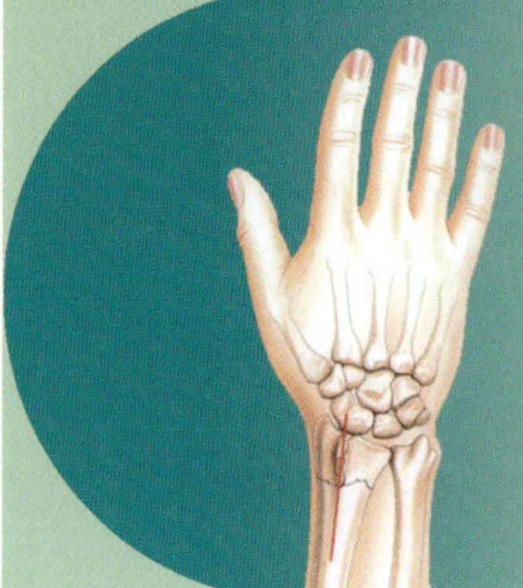

Wrist Denervation

Jessica H. Peelman and Peter J. Stern

Indications

- Painful arthrosis of the wrist, preservation of functional movement. Common etiologic conditions include scaphoid nonunion or scapholunate advanced collapse (SNAC/SLAC), Kienböck disease, inflammatory arthropathies, and post-traumatic arthritis following distal radius fractures or carpal dislocations.
- Patients who require wrist motion for daily function, for example, contralateral upper extremity amputees or dependence on assistive devices for ambulation.
- The patient in Figure 85-1 suffers from chronic wrist pain secondary to Kienböck disease. He is a bilateral above-knee amputee and depends on both upper extremities for ambulation.
- Patient selection is controversial. Local anesthetic blocks with postinjection assessment of pain relief and functional improvement are useful in determining which patients may benefit from the procedure.

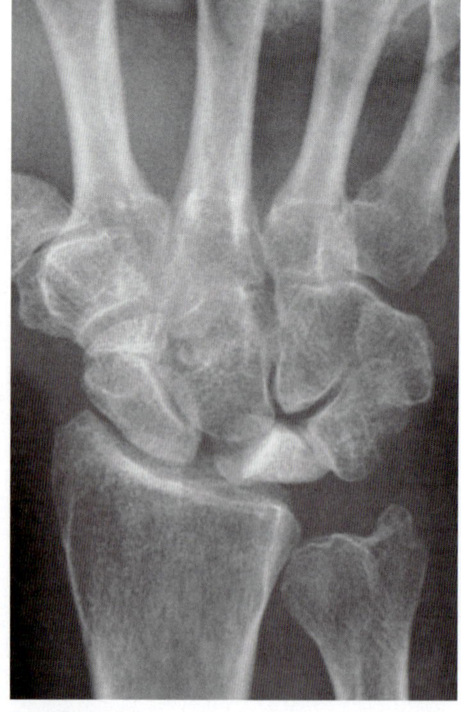

FIGURE 85-1

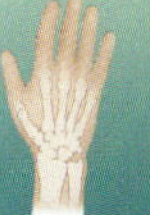

Examination/Imaging

Clinical Examination

- Injection of 1 mL of bupivacaine (Marcaine) 0.5% approximately 1 cm ulnar and 3 cm proximal to the Lister tubercle has been shown to reliably deliver medication to both the posterior interosseous nerve (PIN) and the anterior interosseous nerve (AIN). The needle is inserted; when resistance of the interosseous membrane is felt, the needle is withdrawn slightly, and the medication is injected to anesthetize the PIN. Next, the needle is advanced just through the membrane, and another injection is performed to anesthetize the AIN. Blocking the AIN and PIN helps indicate whether partial denervation will be beneficial (Fig. 85-2A).
- If complete denervation is planned, 1 mL of bupivacaine 0.5% is injected around the remaining nerves, including the palmar branch of the median nerve, branches of the radial nerve, the dorsal cutaneous branch of the ulnar nerve, and the recurrent intermetacarpal branches (Fig. 85-2B to D).
- After injection, pain is expected to be diminished considerably, and work output should at least double.

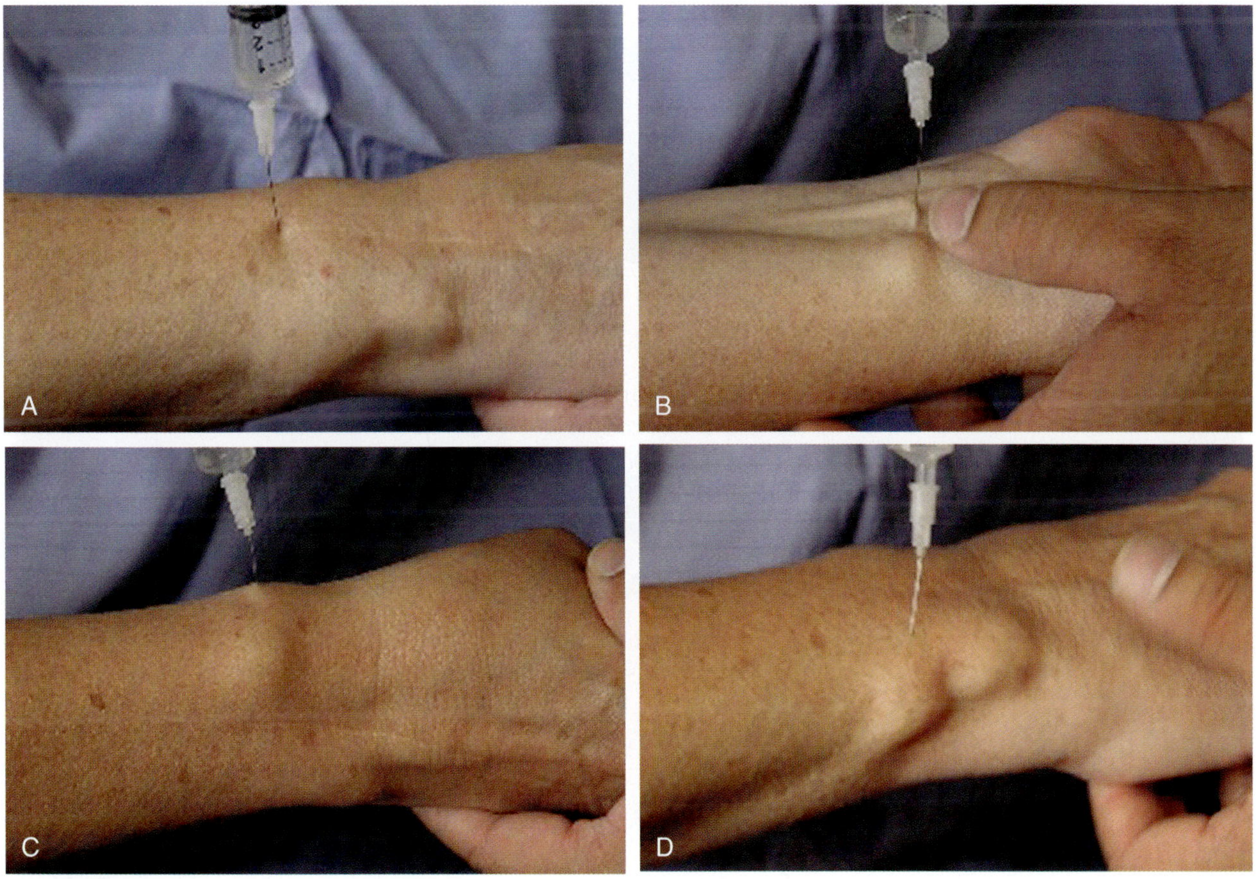

A B C D

FIGURE 85-2

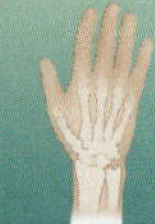

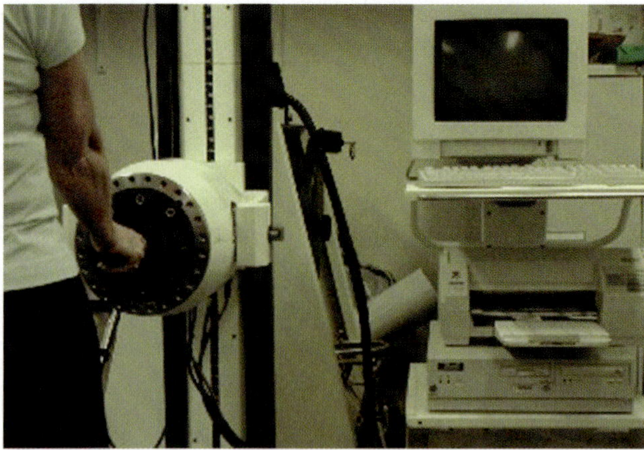

FIGURE 85-3

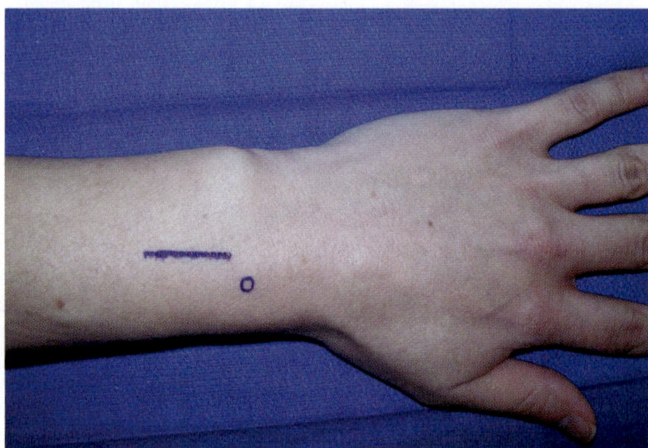

FIGURE 85-4

- A Baltimore Therapeutic Equipment (BTE) Work Simulator (Fig. 85-3) can be used to assess work function before and after bupivacaine injection. Functional assessment provides the most accurate prediction of success following wrist denervation and provides the patient with a good idea of what to expect after surgery.

Surgical Anatomy

- The innervation to the wrist is very rich. The main structures involved are the PIN and AIN. Branches of the radial, ulnar, and median nerves also contribute.

Positioning

- The patient is placed supine with the operative arm outstretched on a hand table. The procedure is performed under tourniquet control.

Exposures

- For partial denervation (PIN and AIN), a single longitudinal or transverse dorsal incision is used. Beginning about 2 cm proximal to the ulnar head, a 2- to 3-cm incision is made over the interval between the distal radius and ulna. The deep antebrachial fascia is incised longitudinally, exposing the extensor pollicis longus (third compartment) and extensor digitorum communis (fourth compartment) (Fig. 85-4).

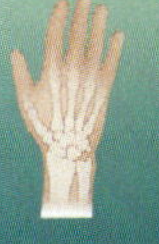

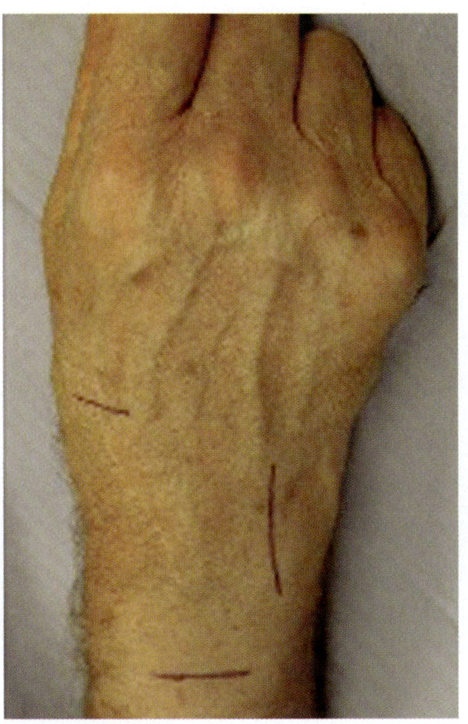

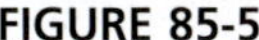

FIGURE 85-5

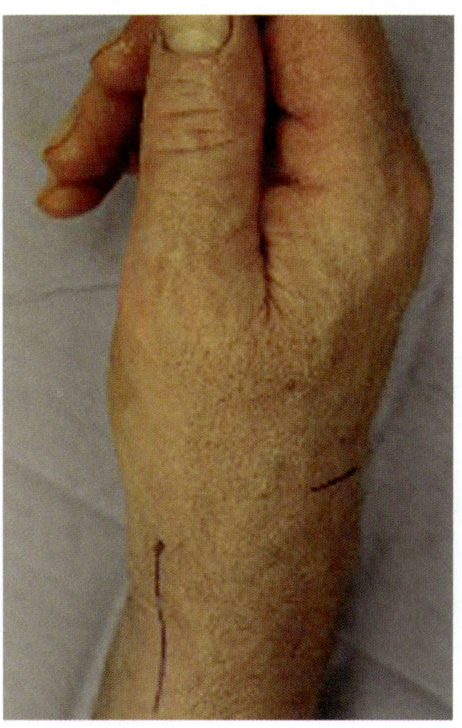

FIGURE 85-6

PEARLS

We prefer a longitudinal dorsal incision as opposed to a transverse incision because it simplifies the approach for possible future wrist reconstruction.

PITFALLS

The AIN and PIN are accompanied by the anterior and posterior interosseous arteries, respectively. Care must be taken to identify and protect these arteries during exposure to avoid injury and postoperative bleeding.

There is controversy regarding the merits of full denervation versus partial denervation. There is some evidence in the literature that suggests the results of partial denervation may deteriorate over time. However, we prefer partial denervation because it is simple, does not require multiple incisions, and has been shown to be effective in multiple reports.

- Full denervation can be done through four incisions. Incision 1: A transverse incision is made 3 to 5 cm proximal from the wrist on the dorsal forearm (Fig. 85-5). If a more distal incision is used, some articular branches from the PIN may not be completely eliminated. The extensor retinaculum over the fourth compartment is partially incised, and the finger extensor tendons are retracted ulnarly. The PIN is visualized on the radial floor of the fourth extensor compartment and isolated. The interosseous membrane is incised next, and branches of the AIN are visualized. Incision 2: A dorsal ulnar incision (see Fig. 85-5) is made over the wrist at the level of the ulnar head with dissection down to the extensor retinaculum. In the skin flap, the dorsal branch of the ulnar nerve is isolated. Incision 3: Through a volar radial incision centered over the radial artery at the level of the wrist and distal forearm, a plane is developed under the radial vessels, the palmar cutaneous branch of the median nerve, and the radial nerve (Fig. 85-6). Incision 4: A transverse incision is made over the dorsal base of the metacarpals and then through fascia to expose recurrent intermetacarpal branches (see Figs. 85-5 and 85-6).

Procedure

Step 1: Partial Denervation

- The extensor pollicis longus (EPL) is retracted radially, and the radial border of the fourth compartment is visualized by partially incising the retinaculum proximally. The digital extensor tendons are retracted ulnarly. The PIN and its vessels are visualized on the radial floor of the fourth dorsal compartment.

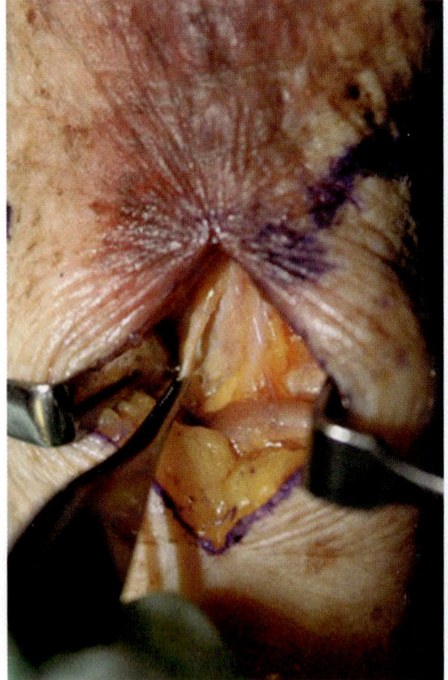
FIGURE 85-7

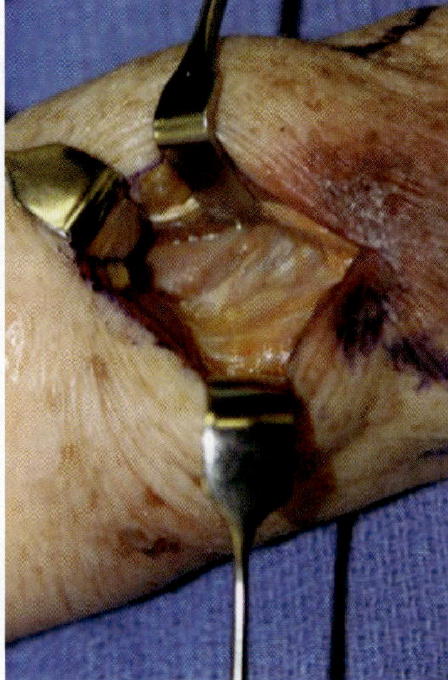
FIGURE 85-8

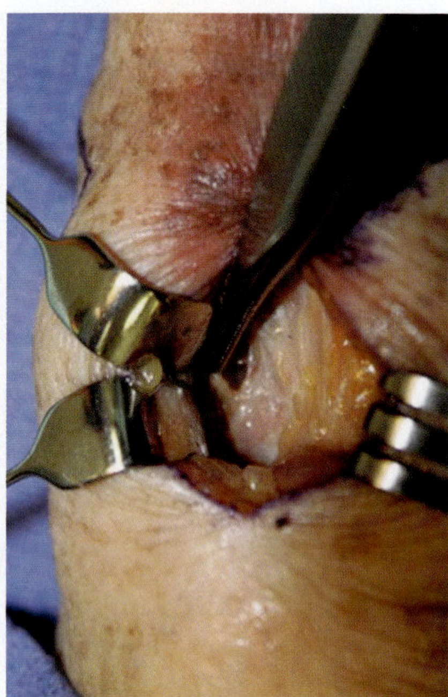
FIGURE 85-9

STEP 1 PEARLS

When performing a full wrist denervation, the PIN and AIN denervation will be performed as described through incision 1.

STEP 1 PITFALLS

The pronator quadratus may be denervated if the AIN is resected too far proximally.

The posterior and anterior interosseous arteries must be identified and protected to prevent postoperative bleeding and hematoma formation.

- The PIN is identified and dissected free using a longitudinal spreading technique. A 1- to 2-cm segment of nerve is resected sharply (Fig. 85-7).
- The interosseous membrane is visible beneath the PIN. The interosseous membrane is carefully incised longitudinally to expose the AIN. The AIN is identified and dissected free using a longitudinal spreading technique. A 1- to 2-cm segment of nerve is resected sharply as far distally as possible (Figs. 85-8 and 85-9).

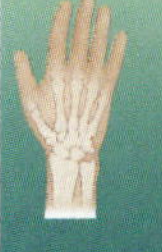

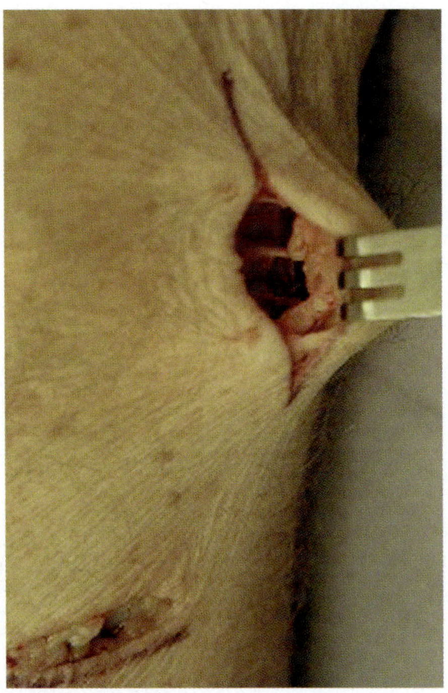

FIGURE 85-10

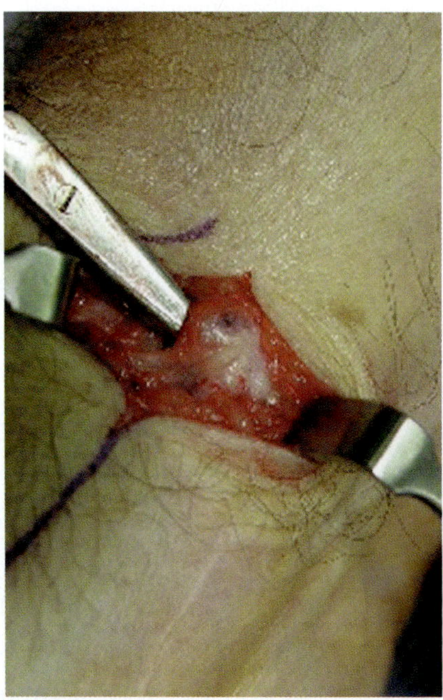

FIGURE 85-11

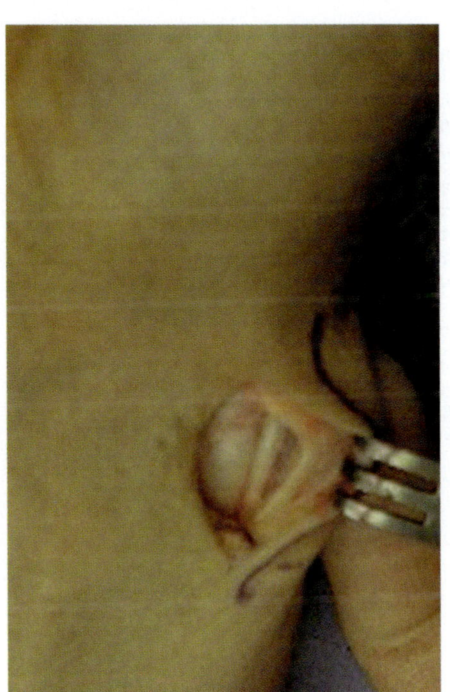

FIGURE 85-12

Step 2: Full Denervation: Incision 2

- PIN and AIN denervations are first performed through incision 1 as described previously.
- The plane between the extensor retinaculum and the subcutaneous fat is developed. The articular perforating fibers of the dorsal branch of the ulnar sensory nerve are isolated, cauterized, and resected (Fig. 85-10).
- Often, the excision of these perforating articular branches is accomplished blindly with dissection of the layer between the ulnar sensory nerve and the fascia. The index finger can be used as a blunt dissector, creating a "controlled degloving" of the skin over the dorsum of the wrist and the base of the ulnar head.

Step 3: Full Denervation: Incision 3

- The radial artery carries sympathetic pain fibers to the wrist joint. A plane is developed deep to the artery and veins, and a segment of periarterial tissue is resected. Sympathetic branches from the artery to the wrist joint are divided (Fig. 85-11).
- A plane is created deep to the palmar cutaneous branch of the median nerve volarly, and the radial sensory nerve dorsally that will meet the plane from incision 2. Again, the index finger can be used to develop these planes (Fig. 85-12).

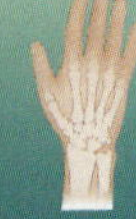

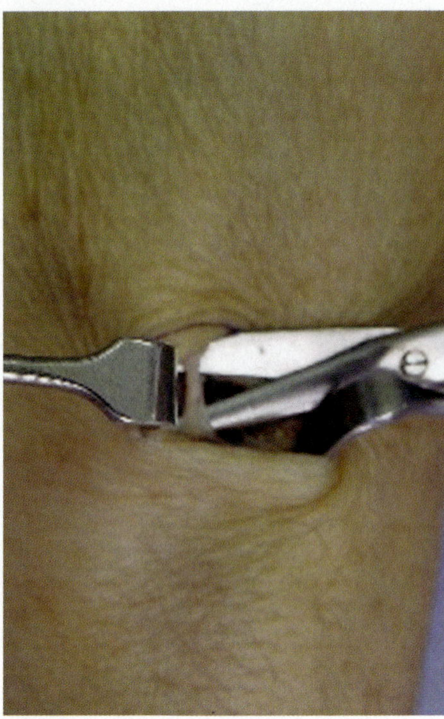

FIGURE 85-13

Step 4: Full Denervation: Incision 4

- The extensor tendons are retracted through the transverse incision over the dorsal base of the metacarpals and through the fascia.
- The recurrent articular fibers, which are seen at the metacarpal base level, are isolated and cauterized (Fig. 85-13).

PEARLS

Patients should be told that if there is no improvement by 4 to 6 weeks, it is unlikely that the procedure will be successful.

Postoperative Care and Expected Outcomes

- A light dressing and short-arm splint are applied for 10 days.
- After that, the splint is removed, and active range of motion is encouraged.
- After 2 weeks, strengthening is initiated.
- Patients should return to work within 2 to 4 weeks.

Acknowledgment

We would like to give a special thanks to the authors of this chapter in the previous edition, Carlos Heras-Palou and Thomas R. Hunt III, because their work served as an excellent foundation and contribution to this chapter.

Evidence

Buck-Gramcko D. Denervation of the wrist joint. *J Hand Surg [Am]*. 1977;2:54-61.
Follow-up studies of 195 patients after wrist denervation. Two thirds had very good results. Average follow-up was 4 years. (Level IV evidence)

Ferres A, Suso S, Foucher G. Wrist denervation: surgical considerations. *J Hand Surg [Br]*. 1995;20:769-772.
Results after partial denervation are worse than results achieved by total denervation. (Level IV evidence)

Grafe MW, Kim PD, Rosenwasser MP, Strauch RJ. Wrist denervation and the anterior interosseous nerve: anatomic considerations. *J Hand Surg [Am]*. 2005;30:1221-1225.
A cadaveric study that suggested division of the anterior interosseous nerve 2 cm proximal to the ulnar head when using a dorsal approach to retain innervation to the pronator quadratus. (Level V evidence)

Lin DL, Lenhart MK, Farber GL. Anatomy of the anterior interosseous innervation of the pronator quadratus: evaluation of structures at risk in the single dorsal incision of wrist denervation technique. *J Hand Surg [Am]* 2006;31:904-907.
This cadaveric study determined that a single dorsal incision for wrist denervation risks complete denervation of the pronator quadratus and suggested resection of the anterior interosseous nerve close to the distal margin of pronator quadratus. (Level V evidence)

Weinstein LP, Berger RA. Analgesic benefit, functional outcome, and patient satisfaction after partial wrist denervation. *J Hand Surg [Am]*. 2002;27:833-839.
Partial wrist denervation is a useful palliative procedure for chronic wrist pain when reconstructive procedures are not feasible or desirable. (Level IV evidence)

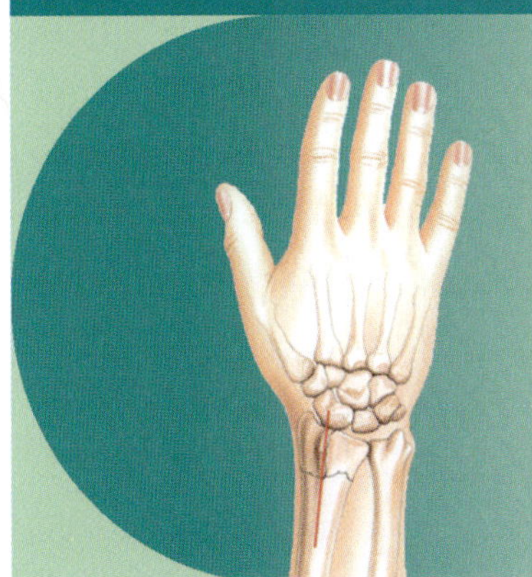

Proximal Row Carpectomy

Jeffrey A. Greenberg

See Video 64: Proximal Row Carpectomy

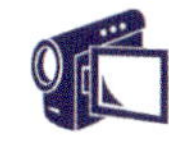

Indications

- Scapholunate advanced collapse (SLAC) or scaphoid nonunion advanced collapse (SNAC) with preserved midcarpal joint (stages 1 and 2).
- Kienböck disease (Stage 3).
- Chronic carpal instability.
- Failed soft tissue reconstruction.
- In general, indications are similar to those for four-corner fusion; however, the midcarpal joint needs to be preserved.

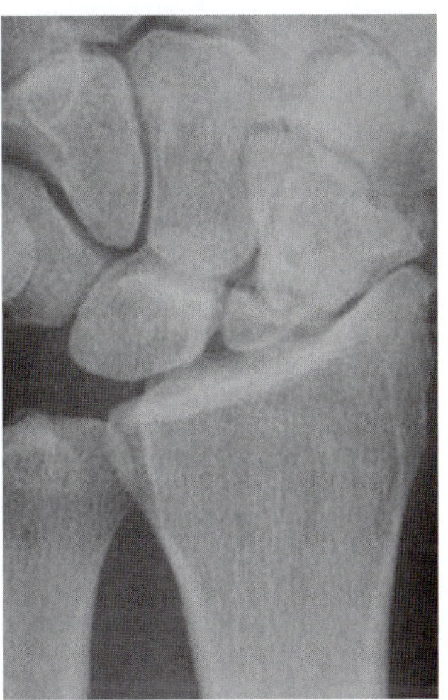

FIGURE 86-1

Examination/Imaging

Clinical Examination

- Radioscaphoid and midcarpal joints may be tender to palpation.
- Visible fullness may be present secondary to hypertrophic synovitis.
- Decreased range of motion.
- Pain with loading of midcarpal joint, particularly with radial and ulnar deviation.
- Pain with extension loading.
- Decreased grip strength.

Imaging

- Plain radiographs are usually sufficient to stage the disease and ensure that the midcarpal joint is preserved (Figs. 86-1 and 86-2).
- Advanced imaging (computed tomography) can be performed to determine the status of the midcarpal joint; however, patients are made aware preoperatively that an intraoperative decision to convert to a limited wrist fusion can be made if there is excessive, unrecognized midcarpal joint degenerative change.

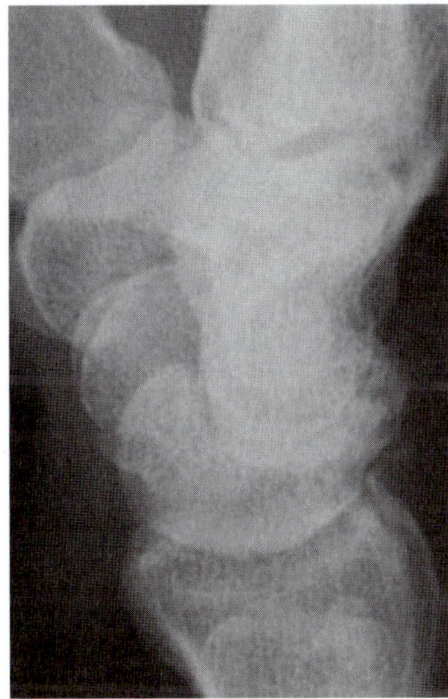

FIGURE 86-2

Surgical Anatomy

- In either SLAC or SNAC, there will be widening at the scapholunate interval.
- Significant scaphoid flexion, lunate extension, and dorsal lunate prominence develop.
- Radioscaphoid degenerative change with styloid prominence or osteophytes.
- Dorsal radial prominence.
- Synovitis.
- Proximal scaphoid pole necrosis and/or arthrosis.
- Scaphotrapeziotrapezoid arthrosis may be present.
- The volar extrinsic ligaments (radioscaphocapitate, short and long radiolunate) originate from the volar radius and extend obliquely to the carpus. These should be intact; insufficiency or iatrogenic damage could lead to ulnar translation and radiocapitate instability after surgery (Fig. 86-3). The dorsal ligaments of the wrist—dorsal radiocarpal (DRC) and dorsal intercarpal (DIC)—have a conjoined insertion on the triquetrum. They provide the capsulotomy landmarks for wrist exposure (Fig. 86-4).

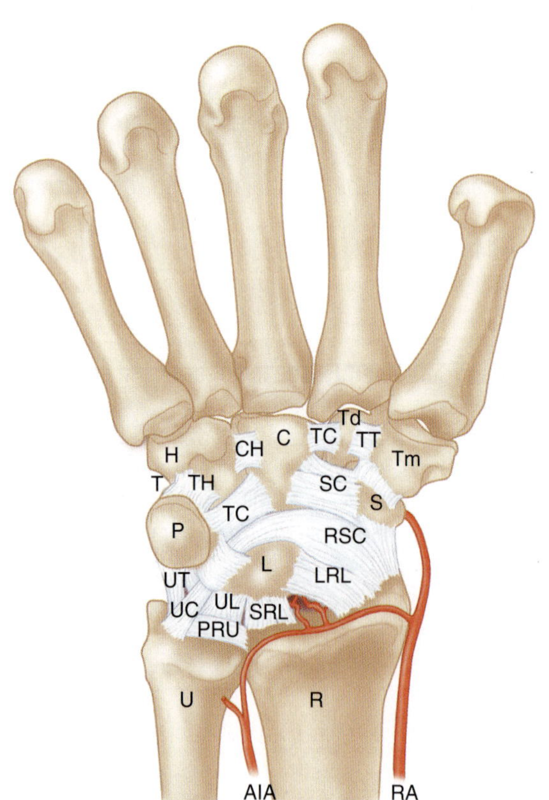

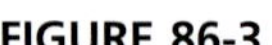
FIGURE 86-3

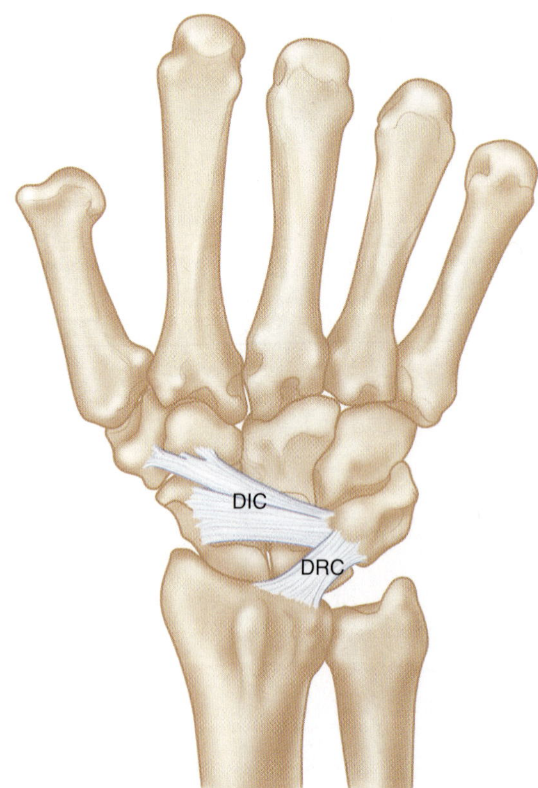

FIGURE 86-4

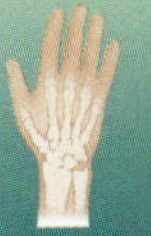

Positioning

- The patient is positioned supine, the hand and forearm are supported on a hand surgery table, and a proximal tourniquet is used.
- Operating on the dorsal wrist is easier if the surgeon is positioned at the head of the patient as opposed to at the axilla.

Exposures

> **PEARLS**
>
> *The dorsal capsular ligaments are more prominent with the wrist in flexion. Placing a "bump" under the wrist facilitates visualization. Fatty perivascular tissue is sometimes prominent on the dorsal capsule. Bluntly dissecting it off the capsule with a sponge also facilitates visualization of the ligaments.*
>
> *Leave a cuff of ligament along the radial rim for closure, but incise the ligament close enough to the radius to visualize the proximal carpal row.*

- A straight dorsal midline incision centered over the radiocarpal joint is used (Fig. 86-5).
- Flap elevation is performed sharply, protecting the cutaneous branches of the superficial radial and dorsal ulnar sensory nerves within the subcutaneous tissue.
- The retinaculum over the third dorsal compartment is incised and the extensor pollicis longus (EPL) retracted (Fig. 86-6).
- Retinacular flaps are raised exposing the second through fifth dorsal compartments.
- Retractors are placed between the second and fourth dorsal compartment tendons.
- A posterior interosseous neurectomy is performed. The PIN is located on the floor of the fourth dorsal compartment
- The capsule is incised along the DIC and DRC ligaments raising a radially based flap (Fig. 86-7).

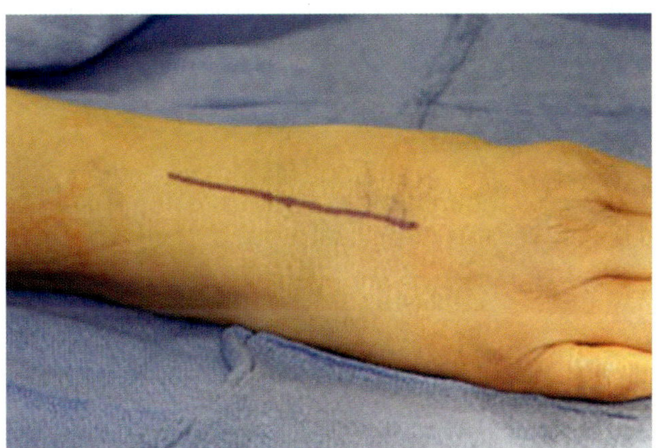

FIGURE 86-5

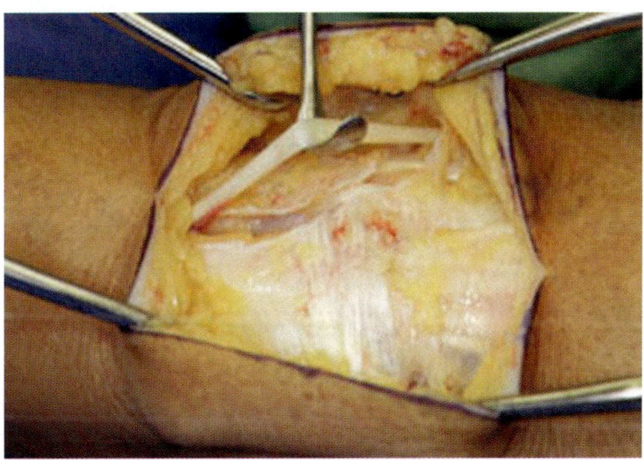

FIGURE 86-6

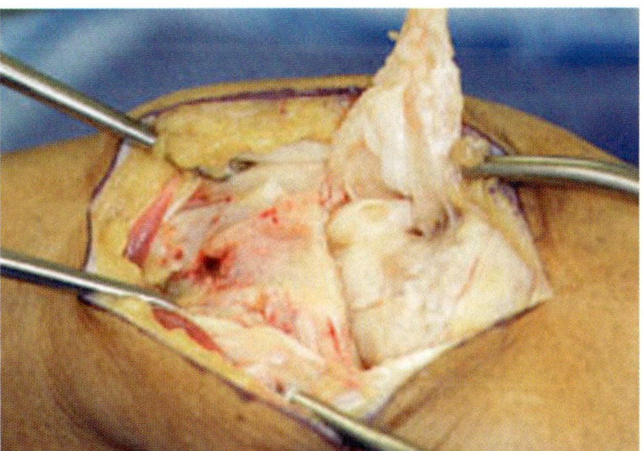

FIGURE 86-7

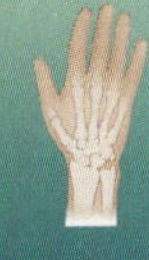

STEP 1 PEARLS

Mild degenerative change at the capitate head or radiolunate joint can be treated with proximal row carpectomy (PRC) and concomitant capsular interposition.

Osteochondral resurfacing has also been described as an adjunctive procedure with PRC for capitate chondrosis. An osteochondral graft is obtained from the excised carpus, usually the lunate, and inserted into the defect created after excising the area of cartilage loss (limited to a single area <10 mm in diameter).

STEP 1 PITFALLS

Significant degenerative change at either the radiolunate or midcarpal joints precludes PRC, and alternative procedures should be performed.

STEP 2 PEARLS

A joystick can be placed in the lunate to facilitate manipulation.

Care is taken to avoid injury to the volar ligaments and cartilage of the distal radius and capitate.

It is easier to completely remove the bone using careful circumferential subperiosteal dissection rather than a piecemeal technique with a rongeur.

STEP 2 PITFALLS

Injuring the volar extrinsic ligaments can lead to late instability and carpal translation.

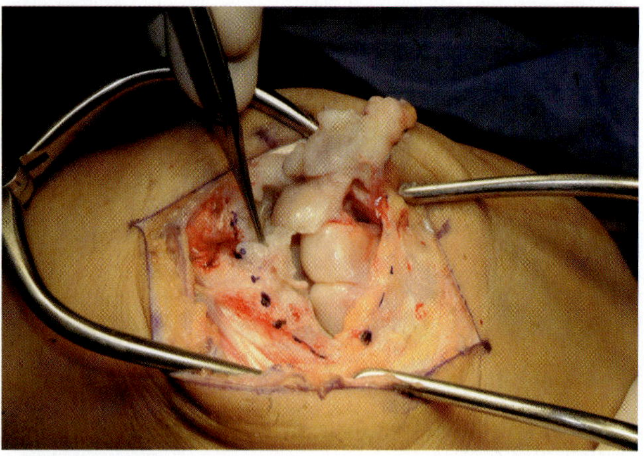

FIGURE 86-8

- If a soft tissue interposition using the capsule is planned, a proximally based, rectangular flap of capsule is harvested instead of using the capsular exposure previously described. The soft tissue interposition procedure is used if there is some articular wear on the capitate.

Procedure

Step 1

- Inspection of the distal radius and midcarpal joint is performed. Ensure that the lunate fossa and proximal capitate are intact. Alternative procedures should be considered if there is damage to the midcarpal or radiolunate articulations (Fig. 86-8).

Step 2

- The lunotriquetral ligament is divided, and the lunate is excised in its entirety by carefully dissecting it off the volar ligament. This technique minimizes the chance of bone attached to the capsule being left behind.
- Avoid injuring the cartilage surface of the radiolunate joint or capitate head.

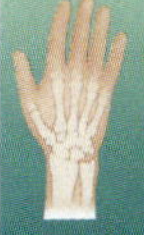

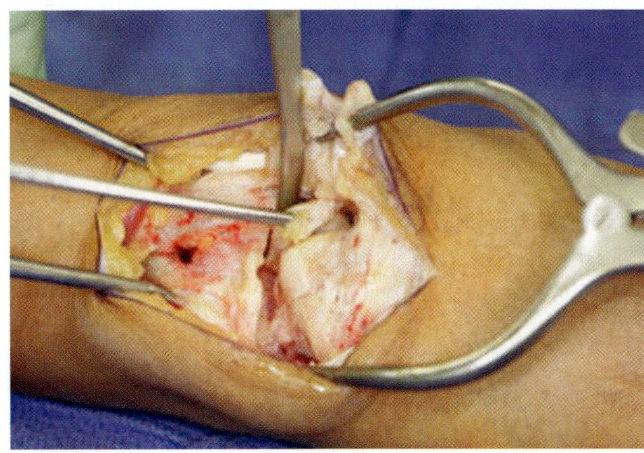

FIGURE 86-9

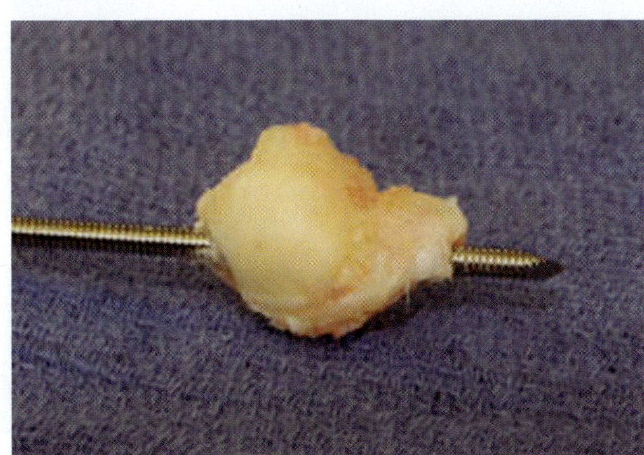

FIGURE 86-10

STEP 3 PEARLS

Similar to the lunate, it is easier to remove the triquetrum in one piece.

STEP 3 PITFALLS

Avoid injury to the ulnar neurovascular bundle or the dorsal sensory branch of the ulnar nerve; both are in close proximity to the triquetrum.

STEP 4 PEARLS

A sharp curved elevator facilitates subperiosteal dissection and complete removal.

STEP 4 PITFALLS

Avoid damage to the volar extrinsic ligaments, radial artery, and head of the capitates.

Step 3

- The triquetrum can be excised in its entirety by careful circumferential subperiosteal dissection.

Step 4

- After removal of the lunate and triquetrum, a joystick should be placed in the scaphoid (Fig. 86-9). Threaded Steinmann pins, Schanz screws, or threaded gimlets can be used. Avoid temptation for piecemeal excision using a rongeur because it is easier to remove the entire scaphoid using careful and deliberate subperiosteal dissection methods (Fig. 86-10).

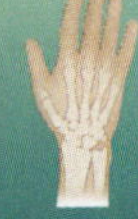

STEP 5 PEARLS

Decompress the radiocarpal joint with radial styloidectomy.

STEP 5 PITFALLS

Excessive bone resection during styloidectomy will compromise the integrity of the volar extrinsic ligaments.

Persistent stylocarpal impingement may persist if the radiocarpal joint is not decompressed.

Step 5

- The capitate should seat in the lunate fossa and be stable. Styloid impingement is assessed, and, if present, a radial styloidectomy should be performed (Fig. 86-11).

Additional Steps

- Anatomic capsular closure using nonabsorbable suture is performed.
- The extensor retinaculum is closed, leaving the EPL transposed (Fig. 86-12).
- Skin is closed with interrupted nonabsorbable suture.
- A well-padded dressing is applied to control edema yet allow digital range of motion.
- A radiograph is taken to ensure that the capitate is reduced on the radius (Figs. 86-13 and 86-14).

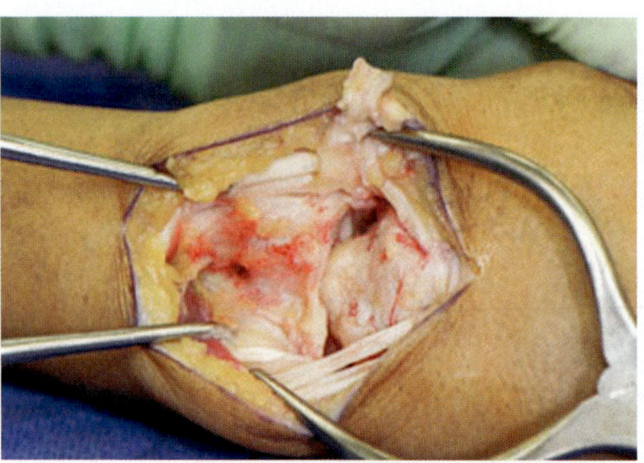

FIGURE 86-11

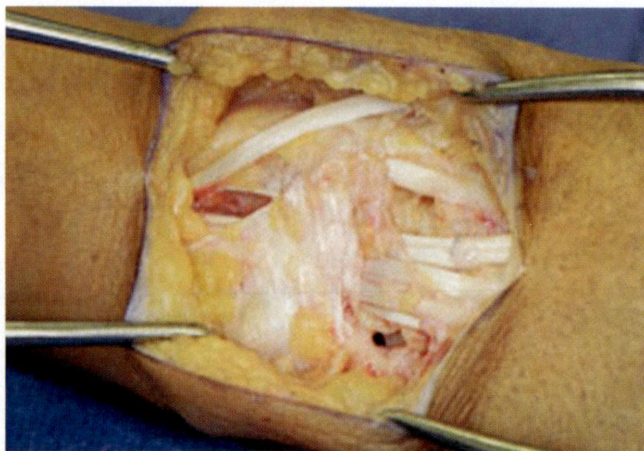

FIGURE 86-12

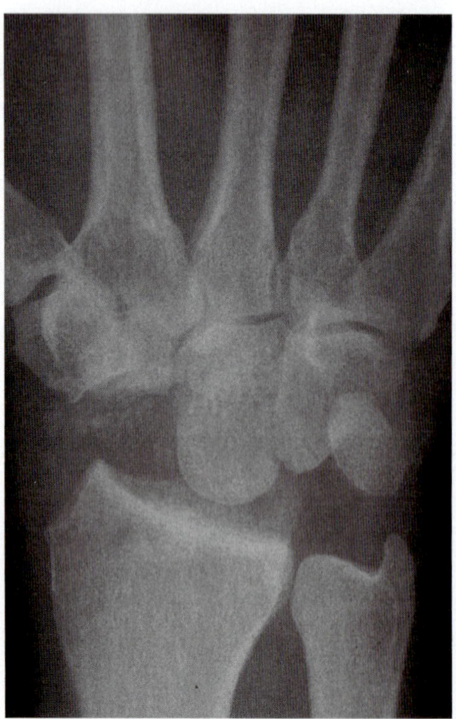

FIGURE 86-13

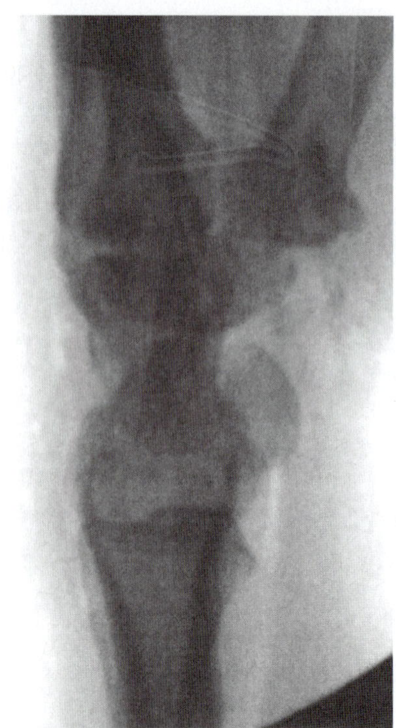

FIGURE 86-14

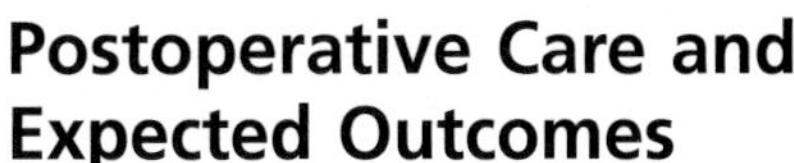

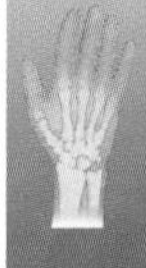

Postoperative Care and Expected Outcomes

- Dressing and suture are removed 2 weeks after surgery.
- A short-arm cast is worn until 6 weeks after surgery.
- A removable splint is applied and range of motion initiated 6 weeks after surgery.
- Strengthening exercises can begin at 10 to 12 weeks.
- Expect 70 degrees of arc of motion and recovery of 70% of grip strength.
- Postoperative swelling can persist.
- Recovery can be prolonged—up to 12 to 18 months.

Evidence

Cohen MS, Kozin SH. Degenerative arthritis of the wrist: proximal row carpectomy versus scaphoid excision and four-corner arthrodesis. *J Hand Surg [Am].* 2001;26:94-104.
This comparative study looked at 19 patients in two groups from two different institutions. No significant differences in motion, grip strength, or function were noted between the groups. (Level III evidence)

Croog AS, Stern PJ. Proximal row carpectomy for advanced Kienböck's disease: average 10-year follow-up. *J Hand Surg [Am].* 2008;33:1122-1130.
This study evaluated 21 patients with Lichtman stage IIIA, IIIB, or IV Kienböck disease who underwent PRC. Eighteen of the 21 patients with an average follow-up of 10 years achieved an average wrist flexion-extension arc of 105 degrees and maximal grip strength of 35 kg, which averaged 87% of that of the contralateral wrist. The average DASH score was 12 points, and the average PRWE score was 17, each representing minimal functional limitation. Two of 3 patients who required a radiocapitate arthrodesis had stage IV disease, and the authors express caution with use of PRC in this population of patients. There was no significant association between postoperative radiographic findings and clinical outcomes. (Level IV evidence)

DiDonna ML, Kiefhaber TR, Stern PJ. Proximal row carpectomy: study with a minimum of ten years of follow-up. *J Bone Joint Surg [Am].* 2004;86:2359-2365.
Twenty-two PRCs in 21 patients were reviewed with an average follow-up time of 14 years. Eighteen of the 22 patients demonstrated satisfactory pain relief, 72 degrees of flexion-extension arc, and recovery of 91% of grip strength of the opposite side. Pain relief was graded as complete in 9, mild in 4, and moderate residual in 5. There were 4 failures, all in patients younger than 35 years old. (Level IV evidence)

Lumsden BC, Stone A, Engber WD. Treatment of advanced-stage Kienböck's disease with proximal row carpectomy: an average 15-year follow-up. *J Hand Surg [Am].* 2008;33:493-502.
Proximal row carpectomy was used to treat 17 patients with advanced-stage (Lichtman IIIA and IIIB) Kienböck disease. Thirteen of the 17 patients with an average follow-up of 15 years were evaluated. Twelve of 13 patients demonstrated excellent or good results. They achieved a total arc of motion of 73% of the uninvolved side and grip strength that averaged 92% of the uninvolved side. All patients demonstrated some degree of degenerative changes. Despite radiographic evidence of radiocapitate degenerative change in nearly all patients, clinical results did not correlate with radiographic degeneration. (Level IV evidence)

Tang P, Imbriglia JE. Osteochondral resurfacing (OCRPRC) for capitate chondrosis in proximal row carpectomy. *J Hand Surg [Am].* 2007;32:1334-1342.
This paper presents a novel approach to the use of PRC in patients with Outerbridge grade II to IV capitate chondrosis. The authors performed osteochondral resurfacing of the capitate in addition to PRC. Eight patients with an average follow-up of 18 months demonstrated improved pain and maintenance of wrist range of motion and grip strength. Mayo wrist scores improved from 51 to 68. DASH score averaged 19.5 postoperatively. Seventy-five percent of patients had mild to no degenerative change on postoperative radiographs, and magnetic resonance imaging 21 months after surgery showed graft incorporation. (Level IV evidence)

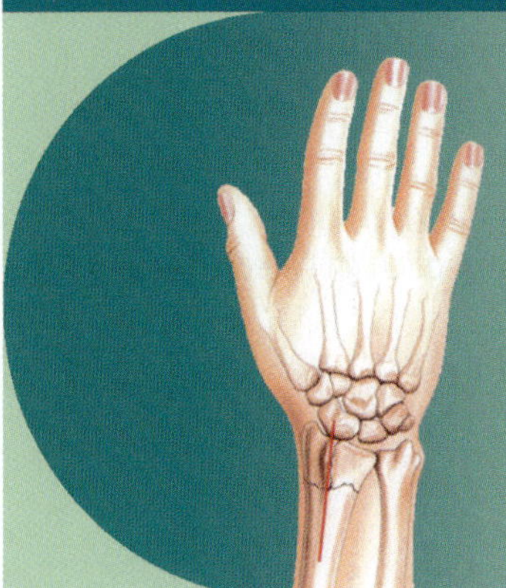

Four-Corner Fusion

Jeffrey A. Greenberg

See Video 65: 4-Corner Fusion Using Kirschner Wires

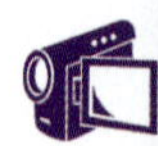

Indications

- Scapholunate advanced collapse (SLAC)
- Scaphoid nonunion advanced collapse (SNAC)
- Radiocarpal arthrosis
- Carpal instability patterns
- Failed soft tissue reconstructions

Examination/Imaging

Clinical Examination

- Radial fullness
- Decreased range of motion
- Decreased grip strength
- Painful range of motion
- Crepitus
- Painful extension loading
- Watson maneuver eliciting pain
- Styloid tenderness
- Carpal tunnel syndrome possible

Imaging

- Plain radiographs are usually sufficient for diagnosis. SLAC wrist, stage 3, demonstrates abnormal position of the scaphoid, scapholunate widening, radioscaphoid degenerative change and midcarpal arthrosis (Fig. 87-1).
- In cases in which there is uncertainty about the status of the radiolunate joint, advanced imaging (computed tomography) may be used.

Surgical Anatomy

- In either SLAC or SNAC, there will be widening at the scapholunate interval.
- Significant scaphoid flexion, lunate extension, and dorsal lunate prominence develop.
- Radioscaphoid degenerative change with styloid prominence and osteophytes is noted.
- Proximal scaphoid pole necrosis and/or arthrosis is present (Fig. 87-2).
- Synovitis is present.
- Scaphotrapeziotrapezoid arthrosis may be present.
- The dorsal ligaments of the wrist—dorsal radiocarpal (DRC) and dorsal intercarpal (DIC)—have a conjoined insertion on the triquetrum. They provide the capsulotomy landmarks for wrist exposure.

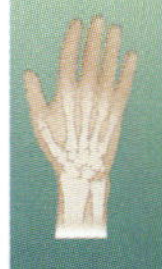

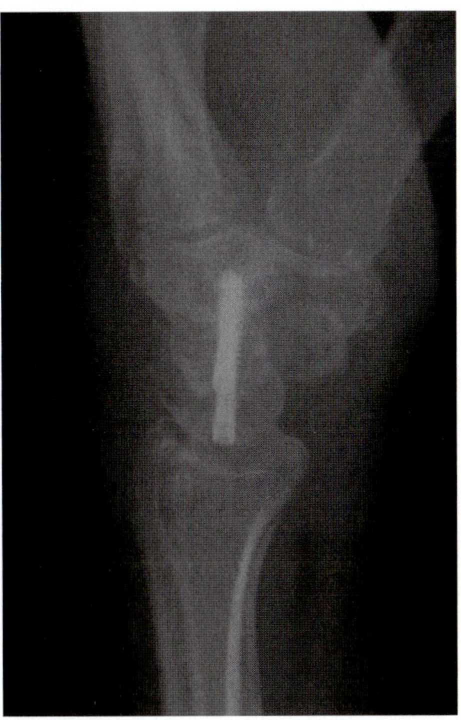

FIGURE 87-1

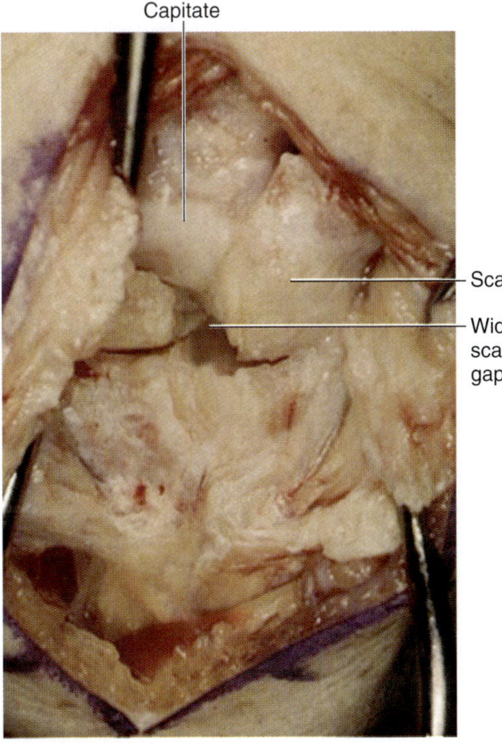

FIGURE 87-2

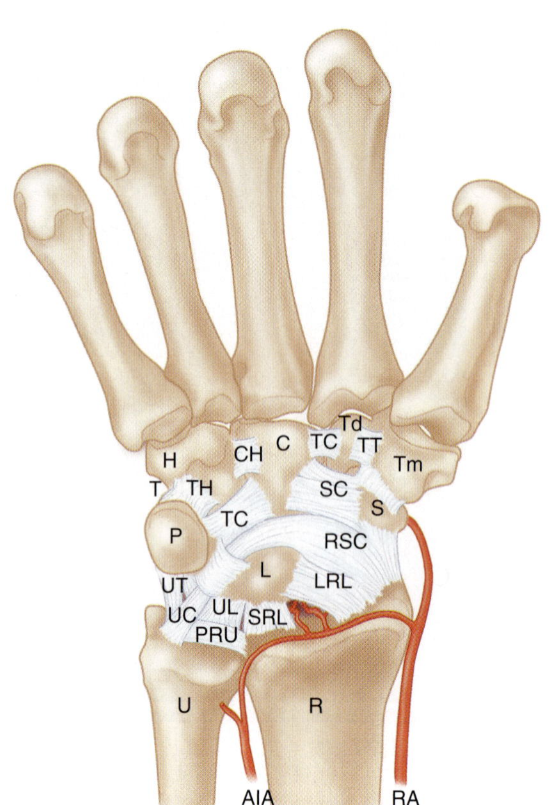

FIGURE 87-3

- The volar extrinsic ligaments (radioscaphocapitate, short and long radiolunate) originate from the volar radius and extend obliquely to the carpus. These should be respected during scaphoid excision (Fig. 87-3).

Positioning

- The patient is positioned supine, the hand and forearm are supported on a hand surgery table, and a proximal tourniquet is used.
- Operating on the wrist is easier if the surgeon is positioned at the head of the patient as opposed to at the axilla.

PEARLS

Wrist flexion and bluntly removing fibrofatty tissue from the dorsal capsule facilitate visualization of the DIC and DRC.

Exposures

- A dorsal midline incision centered over the radiocarpal joint is used.
- Thick flaps are elevated dorsal to the retinaculum, keeping cutaneous nerves within these flaps.
- The retinaculum over the third dorsal compartment is incised.
- Retinacular flaps are raised, exposing the second through fifth compartments (Fig. 87-4).
- The extensor tendons are retracted using retractors placed between the second and fourth compartments.
- A posterior interosseous neurectomy is performed.
- A capsulotomy is performed by dividing the dorsal capsule along the dorsal intercarpal and dorsal radiocarpal ligaments (Fig. 87-5). The flap is elevated off the dorsum of the triquetrum and reflected, keeping it radially based (Fig. 87-6).

PITFALLS

Dividing the DRC too distally makes it difficult to access and work on the lunate.

Failure to expose the capsule between the second and fifth compartments compromises visualization.

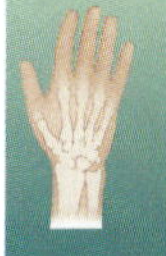

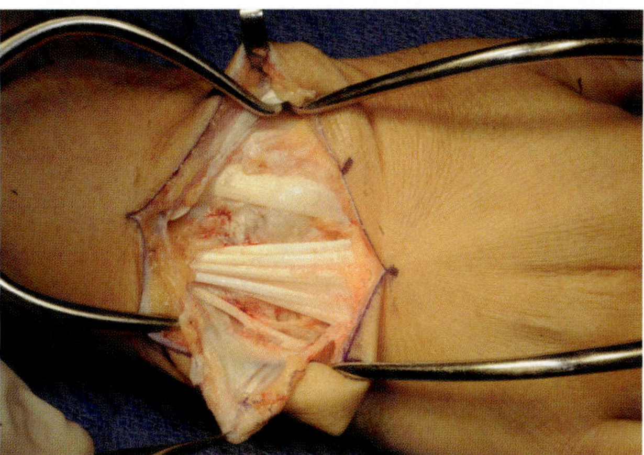

FIGURE 87-4

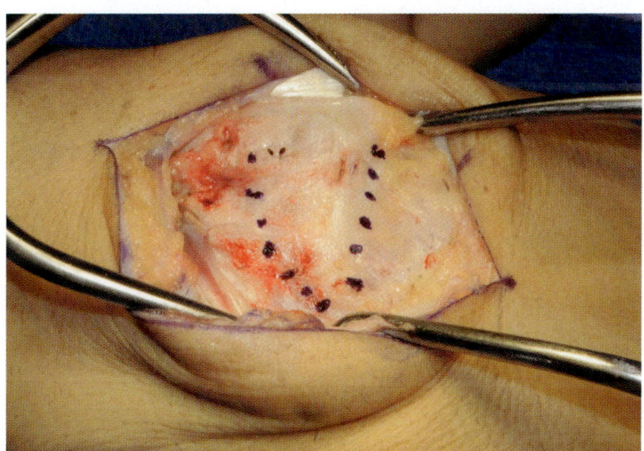

FIGURE 87-5

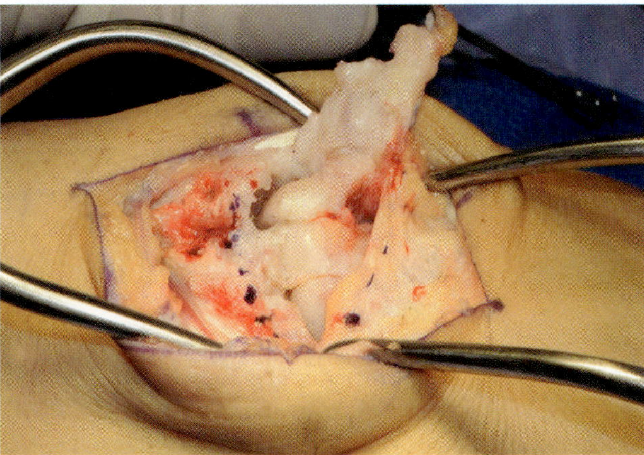

FIGURE 87-6

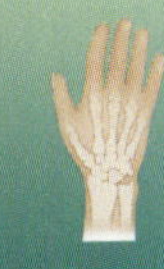

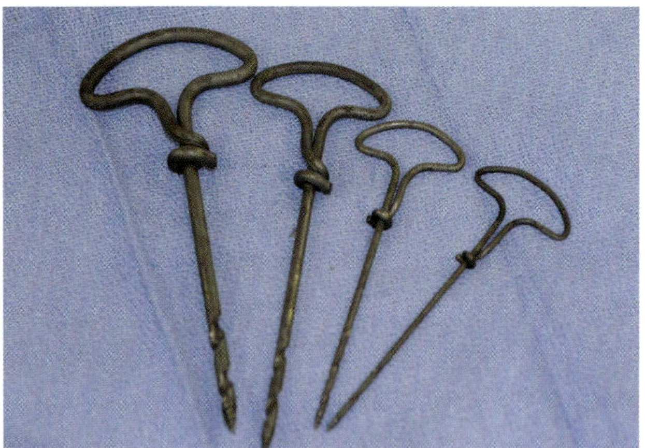

FIGURE 87-7

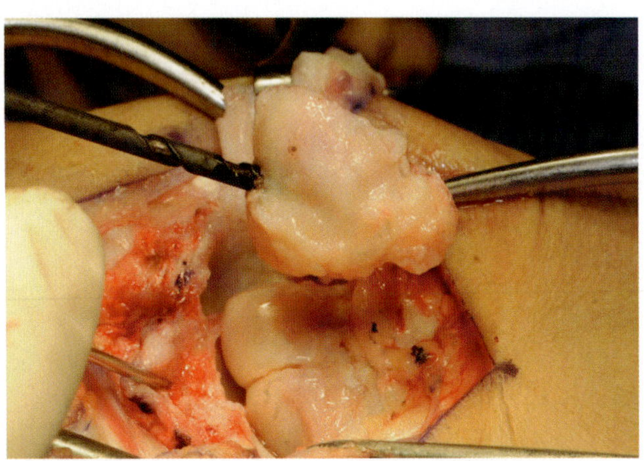

FIGURE 87-8

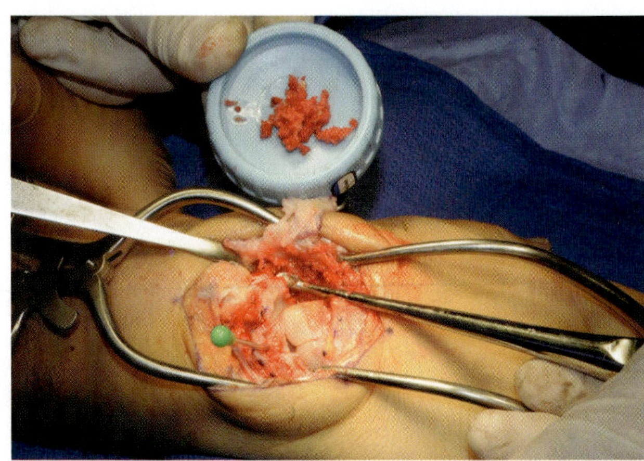

FIGURE 87-9

Procedure

Step 1

- Inspection of the radiolunate joint is performed to ensure that it is free of degenerative change.
- A threaded gimlet, Schanz screw, or Steinman pin is used as a joystick to facilitate removal of the scaphoid (Fig. 87-7).
- The scaphoid is excised in one piece (Fig. 87-8).

Step 2

- After scaphoid removal, a styloidectomy is performed.
- Cancellous bone graft is harvested from the distal radius, accessing cancellous bone through the styloidectomy site (Fig. 87-9).

STEP 1 PEARLS

Avoid the temptation to morselize the scaphoid or remove it piecemeal because it is easier to carefully dissect the bone subperiosteally and remove it in one piece. A curved, sharp Carroll elevator facilitates the deeper dissection.

STEP 1 PITFALLS

Care must be taken to avoid injury to the volar extrinsic ligaments, radial artery, and capsular flap during scaphoid excision.

STEP 2 PITFALLS

Avoid an excessive styloidectomy because this can compromise the volar extrinsic ligaments and lead to ulnar translational instability.

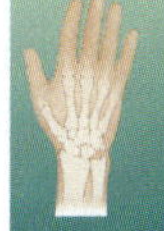

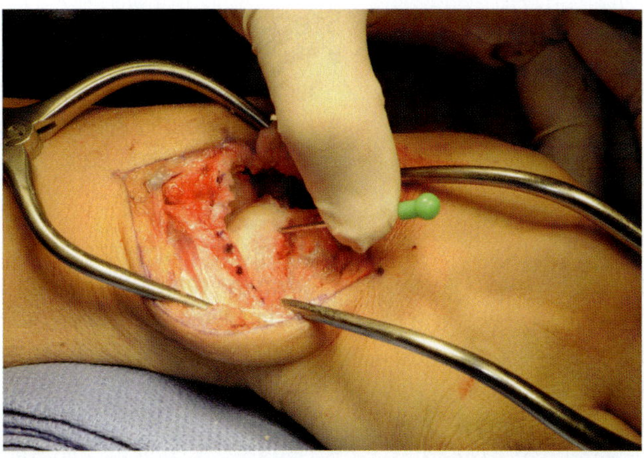

FIGURE 87-10

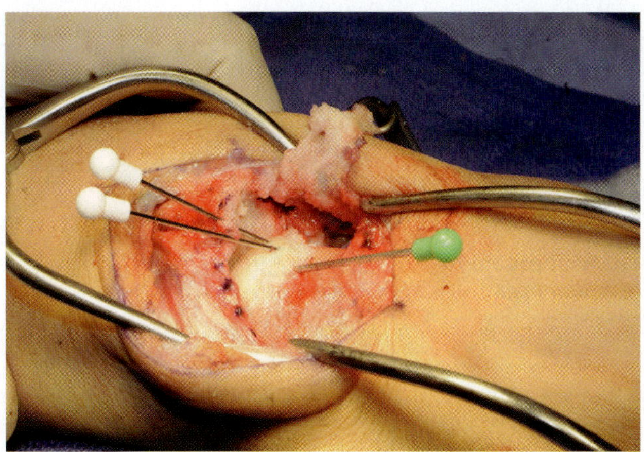

FIGURE 87-11

Step 3

- A 0.062-inch Kirschner wire is placed in the dorsal lunate as a joystick. The lunate is usually in an abnormally extended position, and it must be reduced to a colinear relationship with the capitate (Fig. 87-10). Soft tissue release may be necessary to achieve this relationship.
- After confirming that reduction is possible, the midcarpal joint is exposed, and the cartilage and subchondral bone of the distal lunate and capitate are removed.
- Bone graft is placed, and the lunate is reduced.
- Provisional K-wire fixation holds the lunate, and the capitate is reduced (Fig. 87-11).
- Intraoperative fluoroscopy confirms reduction.

STEP 3 PEARLS

Occasionally a large dorsal lunate osteophyte is present and may be removed to facilitate visualization of the midcarpal joint.

When correctly reduced, the capitate appears to overhang the radial margin of the lunate.

Colinearity of the lunate to the capitate, or even slight lunate flexion, is desirable.

STEP 3 PITFALLS

Malreduction or incomplete reduction of the lunate is the most common error and is associated with poor clinical results.

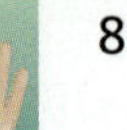

Step 4

- The lunotriquetral, triquetrohamate, and capitohamate intervals are prepared by removing cartilage and subchondral bone.
- Graft is placed in these intervals.
- Provisional fixation from the triquetrum to the capitate is performed.

STEP 4 PEARLS

The capitohamate relationship is relatively immobile and does not need to be completely taken down for fusion preparation.

STEP 4 PITFALLS

Inadequate articular surface preparation can lead to delayed union and/or nonunion.

If power tools are used for surface preparation, it is important to keep heat at a minimum to avoid bone necrosis.

Step 5

- The radiocarpal joint is flexed, and a guidewire for a cannulated screw is placed down the central lunate-capitate axis.
- A cannulated screw is placed compressing the midcarpal joint.
- A second screw is placed obliquely to the first screw, usually from the triquetrum into the capitate (Fig. 87-12).
- Range of motion and stability are checked.
- Fluoroscopy confirms hardware placement (Fig. 87-13).

STEP 5 PEARLS

Screw back-out can be limited by placing two screws obliquely to one another.

No fixation is necessary across the capitohamate interval.

Two screws are usually adequate to secure the entire fusion mass.

STEP 5 PITFALLS

Parallel placement of screws has been associated with screw back-out and potential damage to the distal radial articular surface.

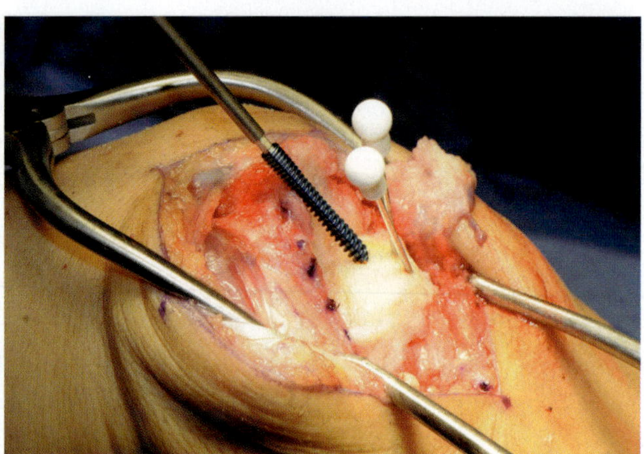

FIGURE 87-12

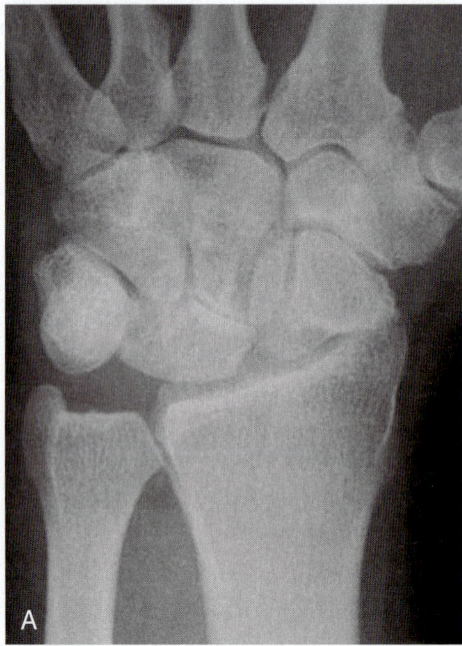

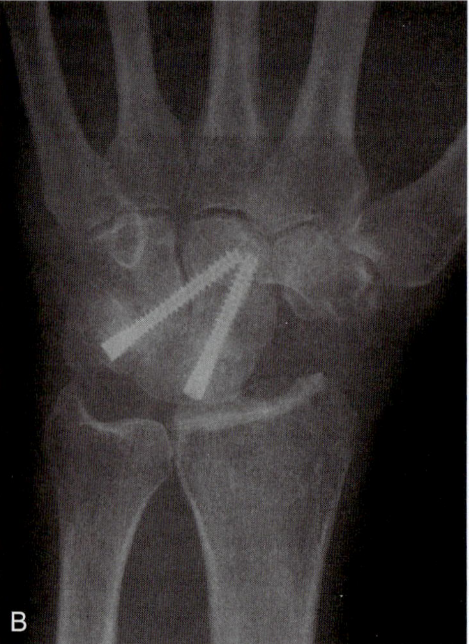

FIGURE 87-13

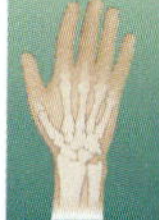

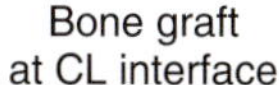

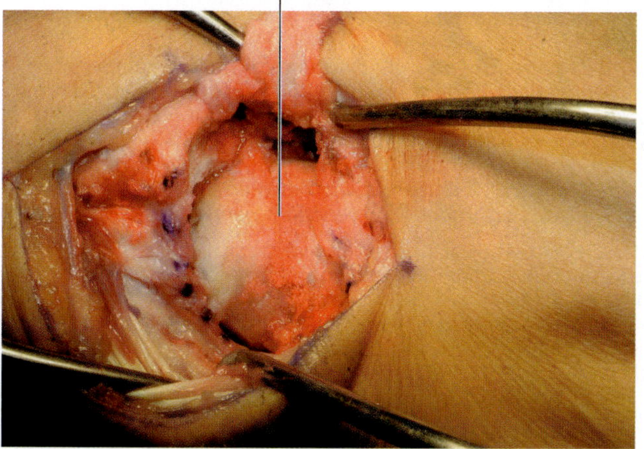

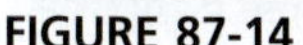
FIGURE 87-14

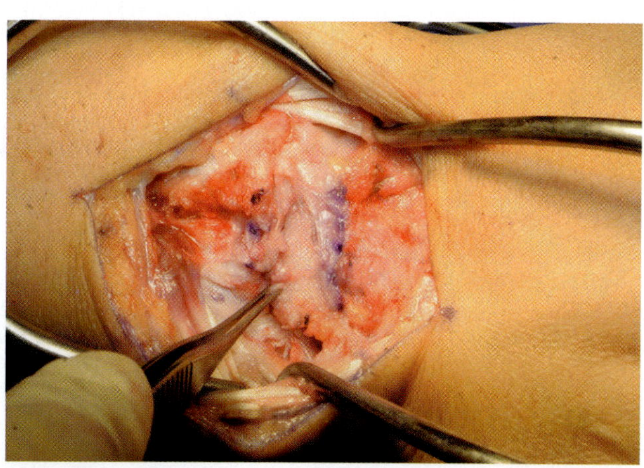

FIGURE 87-15

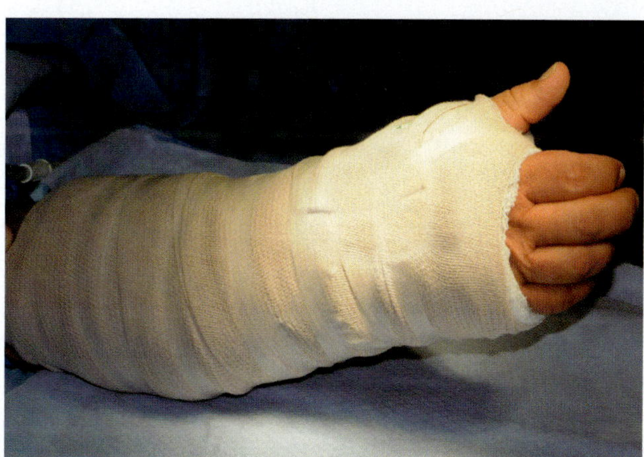

FIGURE 87-16

Additional Steps

- An additional graft is placed to fill the prepared interfaces (Fig. 87-14).
- The capsule is closed anatomically with nonabsorbable suture (Fig. 87-15).
- The retinaculum is closed leaving the extensor pollicis longus (EPL) transposed.
- The skin is closed with nonabsorbable suture.
- A bulky compressive dressing is applied to allow digital range of motion and to help control edema (Fig. 87-16).

PEARLS

If fixation intraoperatively is tenuous, postoperative cast immobilization is recommended.

PITFALLS

Premature range of motion or excessive use in noncompliant patients can lead to hardware failure and nonunion.

Postoperative Care and Expected Outcomes

- The postoperative dressing is maintained for 2 weeks.
- The wrist is then immobilized in a removable custom-molded splint that is worn full time except for bathing.
- Range-of-motion exercises can commence 6 to 8 weeks after surgery.
- Strengthening exercises begin at 12 weeks.
- Patients can expect to lose about 50% of their preoperative range of motion with a total arc of motion of about 60 to 90 degrees.
- Complete recovery can be prolonged—up to 12 to 18 months.

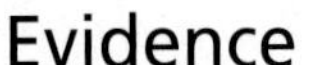

Evidence

Bain GI, Watts AC. The outcome of scaphoid excision and four-corner arthrodesis for advanced carpal collapse at a minimum of ten years. *J Hand Surg [Am]*. 2010;35:719-725.

This study evaluated 31 patients who were available for review from a cohort of 35 patients who underwent scaphoid excision and four-corner arthrodesis. Minimum follow-up was 10 years. Preoperative pain scores of 6/10 decreased to 0/10 at 1 year. A decrease in wrist flexion by an average of 22% was noted. Grip strength did not change significantly. Pain scores, wrist function, patient satisfaction, and arc of motion were maintained between 1 and 10 years. Two patients required total wrist arthrodesis for persistent pain. (Level IV evidence)

Cohen, MS, Kozin SH. Degenerative arthritis of the wrist: proximal row carpectomy versus scaphoid excision and four-corner arthrodesis. *J Hand Surg [Am]*. 2001;26:94-104.

In this comparative retrospective study, 19 patients with an average of 28 months of follow-up achieved a flexion arc that was 58% of the unaffected side and grip strength that was 79% of the unaffected side. (Level III evidence)

Dacho AK, Baumeister S, Germann G, et al. Comparison of proximal row carpectomy and midcarpal arthrodesis for the treatment of scaphoid nonunion advanced collapse (SNAC-wrist) and scapholunate advanced collapse (SLAC-wrist) in stage II. *J Plast Reconstr Aesthet Surg*. 2008;61:1210-1218.

DASH scores improved from 43 preoperatively to 21 postoperatively in this group of 17 patients. They noted 72% grip strength of the opposite side, 56% flexion-extension arc, and an 88% rate of return to previous employment. (Level III evidence)

Vance MC, Hernandez JD, Didonna ML, et al. Complications and outcome of four-corner arthrodesis: circular plate fixation versus traditional techniques. *J Hand Surg [Am]*. 2005;30:1122-1127.

Thirty-one patients with an average of 59 months of follow-up reported recovery of 50% of the flexion-extension arc and 60% of the radioulnar deviation arc as well as 79% of grip strength. DASH scores averaged 8; 30 of the 31 patients were able to return to previous employment activities. (Level IV evidence)

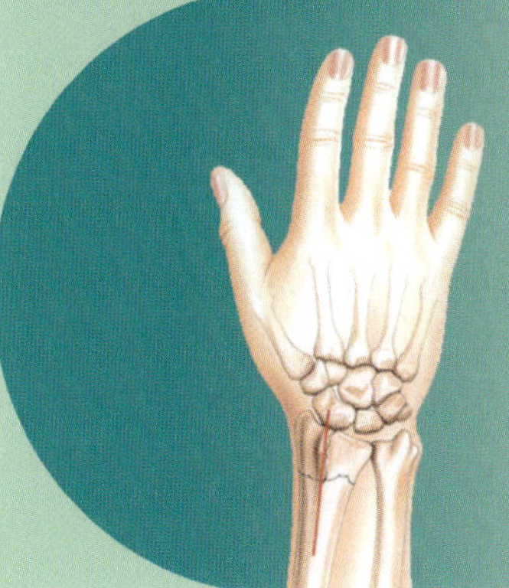

Four-Corner Fusion Using a Circular Plate

Shimpei Ono, Sandeep J. Sebastin, and Kevin C. Chung

See Video 66: 4-Corner Fusion with a Circular Plate

Indications

- Scaphoid nonunion with capitolunate arthritis (SNAC wrist stage III)
- Static scapholunate instability with capitolunate arthritis (SLAC wrist stage III)
- Midcarpal arthritis

Examination/Imaging

Clinical Examination

- A sequential progression of arthritic changes has been described for scaphoid nonunion and static scapholunate instability. They are called the scaphoid nonunion advanced collapse (SNAC) and scapholunate advanced collapse (SLAC), respectively (Fig. 88-1).
- A four-corner fusion involves removal of the scaphoid (only the distal scaphoid may be removed in SNAC) and fusion of the lunate, triquetrum, capitate, and hamate. The other option is a proximal row carpectomy (PRC) that involves removal of the scaphoid, lunate, and triquetrum and allows the capitate to articulate in the lunate fossa of the radius.
- A four-corner fusion is the preferred option in stage III SNAC/SLAC because the capitolunate joint is arthritic and a PRC will result in an arthritic capitate articulating with the lunate fossa.
- In stage II SNAC/SLAC, a PRC or a four-corner fusion may be done. A PRC is simpler and does not rely on fusion of small carpal bones. A four-corner fusion maintains carpal height and provides better hand strength compared with PRC.
- A diagnosis of SNAC or SLAC wrist is often made in patients who seek medical advice for other conditions of the wrist. They are usually minimally symptomatic or asymptomatic, tend to be older, and engage in less physically demanding tasks. This group of patients should be managed conservatively with activity modification, intermittent splintage, and nonsteroidal analgesics. Surgery should be reserved for patients who fail conservative measures or in younger symptomatic patients in whom further progression of arthritis can be prevented.

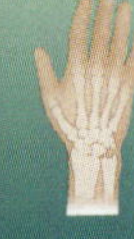

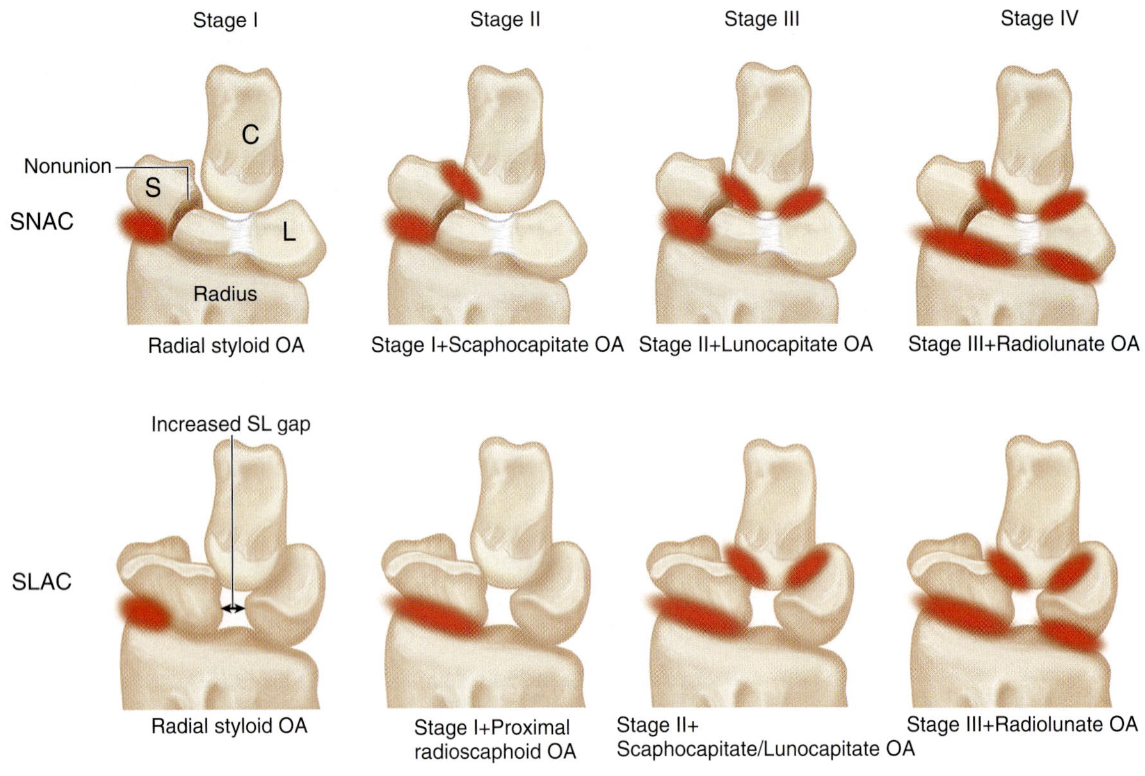

FIGURE 88-1

Imaging

- Standard wrist posteroanterior and lateral views are usually sufficient in SNAC/SLAC wrists. One should be able to determine whether there is arthritis involving the capitate (PRC cannot be done) or arthritis involving the lunate fossa of the radius (both PRC and four-corner fusion cannot be done). If the radiograph shows ulnar translocation of the carpus, it means that the palmar radiocarpal ligaments, especially the radioscaphocapitate, are lax, and a PRC cannot be done.
- If the condition of these joints cannot be clearly assessed by a radiograph, a computed tomography scan or a wrist arthroscopy should be considered.

Surgical Anatomy

- The distal radius has two articular fossae for the scaphoid and lunate. The scaphoid fossa is shaped like a spoon and narrows as it approaches the radial styloid. This results in incongruency between the scaphoid and the scaphoid fossa during positional changes and results in uneven loading of scaphoid fossa, making degenerative changes of the radioscaphoid joint common. On the other hand, the lunate fossa is spherical and remains congruently loaded in all positions of the lunate, making the radiolunate joint highly resistant to degenerative changes.

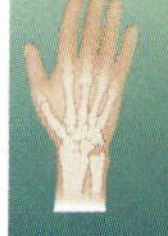

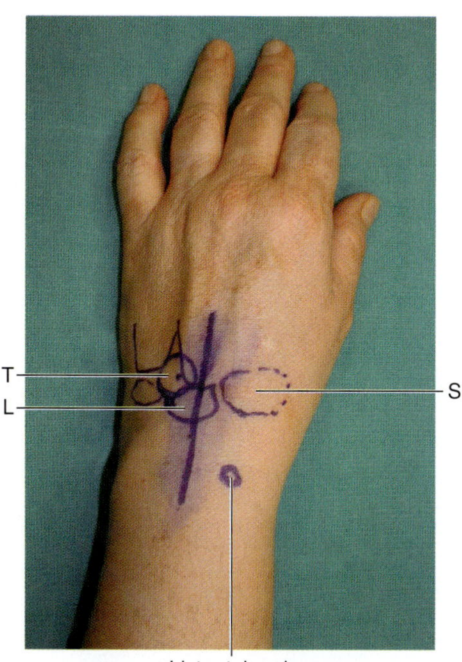

FIGURE 88-2

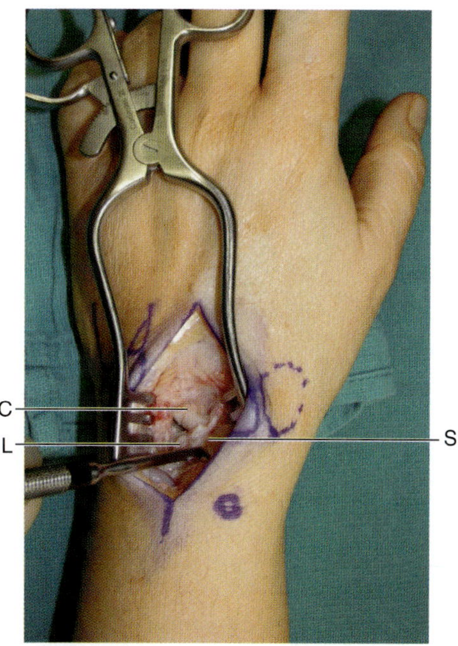

FIGURE 88-3

PITFALLS

Care is taken not to injure the branches of the radial sensory nerve.

STEP 1 PEARLS

A 0.062-inch K-wire inserted into the scaphoid to serve as a joystick can make dissection of the scaphoid from the volar capsule easier.

The entire scaphoid is removed in one piece and not in a piecemeal fashion. This ensures that portions of the scaphoid attached to the volar capsule are not left behind.

STEP 1 PITFALLS

Care is taken to preserve the radioscaphocapitate and long radiolunate ligaments.

Great care must be taken not to scratch the articular surface of the lunate fossa on the radius when dissecting off the volar capsule from the scaphoid.

The scaphoid is used for harvesting cancellous bone graft only if the scaphoid is healthy, for example in scapholunate dissociation. For scaphoid nonunion, the bone is not good quality, so it is preferable to obtain bone graft from the radius or the iliac crest. Artificial bone graft may also be used, but fusion must be ensured by radiograph before initiating wrist motion.

Exposures

- A 6-cm dorsal longitudinal incision centered over the radiocarpal joint in line with the long finger metacarpal is made (Fig. 88-2). Sharp dissection is carried down to the extensor retinaculum. Skin and subcutaneous tissue flaps are raised on both sides. The third dorsal compartment is identified and opened along its entire length. The extensor pollicis longus (EPL) tendon is left in its sheath and not transposed. One must know the location of the EPL when incising the wrist capsule proximally. The wrist capsule is opened longitudinally and dissection performed to elevate the second and fourth compartments such that the second and fourth compartment tendons are maintained within the compartment. This exposes the scaphoid, lunate, triquetrum, capitate, and hamate.
- Figure 88-3 shows a Freer elevator within the SL interval demonstrating a complete rupture of the SL ligament.

Procedure

Step 1: Scaphoidectomy

- The scapholunate ligament is divided, and a sharp-edged Freer or an Obwegeser periosteal elevator is used to separate the scaphoid from the volar capsule. After adequate detachment of the volar capsule, a rongeur is used to hold the scaphoid and using a twisting motion, the surgeon removes the scaphoid as one piece.
- The cancellous bone within the scaphoid is harvested for bone grafting.

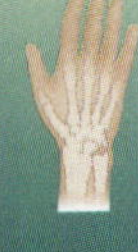

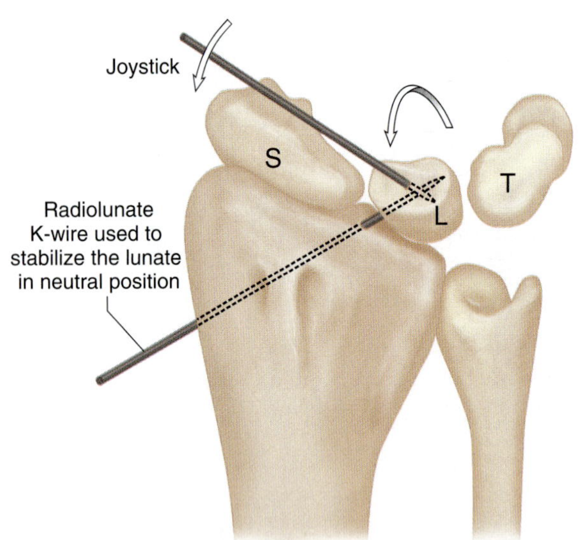

FIGURE 88-4

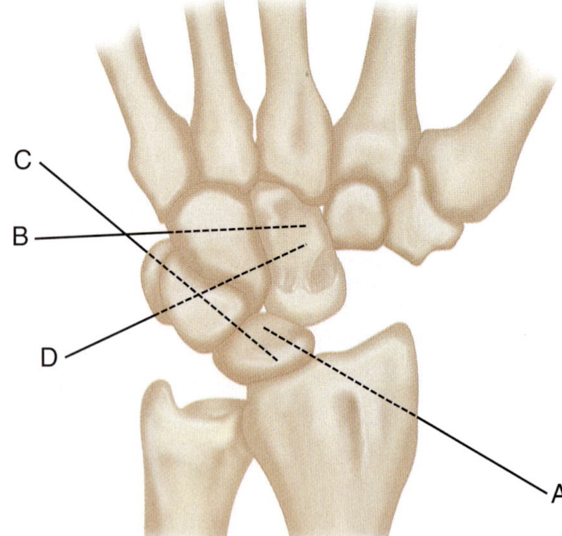

FIGURE 88-5

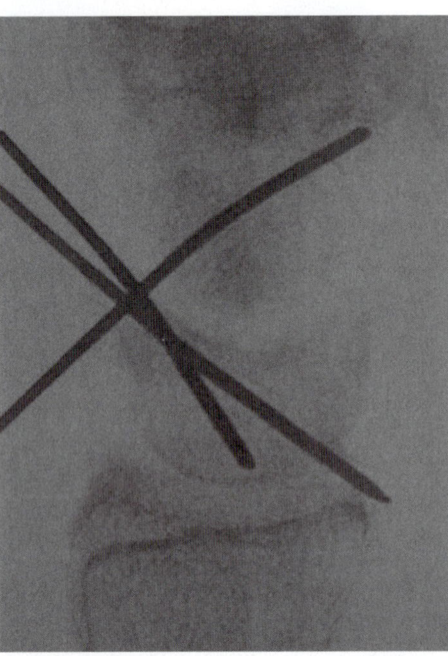

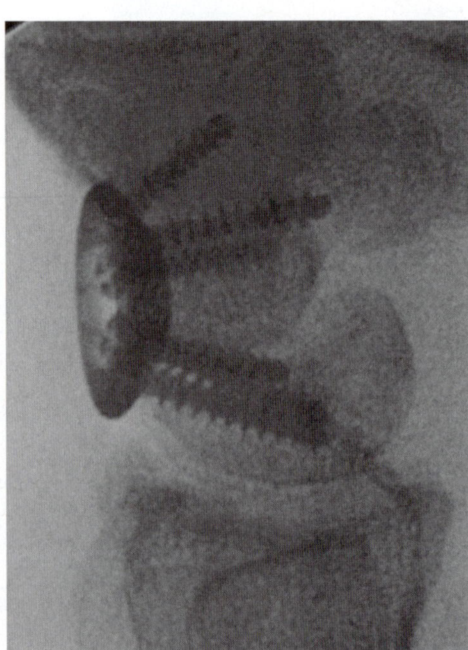

FIGURE 88-6

STEP 2 PEARLS

- The correction of the dorsiflexed lunate is the key step in four-corner fusion because the position of remaining three carpal bones is related to the position of the lunate. It is important to stabilize the corrected lunate to the radius before fusion (Fig. 88-4). Otherwise, the lunate may re-displace to a dorsal position after plate fixation (Fig. 88-6). With the lunate in neutral position, the patient's wrist can move dorsally and volarly with equal ease. If the lunate remains in dorsal posture, wrist flexion will be difficult.

Step 2: The Lunate Is Stabilized in Neutral Position

- A 0.045-inch K-wire is inserted into the lunate as a joystick and used to correct the dorsally flexed position of the lunate (DISI) and bring it into a neutral position. This is confirmed by fluoroscopic examination. Then an oblique K-wire is passed from the distal radius to the lunate to maintain this position. This K-wire must be placed volarly to avoid the circular plate screws from impinging the wire (Fig. 88-4).

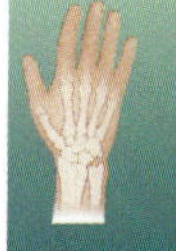

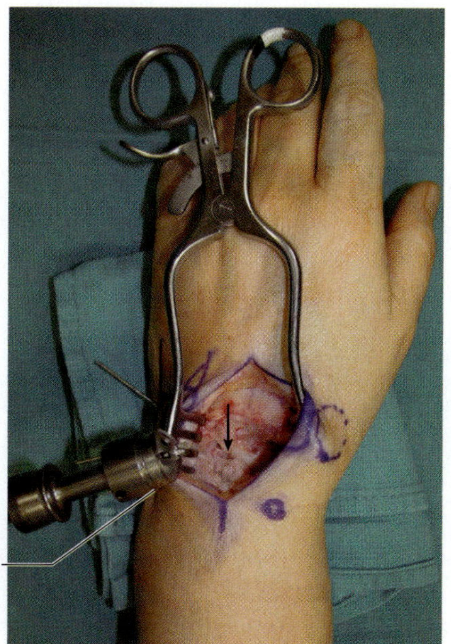

FIGURE 88-7

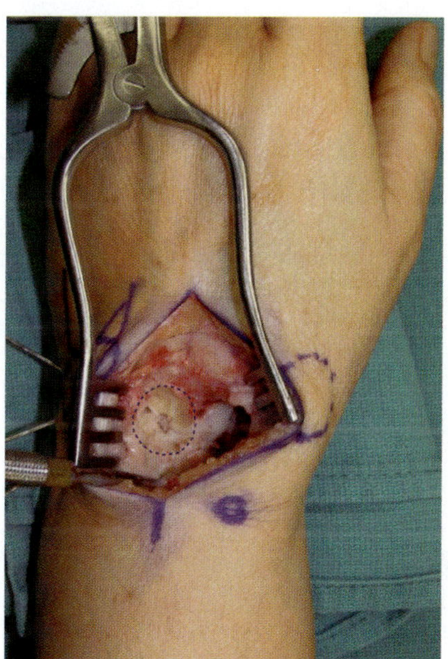

FIGURE 88-8

STEP 3 PEARLS

The K-wires should be placed in the volar half of the carpus to prevent impingement with the reamer for the hub plate.

STEP 4 PITFALLS

It is important to ream to sufficient depth so that the entire circular plate lies under the bony surfaces of the four bones, to prevent postoperative impingement of the plate on the distal radius.

Step 3: Stabilize the Carpal Bones with K-Wires

- Additional K-wires are placed from the ulnar wrist into the hamate-capitate (*B* in Fig. 88-5), the triquetrolunate (*C* in Fig. 88-5), and the triquetral-hamate-capitate (*D* in Fig. 88-5) to stabilize all four carpal bones.

Step 4: Ream the Carpal Bones

- The reamer is centered over the junction of the four carpal bones (Fig. 88-7). We used Hub Cap Limited Wrist Fusion Plate from Acumed LLC.
- The carpal bones are reamed until the dorsal surface of the carpal bones lies between the two lines on the reamer head. This ensures that the fusion plate will sit sufficiently deep within the carpus (Fig. 88-8).

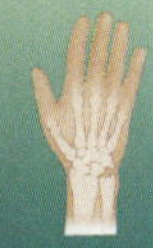

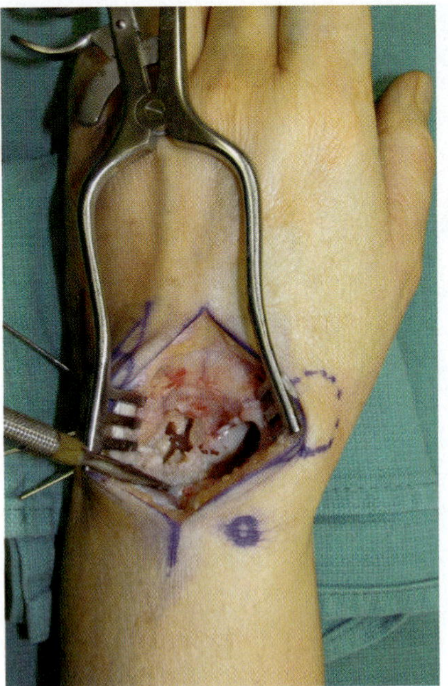

FIGURE 88-9

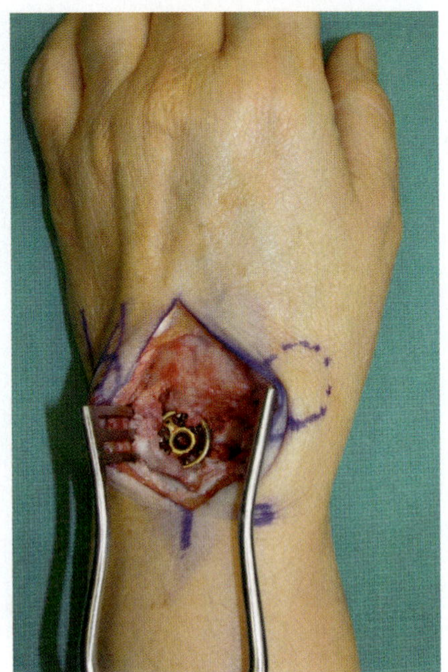

FIGURE 88-10

Step 5: Denude the Cartilage between the Four Bones

- The reamer is removed, and the cartilage between the four bones is denuded with a side-cutting bur. Constant irrigation during burring is important to prevent heat-induced necrosis of the bone in the fusion site. The burring must be meticulous to remove all articular surfaces between the four bones (Fig. 88-9).

Step 6: Fix the Circular Plate

- An appropriate-sized circular plate is placed into the depression, and the circular plate is aligned such that the maximal purchase of all four bones is ensured by the screws. The number of screws and the order of screw placement vary between manufacturers, and the surgeon is advised to check with the manufacturer. We use an Acumed Hub Plate that allows a maximum of seven screws. The single hole slot is directed toward the hamate. The recommended order of screw fixation is hamate, lunate, capitate, and triquetrum. One screw is placed into each bone first, and this is followed by additional screws, if there is space for them (Fig. 88-10).

STEP 6 PEARLS

The Acumed system uses a 2.0-mm drill bit and 2.7-mm self-tapping screws.

The first screw into the hamate should not be fully tightened to avoid the screw from tipping towards the hamate. Rather, the screw is tightened loosely, followed by placing the lunate screw. Both screws are then tightened sequentially to seat the circular plate securely within the four bones.

STEP 6 PITFALLS

Holes should be drilled to within 2 mm of the far cortex. Avoid bicortical drilling.

Step 7: Pack Bone Graft

- Bone graft harvested from the scaphoid is packed into the gap between the joints before the circular plate is placed. Additional bone graft can be harvested from the distal radius or using artificial bone chips.
- All screws are now tightened, and the preliminary K-wires are removed.

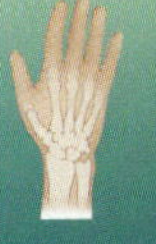

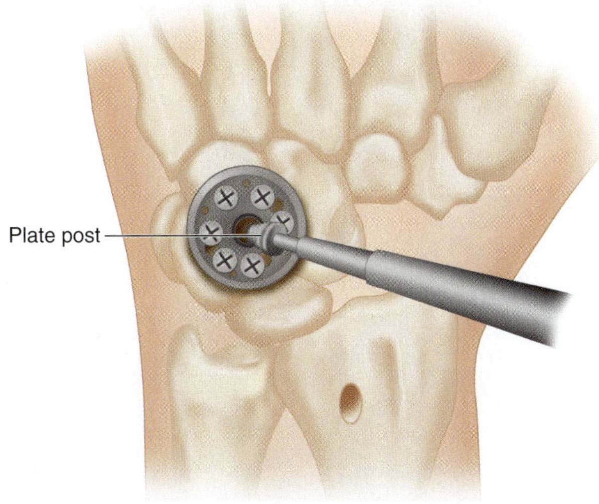

FIGURE 88-11

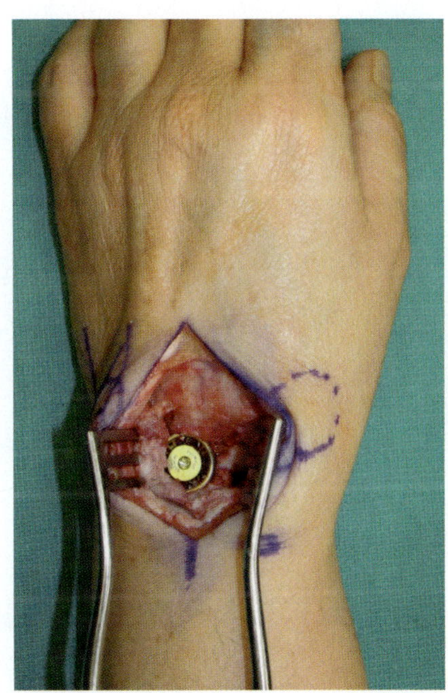

FIGURE 88-12

Step 8: Remove the Plate Post and Apply the Screw Cover

- The Acumed plate has a central plate post. The central hole is packed with bone graft, followed by a screw cover that is locked into the plate to prevent migration of screws, which was a problem in prior designs (Fig. 88-11).
- The screw cover prevents back-out of the carpal screws (Fig. 88-12).

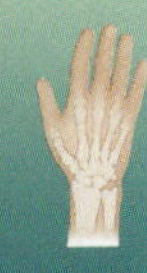

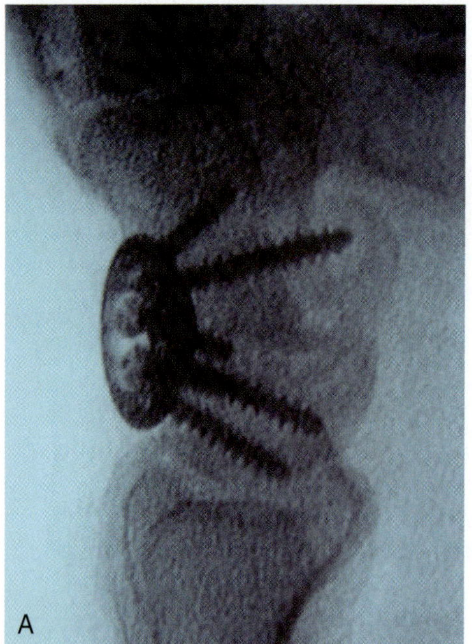

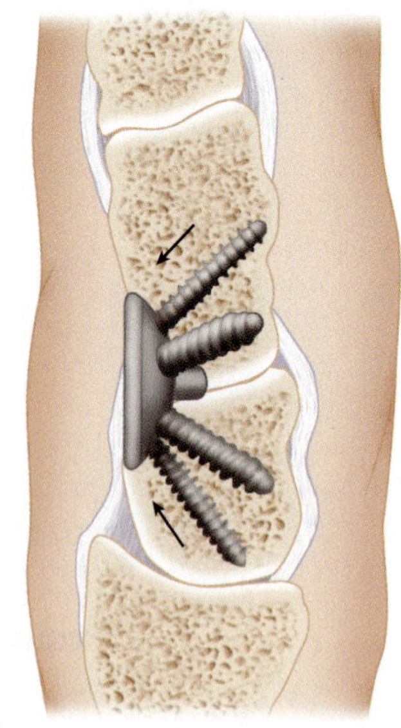

A B

FIGURE 88-13

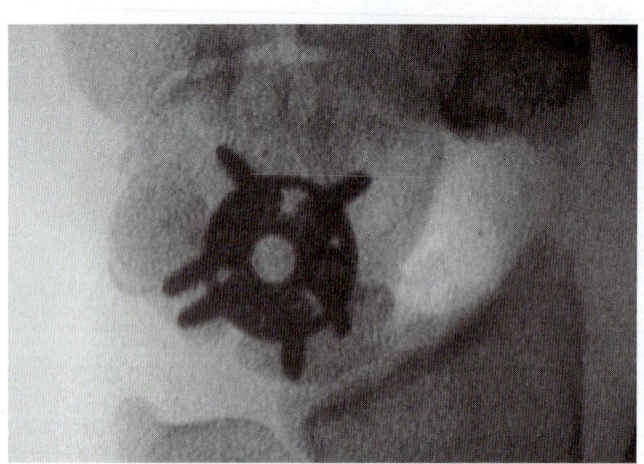

FIGURE 88-14

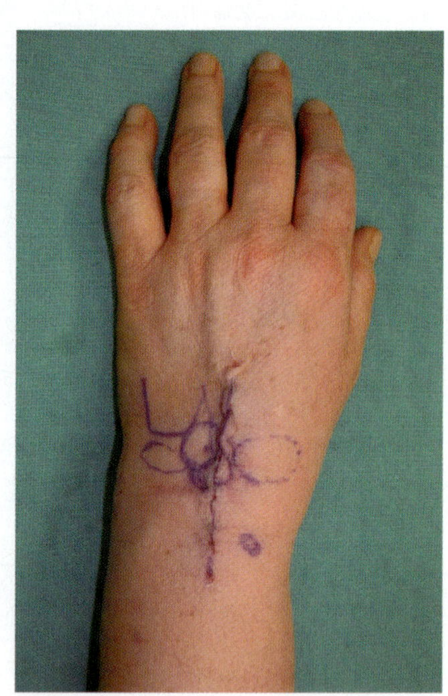

FIGURE 88-15

Step 9: Assess Final Fixation

- A final fluoroscopic examination is done to confirm proper placement of the implant and to check for any impingement during range of motion (Figs. 88-13 and 88-14).

Step 10: Closure

- The wrist capsule is closed with 3-0 Vicryl sutures. The tourniquet is deflated, and all bleeding areas are cauterized.
- The extensor retinaculum that is partially opened is closed with 3-0 Vicryl sutures.
- Skin is closed with 4-0 PDS sutures (Fig. 88-15).

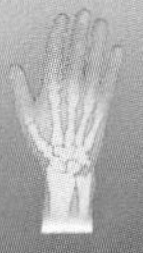

Postoperative Care and Expected Outcomes

- Patients are immobilized in a volar short arm plaster splint for 1 week and then fitted with a removable Orthoplast wrist splint to be worn for the next 5 weeks. Patients are started on active finger exercises at 1 week. Wrist motion is not permitted because prior complications such as screw loosening or breakage were related to early motion in patients who started stressing the wrist before the fusion had healed. Wrist motion is not commenced for at least 6 weeks or even longer, until radiographic fusion is seen.
- Patients are permitted to perform light activities of daily living while wearing the splint.
- The early results using the dorsal circular plating system for four-corner fusion were disappointing and associated with a high incidence of screw fractures and nonunion rates. However, improved implants and prolonged wrist splinting may improve the outcomes. The postoperative range of motion is about 50% of the uninjured side, and the grip strength is about 80% of the uninjured side.

Evidence

Chung KC, Watt AJ, Kotsis SV. A prospective outcomes study of four-corner wrist arthrodesis using a circular limited wrist fusion plate for stage II scapholunate advanced collapse wrist deformity. *Plast Reconstr Surg*. 2006;118:433-442.

This study prospectively evaluated 11 patients who underwent four-corner fusion using a circular plate internal fixation technique. Patients with symptomatic stage II SLAC wrist were treated with scaphoid excision and four-corner fusion using the Spider Limited Wrist Fusion Plate (KMI, San Diego, Calif.). Patients were prospectively evaluated at 6 months and 1 year using a standard study protocol with radiographs, functional tests, and an outcomes questionnaire. Grip strength, lateral pinch strength, and Jebsen-Taylor test scores at 1 year were not significantly different from preoperative values. Mean active ROM was 87 degrees preoperatively and 74 degrees at 1-year follow-up (P = .19). The Michigan Hand Outcomes Questionnaire showed no significant improvement in function, activities of daily living, work, pain, or patient satisfaction. The mean pain scores decreased from 54 preoperatively to 42 1-year postoperatively (P = .30), indicating persistent wrist discomfort. Three patients had broken screws: one was asymptomatic, one required 3 months of strict wrist immobilization, and one was reoperated for symptomatic nonunion. The authors concluded that four-corner fusion using the first-generation Spider plate technique had the advantage of earlier mobility and more patient comfort because of the absence of protruding K-wires; however, patients continued to have disabling pain, functional limitations, work impairment, and low satisfaction scores postoperatively. (Level II evidence)

Merrell GA, McDermott EM, Weiss AP. Four-corner arthrodesis using a circular plate and distal radius bone grafting: a consecutive case series. *J Hand Surg [Am]*. 2008;26:635-642.

The authors performed a retrospective assessment of 28 patients who underwent a standardized four-corner arthrodesis with a second-generation circular plate and distal radius bone grafting for a diagnosis of SLAC, SNAC, or midcarpal arthrosis. Complete data were obtained for 26 of the patients and partial data for the other 2. Follow-up examination included visual analogue scale and activity scores, work status, posteroanterior and lateral radiographs, bone union status, grip strength, range of motion, and complications. Average follow-up was 46 months. Range of motion averaged 45% of the uninjured side (average extension, 35 degrees; average flexion, 26 degrees). Grip strength averaged 82% of the uninjured side. The mean visual analogue scale pain and activity scores were 2.3/10 and 2.4/10. Only 1 patient required job modification because of wrist impairment. Radiographs demonstrated union of the primary capitolunate fusion mass in all of the cases. There was 1 case of probable but not certain peritriquetral nonunion and 1 case of asymptomatic loss of radiolunate joint space; in terms of hardware, there was screw back-out (of one screw) in 1 case, and the plate broke in 1 case. Two patients underwent reoperation, one for radial styloid impingement pain and the other for lack of flexion. The authors concluded that use of a dorsal circular plate and distal radius bone grafting produced excellent and reproducible results in this consecutive series. Notably, there was no development of secondary arthritic changes at the radiolunate joint, indicating a reasonable durability to the procedure. (Level IV evidence)

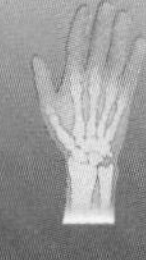

Vance MC, Hernandez JD, Didonna ML, Stern PJ. Complications and outcome of four-corner arthrodesis: circular plate fixation versus traditional techniques. *J Hand Surg [Am]*. 2005;30:1122-1127.

The authors reviewed the clinical and radiographic results of 27 cases of scaphoid excision and four-corner arthrodesis using a circular plate compared with 31 cases of traditional techniques (e.g., wires, staples, screws). Patients were surveyed using the standardized DASH questionnaire and classification scales for pain and satisfaction. Objective measurements included grip strength and ROM. The rate of major complications (nonunion or impingement) was much greater with circular plate fixation (48%) versus traditional fixation techniques (6%). With the plate procedure, the grip strength and arc of motion decreased about 30% and 52%, respectively, compared with decreases of 21% and 50%, respectively, for the traditional fusion methods. Additionally, subjective patient dissatisfaction was 40% in the plate group compared with 0% in the traditional group. The authors concluded that the increased complication and dissatisfaction rates associated with plate fixation may be attributable to possible biomechanical imperfections or increased technical demands with this fusion system. (Level III evidence)

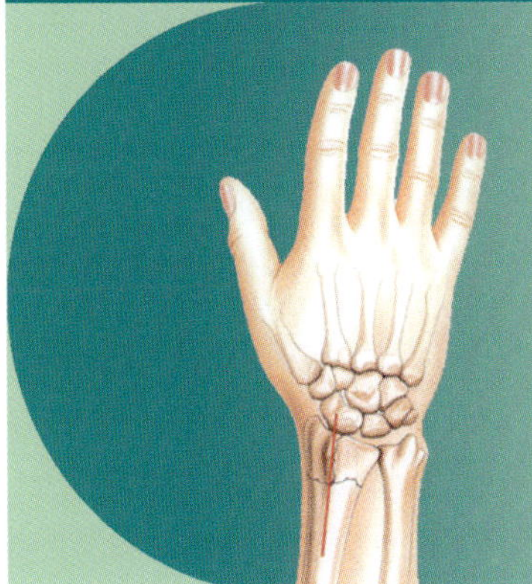

PROCEDURE 89

Total Wrist Fusion

Jeffrey A. Greenberg

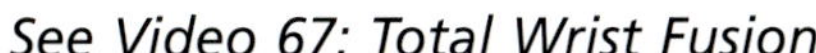

See Video 67: Total Wrist Fusion

Indications

- Painful wrist with limited range of motion (ROM)
- Osteoarthritis, inflammatory arthritis, and posttraumatic arthritis
- Multijoint involvement, radiocarpal and midcarpal
- Failed limited wrist fusions
- Failed soft tissue reconstructions
- Carpal instability patterns
- Patient's desire for definitive, one-stage treatment
- Contraindications for joint arthroplasty
- Failed arthroplasty

Examination/Imaging

Clinical Examination

- Painful ROM
- Limited ROM
- Decreased grip strength
- May have hypertrophic synovitis
- Visible deformity
- Pain, instability, and crepitus with load
- Associated carpal tunnel syndrome

Imaging

- Plain films are usually sufficient to diagnose degenerative changes at the radiocarpal and midcarpal articulations. Fig. 89-1 shows a patient with scaphoid nonunion advanced collapse.

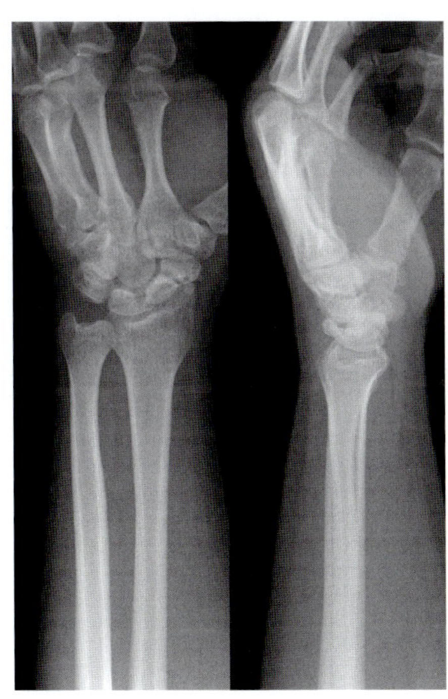

FIGURE 89-1

Surgical Anatomy

- Deformity is frequently encountered.
- Alignment must be corrected, and the wrist must be positioned appropriately.
- Hypertrophic synovitis may obscure bony anatomy.

Positioning

- The patient is placed in a supine position with the affected extremity on a table designed for hand surgery.
- Operative procedures are more easily performed with the surgeon at the head as opposed to being seated at the axilla.

We would like to acknowledge Kevin C. Chung, MD, for providing the clinical pictures for this chapter.

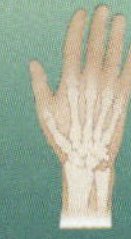

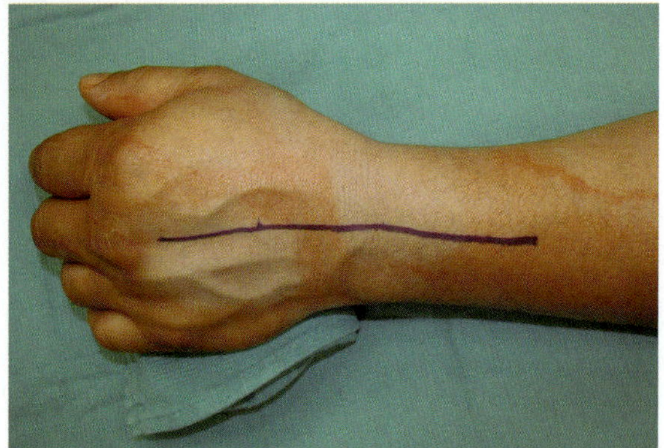

FIGURE 89-2

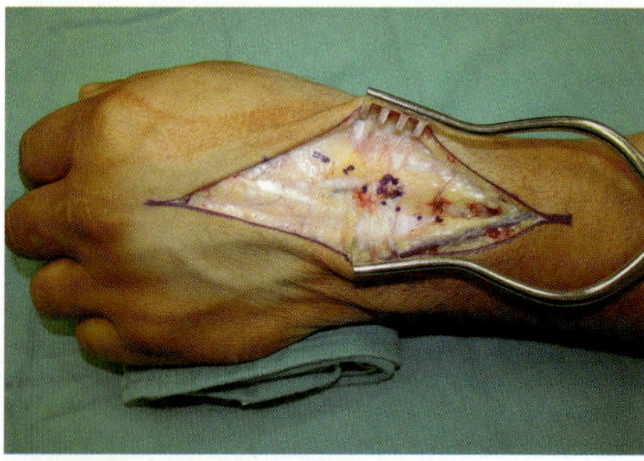

FIGURE 89-3

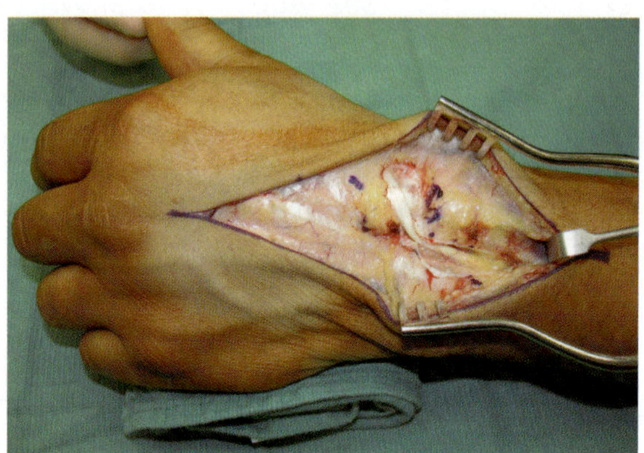

FIGURE 89-4

Exposures

- A dorsal midline incision is used, centered at the radiocarpal joint and extending past the midpoint of the long finger metacarpal and proximally, about 5 cm proximal to the Lister tubercle (Fig. 89-2).
- Flaps are elevated, keeping cutaneous nerves in the flaps (Fig. 89-3).
- Incise third dorsal compartment and retract the extensor pollicis longus (EPL) tendon (Fig. 89-4).
- Raise retinacular flaps, exposing the second to fifth extensor compartments.
- The posterior interosseous nerve (PIN) is located on the floor of the fourth extensor compartment. A PIN excision is performed after retracting the extensor tendons.
- A radially based capsular flap is formed by incising the dorsal intercarpal and dorsal radiocarpal ligaments and elevating them off the dorsal triquetrum (Fig. 89-5).
- Subperiosteal dissection is used to expose the dorsal radius, the carpus, and the long finger metacarpal (Fig. 89-6).

PEARLS

The extensor carpi radialis longus (ECRL) and extensor carpi radialis brevis (ECRB) tendons can be released from the dorsal aspects of index finger and long finger metacarpals, respectively, and used to augment soft tissue coverage of the hardware when closing the capsular flap.

An alternative capsulotomy is straight midline longitudinal (see Fig. 89-6).

PITFALLS

Maintain a thick capsular flap so that it may be used to cover the plate.

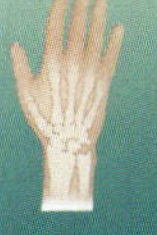

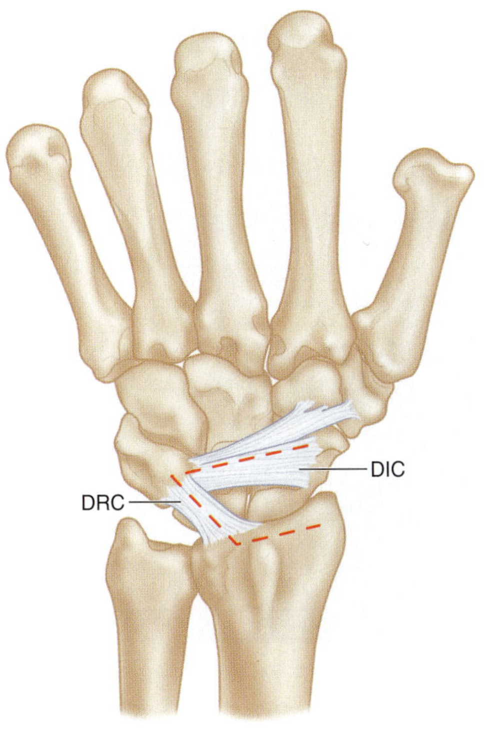

FIGURE 89-5

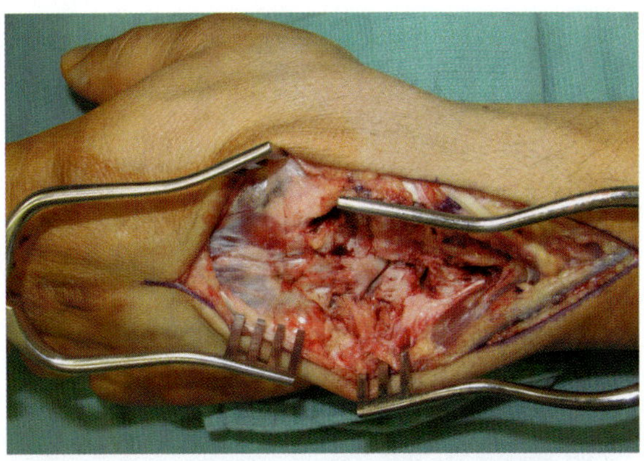

FIGURE 89-6

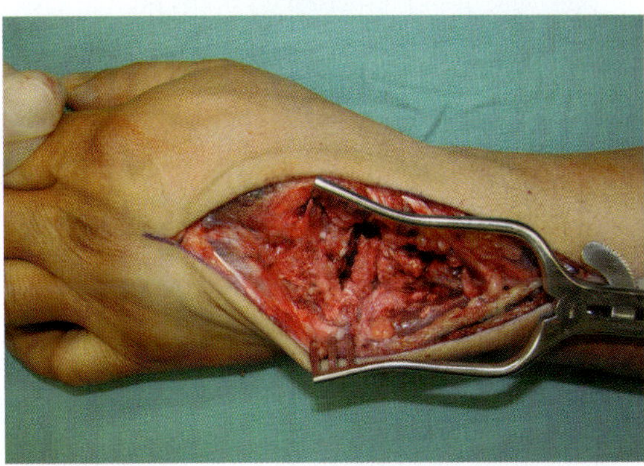

FIGURE 89-7

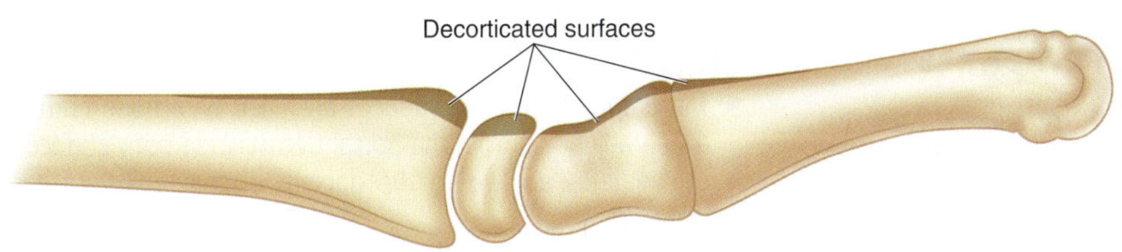

FIGURE 89-8

STEP 1 PEARLS

Ensure that the joint can be reduced and aligned. Soft tissue releases may be necessary to facilitate alignment of the radius, lunate, capitate, and long finger metacarpal.

In chronic cases with severe carpal deformity (e.g., neglected perilunar fracture-dislocations), excision of the proximal carpal row will facilitate alignment before fusion.

The entire joint height should not be taken down for preparation. This ensures that carpal height will be maintained.

Procedure

Step 1

- The dorsal aspect of the radius, carpus, and third carpometacarpal (CMC) joints are decorticated with an osteotome. The dorsal radius, including Lister tubercle, must be contoured by decortication or else it will be difficult to seat the plate on the dorsal radius (Fig. 89-7).
- The joints to be fused are prepared by removing articular cartilage and subchondral bone. These include the radioscaphoid, radiolunate, scaphocapitate, lunocapitate, and third CMC joints (Fig. 89-8).
- The ulnar joints (lunotriquetral, triquetrohamate) are not included in the fusion mass.

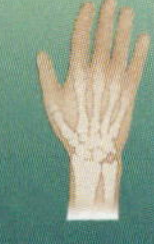

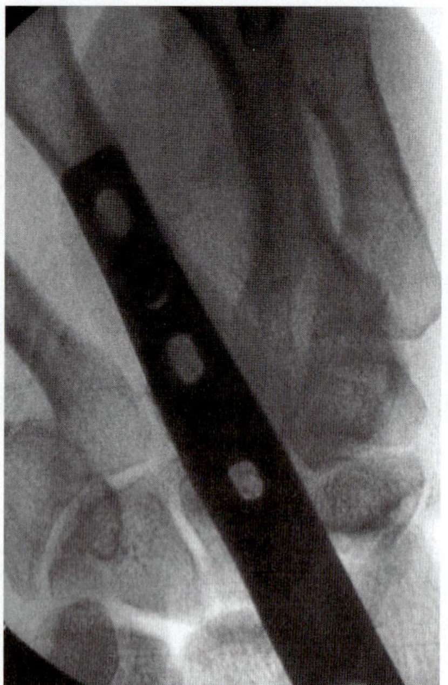

FIGURE 89-9

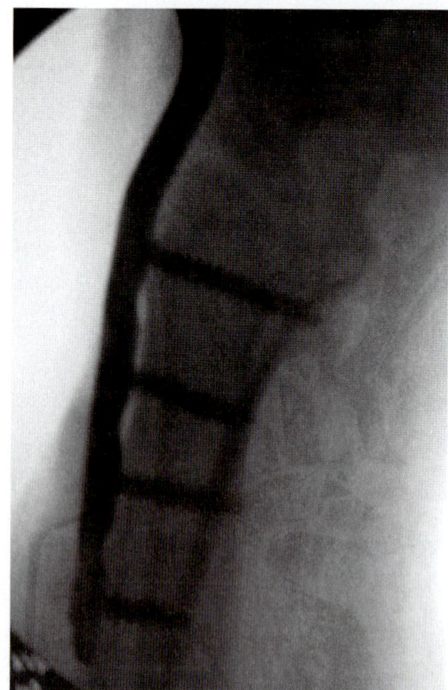

FIGURE 89-10

STEP 1 PITFALLS

Failure to achieve carpal reduction and alignment will make plate application and appropriate positioning difficult.

STEP 2 PEARLS

The wrist fusion fixation plate will not lie on a noncontoured surface of radius. The surgeon needs to resect bone and cartilage to provide an adequate fixation surface for the plate to rest on.

Desired arthrodesis position is 10 degrees of extension and slight ulnar deviation.

STEP 2 PITFALLS

Failure to contour the dorsal radius will result in poor adaptation of the plate to the bone and will compromise fixation.

In addition, a prominent plate that does not lie on the bone will be difficult to cover with soft tissue when closing the capsule and retinaculum. Retinacular deficiency may lead to extensor dysfunction.

Step 2

- Determine the plate location on the dorsal radius, carpus, and metacarpal, paying particular attention to rotation.
- In some cases, a groove in the distal radial articular surface may need to be created to accept the curved portion of the plate.
- Harvest bone graft from the distal radius through a cortical window or drill hole adjacent to the plate.

Step 3

- The prepared articular surfaces are filled with bone graft harvested from the distal radius and from the dorsal decorticated bony surfaces.
- The plate is applied to the dorsum of the radius, carpus, and long finger metacarpal.
- Affix plate to the long finger metacarpal in neutral rotation (Fig. 89-9).
- Affix plate to radius in compression mode (Fig. 89-10).
- Supplement fixation with the oblique carpal screw (Fig. 89-11).
- Use intraoperative fluoroscopy to assess plate and screw position.

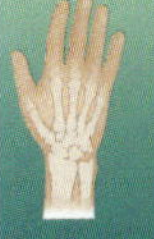

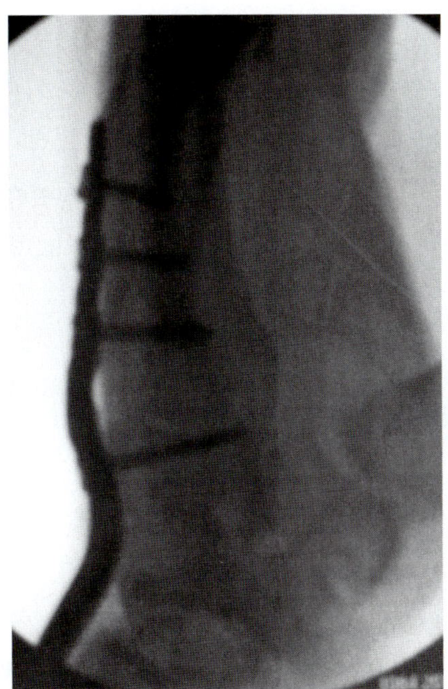

FIGURE 89-11

STEP 3 PEARLS

Expose enough of the metacarpal so that the plate can be centrally positioned and aligned with the appropriate rotational orientation.

The location of the metacarpal screw can be marked with a marker, and with the plate removed, the orientation of the screw can be assessed.

Locking screw fixation can be used in patients with poor bone stock (Fig. 89-12).

Alternative sources of bone graft are iliac crest, olecranon, proximal tibia, and allograft.

STEP 3 PITFALLS

Malrotation is the most common malalignment when performing plate fixation. The wrist position should be neutrally rotated, extended, and slightly ulnar-deviated.

Ensure full forearm rotation and passive digital ROM after plate application.

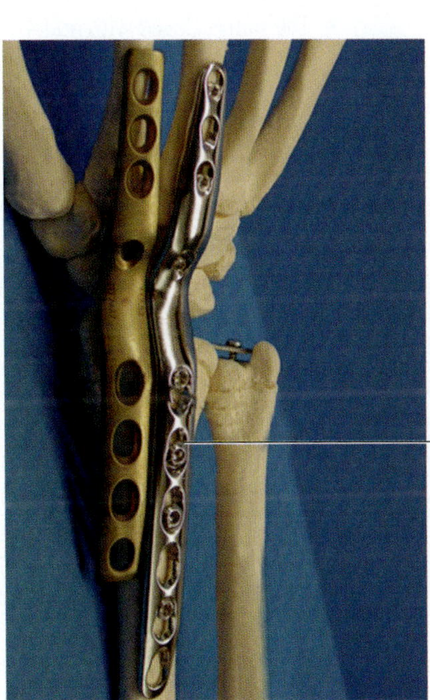

FIGURE 89-12

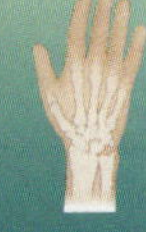

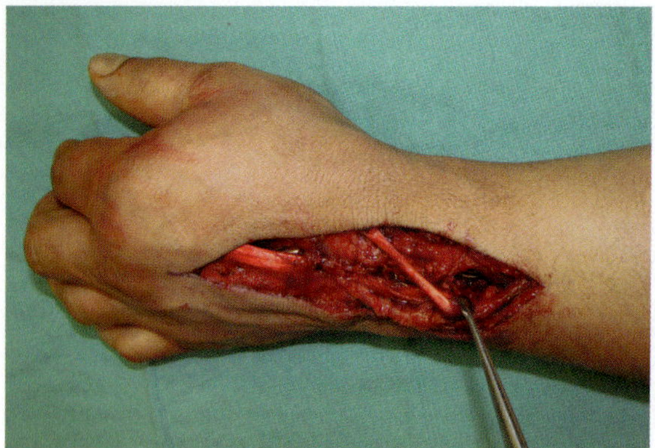

FIGURE 89-13

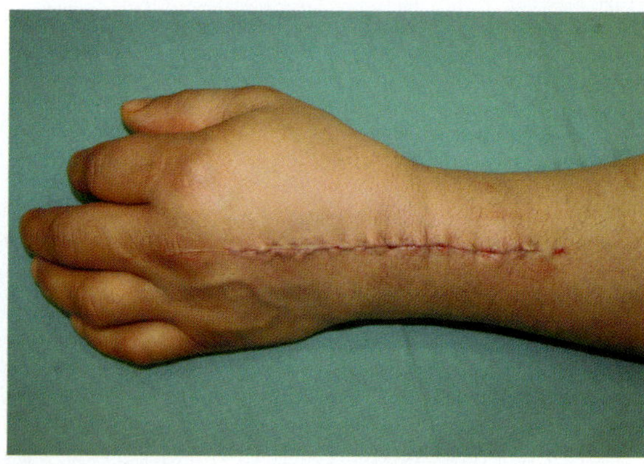

FIGURE 89-14

STEP 4 PEARLS

The ECRL and ECRB tendons can be released from the metacarpals and incorporated into the capsular closure when soft tissue coverage is deficient or limited.

Alternative coverage of the plate can be achieved using a split extensor retinaculum, placing one flap deep to the extensor tendons over the plate and one flap dorsal to the extensor tendons.

STEP 4 PITFALLS

Splinting with the metaphalangeal joints in extension can result in intrinsic tightness and loss of digital ROM.

Step 4

- Once the plate is secured, additional bone graft is packed around prepared joints.
- The capsular flap can frequently be closed over the plate by advancing the ulnar attachment radially.
- The extensor retinaculum is closed leaving the EPL transposed (Fig. 89-13).
- The skin is closed with nonabsorbable suture or a subcuticular absorbable suture (Fig. 89-14).
- A bulky dressing to control edema is applied with a splint supporting the wrist.

Postoperative Care and Expected Outcomes

- If intraoperative fixation is stable, a removable splint can be fitted 2 weeks after surgery. This splint is worn full-time except for bathing.
- If fixation or patient compliance is tenuous, then postoperative cast immobilization is recommended.
- Digital ROM and edema control are emphasized during this timeframe.
- A removable splint is worn until 3 months after surgery.
- Strengthening exercises may begin at 12 weeks after surgery.
- Expected patient outcomes are pain relief, solid fusion, full digital ROM, and full forearm rotation.
- Radiographs should show consolidation of prepared articular surfaces with no hardware loosening or lucency (Fig. 89-15).
- The patient achieves of about 80% grip strength of the dominant hand.
- The patient is able to complete most activities of daily living (Fig. 89-16).
- Perineal care and using the hand and wrist in tight spaces may be limited.
- Recovery can be prolonged.

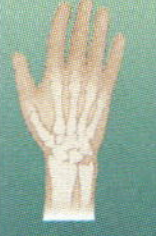

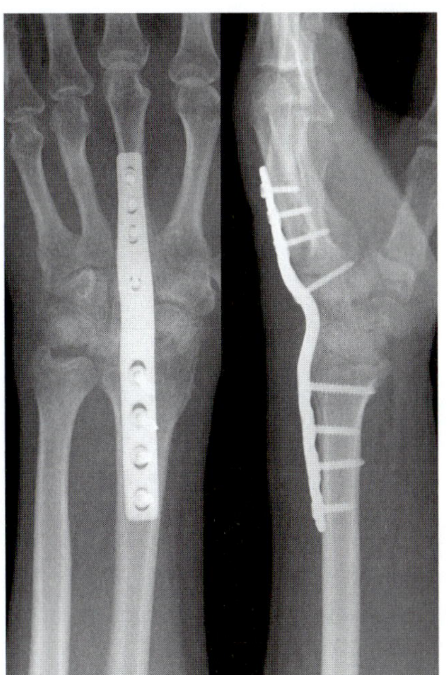

FIGURE 89-15

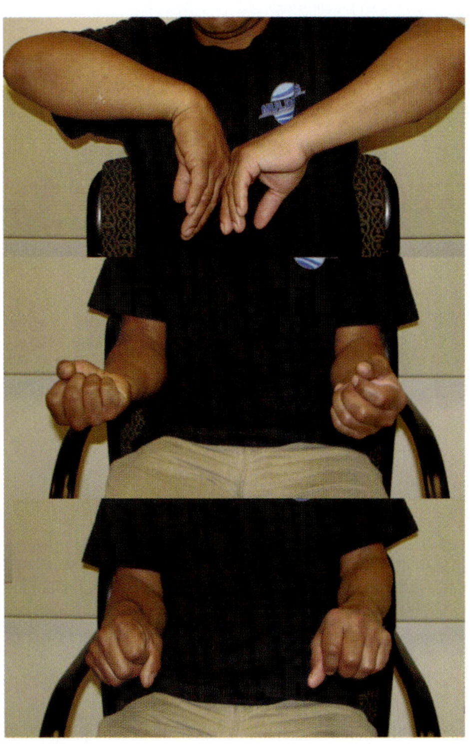

FIGURE 89-16

Evidence

Cavaliere CM, Chung KC. Total wrist arthroplasty and total wrist arthrodesis in rheumatoid arthritis: a decision analysis from the hand surgeons' perspective. *J Hand Surg [Am]*. 2008;33:1744-1755.

Although the emphasis of this decision-analysis study was to look at quality adjusted life-years of arthroplasty versus arthrodesis in rheumatoid wrists, the article supports the effectiveness of wrist arthrodesis for patients with unstable, painful wrists affected by rheumatoid arthritis. (Level IV evidence)

Cavaliere CM, Chung KC. A cost-utility analysis of nonsurgical management, total wrist arthroplasty, and total wrist arthrodesis in rheumatoid arthritis. *J Hand Surg [Am]*. 2010;35:379-391.

Both arthroplasty and arthrodesis were shown to be cost-effective treatments for rheumatoid arthritic patients with painful, stiff, or unstable wrists. (Level IV evidence)

Solem H, Berg NJ, Finsen V. Long term results of arthrodesis of the wrist: a 6-15 year follow up of 35 patients. *Scand J Plast Reconstr Surg Hand Surg*. 2006;40:175-178.

Forty fused wrists in 35 patients, mostly rheumatoid patients, were evaluated at an average of 10.5 years after surgery. The study compared the results between Mannerfelt and plate arthrodesis and showed that pain relief was excellent in 28 of the 40 wrists. Patients with arthrodeses using plate fixation demonstrated better results for all variables studied. Wrists plated in dorsal extension gave the best scores for function and strength. (Level IV evidence)

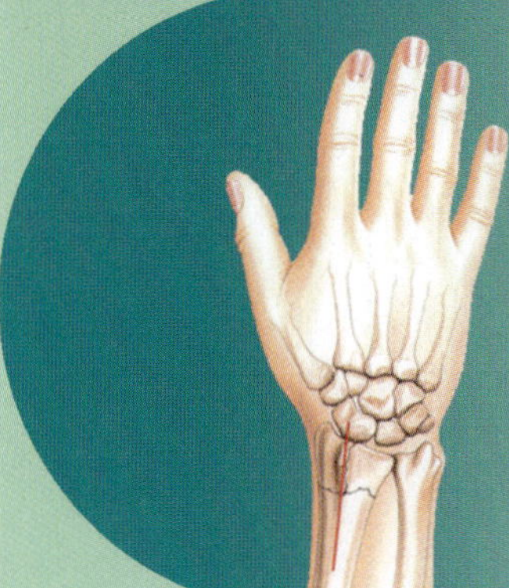

Total Wrist Arthroplasty

Nathan S. Taylor and Kevin C. Chung

Indications

- Destructive and painful wrist conditions resulting from rheumatoid arthritis (RA), osteoarthritis (OA), or trauma
- The procedure is contraindicated in patients with the following conditions:
  - Contractures of the wrist from tendon imbalance or spasticity because of the potential abnormal loading on the implant
  - Prior wrist infections or ongoing infection
  - High demand occupations such as farmers or manual laborers; these patients are better suited for a total wrist fusion
  - Severely osteopenic or osteoporotic bone because poor bone stock will not support the implant
  - Unstable wrists owing to poor soft tissue envelopes because this will not stabilize the implant

Examination/Imaging

Clinical Examination

- One must evaluate active and passive wrist range of motion to determine any presence of carpal subluxation or dislocation and distal radioulnar (DRU) joint stability.
- Additionally, the integrity of the flexor and extensor tendons of the wrist and hand should be assessed.
- One must perform a detailed history of the patient's functional demands, activities, occupation, hobbies, and home circumstances. Patients should be given a trial of splint immobilization, and arthroplasty should be considered for those who find that period of immobilization intolerable.

Imaging

- Posteroanterior, oblique, and lateral radiographs of the wrist are essential to determine extent of wrist destruction. Conditions such as scapholunate advanced collapse (SLAC) and scaphoid nonunion advanced collapse (SNAC) should be noted.
- Additional views of the wrist or computed tomography can be obtained to further evaluate arthritis or to assess less obvious intercarpal arthrosis.
- Wrist arthroscopy may determine whether limited wrist fusion is preferable. Patients with a preserved radiocarpal joint should be considered for motion-sparing wrist procedures such as four-corner bone fusion or proximal row carpectomy. Rheumatoid patients with radiocarpal arthritis but a preserved midcarpal joint may be eligible for radiolunate or radioscapholunate fusion to maintain midcarpal motion.

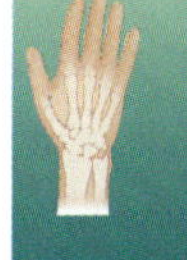

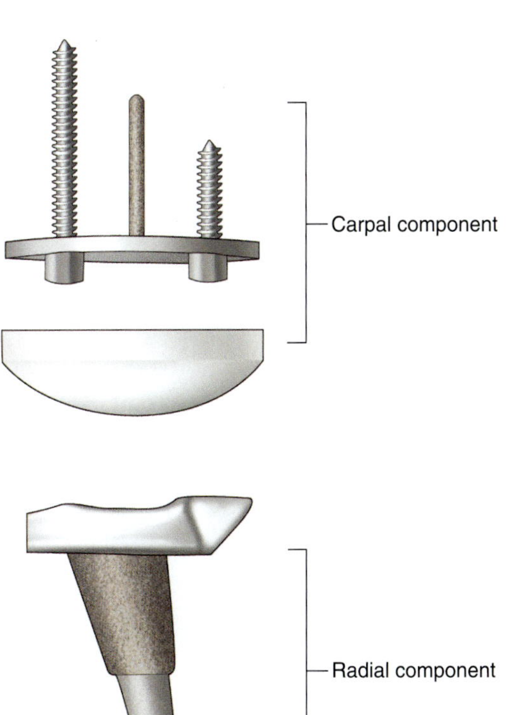

FIGURE 90-1

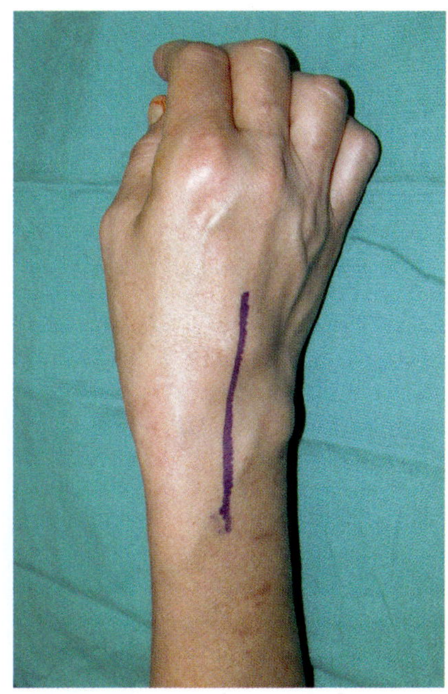

FIGURE 90-2

Surgical Anatomy

- The implant described in this chapter is the Universal II implant design, which is the most popular total wrist arthroplasty implant used in the United States. Other implant designs are available, but comparative or long-term studies are not presented to determine which implant type is most durable and has the lowest complication rate. The implant design consists of two components. The carpal component is fixated with two screws (Fig. 90-1).
- The radial component has an articular inclination of 15 degrees to simulate the anatomy of the distal radius.
- Distal and proximal stems are porous coated, which has the theoretical advantage of allowing osseointegration of the components.
- The size of the implant placed can be estimated preoperatively from the wrist radiograph.

Positioning

- The procedure is performed under tourniquet control with the patient in the supine position and the extremity abducted with the hand on a hand table.
- A mini C-arm is mandatory to check the position of various implant components intraoperatively.

Exposures

- An 8-cm incision is made on the dorsal wrist, centered on the axis of the long finger metacarpal (Fig. 90-2).
- Radial and ulnar skin flaps are elevated, and the extensor retinaculum is visualized.

PEARLS

If there is arthritic change involving the DRU joint, a Darrach procedure is performed by resecting the distal ulna at a 45-degree oblique apex-ulnar angle. RA patients often have DRU disease, and distal ulna excision is performed to alleviate future problems. For OA patients with only radiocarpal disease, the radioulnar joint can be preserved.

The head of the resected ulna should be saved for bone graft.

The ECRB, and preferably the ECRL tendon as well, should be intact or otherwise reconstructible.

A segment of the posterior interosseous nerve can be excised just proximal to the radiocarpal joint.

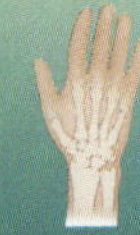

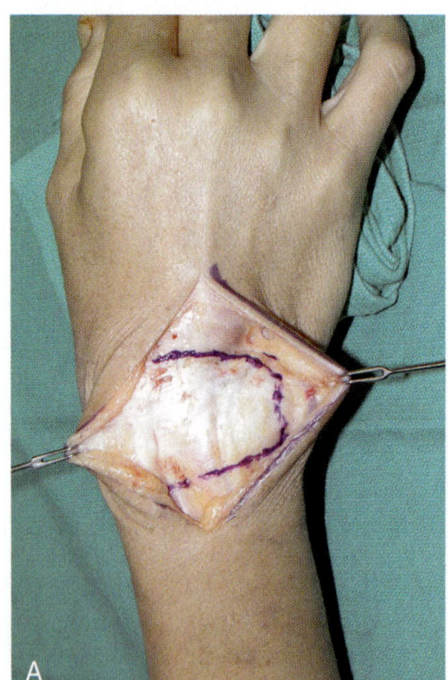

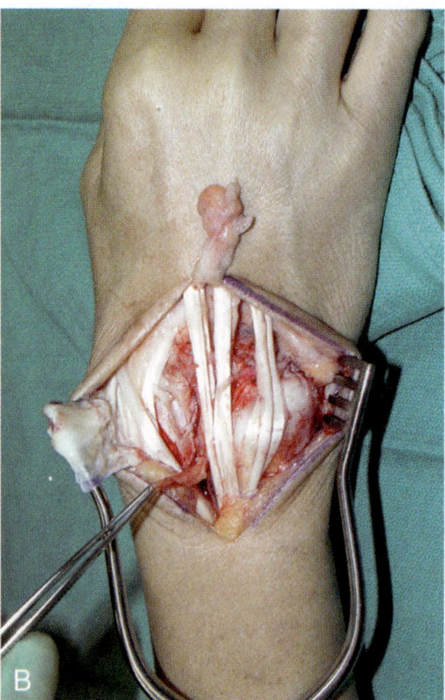

FIGURE 90-3

- The entire extensor retinaculum is elevated from the sixth dorsal compartment all the way to the radial attachment over the first compartment. The septa between the compartments are taken down to create a continuous flap of extensor retinaculum. The elevation of the extensor retinaculum stops between the first and second compartments (Fig. 90-3).
- The extensor tendons are then retracted to expose the wrist.
- The wrist capsule is elevated subperiosteally proximal to the radiocarpal joint as a rectangular, distally base flap (Fig. 90-4A and B). The purpose of the wrist capsular flap is to cover and to provide stout capsular support for the implant.

Procedure

Step 1

- The wrist is flexed to have an end-on view of the radius articular surface. A bone awl is placed 5 mm below the dorsal articular surface of the radius just slightly radial to the Lister tubercle (Fig. 90-5).
- The radial alignment guide is inserted into the cavity created by the awl, and fluoroscopy is used to confirm that the guide rod is centered in the radius, both in the anteroposterior and lateral planes (Fig. 90-6).

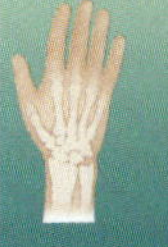

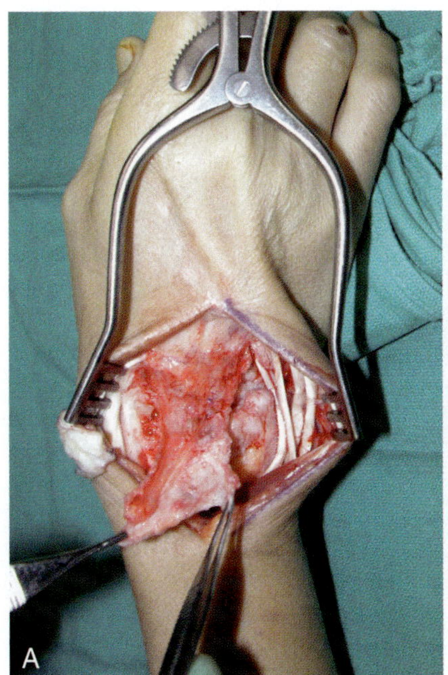

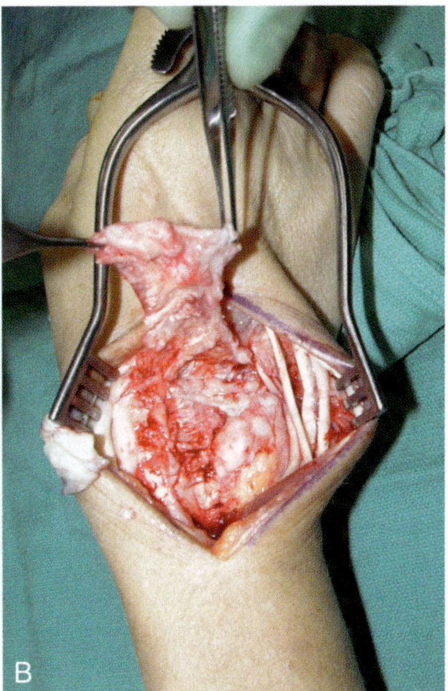

FIGURE 90-4

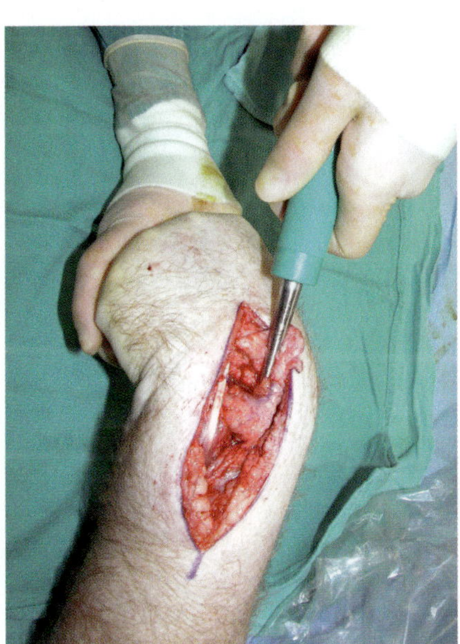

FIGURE 90-5

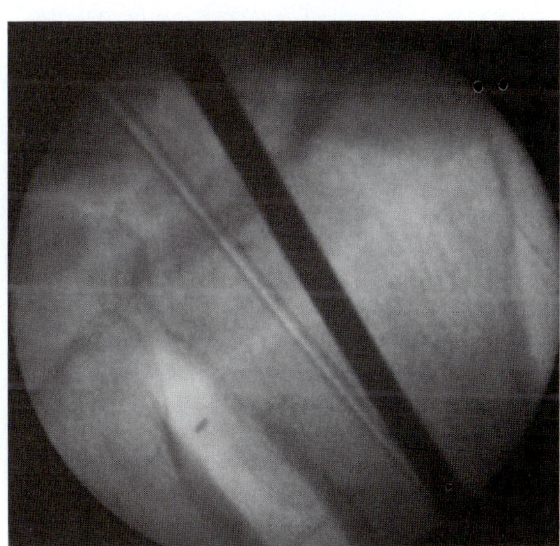

FIGURE 90-6

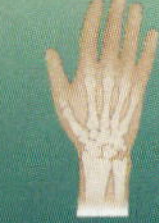

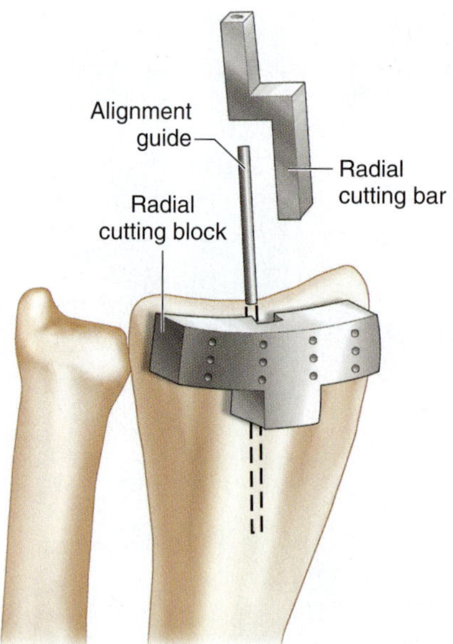

FIGURE 90-7

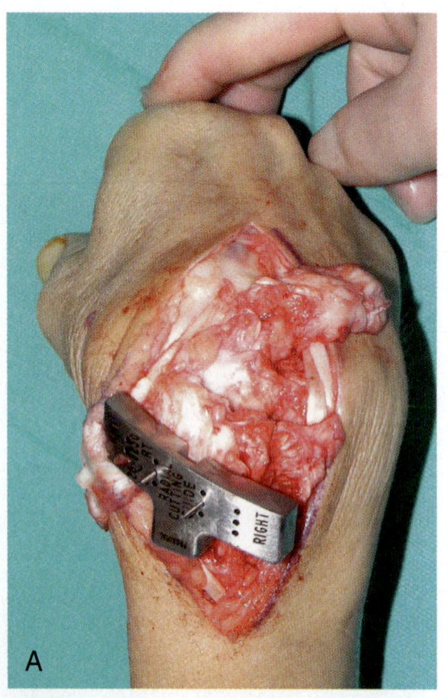

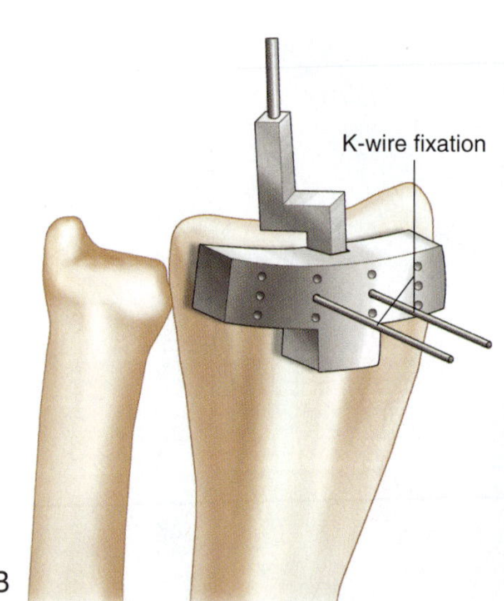

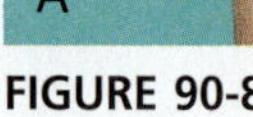

FIGURE 90-8

STEP 2 PEARLS

Remove part of the radial styloid in rheumatoid patients with ulnar translation to facilitate realignment of the wrist.

STEP 2 PITFALLS

The flexor tendons and median nerve are at risk for a saw injury because of their close proximity to the volar aspect of the radius and care should be taken to avoid this.

Step 2

- After confirmation of the position of the alignment guide, the articular surface of the radius is cut. The radial cutting bar is slipped on the alignment guide, and the radial cutting block is then mounted onto the guide bar for positioning (Fig. 90-7). This system requires minimal resection of the articular surface to preserve the stability of the soft tissue envelope around the implant.
- Kirschner wires are used to stabilize the cutting guide block against the radius. There are three rows of K-wire fixation points that correspond to a distance of about 2 mm between the rows. This is to allow placement of the guide bars more proximally or more distally if necessary to achieve the appropriate amount of bone resection (Fig. 90-8A and B). After scoring the dorsal radius with the oscillating saw, the cutting block and the K-wires are removed, and the radius cut is completed (Fig. 90-9A and B).

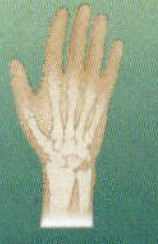

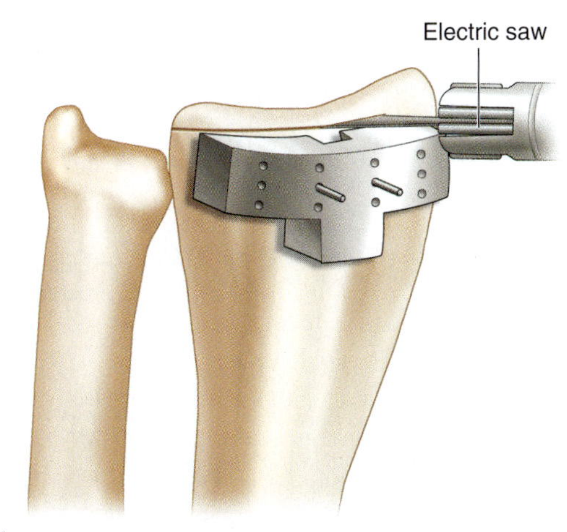

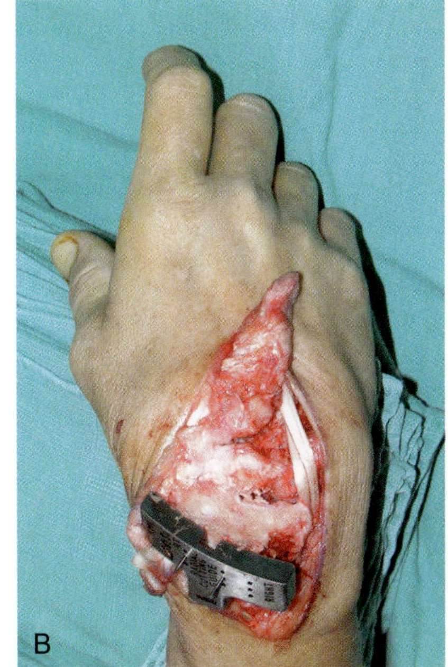

FIGURE 90-9

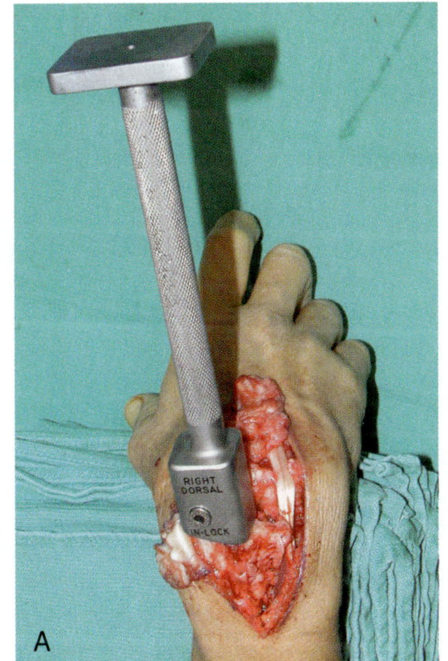

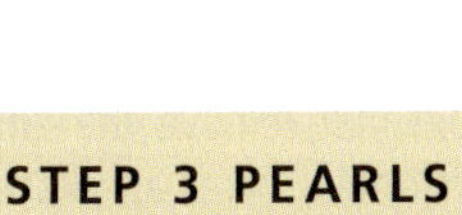

FIGURE 90-10

> **STEP 3 PEARLS**
>
> *To achieve proper implant alignment, the broach is inserted slightly dorsal in the metaphysis to avoid tracking along the palmar metaphyseal flare that will cause palmar tilt of the implant.*

> **STEP 3 PITFALLS**
>
> *A very large lunate fossa defect will result in poor implant support*

Step 3

- The guide bar is again inserted into the medullary cavity, and a broach is used to prepare the cavity (Fig. 90-10A and B). A mallet is used to place the broach flush with the cut surface of the radius. A trial implant is inserted and tapped with an impactor to fully seat it (Fig. 90-11A and B). In most cases, this system is press-fit without the use of cement. An appropriate-sized trial implant should not extend past the radial and ulnar corners of the distal radius.

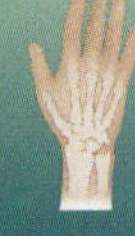

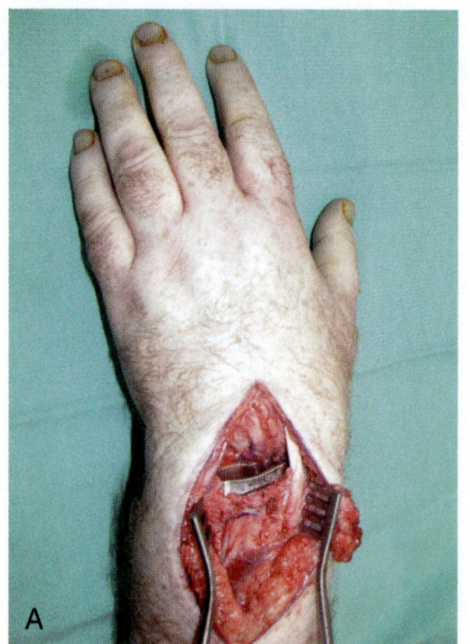

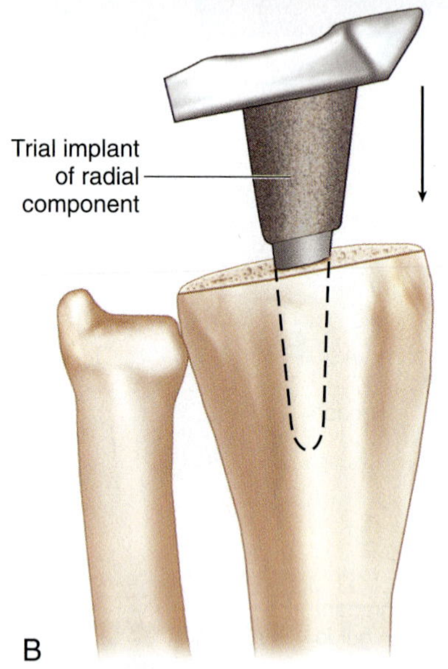

FIGURE 90-11

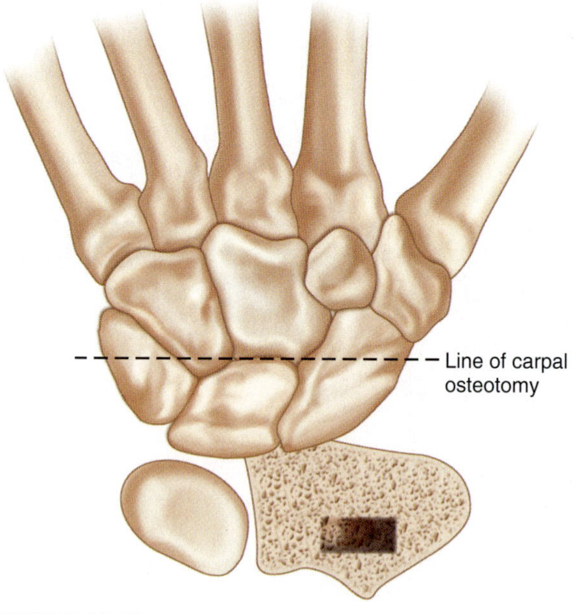

FIGURE 90-12

STEP 4 PEARLS

Minimizing resection of the carpus is vital to successful implant placement.

Step 4

- The carpal osteotomy is now performed at the level of the capitate head and across the waists of both the scaphoid and the triquetrum (Fig. 90-12).
- To facilitate the carpal osteotomy, one should first remove the lunate. If the scaphoid and the triquetrum are mobile, provisional K-wires are placed over the volar cortices of both carpal bones to stabilize them during the procedure and to avoid interfering with the osteotomy (Fig. 90-13).
- An appropriate carpal drill guide corresponding to the chosen implant size is selected. The drill guide plate is placed over the long finger metacarpal, and a 2.5-mm drill bit is drilled into the capitate. The depth of the drill hole corresponding to the implant size is marked on the drill (Fig. 90-14A and B).

Step 5

- The drill guide is removed, and the hole is countersunk. The cutting guide bar is inserted into the hole in the capitate, and the cutting guide block is placed over the cutting guide bar for carpal osteotomy (Fig. 90-15).

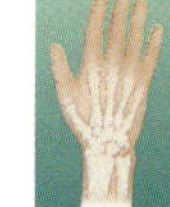

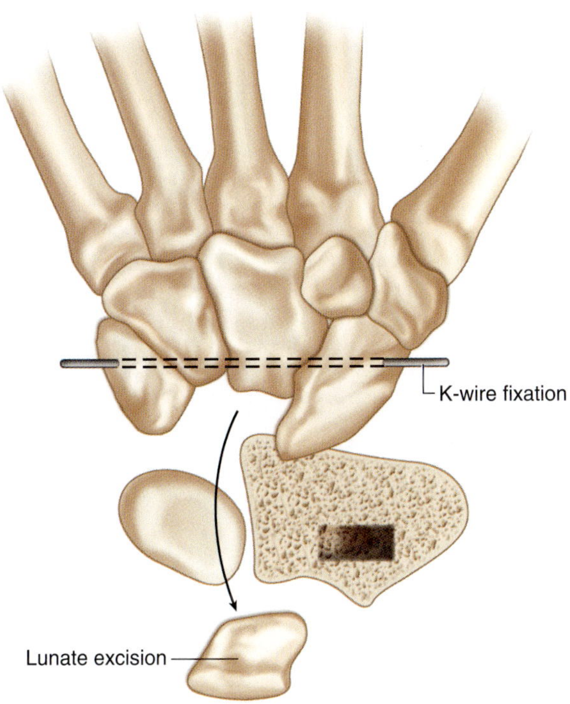

FIGURE 90-13

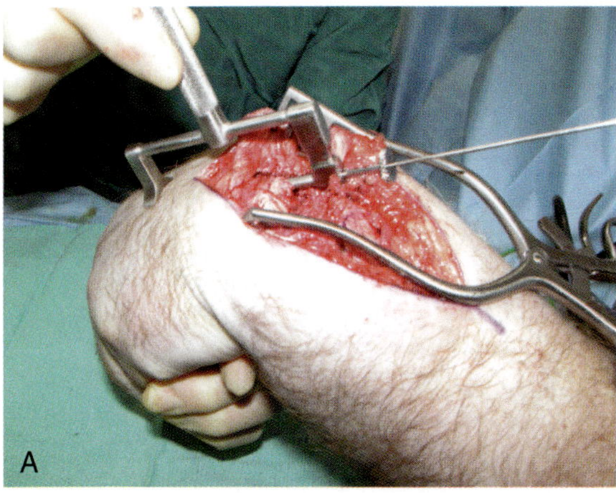

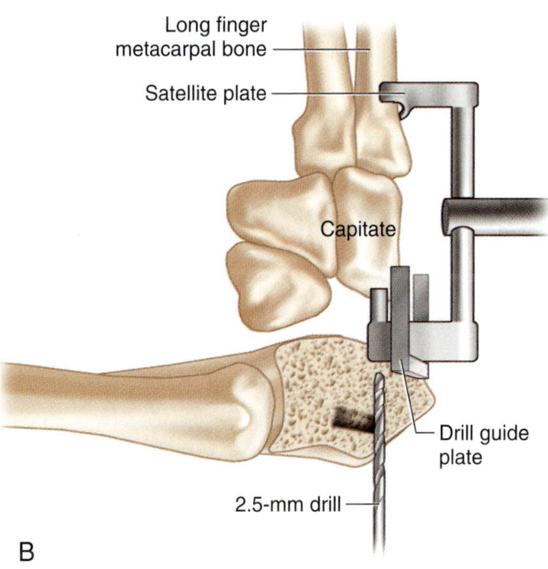

FIGURE 90-14

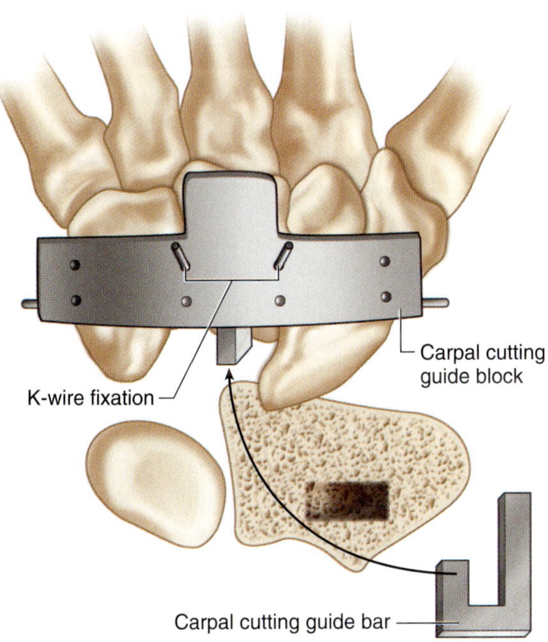

FIGURE 90-15

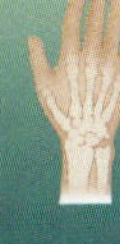

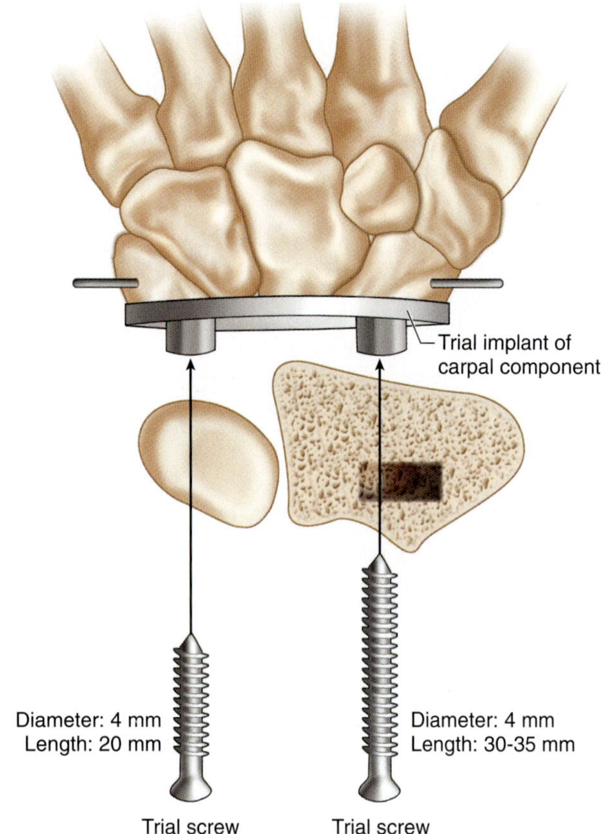

FIGURE 90-16

FIGURE 90-17

Step 6

- K-wires are placed through the cutting guide block to stabilize the carpal bone similarly to the surgical sequence in the radial component. The osteotomy is made a few millimeters distal to the head of the capitate across the waist of the scaphoid and the proximal portion of the hamate. The carpal component is inserted into the capitate hole. The dorsal edge of the carpal component must be flush with the dorsal cortex of the capitate (Fig. 90-16).

Step 7

- Screws are inserted into the radial and ulnar screw holes of the carpal component. A drill guide with the saddle sitting on the index metacarpal will be placed over the radial hole of the carpal component. A 30- to 35-mm long 2.5-mm drill hole is drilled into the trapezoid across the carpometacarpal (CMC) joint of the index metacarpal. A 4-mm screw is inserted into the radial screw hole. The ulnar hole is drilled in similar fashion, but the screw does not cross the CMC joint. The 2.5-mm drill bit is drilled into the triquetrum and the hamate. A 4-mm screw that is 20 mm in length is inserted into the triquetrum and the hamate (see Fig. 90-16).
- A polyethylene trial component is inserted over the carpal component. One should feel a "pop" when the polyethylene component fits snugly over the metal trial component (Fig. 90-17).

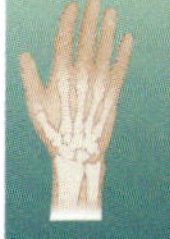

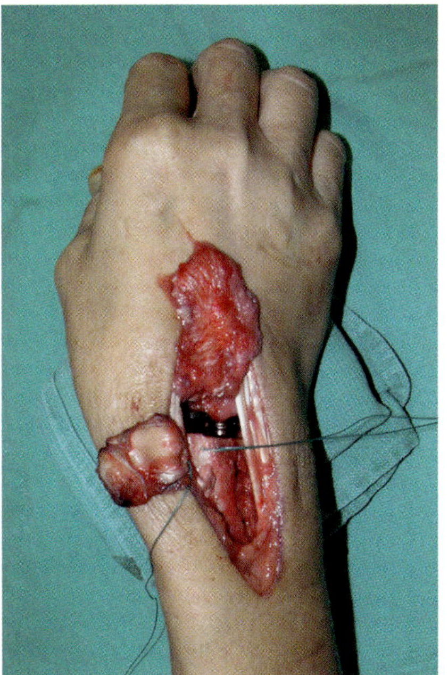

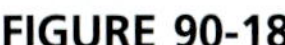

FIGURE 90-18

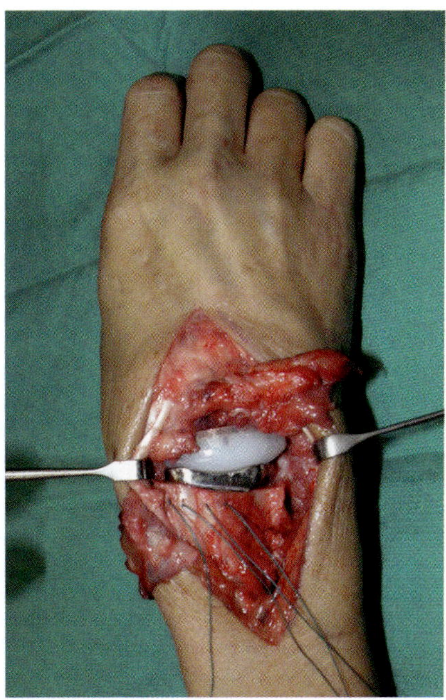

FIGURE 90-19

STEP 8 PEARLS

Step-cut tendon lengthening of the flexor carpi ulnaris and the flexor carpi radialis may be needed to achieve proper balance.

If the prosthesis remains tight, additional bone can be resected from the radius.

It is important to perform axial distraction and evaluate for excessive laxity that may lead to implant dislocation.

Step 8

- Range of motion and stability are evaluated. The wrist should rest in a neutral position, and one should observe 35 degrees of extension and 35 degrees of flexion with about 10 degrees of radial- and ulnar-deviation angles. If the wrist feels lax, a thicker polyethylene implant is inserted to add more volume to the wrist and impart more stability.
- The trial components are removed. We place drill holes on the dorsal cortex of the radius to accommodate three 2-0 braided permanent sutures for dorsal capsular repair to the radius (Fig. 90-18).

Step 9

- The carpal component is then inserted into the capitate, and the appropriate length screws are placed.
- The radial component is press-fit and impacted into the radius. An appropriate-sized polyethylene component is fitted over the carpal component using an impactor (Fig. 90-19). One must feel a "pop" as the polyethylene component fits securely into the groove in the carpal component.
- If there is motion between the carpal bones because these bones have not fused previously, a small bur is used to remove the articular surface between the triquetrum, hamate, capitate, scaphoid, and trapezoid. Previously removed bone graft is packed into the carpal intervals to achieve intercarpal fusion.

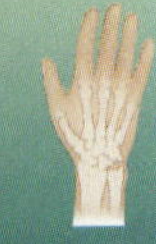

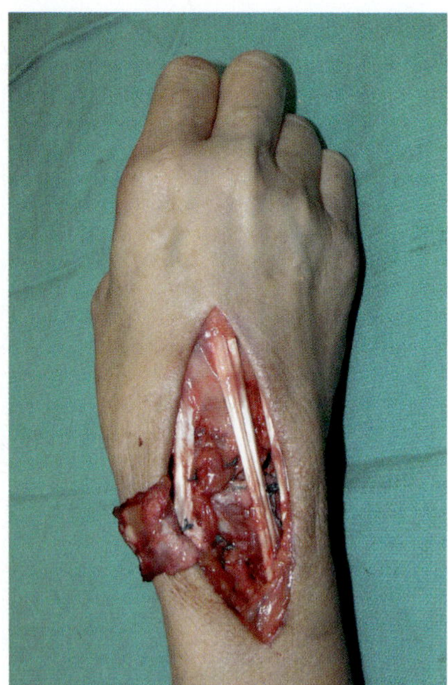

FIGURE 90-20

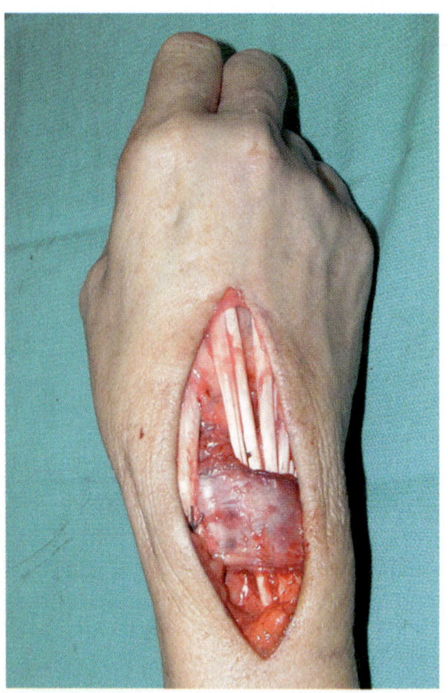

FIGURE 90-21

Step 10

- The dorsal capsule is reattached to the distal margin of the radius (Fig. 90-20).
- The extensor retinaculum is sutured over the extensor tendons and secured either to the remnant of the retinaculum or over drill holes in the distal ulna if the distal ulna was resected (Fig. 90-21). If the dorsal wrist capsular closure is not sufficiently tight, half of the extensor retinaculum can be placed under the extensor tendons to augment the wrist capsular closure.
- Preoperative and postoperative radiographs are shown in Figure 90-22A to D.

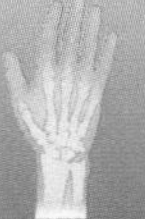

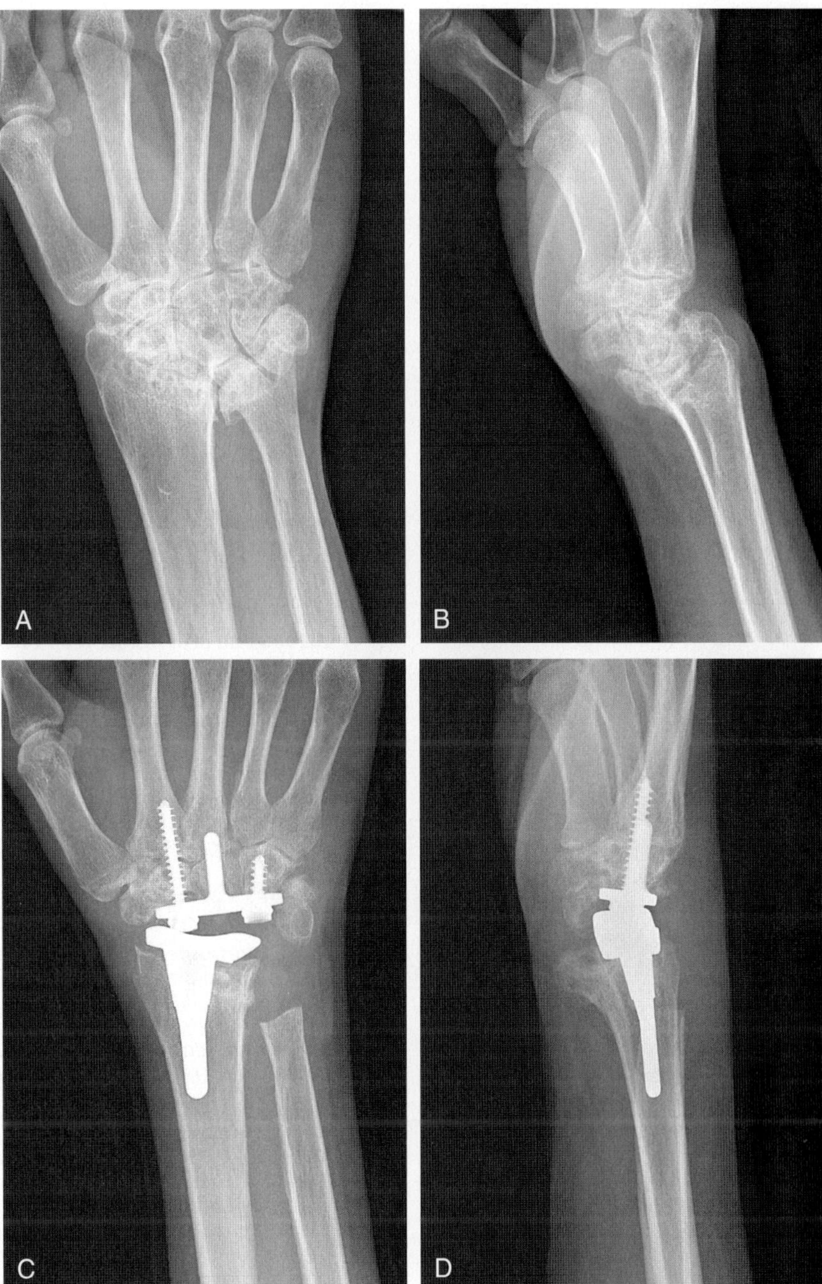

FIGURE 90-22

Postoperative Care and Expected Outcomes

- The wrist is immobilized in a short-arm splint for 2 to 4 weeks depending on stability of the implant. A removable short-arm splint is used for another 2 to 4 weeks.
- During the splinting period, the patient will start active flexion, extension, pronation, and supination exercises several times a day. After 8 weeks, strengthening and passive exercises can be started. After 2 to 3 months, unrestricted exercises are initiated, but the patient is cautioned against repetitive strong loading and hard work.

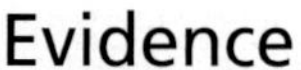

Evidence

Cavaliere CM, Chung KC. A systematic review of total wrist arthroplasty compared with total wrist arthrodesis for rheumatoid arthritis. *Plast Reconstr Surg*. 2008;122:813-825.
The authors performed a systematic review of the existing literature on outcomes of both procedures in rheumatoid arthritis. They found that total wrist fusion provides more reliable relief than total wrist arthroplasty, and complication and revision rates were higher for total wrist arthroplasty, although satisfaction was high in both groups. Functional active arc of motion with total wrist arthroplasty was demonstrated in only 3 of 14 studies reporting appropriate data. The authors concluded that existing data do not support widespread application of total wrist arthroplasty for the rheumatoid wrist. (Level II evidence)

Cavaliere CM, Chung KC. A cost-utility analysis of nonsurgical management, total wrist arthroplasty, and total wrist arthrodesis in rheumatoid arthritis. *J Hand Surg [Am]*. 2010;35:379-391.
The authors performed a cost-utility analysis comparing nonsurgical management, total wrist arthroplasty, and total wrist arthrodesis for the rheumatoid wrist. They surveyed 49 patients with rheumatoid arthritis and 109 hand surgeons and rheumatologists and found that both patients and physicians favored surgical management over nonsurgical treatment. They concluded that total wrist arthroplasty and total wrist arthrodesis are both extremely cost-effective procedures and that total wrist arthroplasty has only a small incremental cost over total wrist arthrodesis. Based on this, total wrist arthroplasty should not be considered cost-prohibitive in the treatment of rheumatoid arthritis. (Level II evidence)

Divelbliss BJ, Sollerman C, Adams BD. Early results of the Universal total wrist arthroplasty in rheumatoid arthritis. *J Hand Surg [Am]*. 2002;27:195-204.
Outcomes of use of the Universal I prosthesis were evaluated in 14 wrists at 1-year follow-up and 8 wrists at 2-year follow-up. All patients were women, and mean age was 48 years. The DASH score decreased from 46 to 22. Complications included three palmar dislocations, and all three patients had active inflammation of the wrists. This paper provided an outcome evaluation of the first-generation prosthesis using the Universal total wrist design. (Level IV evidence)

Murphy DM, Khoury JG, Imbriglia JE, Adams BD. Comparison of arthroplasty and arthrodesis for the rheumatoid wrist. *J Hand Surg [Am]*. 2003;28:570-576.
This is a retrospective study comparing 24 patients with arthrodesis with 23 patients with arthroplasty. Both groups were matched by age and radiographic staging. The outcomes were based on the DASH and PRWE questionnaires. The authors showed that there was no difference in the outcomes questionnaire scores between the two groups. Both groups were equally satisfied, and the complication rates were similar. (Level III evidence)

Radmer S, Andresen R, Sparmann M. Total wrist arthroplasty in patients with rheumatoid arthritis. *J Hand Surg [Am]*. 2003;28:789-794.
This is a second follow-up study of a previous 18-month follow-up study of use of a wrist prosthesis. At 18-month follow-up, the authors reported excellent outcomes in all patients, with minimal complication rates. At 52-month follow-up of 40 patients with this type of wrist prosthesis, all patients had serious complications, and all underwent arthrodesis. This study illustrated the need for long-term follow-up of wrist arthroplasty procedures to establish their effectiveness and complications. (Level IV evidence)

Vicar AJ, Burton RI. Surgical management of the rheumatoid wrist-fusion or arthroplasty. *J Hand Surg [Am]*. 1986;11:790-797.
This is a retrospective review of two groups of patients who underwent wrist fusion or arthroplasty. The authors found that both groups did well with either procedure. The wrist arthroplasty group had 5 degrees of flexion, 30 degrees of extension, and 10 degrees of ulnar and radial deviation. The authors recommended arthroplasty in the dominant wrist when both wrists required treatment. The nondominant wrist should be fused in neutral position. (Level III evidence)

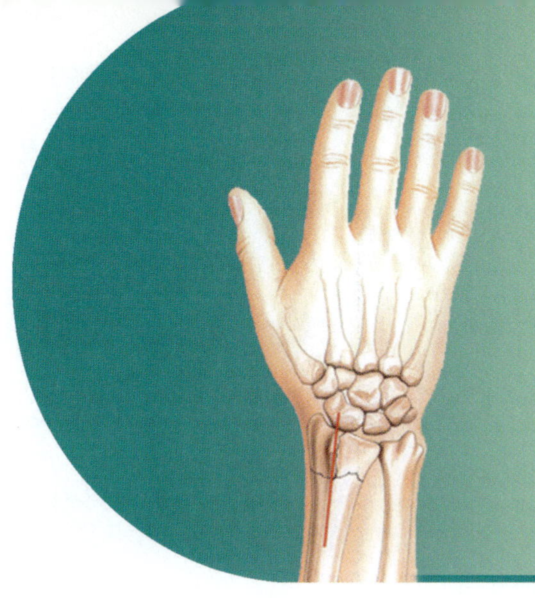

Section XIV

TUMORS

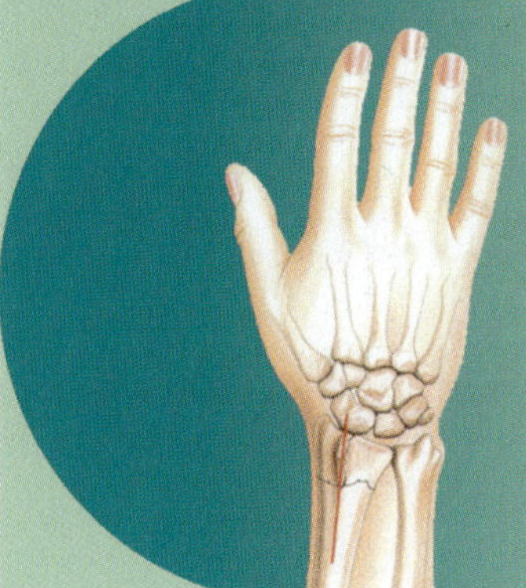

PROCEDURE 91

Treatment of Mucous Cysts of the Distal Interphalangeal Joint

Shimpei Ono, Sandeep J. Sebastin, and Kevin C. Chung

Indications

- Symptomatic mucous cyst
  - Progressive cyst with impending rupture due to thinning of skin (Fig. 91-1)
  - Discomfort or pain due to pressure from the cyst
  - Nail deformity (see Fig. 91-1)
- Asymptomatic mucous cyst
  - Aesthetic appearance
  - Patient desire
- Patients should be advised that cyst excision might not provide complete pain relief in the context of an underlying arthritic joint because pain can be due to either the cyst or the underlying arthritic joint. The only treatment that can ensure a cyst will not recur is distal interphalangeal (DIP) joint arthrodesis.

Examination/Imaging

Clinical Examination

- A mucous cyst is a degenerative cyst of the DIP joint arising as a result of osteoarthritis. It usually occurs between the fifth and seventh decades of life, and patients have DIP joint osteoarthritis including Heberden nodes (Fig. 91-2).
- The cyst may present on the dorsum at the level of the DIP joint on either side between the extensor tendon and the collateral ligament or under the eponychium to cause longitudinal grooving of the nail plate (Fig. 91-3).

Imaging

- Anteroposterior and lateral view radiographs are useful in determining the location of the osteophytes and degree of osteoarthritic change (joint subluxation, deformity, and joint space narrowing) (Fig. 91-4).

Surgical Anatomy

- The mucous cyst originates from the DIP joint in relation to one of the osteophytes, and the stalk of the cyst passes between the collateral ligament and the extensor insertion to present on the dorsum of the DIP joint. Occasionally, the stalk can connect with another mucous cyst on the opposite side of the DIP joint. This cyst may not be clinically obvious (occult cyst), and the entire DIP joint should be examined during surgery.
- The terminal extensor insertion is about 1.2 mm from the proximal edge of the nail matrix (Fig. 91-5).

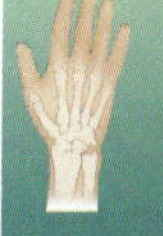

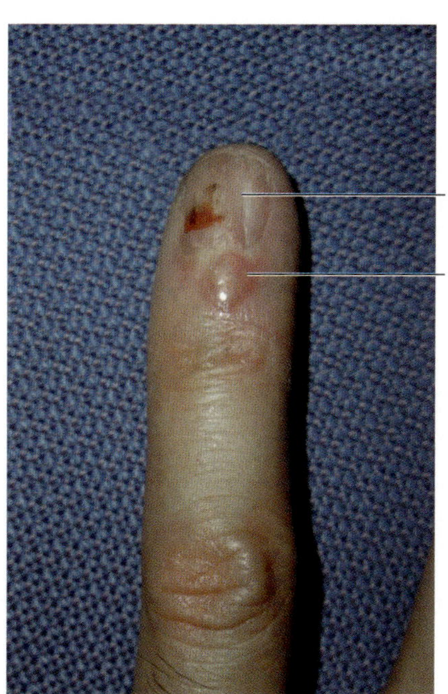

FIGURE 91-1

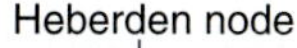

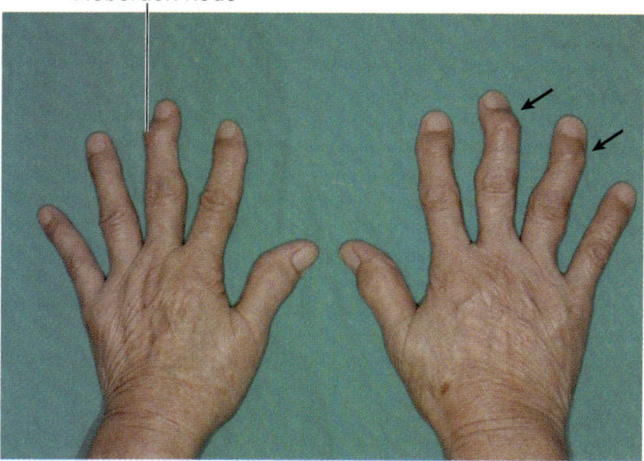

FIGURE 91-2

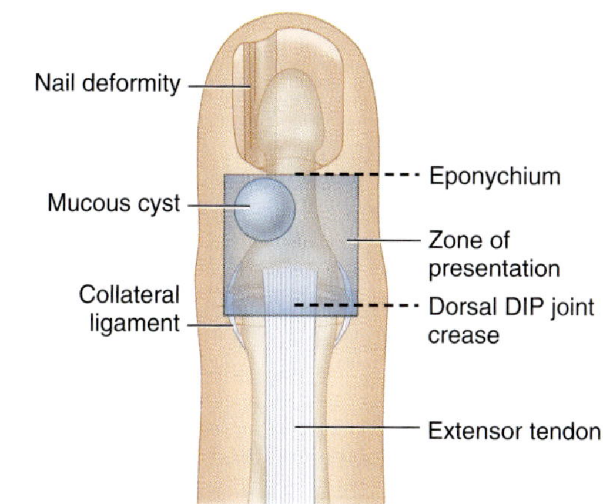

FIGURE 91-3

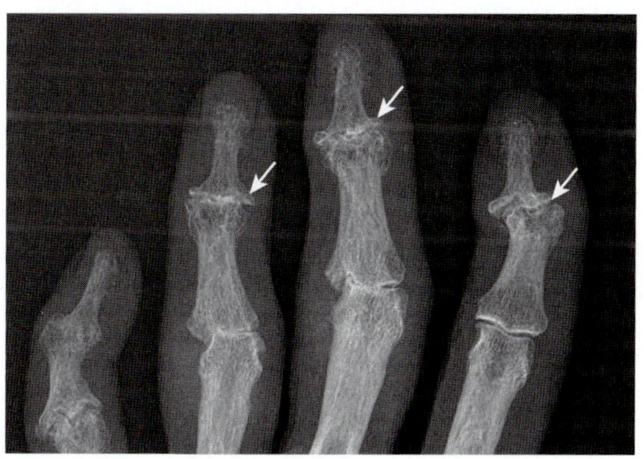

FIGURE 91-4

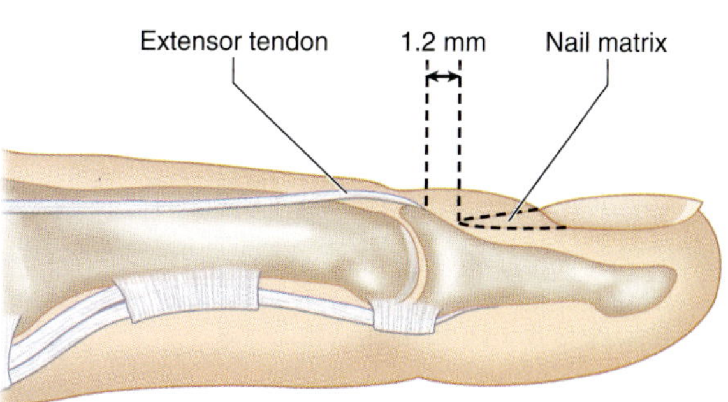

FIGURE 91-5

Positioning

- The procedure can be performed under a digital block using a forearm, arm, or digital tourniquet.

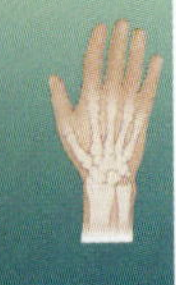

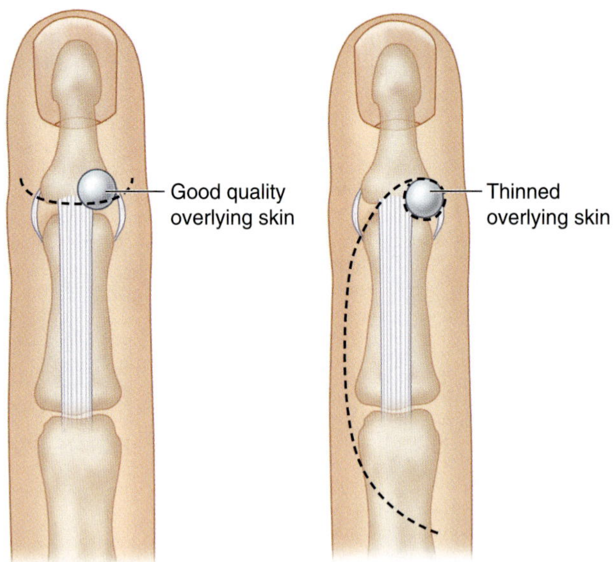

FIGURE 91-6

Exposures

- Mucous cyst with good-quality overlying skin
  - We use a gentle curving transverse incision centered over the DIP joint. A distally based skin flap is elevated in a plane superficial to the cyst (Fig. 91-6).
- Mucous cyst with thinned overlying skin
  - We use a longitudinal elliptical incision that includes the thinned skin. A long rotational flap is designed proximally to cover the resulting skin defect skin (see Fig. 91-6).

PEARLS

Traction sutures can be placed on the skin flaps to provide better exposure.

The proximal extent of the flap depends on the size of the skin defect. Extending the flap to the proximal joint is usually sufficient, and, if required, a back-cut can be added.

PITFALLS

Care must be taken not to injure the nail bed.

The skin flaps need to be elevated in full thickness to maintain the vascularity

Procedure

Step 1: Mobilization of Cyst

- The cyst is separated from the overlying skin and the extensor tendon.
- If a stalk extends under the nail bed, it will have to be carefully dissected to the joint.

STEP 1 PEARLS

The extensor tendon can be retracted laterally to provide better exposure.

Care is taken not to injure the insertion of the extensor tendon or the nail matrix.

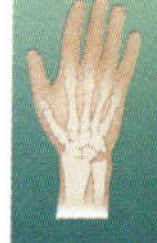

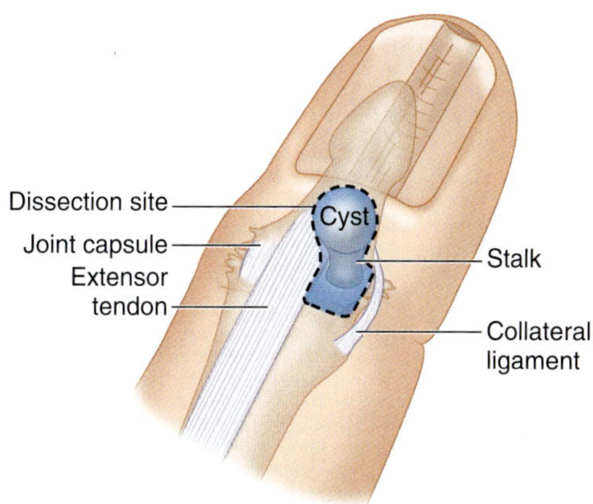

FIGURE 91-7

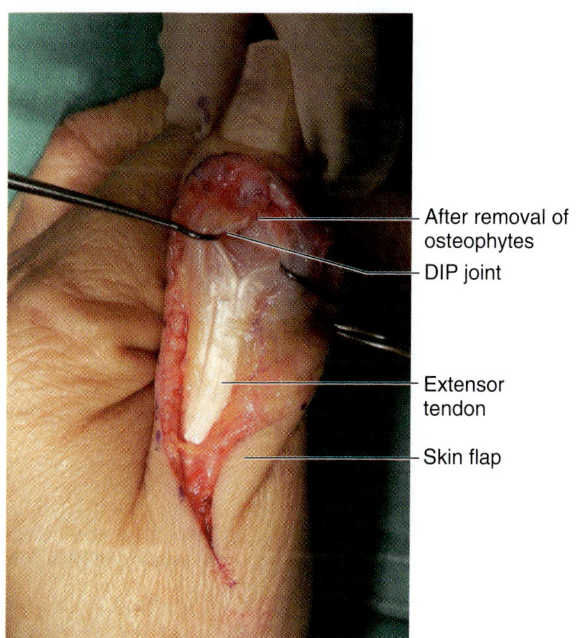

FIGURE 91-8

Step 2: Removal of the Cyst

- The cyst is excised en-mass and includes any thinned overlying skin, the cyst and the stalk, and all soft tissue between the extensor tendon and collateral ligament (synovium and joint capsule). (Fig. 91-7 depicts the soft tissue zone that needs to be excised in the dotted line.)
- Any remaining synovium within the joint is also excised.

STEP 2 PEARLS

It is important to remove all synovium to allow a clear visualization of the DIP joint.

Both sides of the extensor tendon must be examined for any occult cysts.

It is preferable to leave behind a portion of the cyst wall that is in close relation to the nail bed rather than risk injury to the nail bed from an aggressive débridement.

Step 3: Removal of DIP Joint Osteophytes

- All osteophytes of the DIP joint should be removed with a small rongeur.

STEP 3 PEARLS

The removal of the osteophytes is the key to successful excision of a mucous cyst.

One must inspect under the extensor insertion and the collateral ligaments for osteophytes that are seen on the radiograph but cannot be seen in the wound.

Step 4: Flap Elevation

- If required, a rotational flap can be designed to cover the skin defect. The flap is elevated in the loose areolar plane superficial to the extensor tendon paratenon (Fig. 91-8).

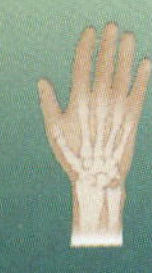

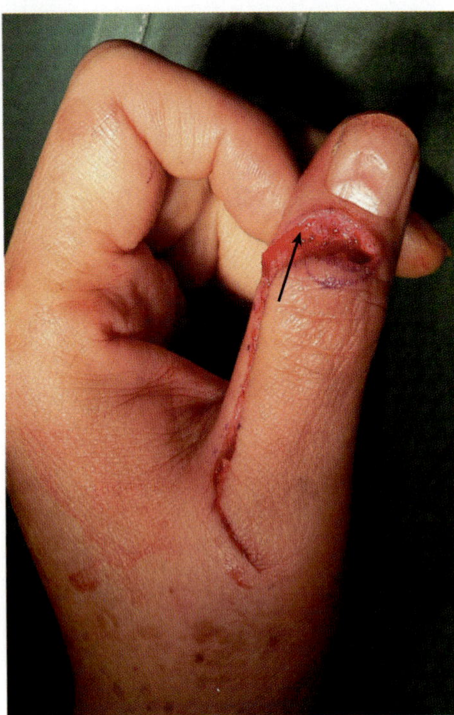

FIGURE 91-9

Step 5: Skin Closure

- The tourniquet is released and hemostasis secured.
- The flap is advanced into the defect (Fig. 91-9) and sutured with a few 5-0 Ethilon sutures.

STEP 5 PEARLS

It is better to close the skin loosely and leave any residual skin defects to heal by secondary intention instead of attempting a watertight closure.

A Xeroform dressing with overlying gauze is applied as a wick to absorb any residual blood. A volar finger splint is applied to keep the DIP joint straight.

STEP 5 PITFALLS

Do not close skin flaps under tension. This will result in partial skin flap necrosis, wound breakdown, and increased risk for infection.

Postoperative Care and Expected Outcomes

- The splint is used to immobilize the DIP joint for 5 to 7 days, and the patient is asked to start gentle active range-of-motion exercises thereafter.
- Surgical excision has a high success rate (>90%) and low recurrence rate (2% to 3%), provided that all osteophytes are removed during surgery. A loss of 5 to 20 degrees of motion, joint stiffness, contour changes of the proximal nail fold, and nail dystrophies occur postoperatively in up to 25% of patients.

Evidence

Fritz GR, Stern PJ, Dickey M. Complications following mucous cyst excision. *J Hand Surg [Br]*. 1997;22:222-225.

The authors reported that 86 mucous cysts in 79 patients were surgically excised along with accompanying osteophytes. Rotation flaps were created in 58 of the 86 (67%). Follow-up was carried out at an average of 2.6 years. Fifteen digits (17%) had a residual loss of extension of 5 to 20 degrees at the IP or DIP joint. One patient developed a superficial infection, and 2 developed a DIP septic arthritis, which eventually required DIP arthrodesis. Nail deformities were present in 25 of 86 digits preoperatively (29%), 15 of which resolved after surgery (60%). Four of 61 digits developed a nail deformity that was not present preoperatively (7%). Three of 86 digits (3%) developed recurrence. Other complications included persistent swelling, pain, numbness, stiffness, and radial or ulnar deviation at the DIP joint. (Level IV evidence)

Kasdan ML, Stallings SP, Leis VM, Wolens D. Outcome of surgically treated mucous cysts of the hand. *J Hang Surg [Am]*. 1994;19:504-507.

The results of a surgical procedure for the treatment of digital mucous cysts are described. In this series, a longitudinal incision was made directly over the mucous cyst, and the cyst was excised with routine removal of osteophytes. One hundred ninety-one mucous cysts from 178 patients were treated from 1973 to 1992. The average age of the study population was 57 years. There were only two recurrences and two postoperative infections. Both patients with recurrences presented more than 40 months after surgery. Sixty-four of the cysts had been previously treated elsewhere. The most common postoperative complaint was tenderness of the joint. Associated nail deformities were corrected in 40 of 46 cases. (Level IV evidence)

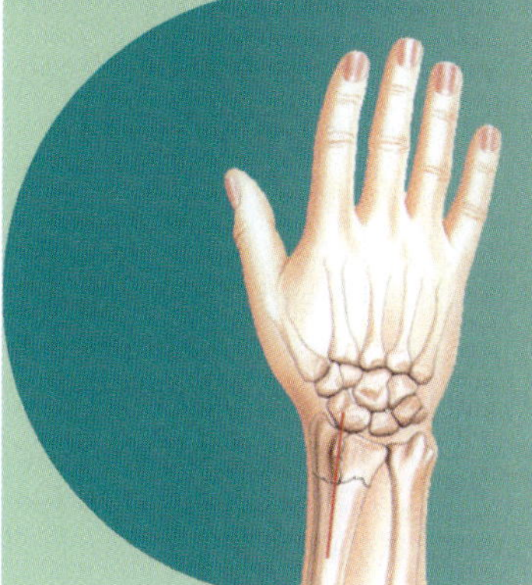

PROCEDURE 92

Excision of a Dorsal Wrist Ganglion

Sandeep J. Sebastin and Kevin C. Chung

See Video 68: Treatment of Dorsal Wrist Ganglions

Indications

- Patient concern about appearance or malignancy (Fig. 92-1)
- Ganglion with associated pain

Examination/Imaging

Clinical Examination

- Patients are usually asymptomatic, and a specific history of antecedent trauma is available only in 10% of patients. Patients with pain or history of trauma should be examined for evidence of scapholunate (SL) instability. This includes tenderness at the SL joint, the Watson scaphoid shift test, and the resisted finger extension test. The resisted finger extension test is done by asking the patient to extend the index and middle fingers against resistance with the wrist partially flexed. These tendons pass over the SL joint, and if there is inflammation of the SL joint with synovitis, resisted extension compresses the area of synovitis, resulting in pain.
- Pain associated with a ganglion may not go away after excision of the ganglion, and patients must be appropriately counseled.
- The clinical diagnosis of a ganglion is relatively simple and can be confirmed by transillumination. The differential diagnosis for swellings on the dorsum of the hand includes extensor tendon ganglion (moves with the tendon), extensor tendon tenosynovitis (diffuse and moves with the tendon), lipoma, and sebaceous and epidermal cysts (do not transilluminate).

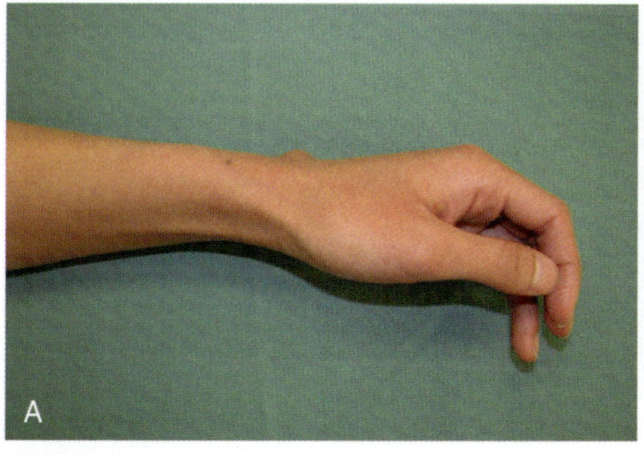

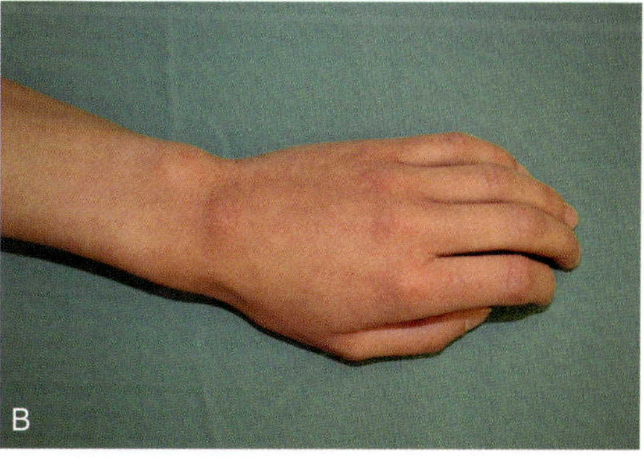

FIGURE 92-1

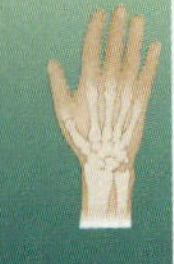

Imaging

- A preoperative radiograph is not required in all dorsal wrist ganglions and needs to be ordered if patients complain of pain or history of antecedent trauma.

Surgical Anatomy

- A dorsal wrist ganglion typically arises from the SL joint and usually presents on the dorsum of the hand over the SL joint (1 to 2 cm distal to Lister tubercle). However, depending on the course of the ganglion and the length of the stalk, it may present anywhere on the dorsum of the hand. Irrespective of anatomic location of the ganglion on the dorsum of the hand, it must be presumed that it is arising from the SL joint and incisions planned accordingly.

PEARLS

For a large ganglion, it is not necessary to make the incision as wide as the ganglion. Mobilization of the ganglion and retraction of skin can help in dissecting the ganglion out through a smaller incision.

Positioning

- The patient is positioned supine, and the procedure is done under tourniquet control.

Exposures

- A transverse incision is preferred because it is more aesthetic and the most common indication for excision of the ganglion is appearance. For dorsal wrist ganglions that present in the typical location over the SL joint, the incision is made directly over the ganglion. However, if the ganglion is not located directly over the SL joint, one must plan the incision in such a manner that the ganglion can be dissected and the stalk followed to the SL joint. Occasionally this may need two transverse incisions or a single longitudinal incision. If a clinical diagnosis of a ganglion is doubtful, a longitudinal incision is preferred because it can easily be extended.
- A 2-cm transverse incision is made over the skin (Fig. 92-2). The capsule of the ganglion is identified.

PITFALLS

Care must be taken to identify any sensory branches of the superficial radial nerve that are occasionally draped and stretched around the ganglion. They must carefully be dissected off the capsule.

Superficial veins must be mobilized and dissected off or divided between ligatures.

Procedure

Step 1: Mobilization of Ganglion Cyst

- The portion of the ganglion superficial to the extensor retinaculum is dissected free from the surrounding soft tissue. This is done by holding the ganglion with a blunt forceps and retracting it to one side, while the assistant retracts the skin to the opposite side (Fig. 92-3).
- Next the extensor retinaculum adjacent to the ganglion needs to be divided to allow deeper mobilization of the cyst.

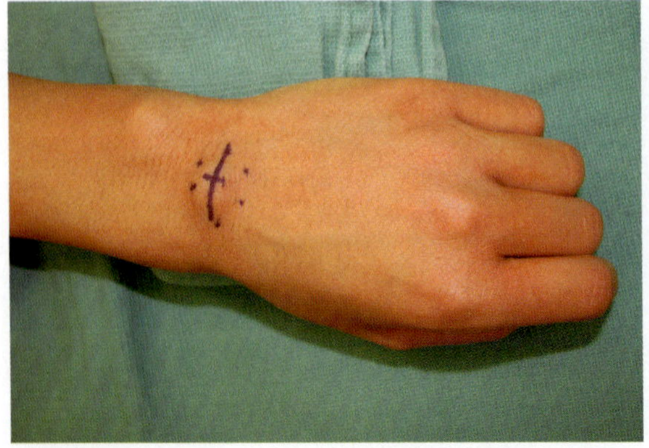

FIGURE 92-2

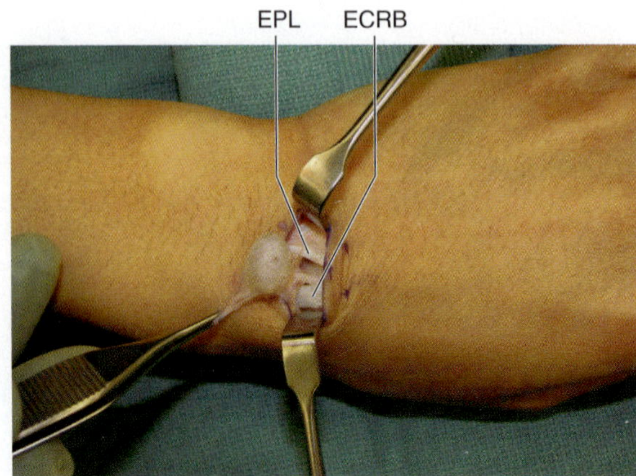

FIGURE 92-3

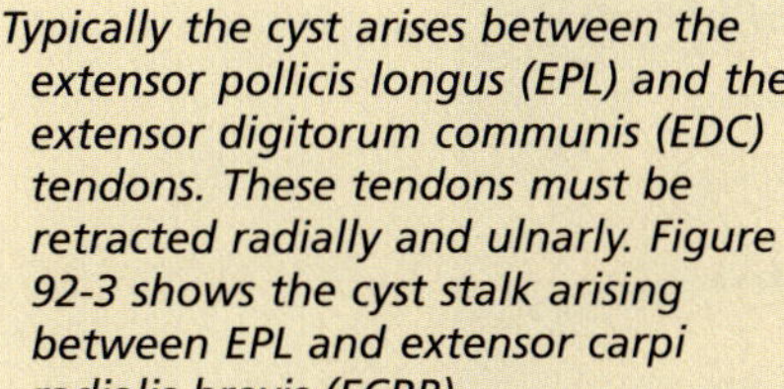

STEP 1 PEARLS

Typically the cyst arises between the extensor pollicis longus (EPL) and the extensor digitorum communis (EDC) tendons. These tendons must be retracted radially and ulnarly. Figure 92-3 shows the cyst stalk arising between EPL and extensor carpi radialis brevis (ECRB).

Although excision of the entire cyst keeping the cyst intact is an admirable goal, it is much easier to dissect a punctured cyst. This is best done after the initial dissection through the retinaculum is complete and the cyst capsule is well defined. The cyst can be punctured, the gelatinous fluid evacuated, and the capsule held for further dissection (Fig. 92-4).

STEP 1 PITFALLS

Care must be taken to prevent inadvertent injury to the extensor tendons.

STEP 2 PEARLS

The rim of capsular tissue usually measures 1.5 cm in diameter.

Any synovitis of the SL joint or adjoining joints should also be excised (Fig. 92-6).

The edge of the capsule should be cauterized with bipolar cautery before releasing the tourniquet because it is very difficult to cauterize it subsequently.

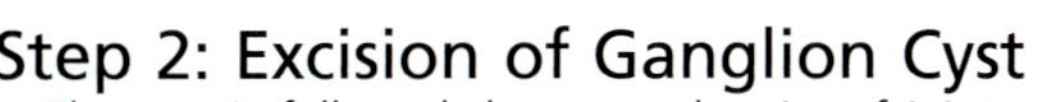

Step 2: Excision of Ganglion Cyst

- The cyst is followed deeper, and a rim of joint capsule is incised around the stalk.
- The capsule is then opened proximal and distal to the stalk.
- The cyst and its stalk along with the rim of joint capsule are dissected down to its attachment on the SL ligament.
- The cyst and the stalk are excised tangentially off the SL ligament, taking a small portion of the ligament with it (Fig. 92-5).

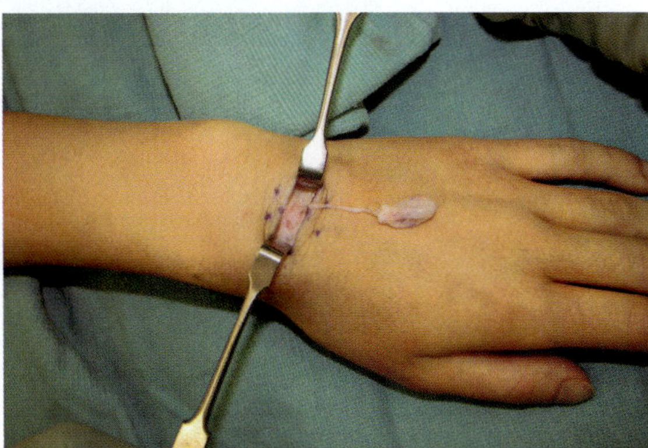

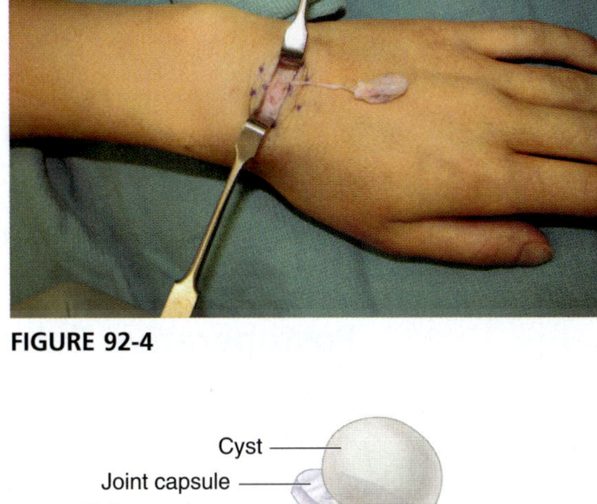

FIGURE 92-4

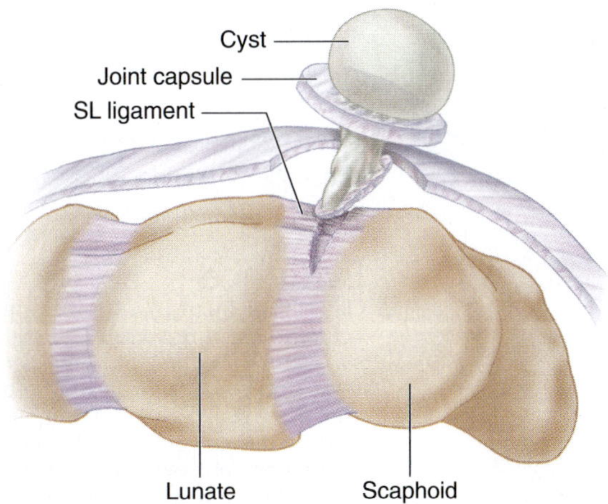

FIGURE 92-5

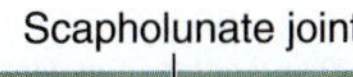

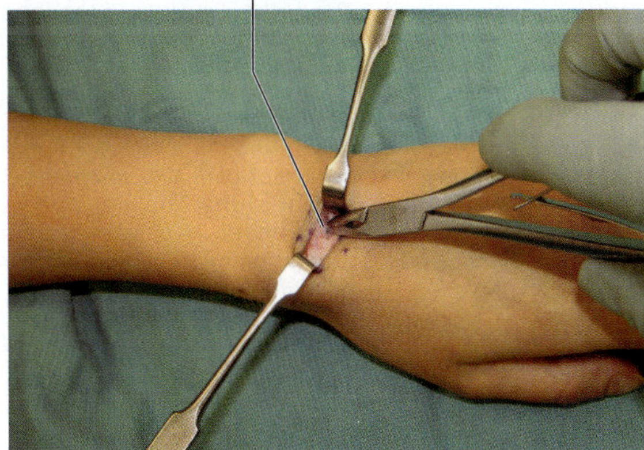

FIGURE 92-6

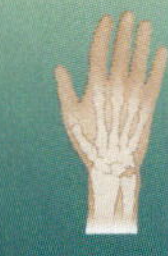

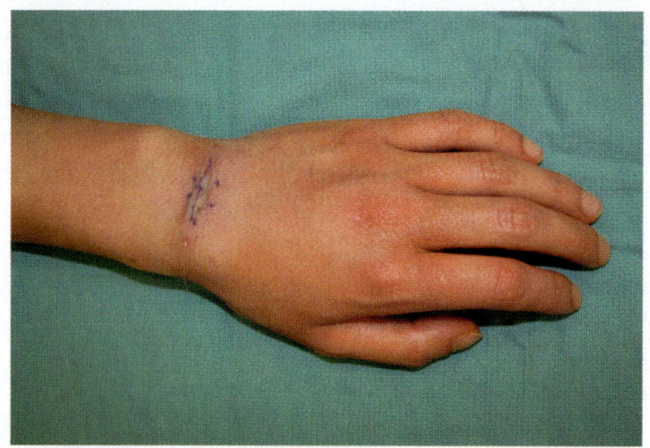

FIGURE 92-7

STEP 3 PEARLS

It is important to achieve meticulous hemostasis because a dead space is created after removal of the cyst. If excellent hemostasis cannot be achieved, it is advisable to leave a small drain that can be removed after 1 to 2 days.

STEP 3 PITFALLS

A repair of the capsule should not be done because it will restrict postoperative wrist flexion.

Step 3: Hemostasis

- The tourniquet is released and hemostasis secured.

Step 4: Skin Closure

- The incision should be closed in layers. A monofilament nonabsorbable subcuticular suture is used for closure of the skin (Fig. 92-7).

Postoperative Care and Expected Outcomes

- Patients should be splinted in slight flexion for a week and can resume normal activities thereafter.
- There is 5% to 10% incidence of recurrence following excision, which usually is a result of incomplete excision. Other complications of surgical treatment of ganglions include wrist stiffness, hypertrophic scar, neuroma formation, and persistent pain.

Evidence

Clay NR, Clement DA. The treatment of dorsal wrist ganglia by radical excision. *J Hand Surg [Br]*. 1988;13:187-191.

The authors followed 62 patients with dorsal wrist ganglia who underwent excision through a transverse dorsal incision. The specimen included a portion of the wrist capsule and any attachments to deeper structures. The authors were able to follow up 51 patients at a mean interval of 28 months. Seventy-three percent were asymptomatic, and 17% had only mild pain. Nine patients complained of weakness of grip. There were two recurrences, and one patient develop SL instability. (Level IV evidence)

Dias JJ, Dhukaram V, Kumar P. The natural history of untreated dorsal wrist ganglia and patient reported outcome 6 years after intervention. *J Hand Surg [Br]*. 2007;32:502-508.

The authors evaluated the long-term outcome of excision, aspiration, and no treatment of 283 dorsal wrist ganglia in 283 patients who responded to a postal questionnaire at a mean of 70 months. The resolution of symptoms was similar between the treatment groups (P > .3). Pain and unsightliness improved in all three treatment groups. The prevalence of weakness and stiffness varied only slightly in all three treatment groups. More patients with a recurrent or persistent ganglion complained of pain, stiffness, and unsightliness (P < .0001). Patient satisfaction was higher after surgical excision (P < .0001), even if the ganglion recurred. Twenty-three of 55 (58%) untreated ganglia resolved spontaneously. The recurrence rates were 58% (45/78) and 39% (40/103) following aspiration and excision, respectively. Eight of 103 patients had complications following surgery. According to this study, neither excision nor aspiration provided significant long-term benefit over no treatment. (Level III evidence)

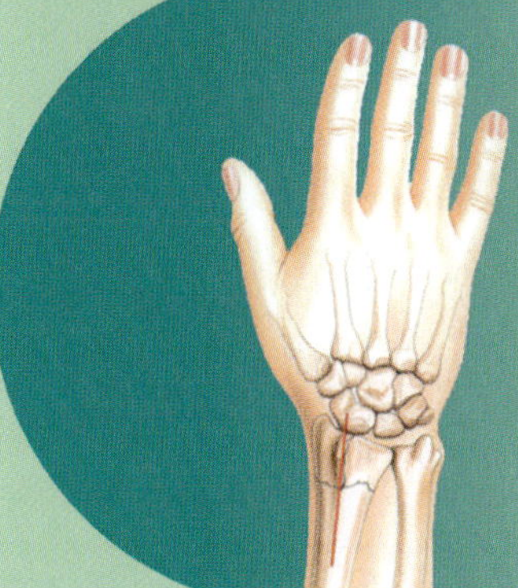

PROCEDURE 93

Digital Ray Amputation

Pao-Yuan Lin, Sandeep J. Sebastin, and Kevin C. Chung

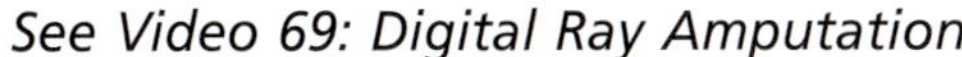
See Video 69: Digital Ray Amputation

Indications

- Traumatic amputation close to the metacarpophalangeal (MCP) joint that leaves a gap in the hand
- Elective procedure in patients with a functionally impaired digit
- Treatment of infection, failure of replantation, vascular disorder, or tumor

Examination/Imaging

Clinical Examination

- In patients undergoing ray amputation for a painful stump, the point of maximal tenderness due to a neuroma (if any) should be identified preoperatively and marked. Figure 93-1 shows a patient with a painful stump.

Imaging

- Radiographs of the hand (Fig. 93-2).

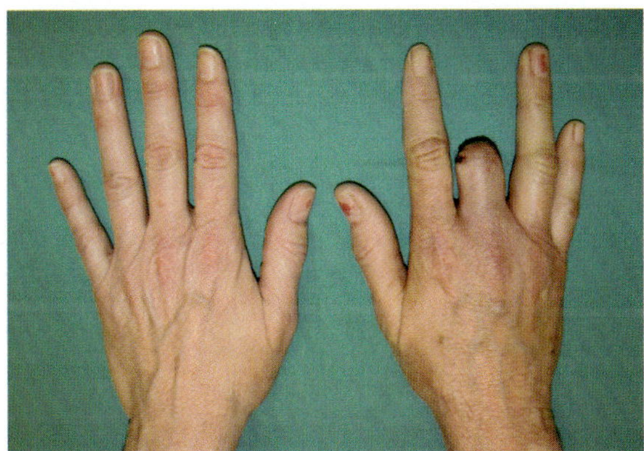

FIGURE 93-1

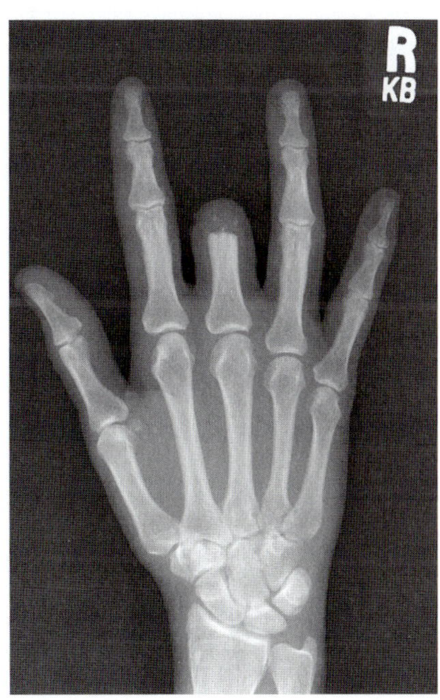

FIGURE 93-2

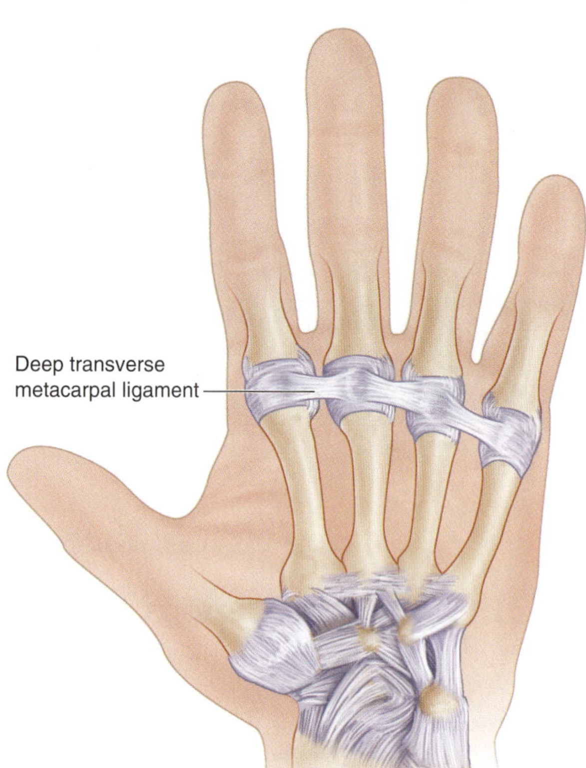

FIGURE 93-3

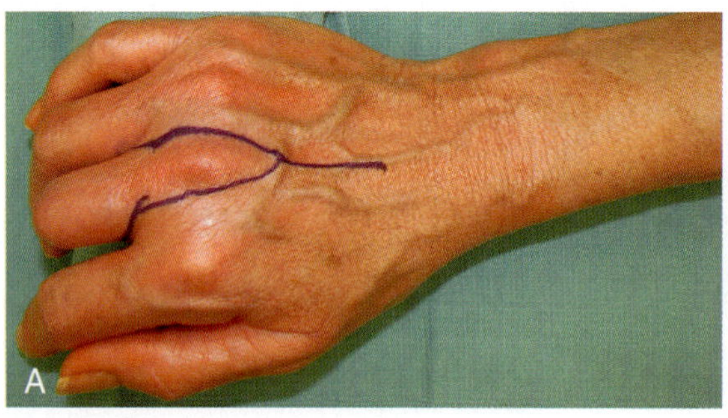

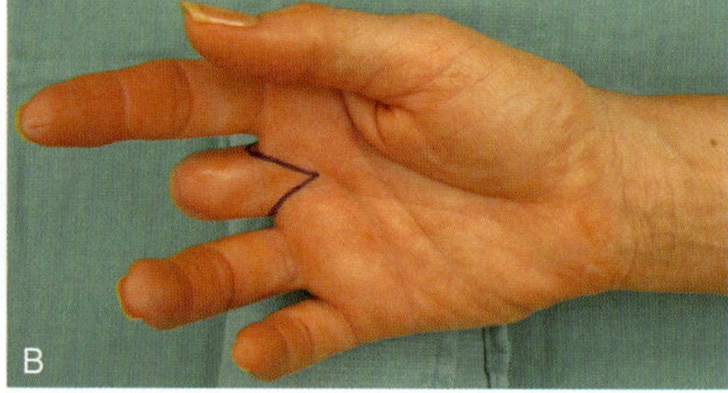

FIGURE 93-4

Surgical Anatomy

- The deep transverse metacarpal ligament connects the volar plates of the MCP joints of the index, long, ring, and small fingers. The flexor tendons, neurovascular bundles, and lumbrical tendon pass palmar to the deep transverse MCP ligament, whereas the interosseous tendon lies dorsal to it (Fig. 93-3).

Positioning

- The procedure is performed under tourniquet control. It can be done under regional or general anesthesia. The patient is positioned supine with the affected extremity on a hand table.

Exposures

- A racket-shaped incision is marked around the base of the finger. On the dorsum, this incision extends over the proximal metacarpal in a longitudinal fashion (Fig. 93-4A). On the palmar aspect, it is designed as a V (Fig. 93-4B).

PEARLS

The incision is made on the finger that is going to be amputated and not into the web. This allows a good repair of the web space after the ray amputation.

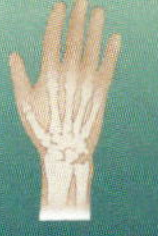

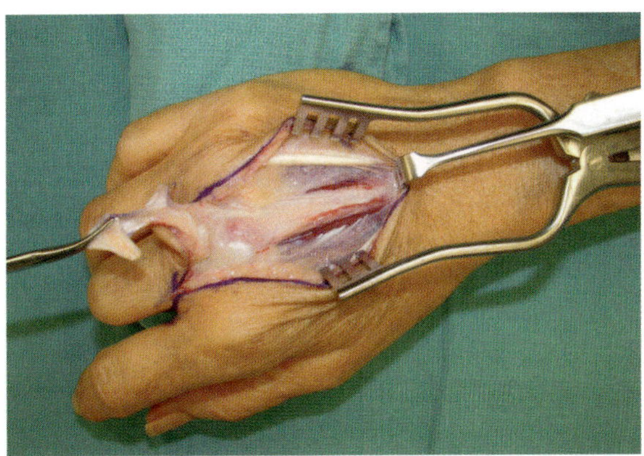

FIGURE 93-5

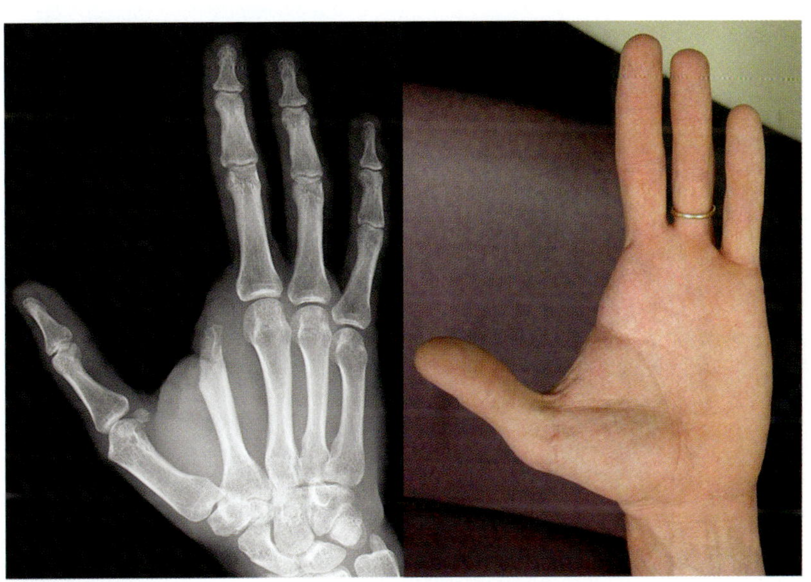

FIGURE 93-6

Procedure

Step 1

- The extensor digitorum communis (EDC) tendon is identified on the dorsum, divided at mid-metacarpal shaft, and raised as a distally based tendon (Fig. 93-5). The juncturae to the adjacent fingers are also divided.

Step 2

- The periosteum is incised longitudinally on the dorsum of the metacarpal, and the interosseous muscle on both sides of the metacarpal shaft is separated from the metacarpal, along with the periosteum, to about 1 cm distal to the respective carpometacarpal (CMC) joint to preserve the insertion wrist flexor or extensor tendons.

Step 3

- A transverse osteotomy of the metacarpal shaft is done using a saw about 1 cm distal to the CMC joint by preserving the insertions of the ECRL, ECRB, or ECU.

STEP 1 PEARLS

The extensor indicis proprius (EIP) or the extensor digiti quinti minimi (EDQM) tendons will have to be divided at the same level as the EDC when a ray amputation of the index or small finger is being carried out.

STEP 2 PITFALLS

Care must be taken not to elevate the extensor carpi radialis longus (ECRL), extensor carpi radialis brevis (ECRB), or extensor carpi ulnaris (ECU) from the base of the index, long, and small metacarpals, respectively.

STEP 3 PEARLS

The osteotomy for the index finger is done more distally at the level of the neck of the metacarpal in an oblique fashion; this allows the new web space to have a more natural slope (Fig. 93-6). In addition, it preserves the transverse width of the palm and the origins of the first dorsal interosseous and the adductor pollicis muscle.

The osteotomy of the small finger metacarpal is also done like the index finger (oblique and distally).

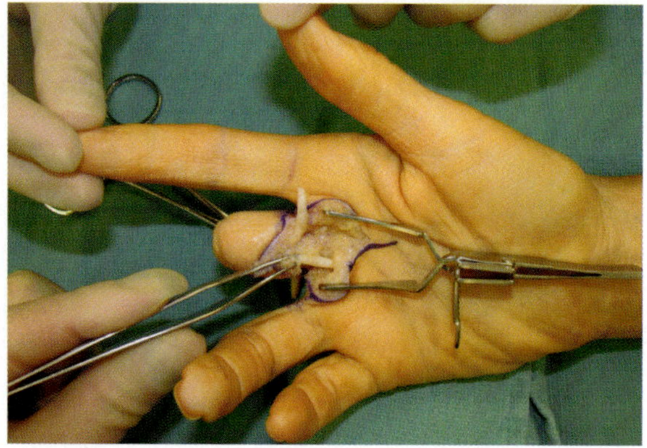

FIGURE 93-7

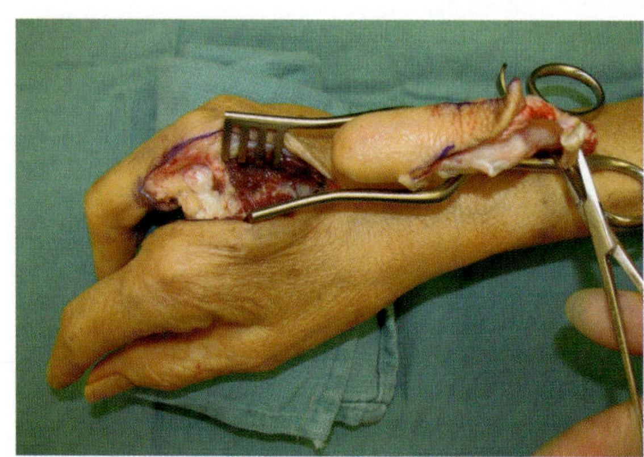

FIGURE 93-8

Step 4

- The common and proper digital arteries and nerves are identified through the palmar incision.
- The A1 pulley and flexor tendons are also identified.

Step 5

- The proper digital nerves to the finger undergoing ray amputation are divided distal to the origin from the common digital nerve using a blade and allowed to retract into the proximal soft tissues (Fig. 93-7).

Step 6

- The proper digital arteries are also ligated and divided distal to their origin from the common digital artery.

Step 7

- The A1 pulley is opened, and the flexor digitorum superficialis and profundus tendons are divided.

Step 8

- The deep transverse intermetacarpal ligament is identified at the neck of the metacarpal and divided close to the metacarpal shaft.

Step 9

- The finger is now freed from any other soft tissue holding it and excised (Fig. 93-8).

STEP 5 PITFALLS

One must ensure that the nerves are correctly identified before dividing them.

The proximal end of the nerve must be handled minimally to prevent any subsequent symptomatic neuroma formation.

One must ensure that the nerve has retracted proximally and that there is good soft tissue overlying it.

STEP 6 PITFALLS

There are interconnecting vessels between the deep and superficial arch at the level of the metacarpal neck. They must be identified and divided. Otherwise they will result in troublesome bleeding, once the tourniquet is released.

STEP 8 PEARLS

It is important to divide the deep transverse intermetacarpal ligament close to the shaft so that enough ligament is available to do a strong repair subsequently.

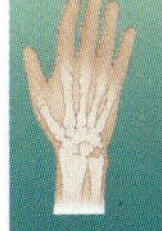

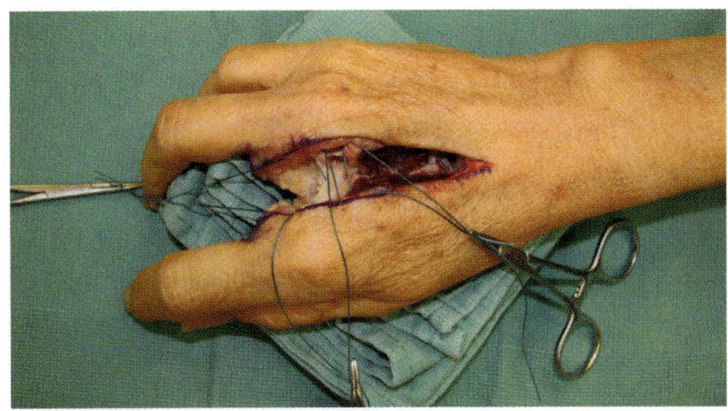

FIGURE 93-9

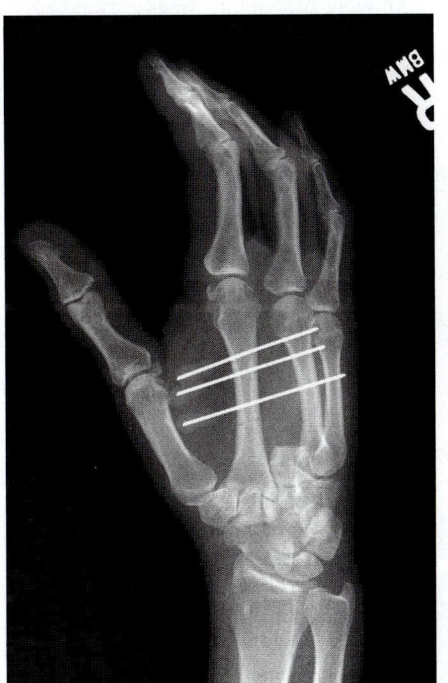

FIGURE 93-10

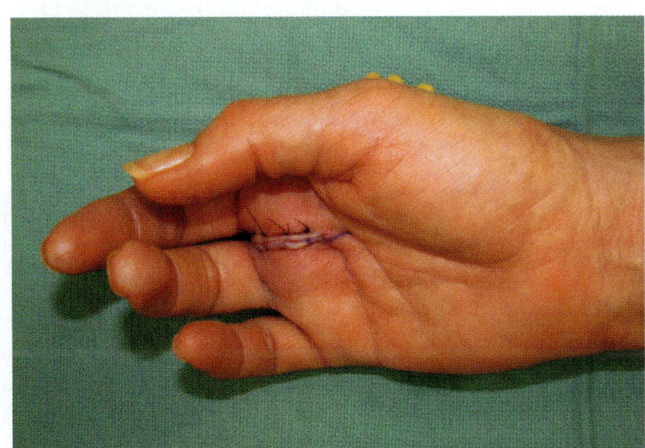

FIGURE 93-11

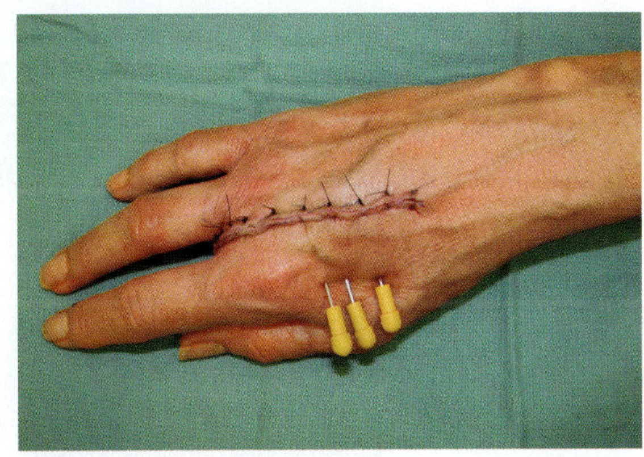

FIGURE 93-12

STEP 10 PEARLS

When setting tension, one must ensure that there is no scissoring of the digits. This is done by passively flexing and extending the wrist (tenodesis) to see whether the fingers fall into a good cascade (Fig. 93-11).

Step 10

- Two or three loops of 2-0 braided sutures (Ethibond or similar) are placed into the ends of the intermetacarpal ligament (Fig. 93-9).
- The gap between the heads of the adjoining metacarpals is reduced manually and maintained using two or three transverse Kirschner wires (Fig. 93-10).
- The intermetacarpal ligament sutures are then tied.

Step 11

- The tourniquet is deflated, and hemostasis is performed.
- The subcutaneous layer of wound is repaired by absorbable suture, and the skin is closed with 3-0 nylon (Fig. 93-12).

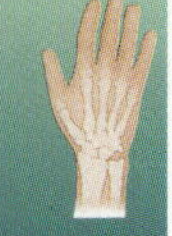

Postoperative Care and Expected Outcomes

- A short-arm plaster of Paris volar splint is applied by immobilizing the wrist and the fingers.
- The wound is inspected, sutures are removed, and a thermoplastic splint applied 10 days after the operation.
- Gentle active finger motion exercises are initiated, with splinting protection for another 4 to 6 weeks.
- The K-wires are removed 4 to 6 weeks later, and the patient is allowed unrestricted motion.
- Figure 93-13 shows the postoperative appearance at 5 months' follow-up.
- Most authors have reported 25% to 30% loss of grip strength following ray amputation. The average time off from work is about 13 weeks.

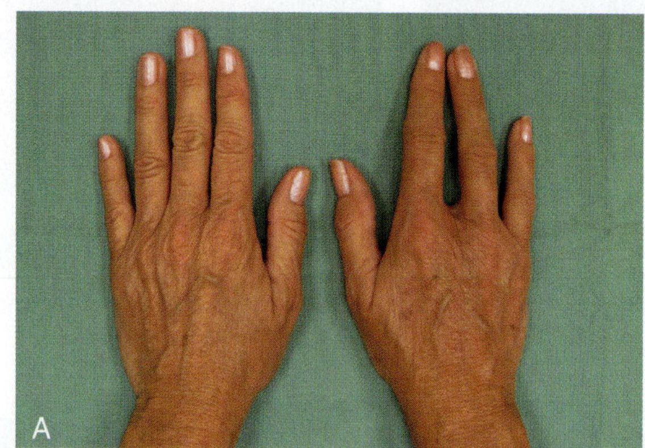

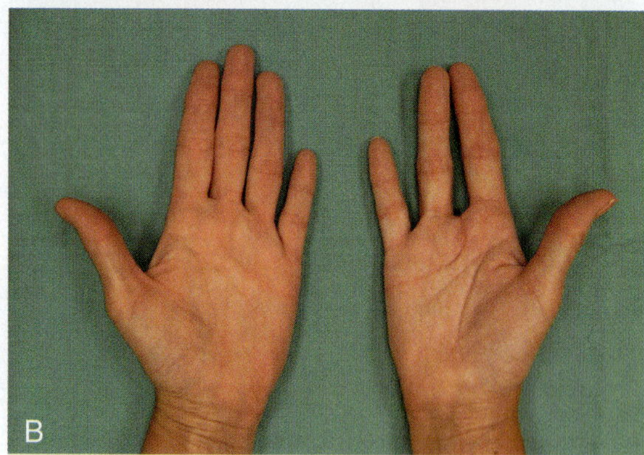

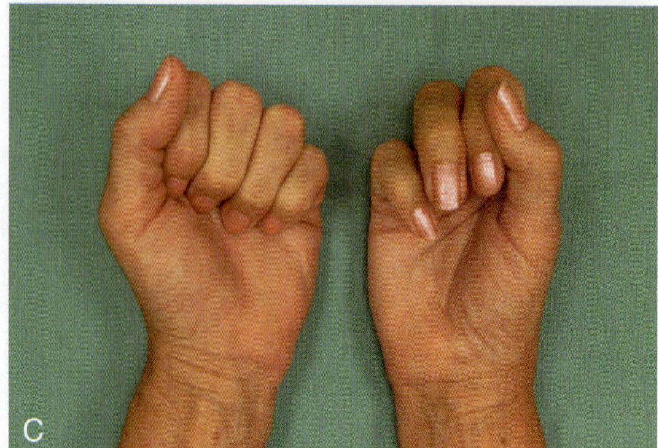

FIGURE 93-13

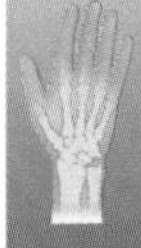

Evidence

Melikyan EY, Beg MSA, Woodbridge S, et al. The functional results of ray amputation. *Hand Surg*. 2003;8:47-51.

A retrospective analysis of 20 patients who underwent ray amputation was done an average of 32 months after the procedure. The authors used the DASH questionnaire, physical examination, and functional testing. They found that patients had lost an average of 27% of their grip strength and 22% of their three-point pinch strength. The DASH function score was 29.2. Nine patients returned to their previous occupations. The authors concluded that the disability caused by ray amputation was acceptable to most patients. (Level IV evidence)

Peimer CA, Wheeler DR, Barrett A, et al. Hand function following single ray amputation. *J Hand Surg [Am]*. 1999;24:1245-1248.

The authors assessed and contrasted the results of primary and secondary reconstructive ray amputation. They demonstrated that primary ray resection is associated with less total cost with respect to the injury itself and subsequent disability. Most patients returned to their preinjury occupation and were subjectively satisfied with the appearance and function of the hand. A very curious finding was the significant differences in grip strength, key pinch, oppositional pinch, and rate of manipulation test results in those patients who had unsettled litigation and compensation issues. These differences could not be explained on a physical or anatomical basis, implicating secondary gain issues. (Level IV evidence)

Index

Page numbers followed by t indicate tables, f indicate figures, and b indicate boxes. Entries followed by *web* indicate supplemental online material.

C

G

R

U